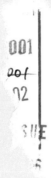

COMPLICATIONS IN
DIAGNOSTIC IMAGING AND
INTERVENTIONAL RADIOLOGY

To my wife Vera for her invaluable support during many editorial crises.
GEORGE ANSELL

For their support and love, to
    my parents, Ernst H. and Hilda K. Bettmann,
    my children, William, Joanna, and Robert
      Bettmann,
    my grandchild Mackenzie, and most importantly,
    my wife, Ellen Hofheimer Bettmann.
MICHAEL A. BETTMANN

For my father, S.A. Kaufman MD.
JOHN A. KAUFMAN

To Kathy Howes for her tireless secretarial and administrative help.
ROBERT A. WILKINS

Complications in Diagnostic Imaging and Interventional Radiology
Third Edition

EDITED BY

George Ansell MD, FRCP, FRCR
Formerly Senior Consultant Radiologist
Whiston Hospital, Merseyside
and Lecturer in Radiodiagnosis
University of Liverpool, UK

Michael A. Bettmann MD
Chief, Cardiovascular and Interventional Radiology
Dartmouth-Hitchcock Medical Center
Lebanon, New Hampshire, USA

John A. Kaufman MD
Assistant Professor of Radiology
Harvard Medical School
Division of Vascular Radiology
Massachusetts General Hospital
Boston, Massachusetts, USA

Robert A. Wilkins FRCR
Consultant Radiologist
Northwick Park Hospital
Harrow, Middlesex, UK

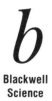

Blackwell Science

© 1976, 1987, 1996 by
Blackwell Science, Inc.
Editorial Offices:
238 Main Street, Cambridge
  Massachusetts 02142, USA
Osney Mead, Oxford OX2 0EL
  England
25 John Street, London WC1N 2BL
23 Ainslie Place, Edinburgh EH3 6AJ
  Scotland
54 University Street, Carlton
  Victoria 3053, Australia
Arnette Blackwell SA,
  224 Boulevard Saint Germain
  75007 Paris, France
Blackwell Wissenschafts-Verlag GmbH
  Kurfürstendamm 57
  10707 Berlin, Germany
  Zehetnergasse 6, A-1140 Wien, Austria

Notice: The indications and dosages of all drugs
in this book have been recommended in
the medical literature and conform to the practices
of the general medical community. The medications
described do not necessarily have specific approval
by the Food and Drug Administration for use
in the diseases and dosages for which
they are recommended. The package insert
for each drug should be consulted for use and
dosage as approved by the FDA. Because standards
of usage change, it is advisable to keep abreast
of revised recommendations, particularly those
concerning new drugs.

First published 1976
Second edition 1987
Third edition 1996

Acquisitions: Christopher Davis
Development: Coleen Traynor
Production: Karen Moore
Manufacturing: Paul Lansdowne
Typeset by: Setrite Typesetters, Hong Kong
Printed and bound in Great Britain by
The Bath Press

96 97 98 99 5 4 3 2 1

DISTRIBUTORS

USA
  Blackwell Science, Inc.
  238 Main Street
  Cambridge, Massachusetts 02142
  (*Telephone orders*: 800 215 1000
                       617 876 7000)
Canada
  Copp Clark Ltd
  2775 Matheson Blvd East
  Mississauga, Ontario
  (*Telephone orders*: 800 263-4374
                       905 238−6074)
Australia
  Blackwell Science Pty Ltd
  54 University Street
  Carlton, Victoria 3053
  (*Telephone orders*: 03 9347 0300)
Outside North America and Australia
  Blackwell Science Ltd
  c/o Marston Book Services Ltd
  PO Box 269
  Abingdon
  Oxon OX14 4YN
  England
  (*Telephone orders*: 44 1235 465500)

Library of Congress
Cataloging in Publication Data

Complications in diagnostic and
  interventional imaging/edited by
  George Ansell . . . [et al.]. — 3rd ed.
      p.   cm.
  Rev. ed. of: Complications in
diagnostic imaging/edited by G. Ansell,
R.A. Wilkins: foreword by Sir Thomas Lodge.
2nd ed. 1987.
    Includes bibliographical references
    and index.
    ISBN 0-86542-243-5
    1. Diagnostic imaging — Complications.
    2. Radiology, Interventional — Complications.
    I. Ansell, G. (George).
    II. Complications in diagnostic imaging.
    [DNLM: 1. Diagnostic Imaging —
    adverse effects.
    2. Radiology, Interventional.
    3. Contrast Media — adverse effects.
    WN 180 C737 1996]
      RC78.7.D53C65   1996
    616.07′54 — dc20   95-41053

Contents

Part 5: Risk Identification and Management

Contributors

David J. Allison MD, FRCP, FRCR, *Director, Department of Diagnostic Radiology, Royal Postgraduate Medical School, Hammersmith Hospital, DuCane Road, London W12 0HS, UK*

Mohamed Amin, MD, *Fellow, Department of Radiology, University of Michigan Medical School, University Hospitals, 1500 E. Medical Center Drive, Ann Arbor, MI 48109-0030, USA*

George Ansell MD, FRCP, FRCR, *Liverpool Medical Institution, 114 Mount Pleasant, Liverpool L3 5SR, UK*

Michael A. Bettmann MD, *Chief, Cardiovascular and Interventional Radiology, Dartmouth-Hitchcock Medical Center, 1 Medical Center Drive, Lebanon, NH 03756, USA*

Anne E. Boothroyd MB, ChB, FRCR, *Consultant Radiologist, Department of Radiology, Royal Liverpool Childrens Trust, Alder Hey Hospital, Eaton Road, Liverpool L12 2AP*

Robert D. Boutin MD, *Co-Director, Musculoskeletal Imaging, Department of Radiology, Beth Israel Hospital, 330 Brookline Avenue, Boston MA 02215, USA*

Helen Carty FRCP, FRCPI, FRCR, *Consultant Radiologist, Department of Radiology, Royal Liverpool Childrens Trust, Alder Hey Hospital, Eaton Road, Liverpool L12 2AP, UK*

Michael Y.M. Chen MD, *Department of Radiology, The Bowman Gray School of Medicine, Wake Forest University, Medical Center Blvd, Winston-Salem, NC 27157-1088, USA*

Paul M. Chetham MD, *Assistant Professor of Anesthesia, University of Colorado Health Sciences Center, Denver, CO 80262, USA*

John F. Cockburn MRCP, FRCR, FFRRCSI, *William Cook Fellow in Interventional Radiology, Royal Postgraduate Medical School, The Hammersmith Hospital, DuCane Road, London W12 0HS, UK*

Richard H. Cohan MD, *Associate Professor, Department of Radiology, University of Michigan Hospitals, University Hospital, 1500 E. Medical Centre Drive, Ann Arbor, MI 48109-0030, USA*

J. Oscar M.C. Craig FRCR, FRCS, FRCP, FRCGP, FRCSI, FFRRCSI (Hon), FHKCR (Hon), *Honorary Consultant Radiologist, St. Mary's Hospital, London; Past President, The Royal College of Radiologists; Member, President's Advisory Board, Medical Protection Society; 18 Sandy Lane, Cheam, Surrey SM2 7NR, UK*

Horacio B. D'Agostino MD, *Associate Professor of Radiology, Chief, Interventional Radiology Service, Department of Radiology, University of California, San Diego, Medical Center, 200 West Arbor Drive, San Diego, CA 92103-8756, USA*

Michael D. Dake MD, *Chief, Department of Cardiovascular and Interventional Radiology, Stanford University Medical Center, Room H-3647, Stanford, CA 94305, USA*

Maria M. Damiano RT, *Director of Education, Department of Radiology, Brigham and Women's Hospital, 75 Francis Street, Boston, MA 02115, USA*

Catherine Dring (lawyer in private practice), *San Diego, CA, USA*

N. Reed Dunnick MD, *Professor and Chairman, Department of Radiology, University of Michigan Hospitals, University Hospital B1G503/0030, 1500 E. Medical Center Drive, Ann Arbor, MI 48109-0030, USA*

Janette D. Durham MD, *Associate Professor of Radiology at the University of Colorado School of Medicine, Interventional Radiology, University of Colorado Health Sciences Center, 4200 E. 9th Avenue (A030), Denver, CO 80262, USA*

Randall J. Enstrom MD, *Assistant Chief, Department of Radiology, Kaiser Foundation Hospital, 2025 Morse Avenue, Sacramento, CA 95825, USA*

Michael S. Feld PhD, *Professor of Physics, Massachusetts Institute of Technology; Director, George R. Harrison Spectroscopy Laboratory, Cambridge, MA, USA*

Geoffrey S. Ferguson MD, *Group Health Cooperative of Puget Sound, Clinical Associate Professor, University of Washington School of Medicine, Group Health Central Hospital, Department of Radiology, 200 15th Avenue East, Seattle, WA 98112, USA*

Robert D.G. Ferguson MD, *Mid South Imaging and Therapeutics, Suite 364, 930 Madison Avenue, Memphis, TN 38103, USA*

Christopher D.R. Flower FRCP(C), FRCR, *Consultant Radiologist, Addenbrooke's Hospital, Hills Road, Cambridge CB2 2QQ, UK*

Roger A. Frost MRCP, FRCR, *Consultant Radiologist, Salisbury District Hospital, Salisbury, Wiltshire SP2 8BJ, UK*

Margaret E. Hansen MD, *Assistant Professor, Department of Radiology, University of Texas Southwestern Medical Center, 5323 Harry Hines Blvd, Dallas, TX 75235-8896, USA*

Shyam B. Hatangadi MD, *Research Fellow, Division of Maternal Fetal Medicine, Department of Obstetrics and Gynecology, St. Peters Medical Center, MOB 4th floor, 254 Easton Avenue, New Brunswick, NJ 08903-0591, USA*

James E. Jackson MRCP, FRCR, *Senior Lecturer in Diagnostic Radiology, Royal Postgraduate Medical School, The Hammersmith Hospital, DuCane Road, London W12 0HS, UK*

Mark D. Jacobson MD, *Interventional Radiologist, Westside Regional Medical Center, 8201 West Broward Blvd, Plantation, FL 33324, USA*

A. Everette James Jr ScM, MD, Esq. *Chair Emeritus, Department of Radiology and Radiological Sciences, Vanderbilt University, Nashville; Senior Policy Advisor, National Academy of Sciences (Institute of Medicine), Visiting Scientist, National Institutes of Health, Washington DC; Adjunct Professor, John Hopkins School of Medicine, Baltimore MD; Special Advisor, Board of Science and Technology, Office of the Governor, Raleigh NC, St James Place, Box 789, Robersonville, NC 27871, USA*

Chester R. Jarmolowski MD, *Director, Pittsburgh Vascular Institute, Department of Radiological Sciences and Diagnostic Imaging, Shadyside Hospital, 5230 Centre Avenue, Pittsburgh, PA 15232, USA*

Emanuel Kanal MD, *Director of MRI, Associate Professor of Radiology, Department of Radiology, University of Pittsburgh, Pittsburgh NMR Institute, Pittsburgh, PA 15261, USA*

John A. Kaufman MD, *Instructor in Radiology, Harvard Medical School, Division of Vascular Radiology, Massachusetts General Hospital, 32 Fruit Street, Boston, MA 02114, USA*

Michael J. Kellett MA, MB, B Chir, FRCR, *Consultant Radiologist, St Peters Hospital and Institute of Urology and Nephrology, University College, London; Department of Uroradiology, St Peter's Hospital, Middlesex Hospital, Mortimer Street, London W1N 8AA, UK*

Brian Kendall MD, *Consultant Neuroradiologist, Neuroradiology Department, Royal Free Hospital, Pond Street, London; Middlesex Hospital, Mortimer Street, London W1N 8AA, UK*

Ducksoo Kim MD, *Director, Vascular and Interventional Radiology, Beth Israel Hospital, Associate Professor of Radiology, Harvard Medical School, 330 Brookline Avenue, Boston, MA 02215, USA*

Robert A. Knuppel MD, MPH, *Professor and Chair, Department of Obstetrics, Gynecology, and Reproductive Sciences, Robert Wood Johnson Medical School, 125 Paterson Street, New Brunswick, NJ 08901-1977, USA*

David A. Kumpe MD, *Director of Interventional Radiology and Professor of Radiology and Surgery at the University of Colorado School of Medicine, Department of Radiology, University of Colorado Health Sciences Center, 4200 E. 9th Avenue (A030), Denver, CO 80262, USA*

Colin R. Lazarus BPharm, PhD, MRPharmS, *Radiopharmacist, Department of Nuclear Medicine, Guy's Hospital, St Thomas Street, London SE1 9RT, UK*

Elsie Levin MD, *Assistant Professor (Clinical), Boston University Medical School; Radiologist, Faulkner-Sagoff Centre 1153 Centre Street, Jamaica Plain, MA 02130, USA*

Robert P. Liddell MS, *Department of Radiology, Stanford University Medical Center, Room H-3647, Stanford, CA 94305, USA*

Leonard J. Lind MD, FCCM, *Associate Professor of Anesthesiology, University of Cincinnati, College of Medicine, Cincinnati, OH 45267-0555, USA*

Gordon Lyons MD, FRCA, *Consultant Anesthetist, St James's University Hospital, Beckett Street, Leeds LS9 7TF, UK*

Michael N. Maisey BSc, MD, FRCP, FRCR, *Professor of Radiological Sciences, Department of Nuclear Medicine, Guy's Hospital, St Thomas Street, London SE1 9RT, UK*

M. Victoria Marx MD, *Assistant Professor of Radiology, University of Michigan Medical Center, B1D502, Box 0030, 1500 E. Medical Center Drive, Ann Arbor, MI 48109-0030, USA*

Iain W. McCall FRCR, *Consultant Radiologist, Department of Diagnostic Imaging, The Robert Jones and Agnes Hunt Orthopaedic Hospital, Oswestry SY10 7AG, UK*

Charles A. McConnell MRCP, FRCR, *Consultant Radiologist, Department of Radiology, Glan Clwyd District General Hospital, North Wales LL18 5UJ, UK*

Hylton B. Meire FRCR, *Consultant Radiologist, King's College Hospital, Denmark Hill, London SE5 9RS, UK*

Satish C. Muluk MD, *Assistant Professor of Surgery, University of Pittsburgh School of Medicine, A-1011 PUH, 200 Lothrop Street, Pittsburgh PA 15213, USA*

Phillip S. Mushlin MD, PhD, *Associate Professor of Anesthesia, Harvard Medical School, Brigham and Women's Hospital, 75 Francis Street, Boston, MA 02115, USA*

Steven B. Oglevie MD, *Assistant Professor of Radiology, University of California, San Diego; Chief of Interventional Radiology, Department of Veterans Affairs Medical Center, 3350 La Jolla Village Drive, San Diego, CA 92161, USA*

Risteard M. O'Laoide MB, FRCR, FFR[RCSI] *Consultant Radiologist, Department of Radiology, Meath and Adelaide Hospitals, Heytesbury Street, Dublin 8, Ireland*

William W. Orrison, Jr MD, *Chief of Neuroradiology, Professor of Radiology, Associate Professor of Neurology, University of New Mexico School of Medicine, 915 Camino de Salud, Albuquerque, NM 87131-5336, USA*

David J. Ott MD, *Department of Radiology, The Bowman Gray School of Medicine, Wake Forest University, Medical Center Blvd, Winston-Salem, NC 27157-1088, USA*

Simon P.G. Padley BSc, MB, BS, MRCP, FRCR, *Consultant Radiologist, Chelsea and Westminster Hospital, 369 Fulham Road, London SW10 9NH, UK*

Yuri R. Parisky MD, *Assistant Professor of Radiology, Director, Outpatient Radiology, University of Southern California Medical Center, 1200 North State Street, Room 3550, Los Angeles, CA 90033, USA*

Philip C. Pieters MD, *Assistant Professor, Department of Radiology, Virginia Commonwealth University, Medical College of Virginia, School of Medicine, MCV Station, Richmond, VA 23298, USA*

C. Christopher Pittman MD, *Clinical Assistant Professor of Radiology, University of South Florida College of Medicine, Tampa; Department of Radiology, Division of Interventional Radiology, Tampa General Hospital, Tampa, FL 33601, USA*

Maurice John Raphael MA, MD, FRCP, FRCR, *Consultant Radiologist, The Middlesex Hospital, Mortimer Street, London W1N 8AA, UK*

Charles E. Ray, Jr MD, *Director, Angiography/ Interventional Radiology, Roswell Park Cancer Institute; Assistant Professor of Radiology, SUNY at Buffalo, Elm and Carleton Sts, Buffalo NY 14263, USA*

Susan Robinson MBBS, *Anesthesiologist, Melbourne, Australia*

Max P. Rosen MD, *Department of Radiology, Beth Israel Hospital, Assistant Professor of Radiology, Harvard Medical School, 330 Brookline Avenue, Boston, MA 02215, USA*

Marilyn A. Roubidoux MD, *Assistant Professor, Department of Radiology, University of Michigan Hospitals, University Hospital, 1500 E. Medical Center Drive, Ann Arbor, MI 48109-0030, USA*

Ross S. Rulli EEN, *Radiology Technician II, Radiology Engineering Department, Children's Hospital, Boston, MA 02115, USA*

Frederick W. Rupp MD, *Assistant Professor of Radiology, University of New Mexico School of Medicine, 915 Camino de Salud, Albuquerque, NM 87131, USA*

Michael S.T. Ruttley MB, FRCP, FRCR, *Consultant Radiologist, University Hospital of Wales, Heath Park, Cardiff CF4 4XW, Wales, UK*

Barry A. Sacks MD, *Clinical Assistant Professor of Radiology, Harvard Medical School and Beth Israel Hospital, Boston; Department of Radiology, MetroWest Medical Center, 67 Union Street, Natick, MA 01760, USA*

Norman L. Sadowsky MD, *Professor of Radiology (Clinical), Tufts University School of Medicine; Director, Faulkner-Sagoff Centre, 1153 Centre Street, Jamaica Plain, MA 02130, USA*

Frank G. Shellock PhD, FACC, FACSM, *Director, Research and Technology Advancement, American Health Services Corporation, Newport Beach; Associate Professor of Radiology, UCLA School of Medicine, Los Angeles; Director, Research and Quality Assurance, Future Diagnostics Inc., 6380 Wilshire Blvd, 900, Los Angeles, CA 90048, USA*

Neil J. Solomon MD, *Interventional Radiologist, Forbes Regional Hospital, 2570 Haymaker Road, Monroeville PA 15146, USA*

James B. Spies MD, *Chief, Interventional Radiology, Department of Radiology, Sibley Memorial Hospital, 5255 Loughboro Road, NW, Washington, DC 20016, USA*

Keith J. Strauss MSc, *Director, Radiology, Physics, and Engineering, Childrens Hospital, 300 Longwood Avenue, Boston, MA 02115, USA*

Amy S. Thurmond MD, *Radiologist, Associate Professor of Radiology and Obstetrics and Gynecology, Oregon Health Sciences University, 12031 S.W. Breyman Avenue, Portland, OR 97219, USA*

Eric vanSonnenberg MD, *Chairman and Professor of Radiology, Professor of Internal Medicine and Surgery, Department of Radiology, University of Texas Medical Branch at Galveston, 301 University Boulevard, Galveston, TX 77555-0709, USA*

Mark H. Wholey MD, *Chairman, Pittsburgh Vascular Institute, Department of Radiological Sciences and Diagnostic Imaging, Shadyside Hospital; Clinical Professor of Radiology, University of Pittsburgh School of Medicine, 5230 Centre Avenue, Pittsburgh, PA 15232, USA*

Robert A. Wilkins MD, *Consultant Radiologist, Northwick Park Hospital, Watford Road, Harrow, Middlesex HA1 3UJ, UK*

Louise S. Wilkinson BA, BM, BCh, *Northwick Park Hospital, Watford Road, Harrow, Middlesex HA1 3UJ, UK*

Rowan Wilson MRCP, FRCA, *Consultant Anesthetist, St James's University Hospital, Leeds LS9 7TF, UK*

Preface to the third edition

Primum non nocere
[First do no harm]

During the nine years since the second edition of this book was published in 1987, imaging has continued to advance at a very rapid rate, producing many clinical benefits for our patients. Nowhere is this more evident than in the field of interventional imaging.

With all the new techniques, however, there is a cost—risk—benefit equation to be considered. We must therefore recognize and contend with any new problems that may arise. Moreover, complications may also continue to occur with the longer established procedures.

This new third edition has been restructured and largely rewritten with many new chapters. It is divided into five parts. The first addresses the major concerns about patient care, including sedation, anesthesia, related medications and resuscitation. These are considerations which apply to all areas of diagnostic imaging, since even with totally noninvasive examinations, the physician may be dealing with distressed or clinically unstable patients. Precautions against infectious complications are also of increasing importance.

The second section addresses relevant technical concerns such as radiation safety, electrical and mechanical considerations with radiologic equipment, and the broad bio-effects of ultrasound, isotopes, magnetic resonance imaging, and lasers. Part three is specifically designated for a comprehensive review of intravascular iodinated contrast media.

The fourth section deals with specific modalities and areas of practice covering all the main organ systems, ranging from complications with vascular procedures to those associated with skeletal and pediatric imaging. Each chapter is organized to provide an overview, first of major complications followed by those that are less important or infrequent. These are analyzed with relation to incidence, etiology, risk factors, prevention, and treatment.

Investigations such as bronchography and lymphography, which are now used infrequently, have been omitted: the reader is referred to earlier editions of the book for information on these subjects. The final section deals with broader but increasingly important topics focussing on liability and risk management issues.

We welcome the expertise of our new contributors, many of whom come from the USA. As in both previous editions, we consider that effective prevention and treatment of complications is dependent on a thorough knowledge of fundamentals. We have therefore aimed to make the book comprehensive but readable.

It will be of particular value to radiologists in training, but we believe that experienced radiologists and indeed other clinicians will also find much of interest to them. The book is also designed to serve as a departmental reference manual with emphasis on rapid accessibility of authoritative information. This is aided by extensive referencing of each chapter, detailed cross referencing, and the inclusion of a comprehensive index.

This book will be published shortly after the 100th anniversary of the discovery of X-rays by Roentgen in November 1895. We would be gratified if it makes a useful contribution to the further advancement of our speciality and to the safety of our patients.

GEORGE ANSELL
ROBERT A. WILKINS

The revered Latin statement that appears at the beginning of the Preface is the basis of this volume. Radiology is an increasingly diverse and complex field. As an example, in the early 1970s, the oral examination of the American Board of Radiology consisted of five sections. Today, there are 10. In the 1970s, ultrasound, as measured against today's capabilities, was primitive. Computed tomography and magnetic resonance imaging (MRI) had not yet been introduced. Neuroradiology included diagnostic angiography, myelography with oil-based, nonwater-soluble contrast agents, and pneumoencephalography. Mammography was relatively infrequently performed and image-guided biopsy was not considered relevant. Cardiovascular radiology was still largely cardiac and diagnostic. The only interventions commonly undertaken were for improved diagnosis of malignancies, and subsequently for treatment of gastrointestinal bleeding. Radiology today is a different, broader, and more complex field than it was when the first edition of this volume was published in the 1970s.

As has always been the case, complications occur. As the field has evolved, so have both the nature and the understanding of complications. Complications are almost certainly unavoidable to some extent. ·Some of those who are ill invariably get sicker, and adverse events such as myocardial infarction in a patient with unstable angina or renal failure in a patient with long-standing severe diabetes mellitus may well occur merely coincidental to a radiologic examination rather than because of it. That is, there is almost certainly an irreducible incidence of some adverse events, and some "complications" will occur whether or not an examination is performed.

On the other hand, it is important to "first do no harm". Some complications are unquestionably due to the examination, be it a diagnostic mammogram or a neurointerventional procedure. To best serve patients, it is important to be as aware of and knowledgeable about such complications as is currently possible. Although the state of knowledge is always incomplete, it is possible to be aware of both common and rare complications, and to attempt to fully understand, prevent, and effectively treat them. That was always the aim of this book, and is the underlying theme of this third edition.

This volume is divided into five sections. The first addresses the major underlying concerns about patient care: analgesia and anesthesia, related medications, infection, and resuscitation. These are considerations which apply to all areas of diagnostic imaging, since even with the totally noninvasive examinations, the physician may be dealing with distressed or clinically unstable patients. The second addresses major technical concerns such as radiation effects, mechanical considerations with radiologic equipment and the broad bio-effects of ultrasound, isotopes, lasers, and MRI. The third section is an extensive review of iodinated contrast agents. The fourth section deals with specific modalities and areas of practice ranging from diagnostic thoracic radiology to specific areas of intervention such as vascular thrombolysis. These chapters are organized to provide an overview, first of major and frequent complications, and then less important and/or less common ones. Within this framework, each chapter addresses the incidence, etiology, risk factors for, means of prevention, recognition, and treatment of the relevant complications. The final section deals with what can be considered broader, but no less important, topics, focussing on liability and risk management issues. Chapters in this section, as benfits the entire book, deal separately with the British and American situations and experiences.

The evolution of diagnostic imaging over the century since the discovery of X-rays by Roentgen in November 1985 has been dramatic. The changes in the last two decades since the first edition of this volume have also been dramatic. This volume has been made possible by the hard work of many individuals from many fields which make up and interact with diagnostic and interventional radiology. In keeping with the complexity of the topic, there are contributions from several different countries.

It is our hope that this volume will prove valuable to individuals at all levels of training in radiology, as well as to others who come in contact with this field — as essentially all in medicine now do! It is also our intent that this volume serve as a reference, providing information prior to examinations as well as a source of knowledge and aid after complications have been encountered. With the thoughtful, energetic contributions of many talented authors we hope that this effort will prove useful in achieving the goal of improved understanding, prevention, and treatment of complications, and will thus lead us closer to the goal of "first do no harm".

MICHAEL A. BETTMANN
JOHN A. KAUFMAN

Preface to the first edition

In recent years there have been spectacular advances in radiology. As in all other spheres of medicine, however, the increased benefit to the patient in diagnostic accuracy must be balanced against the inevitable small but significant risk of complications which may ensue. Because of the rarity of many of these complications, an individual radiologist will fortunately witness few of them during his career. Nevertheless, every radiologist must be conversant with these possibilities so that if a complication does arise, he will be able to diagnose this promptly and institute appropriate treatment. This book provides a comprehensive and authoritative review of the subject. Particular emphasis has been placed on techniques and fundamental principles, thereby providing a rational approach to prevention and treatment.

I am grateful to my colleagues, all acknowledged experts in their fields, who so readily agreed to contribute to the book. Radiologists will mourn the sad loss of Professor Arne Engeset and the chapter written in collaboration with Professor Lundervold will be a lasting tribute to his memory.

I should also like to thank the many radiologists who participated in the UK National Radiological Survey for the valuable information derived from their reports. Much of this material has been incorporated into the book where it provides an important and easily accessible source of reference.

Finally, I should like to pay tribute to the publishers for their helpful co-operation and for the excellent reproduction of the illustrations.

GEORGE ANSELL

Part 1
Care of the Patient

CHAPTER 1

Sedation

Gordon Lyons and Rowan Wilson

Introduction

Radiologists use sedative techniques for: (i) invasive diagnostic or therapeutic procedures in adults and children; and (ii) computed tomography (CT) and magnetic resonance imaging (MRI) in children, and may well regard sedation as a means to an end. Sedative regimens are infrequently evaluated by radiologists; reports generally take the form of uncritical descriptions of a single technique, although perhaps with large numbers of patients [1–7]. Studies involving randomization, controls, and blinding are almost never done by radiologists, but feature regularly in the published work of gastrointestinal (GI) endoscopists [8–15]. Since much of this work is of direct relevance to any doctor who administers sedative drugs, it has been incorporated into this review. Complications of sedative techniques in general, and of specific drugs, will be dealt with, as will problems associated with the sedation of children. A study of the latter reveals an unexpected difference between North American and UK practice, which may have its roots in the definitions of anesthesia and sedation used in each country. Since anesthesia may be regarded as a complication of a sedative technique, and is associated with complications in its own right, an understanding of the end point of a technique is fundamental to safe practice. It is therefore necessary to begin with an examination of the definitions and guidelines produced for medical staff who are involved in the practice of sedation.

Definitions and guidelines

In the UK, problems with the training of dentists in anesthesia and sedation led, in 1978, to the formation of the Wylie working party. This defined simple sedation as:

> A technique in which the use of a drug or drugs produces a state of depression of the central nervous system enabling treatment to be carried out, but during which verbal contact with the patient is maintained throughout the period of sedation. The drugs and techniques used should carry a margin of safety wide enough to render unintended loss of consciousness unlikely [16].

The term "simple sedation" has been replaced by "conscious sedation". Although intended for dentists, this definition has been adopted by the Joint Working Party of the Royal Colleges of Radiologists and Anaesthetists, and is included in their report *Sedation and Anaesthesia in Radiology* [17]. This report goes on to state that: "The terms and concepts of heavy sedation and basal narcosis should be abandoned. Sedation under these circumstances carries a significant risk of unconsciousness, and so produces a state of anaesthesia with all its attendant risks" [17].

The nearest North American equivalent is the "Guidelines for the elective use of conscious sedation, deep sedation and general anesthesia in pediatric patients", published by the Section on Anesthesiology of the American Academy of Pediatrics (AAP) [18]. The definition of conscious sedation given here is that of Wylie, paraphrased. Both definitions require maintenance of protective reflexes and response to verbal command. The latter functions as a clinical test, which allows an observer to differentiate between sedation and general anesthesia.

Deep sedation is defined as:

A controlled state of consciousness or unconsciousness from which the patient is not easily aroused, which may be accompanied by partial or complete loss of protective reflexes, including the ability to maintain a patent airway independently and respond purposefully to physical stimulation or verbal command [18].

General anesthesia is defined as:

A controlled state of unconsciousness accompanied by a loss of protective reflexes, including the ability to maintain a patent airway independently and respond purposefully to physical stimulation or verbal command [18].

Key points to note here are that there is no clinical test by which an observer can differentiate between deep sedation and general anesthesia. The difference between the two has become a problem of semantics. Also, deep sedation is synonymous with heavy sedation, which the Royal Colleges recognize as a form of anesthesia [17]. The importance of clearly defining the dividing line between sedation and anesthesia lies in the ability to identify the personnel who are qualified to perform such procedures. Whereas anesthesia is a distinct discipline with an easily recognized province of activity, the practice of sedation is open to all disciplines. Certification is not required. Consequently, the USA experience details many instances of radiologists and their technicians, with no formal training in sedation or anesthesia, giving what would pass in the UK as a general anesthetic, to small children [1–5,19–21].

The AAP guidelines form the only recommendation for the management of children, and if they encourage non-anesthetists to practice beyond their remit, the practice of pediatric sedation might be expected to attract a notable morbidity and mortality. This is indeed the case [4,5, 19–23]. These problems seem confined to North America, and will be considered elsewhere.

The AAP guidelines fortunately have not gained credence in the UK, and are being abandoned in the USA. In recognition of the problems, some hospitals are formulating their own definitions in terms that correspond to Wylie's [23].

Mortality

Mortality totally attributable to anesthesia is less than 1: 100 000 [24]. There are no figures to suggest what the mortality for radiologic sedation might be. However, estimates of mortality from upper GI endoscopy range from 1:7500 to 1:20 000 [25,26]. Cardiopulmonary problems account for 50% of the morbidity and 60% of deaths [27].

While the complication rate of gastroscopy has decreased by 40% over the past 15 years, from 0.13 to 0.08%, there has been a small increase in the mortality and cardiopulmonary complication rate, which correlates well with the increasing number of elderly and compromised patients [28].

Sedative techniques contribute to mortality through drug-induced respiratory depression, and it can be argued that mortality from anesthesia alone is not comparable with that of upper GI endoscopy because of the contribution to upper airway obstruction from the endoscope [8]. Apnea and oxygen desaturation occur with insertion of the endoscope, but after this, desaturation is not related to respiratory pattern [9]. On the other hand, desaturation has been observed in a group of patients, irrespective of whether the endoscopy was performed on the upper or lower GI tract, and independent of the use of sedation [29]. It would seem safe to assume that the presence of an upper GI endoscope, and the performance of any invasive procedure, might have a negative effect on oxygen saturation [28] (Fig. 1.1).

Cardiopulmonary risk

The first recorded death during GI endoscopy occurred in the 1950s, and was attributed to ventricular fibrillation [28]. In a more recent questionnaire survey, 48 correspondents reported 52 deaths, 119 respiratory arrests, and 37 cardiac arrests. Of responding doctors, 40% had experience of severe respiratory depression in the previous 2 years, and 11% had seen it on more than three occasions. Over 50% only gave oxygen once a year [25]. Reviewing complications of upper GI endoscopy, Hart and Classen [28] reported a cardiac complication rate of 0.047%, and a respiratory complication rate of 0.026%, in 175 000 sedated endoscopy patients. Among the cardiac complications were arrhythmias (17%), myocardial infarction (6%), and cardiac arrest (4%). The two major pulmonary complications were apnea (40%), and aspiration pneumonia (52%). In 75 000 examinations conducted without intravenous (IV) sedation, aspiration pneumonia did not occur, and there was only one cardiac arrest [28].

Respiratory factors

Contributing factors in oxygen desaturation during endoscopic cholangiopancreatography (ECP) are advancing age, preexisting lung disease, increasing IV sedation, and diameter of the endoscope [8]. During ECP 44% of patients may become hypoxic [10]. Chronic obstructive airway disease in patients requiring IV sedation has been identified as a particular risk factor by some [8,28], but others have found that age, sex, dose of midazolam, and preendoscopy respiratory function tests failed to identify those patients at risk of hypoxia [31,32]. While the use of IV sedatives is associated with significant oxygen desaturation [8,9,31,32], when

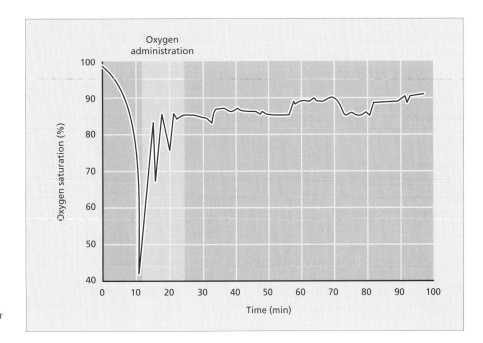

Fig. 1.1 Severe oxygen desaturation occurring during upper GI endoscopy. This patient had a short respiratory arrest requiring manual ventilation for approximately 3 minutes. Oxygen was then administered by nasal cannulae for the remainder of the examination [30].

effective sedation improves patient tolerance the degree of desaturation may be reduced. Other risk factors include the duration of the procedure, the inexperience of the operator [11], and the use of IV contrast media which, by shifting the oxyhemoglobin dissociation canal to the left, can exacerbate the effects of desaturation. However, the shift is short lived, and may not be of clinical significance [33].

Cardiac factors

An electrocardiogram (EKG) is required in order to show rhythm disturbances during GI endoscopy. At the beginning of the procedure an increase in rate is commonly seen, and, in some patients, ST wave changes and ventricular extra-systoles [8,28], but supraventricular tachycardia is rare. The incidence of serious arrhythmias in patients with cardiac histories is 30%, compared with 6% in those without. Arrhythmias are more likely in the presence of oxygen desaturation and poor patient tolerance [8] (Fig. 1.1).

Sedative techniques

In their nationwide survey of sedation for upper GI tract endoscopy, Daneshmend *et al.* [25] estimated that 40 000 GI endoscopies are performed in the UK every year. Of those using IV sedation, one-third use midazolam, and less than 20% use additional IV drugs. Severe hypoventilation was reported by 47% of doctors who titrated drugs, compared with 37% of bolus givers. Of those using additional drugs, 52% reported severe hypoventilation, compared with 40% using one drug. The additional drug commonly used was pethidine. The authors question the safety of pethidine

when used in combinations, but feel that problems associated with titration come from more alert respondents, and do not represent a causal relationship. There was no difference in the number of incidents between users of midazolam and diazepam [25]. When IV sedative drugs are being given, it is likely that one or other of these drugs will be involved.

Midazolam and diazepam

Midazolam is favored for short procedures because its pharmacologic profile is more suitable. Diazepam is burdened with longer distribution and elimination half-lives, and a slower total body clearance. At equivalent doses, midazolam produces more amnesia [12]. Both drugs induce modest hypotension, which remains stable. In contrast to diazepam, midazolam does not reduce systemic vascular resistance. The reduction in blood pressure is related to a reduced cardiac output, and is commonly associated with an increase in heart rate. Myocardial oxygen demand is reduced, but coronary autoregulation remains unaltered [34,35].

Concern in the USA over the safety of midazolam prompted a call to ban its use for conscious sedation in the over 60s. Dose recommendations in the USA were thought to be inappropriately large, and responsible for significant cardio-respiratory side-effects, especially in the elderly, who are less able to distribute and eliminate midazolam, and therefore more sensitive. Early dose-finding studies in the UK showed that in excess of 0.1 mg/kg resulted in oversedation. Eighty-eight per cent of patients were satisfied with 0.07 mg/kg, although amnesia decreased from 88 to 64%. UK recommendations are for 2.5 mg (0.036 mg/kg) to 7.5 mg (0.1 mg/kg) for 70 kg adults, with lower doses for the elderly.

In December 1985, the Food and Drugs Administration (FDA) approved 0.1–0.15 mg/kg (rarely, 0.2 mg/kg) for adults, and for the elderly, 0.07–0.1 mg/kg, which is similar to the dose range for diazepam. In May 1986, midazolam was released in the USA, and by November 1986, 13 fatalities had been reported due to respiratory depression and cardiac arrest, mainly in elderly patients for conscious sedation. In 1987, the USA dose was revised to 0.07 mg/kg for adults, and 0.05 mg/kg for the elderly. By January 1988, 66 deaths had been reported. By contrast, in the UK, four deaths had been reported to the Committee of Safety of Medicines and, in addition, nine reports of respiratory depression, two of respiratory arrest, two of hypotension, and one instance of heart block. The majority of these reports followed the use of midazolam for conscious sedation, and probably represent significant underreporting. Recommendations for the safe use of midazolam include ensuring the dose is correct, making allowance for age, titrating to take account of individual variation, and using the more dilute 2 mg/ml formulation [36]. Not only does the dose requirement of both benzodiazepines decline with age, but in those over 60 years old the relative potency of midazolam increases to the extent that diazepam has been recommended for the elderly [37] (Fig. 1.2).

Midazolam produces more retrograde amnesia than diazepam [13], and has greater acceptance when given for endoscopic sedation in children [38]. While it is generally reckoned to cause less phlebitis and pain on injection [14], this is not a constant finding [13].

Benzodiazepines and opioid combinations

The capacity of opioids to enhance the hypnotic effect of benzodiazepines is greater than their analgesic potency. Subanalgesic doses of alfentanil can double the potency of midazolam [39]. Synergism has also been shown with fentanyl [40]. When used in conjunction with an opioid, midazolam 0.15–0.2 mg/kg can induce anesthesia [41]. Pethidine is commonly used with benzodiazepines for endoscopic procedures. A review of its use with diazepam (53 mg pethidine/8.4 mg diazepam per 70 kg body weight), for 758 endoscopic procedures, found a 1% complication rate, and 2.5% needed naloxone [42]. Similar doses were given to 55 colonoscopy patients without incident, but an equivalent dose of midazolam in combination with pethidine rendered 8% of patients unrousable [14]. Midazolam in combination for GI endoscopy was associated with significant oxygen desaturation in 20%, and apnea in 10% [30].

One alternate to pethidine is the partial agonist nalbuphine. As an agonist for the κ-receptor, it combines analgesia with sedation, and has dose-limited respiratory depression. It has no cardiovascular effects and is reversed by naloxone [43]. It has been used as the sole sedation in hundreds of patients undergoing endoscopy, angiography, and angioplasty. Failure

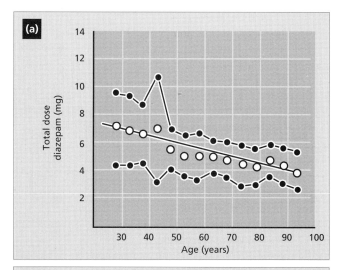

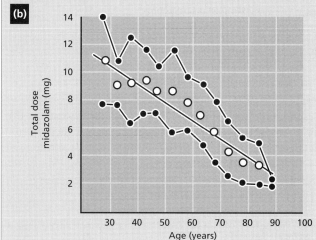

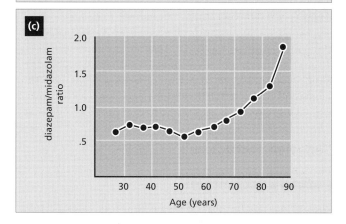

Fig. 1.2 Smaller doses of diazepam (a) and midazolam (b) are required with advancing age. Over the age of 60 years, midazolam becomes increasingly potent when compared with diazepam (c) [37].

rate was less than 0.5%, and the only complication was occasional pain on injection [6]. When combined with midazolam in volunteers, no severe respiratory depression was noticed, but minor respiratory changes persisted for up to 2 hours, and there was an appreciable incidence of movement-related nausea [44]. A nalbuphine/midazolam combination for fiberoptic bronchoscopy produced more sedation and greater comfort than midazolam alone, but also more nausea, dizziness, and longer recovery. Two patients became apneic after nalbuphine [35]. When compared with pentazocine in combination with diazepam, for aortography, complication rates were the same [43].

Use of opioids in combination with benzodiazepines may improve patient comfort, but risk of apnea and significant hypoventilation is greatly increased [25].

Reversing benzodiazepines

Flumazenil reversal of midazolam sedation following endoscopy will ensure that the majority of patients are awake 5 minutes after the procedure ends, with the apparent potential for earlier discharge [12]. Any advantage in alertness and psychomotor performance has gone within 4 hours [15]. Because the half-life of flumazenil (<1 hour), is significantly shorter than that of the drugs it is being used to reverse, resedation is a danger [36]. Although the cardiac effects of midazolam are reversed [34], the respiratory effects may not be [45]. It could be argued that the use of flumazenil is an indication for longer observation, and warnings about inducing a false sense of security with its use are appropriate [36]. Titration of small doses at 1-minute intervals to a maximum of 1–2 mg is recommended [41]. It may cause pain on injection [12].

Local anesthetic throat spray

Mucosal absorption of tetracaine 20–25 mg was responsible for convulsion in two patients and collapse in a third, with one fatality [46].

Sedative techniques for children

Chloral hydrate is the most commonly used sedative drug [19,47], followed by a cocktail comprising pethidine, promethazine, and chlorpromazine (PPC). Barbiturates are used in 15% of pediatric sedations. Reports list 25 different pairs of drugs used in the sedation of toddlers [19], with some children receiving up to five different depressant drugs, a factor associated with increased risk [48].

There is no consensus for the best sedation protocol [19], and although some detail critical incidents [4,5,7,21,48–52], dramatic underreporting is suspected [19]. The Pediatric Drug Surveillance Service of the Harvard Children's Hospital report four times as many life-threatening reactions in children sedated for imaging procedures than in the general population [48]. Nine deaths are reported by 129 pediatric radiologists, with a further 18 incidents of respiratory arrest, all associated with the sedation of children [22]. Given that deep sedation as practiced in North America is indistinguishable from anesthesia as recognized in the UK, airway problems might be expected. Keeter *et al.* [19] reported that emergency airway care is thought to be indicated by 11% of replying hospitals, when snoring is not wholly relieved by neck extension. Fifty-four per cent recognized that hypoventilation required intermittent positive pressure with bag and mask, and 75% would do so for apnea. The fate of children sedated in the remaining 25% of hospitals is unenviable! This information was collected from a 13-page questionnaire sent to 834 hospitals in the USA [19]. One optimistic interpretation of this data is that rather than signifying ignorance of the most fundamental aspect of resuscitation, it might represent questionnaire fatigue.

Different protocols produce different problems, and these will be considered individually below.

Chloral hydrate

Chloral hydrate is favored because it has little potential for toxicity [47], but some regard it as unreliable [2]. It is easy to administer, and because of its relatively long onset time — up to 1 hour [21] — could be given on the ward or in a waiting area. The recommended dose for children is given as 30–50 mg/kg, up to a maximum single dose of 1 g [53]. In practice, doses given range from 30 to 100 mg/kg in a single dose [2,20,21,51,52], and some quote a ceiling dose of 2 g [21,51]. Smaller doses are suggested for children with liver, renal, respiratory, and central nervous system disorders [51]. Undisguised, it has an unpleasant taste, and can cause gastric irritation. An alternate is triclofos sodium, a derivative of chloral but with fewer GI upsets, and no reduction in oxygen saturation [54]. The recommended dose is 10–25 mg/kg [53].

Greenberg *et al.* [51] evaluated high dose chloral hydrate given to 295 children for 326 CT scans, and 111 children with medical problems, for 124 CT scans, who received a lower dose. In those given the higher dose, five required supplementation with diazepam 0.1 mg/kg. Ninety-three per cent of scans were considered satisfactory, and 1.2% were regarded as total failures. Five children became hyperactive, 14 vomited, and four had respiratory problems. Of the latter, one was associated with asthma, one child with learning difficulties inhaled secretions, and two required intubating for airway obstruction; one of these also had learning difficulties. There were 10 times as many failed scans in the low-dose group [51].

Strain *et al.* [2] retrospectively examined the management of 5134 children undergoing CT in Denver between 1983 and 1985. Of the 749 who required sedation, 12% received high-dose chloral hydrate. There was a trend towards the use of IV barbiturate because the use of chloral hydrate was associated with a 13% failure rate, and required up to 2 hours for recovery [2].

Thompson *et al.* [21] conducted the only prospective comparative study, but because some patients were randomized and others were not, any scientific merit is submerged in confused design. Children undergoing sedation for the first time were deprived of sleep, and then given either high-dose chloral hydrate, or a cocktail consisting of atropine, pethidine, and promethazine, by two intramuscular (IM) injections. IV access was established, and supplements of secobarbitone were given if required. Of examinations in the chloral group 15%, compared with 12% in the cocktail group, failed. This was not statistically significant. A similar number in both groups (10%) required secobarbitone supplements. The IM injections were unpopular. The authors reported no deaths, but there were seven life-threatening complications in 898 CT scans. Two instances of "asphyxia", one apnea, one airway obstruction, and one problem with secretions, were seen in sedated children. The other two problems were complications of general anesthesia [21].

PPC

First used in children for cardiac catheterization [20], PPC has also been recommended as sedation for CT in a dose of 0.1 ml/kg. Each milliliter contains pethidine 25 mg, promethazine 6.25 mg, and chlorpromazine 6.25 mg [3]. This is equivalent to giving a 70-kg adult pethidine 175 mg, promethazine 45 mg, and chlorpromazine 45 mg [50], although a ceiling dose of 2 ml has been quoted. It has been given to children over a wide range of ages [48,50], and recommended for those aged 1 month to 5 years [3]. It has proved effective in 86–95% of scans [3,20]. Undesirable effects include lethargy, agitation, urinary retention, and respiratory depression. Doses as low as 0.07 ml/kg have caused respiratory arrest, and 7 hours or more are required for recovery [50,55]. PPC has also been criticized on the grounds that it lowers seizure threshold, and that promethazine is antianalgesic [55]. Nahata *et al.* [50] believe that no dose is safe. They point out that it is impossible to optimize doses of a three-drug cocktail, that there is potential synergism for central nervous, respiratory, and cardiovascular depression, and that there is no rationale for combining phenothiazines [50]. Techniques with prolonged recovery times are potentially dangerous in out-patient settings [5,20].

Barbiturates

Two studies performed by anesthetists describe the use of *methohexitone* for sedation in CT and MRI. Varner *et al.* [56], in a randomized comparison of IM methohexitone, gave either 3.5% or 5% in a dose of 10 mg/kg, to 50 children aged between 2 months and 5 years. Adequate sedation was achieved in 92%. Both groups were asleep in 3–4 minutes, were arousable after 45–50 minutes, and alert by 80–90 minutes. There were no differences between the groups. The IM injection was painful. The authors concluded that this technique compared favorably with other reported sedative techniques [56].

Griswold and Liu [57] gave methohexitone 30 mg/kg to 40 children aged between 10 weeks and 7 years, by the rectal route. The children were assessed separately according to whether they were chronic phenobarbitone users, whether they were on other therapy, or no therapy at all. They found that 30 mg/kg was adequate for most children, but was not effective for children on chronic barbiturate therapy. Five patients slept for more than 100 minutes [57].

Before being advocated for CT, *pentobarbitone* had a moderate vogue in the practice of anesthesia in the 1920s and early 1930s, but when given IV was often unpredictable and unsatisfactory, and was superseded [58]. Doses varying from 5 to 6 mg/kg IM and 2 to 6 mg/kg IV have been given to children from 6 weeks or less, to 5 years of age [1–4]. Failure rates are of the order of 1–2%. It is effective for 60 minutes [1,4]. Sanders and Lo [5] reported five critical incidents in 895 examinations. Two premature infants experienced transient apnea or hypopnea, two premature infants experienced temporary bradycardia, and one infant suffered a fatal cardiac arrest. This child was sedated 2 days after correction of tetralogy of Fallot, and was given phenytoin 30 mg/kg immediately before CT. This gives a complication rate of 0.6%, and a mortality rate of 1:1000 [5].

Strain *et al.* [4] studied the respiratory and cardiac effects of IV pentobarbitone given to 255 children aged 6 weeks to 3 years, undergoing CT. Cardiac and respiratory rates, and oxygen saturation were monitored, as was breath flow and chest wall excursion. The latter allowed observers to differentiate between apnea and loss of airway. No cardiac problems were detected, but oxygen saturation dropped to 80%, or less, of baseline values in 17 children (7%). Three children (1.5%) developed partial obstruction, and in 14 (6%) an altered respiratory pattern was observed. In one instance, desaturation stabilized at 75%, until the end of the 7-minute examination. At this point, the head was turned and the oxygen saturation rose immediately to 85%. Another child was cyanosed with a saturation of 50%. This rose to 85% on stimulation. Most children who desaturated did so within the first 5 minutes. No resuscitation, intubation, or ventilation was required. The authors justify the desaturation observed by comparing it with lobar pneumonia, when oxygen saturation may fall to 70% for prolonged periods. If it is permissible to compare the hypoxia caused by two quite distinct sets of circumstances, it should be remembered that lobar pneumonia is not a benign condition. In addition, barbiturate-induced hypoxia is avoidable, either by the appropriate degree of respiratory support, or by using a less depressant technique.

Another case report featured in this study is further cause for concern. A child with learning difficulties with mandibular hypoplasia, mandibular fracture with osteomyelitis, parotid inflammation, and retropharyngeal abscess, who had been hospitalized previously for apnea and airway obstruction, was given IV pentobarbitone. Although desaturation occurred, this was relieved by adjusting the head. This child had three separate potential sources of airway obstruction that would tax most anesthetists [59]. In particular, the use of IV barbiturates in the presence of inflammation of the mouth and jaw has a recognized mortality [60]. Strain *et al.* [4] call their paper "Safe sedation for children undergoing CT".

Opioids

Drugs in this section include morphine, pethidine [2,20,48], and fentanyl. The latter is recommended when IV pentobarbitone fails [1], but Fisher [47] feels that fentanyl is unsuitable for use by radiologists because of its potential for profound respiratory depression and chest wall rigidity.

Mitchell *et al.* [48] describe life-threatening complications, including respiratory arrest and central nervous system depression, in four infants aged between 2 days and 2 months. Two had been given morphine, one pethidine and promethazine, and one pethidine and diazepam. Multiple doses of naloxone were required [48]. Neonates are unduly sensitive to morphine, and it is not recommended for children under 1 year of age [61].

Benzodiazepines

Midazolam is commonly used, either alone [7,22], or with pethidine [49]. Diazepam [2] and temazepam [52] have also been used. Blumer *et al.* [7] studied the pharmacokinetics and pharmacodynamics of midazolam in 20 children, aged 2–6 years, undergoing CT. Initial bolus doses of 0.1 mg/kg, 0.15 mg/kg, 0.2 mg/kg, and 0.25 mg/kg were each given to five children. Four children slept after 0.2 mg/kg. Efficacy in the other groups ranged from 20 to 60%. Metabolite accumulated more rapidly in nonresponders, and elimination ranged from 10 to 120 minutes. Adverse reactions included transient hypotension in four, hiccoughs in three, nystagmus in nine, and dose-dependent agitation in five. The authors concluded that the pharmacokinetics and pharmacodynamics differ from adults [7].

Propofol

Valtonen [62] compared propofol, an IV anesthetic used for sedation, with thiopentone, in 30 children aged 3–10 years. All were given diazepam 0.2 mg/kg before the procedure, and then either propofol 1.5–2 mg/kg, or thiopentone 3–4 mg/kg. Anesthesia was achieved when children no longer responded to command, and kept still. This falls within the AAP definition of deep sedation [18]. Apnea was defined as 15 seconds without spontaneous respiration, but none was recorded, and there was no hypercapnia. Both drugs were satisfactory, but the propofol group woke up quicker [62].

Many of the studies above have claimed to evaluate safety, but without defining limits. As a result, the authors' conclusions are invalid. More general criticisms can be applied to the use of retrospective data, the lack of controls and blinding, varying definitions of efficacy, and lack of standardization. Consequently, comparative evaluations are impossible [20]. Conscious sedation is the only safe form of sedation for nonanesthetists, and from the above regimens only chloral hydrate and the benzodiazepines are suitable. Barbiturates are general anesthetics and should be reserved for anesthetists; PPC and opioids have too high a morbidity. There is a reluctance to accept the risks of general anesthesia for pediatric imaging [21], and it tends to be looked upon as a last resort [22].

It can be argued that a general anesthetic in the hands of an anesthetist is safer than a pediatric sedation in the hands of a radiologist. Moves to involve anesthetists in the practice of sedation have significantly reduced critical incidents [23].

Avoiding complications

Measures have been advocated for improving the standard of care on a number of fronts.

Patient selection

It is important that risk is assessed for each individual, and this can be done either by a grading system such as the American Society of Anesthesiologists Physical Status (ASA PS) classification [63], or a checklist similar to that used by day care units, or both. The Royal Colleges [17] approve the list recommended for endoscopy patients [26]. The ASA PS classification is suggested for endoscopy patients [26] and by the AAP in their guidelines for children [18]. The need for sedation in individual children should be questioned. Strain *et al.* [2] reduced the overall requirement for sedation from 21% to 10%, but in other centers up to 93% of children are sedated or anesthetized [21]. Giving adequate information, psychologic counseling, allowing a child gradually to familiarize with the enclosed space, the prone position, and the presence of a parent, may make sedation unnecessary, and should be encouraged [1,17,52].

Patients identified as high risk by virtue of their ASA PS classification 3 or 4, or by positive answers to the questions in the checklist, should be assessed by an anesthetist to establish if a general anesthetic is indicated, or whether sedation should be performed in the presence of an anesthetist. Wherever there is any doubt about suitability for sedation, the opinion of an anesthetist should be sought.

Personnel

In their survey of pediatric sedation, Keeter *et al.* [19] reported that in 47% of hospitals the radiologist took responsibility for the sedation regimen; in 37% a primary care physician took charge; and in 1% anesthetists were involved. Only rarely is one person solely responsible for staying with and monitoring the patient, and even more rarely is that person skilled in dealing with a complication. Reports mention periodic observation of the patient or monitors, and even advice not to leave the patient unattended for too long [1,7]. Patient monitoring is at a disadvantage when it has to compete for the attention of the radiologist, and in recognition of this an assistant dedicated to the patient is recommended. Both the supervising radiologist and the monitoring assistant should have received appropriate training, and be capable of cardiopulmonary resuscitation [17,26]. Currently, established recognized training does not exist, and standards are undefined. Eventually, these deficiencies

will be corrected, and it is likely that management of sedated patients will be limited to certificated individuals.

Oxygen

The case for giving oxygen has been convincingly argued [2,10,26,33,47]. While much morbidity is directly due to hypoxemia, administration of oxygen is of little benefit if apnea goes unrecognized. Oxygen reserves are more limited in children; in part due to increased oxygen consumption, and in part to a reduced residual volume. Administration of oxygen increases reserves and, hence, the safety margin in the event of apnea or airway obstruction. A lightweight mask or nasal cannulae should be used routinely, with an oxygen flow rate of 1–4 l/min (Fig. 1.3).

Pulse oximetry

It has been suggested that the introduction of a mandatory minimal monitoring requirement into anesthesia in Australia and the USA has not influenced the incidence of death or brain damage [64]. On the other hand, anesthetists in Massachusetts who undertake to use both capnograph and pulse oximeter can expect a 20% insurance discount.

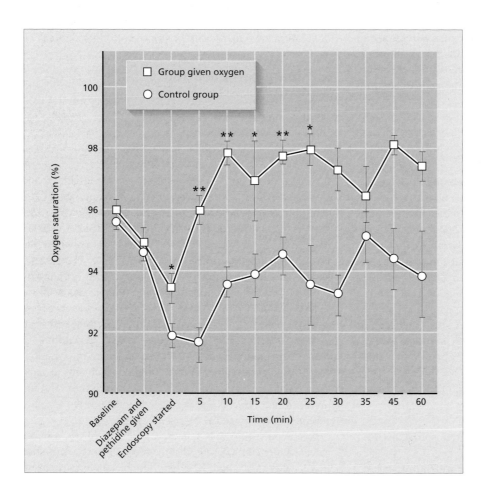

Fig. 1.3 Mean (standard error of the mean) oxygen saturation in 39 patients given intranasal oxygen, and 41 controls during retrograde ECP [10].

Youngson [65] argues that respiratory monitoring of this kind has decreased the mortality of anesthesia, and is cost effective. The same arguments apply to sedation in radiology. Visual inspection of the patient is inadequate when sophisticated electronic equipment is available automatically to monitor a wide range of physiologic parameters; devices capable of early warning of respiratory depression should be mandatory. One such device is the pulse oximeter, which can detect falls in saturation not apparent clinically, and also gives useful information about pulse rate, rhythm, and peripheral perfusion. Alarm limits for minimum saturation can be set, and an audible beep, the pitch of which can vary as saturation changes, can be listened for continuously. Once the oxygen saturation has fallen below 95% — onto the steep part of the oxyhemoglobin dissociation curve — oxygen reserves will be depleted, and further desaturation will require urgent remedial action. Pulse oximetry is recommended during GI endoscopy [26], and by the Royal Colleges [17], and other authorities [10,28,42].

Capnography

A capnograph measures expired carbon dioxide, and provides the most sensitive assessment of airway patency and respiratory depression. Apnea can be detected before the pulse oximeter registers desaturation, so that prompt action can prevent hypoxemia occurring. However, a waveform needs to be visualized, and a certain degree of familiarity with the device is recommended. Values can either increase or decrease during hypoventilation, and carbon dioxide can often still be detected during severe airway obstruction [47]. Reliably detecting and recording oral or nasal airflow in a sedated patient with a supplementary oxygen device attached may not be easy. Sampling from a nasal catheter or one limb of nasal oxygen prongs, can be effective, but the remote monitoring required in scanning rooms causes a long lag time, which tends to disfigure the waveform. Daily use has made capnography popular with anesthetists. Currently, it does not feature among recommendations for monitoring; nevertheless, it deserves the same kind of critical evaluation that pulse oximetry has experienced.

EKG

Because arrhythmias do not appear until hypoxemia is relatively severe, the EKG does not provide an early warning, although in infants bradycardia has an earlier onset. It is useful for monitoring heart rate, and is essential for resuscitation. It is recommended for GI endoscopy [26], and by the Royal Colleges [17], and other authorities [18,28,42].

Blood pressure

An automatic device will display systolic, mean, and diastolic pressures every few minutes, and is the easiest system to use. It will not provide early warning, but is recommended by the Royal Colleges [17].

Recovery

Recovery areas are recommended in endoscopy suites [26], and in departments of radiology [17]. In a dedicated area equipped with suction and oxygen, patients should continue to be monitored by trained staff, until fit for discharge. Criteria for discharging day care patients should include normal vital signs, alertness, and the ability to walk with minimal assistance [18,25]. Patients should be accompanied from the radiology department by a responsible adult with instructions as to what to do, and whom to contact, in the event of problems.

Resuscitation

When sedation goes wrong the means of achieving a secure airway and assisting ventilation must be to hand. An oxygen supply, stethoscope, tipping trolley, emergency drugs, suction, defibrillator, intravenous fluid, and administration sets, together with the recommended monitoring devices should be available, and subject to regular maintenance checks. Where a pediatric population is served, drug dosage charts are advisable, and a range of sizes must be catered for [17,18,26,46] (see also Chapter 4, p. 47).

Effects of policing

Concern over "accidents" associated with the practice of conscious sedation by nonanesthetists in the USA resulted in a department of anesthesiology assuming responsibility for all administrations of drugs likely to produce loss of "protective reflexes". This was defined as the need to assist ventilation with bag and mask, the occurrence of oxygen desaturation, the need for opioid reversal, and hemodynamic instability. These were made notifiable events which were monitored to assess competence of the practitioner and justification of the use of sedation. Privileges for conscious sedation were only granted when appropriate. The recommendations for personnel, monitoring, and resuscitation became mandatory. As a result of this policy, the reporting of incidents reduced to near zero [23]. Radiologists may choose to meet standards set by anesthesia, or they may be obliged to do so.

References

1 Kaufman RA. Technical aspects of abdominal CT in infants and children. *Am J Roentgenol* 1989;153:549–554.
2 Strain JD, Harvey LA, Foley LC, Campbell JB. Intravenously administered pentobarbital sodium for sedation in pediatric CT.

Radiology 1986;161:105−108.

3 Berger PE, Kuhn JP, Brusehaber J. Techniques for computed tomography in infants and children. *Radiol Clin N Am* 1981;19: 399−408.

4 Strain JD, Campbell JB, Harvey LA, Foley LC. IV Nembutal: safe sedation for children undergoing CT. *Am J Roentgenol* 1988;15: 975−979.

5 Sanders JE, Lo W. Computed tomography premedication in children. *J Am Med Assoc* 1983;249:263.

6 Glanville JN. Technical report: nalbuphine hydrochloride (nubain, DuPont) as premedication for radiological procedures. *Clin Radiol* 1990;42:212−213.

7 Blumer J, Weissman B, Horwitz S, Myers C, Reed M. Midazolam sedation for computerized tomography (CT) in children: pharmacokinetics and pharmacodynamics. *Acta Pharmalog Toxicol* 1986;59(Suppl. 5):75.

8 Lieberman DA, Wuerker CK, Katol RM. Cardiopulmonary risk of esophagogastroduodenoscopy. Role of endoscope diameter and systemic sedation. *Gastroenterology* 1985;88:468−472.

9 Rimmer KP, Graham K, Whitelaw WA, Field SK. Mechanisms of hypoxaemia during panendoscopy. *J Clin Gastroenterol* 1989;11: 17−22.

10 Griffin SM, Chung SCS, Leung JW, Li AKC. Effect of intranasal oxygen on hypoxia and tachycardia during endoscopic chol-angiopancreatography. *Br Med J* 1990;300:83−84.

11 Lavies NG, Creasy T, Harris K, Hanning CD. Arterial oxygen saturation during upper gastrointestinal endoscopy: influence of sedation and operator experience. *Am J Gastroenterol* 1988;83: 618−622.

12 Pearson RC, McCloy RF, Morris P, Barhan KD. Midazolam and flumazenil in gastroenterology. *Acta Anaesthesiol Scand* 1990; 34(Suppl. 92):21−24.

13 Gilvaney JM, Craig M, Fielding JF. Short report: sedation for upper gastrointestinal endoscopy — diazepam versus midazolam. *Aliment Pharmacol Ther* 1990;4:423−425.

14 Lewis BS, Shlien RD, Wayne JD, Knight RJ, Aldoroty RA. Diazepam versus midazolam (versed) in outpatient colonoscopy: a double blind randomised study. *Gastrointest Endosc* 1989;35: 33−36.

15 Andrews PJD, Wright DJ, Lamont MC. Flumazenil in the out-patient. *Anaesthesia* 1990;45:445−458.

16 The Wylie report: report of the working party on training in dental anaesthesia. *Br Dent J* 1981;151:385−388.

17 The Royal College of Radiologists, the Royal College of Anaes-thetists. *Sedation and Anaesthesia in Radiology*. Report of a joint working party, 1992.

18 Committee on Drugs, Section on Anesthesiology, American Academy of Pediatrics. Guidelines for the elective use of con-scious sedation, deep sedation, and general anesthesia in pediatric patients. *Pediatrics* 1985;76:317−321.

19 Keeter S, Benator R, Weinberg SM, Hartenburg MA. Sedation in pediatric CT: national survey of current practice. *Radiology* 1990; 175:745−752.

20 Nahata MC. Sedation in pediatric patients undergoing diagnostic procedures. *Drug Intel Clin Pharm* 1988;22:711−715.

21 Thompson JR, Schneider S, Ashwal S, Holden BS, Hinshaw DB, Hasso AN. The choice of sedation for computed tomography in children. A prospective evaluation. *Radiology* 1982;143: 475−479.

22 Cohen MD. Pediatric sedation. *Radiology* 1990;175:611−612.

23 Schares T. *Administration of Conscious Sedation by Non Anesthesio-logists*. The Hague: Abstracts of the 10th World Congress of Anesthesiologists, 1992:678.

24 Buck N, Devlin HB, Lunn JN. *Report of a Confidential Enquiry into Perioperative Deaths*. London: Nuffield Provincial Hospital Trusts, 1987.

25 Daneshmend TK, Bell GD, Logan RFA. Sedation for upper gastrointestinal endoscopy: results of a nationwide survey. *Gut* 1991;32:12−15.

26 Bell GD, McCloy RF, Charlton JE et al. Recommendations for standards of sedation and patient monitoring during gastro-intestinal endoscopy. *Gut* 1991;32:823−827.

27 Bell GD, Brown S, Morden A, Coady T, Logan RFA. Prevention of hypoxaemia during upper airway gastrointestinal endoscopy by means of oxygen via nasal cannula. *Lancet* 1987;1:1022.

28 Hart R, Classen M. Complications of diagnostic gastrointestinal endoscopy. *Endoscopy* 1990;22:229−233.

29 Fassoulaki A, Mihas A. Changes in arterial blood gases associated with gastrointestinal endoscopies. *Acta Anaesthesiol Belgica* 1987; 38:127−131.

30 Murray AW, Morran CG, Kenny GNC, Anderson JR. Arterial oxygen saturation during upper gastrointestinal endoscopy: the effects of a midazolam/pethidine combination. *Gut* 1990;31: 270−273.

31 Bell GD, Reeve PA, Moshin M et al. Intravenous midazolam: a study of the degree of oxygen desaturation occurring during upper gastrointestinal endoscopy. *Br J Clin Pharmacol* 1987;23: 703−708.

32 Dark DS, Campbell DR, Wesselius LJ. Arterial oxygen desatu-ration during gastrointestinal endoscopy. *Am J Gastroenterol* 1990;85:1317−1321.

33 Kim SJ, Salem MR, Joseph NJ, Madayag MA, Cavallino RP, Crystal GJ. Contrast media adversely affect oxyhaemoglobin dissociation. *Anesth Analg* 1990;71:73−76.

34 Marty J, Nitenberg A. The use of midazolam and flumazenil in cardiovascular diagnostic and therapeutic procedures. *Acta Anaesthesiol Scand* 1990;34(Suppl. 92):33−34.

35 Sury MRJ, Cole PV. Nalbuphine combined with midazolam for outpatient sedation. An assessment in fibreoptic bronchoscopy patients. *Anaesthesia* 1988;43:285−288.

36 Anonymous. Midazolam — is antagonism justified? *Lancet* 1988; 2:140−142.

37 Scholer SG, Schafer DF, Potter JF. The effect of age on the relative potency of midazolam and diazepam for sedation in upper gastrointestinal endoscopy. *J Clin Gastroenterol* 1990;12: 145−147.

38 Tolia V, Fleming SL, Kauffman RE. Randomised double blind trial of midazolam and diazepam for endoscopic sedation in children. *Develop Pharmacol Ther* 1990;14:141−147.

39 Kissin I, Vinik HR, Castillo R, Bradley EL. Alfentanil potentiates midazolam induced unconsciousness in subanalgesic doses. *Anesth Analg* 1990;71:65−69.

40 Ben-Schlomo I, Abd-El-Khalim H, Ezry J, Zohar S, Tverskoy M. Midazolam acts synergistically with fentanyl for induction of anaesthesia. *Br J Anaesthes* 1990;64:45−47.

41 Amrein R, Hetzel W. Pharmacology of midazolam and flumazenil. *Acta Anesthesiol Scand* 1990;34(Suppl. 92):6−15.

42 Andrus CH, Dean PA, Ponsky JL. Evaluation of safe effective intravenous sedation for utilisation in endoscopic procedures. *Surg Endosc* 1990;4:179−183.

43 Graham JL, McCaughey W, Bell PF. Nalbuphine and pentazocine in an opioid/benzodiazepine sedative technique: a double blind

comparison. *Ann Roy Col Surg Engl* 1988;70:200−204.

44 Sury MRJ, Cole PV. Nalbuphine combined with midazolam for outpatient sedation. An assessment of safety in volunteers. *Anaesthesia* 1988;43:281−284.

45 Carter AS, Bell GD, Coady T, Lee J, Morden A. Speed of reversal of midazolam induced respiratory depression by flumazenil — a study in patients undergoing upper gastrointestinal endoscopy. *Acta Anaesthesiol Scand* 1990;92:59−64.

46 Patel D, Chopra S, Berman MD. Serious systemic toxicity from use of tetracaine for pharyngeal anaesthesia in upper endoscopic procedures. *Digest Dis Sci* 1989;34:882−884.

47 Fisher DM. Sedation of pediatric patients: an anesthesiologist's perspective. *Radiology* 1990;175:613−615.

48 Mitchell A, Louik C, Lacouture P, Stone D, Goldman P, Shapiro S. Risks to children from computed tomographic scan premedication. *J Am Med Assoc* 1982;247:2385−2388.

49 Diament MJ, Stanley P. The use of midazolam for sedation of infants and children. *Am J Roentgenol* 1988;150:377−378.

50 Nahata MC, Clotz MA, Krogg EA. Adverse effects of meperidine, promethazine and chlorpromazine for sedation in pediatric patients. *Clin Pediat* 1985;24:558−560.

51 Greenberg SB, Faerber EN, Aspinall C. High dose chloral hydrate sedation for children undergoing CT. *J Comput Ass Tomog* 1991;15:467−469.

52 Peden CJ, Menon DK, Hall AS, Sargentoni J. Magnetic resonance for the anaesthetist. *Anaesthesia* 1992;47:508−517.

53 British Medical Association and Royal Pharmaceutical Society of Great Britain. *British National Formulary*, No. 24. London: BMA, RPSGB, 1992:140.

54 Schreiner MS, Nicholson SC, Martin T, Whitney L. Should children drink before discharge from day surgery? *Anesthesiology* 1992;76:528−533.

55 Wong D. Pedicocktail not recommended. *Pediat Nurs* 1991;17:304,320.

56 Varner PD, Elbert JP, McKay RD, Nail CS, Whitlock TM. Methohexital sedation of children undergoing CT scan. *Anesth Analg* 1985;64:643−645.

57 Griswold JD, Liu MP. Rectal methohexital in children undergoing computerised cranial tomography and magnetic resonance imaging scans. *Anesthesiology* 1987;67:3A,A494.

58 Vickers MD, Schieden H, Wood Smith FG. *Drugs in Anaesthetic Practice*, 6th edn. London: Butterworths, 1984:99.

59 Latto IP, Rosen M. *Difficulties in Tracheal Intubation*. Eastbourne: Bailliere Tindall, 1985.

60 Atkinson RS, Rushman GB, Lee JA. *A Synopsis of Anaesthesia*, 10th edn. Bristol: Wright, 1987:236.

61 Steward DJ. *Manual of Pediatric Anesthesia*, 3rd edn. New York: Churchill Livingstone, 1990.

62 Valtonen M. Anaesthesia for computerised tomography of the brain in children: a comparison of propofol and thiopentone. *Acta Anaesthesiol Scand* 1989;33:170−173.

63 Keats AS. The ASA classification of physical status — a recapitulation. *Anesthesiology* 1979;49:233−236.

64 Aitkenhead AR. Risk management in anaesthesia. *J Med Defence Union* 1991;4:86−90.

65 Youngson R. Why anaesthesia can still kill. *New Sci* 1991;1755:53−56.

Analgesia and anesthesia

Phillip S. Mushlin, Paul M. Chetham, Susan Robinson and Leonard J. Lind

Introduction

Radiologists increasingly explore anesthesia options to provide their patients with sedation, analgesia, or anesthesia during diagnostic and interventional procedures. Conscious sedation is often sufficient to relieve anxiety and minimize patient discomfort, but regional or general anesthesia may be preferable or necessary for prolonged or painful procedures. In this chapter, we discuss risks and complications of various anesthetic approaches and focus on concerns related to patient preparation, monitoring, and dismissal from the radiology suite [1].

One should appreciate that any anesthetic approach imposes an element of risk. But, complications attributable to anesthesia that are most likely to lead to major morbidity and death are primarily respiratory events: inability to maintain an airway, laryngospasm, pulmonary aspiration of gastric contents, failure of tracheal intubation, bronchospasm, and postanesthetic respiratory depression [2]. Circulatory failure can also occur in the perianesthetic period, often as a result of ongoing respiratory insufficiency or failure. Other notable complications associated with anesthesia include drug overdose, idiosyncratic drug reactions (e.g., anaphylaxis), myocardial ischemia, and acute pulmonary edema.

Hospital operating room anesthesia has become much safer over the past decade [3]. The reduction in risk to patients has resulted from many factors, including introduction and institution of standards of practice, improved training of anesthetists, advances in monitoring, and creation of an environment wherein safety issues are of paramount concern to the entire health care team [3–6]. A recent retrospective review of anesthesia risk to "healthy" patients at Harvard Medical School revealed a striking reduction in intraoperative accidents (from 1:75 000 to 1:392 000) and associated deaths (from 1:151 400 to 0:392 000), following adoption of the monitoring standards [5]. For critically ill patients and emergency procedures, however, rates of complication and death remain high [2].

The task of reducing risk begins with a thorough, preprocedural evaluation of the patient, which should focus on the medical history and physical examination. Important predictors of adverse cardiac and respiratory outcome, in patients undergoing general anesthesia, include congestive heart failure, ventricular arrhythmias, atrial fibrillation, and myocardial infarction occurring during the prior 12 months [7,8]. Smoking and chronic obstructive pulmonary disease are also well-documented causes of increased perioperative respiratory morbidity and mortality [9,10].

In addition, advanced age imposes risks, owing to decreased physiologic reserve and enhanced sensitivity to respiratory depressant effects of sedative and analgesic agents. Untutored physicians may inadvertently administer inappropriately high doses or combinations of drugs (e.g., scopolamine and lorazepam), that predispose to major morbidity or death in unmonitored, elderly patients [9,11]. Hepatic or renal disease can similarly increase anesthetic risk, in part by altering patient responses to sedative and opioid medication.

Lastly, a complete medication history, including assessment of usage patterns, patient compliance, and adverse reactions to drugs, is essential for safe patient care. Failure to obtain information on use of psychotropic drugs — opioids, benzodiazepines, or ethanol — may lead to inadvertent discontinuation of the drugs, precipitating signs of substance withdrawal, including elevated blood pressure, tachycardia, diaphoresis, agitation, and seizures. In general, chronic ingestion of opioids, benzodiazepines, or ethanol increases dose requirements for similar drugs, whereas acute ingestion actually decreases the dose requirement.

Some drugs may be discontinued on the day of surgery, but others should not. For example, perioperative cardiovascular instability appears to be more common following abrupt discontinuation of antianginal or antihypertensive drugs.

Caution should be the rule when prescribing drugs that have previously caused untoward effects (e.g., hypotension with vancomycin or vomiting with opioids) in a patient. Patients often report "allergic" reactions to local anesthetics (anxiety, chest discomfort, palpitation), although such reactions actually arise from inadvertent intravascular injection or rapid vascular absorption of the epinephrine contained in the local anesthetic solution. True allergies to the benzodiazepines (diazepam and midazolam) or amide local anesthetics (lidocaine and bupivacaine) are rare; aminoesters (procaine, cocaine, and 2-chloroprocaine) more commonly produce allergic-type reactions because they are derivatives of para-aminobenzoic acid. When uncertainty exists about an allergic reaction to a local anesthetic, skin testing may be helpful. A negative skin test to the anesthetic in a nonanergic patient provides a reasonable basis for using the agent [12].

As any patient receiving sedative or hypnotic drugs may be at risk for aspiration pneumonitis or life-threatening airway obstruction, he or she is generally required to refrain from eating or drinking for at least 8 hours prior to anesthetic intervention [1]. An 8-hour fast, however, does not ensure an empty stomach, especially in obese, diabetic, or pregnant patients, or those with intraabdominal pathology (peritonitis, gastric outlet, or bowel obstruction).

Another important step in risk reduction is choice of anesthetic technique, which must be selected to meet the needs of the patient, the experience of the radiologist, and the complexity of the procedure. Intuitively, an anesthetic approach that maximizes patient comfort, minimizes stress, and poses the least physiologic trespass would appear to be the best plan for any patient. Nonetheless, numerous studies have failed to provide clear evidence that risk of mortality differs among anesthetic techniques [13].

Anesthetic techniques: general overview

For brief diagnostic procedures in cooperative patients, local anesthesia without sedation provides the simplest approach. But, supplemental sedation, which can be administered by the radiology care team, may improve patient satisfaction during routine diagnostic and interventional procedures. An anesthesia consult (for choice and dosage of drug)

may be helpful for difficult procedures, or when working with medically compromised or pregnant patients (e.g., benzodiazepines given during the first trimester of pregnancy may increase the possibility of congenital malformation). At times, management of a patient by an anesthesia care team may be indicated, even for procedures performed under local anesthesia (high-risk, critically ill, or uncooperative patients; procedures requiring deep levels of sedation or performed in a position that compromises the airway).

Airway obstruction and major respiratory depression may occur when a well-intentioned care team aggressively administers sedatives or analgesics to compensate for inadequate infiltration of local anesthetic. When structures are difficult to anesthetize by tissue infiltration, or if muscle relaxation is desired at the operative site, regional anesthesia should be considered. This method is also useful to minimize patient discomfort from a disease affecting an area of the body remote from the radiologic procedure; for example, spinal anesthesia will eliminate pain caused by an ischemic lower extremity, helping a patient to remain supine and motionless over extended periods.

General anesthesia is preferable for uncooperative patients or during prolonged, complex procedures, wherein other techniques would fail to provide adequate analgesia. Also, for procedures that predispose to abrupt airway compromise, such as deliberate embolization of arteriovenous malformations of head and neck, general anesthesia may be the choice, with use of a cuffed tracheal tube to ensure protection and patency of the airway.

Conscious sedation (Table 2.1)

Sedation is a state associated with mood alteration, decreased anxiety, drowsiness, perhaps analgesia, and a depressed level of consciousness, wherein a patient retains the ability to maintain an airway and to respond appropriately to verbal commands [14]. Sedatives and opioids enhance patient acceptance of procedures performed with regional techniques or cutaneous infiltration of anesthetics [1,15]. Careful titration of agents is essential as inadequate sedation predisposes patients to agitation, tachycardia, and elevated blood pressure, while excessive sedation can render a patient semicomatose, increasing susceptibility to airway obstruction and hypoxia, as well as prolonging recovery from anesthesia [16].

Complications

Respiratory

Both sedatives and opioids inhibit pulmonary ventilation and predispose patients to airway obstruction. Opioids impair the respiratory response to hypercarbia, while benzodiazepines (midazolam and diazepam) decrease ventilatory

Table 2.1 Complications associated with conscious sedation

Procedure	Major complications	Minor complications
Local anesthetics	Seizures Coma Respiratory depression (apnea) Hypotension Cardiovascular collapse	Pain on injection Tachycardia/hypertension Altered mental status
Sedatives and analgesics	Respiratory depression (hypoxia and hypercarbia) Cardiovascular depression (bradycardia, hypotension)	Pain on injection, subsequent phlebitis Agitation, confusion Amnesia Dysphoria Chest wall rigidity Nausea and vomiting Pruritis Biliary spasm Delayed time to discharge

responses to both hypercarbia and hypoxia [17,18]. The incidence of hypoxia (oxygen desaturation <90%) has been reported to range from 0 to 38% in patients having conscious sedation during regional or local anesthesia [16,19−22]. The variability in incidence of hypoxia undoubtedly relates to patient characteristics: age, coexisting disease, the drugs used to produce sedation, use of supplemental oxygen, method and rate of drug administration (bolus versus infusion), and depth of sedation.

A large initial bolus dose of midazolam often produces apnea or partial airway obstruction [23]. But, even low doses (1−2.5 mg, intravenous (IV) bolus), administered to relatively healthy patients breathing room air, have been known to produce moderate to severe hypoxia ($S_pO_2 = 75-88\%$) in many a patient [19]. Slow administration of drug (as by infusion) is less likely to precipitate hypoxia [20].

Upper airway obstruction is frequently responsible for the hypoxia that occurs during conscious sedation. Obstruction can usually be relieved by maintaining patient alertness through verbal encouragement or tactile stimulation; when consciousness is markedly depressed, a chin lift, forward jaw thrust, or even placement of an oral or nasal airway may be required to ensure airway patency [16,21,24].

Specific pharmacologic antagonists can also be used to ameliorate severe respiratory depression or airway obstruction during IV administration of benzodiazepines or opioids. An opioid antagonist, such as naloxone, effectively reverses most opioid effects, including respiratory depression and sedation. Flumazenil, a specific benzodiazepine antagonist, reverses benzodiazepine-induced sedation, but cannot be relied upon completely to reverse ventilatory depressant effects [25]. Recurrent sedation and respiratory depression may be a problem when using single, IV doses of either naloxone or flumazenil, owing to their short durations of action. Thus, when used to reverse effects of large doses of long-acting agonists, patients must be carefully observed for at least 2 hours after treatment with these short-acting antagonists.

Sedatives (benzodiazepines) and opioids, administered concomitantly, interact synergistically to cause periodic apnea and hypoxia [16,24]. This was amply demonstrated in a study by Bailey *et al.* [24] on 12 healthy volunteers treated with IV bolus doses of midazolam (0.05 mg/kg), fentanyl (2.0 μg/kg), or a combination of the two. Volunteers breathed room air during the study. No subject receiving midazolam or fentanyl alone developed apnea. Subjects receiving both drugs, in contrast, experienced profound respiratory depression; within 5 minutes of drug administration, 50% became apneic and 92% became hypoxemic (versus 0% hypoxia with midazolam and 50% hypoxia with fentanyl alone).

Another problem associated with opioids is chest wall rigidity. Rigidity is more common with highly potent (fentanyl or sufentanyl) than less potent (meperidine or morphine) opioids, especially when the agents are administered rapidly in large doses. Severe rigidity, which is fortunately rare during conscious sedation, significantly impairs breathing, mandating treatment with naloxone or muscle relaxants followed by tracheal intubation [1].

Cardiovascular

Patients receiving sedation plus infiltration of local anesthetics experience minimal alteration of their cardiovascular status, less than associated with regional anesthesia coupled with sedation [26]. Onset of sedation tends to decrease blood pressure and pulse rate, primarily by diminishing anxiety and the accompanying autonomic response. In one study, hypotensive episodes (blood pressure reduction by more than 30% of baseline) occurred in 10% of healthy patients, most commonly after an initial dose of midazolam or fentanyl [16]. While most sedatives and opioids lower blood pressure by lessening sympathetic tone, some opioids decrease pressure by releasing histamine (e.g., morphine, meperidine) and lowering systemic vascular resistance [1,20]. Normal blood pressure is usually restored rapidly by administration of a bolus of a balanced salt solution or a low dose of a vasopressor.

Local anesthetics, especially following inadvertent, intravascular injection, can cause hypotension by a variety of mechanisms, including myocardial depression, vasodilatation, bradycardia, and arrhythmias. Fortunately, neurologic disturbances (described below) usually precede life-threatening cardiotoxic effects of local anesthetics. But, sedative drugs may mask neurotoxicity, allowing cardiovascular collapse (CC) to occur without warning. This was demonstrated in a cogent study by Bernards *et al.* [27]. The earliest manifestation of bupivacaine toxicity (given via IV infusion) in animals premedicated with benzodiazepines was CC. Unpremedicated animals, in contrast, exhibited premonitory neurologic signs long before developing cardiovascular impairment [27].

Elevation of blood pressure and heart rate often result from inadequate analgesia or apprehension [16]. But, such elevations can also result from hypercarbia (respiratory depression, airway obstruction), urinary bladder distention, or intravascular injection of local anesthetic solution, owing to either neuroexcitatory effects of the anesthetic or to epinephrine contained in the solution [16,27].

While drugs such as fentanyl or sufentanil can cause bradycardia, a slowing heart rate may also result from severe hypoxia and indicate impending cardiac arrest [28]. Thus, progressive bradycardia during conscious sedation must be immediately evaluated for evidence of respiratory insufficiency.

Neurologic

The goal of IV drugs to supplement local anesthesia is to produce a calm, relaxed patient. Paradoxically, agitation, hostility, and confusion are occasionally observed in sedated patients. In one study, such behavioral disturbances accounted for 8% of adverse reactions to midazolam [24]. In another study, agitation or excitement occurred in 9% of patients receiving midazolam and fentanyl during lengthy dental procedures [16]. The excitation appeared to result from presentation of a painful stimulus (operative site or distended urinary bladder) to a disoriented patient. One should keep in mind that the most serious cause of agitation and confusion in sedated patients is hypoxemia, which should always be ruled out as a contributing factor.

Intuitively, it might seem that patients should recover more rapidly from conscious sedation than from general anesthesia, but this is not always the case. Midazolam, a short-acting benzodiazepine, may yield residual sedation

and difficulty with ambulation (dizziness) for hours following completion of an operation, depending largely upon the age of the patient and total dose administered [16]. In such circumstances, flumazenil is useful for antagonizing somnolence and may expedite discharge of the patient [29].

Local anesthetics have been implicated in causing prolonged somnolence following radiologic procedures, presumably owing to neurodepressive effects [30]. In rare instances, profound neurologic dysfunction results from intravascular injection or rapid absorption of local anesthetic during conscious sedation. Early symptoms of systemic local anesthetic toxicity include lightheadedness, dizziness, tinnitus, and disorientation. The most frequently observed signs are excitatory: shivering, twitching of facial musculature and tremors of the hands. Generalized convulsions, followed by central nervous system (CNS) depression, occur when initial signs and symptoms are unheeded or go undetected, and additional anesthetic is injected following an already toxic dose [12]. Repeated aspiration during injection is the most important measure in preventing intravascular injection. Limiting total doses of local anesthetics (maximum 500 mg lidocaine, 250 mg bupivacaine for a 70 kg adult) will minimize absorption-related toxic reactions; for example, blood levels of lidocaine are very low following subcutaneous infiltration of 200 mg of lidocaine (10 ml, 2% solution) in adults undergoing cardiac catheterization [31].

Vascular and cutaneous

Local anesthetics, when infiltrated into skin and subcutaneous tissue, typically cause transient pain at the injection site; to diminish pain, consider adding sodium bicarbonate to the anesthetic solution [32]. Pruritis and urticaria may result from injection of histamine-releasing drugs, such as morphine and meperidine. Pain, burning, pruritis, and phlebitis are associated with parenteral administration of drugs such as lorazepam, diazepam, or hydroxyzine, owing largely to tissue irritation caused by the chemicals (propylene glycol) used pharmaceutically to prepare these water-insoluble drugs [1]. To minimize venous irritation, use a large bore catheter (e.g., No. 16 or 18 gage), a larger vein (forearm), and rapid flow of fluids via the IV line.

Gastrointestinal

Most opioids increase biliary smooth muscle tone and constrict the sphincter of Oddi, resulting in high intrabiliary pressure and a large resistance to bile flow [33]. Morphine, meperidine, and fentanyl may elevate common bile duct pressure 10-fold within 15 minutes following injection; the effect may persist for 2 hours, producing typical biliary colic, complicating diagnostic evaluation of biliary pathology, and impeding placement of biliary stents and drainage devices (1,34). When opioids are indicated during biliary procedures, agonist—antagonists (butorphanol, nalbuphine), which exert little or no effect on biliary smooth muscle tone, may be preferable to agents that selectively stimulate the μ-subtypes of opioid receptors (fentanyl, meperidine, and morphine) [34—36].

Other drugs that decrease sphincter of Oddi pressure and antagonize biliary spasm include glucagon, atropine, nitroglycerin, amyl nitrate, or nifedipine [33]. Naloxone can relieve biliary spasm resulting from opioids, but is often unacceptable as it also reverses opioid-induced analgesia. Thus, when analgesia is needed, but opioid-induced biliary spasm must be avoided, regional anesthesia (epidural or intercostal nerve blocks) or general anesthesia should be considered [1].

Nausea and vomiting are well-known, untoward effects of opioids and certain sedative-hypnotics, such as methohexital and etomidate [21]; antiemetics (droperidol, metoclopramide) provide effective treatment and appear to diminish the incidence of nausea and vomiting when administered prior to an anesthetic or procedure [1].

Recommendations to avoid complications

Patients undergoing conscious sedation should receive supplemental oxygen. Hypoxia, excessive sedation, or distention of the urinary bladder can lead to patient agitation and confusion. Medications should be titrated to the desired end point. Opioids should be used primarily during procedures requiring analgesia. Ventilation should be assessed continuously by a qualified individual who is not involved in performing the radiologic procedure; the observer should note and record respiratory rate, adequacy of chest wall movement, and degree of oxygen saturation of hemoglobin using pulse oximetry. Equipment (e.g., artificial airways, ambu bags) and pharmaceutical agents (e.g., naloxone, flumazenil, epinephrine) should be available for immediate use.

Regional anesthesia (Table 2.2)

Regional anesthesia, often applied for complex operative procedures limited to the lower abdomen or to an extremity, can provide profound analgesia and skeletal muscle relaxation without impairing the ventilatory, circulatory, or cognitive status of a patient. Local anesthetics are administered via bolus doses or through catheters positioned in the proximity of peripheral nerves, nerve plexuses, or in the epidural space. Catheters offer advantages over single injection techniques, being useful not only for unexpectedly protracted procedures, but also for management of postoperative pain. Certain operations such as thoracotomies or extensive hepatobiliary procedures may best be performed using a combination of regional techniques and general anesthesia, allowing for control of ventilation and minimizing patient movement during procedures.

Which radiologic interventions should be performed utilizing regional anesthetic techniques? [1] Regional methods are preferable for procedures associated with significant discomfort. Continuous catheter techniques (brachial plexus or epidural) can be used to provide long-term analgesia and should be considered when multiple procedures are anticipated over the course of several days.

Table 2.2 Complications associated with regional anesthesia

Procedure	Major complications	Minor complications
Intercostal nerve block	Local anesthesia toxicity Pneumothorax Hemothorax	Injection site hematoma
Brachial plexus block: axillary or interscalene	Local anesthesia toxicity Persistent neuropathy (motor or sensory)	Injection site hematoma Postprocedural motor impairment
Interscalene block	Pneumothorax Local anesthetic toxicity	Phrenic nerve paralysis (unilateral)
Central neuraxis block: subarachnoid and epidural	Hypotension (precipitous) Cardiac arrest Respiratory paralysis (high level) Epidural abscess or hematoma Lower extremity paralysis Cauda Equina syndrome Persistent paresthesia	Back pain Postural headache Bradycardia Hypotension Urinary retention
Epidural	Local anesthetic toxicity	

Major complications

Cardiovascular

Spinal and epidural anesthetics decrease blood pressure by different mechanisms [37]. Spinal anesthesia, employing very low doses of local anesthetic, lowers pressure primarily through sympathetic denervation. Counterbalancing the tendency of sympathetic denervation to dilatate arterioles (reduction of afterload) is the autonomous tone of arteriolar smooth muscle; thus, healthy, nonpregnant patients often exhibit only modest decreases in pressure [37]. Major hypotension results when venous return becomes inadequate, secondary to venodilatation and increased venous capacitance from diminished sympathetic tone. With sympathetic blockade, venous return is highly dependent on patient positioning; a patient in a supine position, or with legs elevated, experiences less hypotension than when sitting.

Hypovolemia prior to induction of spinal anesthesia increases susceptibility to an abrupt, precipitous drop in blood pressure with onset of the block. A decrease in heart rate may result from epidural or spinal anesthesia, owing to inhibition of cardioaccelerator activity (T1–T4), or to enhancement of vagal tone, as intrinsic chronotropic stretch receptors in the right atrium and adjacent great vessels respond to a decrease in venous return [38].

The mechanism of cardiovascular depression associated with epidural anesthesia is more complex [37]. Onset of sympathetic denervation is relatively slow compared to spinal anesthesia, allowing sufficient time for compensatory vasoconstriction in unblocked segments; thus, epidural anesthesia lowers pressure more gradually than spinal anesthesia. With an epidural, effects of local anesthetics on the cardiovascular system are germane since the doses needed are much greater than those used for spinal anesthesia. Also, amounts of epinephrine (usually varying from 15 to 150 µg) employed during epidural anesthesia (to minimize intravascular absorption of local anesthetics) may be sufficiently high to cause tachycardia, hypotension (β-effect), or elevated blood pressure (α-effect).

Local anesthetic toxicity is more likely to occur with a regional anesthetic technique than during cutaneous infiltration. The former often involves injection of anesthetics into highly vascular tissues, and occasionally, inadvertent injections into the major blood vessels that accompany nerve plexuses (intercostal, axillary, interscalene, and epidural). High blood levels of local anesthetic can cause sinus bradycardia, sinus arrest, cardiac contractile dysfunction, and malignant ventricular arrhythmias [12]. But, low doses of a local anesthetic can also cause problems. For example, 15 mg of lidocaine or 5 mg of bupivacaine have precipitated seizures after inadvertent injection into the internal carotid or vertebral artery, during attempts to anesthetize structures in the neck [39].

Bupivacaine, often used because of its long duration of action, is considerably more toxic than lidocaine. Moreover, the ratio of the dose that produces cardiovascular collapse (CC) to the dose that produces seizures (CC:CNS ratio) is lower for bupivacaine than for lidocaine [40]. In other words, when neurotoxicity becomes apparent, patients are closer to experiencing CC with bupivacaine versus lidocaine. Furthermore, successful resuscitation from bupivacaine toxicity may be relatively difficult, in part because bupivacaine, unlike lidocaine, often produces intractable arrhythmias [12].

Respiratory

Respiratory complications may be associated with regional anesthesia. For example, a pneumothorax can result from a needle puncture of the pleura or lung during performance of an interscalene or intercostal nerve block; thus, bilateral blocks of this type are not recommended. The incidence of pneumothorax is 1–2% [41], even in experienced hands. Diaphragmatic paralysis (unilateral) often results with interscalene block as the phrenic nerve becomes paralyzed. In some cases, spinal or epidural anesthesia (mid–upper thoracic levels) will lead to respiratory difficulty in patients with severe asthma or chronic obstructive pulmonary disease via paralysis of accessory muscles of breathing.

Hematologic

Bleeding or hematoma formation are well-known complications of regional anesthesia, especially involving perivascular placement of needles and catheters [41]. Hematoma formation in the epidural space, as a result of spinal or epidural anesthesia, is a dangerous complication that occurs very rarely (fewer than 1:100 000). In a study of more than 4000 patients, there was no clinical evidence of hematoma formation after vascular operations performed with epidural anesthesia, despite intraoperative anticoagulation with heparin, which produced partial prothrombin time (PTT) values approximately two times higher than control PTT [42]. A regional technique is not necessarily contraindicated in patients with slight abnormalities of platelet function or coagulation profile; the risk–benefit analysis must be considered in such cases. Medical personnel involved in caring for patients at risk for an epidural hematoma must be able to recognize its manifestations (severe, progressive back pain, ascending muscle weakness, bladder/bowel incontinence, and persistent bilateral sensory deficit), and ensure that patients receive immediate diagnostic evaluation and treatment (magnetic resonance imaging (MRI) or computed tomography (CT scan); emergent decompression laminectomy).

Neurologic

In general, neurologic complications resulting from regional techniques are primarily related to either systemic toxicity of a local anesthetic, local toxic effects of the anesthetic, needle punctures, infection, or compression by a hematoma [41].

Systemic toxicity of local anesthetics is manifest initially by tinnitus, visual disturbance, lightheadedness, numbness of the tongue, and drowsiness; progression leads to seizures, coma, and apnea. The likelihood of a patient experiencing a toxic reaction to a local anesthetic depends upon a number of factors, including site of injection, vascularity of the site, and presence or absence of vasoconstrictor in the solution. During properly performed regional procedures, blood concentrations of local anesthetic are highest with intercostal nerve block, lower during epidural and brachial plexus blockade, and lowest following subcutaneous infiltration [12].

Nerve injury, a common cause of litigation, was found to represent 15% of all claims in the Closed Claims Study by the American Society of Anesthesiologists (ASA) [43]. Despite the frequency of the problem, the exact mechanism of nerve injury is often unclear (trauma versus neurotoxicity of anesthetic). In patients undergoing regional anesthesia, lumbosacral nerve roots are the most commonly injured structures, followed in frequency by brachial plexus injuries. Spinal or epidural anesthesia rarely causes serious injury. In a review of over 110 000 cases, four patients were found to have permanent paralysis or paresis [44]. The most feared complications of epidural or spinal anesthesia are epidural abscess and hematoma. Thus, anesthetists exercise great care to prevent such complications, including use of aseptic technique, avoidance of paresthesia, identification of potential bleeding tendencies, and use of appropriate local anesthetics and vasoconstrictors.

Minor complications

Minor complications of regional techniques include pain or hematoma at the injection site, and backache or mild headache following spinal or epidural anesthesia. Dural punctures, however, can produce severe postural headache (postdural puncture headache, PDPH): the headache is typically frontal, made worse by an erect position, alleviated by the supine, and occasionally accompanied by photophobia, nausea, diplopia, and auditory disturbance. Risk factors for development of a PDPH include use of large bore needles (17 versus 25–26 gage), inadvertent dural puncture during epidural placement, female gender, and young age. Treatment of PDPH should initially employ conservative measures such as hydration, bed rest, mild analgesics, and caffeine or theophylline. When conservative management fails, an epidural blood patch (with autologous blood) should be placed; this usually provides rapid relief of even the most severe PDPH.

Urinary retention, necessitating bladder catheterization, may accompany spinal or epidural anesthesia, especially when blood volume is expanded intentionally (balanced salt solutions) to avoid hypotension from sympathetic blockade. Urinary bladder distention following epidural or spinal anesthesia can be an unexpected cause of profound bradycardia and hypotension that is unresponsive to the usual resuscitative interventions. In this setting, drainage of the urinary bladder can avert a crisis [45].

Recommendations to avoid complications

Patients who receive a regional anesthetic during radiologic procedures must be well monitored (pulse oximetry, electrocardiography, blood pressure) and adequately hydrated. Careful needle placement is required to avoid intravascular injection or permanent neurologic injury. Appropriate dosing of local anesthetic minimizes the occurrence of neurologic and cardiovascular complications of the anesthetics.

General anesthesia (Table 2.3)

General anesthesia is often required for patients who are highly anxious, uncooperative, disoriented, obtunded, or

Table 2.3 Complications of general anesthesia

Life-threatening incidents or complications	
Respiratory	Unrecognized esophageal intubation
	Inability to intubate the trachea or ventilate the lungs
	Unrecognized, inadvertent tracheal extubation or disconnection from the anesthesia circuit
	Severe bronchospasm, refractory to usual therapy
	Aspiration of gastric contents, especially when the fluid is highly acidic, particulate in nature, or infectious
	Postprocedural respiratory insufficiency or apnea
Cardiac	Hypotension
	Hypertension
	Arrhythmia
	Myocardial ischemia
	Myocardial infarction
	Cardiac arrest
Drug related	Anaphylaxis
	Malignant hyperthermia
Neurologic	Hypoxic brain damage
	Nerve injuries
Minor complications	
	Nausea and vomiting
	Headache
	Prolonged recovery
	Unanticipated hospital admission
	Oral and dental trauma
	Recall of events or pain during a procedure
	Sore throat
	Phlebitis at site of catheter placement

adamantly opposed to sedation or regional techniques. General anesthesia should also be considered when airway protection is needed during the procedure.

The risk of major morbidity and mortality from anesthesia has been estimated to be between 1:850 and 1:8000 [2,46,47]. Various classification schemes (Goldman Cardiac Risk Index [7]; ASA classification) have been devised to help identify surgical patients at high risk for perioperative complications. Factors associated with enhanced mortality include age greater than 80 years, emergency procedures, renal failure, diabetes, recent myocardial infarction, and congestive heart failure [7,47–50]. Although the importance of any particular risk factor is debatable, it seems clear that patients with severely limited physiologic reserve involving at least one major organ system (ASA 3,4,5) have greatly increased rates of morbidity and mortality [48].

One must recognize that major anesthesia complications are not only limited to high-risk patients. In fact, the largest percentage of the morbidity from general anesthesia occurs in relatively healthy patients (ASA 1 or 2; in whom most anesthesias are performed), as demonstrated by two recent prospective studies [2,47]. The studies indicate that most serious adverse events are often not "predictable" and include acute compromise of the respiratory (airway obstruction, apnea, hypoxemia, bronchospasm) and cardiovascular (hypotension, myocardial ischemia, bradycardia, arrhythmia) systems. The majority of complications occur during conduct of anesthesia (28% at induction, 30% during maintenance), but incidents arising during the recovery period are not infrequent (42%) and carry a more ominous prognosis [2].

Assessments of anesthesia risk have been based on experiences in an operating room environment; a familiar setting for anesthetists. Administration of general anesthesia beyond this setting may create special problems. Colleagues may not be present to assist when unanticipated complications arise, and technical support personnel may not be available to troubleshoot or replace malfunctioning equipment. Thus, safe conduct of general anesthesia in areas remote from an operating suite requires experienced anesthetists, strict adherence to standards of patient monitoring, and scrupulous maintenance of anesthesia equipment. Transportation of patients to and from a radiology suite also requires appropriately trained personnel who can attend to patient needs during transport.

Any patient having a radiologic intervention for which general anesthesia is contemplated, needs a preprocedural consultation with an anesthetist. Anesthetic options and risks are typically discussed after the anesthesia consultant has evaluated reported allergies or sensitivities to drugs, investigated difficulties with prior anesthetics, identified and addressed significant medical problems requiring prompt attention, and assessed the need for special techniques and equipment to manage the patient's airway. Emergency procedures often preclude detailed preanesthetic evaluation; in such cases, radiologists should provide anesthetists with the essential information (e.g., medical and anesthesia history, current drugs, allergies, and laboratory data) prior to induction of anesthesia.

Major complications

Respiratory

Respiratory complications comprised the largest class of serious injuries (34%) reported in the ASA Closed Claims Study [51]. In 85% of claims examined, a patient died or suffered hypoxic brain damage. Difficulty in performing tracheal intubation, inability to ventilate the lungs, and failure to recognize esophageal intubation accounted for 75% of adverse respiratory events [51].

Evaluation of a patient's airway, including a review of previous anesthesia records, is essential to detect and manage a potentially difficult tracheal intubation. Difficulties should be anticipated in patients having a short, thick neck, full dentition with limited mouth opening, redundant oral–pharyngeal soft tissue, or limited neck extension [52]. Patients with systemic diseases, such as rheumatoid arthritis or ankylosing spondylitis, may have limited mobility of the cervical spine and temporomandibular joints, which can make routine airway management impossible. In such cases, tracheal intubation may require fiberoptic laryngoscopy or bronchoscopy, a nasotracheal approach or, rarely, a surgical airway (cricothyroidotomy or tracheostomy).

Aspiration of gastric contents following induction is a rare occurrence (0.05%), but carries a 5% mortality rate [53]. Emesis containing large quantities of fluid or solid materials can rapidly obstruct airways causing death; smaller volumes may produce pneumonitis. Factors associated with an increased risk of aspiration include emergency procedures, history of delayed gastric emptying or esophageal reflux, obesity, elevated intracranial pressure, small bowel obstruction, and pregnancy. Current recommendations for prevention of aspiration of acidic gastric contents include having the patient fast for a minimum of 4–6 hours, treating with H_2 blockers (oral or parenteral; cimetidine, famotidine) 8 hours prior to the procedure, and giving oral, nonparticulate antacids (30 ml of 0.3 mol/l sodium citrate) within 30 minutes of the induction of anesthesia.

In patients with acute abdominal disease (bowel obstruction), a nasogastric tube should be placed and suctioned prior to anesthetization. Protection of the airway sometimes mandates awake tracheal intubation, but use of cricoid pressure during rapid induction of general anesthesia is usually sufficient to prevent regurgitation and aspiration.

After successful tracheal intubation, vigilance is still necessary. Positioning a patient for radiologic procedures, e.g., may lead to inadvertent endobronchial intubation (head flexion), obstruction (kinking of the tracheal tube), accidental extubation, or disconnection of the tube from the anesthesia circuit. Thus, constant attention must be paid to pulmonary ventilation and oxygenation, frequently checking on the breathing circuit, evaluating chest wall motion, and listening for breath sounds bilaterally. Pulse oximetry, currently a standard for anesthesia monitoring, and capnography can provide early detection of major airway or ventilatory incidents and supply information, that when properly interpreted, should decrease the likelihood of serious morbidity and mortality [2,54].

During general anesthesia, bronchospasm can be life-threatening [47]. This complication may be expected in asthmatics, but also occurs occasionally in patients with no history of reactive airway disease. Vulnerability to bronchospasm is greatest immediately following laryngoscopy, intubation, or extubation of the trachea, or upon instrumentation (endoscopy or suctioning) of the airway during light planes of anesthesia. No patient with acute bronchospasm should receive a general anesthetic for an elective procedure; medical therapy should be optimal before the patient presents to the radiology suite. Prophylactic measures to minimize intraoperative ventilatory complications in patients with bronchospastic disease include treatment with an aerosolized bronchodilator, avoidance of histamine-releasing drugs (morphine, meperidine), and maintenance of deeper planes of anesthesia during airway manipulation or instrumentation. Bronchospasm refractory to aerosolized bronchodilators may indicate an anaphylactic reaction, requiring treatment with parenteral epinephrine [55].

Perioperative ventilatory complications are not uncommon in patients with obstructive pulmonary disease, hepatic or renal insufficiency, neuromuscular diseases, morbid obesity, and advanced age.

Residual effects of anesthetics (opioids, inhalation agents, or neuromuscular blockers), which are often responsible for ventilatory insufficiency during recovery from general anesthesia, must be rapidly detected and treated. Discharge of patients from the recovery area should be in accordance with established guidelines [1].

Cardiovascular

Cardiovascular depression usually occurs during induction of general anesthesia. This is typically followed by an increase of blood pressure and heart rate, caused by laryngoscopy and tracheal intubation. In hypertensive patients, or in those who abruptly discontinue cardiac medications (β-adrenergic blockers), anesthesia-related hemodynamic instability can be quite pronounced. Arrythmias (sinus tachycardia, sinus or nodal bradycardia, atrial and ventricular ectopic beats) have been noted in up to 60% of patients during general anesthesia but are generally benign.

Intravascular volume depletion can exacerbate anesthesia-induced hypotension (systolic blood pressure less than 90 mmHg or a 30% reduction from the baseline value). Significant fluid deficits are often caused by protracted

diarrhea or vomiting, aggressive therapy with cathartics (bowel preparation), large third-space sequestration (burns, small bowel obstruction), or prolonged abstention from fluid intake. IV fluid administration prior to induction of anesthesia (500−1000 ml) can reduce the severity and duration of the hypotension that frequently occurs upon induction of anesthesia. But, even in the absence of hypovolemia, anesthetic agents often markedly lower blood pressure via peripheral vasodilatation or direct cardiac depression (e.g., benzodiazepines plus opioids, inhalational anesthetics). Thus, frequent blood pressure measurements (every 1−5 minutes) are mandatory. This is easily accomplished with an automatic, noninvasive blood pressure monitoring device. However, continuous arterial pressure measurements may be needed in critically ill patients.

Major elevations in blood pressure (systolic blood pressure greater than 160 mmHg or a 30% elevation in baseline pressure), at least for brief periods of time, are not infrequent with general anesthesia, especially during airway instrumentation or emergence from anesthesia. Patients with chronic hypertension are the most likely to exhibit pressure elevation perioperatively [56]; the elevations usually result when the level of anesthesia is insufficient to antagonize adrenergic responses to a noxious stimulus (pain, hollow viscus distention, surgical incision, or manipulation). Adjusting the depth of anesthesia usually suffices, but treatment with adrenergic blocking agents (esmolol, labetolol, or propranolol), peripheral vasodilators, or a calcium entry blocker (nifedipine, nicardepine) is required when persistently elevated blood pressure threatens onset of myocardial ischemia or cerebrovascular injury. One must always be aware that hypercarbia or hypoxia, which increase sympathetic outflow, can elevate heart rate or blood pressure; arterial blood gases and adequacy of pulmonary ventilation may need to be evaluated immediately.

Electrocardiographic abnormalities commonly occur during general anesthesia. Sinus tachycardia often results from insufficient depth of anesthesia or hypovolemia, and is a major risk factor for myocardial ischemia [47]. Sinus bradycardia may be caused by traction or distention of abdominal viscera, but it can also signal severe hypoxia and impending cardiac arrest [28].

Atrial arrhythmias are often benign and can arise from atrial distention during rapid hydration of a patient. Ventricular ectopic beats may be seen in healthy individuals during light planes of anesthesia, provoked by intense stimulation. But, progression of ventricular ectopy should alert the anesthetist to the possibility of inadequate ventilation (hypoxia, hypercarbia) or myocardial ischemia; high-grade ventricular ectopy is often associated with an adverse cardiovascular outcome following general anesthesia [47].

Myocardial ischemia in the perioperative period is most commonly associated with known coronary disease, congestive heart failure, or previous myocardial infarction (MI)

[7,49,50,57]. Intraoperative risk factors for MI include tachycardia, hypertension, and profound hypotension [50,57]. Patients who have had a recent MI (0−3 months) have the greatest risk of reinfarction (6−36%); the risk is decreased by 4 6 months (3 26%), and further diminished by 6 months (1−5%) [49,50]. Reinfarction in the perioperative period is associated with a very high mortality rate (26−50%). Recent studies indicate a lower incidence of reinfarction and subsequent mortality, which appears to be related to improved preparation of patients preoperatively, frequent use of invasive monitoring, and/or liberal use of inotropes and vasodilators to treat decreased cardiac output states [50,57].

Cardiac arrest from anesthesia carries an incidence of 1.5−1.7/10 000 anesthetics [28]; bradycardia precedes the arrest in a majority of cases. Failure to ventilate the lungs (inability to intubate, esophageal intubation, severe bronchospasm) and overdose of inhalation agents are commonly associated factors. Emergency surgery (versus elective) is associated with a sharply increased incidence of cardiac arrest related to anesthesia [28].

Drug-related

Ability to promote mast-cell degranulation and to release histamine is a well-described property of several commonly used anesthesia drugs, including tubocurarine, succinylcholine, thiopental, morphine, and meperidine. Of much greater concern is anaphylaxis, a dramatic hypersensitivity reaction provoked by pharmacologic agents. It occurs with an incidence estimated at 1:3000 hospitalized patients, and is probably responsible for up to 500 deaths annually [55]. Anaphylactic reactions usually require previous exposure to the offending agent, and result when an antibody (immunoglobulin E, IgE) to the drug interacts with the drug to produce mast-cell degranulation and release of vasoactive compounds. Neuromuscular blocking drugs can actually precipitate anaphylaxis during an initial exposure, especially in patients sensitized to household products having quaternary ammonium groups (cosmetics or detergents). Antibodies to these products will occasionally crossreact with neuromuscular relaxants. Anaphylactoid reactions require no prior exposure to an offending agent, and occur when the chemical complexes with IgG or IgM, and complement. Anaphylactic and anaphylactoid reactions are clinically indistinguishable, commonly presenting with urticaria, severe bronchoconstriction, acute pulmonary hypertension, respiratory failure, and CC.

When a history of drug allergy or atopia is elicited, one can simply avoid using the reported allergens, as well as anesthetics that directly release histamine. Difficulty arises when the history suggests the possibility of a drug allergy, but the offending agent is unknown. For many drugs, skin testing is not helpful. Thus, when a suspected allergen is indicated for diagnostic or therapeutic reasons (protamine, contrast dyes), the patient is often given H_1 and H_2 antagonists plus corticosteroids, prior to receiving the agent in question. Severe anaphylactic or anaphylactoid reactions require immediate treatment with IV epinephrine, 100% oxygen, and may occasionally necessitate cardiopulmonary resuscitation [55].

Malignant hyperthermia (MH) is a potentially fatal syndrome characterized by a disorder of sarcoplasmic calcium metabolism in skeletal muscle, associated with muscle contracture and accelerated glycolysis (marked elevation in oxygen consumption, carbon dioxide production, and core temperature) [58]. Patients exhibit manifestations of an acutely developing, hypermetabolic state (up to 10 times normal), often presenting with sudden unexplained tachycardia, tachypnea, hyperpnea, cyanosis, fever, arrhythmia, and muscle rigidity. Characteristic laboratory findings include respiratory and metabolic acidosis, hyperkalemia, and arterial hypoxemia. Late complications include renal failure, disseminated intravascular coagulopathy, and cardiac failure.

MH is a pharmacogenetic disease, with a polygenic mode of inheritance, and an estimated incidence of 1:12 000 pediatric anesthetics and 1:20 000 adult anesthetics. Individuals genetically predisposed to develop the disorder do so only when confronted with drugs or stressful environmental factors which trigger the disease. But, MH does not invariably occur in genetically predisposed individuals, even when they receive "triggering" agents such as succinylcholine or a volatile anesthetic (halothane, enflurane, and isoflurane).

Mortality from MH prior to availability of IV dantrolene was over 70%. It now ranges from 7 to 20% [58]. Since dantrolene is life-saving during fulminant episodes of MH, all anesthetizing areas must have a readily available supply of dantrolene. Patients at risk for MH (family history, myopathic syndromes, Duchenne muscular dystrophy), or with a definite history of MH are still candidates for general anesthesia, but only with agents that do not trigger the syndrome. Presentation of MH may be delayed in some patients, not becoming apparent until early in the postoperative period. Thus, whenever a diagnosis of MH is suspected, patient vital signs must be closely monitored for at least 24 hours following anesthesia.

Neurologic

Hypoxic brain damage is the most feared complication of general anesthesia. As discussed previously, airway and ventilatory problems are the most common causes. Unfortunately, the first, irrefutable indication of prolonged, unrecognized severe arterial hypoxemia during anesthesia is often cardiac arrest. In such instances, major neurologic impairment will result despite rapidly effective cardiopulmonary resuscitation [28]. Improved training of anesthesia care providers and better monitoring of patients is necessary to decrease the incidence and severity of these events [54].

Nerve injuries account for up to 15% of anesthesia-related injuries, with over 66% occurring during general anesthesia [43]. The anesthetized patient is particularly susceptible to injury from prolonged, improper positioning of limbs, which can lead to excessive traction on major nerve plexuses or roots (brachial, lumbosacral), or compression injuries related to hard, unpadded surfaces or metal edges of the operating table. Ulnar neuropathy is the most common injury attributable to improper positioning or inadequate protection [43]. To avoid brachial plexus injury, the arms should not be abducted more than 90°, and the patient's head should be maintained in a neutral position whenever possible. Proper patient positioning and padding of areas susceptible to pressure damage are required to minimize injury to peripheral nerves and the skin.

Minor complications

Minor complications following general anesthesia include prolonged recovery, headache, nausea and vomiting, sore throat, oral and dental trauma, recall of intraoperative events, and phlebitis. Although not life-threatening, these complications are responsible for most postoperative morbidity. Most radiologic procedures are relatively nonstimulating to patients, so large doses of anesthetic agent are not needed. Nonetheless, some patients, particularly the elderly, may experience delayed emergence and recovery from anesthesia. Headache often results from stress and anxiety, as well as long periods of fasting on the day of the procedure.

Nausea and vomiting are frequent during recovery from general anesthesia. In most cases, gastrointestinal upset results from gastric distention during anesthesia and surgery, perioperative stress, or agents used for anesthesia or postoperative analgesia (opioids). Incidence of postoperative vomiting may be diminished by emptying gastric contents (intraoperative nasogastric tube), avoidance of large doses of opioids, and prophylactic administration of antiemetics (e.g., droperidol, phenergan, metachlopramide). In a minority of cases, antiemetics do not relieve postoperative nausea and vomiting. This problem continues to be a common reason for delayed discharge of patients from the recovery area and for unanticipated hospital admissions [59].

Sore throat often results from orotracheal intubation. Oral and dental injuries are responsible for a large proportion of legal claims against anesthetists. While careful laryngoscopy and tracheal tube placement help to avoid trauma in most patients, poor dentition and peridontitis predispose to injury, mandating dental consultation before a procedure, whenever feasible.

Recall of events during anesthesia occurs in 0.2–25% of patients, with a higher incidence of unpleasant dreams postoperatively [60]. Situations most commonly associated with recall include cardiac operations (cardiopulmonary bypass), Cesarean delivery, brief interventions (bronchoscopy, radiologic procedures) utilizing "light" planes of anesthesia, total IV anesthesia without benzodiazepines, and emergency surgery, especially during prolonged hypotensive episodes when anesthetics are discontinued to prevent further hemodynamic compromise [61].

Volatile anesthetics and benzodiazepines, having relatively good amnestic properties, minimize, but do not eliminate the possibility of recall [61]. Identifying patients who experienced awareness under anesthesia is not invariably straightforward; during the postoperative visit, one needs to ask questions about specific intraoperative events. The emotional and psychologic response of the patient to awareness under anesthesia should be evaluated. In rare instances, psychiatric consultation may be needed.

Phlebitis at the site of IV cannulation can create localized pain lasting for days to weeks following removal of the catheter. Phlebitis caused by cannulation and administration of drugs occurs more frequently in small veins of the hand than in larger veins (antecubital). Hyperosmolar drugs and agents formulated in organic solvents (diazepam) rather than aqueous solvents (midazolam) often contribute to phlebitis. Treatment is symptomatic, with local heat, elevation, and use of analgesics.

Unanticipated hospital admissions following ambulatory procedures result from excessive pain, bleeding, intractable vomiting, urinary bladder retention, postoperative somnolence, airway obstruction, aspiration pneumonitis, or suspected myocardial infarction. Hospital admissions are more commonly associated with general anesthesia than with conscious sedation, especially when the procedure lasts for more than 1 hour [59].

Recommendations to avoid complications

General anesthesia should be reserved for the few radiologic procedures and patients requiring this method of anesthesia. Prior to the actual scheduling of cases, anesthesia personnel should inspect and evaluate the suitability of radiology suites for the administration of general anesthesia. An adequate amount of time must be allowed for patient evaluation, preparation of monitors and equipment, and induction of anesthesia. Hurriedly processing patients through the radiology suite can have dire consequences. Proper positioning and careful movement of anesthetized patients during radiologic interventions will help prevent airway compromise and peripheral neurologic injury.

References

1 Lind LJ, Mushlin PS. Sedation, analgesia, and anesthesia for radiologic procedures. *Cardiovasc Intervent Radiol* 1987;10: 247–253.

2 Tiret L, Desmonts JM, Hatton F *et al.* Complications associated with anaesthesia: a prospective survey in France. *Can Anaesth Soc J* 1986;33:336−344.

3 Eichhorn JH. Risk management. In: Benumof JI, Saidman LJ, eds. *Anesthesia and Perioperative Complications.* St Louis: CV Mosby, 1991:648−666.

4 Eichhorn JH, Cooper JB, Cullen DH *et al.* Standards for patient monitoring during anesthesia at Harvard Medical School. *J Am Med Assoc* 1986;256:1017−1020.

5 Eichhorn JH, Cooper JB, Cullen DH *et al.* Anesthesia practice standards at Harvard: a review. *J Clin Anesth* 1988;1:55−65.

6 Eichhorn JH. Prevention of intraoperative anesthesia accidents and related severe injury through safety monitoring. *Anesthesiology* 1989;70:572−577.

7 Goldman L, Caldera DL, Nussbaum SR *et al.* Multifactorial index of cardiac risk in noncardiac surgical procedures. *New Engl J Med* 1977;297:845−850.

8 Forrest JB, Rehder K, Cahalan MK *et al.* Multicenter study of general anesthesia. Predictors of severe perioperative adverse outcomes. *Anesthesiology* 1992;76:3−15.

9 Cheng EY, Cheng RM. Impact of aging on preoperative evaluation. *J Clin Anesth* 1991;3:324−343.

10 Pearce AC, Jones RM. Smoking and anesthesia: preoperative abstinence and perioperative morbidity. *Anesthesiology* 1984;61:576−584.

11 Greenblatt DJ, Sellers EM, Shader RI. Drug disposition in old age. *New Engl J Med* 1982;306:1081−1088.

12 Strichartz GR, Covino BG. Local anesthetics. In: Miller RD, ed. *Anesthesia,* 3rd edn. New York: Churchill Livingstone, 1987: 437−440.

13 Forrest JB. Risk factors of importance: the anesthetic. In: Duncan PG, ed. *Anesthetic Risk and Complication.* Philadelphia: JP Lippincott, 1992:228−240.

14 Concensus Conference. Anesthesia and sedation in the dental office. *J Am Med Assoc* 1985;254:1073−1976.

15 Philip BK. Supplemental medication for ambulatory procedures under regional anesthesia. *Anesth Analg* 1985;64:1117−1125.

16 Lind LJ, Mushlin PS, Schnitman PA. Monitored anesthesia care for dental implant surgery. *J Oral Implant* 1990;16:106−113.

17 Reves JG, Frangen RJ, Vinik HR, Greenblatt FJ. Midazolam: pharmacology and uses. *Anesthesiology* 1985;62:310−324.

18 Alexander CM, Gross JB. Sedative doses of midazolam depress hypoxic ventilatory responses in humans. *Anesth Analg* 1988; 67:377−382.

19 Smith DC, Crul FJ. Oxygen desaturation following sedation for regional anesthesia. *Br J Anaesth* 1989,62.206−209.

20 White PF, Negus JB. Sedative infusions during local and regional anesthesia: a comparison of midazolam and propofol. *J Clin Anesth* 1991;3:32−39.

21 Urquhart ML, White PF. Comparison of sedative infusions during regional anesthesia − methohexital, etomidate and midazolam. *Anesth Analg* 1989;68:249−254.

22 de Bruijn NP, Hlatky MA, Jacobs JR *et al.* General anesthesia during percutaneous transluminal coronary angioplasty for acute myocardial infarction. *Anesth Analg* 1989;68:201−207.

23 Aun C, Flynn PJ, Richards J, Major E. A comparison of midazolam and diazepam for intravenous sedation in dentistry. *Anaesthesia* 1984;39:589−593.

24 Bailey PL, Pace NL, Ashburn MA *et al.* Frequent hypoxemia and apnea after sedation with midazolam and fentanyl. *Anesthesiology* 1990;73:826−830.

25 Gross JB, Weller RS, Conard P. Flumazenil antagonism of midazolam-induced ventilatory depression. *Anesthesiology* 1991; 75:179−185.

26 Popat MT, Giesecke AH. Midazolam infusion for sedation in day surgery patients. In: Reves JG, Sladen RN, eds. *Anesthesia and Sedation by Continuous Infusion.* Princeton: Exerpta Medica, 1992:40−43.

27 Bernards CM, Carpenter RL, Rupp SM *et al.* Effect of midazolam and diazepam premedication on central nervous system and cardiovascular toxicity of bupivacaine in pigs. *Anesthesiology* 1989;70:318−323.

28 Kenan RL, Boyan CP. Cardiac arrest due to anesthesia. *J Am Med Assoc* 1958;253:2373−2377.

29 White PF. Use of sedative infusions during outpatient local and regional anesthesia. In: Reves JF, Sladen RN, eds. *Anesthesia and Sedation by Continuous Infusion.* Princeton: Exerpta Medica, 1992:33−39.

30 Palmisano JM, Meliones JN, Crowley DC *et al.* Lidocaine toxicity after subcutaneous infiltration in children undergoing cardiac catheterization. *Am J Cardiol* 1991;67:647−648.

31 Schwartz ML, Covino BG, Narang RM *et al.* Blood levels of lidocaine following subcutaneous administration prior to cardiac catheterization. *Am Heart J* 1974;88:721−723.

32 McKay W, Morris R, Mushlin P. Sodium bicarbonate attenuates pain on skin infiltration with lidocaine, with or without epinephrine. *Anesth Analg* 1987;66:572−574.

33 Goff JS. The human sphincter of Oddi. *Arch Int Med* 1988;148: 2673−2677.

34 Radnay PA, Duncalf D, Novakovic M. Common bile duct pressure changes after fentanyl, morphine, meperidine, butorphanol and naloxone. *Anesth Analg* 1984;63:441−444.

35 Arguelles JE, Franatovic Y, Romos-Salas F *et al.* Intrabiliary pressure changes produced by narcotic drugs and inhalation anesthetics in guinea pigs. *Anesth Analg* 1979;58:120−123.

36 McCammon RI, Stoelting RK, Madura JA. Effects of butorphanol, nalbuphine and fentanyl on intrabiliary tract dynamics. *Anesth Analg* 1984;63:139−142.

37 Covino BG. Cardiovascular effects of spinal and epidural anesthesia. *Regional Anaesthesiol* 1978;12:23−26.

38 Baron FJ, Decaux-Jacolot A, Edouard A *et al.* Influence of venous return on baroreflex control of heart rate during lumbar epidural anesthesia in humans. *Anesthesiology* 1986;64: 188−193.

39 Korevaar WC, Burney RG, Moore PA. Convulsions during stellate ganglion block: a case report. *Anesth Analg* 1979;58; 329−330.

40 Albright GA. Cardiac arrest following regional anesthesia with etidocaine or bupivacaine. *Anesthesiology* 1979;51:285−287.

41 Bridenbaugh PO. Complications of local anesthetic neural blockade. In: Cousins ML, Bridenbaugh PO, eds. *Neural Blockade,* 2nd edn. Philadelphia: JB Lippincott, 1988:695−717.

42 Rao TLK, El-Etr AA. Anticoagulation following placement of epidural and subarachnoid catheters. *Anesthesiology* 1981;55: 618−620.

43 Kroll DA, Kaplan R, Posner K *et al.* Nerve injury associated with anesthesia. *Anesthesiology* 1990;73:202−207.

44 Kane RE. Neurologic deficits following epidural or spinal anesthesia. *Anesth Analg* 1981;60:150−161.

45 Beardsworth D, Lind LJ. Bladder distention and cardiovascular depression during recovery from epidural anesthesia. *Regional Anesth* 1985;10:184−186.

46 Forrest JB, Rehder K, Goldsmith CH *et al*. Multicenter study of general anesthesia. 1. Design and patient demography. *Anesthesiology* 1990;72:252–261.

47 Forrest JB, Cahalan MK, Rehder K *et al*. Multicenter study of general anesthesia. 2. Results. *Anesthesiology* 1990;72:262–268.

48 Cohen MM, Duncan PG, Tate RB. Does anesthesia contribute to operative mortality? *J Am Med Assoc* 1988;260:2859–2863.

49 Tarhan S, Moffitt EA, Taylor WF, Giuliam ER. Myocardial infarction after general anesthesia. *J Am Med Assoc* 1972;220:1451–1454.

50 Rao TL, Jacobs KH, El-Etr AA. Reinfarction following anesthesia in patients with myocardial infarction. *Anesthesiology* 1983;59:499–505.

51 Caplan RA, Posner KL, Ward RJ *et al*. Adverse respiratory events in anesthesia: a closed claim analysis. *Anesthesiology* 1990;72:828–833.

52 Mallampati SR, Gatt SP, Gugino LD *et al*. A clinical sign to predict difficult intubation: a prospective study. *Can Anaesth Soc J* 1985;32:429–434.

53 Olsson GL, Hallen B, Hambraeus-Jonzon K. Aspiration during anesthesia: a computer aided study in 250,543 anesthetics. *Acta Anaesthesiol Scand* 1988;32:653–664.

54 Tinker JH, Dull DL, Caplan RA *et al*. Role of monitoring devices in prevention of anesthetic mishaps: a closed claims analysis. *Anesthesiology*, 1989;71:541–546.

55 Bochner BS, Lichtenstein LM. Anaphylaxis. *New Engl J Med* 1991;324:1785–1790.

56 Gal TJ, Cooperman LH. Hypertension in the immediate post-operative period. *Br J Anaesth* 1975;47:70–74.

57 Mangano DI. Perioperative cardiac morbidity. *Anesthesiology* 1990;72:153–184.

58 Gallant EM, Ahern CP. Malignant hyperthermia: responses of skeletal muscles to general anesthetics. *Mayo Clin Proc* 1983;58:758–763.

59 Gold BS, Kitz DS, Lecky JN *et al*. Unanticipated admission to the hospital following ambulatory surgery. *J Am Med Assoc* 1989;262:3008–3010.

60 Ghoneim MM, Block RJ. Learning and consciousness during general anesthesia. *Anesthesiology* 1992;76:279–305.

61 Mark JB, Greenberg LM. Intraoperative awareness and hypertensive crisis during high dose fentanyl-diazepam oxygen anesthesia. *Anesth Analg* 1983;62:698–700.

Drugs used in the imaging department

Charles A. McConnell

A considerable number of drugs are administered in X-ray departments at the instigation of a radiologist; some of these will be aids to diagnostic procedures, others will be aids to therapeutic procedures, and others will be used to treat a collapsed patient. The uses, acute complications, and contra-indications to a selection of these drugs will be considered. The dosage quoted will be that for an average-sized adult.

The drugs included in this chapter are a selected, limited list and readers should be fully conversant with manufacturers' current literature for any drugs they may prescribe. Antibiotics have been excluded from consideration because of the great number available, rapidly changing fashions, and the role of personal preference in their selection.

Drugs are classified by their site of action and application.

Drugs acting on the gastrointestinal system

Drugs increasing gastrointestinal motility

Ceruletide

A synthetic decapeptide similar in action to cholecystokinin, but three times as potent. Ceruletide stimulates contraction of the gall bladder, small-bowel peristalsis, and causes relaxation of the sphincter of Oddi.

Indications

1 To produce gall bladder contraction in oral cholecystography.
2 To accelerate small-bowel transit during follow-through contrast studies.
3 As an adjunct to the passage of retained calculi from the common bile duct, while flushing through a T-tube [1].

Dosage

Intramuscular injection of 0.3 mg/kg.

Side-effects

Nausea, vomiting, colic, and diarrhea may occur. Overdosage may cause spasm of the cystic duct, severe pain, and hypotension.

Metoclopramide (Maxolon, Primperan, Regulan)

A dopamine antagonist producing a positive effect on gastrointestinal motility, thus accelerating gastric emptying and small-bowel transit.

Metoclopramide also increases the tone of the esophageal sphincter mechanism to counteract reflux and has a central antiemetic action.

Indications

1 To hasten small-bowel transit, thus reducing the duration of small-bowel contrast studies [2].
2 To aid duodenal intubation.
3 To prevent or treat nausea and vomiting.

Dosage

Orally, 10–20 mg 20 minutes before the procedure, or by intramuscular or intravenous injection at the time of the procedure.

Side-effects

Extrapyramidal side-effects may occur, particularly in the young and elderly, due to alteration of dopamine transmission. They present as trismus, torticollis, oculogyric crisis, dyskinesia, or fatigue. Such side-effects may follow a single dose of metoclopramide, but their frequency rises with increasing dosage. Severe extrapyramidal side-effects may be treated with antiParkinsonian agents, such as procyclidine hydrochloride, or certain antihistamines, such as diphenhydramine.

Contraindications

Hypertensive crisis may occur in patients with pheochromocytoma.

Drugs reducing gastrointestinal motility

Glucagon

A synthetic polypeptide originally isolated from the α-cells of the islets of Langerhans in the pancreas. Glucagon stimulates cyclic adenosine monophosphate (cAMP), mobilizing hepatic glycogen, producing relaxation of the smooth muscle of the gastrointestinal tract, and has a positive inotropic effect on cardiac muscle.

Indications

1 Hypotonic examination of the gastrointestinal tract during contrast examination [3].
2 Relaxation of esophageal tone to aid the passage of an impacted foreign body or food bolus.
3 To reduce biliary spasm, relieve biliary colic, and aid the passage of calculi.
4 To enhance intravenous cholangiography.
5 To relieve ureteric colic and aid the passage of urinary calculi.
6 As an adjunct to hysterosalpingography.
7 To reverse hypoglycemic states in patients with diabetes mellitus.

8 To reverse hypotension in anaphylactic shock in patients refractory to β-adrenergic agonists because of prior administration of β-adrenergic blocking agents [4].

Dosage

As an adjunct to gastrointestinal contrast examination, 0.2 mg by intramuscular or intravenous injection. The onset of action on the bowel is 10 minutes after intramuscular injection or 1 minute after intravenous injection. For the treatment of hypoglycemia or hypotension, 1–2 mg repeated after 15 minutes if required.

Side-effects

In high dosage, nausea and vomiting is common. Allergic reactions may occur including the development of erythema multiforme [5], and arthralgia.

Contraindications

Glucagon should be used with caution as a diagnostic aid in patients with diabetes mellitus. Hypertensive crisis may be precipitated in patients with pheochromocytoma, and hypoglycemia may occur in patients with insulinoma.

Hyoscine butylbromide (Buscopan)

An anticholinergic agent particularly suited for use in the X-ray department because of its short duration of action.

Indications

1 Hypotonic examination of the upper and lower gastrointestinal tract.
2 The relief of tubal spasm during hysterosalpingography.

Dosage

Intramuscular or intravenous injection of 20 mg immediately before the examination

Side-effects

These are relatively mild and anticholinergic in type: dry mouth, tachycardia, blurred vision due to lack of accommodation and precipitation of closed-angle glaucoma, or urinary retention in susceptible patients (see also p. 38).

Contraindications

Care must be exercised with elderly patients suffering from prostatism or visual problems.

Propantheline bromide (Pro-Banthine)

A quaternary ammonium anticholinergic agent which has a 6-hour duration of action, but is otherwise similar to hyoscine butylbromide.

Indications and side-effects

As for hyoscine butylbromide.

Dosage

Intramuscular or intravenous injection of 10–30 mg immediately before the examination.

H₂-histamine antagonists

H₂-receptor antagonists reduce both the acidity and volume of gastric secretion.

Cimetidine (Tagamet)

Indications

Cimetidine is primarily used in peptic ulcer prophylaxis and therapy, but it may be used as an adjunct to radioisotope scanning with pertechnetate in the diagnosis of Meckel's diverticulum [6]. The value of combined H_1 and H_2 antagonists in the prophylaxis and treatment of contrast-media allergy is controversial. Cimetidine may have a place in the treatment of refractory anaphylactic shock (see p. 285).

Dosage

In the investigation of Meckel's diverticulum, 300 mg 6 hourly for 48 hours before the examination via the oral, intramuscular, or intravenous routes (children receive 20 mg/kg of body weight/day).

Side-effects

Mental confusion, dizziness, and drowsiness may occur. The Stevens–Johnson syndrome [7], a rise in serum creatinine, and cardiac arrhythmia [8] have all been recorded.

Contraindications

A reduced dosage is required in renal failure or cardiovascular disease. The actions of phenytoin, warfarin, and other drugs subject to hepatic secretion may be prolonged by cimetidine.

Drugs used in arterial catheterization and interventional procedures

Agents affecting blood coagulation (see also p. 372)

Alteplase (Actilyse, Activase)

A recombinant human tissue type, plasminogen activator which is relatively inactive until it binds to fibrin. This binding activates the conversion of plasminogen to plasmin, inducing clot lysis.

Indications

As for streptokinase (see p. 31).

Dosage

Intraarterial administration of 0.5–1 mg/h for a few hours, the effects being monitored clinically, angiographically, and by fibrinogen titer. The arterial catheter should be placed directly into the thrombus.

Side-effects

Alteplase has a low antigenic potential and side-effects are generally minimal. Hemorrhage may occur but the risk is reduced by the high binding capacity to fibrin and its 5 minute half-life in plasma. If serious bleeding occurs, treatment should be discontinued and, if necessary, fresh frozen plasma, fresh whole blood, or synthetic antifibrinolytic agents administered.

Contraindications

Severe hypertension, coagulation defects, peptic ulcer, major surgery, and liver disease. Alteplase should be used with caution in renal failure, pregnancy, and in association with anticoagulants.

Aminocaproic acid (Amicor)

An antifibrinolytic agent inhibiting plasminogen activators.

Indications

Aminocaproic acid may be beneficial in hemorrhage resulting from the administration of streptokinase or urokinase (see p. 31).

Dosage

Oral administration produces peak plasma concentration after 2 hours, or alternately a slow intravenous infusion in dextrose or saline may be employed: 3–6 g, 4–6 hourly is used to control hemorrhage.

Side-effects

Diarrhea, headache, hypotension, skin rashes, muscle pain, and weakness may all occur. Hemorrhage may supervene if excessive fibrinolysis is produced, but conversely a thrombotic angiopathy may occur including intracranial thrombosis. Muscle necrosis producing myoglobinuria and renal failure may also supervene.

Contraindications

Concomitant administration of an oral contraceptive or impaired renal function (see also p. 280).

Aspirin

Indications

Aspirin may be used as a simple analgesic or antiinflammatory agent. The antiplatelet effect may be used in the prevention of myocardial infarction and stroke, to reduce restenosis following angioplasty, and in the prophylaxis of deep vein thrombosis.

Dosage

An oral dose of 300–900 mg, 4–6 hourly may be used for analgesic and antipyretic effects. Doses of 4–8 g/day may be used to produce optimal antiinflammatory effects, achieving a plasma salicylate level of 150–300 µg/ml. A dose of 75–325 mg daily is effective in achieving an antiplatelet effect.

Side-effects

Gastrointestinal symptoms are common and may be minimized by giving aspirin with food. Peptic ulceration may result in occult or frank blood loss and perforation; these effects may be reduced by the use of enteric coated preparations and administration of histamine H_2 antagonists or high-dose antacids. Allergic reactions may occur causing urticaria, angiedema, rhinitis, and bronchospasm. Aspirin has been implicated in the etiology of Reye's syndrome, and use in children should be restricted to the treatment of juvenile rheumatoid arthritis.

Mild chronic overdosage causes dizziness, tinnitus, deafness, nausea, vomiting, and confusion, and may be controlled by reducing the dose. Acute overdosage causes hyperventilation, fever, ketosis, metabolic acidosis, coma, and cardiopulmonary collapse.

Aspirin increases the bleeding time and may cause hepatotoxicity.

Contraindications

Caution is necessary when administering aspirin to patients with a history of dyspepsia, or when renal or hepatic function is impaired. It should not be used in patients with a history of allergy to aspirin and other nonsteroidal antiinflammatory drugs (NSAIDs), or in patients with hemorrhagic disorders. It should be avoided in children under the age of 12 years.

Dipyridamole (Persantin)

See p. 41.

Heparin

Heparin produces its anticoagulant action by inhibiting the formation of factor X, the transformation of prothrombin to thrombin, and fibrinogen to fibrin. Heparin has a rapid action and an effective half-life of 100 minutes. The anticoagulant effects are effectively reversed by protamine sulfate (see below).

Indications

Heparin may be added to the flushing solution during catheterization procedures to prevent thrombus, or be given subcutaneously as prophylaxis for deep venous thrombosis. Increased systemic dosages produce effective anticoagulation.

Dosage

Subcutaneous injection of 5000 U 8–12 hourly for prophylaxis against venous thrombosis. Effective anticoagulation produced by daily intravenous infusion of 20 000–40 000 U, but the dose should be adjusted in accordance with coagulation tests.

Side-effects

Effective heparin anticoagulation has a risk of hemorrhage varying from 4.9 to 17.7% (average 9%), the peak incidence occurring on the third day [9]. Hemorrhage may occur at various sites, but it most commonly presents as hematemesis, melena, or hematuria. Cerebral hemorrhage may have particularly severe consequences. Heparin resistance may be caused by concomitant administration of intravenous nitroglycerin, with increased sensitivity when discontinuing the nitroglycerin [10]. Spontaneous arterial emboli due to heparin-induced thrombocythemia is a rare but potentially fatal complication [11]. Hypersensitivity reactions may occur including sneezing, conjunctivitis, bronchospasm, and hypotension.

Contraindications

A bleeding diathesis or peptic ulcer. Aspirin administration and recent or imminent surgery are relative contraindications.

Protamine sulfate

Protamine sulfate neutralizes the effects of heparin (see above) by combining with it to form a stable inactive complex.

Indications

To counteract the anticoagulant effect of heparin.

Dosage

Slow intravenous injection of a maximum of 50 mg, the actual dose being calculated on the basis of 1 mg of protamine sulfate neutralizing 100 U of heparin.

Side-effects

Rapid administration may produce flushing, dyspnea, hypotension, and bradycardia. Urticaria and bronchospasm may occur, possibly related to the fish antigens from which protamine is derived. Overdosage may cause an anticoagulant effect.

Contraindications

Combination with diatrizoic acid will produce a precipitate: protamine sulfate should *not* be injected via the angiographic catheter.

Streptokinase (Kabikinase, Streptase)

A thrombolytic agent obtained from the filtrate of certain hemolytic streptococci. Streptokinase activates plasminogen to plasmin, which produces clot lysis.

Indications

Lysis of recent arterial or venous thrombus and of pulmonary emboli.

Dosage

Intraarterial administration of 5–10 000 IU/h for a few hours, the effects being monitored clinically, angiographically, and by estimation of thrombin time and fibrinogen titer. Alternately intravenous administration of a loading dose of 500 000 IU followed by 2 500 000 IU/day may be used.

Side-effects

Fever or anaphylactoid reactions may occur in more than 50% of patients, but a prophylactic dose of steroid (equivalent to 100 mg of hydrocortisone) considerably reduces this risk. Hemorrhage may occur. This is particularly dangerous in the central nervous system, but rupture of the liver and spleen may occur. The patient's clinical state and clotting factors must be closely monitored: if severe hemorrhage occurs it should be controlled by steroids, fresh blood, fibrinogen, and aminocaproic acid. The incidence of serious bleeding and systemic effects is considerably reduced using low-dose intra-arterial administration in comparison with larger intravenous dosages.

Contraindications

Severe hypertension, coagulation defects, pregnancy, peptic ulcer, recent surgery, or oral anticoagulation.

Tranexamic acid (Cyklokapron)

Indications

Tranexamic acid has a similar action to aminocaproic acid (see p. 29), but in particular it may prevent and treat hereditary angioneurotic edema.

Dosage

One gram 6 hourly for 48 hours before and after exposure to the risk factor, such as contrast media. Administration may be by the oral route or slow intravenous injection.

Side-effects

Similar, but claimed to be less severe than those of aminocaproic acid. The dose should be reduced in renal failure.

Urokinase (Abbokinase, Breokinase)

A thrombolytic agent with a similar action to streptokinase (see above), which possesses the same risk of hemorrhage. Urokinase is claimed to be less antigenic because it is derived from human urine.

Indications and side-effects

As for streptokinase.

Dosage

Approximately 1000–4000 IU/min via an arterial catheter placed directly into the thrombus [12].

Arterial vasodilators

Nifedipine

A calcium channel blocker with peripheral and coronary vasodilator properties.

Uses

Most commonly used for the treatment of hypertension, heart failure, and angina pectoris, but in the radiology department it may be used for coronary, peripheral and renal artery vasodilatation, and in Raynaud's disease.

Dosage

A single dose of 10–20 mg given sublingually may be used for prophylaxis or in the acute situation for arterial spasm or hypertension. Transcatheter intra-arterial administration of 100–200 µg over 120 seconds may be used for coronary artery spasm. The maximum recommended dose is 1200 µg in 3 hours.

Side-effects

Dizziness, flushing, headache, and hypotension are common. Gastrointestinal disturbance or urinary frequency may occur. Severe hypotension may precipitate myocardial or central ischemia. There is a possibility of hemorrhagic complications during surgical procedures [13].

Precautions

Caution should be exercised in patients with hypotension and poor cardiac function. Nifedipine may precipitate heart failure in patients with aortic stenosis.

The dose should be reduced in hepatic and renal failure. Although usually well tolerated in combination with β-blockers, severe hypotension may occasionally be precipitated.

Papaverine sulfate (Cerebid)

See p. 42.

Tolazoline (Priscol, Priscoline)

See p. 42.

Therapeutic vasoconstrictors

Vasopressin (Pitressin)

A synthetic preparation of antidiuretic hormone with a half-life of 10 minutes and the ability to produce smooth-muscle spasm and vasospasm.

Indications

The control of gastrointestinal hemorrhage.

Dosage

Selective intraarterial infusion of 0.1–0.4 U/min is usually effective in controlling gastrointestinal hemorrhage. The more selective the infusion the better the result, with the exception of bleeding esophageal varices, in which circumstances an intravenous infusion of 0.2–0.8 U/min is as effective as intraarterial infusion [14].

Side-effects

Pallor, nausea, and a desire to defecate are common. Local gangrene [15] and myocardial ischemia may result from arteriolar spasm in the peripheral vessels and coronary circulation, respectively. Hypersensitivity reactions are also described.

Contraindications

Myocardial ischemia, peripheral vascular disease, hyponatremia, and water intoxication may occur in renal failure.

Gallstone dissolution

Monooctanoin

Uses

Monooctanoin is an effective agent for the dissolution of cholesterol gallstones [16]. Retained calculi may be dissolved in the postoperative period by an infusion via a cholecystostomy tube or T-tube.

Dosage

Begin with 5 ml/h, and increase to 10 ml/h [17].

Side-effects

Nausea, vomiting, diarrhea, and duodenal ulceration may occur. Impaction of a stone producing pain may result if the infusion rate is too high.

Local anesthetic, sedative, and analgesic agents

Chloral hydrate

Uses

As a sedative or hypnotic, therapeutic doses have little effect on respiration and blood pressure.

Dosage

As an oral hypnotic 0.5−2.0 g at night in adults and 20−50 mg/kg body weight in children. The adult sedation dose is 250 mg, three times daily, up to a maximum of 2 g. It should be taken well diluted with water or milk.

Side-effects

Chloral hydrate is corrosive to skin and mucous membranes, unless well diluted or in gelatin capsules. The most common adverse effect is gastric irritation. It may produce ataxia, drowsiness, paradoxical excitement, and confusion. Overdosage causes coma and respiratory depression, and the irritant effect may cause vomiting and gastric necrosis. Cardiac arrhythmias, hepatic and renal drainage may occur. Tolerance and dependence may develop with prolonged or high dosage.

Contraindications

Chloral hydrate should not be used in patients with hepatic or renal impairment, or with severe cardiac disease. It should be used with caution in patients with porphyria and may enhance the effects of warfarin. Patients should not drive or operate machinery after its administration.

Diazepam (Valium, Diazemuls)

Diazepam is typical of the benzodiazepine group of tranquillizers and has active metabolites, the principal of which (desmethyldiazepam) has a half-life of 2−5 days.

Indications

Diazepam may be used for premedication, sedation, or to control an epileptic seizure.

Dosage

Use 2−20 mg by oral or intravenous route. Intravenous injection should be slow, using a large vein, and the dose titrated against response. Intramuscular injection is unreliable and slow in onset.

A preparation containing diazepam in an oil-in-water base (Diazemuls) reduces the incidence of thrombophlebitis and is preferred for intravenous usage. Rare cases of diazepam allergy have occurred [18,19].

Side effects

The most common side-effects are drowsiness, ataxia, and incoordination; great care must be exercised with out-patients whose ability to drive a vehicle or operate machinery may be impaired. Overdosage produces respiratory depression, apnea, and coma: assisted ventilatory support may be required. Occasionally, benzodiazepines produce a paradoxic effect causing excitement instead of sedation. Intravenous injection should be slow to reduce the risk of hypotension or apnea. Local thrombophlebitis and pain commonly follow intravenous injection.

Contraindications

Elderly and debilitated patients should receive half the normal adult dose. Patients with liver disease or chronic pulmonary dysfunction may require reduced dosage. *Intraarterial administration must be avoided.*

Lignocaine (Lidocaine, Xylocaine)

The most widely used local anesthetic agent of the amide type. Lignocaine prevents both the generation and transmission of nerve impulses. Administration may be via topical application, local infiltration, or as a regional anesthetic agent. Lignocaine is also a class I antiarrhythmic agent and is used intravenously to treat ventricular arrhythmias.

Indications

Local anesthesia. The prophylaxis and control of ventricular premature contractions and ventricular fibrillation.

Dosage

When used as an anesthetic agent, the dose must not exceed 200 mg (3 mg/kg body weight). Solutions of 0.5 and 1% are sufficient for local infiltration, 1−2% for endotracheal use, or 2−4% solution for topical anesthesia in the pharynx and larynx. When used as an antiarrhythmic agent, 50−150 mg by slow intravenous injection acts as a loading dose followed by an infusion of 1−4 mg/min.

Side-effects

Systemic toxicity is the most common cause of side-effects and is usually due to overdosage or inadvertent intravascular injection. Systemic effects involve predominantly the central nervous and cardiovascular systems, producing dizziness, muscle twitching, paresthesia, and confusion, progressing to convulsions, respiratory depression, cardiac arrhythmia, and arrest as the dose is increased. Convulsions may be controlled by diazepam. Adequate oxygenation is important as a prophylactic and therapeutic measure in the management of the cardiovascular and central nervous system side-effects. Allergy accounts for less than 1% of side-effects; however, contact dermatitis may occur (see also p. 18).

Midazolam (Hypnovel)

A powerful benzodiazepine having a half-life of only 2 hours, available only in solution. Generally, its indications and side-effects are similar to diazepam, but midazolam may be administered by intramuscular injection since it is very rapidly absorbed and well-tolerated locally.

Dosage

Intravenous or intramuscular route of 2–10 mg. When used intravenously, the dose should be in 2 mg increments over 30 seconds, titrated against the clinical response.

Morphine sulfate

The principal alkaloid of opium acting mainly on the central nervous system and smooth muscle.

Indications

Commonly used to provide analgesia and anesthesia in the preoperative, operative, and postoperative periods. Morphine also has a valuable role in the management of acute left ventricular failure.

Dosage

Administered by subcutaneous, intramuscular, or slow intravenous injection. A dose of between 5 and 15 mg is common.

Side-effects

Morphine exhibits the usual opioid-induced side-effects of nausea, vomiting, constipation, drowsiness, and miosis. Urinary retention and biliary colic may occur. Larger doses produce respiratory depression, hypotension, and circulatory collapse which may be fatal. Long-term administration may lead to physical and psychologic dependence on the drug. Anaphylactic reactions and urticaria have occasionally been reported. The effects of morphine are rapidly reversed by the administration of naloxone (see p. 43).

Contraindications

Great care should be exercised when morphine is administered to patients with preexisting liver disease or respiratory depression. The depressant effects of morphine may be enhanced by other central nervous system depressants. Morphine is contraindicated during treatment with antidepressants, particularly monoamine oxidase inhibitors.

Pentazocine (Fortral)

An analgesic with similar actions to morphine, but, in addition, it has weak narcotic antagonist actions.

Indications

As for morphine (see above).

Dosage

By mouth 20–100 mg, 30–60 mg by subcutaneous, intramuscular, or slow intravenous injection.

Side-effects

These are generally similar to those of morphine, but in particular hallucinations may be troublesome. The weak narcotic antagonist action may precipitate withdrawal symptoms in patients who have recently received other narcotic agonist analgesics. Naloxone (see p. 43) is a specific antidote for the depressant effects of pentazocine.

Pethidine (Demerol, Meperidine)

Although it is structurally unlike morphine, pethidine has many similar properties and actions.

Indications

As for morphine (see above).

Dosage

Use 50–150 mg by the oral, subcutaneous, intramuscular, or slow intravenous routes.

Side-effects

These are generally the same as those for morphine except that miosis does not occur, constipation and cough suppression are less marked, and there is less hypnotic effect. Severe reactions including convulsions, hyperpyrexia, coma, and death have occurred when pethidine was administered to patients receiving monoamine oxidase inhibitors.

Contraindications

As with morphine, care must be taken when pethidine is administered to patients with liver disease or respiratory depression but, in addition, particular caution must be exercised in patients with supraventricular tachycardia or those receiving monoamine oxidase inhibitors [20].

Temazepam

A benzodiazepine with a similar action to diazepam but having a shorter half-life of 8 hours and only being available for oral administration. Side-effects and contraindications are also similar to those for diazepam.

Dosage

For premedication, 20–40 mg is administered 0.5–1.0 hour prior to the procedure.

Drugs used in the treatment of allergic reactions and cardiovascular collapse

Antihistamines

Chlorpheniramine maleate (Piriton)

Indications

The prophylaxis and treatment of allergic reactions including sneezing, urticaria, and angioneurotic edema.

Dosage

As an oral preparation, 4 mg four times daily. In severe allergy, 10–20 mg may be administered by subcutaneous, intramuscular, or slow intravenous injection. For the intravenous route it should be diluted in the syringe with 5–10 ml of blood and injected over 1 minute.

Side-effects

Chlorpheniramine is an H_1-receptor *antagonist* and shows the general complications of this group: sedation, inability to concentrate, and muscular incoordination are relatively common; out-patients must be warned of the hazards of alcohol consumption and driving. Central nervous system stimulation is rare, but it may occur leading to insomnia, tremors, and nightmares. The effects of anticholinergic drugs, antidepressants, and alcohol are all potentiated by chlorpheniramine. Dermatologic reactions may occur, but these are very rare with systemic administration and usually result

from topical administration. Hypotension following intravenous injection is usually transitory.

Contraindications

Chlorpheniramine maleate is incompatible with calcium chloride; it should not be mixed with corticosteroids or contrast media. A precipitate has been recorded on mixing with meglumine iodipamide [21]. Chlorpheniramine should *not* be injected intraarterially.

Cimetidine

See p. 29.

Clemastine fumarate (Tavegil, Tavist)

Indications and side-effects

As for chlorpheniramine (see above) and other antihistamines, although clemastine fumarate is claimed to have less of a sedative effect.

Dosage

Use 1 mg twice daily by oral or intramuscular route.

Diphenhydramine hydrochloride

Indications

As for chlorpheniramine (see above). Contrast-media prophylaxis and treatment.

Dosage

Use 50 mg 6 hourly by oral, intramuscular, or intravenous routes.

Side-effects

Diphenhydramine exhibits similar side-effects to chlorpheniramine and has a pronounced sedative action necessitating caution when it is administered to out-patients. An increased incidence of cleft palate has been reported in babies born to women who received diphenhydramine in pregnancy [22].

Contraindications

Diphenhydramine is incompatible in solution with many barbiturate anesthetic agents, hydrocortisone sodium succinate, iodipamide salts, and some concentrations of diatrizoate salts.

Corticosteroids

The relative potency of some corticosteroids is shown in Table 3.1.

Table 3.1 Relative potency of corticosteroids

Preparation	Relative antiinflammatory potency	Relative sodium-retaining potency
Hydrocortisone	1	1.0
Prednisone/prednisolone	4	0.8
Methyl prednisolone	5	0.5
Dexamethasone	25	0.0

Dexamethasone (Decadron, Dexacortisyl, Hexadrol)

A potent glucocorticoid having little or no mineralocorticoid action.

Indications

As for hydrocortisone (see below), but dexamethasone is particularly useful when high doses of steroids are required in such circumstances as cerebral edema.

Dosage

A standard regimen of an initial dose of 10 mg followed by 4 mg 6 hourly by oral, intramuscular, or intravenous routes. Intravenous injection of corticosteroids should be given slowly.

Side-effects

As for hydrocortisone (see below). The intravenous preparation utilizes the sodium phosphate salt and, following large doses, itching and tingling may occur [23].

Hydrocortisone sodium succinate

Indications

Steroid therapy with hydrocortisone is indicated in the prophylaxis and treatment of severe allergic reactions including urticaria, bronchospasm, angioneurotic edema, anaphylaxis, and cardiovascular collapse. The onset of action is usually too slow for steroids to be immediately effective in life-threatening laryngeal edema or anaphylaxis, but they are used as an adjunct to the appropriate symptomatic treatment, e.g., epinephrine.

Dosage

For emergency contrast-media prophylaxis in high-risk patients, Greenberger *et al.* [24] recommend hydrocortisone 200 mg (slowly) intravenously as soon as the procedure is anticipated and every 4 hours until the procedure has been completed.

Side-effects

The vast majority of these are attributed to long-term administration, producing adrenal suppression and Cushing's syndrome. Severe myopathy has been reported following high dosage of hydrocortisone over a 14-hour period. Generalized urticaria and facial edema have occurred following a single dose of hydrocortisone [25]. Peptic ulceration, hemorrhage, and perforation may complicate steroid therapy. Hydrocortisone sodium succinate is unstable in aqueous solution and must be mixed immediately before use, unlike hydrocortisone sodium phosphate which is stable in solution; despite this inconvenience, hydrocortisone sodium succinate has been recommended for intravenous administration because it does not produce paresthesia on injection [26]. It should *not* be mixed in the syringe with antihistamines (see also p. 279).

Methylprednisolone (Medrone, Urbason)

This has similar properties to hydrocortisone (see above), but has less sodium-retaining properties and is therefore not suitable for adrenal replacement therapy.

Indications and side-effects

As for prednisone (see p. 37).

Dosage

Use 4–48 mg daily. In 1985, Lasser recommended 32 mg orally, 12 and 2 hours prior to the examination for the prophylaxis of contrast-media reactions [27].

Prednisolone (Deltacortril enteric, Delta cortef)

This is the active metabolite of prednisone (see below) following transformation by the liver. The bioavailability of prednisolone is more reliable and it is preferred to prednisone. An enteric coating reduces the risk of peptic ulceration.

Indications and side-effects

As for prednisone (see below).

Dosage

As for prednisone (below).

Prednisone (Decortisyl, Deltacortone, Meticorten)

A steroid preparation with high glucocorticoid activity but little mineralocorticoid activity.

Indications and side-effects

As for hydrocortisone, but prednisone is particularly useful in the prophylaxis of contrast-media reactions due to its good gastrointestinal absorption.

Dosage

For contrast-media prophylaxis in high-risk patients, Greenberger and Patterson [28] advise prednisone 50 mg orally 13, 7, and 1 hour prior to use of a nonionic contrast medium, with diphenhydramine 50 mg orally 1 hour before contrast. If there is no cardiovascular or other contraindication, ephedrine 25 mg orally may also be given (see pp. 39, 279). Zweiman and Hildreth [29] have suggested that 150 mg prednisone should also be administered in the 12 hours after contrast.

Cardiac stimulants, bronchodilators, and atropine

Adrenalin (epinephrine)

Epinephrine is a naturally occurring α- and β-sympathomimetic agent. Its major effects are stimulation of the heart, inhibition of the smooth muscle in the bronchial tree producing bronchodilatation, and smooth-muscle stimulation in the peripheral cutaneous blood vessels producing vasoconstriction. Epinephrine also stimulates the central nervous system and metabolic rate (see also pp. 48, 80, 284).

Indications

Epinephrine is the primary drug in the treatment of angioneurotic edema, severe bronchospasm, anaphylactic shock, and cardiac asystole. It may also be used as an adjunct to renal angiography, improving the visualization of a neoplastic circulation [30].

Dosage

In bronchospasm, 0.1 ml increments of a 1:1000 solution up to a maximum of 2 ml in 5 minutes may be given subcutaneously, providing an adequate circulation is maintained.

In cases of severe shock, intravenous epinephrine may be required, but a dilute solution of 1:10 000 must then be used with extreme caution. In cardiac asystole, 5 ml of a 1:10 000 solution may be given intravenously, intratracheally, or in special cases, by direct intracardiac injection.

An intraarterial injection of 5 μg immediately before the contrast medium, enhances renal angiography with a neoplastic circulation (see Contraindications below).

Side-effects

Palpitations, extrasystole, hypertension, cerebral hemorrhage, ventricular fibrillation, hyperglycemia, and pulmonary edema may occur: their frequency is dose related. It may be inappropriate to administer epinephrine, either subcutaneously or intramuscularly, to patients with severe circulatory collapse because, in such circumstances, a subsequent improvement in the circulation may cause further absorption of epinephrine into the circulation, producing overdosage. Complex interactions between epinephrine and α- and β-blocking agents may occur, reducing the effects of epinephrine in patients already receiving β-blocking agents (see pp. 48, 284).

Contraindications

Simultaneous administration of epinephrine and a β-blocker may result in cardiac arrhythmia [31]. Thyrotoxicosis or anesthetic agents, such as halothane, increase sensitivity to epinephrine, while concurrent administration of either tricyclic antidepressants or monoamine oxidase inhibitors [32] may induce dangerous cardiac arrhythmias and hypertension. Myocardial ischemia is a contraindication to epinephrine, except in a life-threatening situation. Myocardial ischemia has occurred in apparently healthy individuals after intravenous injection of epinephrine [33]. There may be a potential pH incompatibility between epinephrine and contrast media [34].

Albuterol (salbutamol)

See p. 40.

Aminophylline

The active constituent of aminophylline is theophylline, which relaxes smooth muscle and stimulates the myocardium and respiration. Ethylenediamine is added to enhance solubility and is physiologically inert, but it may produce hypersensitivity reactions [35].

Indications

The relief of bronchospasm, cardiac asthma, and cardiac failure.

Dosage

A slow intravenous injection of 250–500 mg over 10 minutes, followed, if required, by an infusion of 500 µg/kg per hour.

Side-effects

Hypotension and death may follow too rapid an administration. The cardiovascular effects are dose related, but theophylline has a narrow therapeutic range and side-effects generally occur with blood levels above 20 µg/ml. The common side-effects experienced are nausea, vomiting, headache, palpitation, agitation, and convulsions. Both the young and elderly are at increased risk, and in such cases, the dose should be reduced by 25%. Hypersensitivity is probably due to the ethylenediamine component and comprises urticaria, bronchospasm, and thrombocytopenia.

Contraindications

Patients receiving oral aminophylline are at risk of overdosage from additional parenteral administration.

Atropine

A naturally occurring anticholinergic alkaloid exerting its action by competitive inhibition with acetylcholine.

Indications

As a premedication, atropine reduces bronchial, gastric, and salivary secretions: atropine has a central stimulant action on the central nervous system in clinical dosage. Acute vagal syncope usually responds to simple postural therapy but, occasionally, atropine is required to restore the circulation. Patients with bradycardia whether related to primary cardiac disorders, coronary ischemia, or vagal activity may respond to atropine. Colic due to smooth-muscle spasm in the urinary and gastrointestinal tracts may be relieved by atropine, but biliary colic is not effectively counteracted.

Dosage

For premedication, 0.3–0.6 mg by intramuscular injection 1 hour prior to the procedure. For bradycardia, 0.6–1.2 mg by intravenous injection. This may be repeated at 5-minute intervals up to a total dose of 3 mg.

Side-effects

Anticholinergic effects similar to those exhibited by hyoscine butylbromide occur (see p. 28), but they are more prolonged. With increasing dosage, tachycardia, dry mouth, dilatation of pupil and blurred vision, difficulty in swallowing, and acute retention may occur. Overdosage produces the classical clinical state of belladonna poisoning. Patients with myocardial ischemia may develop ventricular fibrillation following atropine [36].

Contraindications

Prostatic enlargement, closed-angle glaucoma, and the concomitant administration of other anticholinergic agents are all contraindications to atropine administration.

Calcium chloride

Calcium chloride increases myocardial contractility and enhances ventricular excitability.

Indications

To improve myocardial action in profound cardiovascular collapse with asystole or ventricular fibrillation, and to enhance the response of the heart to electric defibrillation.

Dosage

Use 2.5–5.0 ml of a 10% solution by intravenous injection, repeated as required at 10-minute intervals.

Side-effects

The solution is extremely irritant and care must be taken to avoid extravasation which may cause muscle necrosis. Nausea, vomiting, vasodilatation, sweating, and hypotension may occur following calcium chloride administration.

Contraindications

The addition of calcium chloride to sodium bicarbonate solution produces a precipitate of calcium carbonate.

Dopamine hydrochloride (Intropin)

Dopamine is a naturally occurring sympathomimetic agent with direct β-adrenergic effects and indirect α-adrenergic effects. Dopamine also acts to increase renal and mesenteric blood flow. This effect is believed to be due to a direct dopaminergic mechanism.

Indications

Patients with severe shock and congestive heart failure may benefit from a dopamine infusion, due to the rise in blood pressure and positive inotropic effect on the heart.

Dosage

An initial infusion rate of 2—5 µg/kg body weight per min is gradually increased depending on the clinical response up to a maximum of 50 µg/kg per min in seriously ill patients.

Side-effects

There is a risk of local tissue necrosis, as with norepinephrine (see below), and a central venous catheter is the preferred route of administration. Extravasation should be treated by infiltrating the affected area with 10—15 ml saline, containing 5—10 mg phentolamine mesylate to reverse local vasoconstriction. Similar sympathomimetic side-effects to those experienced with epinephrine (see p. 37) also occur.

Contraindications

Treatment with monoamine oxidase inhibitors may cause excessive response. Reduce initial dose.

Ephedrine sulfate

A sympathomimetic agent with α- and β-activity which has slower, less profound but more prolonged action than epinephrine. Ephedrine is well absorbed orally and its effects include raising cardiac output, peripheral vasocontraction, and bronchodilatation.

Indications

Ephedrine may be used to raise cardiac output and blood pressure, and to produce bronchodilatation. Greenberger *et al.* [37] suggested the use of ephedrine in the prophylaxis of contrast-media reactions (p. 279).

Dosage

Oral administration of 15—60 mg three times daily may be prescribed for bronchodilatation. Subcutaneous administration of 15—50 mg or intravenous injection of 20 mg is required for hypotension.

Side-effects

In high doses, ephedrine produces giddiness, headache, nausea, tachycardia, and central nervous system stimulation. Hypertension and ventricular tachycardia are less common than with epinephrine, but they may follow intravenous injection. Convulsions may also occur.

Contraindications

Anesthetic agents, antipsychotic drugs, cardiovascular disease, hypertension, and hyperthyroidism are contraindications. Ephedrine is incompatible in solution with hydrocortisone and sodium bicarbonate.

Epinephrine (adrenalin)

See p. 37.

Norepinephrine acid tartrate (noradrenalin, Levophed, Levarterenol)

A naturally occurring sympathomimetic agent with predominant α-receptor stimulation. Norepinephrine has powerful vasoconstrictor properties, making it unsuitable for subcutaneous or intramuscular injection: for a systemic effect it must be given intravenously. The major effect of norepinephrine is to increase blood pressure by producing peripheral vasoconstriction and a positive inotropic action on the heart.

Indications

Norepinephrine may be used to treat hypotension in patients who have an adequate circulating blood volume. Norepinephrine may be used in myocardial infarction, although animal studies have suggested it may extend the size of the infarct in normotensive patients [38].

Dosage

Norepinephrine is usually administered by an intravenous infusion equivalent to 4 µg/ml; this solution being prepared by diluting strong sterile norepinephrine solution 250 times as recommended by the manufacturer's literature. An initial infusion rate of 2—3 µg/min is subsequently adjusted as required, to maintain a satisfactory blood pressure; the average maintenance dose is 0.5—1.0 µg/min. At the end of therapy, the infusion rate should be gradually reduced to prevent sudden rebound hypotension.

Side-effects

Norepinephrine is extremely irritant, and extravasation produces severe vasoconstriction and tissue necrosis (see Dopamine, above). This risk is reduced by injecting via a plastic cannula inserted into a large vein. Anxiety, transient headache, respiratory difficulty, and hypertension may all occur; the latter may precipitate cerebral hemorrhage. The hypertensive effects are more likely to occur with concomitant administration of adrenergic neuron-blocking agents or antidepressants. Retrosternal pain and transient engorgement of the thyroid may occur.

Phenylephrine

A sympathomimetic agent with predominantly α-adrenergic effects. It produces peripheral vasoconstriction and increased arterial pressure.

Indications

The reversal of hypotension.

Dose

Use 2–5 mg subcutaneously or intramuscularly; or 100–500 µg by slow intravenous injection as a 0.1% solution, repeated as necessary after at least 15 minutes.

Side-effects

As for epinephrine (see p. 37).

Salbutamol (Albuterol, Ventolin)

A direct acting sympathomimetic agent with a predominantly β-effect, thus producing a more prominent bronchodilating action than cardiac action. It has a more prolonged action than epinephrine and is preferred in the treatment of bronchospasm.

Indications

The treatment of severe bronchospasm or anaphylaxis.

Dosage

May be administered in aerosol form in the acute episode using a dose of 200 µg. In more seriously ill patients, administration is more appropriate in a dose of 500 µg by subcutaneous or intramuscular injection, or by slow intravenous injection of 250 µg. It may also be used as a solution containing 10 µg/ml as an infusion in glucose or sodium chloride.

Side effects

General effects as with other sympathomimetics (see epinephrine, p. 37). Tremor, headache, tachycardia, vasodilatation, hypotension, hyperglycemia, hypokalemia. Intramuscular injection may produce local pain. Hypersensitivity reactions producing angiedema, urticaria, and bronchospasm have been reported.

Contraindications

Albuterol should be used with caution in patients with thyrotoxicosis. The actions of albuterol may be interrupted by the use of a β-blocking agent.

Sodium bicarbonate intravenous infusion

Indications

A sodium bicarbonate solution of 4.2% (0.5 mmol/ml) or 8.4% (1 mmol/ml) is administered intravenously to correct the metabolic acidosis caused by prolonged cardiac arrest.

Dosage

An intravenous infusion of 50 mmol after prolonged cardio-pulmonary arrest, with pH monitoring as soon as possible. Further administration should be indicated by pH values.

Side-effects

The solution is extremely irritant to the soft tissues and may produce local necrosis if extravasation occurs [39]. Hyperosmolality, cerebral edema, and hypernatremia may occur with overdosage, particularly in small children.

Contraindications

The solution is incompatible with many other agents, but of particular importance are norepinephrine, dopamine, calcium chloride, and calcium gluconate.

Vasodilators

Captopril (Acepril, Capoten)

Captopril inhibits the conversion of angiotension I to the active angiotension II (angiotensin-converting enzyme (ACE) inhibitor), and thus lowers systemic arterial resistance and reduces the glomerular filtration rate in the kidney with renal artery stenosis.

Indications

As an adjunct to isotope renography in the investigation of renal artery stenosis. A baseline study without ACE inhibitor is necessary for comparison purposes.

Dosage

Use 25–50 mg orally 1 hour before administration of the radionuclide. The patient should be well hydrated and an intravenous infusion of normal saline established.

Side-effects

Hypotension may occur particularly in hypertensive patients on combination therapy regimens, including diuretics. The incidence of adverse reactions is associated with renal impairment and proteinuria. Idiosyncratic angiedema may occur, and when the airway is compromised, subcutaneous epinephrine (0.5 mg 1:1000) should be administered. Blood dyscrasias may occur, but these are usually dose related in patients with renal impairment.

Contraindications

A history of previous hypersensitivity; pregnancy. Care should be exercised in patients with aortic stenosis, congestive heart failure, hyponatremia, and in those receiving diuretics.

Dipyridamole (Persantin)

Dipyridamole is a phosphodiesterase inhibitor, stimulating adenyl cyclase formation, producing an antiplatelet action and vasodilatation.

Indications

May be used for its antiplatelet action in arterial disease and as adjunct to angioplasty. Dipyridamole may also be used as a coronary vasodilator with thallium-201 during myocardial perfusion imaging.

Dosage

For an antithrombotic effect, 300–600 mg daily in three doses by the oral route. For myocardial vasodilatation in conjunction with thallium, a dose of 0.6 mg/kg in 50 ml of normal saline by intravenous injection over 4 minutes.

Side-effects

During myocardial scanning, up to 47% of patients experienced side-effects [40], mostly limited to headache, dizziness, chest pain, and ST changes on the electrocardiogram. Serious complications include myocardial failure or myocardial stunning. Acute bronchospasm may occur. Most of these symptoms are relieved by 250 mg of aminophylline intravenously. Myocardial infarction and death have also been reported.

Contraindications

A known hypersensitivity to dipyridamole, supravalvar aortic stenosis, aortic disease, hypotension associated with recent myocardial infarction, uncompensated heart failure, or arrhythmias.

Enalaprilic acid (Enalaprilat)

Indications and side-effects

As for captopril (see p. 40).

Dosage

Use 50 μg/kg by intravenous injection 15 minutes before administration of the radionuclide.

Glyceryl trinitrate (nitroglycerin, Tridil)

Glyceryl trinitrate has a complex action, the most important components of which are: (i) decrease in the preload and afterload of the heart, thereby reducing oxygen consumption; and (ii) coronary vasodilation, thus increasing the supply of oxygen to the heart.

Indications

The treatment of choice in acute angina pectoris and also of value in prophylaxis. Glyceryl trinitrate is also of benefit in the relaxation of diffuse esophageal spasm [41] and achalasia of the gastric cardia. The peripheral vasodilator effect of glyceryl trinitrate may be useful in countering arterial spasm during arterial catheterization or angioplasty; in such circumstances intraarterial administration is preferred. An intravenous infusion may be of benefit in heart failure; the reduction in cardiac load helping to improve the circulation.

Dosage

Administration for angina pectoris and esophageal spasm is via the sublingual route with 500 μg tablets. The effect is experienced in 30 seconds to 2 minutes and lasts for 30–60 minutes. The tablets have a shelf-life of only 8 weeks [42]. For peripheral vasodilatation, an infusion of 15–20 μg/min is used, increasing in steps up to a maximum of 400 μg/min, or until the desired effect is achieved.

Side-effects

Too rapid an infusion of glyceryl trinitrate produces hypotension. Flushing, dizziness, tachycardia, and throbbing headaches frequently occur. Less commonly, syncope and transient cerebral ischemic attacks are encountered. Transient hypoxemia [43] and methemoglobinemia have been recorded. Intravenous glyceryl trinitrate may produce heparin resistance (see p. 30).

Labetalol

Labetalol is a noncardioselective β-blocker, which also has α-blocking activity, decreasing peripheral vascular resistance.

Indications

The treatment of hypertension and angina pectoris. The antihypertensive effect is more rapid than that produced by other β-blockers, and labetalol may be considered the drug of choice in the treatment of aortic dissection [44], and as a first-line drug in the treatment of pheochromocytoma [45].

Dosage

In the treatment of hypertension, the initial oral dose is 100 mg twice daily increasing to 400 mg twice daily as required. In the elderly, a starting dose of 50 mg twice daily is suggested. In an emergency situation, a slow intravenous injection of 50 mg may be administered, repeated at 5-minute intervals to a maximum of 200 mg. An infusion of 2 mg/min may also be used.

Side-effects

All the classical side-effects of β-blockade may be produced, including heart failure, heart block and bronchospasm. The symptoms of peripheral vascular disease may be exaggerated. Central nervous system effects include depression, confusion, sleep disturbances, and fatigue. Ocular symptoms and hematologic reactions including blood dyscrasias may occur. Skin rash and scalp tingling, nasal congestion, weakness, and hepatitis have been described, and sexual function may be impaired.

The combined β- and α-action may produce profound postural hypotension: blood pressure should be monitored and the patient remain supine for 3 hours after intravenous administration.

Contraindications

Labetalol should not be given to patients with bronchospasm, metabolic acidosis, or heart block. Care should be exercised in patients with heart failure. Symptoms of hyperthyroidism and hypoglycemia may be masked. Abrupt withdrawal may precipitate angina pectoris and ventricular fibrillation. Particular care must be taken when administering labetalol to elderly patients or those with cardiac failure.

Papaverine sulfate (Cerebid)

Indications

A direct smooth-muscle relaxant, of benefit in acute ischemia and arterial spasm.

Dosage

Intraarterial injection of 30−60 mg, followed by an infusion of 30−60 mg/h.

Side-effects

Gastrointestinal disturbance, headaches, and flushing may all occur. Hypersensitivity involving the liver may produce

jaundice [46]. Cardiac arrhythmias can occur. Papaverine precipitates ioxaglate [47].

Phentolamine mesylate (Rogitine, Regitine)

An α-adrenoreceptor blocking agent with a rapid, short-lived effect to lower arteriolar resistance and increase cardiac output.

Indications

Hypertensive crises in patients with pheochromocytoma, or those receiving monoamine oxidase inhibitors, may be treated with phentolamine (see also p. 41).

Dosage

Intravenous injections of 5−10 mg for hypertensive crises, followed by an infusion of 0.5 mg/min if required.

Side-effects

Hypotension, tachycardia, and angina pectoris may occur. Nausea, vomiting, diarrhea, weakness, and dizziness may also be experienced.

Tolazoline (Priscol, Priscoline)

An α-adrenoreceptor blocking agent that has a direct effect on the small peripheral vessels, increasing blood flow.

Indications

To reverse arterial spasm occurring during arterial catheterization, or as an adjunct to the angiographic demonstration of polyarteritis nodosa [48], or bone and soft tissue tumors [49].

Dosage

Administer 25−50 mg by subcutaneous, intravenous, or intraarterial routes.

Side-effects

Tolazoline may cause nausea, vomiting, and diarrhea; it also stimulates gastric acid secretion. Flushing, sweating, and piloerection are particularly common after intraarterial injection. Palpitations and angina may occur, and tolazoline has been implicated in precipitating myocardial infarction. Priscol precipitates ioxaglate [50].

Diuretic

Furosemide, Frusemide (Lasix)

A powerful fast-acting diuretic.

Indications

Furosemide may be used as an adjunct to intravenous urography and isotope renography in diuresis studies. An intravenous injection of 20 mg immediately before the contrast or radioisotope is effective. It may also be used in cases of acute or chronic heart failure to reduce peripheral and pulmonary edema.

Dosage

For radiologic procedures 20 mg is satisfactory; 80–120 mg may be used in the therapy of heart failure, but doses up to 1 g may be used in renal failure. Oral, intramuscular, and intravenous preparations are available; intravenous injections should be diluted and must be given slowly.

Side-effects

Fluid and electrolyte depletion can lead to cardiovascular collapse and death. At high serum concentrations ($>50 \mu g/ml$), tinnitus and deafness may occur [51]. Toxic skin rashes including exfoliative dermatitis may occur, but they are rare. Agranulocytosis and thrombocytopenia have also been reported. The rapid onset of the diuresis may precipitate acute retention in elderly patients with prostatism, and prophylactic bladder catheterization may be considered.

Drugs used in respiratory depression

Flumazenil (Anexate)

This is a specific antidote for the central sedative effects of benzodiazepines, acting by competitive inhibition. It has a rapid but short-lived effect. Due to the long action of some benzodiazepines, sedation may recur, requiring further administration of flumazenil.

Indications

The complete or partial reversion of the sedative effects of benzodiazepines.

Dosage

Initially 200 µg administered intravenously over 15 seconds repeated in 100 µg increments at 60-second intervals as clinically indicated up to a maximum of 1 mg. If sedation recurs, an intravenous infusion of 100–400 µg/h should be established.

Side-effects

Flumazenil may cause overstimulation in patients receiving long-term high-dose benzodiazepine treatment; this effect is reversed by a titrated intravenous dose of diazepam or midazolam. It is, however, generally well tolerated, although occasionally producing flushing, nausea, or a transient increase in blood pressure.

Contraindications

A known hypersensitivity to benzodiazepines. Care should be exercised in patients receiving long-term benzodiazepine therapy. In particular, there is a risk of convulsions in epileptics when the protective effect is suppressed.

Naloxone (Narcan)

A narcotic antagonist with little pharmacologic activity except for its reversal of the effects of narcotic agents.

Indications

The drug of choice in the reversal of respiratory depression produced by narcotic analgesics.

Dosage

Administer 0.4–0.8 mg by subcutaneous, intramuscular, or intravenous injection; due to its short duration of activity, repeated doses may be required as clinically indicated.

Side-effects

Naloxone may induce a rise in blood pressure, cardiac arrhythmias, pulmonary edema [52], nausea, or vomiting. If administered to a narcotic addict, it may precipitate an acute withdrawal syndrome. Naloxone interferes with the endorphin system and therefore also blocks the pain-relief effects of narcotic analgesics.

Drugs used in malignant hyperpyrexia

Dantrolene sodium (Danlene, Dantramacrin)

A muscle relaxant with direct action on skeletal muscle.

Indications

Used by mouth for the symptomatic relief of spasticity. Given intravenously in the treatment of malignant hyperpyrexia and neuroleptic malignant syndrome [53].

Dosage

Used orally for spasticity. A starting dose of 25 mg daily increasing over 7 weeks to a maximum of 100 mg four times daily as clinically appropriate. In malignant hyperpyrexia, a rapid intravenous injection of 1 mg/kg body weight is continued until symptoms subside, to a maximum of 10 mg/kg.

Side-effects

Short-term intravenous administration does not produce serious side-effects. Minor side-effects occur at the start of treatment and are usually transient, including drowsiness, fatigue, malaise, and gastrointestinal symptoms. Hepatotoxicity and pleural effusion with pericarditis may be severe.

Agent to disperse extravasated contrast media

Hyaluronidase (Hyalase)

An enzyme that depolymerizes the mucopolysaccharide hyaluronic acid, increasing the dispersal and subsequent absorption of substances through the soft tissues.

Indications

It is suggested by Elam et al. [54] that hyaluronidase may speed the dispersal of extravasated high-osmolar contrast media, reducing the risk of ulceration: this work has yet to be confirmed in humans. The dispersal of hematoma. See also p. 249.

Dosage

Administer 1500 U in 20–40 ml of saline by local injection at the site of extravasation.

Side-effects

Sensitivity reactions may occur.

Contraindications

Should not be used by intravenous injection or at the site of malignancy or infection.

Agent for chemonucleolysis

Chymopapain (Chymodiactin)

Indications

Used in the treatment of lumbar intervertebral disk prolapse.

Administered under local anesthesia as an injection into the disk.

Dosage

Recommended dose is 2–4 nKat/disk with a maximum dose of 8 nKat/patient.

Side-effects [55]

Anaphylaxis may occur in 1% of patients. Symptoms include angiedema, hypotension, bronchospasm, shock, and cardiac arrest. Allergic skin reactions may occur. Severe back pain, discitis, paralysis, acute transverse myelitis, and cerebral hemorrhage have occurred.

Contraindications

Because of the high risk of anaphylaxis it may only be used for one treatment session per patient. It should not be used in cases of known sensitivity to papaya protein, paralysis, tumors of the spinal canal, and severe spondylolisthesis. It should not be used in patients with severe cardiorespiratory problems, or on β-blockers, who may be at increased risk if anaphylaxis occurs.

Drug index

Drugs for allergic reactions, cardiac resuscitation and arrhythmias, see also pp. 35 and 77.
For selected drug interactions, see pp. 48–49.

References

1 Cuschieri A. Management of retained biliary calculi: relaxation of sphincter induced by ceruletide. *Br Med J* 1984;289:1582.

2 Howarth FH, Cockel R, Hawkins CF. Effects of metoclopramide upon gastric motility and its value in barium progress meals. *Gut* 1967;8:635–636.

3 Bertrand G, Linscheer WG, Raheja KL. Double blind evaluation of glucagon and propantheline bromide (probanthine) for hypotonic duodenography. *Am J Roentgenol* 1977;128:197–200.

4 Zaloga GP, Delacey W, Holmboe E, De Chernow B. Glucagon reversal of hypotension in a case of anaphylactoid shock. *Ann Intern Med* 1986;105:65–66.

5 Edell SL. Erythema multiforme secondary to intravenous glucagon. *Am J Roentgenol* 1980;134:385–386.

6 Baum S, d'Aignon MB, Locko RC, Latshawe RF, Rohrer GV, Petrokub RJ. Pertechnetate/cimetidine abdominal imaging. *Int J Nucl Med Biol* 1981;8:185–186.

7 Ahmed AH, McLarty DG, Sharma SK, Masawe AE. Stevens–Johnson syndrome during treatment with cimetidine. *Lancet* 1978;ii:433.

8 Cohen J, Weetman AP, Dargie HJ, Krikler DM. Life threatening arrhythmias and intravenous cimetidine. *Br Med J* 1979;2:768.

9 Nelson PJ, Moster KM, Stoner C, Moser KS. Risk of complications during intravenous heparin therapy. *W J Med* 1982;136:189–197.

10 Habbab, MA, Haft JI. Heparin resistance induced by intravenous nitroglycerin. *Arch Intern Med* 1987;147:857–860.

11 White PW, Sadd JR, Nensel RE. Thrombotic complications of heparin therapy. *Ann Surg* 1979;190:595.

12 McNamara TO, Fisher JR. Thrombolysis of peripheral arterial and graft occlusions: improved results using high dose urokinase. *Am J Roentgenol* 1985;144:769–775.

13 Berker RG, Alpert JS. The impact of medical therapy on haemorrhagic complications following coronary artery bypass grafting. *Arch Intern Med* 1990;150:2016–2021.

14 Johnson WC, Widrich WC, Ansell JE. Control of bleeding varices by vasopressin: a prospective randomised study. *Ann Surg* 1977;186:369–376.

15 Colombani P. Upper extremity gangrene secondary to superior mesenteric artery infusion of vasopressin. *Digest Dis Sci* 1982;27:367–369.

16 Thistle JL, Carlson GL, Hofmann AF. Monooctanoin, a dissolution agent for retained cholesterol bile duct stones: physical properties and clinical application. *Gastroenterology* 1980;78:1016–1022.

17 Shortsleeve MJ, Schatzki SG, Lee DL. Monooctanoin dissolution of gall stones via a cholecystostomy tube. *Radiology* 1984;153:547.

18 Blumberg MZ, Young S. Diazepam-associated asthma. *Pediatrics* 1974;54:811–812.

19 Milner L. Allergy to diazepam. *Br Med J* 1977;144:15.

20 Clark B, Thompson JW, Widdrington G. Analysis of the inhibition of pethidine N-demethylation by monoamine oxidase inhibitors and some other drugs with special reference to drug interactions in man. *Br J Pharmacol* 1972;44:89–99.

21 Marshall TR, Ling JT, Follis G, Russell M. Pharmacological incompatibility of contrast media with various drugs and agents. *Radiology* 1965;84:536–539.

22 Saxen I. Cleft palate and maternal diphenhydramine intake. *Lancet* 1974;i:407–408.

23 Czerwinksi AW, Czerwinski AB, Whitsett TL. Effects of a single large intravenous injection of dexamethasone. *Clin Pharmacol Ther* 1972;13:638–642.

24 Greenberger PA, Halwig JM, Patterson R, Wallemark CB. Emergency administration of radiocontrast media in high risk patients. *J Allergy Clin Immunol* 1986;77:630–634.

25 Ashford RF, Bailey A. Angioneurotic oedema and urticaria following hydrocortisone. *Postgrad Med J* 1980;56:437.

26 Editorial. Which forms of intravenous hydrocortisone? *Drugs Ther Bull* 1979;17:71–72.

27 Lasser EC. Etiology of anaphylactoid responses. The promise of non ionics. *Invest Radiol Suppl* 1985;20:579–583.

28 Greenberger PA, Patterson P. The prevention of immediate generalized reactions to radiocontrast media in high-risk patients. *J Allergy Clin Immunol* 1991;87:867–872.

29 Zweiman B, Hildreth EA. An approach to contrast studies in reactive humans. *J Allergy Clin Immunol* 1974;53:97.

30 Pollard JJ, Nesbesar RA. Abdominal angiography. *New Engl J*

Med 1968;279:1035−1041.

31 Lampman RM, Santinga JT, Basset DR, Savage PF. Cardiac arrhythmias during epinephrine−propranolol infusion for measurement of *in vivo* insulin resistance. *Diabetes* 1981;30: 618−620.

32 Risch SC, Groom GP, Janowsky DS. The effects of psychotropic drugs on the cardiovascular system. *J Clin Psychiatr* 1982;43: 16−31.

33 Horack A, Raine R, Opie LH, Lloyd EA. Severe myocardial ischaemia induced by intravenous adrenaline. *Br Med J* 1983; 286:519.

34 Holman BL, Dewangee MK. Potential pH incompatibility of pharmacologic and isotopic adjuncts to arteriography. *Radiology* 1974;110:722−723.

35 Editorial. Allergy to aminophylline. *Lancet* 1984;ii:1192−1193.

36 Massumi RA, Mason DT, Amsterdam EA. Ventricular fibrillation and tachycardia after intravenous atropine for treatment of bradycardias. *New Engl J Med* 1972;287:336−338.

37 Greenberger P, Patterson R, Kelly J, Stevenson DD, Simon R, Lieberman P. Administration of radiographic contrast media in high risk patients. *Invest Radiol* 1980;15:540−543.

38 Lesch M. Inotropic agents and infarct size. Theoretical and practical considerations. *Am J Cardiol* 1975;37:508−513.

39 Gaze NR. Tissue necrosis caused by commonly used intravenous infusions. *Lancet* 1978;ii:417−419.

40 Kaul S, Villaneuva FS. Editorial − dipyridamole/thallium 201 imaging: how safe is it? When should it be used? *J Nucl Med* 1991;32:2115−2117.

41 Orlando RC, Bozymski EM. Clinical and manometric effects of nitroglycerin in diffuse oesophageal spasm. *New Engl J Med* 1973;289:23−25.

42 The Council of the Pharmaceutical Society. Glyceryl trinitrate tablets. *Pharmaceut J* 1980; October 11th: 405.

43 Kopman EA, Wegandt GR, Bauer S, Ferguson TB. Arterial hypoxaemia following the administration of sublingual nitroglycerin. *Am Heart J* 1978;96:444−447.

44 Banning AP, Ruttley MST, Musumeci F, Fraser AG. Acute dissection of the thoracic aorta. *Br Med J* 1995;310:72−73.

45 Hull CJ. Phaeochromocytoma. *Br J Anaesth* 1986;58:1453−1468.

46 Pathy MS, Reynolds AJ. Papaverine and hepatotoxicity. *Postgrad Med J* 1980;56:488−490.

47 Pilla TJ, Beshany SE, Shields JB. Incompatibility of Hexabrix and Papaverine. *Am J Roentgenol* 1986;146:1300−1301.

48 Bron KM, Stilley JW, Shapiro AP. Renal arteriography enhanced by tolazoline. Value in the diagnosis of polyarteritis nodosa complicated by perinephric haematoma. *Radiology* 1971;99: 295−301.

49 Hawkins IF, Hudson T. Priscoline in bone and soft tissue angiography. *Radiology* 1974;110:541−546.

50 Fischer HW. Incompatibility between contrast media and pharmacological agents. *Radiology* 1987;162:875.

51 Plumb VJ, James TN. Clinical hazards of powerful diuretics. Furosemide and ethacrynic acid. *Mod Concepts Cardiovasc Dis* 1978;74:91−94.

52 Prough DS, Roy R, Bumgarner J, Shannon G. Acute pulmonary oedema in healthy teenagers following conservative doses of intravenous naloxone. *Anaesthesiology* 1984;60:485−486.

53 Ward A, Chaffman MO, Sarkin EM. Dantrolene. A review of its pharmacodynamic and pharmacokinetic properties and therapeutic use in malignant hyperthermia, the neuroleptic malignant syndrome and an update of its use in muscle spasticity. *Drugs* 1986;32:130−168.

54 Elam EA, Dorr RT, Lagel KE, Pond GD. Cutaneous ulceration due to contrast extravasation. *Invest Radiol* 1991;26:13−16.

55 Agre K, Wilson RR, Brim M, McDermott DJ. Chymodiactin post marketing surveillance. Demographic and adverse experience of data in 29 075 patients. *Spine* 1984;9:479−485.

Further reading

ABPI Data Sheet Compendium 1993−94. London: Datapharm Publications Ltd.

Dukes MNG (ed.). *Meyler's Side Effects of Drugs*, 12th edn. Amsterdam: Elsevier, 1992.

Goodman AG, Gilman LS, Rall TW, Nies AS, Taylor P (eds). *Goodman and Gilman's The Pharmacological Basis of Therapeutics*, 8th edn. Pergamon Press, 1990.

The Joint Formulary Committee. *British National Formulary, Number 28*. British Medical Association and the Pharmaceutical Society of Great Britain, 1994.

Reynolds JEF (ed). *Martindale. The Extra Pharmacopoeia*, 30th edn. London: The Pharmaceutical Press, 1993.

CHAPTER 4

Patient care considerations and resuscitation

Geoffrey S. Ferguson

Introduction

The American College of Radiology estimates that in 1990 there were some 1 036 602 Medicare reimbursements to USA radiologists for performance of "interventional" procedures involving some kind of imaging guidance, and that roughly three times that many were actually performed [1]. Assuming a "generic" 1–3% complication rate, it is possible to estimate that approximately 10 000–30 000 adverse events of some kind occurred in 1990 associated with interventional procedures. As radiologists perform increasingly difficult and hazardous procedures, they must also accept the clinical responsibility for both successful and adverse outcomes. This philosophy is shared by the Society of Cardiovascular and Interventional Radiology: "The radiologist cannot rely on others to recognize and manage the problems that arise in his patient's care" [2]. While the majority of these events will be minor, many will be significant, and some life-threatening. In addition, there is a significant comorbidity in these populations, particularly cardiovascular and pulmonary disease. In a study of factors influencing long-term percutaneous transluminal angioplasty (PTA) success, Capek et al. [3] found that at the time of presentation for femoral–popliteal PTA, 50% of patients were hyperten-

sive, 90% smoked more than one pack of cigarettes per day, 33% were diabetic, and 18% had evidence of generalized cardiovascular disease. In patients presenting with intermittent claudication, Hertzer [4] found that 27% had severe coronary artery disease (CAD), as did 29% of those presenting with rest pain or gangrene. In addition, some procedures are performed on not infrequently critically ill patients, e.g., transcutaneous intrahepatic portosystemic shunt (TIPSS), bronchial arterial embolization, inferior venacaval filters (IVC) filters, pulmonary angiography, etc. Thus, it becomes increasingly important for interventional radiologists to become familiar with not only the specific complications that may be encountered during these procedures, but with some basic principles dealing with the recognition and treatment of associated adverse events. The importance of early recognition and treatment of prehospital sudden cardiac arrest, and an integrated "chain of survival" concept has significantly improved survival rates in out-of-hospital cardiac arrest [5–10], and many of these principles can be applied to radiology departments. This chapter will deal with some general concepts relating to identification and treatment of complications relating to performance of interventional radiologic procedures.

History

Perhaps the most important element in evaluating the patient's potential for complication is the history, particularly with peripheral vascular disease and cerebrovascular disease. Access to the patient's chart prior to preprocedural discussion should not preclude obtaining an adequate history, but can often facilitate the interview and allows directed questioning. For example, some patients may not spontaneously volunteer a history of myocardial infarction, hypertension, angina, or transient ischemic attacks, but this information may be in the medical record. Some cancer patients may consider themselves "cured" despite high potential for recurrent or metastatic disease, and may not include that information in a review of systems. On the other hand, other items of history may be obvious at the time of interview, e.g., amputation, chronic obstructive pulmonary disease (COPD), etc.

Cardiovascular disease affects the potential for complications in several ways. Hypertensives not only have a higher propensity for puncture-site complications such as bleeding and hematoma, but have a higher myocardial oxygen demand because of the increased afterload. The latter may be associated with angina in the presence of CAD. Additionally, hypertensive patients with CAD may be poor candidates for systemic epinephrine, which may be used in an attempt to treat a contrast reaction. As noted above, a history of claudication is sufficient evidence to presume CAD until proven otherwise [3]. Previous myocardial infarction, obviously, indicates significant CAD. A history of congestive failure or cardiomyopathy should indicate caution with intravenous (IV) fluid therapy. For example, vigorous IV hydration prior to contrast injection for prophylaxis of contrast-induced nephropathy is advocated [11], and it has been shown that aggressive IV fluid replacement therapy in the management of contrast reaction is beneficial [12]. Both of these situations could lead to exacerbation of congestive failure, or possibly pulmonary edema in patients with uncompensated congestive failure. Atrial fibrillation, dilated cardiomyopathy, and mitral valvular heart disease may predispose to embolic complications, unrelated to peripheral arterial catheter manipulations, but temporally associated. Atrial or ventricular septal defects, although uncommon, could allow paradoxical emboli from venous manipulations. The importance of a thorough cardiovascular history becomes more important as the complexity, risk, and duration of the procedures increase.

Historical evidence of pulmonary disease should also be sought. COPD results in chronically elevated arterial partial pressure of carbon dioxide (P_{CO_2}). The respiratory center in the medulla can become "desensitized" to these high levels of CO_2, and the primary stimulus to ventilate may be hypoxia [13] (see Airway management section, p. 54). Asthmatics have a raised risk of experiencing anaphylactoid contrast reaction [14, 15] and may benefit from low-osmolar contrast agent and/or premedication. In this regard, long-standing bronchodilator inhaler use can result in relative "tolerance" to adrenergic agents, rendering the patient less responsive to β-adrenergic agonists, again becoming an issue if there should be a contrast reaction. A history of pulmonary embolic disease (or deep vein thrombosis (DVT)) may be useful if venous access and/or intervention is planned, and may be a clue to a hypercoagualable state (e.g., nephrotic syndrome, glioblastoma).

Knowledge of the patient's current drugs and dosage can help in avoidance of complications or adverse drug–drug interaction. Monoamine oxidase inhibitors (MAOIs) and tricyclic antidepressants significantly increase the effects of adrenergic agonists (e.g., epinephrine, dopamine), and therefore pressors should be used with extreme caution in these patients [16]. Lang *et al.* [15] have found that patients receiving β-adrenergic blocking agents may have a higher incidence of anaphylactoid contrast reactions. In addition, β-blocked patients can experience relatively unopposed α-adrenergic stimulation if given systemic epinephrine, with its profound α- and β-adrenergic effects [17]. Nifedipine (often given as a premedication to help prevent arterial spasm in PTA) may work in synergism with other antihypertensives, and hypotension may ensue. In general, patients on calcium channel antagonists will have decreased peripheral vascular tone, and may be more susceptible to contrast-induced hypotension or hypovolemia, as might be encountered with bleeding, third spacing, or sepsis. Anticoagulated patients will be at increased risk for bleeding complications. See Table 4.1 for a listing of selected drug interactions. (Reference [18] is suggested for complete coverage of drug interactions and their mechanisms.)

Finally, the radiologist can occasionally uncover disease states that may be overlooked in a review of systems by examination of the current drugs. For example, the patient may deny "angina", but carry nitroglycerin for chest pain, thereby revealing CAD. Coumadin therapy may be a clue to previous episodes of arterial embolization from chronic atrial fibrillation, a prosthetic cardiac valve, or other vascular disorder. Oral hypoglycemic agents are a clue to borderline diabetes. Digitalis may be used for congestive failure and/or control of atrial fibrillation with fast ventricular response. Other examples are possible, but the principle remains the same: the medication history can provide valuable clues to past and current medical problems.

In summary, a systemic approach to obtaining pertinent history should include questions that will reveal current state of health (review of systems), past medical problems, previous surgeries, allergies, and current drugs with dosage. Particular attention should be directed to cardiovascular disease, respiratory status, renal disease, and current drugs, as these will often have a direct influence on both the occurrence and outcome of procedure-related complications. Some selected historical items and drugs of interest are presented in Table 4.2.

Table 4.1 Selected drug–drug interactions. (From Hansten and Horn [18])

Adenosine/dipyridamole
Dipyridamole inhibits cellular uptake and metabolism of adenosine, leading to increased serum concentration of adenosine. Patients on dipyridamole should receive decreased doses of adenosine

Atropine/verapamil
Verapamil pretreatment increases the tachycardia produced by atropine. The clinical importance of this is not clear

Cimetidine/β-blockers
Cimetidine decreases the activity of microsomal enzymes that metabolize propanolol and similar β-blockers, leading to increased serum concentrations

Epinephrine/β-blockers
Noncardioselective β-blockers enhance the pressor response to epinephrine, resulting in hypertension and tachycardia

Digoxin/verapamil
Verapamil increases the serum concentration of digitalis in nearly all patients taking this combination

Isoproteronol/β-blockers
β-Blockers, especially nonselective agents may reduce the effectiveness of isoproteronol

Lidocaine/β-blockers
Lidocaine concentrations may become excessive during concomitant β-blocker administration

MAOI/demerol
Some patients on MAOIs may develop severe adverse reactions to demerol, including excitation, sweating, rigidity, hypertension, and coma

Tricyclic antidepressants/epinephrine
The pressor response to IV epinephrine may be markedly enhanced in patients receiving tricyclic antidepressants

Table 4.2 Selected items of interest in history and medications

History
Cardiovascular
  Hypertension
  Angina
  Previous myocardial infarction
  Transient ischemic attack, CVA
Pulmonary disease
  Smoking
  COPD
  Asthma
Renal disease
  Dialysis
  Insufficiency
Coagulopathy
  Spontaneous nose/mucous membrane bleeding
  Easy bruising
  Prolonged bleeding
Allergies
  Drug
  Contrast
  "Atopic" individuals
General
  Weight loss
  Fever, chills
  Malaise

Drugs
Antihypertensives
  β-Blockers may influence contrast reaction treatment
  Puncture site problems
Antibiotics
  Aminoglycosides: risk of renal insufficiency
Anticoagulants
  Bleeding risks
Cardiotropic agents
  Risk of volume excess
Nonsteroidal antiinflammatory drugs
  Risk of renal insufficiency
MAOIs
  Use pressors with caution

Physical examination

Patients about to undergo interventional radiologic procedures should have a physical examination commensurate with the nature of the procedure, its risks, and the patient's state of health. This may be modified by local hospital regulations and physician practices. For example, a complete history and physical for overnight hospital admissions may be required by the admitting/attending physician, or could be performed in advance of an elective procedure by the referring physician. In general, the physical examination should be designed to address the current illness, as well as to detect other conditions that may affect the performance or outcome of the procedure. Examples might include hypertension, congestive failure, pneumonitis, unsuspected infection, respiratory insufficiency, abdominal masses, petechiae, etc. For neuroangiography and especially neurointerventional procedures, a baseline neurologic examination may be desirable. For peripheral angiography, a more detailed examination of the vascular system is appropriate, and is often an integral part of the referral process. In addition to notation of generalized features of peripheral ischemia such as hair loss, pallor, ischemic ulcers, and delayed capillary filling time, there should be an evaluation of the strength and character of the carotid, brachial, radial, femoral, popliteal, and dorsalis pedis/posterior tibial pulses. Aneurysmal femoral or popliteal arteries should be noted. Blood pressure should be checked in both arms, and the ankle/brachial index (ABI) calculated. Presence and character of bruits should be recorded. The abdominal aorta is amenable to palpation in nonobese patients, and its size may be estimated [19]. The abdomen and flanks may be auscultated for the presence of bruits, which may be of aortic, renal, or visceral origin.

Because the physical examination is somewhat procedure-specific, establishing a "routine" examination is somewhat difficult, but a basic general examination might include the following.

1 *Vital signs*: heart rate, respiratory rate, temperature, blood pressure (both arms).

2 *Head and neck*: contact lenses, hearing aids, dentures, neck mobility, carotid pulses, mucous membranes for petechiae.

3 *Chest*: depth of respirations, use of accessory muscles, retraction, auscultation, heart tones.

4 *Abdomen*: tenderness (direct and rebound), masses, bowel tones, bruits, aortic size and character of pulsations, splenomegaly, hepatomegaly.

5 *Extremities*: skin texture and color, capillary fill, petechiae, bruises, sensation, symmetry, peripheral pulses (including Doppler if necessary).

Laboratory tests

As in other medical specialties, the use of laboratory tests needs to be adjusted to fit the needs of the particular problem at hand. The goal of "routine" preprocedural laboratory testing is to discover evidence of clinically unsuspected disease that might adversely affect the outcome of a particular procedure. Murphy *et al.* [20] conducted a survey of the members of the Society of Cardiovascular and Interventional Radiology (SCVIR), regarding their existing patterns of routine preprocedural testing, reviewed the literature, and offered proposed screening tests for selected interventional radiologic procedures. Using this approach, they estimated annual savings of $20.0–$34.9 million among SCVIR members alone. Their proposed screening tests are:

Procedure	Screening tests
1 Peripheral angiography	BUN, Creat
2 Neuroangiography	None
3 Transluminal angioplasty	BUN, Creat
4 Intraarterial thrombolysis	PT, PTT, CBC, BUN, Creat, fibrinogen
5 Percutaneous needle biopsy	
(a) Superficial/small bore	None
(b) Deep/large bore	PT, PTT, CBC, platelet count
6 Percutaneous abscess drainage	PT, PTT
7 Percutaneous nephrostomy	PT, PTT
8 Percutaneous biliary drainage	PT, PTT
9 Myelography	None
10 Venography	BUN, Creat

These are, of course, intended for those patients with no physical findings or historical evidence to suggest underlying disease that might require additional laboratory investigation. If history and physical suggest the possibility of a particular organ system abnormality, then further work-up is indicated.

Preanesthesia assessment

If sedation or anesthesia is planned for the procedure, the Joint Commission on Accreditation of Healthcare Organization (JCAHO) [21] has stated that "a preanesthesia assessment of the patient is performed before the operation and other invasive procedures", and that "the plans are documented or referred to in the medical record". This can be accomplished by completion of a preprocedural assessment form, which can include historical items that the patient can fill out prior to interview by the practitioner.

Room design

While most angiographic facilities are well equipped with ancillary patient care devices, interventional procedures are occasionally performed in rooms not originally intended for invasive work. Minimum patient care requirements should include:

1 piped-in oxygen (not cylinders);

2 wall suction (or efficient portable suction device);

3 communication equipment (intercom, telephone);

4 physiologic monitoring: electrocardiogram (EKG), pulse oximetry, and blood pressure;

5 access to the patient's head and chest;

6 immediate access to monitor/defibrillator and "crash cart";

7 airway management equipment (Table 4.3);

8 cardiopulmonary resuscitation (CPR) board and adequate table support for CPR;

9 sufficient space for patient, attendants, monitors, pumps, lines, etc.

Patient preparation

Preprocedural discussion with the patient regarding what he/she will be experiencing is not only an integral part of informed consent, but is an important part of preparation. A candid, complete discussion of the procedure and its goals can often reduce anxiety, improve cooperation, and (importantly), inform the radiologist about the patient's concerns and expectations. For example, many patients gather sometimes incorrect information from family and

Table 4.3 Airway management/oxygenation equipment

Airway	Oxygenation
Suction apparatus	Nasal cannulae
Oral airway	Simple face mask
Nasal airway	Nonrebreathing mask
"Pocket" mask (with long tube)	Transtracheal jet ventilation apparatus
Bag–valve–mask	
Intubation equipment	

friends who may have had similar experiences and, thus, become unnecessarily anxious. Providing the patient with a calm, professional, and realistic discussion of what is about to occur will enhance patient acceptance and compliance.

Venous access

All patients undergoing invasive procedures should have adequate IV access. If possible, this should be a 16-gage cannula in a peripheral vein, with IV solution running at a rate appropriate for the particular patient. Smaller gage lines may be used for drug delivery, but in the event of the need for rapid volume infusion, a large bore peripheral line is desirable [22]. Injection ports for drugs should be readily available. If IV access has previously been established, it should be checked for patency, inflammation at the insertion site, and adequate flow rates. One should remember that flow rates are inversely proportional to the length of the cannula, so that for a given diameter, there will much greater flow rates in short peripheral cannulae than long central ones [23]. This has particular importance in the patient who needs rapid volume expansion (e.g., anaphylactic, septic, or hypovolemic shock), for whom a short fat peripheral line is preferable to a long skinny central one.

In the event of inadequate peripheral veins for large bore cannulae, other sites must be considered. While technically a peripheral vein, the external jugular offers brisk flow to the central circulation, and is often quite large. With the patient in a supine position and legs elevated, the head is turned to the opposite side and digital pressure to the vein just above the clavicle can be applied. Using conventional techniques, a suitable entry point to the vein (Fig. 4.1) is chosen and a

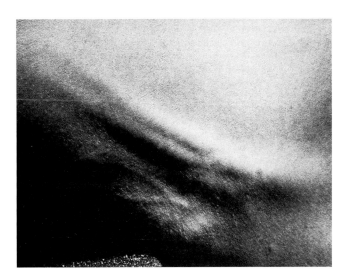

Fig. 4.1 External jugular vein. Distension is facilitated by Trendelenburg positioning. Conventional peripheral venous cannulation materials and techniques can be used if access to the central circulation is not required.

large bore cannula is inserted. Longer catheters may be used to access the central circulation from this approach, but increased resistance to flow over a longer catheter should be kept in mind. Additionally, there is often an acute bend in the external jugular vein as it passes lateral to the sternomastoid muscle and deep to the clavicle, which may impede passage of long lines.

For central venous access, the internal jugular (IJV), subclavian, and femoral veins are possible routes. Radiologists are familiar with the femoral route, which can be used for short-term large bore central access, but is not suitable for long-term use because of its higher propensity for infection. However, the femoral vein is an excellent choice during resuscitation, as it can be rapidly accessed with little if any disruption of resuscitation efforts. Unless the patient is obese, standard peripheral IV cannulae can be used. The IJV provides central access, and is often used for IVC filter placement. The right side is favored because the dome of the lung and pleura are lower on this side, and it is generally a straight line to the right atrium [24]. A frequently recommended technique is the "central" approach with the insertion site at the apex of the triangle formed by the two heads of the sternocleidomastoid muscle. The needle is then advanced at a 45° angle to the skin towards the ipsilateral nipple [23].

An alternate technique (termed "anterior" approach) takes advantage of the constant relationship between the carotid artery and the IJV, analogous to the femoral vein and artery, except that the IJV is lateral to the carotid artery. As these two vessels emerge from the thoracic inlet (along with the vagus nerve) they are enclosed in a fibrous sheath that maintains the IJV lateral to the carotid artery. From the clavicle to the level of the thyroid cartilage the vein is slightly anterior and lateral to the artery, swinging posterior to the artery at the level of the thyroid cartilage [25]. Palpation of the carotid artery at the level of the cricoid cartilage (about half way between the tip of the mastoid and the suprasternal notch) will define a level at which the IJV is just lateral and slightly anterior to the carotid artery [25]. This point is usually 2–3 cm caudal to the angle of the mandible. Puncture of the IJV at this point is analogous to femoral venous puncture in the groin, with the palpating finger(s) on the artery, and the needle directed at the vein, except that in the neck the vein is lateral to the artery (Fig. 4.2). Realtime high-resolution ultrasound, hand-held Doppler, or Doppler-assisted needles may also be employed to assist venous puncture and avoid arterial injury. Standard Seldinger technique and fluoroscopy is then employed for catheter placement. Trendelenburg positioning is critical to distend the vein and avoid air embolism. Keeping the neck musculature relaxed with the head turned to the left will facilitate palpation of the carotid pulse. Wide skin preparation with povidone–iodine solution and careful sterile technique is imperative. Hematoma formation is a potential complication of IJV

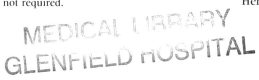

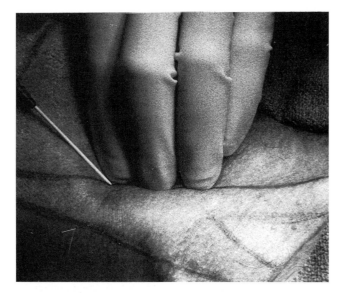

Fig. 4.2 IJV puncture. Trendelenburg positioning distends the vein and decreases the chance of air embolism, Palpating fingers are on the carotid arterial pulse. Needle is directed towards the ipsilateral nipple at about 45° to the skin. Gentle suction applied to a small syringe with 1−2 ml of saline or lidocaine, aids identification of vein entry. Vigorous pulsatile return with the syringe removed indicates arterial entry.

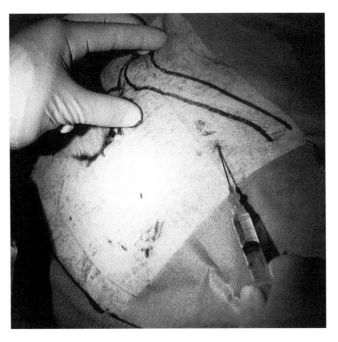

Fig. 4.3 Infraclavicular subclavian vein puncture. Trendelenburg positioning distends the vein and decreases the chance of air embolism. Entry point is 1−2 cm below the clavicle at approximately the junction of its middle and distal thirds. Needle is advanced in the coronal plane, posterior to the clavicle, aiming towards the palpating fingers in the suprasternal notch. Vein entry may occur during advance or withdrawal of needle.

puncture, usually well controlled with 10−20 minutes of manual pressure. The left IJV should not be attempted if the right has developed a hematoma because of the possibility of bilateral hematomas resulting in tracheal compression [23].

The subclavian vein is generally not used as emergency access because of the necessity to interrupt CPR, but does provide good access to the central circulation, usually for purposes of long-term therapy. It can be entered from either infraclavicular or supraclavicular [26,27] approaches. At the author's institution, the left side is favored for infraclavicular subclavian catheterization because of the lower incidence of malpositioned catheters (e.g., up into the jugular vein or into the contralateral subclavian vein). This view is supported by Matthews and Worthley [28] who reported a 15% incidence of malpositioned subclavian catheters from the right, but only 2% on the left, with the same immediate complication rate on both sides: 4% pneumothorax and 2% subclavian artery puncture.

The needle entry point for the infraclavicular approach is 1−3 cm below the clavicle, near the junction of its middle and distal thirds. The needle is advanced posteromedially and slightly cephalad towards the posterior−superior aspect of the sternal end of the clavicle [24] (Fig. 4.3). The reported complication rates vary widely from 0.4 to 11% [27], and include pneumothorax, hemothorax, arterial puncture, and infection [23,24,26,27]. The subclavian artery is posterior (deep) to the vein and clavicle in this location, and is not

accessible to compression if inadvertent arterial puncture and hematoma should develop. With left-sided subclavian approaches, the thoracic duct can be injured [23,24]. A 1% incidence of catheter fracture and embolization to the central circulation has been reported [29], but this seems to be confined to catheters used for long-term therapy, and often with chemotherapeutic agents. Radiologists enjoy the advantage of fluoroscopy to direct the wire and catheter into the superior vena cava, and as with the IJV, ultrasound imaging or audible Doppler can be used to locate the vein for guided puncture.

Monitoring

This section will discuss some principles of patient monitoring as they relate to interventional radiologic procedures. While often less invasive and generally better tolerated than the surgical alternates, these procedures are regularly performed on sedated patients with underlying cardiovascular and pulmonary disease, usually in a darkened room, often with the patient completely draped, sometimes in a prone position, and only rarely in an operating room with an anesthesiologist in attendance. Subtle changes in the patient's condition can and do occur, and unless these are recognized and corrected early on, rapid progression to more significant problems or fatality may ensue. It is therefore important that a radiology team member be assigned the primary task of administering medication and monitoring the patient's status throughout the case. This can be summarized as: "Whoever sedates, monitors". While often evoking visions of high-technology equipment, it is imperative to remember that "patient monitoring" is first and foremost a clinical activity, and that various machines, however sophisticated, should be thought of as merely extensions of the practitioner's senses [30].

Clinical observation

It cannot be overemphasized that continuous visual, verbal, and tactile contact with the patient is the hallmark of effective monitoring during conscious sedation. The boundary between conscious sedation and deep sedation has been crossed when the patient becomes unarousable [13,30], thus increasing the possibility of aspiration, airway compromise, and hypotension. Accordingly, there must be frequent assessment of mental status, skin color, respiratory pattern (rate, tidal volume, thoracic and abdominal excursion), and pulse rate. The practitioner must be constantly alert for early indications of hypoventilation, partial or complete airway obstruction (see Airway management section, p. 54), and emesis. Use of a precordial stethoscope can greatly facilitate these tasks.

EKG

Continuous EKG monitoring during interventional procedures is desirable from a number of standpoints. Increasing pain and the need for additional analgesics can often be predicted by a rise in pulse rate. Unexplained tachycardia may be the harbinger of septic shock. Bradycardia due to excess vagal tone is a common occurrence, and readily treated with atropine. More severe arrhythmias can also be detected, and results of therapy evaluated. Myocardial ischemia can be inferred from ST segment changes, particularly if a baseline rhythm strip in the same lead and/or a 12-lead EKG has been obtained. See Cardiac arrhythmia section, p. 61, for further discussion.

Pulse oximetry

This widely accepted technology continuously and non-invasively displays the percentage of functional arterial hemoglobin that is saturated with oxygen, i.e., the percentage of available hemoglobin that is bound with oxygen [31]. In general, two light-emitting diodes (LEDs) operating at different wavelengths are arranged so that they illuminate a pulsatile tissue bed. A photodetector measures the intensity of each wavelength transmitted by the pulsatile tissue, and a microcomputer calculates the per cent saturated hemoglobin

according to algorithms programmed into the machine's software [32]. In general, these are reliable devices when used with appropriate precautions, failing to give usable readings in only approximately 1% of cases [33]. It should also be noted that pulse oximetry may lose some of its accuracy with profound arterial desaturation (below about 60% S_aO_2), but fortunately, the error tends slightly to underestimate the true value [34]. In order to use pulse oximetry effectively, the practitioner needs to understand some of the assumptions upon which the calculations are based, and what clinical situations might violate these assumptions and lead to misleading data.

The hemoglobin concentration is assumed to be adequate when the user concludes that a given S_aO_2 value is a representation of tissue oxygenation. This assumption is invalid in settings of severe anemia. Although the hemoglobin that passes through the measured pulsatile tissue bed may be well saturated with oxygen, the total oxygen carrying capacity of the blood will be diminished because of the low total hemoglobin. Therefore, in anemic patients, the practitioner should not accept S_aO_2 values in the 92–95% range as satisfactory, but aim for 98–100%.

The pulse oximeter is looking for rhythmic variations in light intensity seen by the photodetector, and assumes that all such variations represent pulsatile arteriolar blood flow. This is violated when there is motion of the detector or the vascular bed, or when venous pulsations are present in the vascular bed. Some machines offer EKG gating to minimize motion artifact, but venous pulsations can still be a problem. In this case, some of the pulsatile blood will be venous, and therefore desaturated after passing through the capillary bed. Since the pulse oximeter's algorithms are based on arteriolar blood, the reading will then be erroneous. When the fingerprobe is being used, venous pulsations can be seen in the finger with tight arm/hand restraints, when the blood pressure cuff inflates on that arm, with the patient lying on the same arm, and occasionally in settings of congestive heart failure.

Pulse oximetry also assumes that all light seen by the photodetectors has passed through a pulsatile tissue bed. This may not be the case when some ambient room light reaches the detector, when the probe is partially off the finger (the LED shines directly on the detector), or when there is peripheral vasoconstriction. The latter may be seen in shock, hypothermia, or with vasoconstrictive medications such as epinephrine which might be given for contrast reaction. Of interest to vascular radiologists, severe peripheral vascular disease may also result in a lack of pulsation in the measured tissue bed.

Other errors in S_aO_2 display can occur with colored vascular dyes such as methylene blue or indocyanine green — agents not commonly encountered in interventional radiologic procedures. Colorless iodinated contrast agents, of course, have no direct effect on pulse oximetry. High levels of carboxyhemoglobin will produce a falsely high S_aO_2 value, of concern in heavy smokers or those recently exposed to smoke inhalation [35]. As noted above, there may be inaccuracies in display when the patient becomes severely hypoxemic, but the primary value of pulse oximetry is not so much its precise correlation with arterial blood gases, but in detecting a trend towards developing hypoxia that can be corrected early before an adverse outcome ensues [31]. In cases where precise knowledge of arterial oxygenation is required, arterial blood gas determination is advised.

With the above in mind, pulse oximetry is an extremely useful tool in the interventional radiologist's armamentarium, allowing much earlier detection of hypoxemia than can be detected with clinical evaluation, where cyanosis and altered mental status are relatively late manifestations. This technology has gained wide acceptance, and is useful for monitoring sedation and those with altered levels of consciousness or impaired ventilation. It should be remembered that although pulse oximetry is a reliable tool for the recognition of hypoxemia due to respiratory depression, it does not detect hypoventilation, characterized by carbon dioxide retention (see Physiology of ventilation, below).

Blood pressure monitoring

Frequent blood pressure determination during the procedure is valuable for detecting adverse trends and events. For example, rising blood pressure and pulse may indicate a need for further analgesia or sedation, vagal episodes can be confirmed, results of therapy monitored, etc. Available techniques include manual determination (with sphygmomanometer and stethoscope or Doppler), automated Doppler, transcatheter invasive, automated noninvasive blood pressure (NIBP), and the servoplethysomomanometer, which offers continuous NIBP display [36]. NIBP has enjoyed widespread use in interventional radiology departments, allowing the practitioner some freedom to perform other duties, reproduce results, the ability to compute and display mean arterial pressure (MAP), report trends, and trigger alarms set at user-definable systolic and diastolic limits. Good correlation with direct arterial methods has been reported [37]. Care must be exercised to avoid frequent repetitive inflations that may lead to upper extremity ischemia, thrombophlebitis, ulnar nerve paralysis, and compartment syndromes [25].

In summary, common monitoring techniques used in interventional radiologic procedures include clinical observation, EKG, NIBP, and pulse oximetry. It is worth emphasizing again that patient monitoring is a clinical activity whose mainstay is frequent visual, verbal, and tactile patient contact, supplemented by various electronic devices. Early identification of adverse trends may allow simple interventions that often will prevent or minimize subsequent complications.

Most radiologists are performing conscious sedation, and the principles of "Monitored anesthesia care" as put forward by the American Society of Anesthesiologists [30,38] can be applied to these procedures. The JCAHO [21] stipulates that when the *medical staff* determines that there is a "reasonable expectation" that sedation "will result in the loss of protective reflexes for a significant percentage of a group of patients", then the patient's physiologic status should be "measured and assessed" during the procedure. At the author's institution, this is performed as:

1 continuous EKG monitoring;
2 continuous pulse oximetry;
3 blood pressure every 10 minutes or more frequently prn;
4 respiratory rate every 10 minutes or more frequently prn.

Airway management

Recognition and management of airway problems is paramount in the prevention of many complications relating to interventional radiology. This section will deal with aspects of ventilation, respiration, airway management, and oxygen delivery systems that will help prevent and correct certain complications.

Physiology of ventilation

A review of the physiology of ventilation is in order. Ventilation can be considered as the process of moving atmospheric air into the alveoli and carbon dioxide from the alveoli back into the atmosphere. The involuntary control of ventilation originates from a chemosensitivity of the respiratory center, located in the ventral portion of the medulla [13]. When stimulated, this area sends impulses a short distance to a slightly more dorsally located inspiratory area, which in turn sends descending neural impulses to muscles of respiration. The respiratory center is sensitive to arterial levels of hydrogen ion concentration, in part derived from carbon dioxide which is present in blood both as physical solution and as hydrogen carbonate (H_2CO_3):

$$H_2O + CO_2 \longleftrightarrow H_2CO_3 \longleftrightarrow H^+ + HCO_3^-.$$

In erythrocytes, the latter reaction is catalyzed by carbonic anhydrase, moving the reaction to the right at a rate 1000 times faster than in plasma, resulting in 99.9% of hydrogen carbonate dissociating to bicarbonate and hydrogen ion [39]. Because of this reaction and the extreme sensitivity of the respiratory center to small increases in arterial hydrogen ion concentration, elevated arterial carbon dioxide tension (P_aCO_2) becomes the primary central stimulus for involuntary ventilation.

Additional stimuli to the inspiratory region of the respiratory center come from "irritant" receptors in the lung and chest wall which respond to stretching and noxious stimuli, and chemoreceptors located in the carotid and aortic bodies which are sensitive to low arterial oxygen tension (P_aO_2) [13,39]. These receptors send ascending impulses to the inspiratory region of the respiratory center via cranial nerves IX and X, and have their greatest influence at P_aO_2 levels less than 60 mmHg [13]. Because normal arterial oxygen tensions are 95–99 mmHg, these peripheral "hypoxia" chemoreceptors can be considered a "back-up" mechanism for the central hypercarbic control of involuntary ventilation.

Although most COPD patients will have a normal hypercarbic drive to ventilate, it is possible for the chemosensitive area in the respiratory center in some severe COPD patients to be rendered tolerant of elevated P_aCO_2. Given the very high incidence of smoking in patients with peripheral vascular disease [3], this situation will occasionally arise in typical interventional practices. In these rather uncommon patients, there may be such tolerance of elevated arterial carbon dioxide that hypoxia rather than hypercarbia becomes the primary stimulus to breathe. The practitioner may remove this hypoxic drive to ventilate by giving supplemental oxygen (which will raise S_aO_2), particularly with high flow rates. If this is done prior to sedation, the respiratory depressive effect of the sedative drug on the respiratory center may go unnoticed if only S_aO_2 is monitored, and the combination of a depressed respiratory center and tolerance of long-standing hypercarbia may lead to significant respiratory acidosis. A fall in respiratory rate and decreased depth of respirations will alert the practitioner to the possibility of hypercarbia, even in the face of adequate arterial oxygenation. This is the physiologic basis for baseline and subsequent serial monitoring of respiratory depth and rate when sedative drugs are administered.

In summary, the central control of ventilation resides in the respiratory center, and hypercarbia is the dominant stimulus to ventilate, with hypoxemia as a secondary mechanism. The respiratory center is depressed with sedatives and narcotic analgesics, and may be rendered less sensitive to elevated P_aCO_2 in some patients with COPD (Fig. 4.4).

Management

The "A" of the ABCs of emergency care is justifiably first on the list of priorities. Without a patent airway and adequate alveolar ventilation, the administration of supplemental oxygen by various adjunctive techniques, attempts to establish a perfusing cardiac rhythm, and maintenance of adequate blood pressure may all be futile. This section will deal with techniques used to identify and treat airway obstruction.

Patients with airway compromise at any level will share some common clinical manifestations, which may include tachycardia, agitation, air hunger, and noisy respirations (unless totally obstructed). As with hypoxemia of any cause, cyanosis is a late finding. Airway obstruction can be divided into extrathoracic- and intrathoracic levels. Extrathoracic causes include oropharyngeal obstruction, either from the tongue or foreign body, and laryngeal obstruction, as may be seen with laryngeal edema in a contrast reaction or laryngospasm in aspiration. The level of airway compromise can be

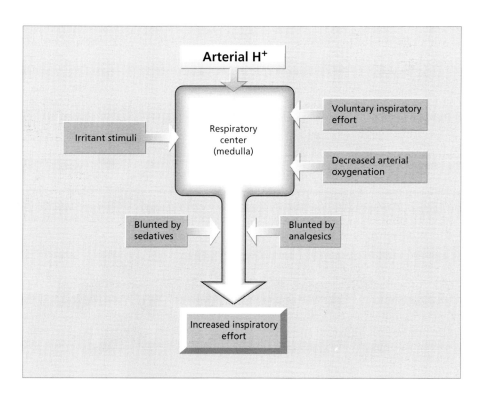

Fig. 4.4 Respiratory regulation. The primary stimulus to increased ventilation is arterial hydrogen ion concentration, with other input from voluntary effort, irritants, and hypoxia. The respiratory center's response to these stimuli is depressed by sedatives and analgesics. See text.

quickly determined with physical examination. With intra-thoracic airway compromise, there will be a tendency for increased airway noises during the exhalation phase of ventilation, because an already narrowed intrathoracic airway will be further narrowed with the raised intrathoracic pressure that occurs during exhalation (Fig. 4.5). For example, the hallmark of bronchospasm is expiratory wheezing. Extrathoracic airway compromise, on the other hand, is characterized by noisy breathing during the inspiratory phase of respiration. The classic example is snoring, caused by relaxation of the jaw and tongue such that the tongue and epiglottis approximate the posterior wall of the oropharynx. Noisy breathing occurs during inspiration as the negative intrathoracic pressure is transmitted to the upper airway and pulls the tongue and epiglottis further down into the throat and closer to the posterior oropharyngeal wall. Laryngeal airway compromise can be differentiated from oropharyngeal by the lack of clinical response of the former to a chin lift or jaw thrust (assuming that obstructing foreign bodies have been excluded or removed). Table 4.4 summarizes recognition and management of airway obstruction.

Chin lift

This maneuver is designed to lift the obstructing tongue away from the posterior wall of the oropharynx. The practitioner stands either at the patient's side or above the head. Placing the fingers of one hand under the apex of the mandible, the chin is lifted anteriorly, while the thumb of the same hand may be used to depress the lower lip in order slightly to open the mouth (Fig. 4.6). This position allows the other hand to be free in order to pinch the nostrils in the

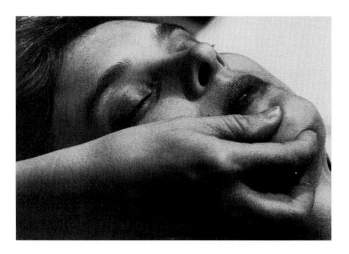

Fig. 4.6 Chin lift. The mandible is lifted anteriorly and superiorly. In the absence of cervical spine injury, the airway may be straightened somewhat by extending the neck. See text.

event of mouth to mouth ventilation or CPR (see below). In the absence of cervical spine injury, the upper airway may be straightened by slightly tilting the head back, placing the palm of the other hand on the patient's head, and pushing down while the fingers under the mandible lift the chin. This maneuver should not be performed in an unconscious patient whose cervical spine status is unknown.

Jaw thrust

This is the procedure of choice to open the upper airway in an obtunded patient when the possibility of cervical spine injury exists [22,24]. It also allows the practitioner to support

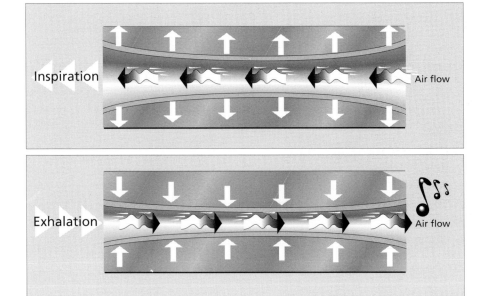

Fig. 4.5 Intrathoracic airway compromise. The decreased intrathoracic pressure during inspiration will tend to expand the airway, while increased intrathoracic pressure during exhalation will tend diffusely to narrow the airway. If regions of intrathoracic airway compromise are present, these will become further narrowed and produce more noise (wheezing), predominantly during the exhalation phase.

Table 4.4 Airway obstruction: recognition and management

Site	Cause	Signs/symptoms	Treatment
Oropharynx Mechanical	Foreign body Vomitus Blood	Noisy inspirations Apnea (obstructed) ↓ Tidal volume Accessory muscles ↑ HR, ↑ RR	Finger sweep Suction Oxygen
Anatomic	Obtundation Sedation (tongue/epiglottis approximate posterior oropharyngeal wall)	Same as above plus responds to chin lift or jaw thrust	Chin lift Jaw thrust Nasal/oral airway Ventilate Intubate Reverse sedation Oxygen
Laryngeal	Edema (e.g., contrast reaction) Spasm (e.g., aspiration, airway insertion)	Stridor No response to chin lift or jaw thrust	Remove stimulus Treat reaction ↑ Airway pressure Oxygen Tracheal jet ventilation Tracheostomy
Bronchial	Asthma Contrast reaction Allergy Aspiration	Exhalation wheezing ↑ HR, ↑ RR Agitation	Bronchodilators Remove allergen Treat reaction Oxygen

HR, Heart rate; RR, respiratory rate.

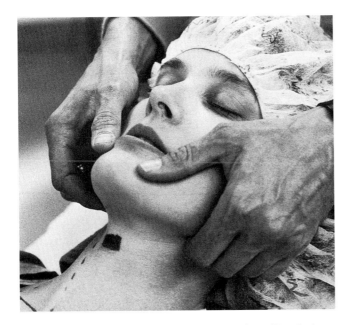

Fig. 4.7 Jaw thrust. The jaw is displaced anteriorly, pulling the base of the tongue away from the posterior wall of the oropharynx and opening the airway.

the head and stabilize the neck in a neutral position while maintaining a patent airway. Additionally, a face mask can be tightly applied, facilitating bag−valve−mask (BVM) or mouth to mask ventilation. The practitioner stands above the patient's head, looking down at the anterior aspect of the chest. The basic jaw thrust maneuver is performed by placing one hand on each side of the face and displacing the angle of the mandible anteriorly with the middle or index fingers (Fig. 4.7). With practice, one hand may be used to apply a face mask and elevate the jaw (Fig. 4.8). If two-rescuer CPR is required, a combined face mask/jaw thrust maneuver can be performed by using two hands to apply the mask with the thumbs and index fingers, while the remaining fingers elevate the jaw (Fig. 4.9). This places the ventilating practitioner in an ideal position to view the compressing hands, thereby timing the ventilations with chest compressions, and simultaneously assessing adequacy of chest expansion in response to the ventilations.

Oropharyngeal airway

The chin lift and jaw thrust are primarily used in obtunded or sedated patients whose jaw and neck musculature is so relaxed that the tongue and epiglottis move posteriorly with

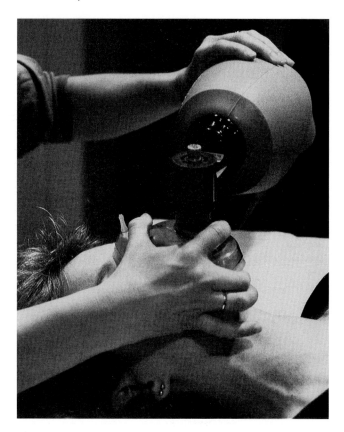

Fig. 4.8 Jaw thrust with BVM. One hand elevates the mandible and seals the mask against the face. The other hand is free to compress the bag.

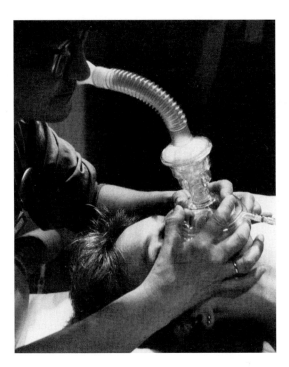

Fig. 4.9 Jaw thrust with mouth to face mask ventilation. Airway control and face mask seal are maintained with both hands. Ventilations for two-person CPR are facilitated. See text.

the mandible, and approximate the posterior wall of the pharynx. If the patient is obtunded to the point of unconsciousness, the gag reflex may be depressed enough to allow placement of an oropharyngeal airway. There are two basic methods of placement. The most expedient is to insert the airway "upside down" into the mouth with the curved end oriented cephalad. It is then advanced along the roof of the mouth until some resistance is felt at the soft palate. The device is then rotated 180° so that the curve is oriented caudad, and is slipped behind the tongue into the posterior pharynx. This method should not be used in children because of the risk of damage to the teeth [22]. The second technique utilizes a tongue blade to depress the tongue while the airway is inserted with the curved tip oriented caudad. The tip is then advanced over the posterior surface of the tongue and down into the posterior pharynx. The correct size of airway can be estimated by approximating the distance from the corner of the mouth to the angle of the mandible, and choosing an oral airway of this length. When correctly placed, the flange of the airway will rest comfortably on the lips. If the device is pushed repeatedly out of the mouth, it may be resting on the back of the tongue, thereby compressing it against the pharyngeal wall rather than elevating it.

Nasopharyngeal airway

Sometimes called a "nasal trumpet", this device is a compliant rubber tube some 15-cm long that is inserted with 2% lidocaine gel into one of the nares. It is carefully advanced posteriorly until the tip lies between the tongue and posterior pharyngeal wall. Forceful introduction may lacerate the nasal mucosa and should be avoided. If resistance is felt, the other naris can be tried. While not providing as much cross-sectional area for ventilation as the oropharyngeal airway, the principle advantage of the nasopharyngeal airway is that it is better tolerated by obtunded or semiconscious patients who may still have an intact gag reflex.

Face masks

As mentioned above, a face mask with a soft compliant seal against the patient's face can be effectively applied in combination with a jaw thrust. The thumb and index finger can keep the mask sealed against the face while the middle, ring, and small fingers anteriorly displace the mandible. Two hands are more effective for those less skilled in airway management, and mouth to mask ventilation is facilitated. These devices are sometimes called "pocket masks," and some have a side port for oxygen administration, and one-way valves to protect the rescuer from emesis. A variation on this theme is provision of a long clear tube with a mouthpiece leading from the mask to the rescuer (Fig. 4.9), allowing for a more comfortable stance and greater protection from emesis.

BVM

These devices are commonly used in airway emergencies, but require somewhat greater skill than other techniques. A tight seal between the mask and face, and a patent upper airway are required. With one hand, the thumb and index finger hold the mask against the mouth, with the thumb over the nasal part of the mask and the index finger over the chin portion. The remaining fingers of this hand are used to perform a jaw thrust and to position the head and neck to optimize a patent airway. The other hand is used to squeeze the bag (see Fig. 4.8). If sufficient personnel are available, it is advantageous to use one rescuer to apply the mask and control the airway, and the other to squeeze the bag, particularly if they are not skilled in BVM use. Supplemental oxygen delivery with BVMs is important. With an oxygen reservoir bag and flow rates of $10-15 l/min$, a fractional oxygen in inspired gas (F_1O_2) of up to 90% may be achieved [24].

Endotracheal intubation

Endotracheal intubation is the definitive means of controlling the airway. Interventional radiologists are unlikely to encounter situations in which they would be called upon to intubate a patient, as most interventional radiologic procedures are performed in a hospital environment with anesthesia and "code team" back-up. Nonetheless, a working knowledge of intubation serves two purposes: (i) preparing for and assisting the intubating practitioner; and (ii) being able to intubate if called upon. Experience in intubation can often be arranged with the cooperation of the anesthesia department in the hospital in which the interventional radiologic procedures are being performed.

Prior to intubation, the laryngoscope light should be checked for proper operation (this should be done routinely at frequent intervals in conjunction with defibrillator checks). As a rule, $7.5-8.0 mm$ internal diameter (ID) tubes are used in adult females, and $8.0-8.5 mm$ ID tubes for males [24,36] The endotracheal tube cuff should be checked for leaks. When possible, the patient should be ventilated on 100% F_1O_2 with a BVM prior to intubation. Intubation should be accomplished within $15-20$ seconds, or as a rough guideline, about the length of time that the intubating practitioner can hold her/his breath. If the tube cannot be placed in this time frame, it should be withdrawn, the patient ventilated on 100% F_1O_2, and then another attempt at intubation be made.

Orotracheal intubation is the usual method for rapid placement of an endotracheal tube under urgent circumstances. In the absence of contraindication to neck extension,

the head is placed in the "sniffing" position. This aligns the longitudinal axis of the oral cavity, pharyngeal airway, and larynx so that there is a fairly straight line from the mouth to the larynx. This position can be achieved by placing an approximate 10-cm pad under the occiput and extending the neck (Fig. 4.10). Either a curved (e.g., Macintosh) or straight blade can be used, although it is customary for the novice to use a curved blade [40]. Wearing gloves, the laryngoscope is held in the left hand, while the right hand gently opens the mouth. The blade is inserted into the right side of the mouth, avoiding the incisors, and advanced along the tongue, visualizing the hard palate and uvula until the posterior pharynx is reached. The curved blade tip is placed in the space between the base of the tongue and the epiglottis. This recess is the vallecula, which is not as deep in the throat as commonly thought, so that it is not usually necessary to place the entire length of the laryngoscope blade in the patient's mouth for successful intubation. Once this position has been reached, the laryngoscope is lifted up and away from the practitioner (imagine your left hand moving towards the junction of the ceiling and the wall you are facing), without using the teeth as a fulcrum and avoiding pressure on the lips (Fig. 4.11). With this upward movement of the blade, the epiglottis is displaced anteriorly, revealing the glottic opening and the pale white vocal cords on either side. The straight blade is used in a similar fashion, except that its tip is usually advanced just beyond the epiglottis, which is then lifted by the tube tip, rather than with the vallecula when the curved blade is used.

Once the glottic opening is clearly in view, the endotracheal tube is grasped in the right hand and advanced through the right side of the oral cavity and through the

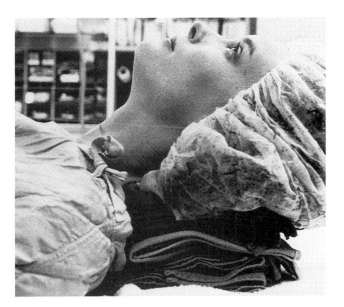

Fig. 4.10 "Sniffing" position for intubation. The occiput is elevated approximately 10 cm to align the airway in preparation for oral intubation.

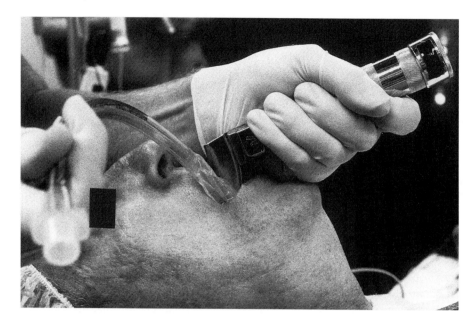

Fig. 4.11 Orotracheal intubation. See text.

vocal cords under direct vision. This may be facilitated by having an assistant pull the right side of the mouth open for better visualization. Visualization may also sometimes be improved by turning the patient's head slightly to the left [36]. A malleable curved stylet may be used to direct the tip of the tube through the cords, taking care to keep the stylet about 1 cm inside the endotracheal tube tip in order to protect the larynx from damage. The tube is carefully observed as it passes through the cords until the top end of the cuff is about 2 cm below the cords. The laryngoscope blade is removed, taking care not to damage teeth, gums, or lips. The cuff is inflated with 5–10 ml of room air. The lung fields and epigastrium are auscultated during ventilations with the bag. If gurgling sounds are heard in the epigastrium and there are no audible breath sounds, the tube is likely to be in the esophagus, and intubation must be repeated. When the tube is in the trachea, there should be good bilateral breath sounds with symmetric chest excursions. The right mainstem bronchus tends to be the one selectively intubated because of its relatively straight alignment with the trachea. In this case, there are decreased breath sounds and diminished chest wall expansion on the left. This is usually corrected by deflating the cuff and withdrawing the tube a short distance until the breath sounds become equal.

The *Sellick maneuver* is application of cricoid pressure to facilitate glottic visualization and prevent regurgitation of gastric contents by compressing the esophagus against the cervical spine (Fig. 4.12). The cricoid cartilage is identified as the next palpable firm structure caudal to the thyroid cartilage (Adam's apple). It forms the inferior margin of the cricothyroid membrane. An assistant places the thumb and index finger on either side of the midline on the cricoid cartilage and applies firm posterior pressure until *after* the endotracheal tube has been placed and the cuff inflated [40].

Blind nasotracheal intubation is a technique that may be used for definitive airway control in a patient who has spontaneous but inadequate ventilations, a tightly clenched mouth, and who may still have an intact gag reflex. A slightly smaller (6.5–7.0 mm) endotracheal tube is chosen than for orotracheal intubation. The technique is similar to nasopharyngeal airway placement, with the tube well lubricated with 2% lidocaine gel, and the bevel against the nasal septum. The tube is gently advanced through the posterior nasopharynx, taking care to avoid trauma to the posterior mucosa (resistance may be felt, which may be improved

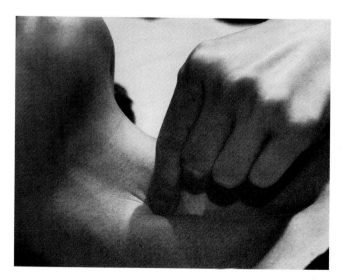

Fig. 4.12 Sellick maneuver. The cricoid cartilage is posteriorly displaced to compress the esophagus against the cervical spine to prevent regurgitation during tracheal intubation. Compression is maintained until the tube is placed and the cuff is inflated.

by withdrawing the tube and trying again with the head extended). As the tube passes into the posterior oropharynx, the practitioner begins to listen carefully to the breath sounds through the endotracheal tube. As the larynx is approached, the breath sounds will become louder. Repositioning the head and tube may be periodically necessary to facilitate this process. When breath sounds are the loudest, the tip of the tube should be just above the glottic opening. The practitioner then anticipates the next inspiratory effort, and times the advance of the tube through the glottic opening with the next inspiration. This may momentarily stimulate the cough reflex. A successful attempt results in rhythmic audible inspiration and exhalation breath sounds through the tube, with final tube position assessed as with orotracheal intubation.

Suction

As with all other aspects of emergency medical equipment, suction apparatus should be routinely tested and inspected prior to its use in an emergency situation. Suction equipment may be fixed (attached to wall suction) or portable, some being battery operated. The unit should be capable of generating at least 300 mmHg of negative pressure, with a clear collection chamber to allow visualization of the contents [23,24]. When suctioning the oropharynx, the use of a large bore catheter such as a "tonsil tip" and large bore suction tubing is recommended to ensure that all large particulate matter will be removed and the tube will not obstruct. Suctioning of endotracheal or tracheostomy tubes and the nasopharynx is generally accomplished with a small-bore flexible catheter that is advanced without suction applied, and then withdrawn with intermittent suctioning on the way out. Before suctioning, the patient should be hyperventilated, preferably with high-concentration oxygen, and suction should not be applied for more than about 15 seconds in order to minimize hypoxia.

Cardiac arrhythmias

Basic physiology

A complete discussion of cardiac electrophysiology is well beyond the intent or scope of this chapter. However, a basic understanding of some of the principles involved will help the practitioner to understand and appropriately prevent and treat some commonly encountered cardiac arrhythmias. This section will discuss some basic physiologic features of the heart that will form a basis for arrhythmia recognition and management.

All living cells manifest a voltage difference across the cell membrane. For the majority of cardiac cells, the interior of the cell carries a resting negative charge of 80–90 mV, with respect to the outside. This charge is maintained by an active transport process known as the sodium–potassium pump. Typical selected ion concentrations in mEq/l are:

	Extracellular	Intracellular
Sodium	145	30–32
Potassium	4	150–160
Calcium	5	0.00007

Without the presence of an active exchange pump process, these concentration gradients would not exist, as diffusion across the cell membrane would rapidly establish ion equilibrium. The cells of the heart can be divided into two main groups: (i) working myocardial cells; and (ii) the electric system. The working cells constitute the majority of the heart, and are able to contract in response to electric stimulation (depolarization). Cells of the electric system do not contract, but initiate and distribute an electric current to the working myocardial cells, causing an orderly sequence of contraction throughout the heart. Within the electric system, there are "pacemaker" cells that are able spontaneously to depolarize without external electric stimulation, a process known as automaticity. These are found: (i) in the sinus node; (ii) the atria; (iii) near the AV node (AV junction); (iv) the bundle of His; and (v) the Purkinje system. Once an impulse is generated by a pacemaker cell, it is distributed to the rest of the heart via the specialized cells of the conduction system (Fig. 4.13). As a rule, the "higher" in the conduction system a pacemaker focus is found, the faster the rate of spontaneous discharge: the SA node fires at 60–100/min, the AV junction at 40–60/min, and "escape" pacemakers in the bundle of His at less than 40/min [23,24]. Under normal conditions, the sinus node exhibits the fastest rate of automaticity, and thus is the dominant pacemaker. Vagal stimulation produces acetylcholine release, resulting in an increase

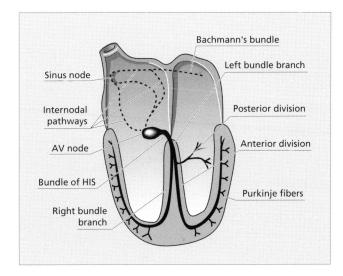

Fig. 4.13 Cardiac conduction system. Pacemaker foci are found in the sinus node, the atria, the AV node, the bundle of His, and in the Purkinje system. See text. (From American Heart Association [24].)

in electronegativity, and in addition an increase in potassium ion conductivity. These combined effects result in a decreased rate of spontaneous diastolic depolarization and a reduction in sinus node firing (bradycardia). Adrenergic stimulation results in an increased rate of sinus node discharge. Pacemaker foci located at lower sites in the conduction system and firing at a slower rate than the SA node can be thought of as back-up centers that continue impulse formation in the event of temporary or permanent loss of the dominant (fastest) pacemaker.

As a cardiac cell's resting potential becomes less negative and approaches zero, a point known as the threshold potential is reached, and the cell completely depolarizes in a very rapid fashion. This rapid depolarization is termed an action potential (Fig. 4.14), and if of sufficient magnitude, will cause adjoining cells to reach their threshold potential, thus causing another depolarization and action potential. In this fashion, a wave of depolarization spreads throughout the entire heart until the entire organ has depolarized. This process is referred to as a propagating impulse, and it is this three-dimensional electric activity that is recorded on the skin surface as the EKG.

There are two basic mechanisms of impulse formation: (i) automaticity, and (ii) reentry. Automaticity is responsible for the normal impulse formation in the SA node, but may be seen in abnormal situations in which a focus of activity arises in some other portion of the heart, perhaps at a faster rate. Reentry is a mechanism of impulse formation that can occur when a local "dual conduction" pathway exists: one branch has a unidirectional block or a longer refractory period, and the other has slow conduction. With reference to Fig. 4.15, consider an impulse traveling down a fiber of the conduction system as it is about to join a muscle fiber. Because there is a block to antegrade conduction in path A, the impulse will reach the muscle fiber via branch B, travel

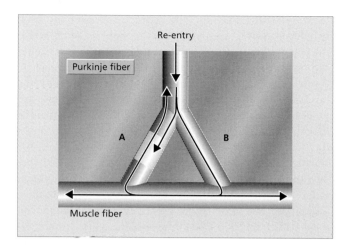

Fig. 4.15 Recently. See text. (From American Heart Association [24].)

in both directions in the muscle fiber, and then retrograde back up branch A (because only a unidirectional block was present). When it reaches the branch point, it is then possible for the impulse to reenter the conduction system. For example, if this were the Purkinje system, then this reentrant impulse could initiate an ectopic propagating action potential beginning in the ventricle: a premature ventricular contraction (PVC).

Normal cardiac impulse conduction

As mentioned above, the SA node, located at the junction of the superior vena cava and right atrium, is the normal site of impulse formation. Propagation through the atria occurs rapidly through three internodal pathways, stimulating atrial contraction in the process. As the impulse reaches the AV

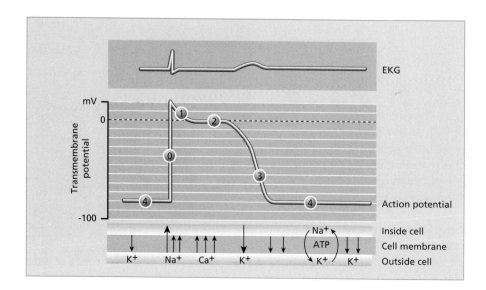

Fig. 4.14 Action potential. See text. (From American Heart Association [24].)

node (located in the inferior aspect of the right atrium), the speed of conduction is markedly slowed from about 1000 mm/s in the atria to some 200 mm/s in the AV node. Emerging from the inferior margin of the complex latticework of fibers that compose the AV node, the propagating action potential enters the bundle of His, a discrete bundle of fibers that passes through the annulus fibrosis and divides into the right and left bundle branches at the upper margin of the interventricular septum. The left bundle is further divided into anterior and posterior divisions, which break up into the Purkinje system, spreading the impulse to the left ventricle and portions of the interventricular septum. The right bundle proceeds down the rightward aspect of the septum, contributing Purkinje fibers to the apex of the septum and the right ventricle, The speed of conduction through the ventricular Purkinje system is even faster than in the atria, being some 4000 mm/s. As will be discussed below, the varying speeds and direction of conduction through the heart are reflected in the EKG.

Arrhythmia origins

Cardiac arrhythmias can be thought of as disturbances of impulse formation (disturbed automaticity), alterations of conduction, or combinations of these two [23]. Examples of disturbed automaticity might include acceleration or deceleration of the SA node (sinus tachycardia, sinus bradycardia), as well as impulses arising from ectopic foci. Examples of the latter would include premature beats in the atria, AV junction, or ventricles. Atrial and ventricular tachycardias can also be considered as disturbances of automaticity, with rapid firing of an ectopic pacemaker focus as the underlying mechanism. Conduction disturbances can be seen with slowed conduction, especially through the AV node, where varying degrees of atrioventricular block occur. Reentry can also be viewed as an alteration of conduction, but on a more local level. Atrial flutter with 3:1 block and premature atrial contraction with first-degree AV block are examples of combined alterations of automaticity and conduction.

EKG

The EKG records the complex electric events occurring in the heart with each cardiac cycle, by assuming that the body can be considered as a giant conductor of electric currents. Any two points on the body surface can be connected to positive and negative "leads", with current flowing towards the positive electrode, producing an upward deflection on the EKG trace. The 12-lead EKG "looks" at the electric activity in 12 different directions, any one of which could be used to evaluate the rhythm, with the standard limb leads being conveniently selectable on most cardiac monitors by using only three leads connected to the patient (Fig. 4.16). By convention, the resulting complexes are labeled the P

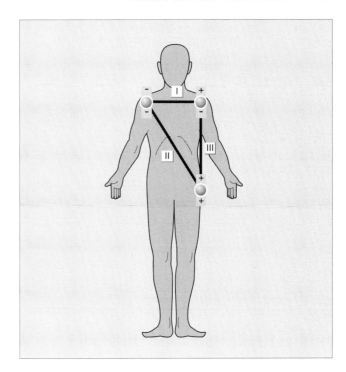

Fig. 4.16 Standard limb leads. Lead II is most commonly used to display rhythm strips. If patch placement interferes with the procedure, they can be applied directly to the limbs.

wave, the QRS complex, and the T wave (Fig. 4.17). Atrial depolarization produces the P wave, which is normally upright in lead II. The PR interval represents the normally slower conduction through the AV node, and should not exceed 0.20 seconds. The QRS complex represents ventricular depolarization, with the Q wave (the first negative deflection) not always visible. As viewed in lead II, the R wave is the next positive (upward) deflection, followed by a negative S wave. Because ventricular depolarization is a rapid event, the normal QRS is narrow and should not exceed 0.10 seconds. Atrial repolarization is obscured by the QRS complex. The ST segment represents the time from complete depolarization of the ventricles to the beginning of repolarization. Since no net electric activity is occurring during this recovery phase of the cardiac cycle, the ST segment is normally flat. With ischemia or injury, the ST segment may be elevated or depressed. Ventricular repolarization results in the T wave, which is usually upright in lead II.

Basic rhythm strip interpretation

Two basic questions need to be answered when performing arrhythmia interpretation: (i) what is the rate?; and (ii) what is the rhythm? Rate determination will be considered first.

By convention, the EKG paper runs at 25 mm/s, resulting

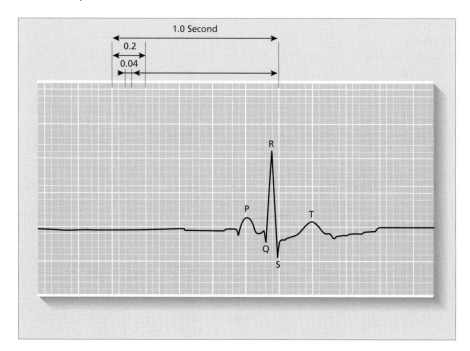

Fig. 4.17 Timing conventions on standard EKG paper and labeled EKG trace. See text.

in each small box representing 0.04 seconds and each large box 0.20 seconds (Fig. 4.17) [23,24]. There are many methods for rate determination; one is to divide the number of large boxes in the RR interval into 300 (Fig. 4.18). An aid to this approach is to memorize the descending "300−150−100−75−60−50" sequence. Rates that fall between these values can be interpolated. A faster but less accurate method is simply to count the number of R waves in 6 seconds (there are 1-second "tic-marks" at the top of the strip) and multiply by 10.

Once the rate is determined, rhythm analysis begins with assessing regularity. This is usually apparent from visual inspection, but in borderline cases, measurement of successive RR intervals with calipers or paper and sharp pencil may be required. To analyze the P waves, one should remember that the normal P wave is upright in lead II, and all the P waves should look identical. If the P waves vary in their morphology, the impulses are arising from different locations within the atria. The next step is to analyze the relationship between the P waves and QRS complexes, which should be 1:1. Each QRS complex should be preceded by a P wave, and the PR interval should be constant and less than 0.20 seconds (one big box). Finally, the QRS complex should be narrow: 0.11 seconds is borderline, and 0.12 seconds (three small boxes) is prolonged. This is an important determination, because with a QRS of normal duration, the impulse must originate above the bundle of His (SA node, atria, or AV junction). With a wide (prolonged, greater than 0.12 seconds) QRS, the impulse formation is either in the ventricles or there is altered ventricular conduction of a supraventricular impulse.

Sinus and atrial arrhythmias

This section is intended to summarize some of the major features of commonly encountered sinus and atrial arrhythmias. Those wishing to acquire cardiac resuscitative skills are encouraged to complete the America Heart Association's Advanced Cardiac Life Support (ACLS) course. Rhythms to be covered in this section are:

1 sinus bradycardia;
2 sinus tachycardia;
3 paroxysmal supraventricular tachycardia (PSVT);
4 multifocal atrial tachycardia (MAT);
5 premature atrial contraction (PAC);
6 atrial flutter;
7 atrial fibrillation (AF).

Sinus bradycardia (Fig. 4.19)

Etiology

Slowing of the sinus node from intrinsic nodal disease (e.g., ischemia), increased parasympathetic tone (pain, anxiety), athletic conditioning, drugs (e.g., propranolol, digitalis).

Identifying characteristics

The rate is less than 60 beats/min (bpm), but usually greater than 40 bpm. Both atrial and ventricular rhythms are regular. P waves are normal. The PR interval is normal or slightly prolonged. The QRS complex is normal. Conduction is normal.

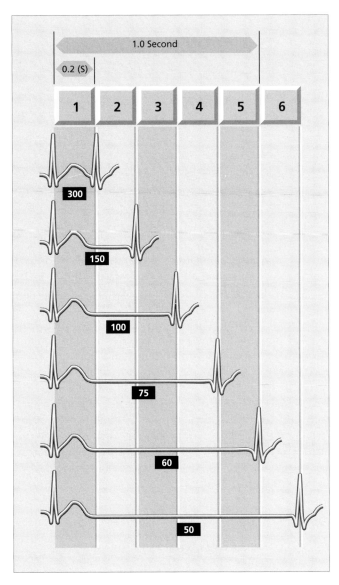

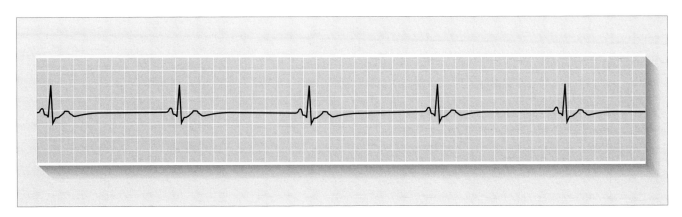

Fig. 4.18 Rate determination. See text. (From Grauer and Cavallaro [23].)

Risk

Because of decreased cardiac output, syncope and angina may occur. Junctional or ventricular escape beats may occur.

Precautions

Avoid negative chronotropic agents such as propranolol and digitalis. Maintain blood pressure (volume expansion, Trendelenburg). Be alert for PVCs.

Treatment

Treatment may not be required if the patient is asymptomatic. If there is hypotension, angina, ventricular escape beats, or a rate less than 30 bpm, IV atropine is the treatment of choice. If unsuccessful, chronotropic support with dopamine or isoproteronol may be necessary. Under extreme circumstances, a pacemaker may be needed.

Sinus tachycardia (Fig. 4.20)

Etiology

Accelerated firing of the sinus node, with a multitude of causes, including pain, anxiety, fever, hypovolemia, exertion, drugs (e.g., epinephrine), hypoxia, or need for increased cardiac output.

Identifying characteristics

The rate is usually 100−160 bpm. Atrial and ventricular rates are regular. The P wave is normal, but may be difficult to find because of the rapid rate; it may be superimposed on the T wave. The PR interval may be at the lower limits of normal. The QRS is normal. Conduction is normal.

Fig. 4.19 Sinus bradycardia.

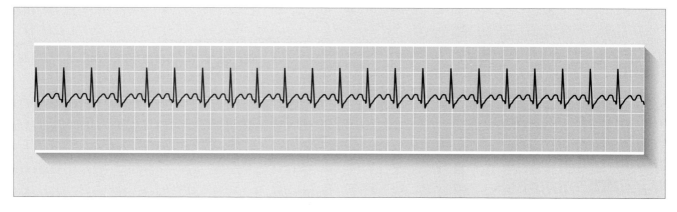

Fig. 4.20 Sinus tachycardia.

Risk

The increased rate may precipitate cardiac decompensation in those with borderline cardiac function. Myocardial oxygen consumption may rise high enough to unmask angina, particularly with underlying CAD.

Precautions

Observe for signs of left ventricular failure (orthopnea, cough, dyspnea, restlessness). Minimize anxiety if possible.

Treatment

Treat underlying cause.

PSVT (Fig. 4.21)

Etiology

PSVT should be distinguished from the more generic term supraventricular tachycardia, which includes *any* tachycardia due to rapid impulse formation above the level of the AV node (sinus tachycardia, paroxysmal atrial tachycardia (PAT),

atrial flutter, atrial fibrillation, etc.). *Paroxysmal* is the key word. Two forms of PSVT are recognized: (i) AV nodal reentrant tachycardia; and (ii) orthodromic AV reentrant tachycardia [16].

AV nodal reentrant tachycardia is the most common form of PSVT in the older population, and is due to a reentrant circuit at the AV nodal level resulting from a dual conduction pathway; one fast and the other slow. Orthodromic AV reentrant tachycardia is usually seen in patients under 35 years old [16], and requires the presence of an accessory pathway. An impulse traverses the AV node in the normal fashion, resulting in a narrow QRS, but then returns to the atrium via an accessory conduction pathway. As this impulse again traverses the AV node, a "circus movement tachycardia" is set up.

Identifying characteristics

Three key features characterize PSVT:
1 it starts abruptly;
2 it ends abruptly;
3 there is 1:1 conduction — the ventricles respond to every impulse created by the supraventricular focus.

The rate is usually 150–250 bpm, both atrial and ventri-

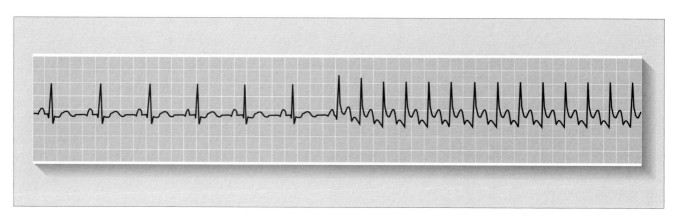

Fig. 4.21 Paroxysmal supraventricular tachycardia.

cular. The rhythm is perfectly regular. P waves are present, but may be very hard to identify, and may not have the normal rounded shape, since they are not originating in the SA node. If a PR interval can be measured, it is usually within normal limits. The QRS complex is normal, except in the presence of an accessory pathway. (See reference [16] for a complete discussion of differentiating the two major forms of PSVT.)

Risk

Uncontrolled rapid ventricular rate may lead to myocardial ischemia and, eventually, cardiac decompensation.

Precautions

As with sinus tachycardia, observe for signs of cardiac decompensation or myocardial ischemia. Provide oxygen as needed.

Treatment

Vagal stimulation such as coughing, unilateral carotid sinus massage, and Valsalva maneuver are simple and often effective measures [41]. Adenosine is a highly effective IV medication for terminating PSVT, although its effect is short lived, and may also transiently increase the degree of AV block enough to uncover underlying atrial activity [42]. IV verapamil is also effective, but should never be given to patients with wide complex tachycardias [16,43]. If the patient becomes symptomatic (angina, diaphoresis, hypotensive), synchronized cardioversion may be used immediately, and almost always terminates the tachycardia, with energy levels of 100 J [41].

Multifocal atrial tachycardia

Etiology

This rhythm is most commonly seen in hypoxic patients with COPD [24,41]. Atrial foci from multiple different sites initiate impulse formation, resulting in an irregularly irregular rhythm that resembles atrial fibrillation in this regard. A high index of suspicion in a clinical setting of COPD may help in the diagnosis.

Identifying characteristics

The atrial and ventricular rates are 100–180 bpm [41]. The rhythm is irregularly irregular. P waves are present, but vary in morphology. PR interval is variable. The QRS complex is normal. As above, this rhythm is most often seen in COPD patients.

Risk

The main problem with this rhythm is confusing it with atrial fibrillation, and treating it as such with digitalis, to which it is notoriously resistant.

Precautions

In a setting of COPD, examine the rhythm strip carefully in multiple leads for evidence of multiformed P waves. Evaluate the patient for clinical signs of hypoxia.

Treatment

Treatment of this rhythm is directed at correcting the underlying hypoxia and any associated metabolic abnormalities.

PAC (Fig. 4.22)

Etiology

This single beat arrhythmia is the result of spontaneous depolarization of a temporary pacemaker focus somewhere in the atria other than the SA node. For the beat on which it occurs, it precludes firing of the SA node because it fires

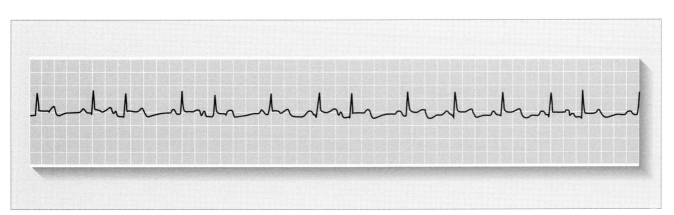

Fig. 4.22 Premature atrial contraction.

before the SA node's next expected beat, hence "premature". PACs may occur without apparent cause, although they are associated with a number of factors, including caffeine, sympathomimetic medications, alcohol, hypoxia, and elevation of atrial pressures.

Identifying characteristics

The underlying rate is usually normal (60–100 bpm), but PACs may occur with any sinus rate. The rhythm is momentarily irregular due to the early firing of the atrial focus. Because the PAC depolarizes the SA node along with the rest of the atria, the SA node begins the generation of another impulse later than it normally would, due to the extra conduction time from the ectopic atrial focus to the SA node. Thus, the next normal sinus beat (P) occurs after a brief noncompensatory pause. The premature (P') wave will have a different shape than the P waves of the sinus beats because of its abnormal location. The P'R interval is variable but often prolonged. The QRS complex is normal unless there is aberrant ventricular conduction. There may also be variable AV block of the premature beat.

Risk

There is no significant risk from occasional PACs. If frequent (more than 8/min), there may be a somewhat increased chance of atrial flutter or fibrillation.

Precautions

If anxiety is present, reassurance should be given. Monitor for frequency of PACs.

Treatment

Correction of the underlying cause (removal of caffeine, sympathomimetic drugs, etc.) is the mainstay of treatment.

Atrial flutter (Fig. 4.23)

Etiology

An atrial focus, probably the result of reentry at the atrial level, supersedes the SA node because of its faster rate. This rhythm may be seen in association with mitral or tricuspid valvular heart disease, CAD, or cor pulmonale.

Identifying characteristics

The atrial rate is rapid, usually 250–350 bpm. Atrial rhythm is regular. The ventricular rhythm varies with the number of impulses transmitted through the AV node. The P waves resemble a "picket fence", or "sawtooth" in lead II, often referred to as "flutter waves". At slower rates (e.g., atrial rate 220 bpm), it is possible to have 1:1 conduction, but most often there is a physiologic second-degree block at the AV node, resulting in 2:1 or 3:1 conduction [23]. The QRS is normal.

Risk

Severe hemodynamic compromise may occur within minutes with 1:1 conduction and rapid ventricular rates. Cardiac output can fall dramatically with insufficient filling time. Even if systemic perfusion is adequate, there may be severe demands on myocardial oxygen consumption, and angina or left ventricular failure may ensue.

Precautions

Monitor EKG for ventricular rate. Observe for clinical signs of hemodynamic compromise.

Treatment

With 3:1 or 4:1 conduction, ventricular rates may be slow

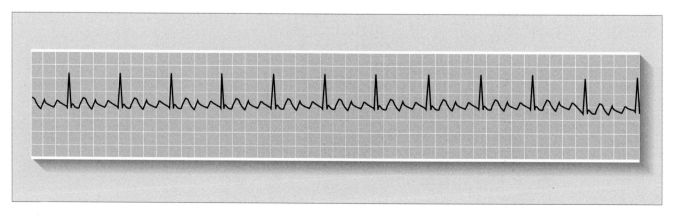

Fig. 4.23 Atrial flutter.

enough that treatment is not necessary. For fast ventricular rates with hemodynamic compromise, synchronized cardioversion at low (25–50 J) energy is the therapy of choice [23,41]. For rapid rates without hemodynamic compromise, digoxin, verapamil, and propranolol can be used.

AF (Fig. 4.24)

Etiology

Possibly the result of multiple ectopic foci or multiple areas of atrial reentry, this rhythm produces a chaotic atrial electric and mechanical process, with no organized atrial contraction. There is usually underlying organic heart disease.

Identifying characteristics

The atrial rate cannot be measured. There are no P waves. The ventricular rate is variable, indeed random. The ventricular rhythm is described as irregularly irregular. There is a physiologic block of variable degree in the AV node. Some of the atrial impulses are conducted into but not through the AV node, where they depolarize the node and contribute to its overall "refractoriness". Thus, ventricular rates with AF are often lower than seen with PSVT or atrial flutter [23]. The QRS is normal, unless there is associated aberrant conduction.

Risk

With uncontrolled fast ventricular rates, there is the potential for hemodynamic compromise, angina, pulmonary edema, and cardiogenic shock. Atrial thrombi may form, with risk of systemic embolization.

Precautions

Observe for clinical evidence of hemodynamic compromise or angina.

Treatment

If chronic AF is present and the patient is asymptomatic with no hemodynamic compromise, and the ventricular rate is 50–100 bpm, no therapy may be required. At the other end of the spectrum, the therapy of choice for acute onset AF with hemodynamic compromise is synchronized cardioversion with 200–300 J [41]. For AF with rapid ventricular response, digoxin is the first line drug, with verapamil and propranolol for resistant cases [44]. If AF with rapid ventricular response deteriorates to hemodynamic compromise within the first 72 hours of onset, synchronized cardioversion may be required to slow the ventricular rate. After 72 hours, there may be increased risk of systemic embolization due to potential atrial thrombus formation [23,24].

Conduction defects and ventricular arrhythmias

The major arrhythmias originating above the AV node were covered above. This section will discuss abnormal rhythms that are associated with altered conduction through the AV node, and those of ventricular origin.

First-degree AV block (Fig. 4.25)

Etiology

This is simply delayed conduction through the AV node. It may be due to drugs (especially digitalis, quinidine, or procainamide), nodal injury as might occur in infarction, or nodal ischemia.

Identifying characteristics

The rate is normal. The rhythm is regular. P waves are normal. The PR interval is prolonged to greater than 0.20 seconds (one big box). Conduction is otherwise normal. The QRS complex is normal.

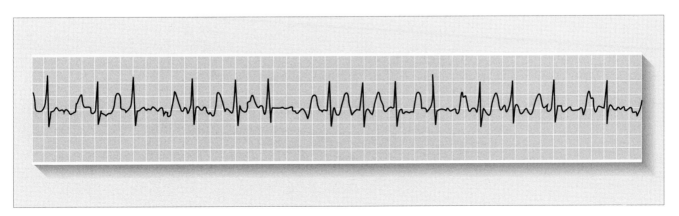

Fig. 4.24 Atrial fibrillation.

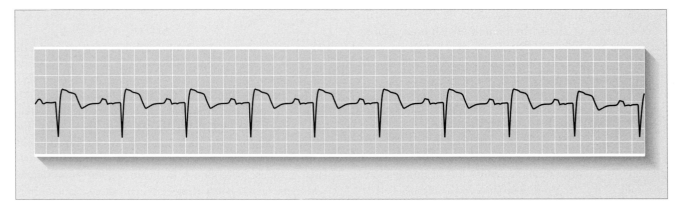

Fig. 4.25 First-degree AV block.

Risk

No particular risk is associated with this rhythm.

Precautions

In a setting of myocardial infarction, monitor for possible progression to second- or third-degree AV block.

Treatment

First-degree block of greater than 0.26 seconds may be treated with atropine to increase AV nodal conduction.

Second-degree AV block: type I (Fig. 4.26)

Note: this is sometimes called Mobitz I or Wenckebach.

Etiology

With AV nodal injury or ischemia, it becomes progressively more difficult for succeeding impulses to pass through the node until a beat is blocked entirely. This may also be seen in association with increased parasympathetic tone and drugs such as propranolol and digoxin.

Identifying characteristics

The atrial rate may be normal. The ventricular rate is slower than atrial because of the blocked beats. Atrial rhythm is regular, while the ventricular rhythm is irregular. P waves are normal. *The PR interval becomes progressively prolonged with a decreasing RR interval, until a P wave is not conducted* [23,24]. Usually, only a single impulse is blocked, and the cycle is then repeated. As a result, there is "group beating", characterized by QRS complexes (and, hopefully, peripheral pulses!) that come in groups until one is lost. The QRS is normal.

Risk

As a rule, the outlook is good, with this often a transient arrhythmia following myocardial infarction. It should be considered potentially dangerous in that there may be progression to third-degree block (see below).

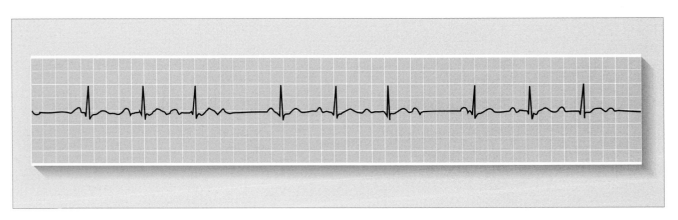

Fig. 4.26 Second-degree AV block; type I.

Precautions

Monitor for progression to third-degree block.

Treatment

Usually, no therapy is needed. If the ventricular rate becomes excessively slow, and the patient is symptomatic from this, atropine may be used.

Second-degree AV block: type II (Fig. 4.27)

Note: an alternate term is Mobitz II.

Etiology

This block is associated with an organic lesion (e.g., infarct, ischemia) just below AV node, either in the bundle of His or a bundle branch. Unlike type I second-degree block, it is not due to drugs or increased parasympathetic tone. One or more impulses are not conducted through the lesion, resulting in dropped beats.

Identifying characteristics

The atrial rate may be normal. The ventricular rate depends on the frequency of the block. The atrial rhythm is regular, but the ventricular rhythm is irregular. The P waves are normal. Unlike type I block, *the PR interval does not lengthen prior to a dropped beat* [23,24]. Nonconducted beats may be random, or with 2:1, 3:1, or 4:1 conduction ratios. If the block is occurring in the bundle of His, the QRS complex will be normal. More often, the block is in one of the bundle branches, and as a result, the usual type II block is associated with a widened QRS complex.

Risk

Unlike type I second-degree block, this rhythm represents a

significant risk because of its propensity unpredictably to deteriorate to third-degree (complete) heart block [23]. This is especially common in a setting of acute myocardial infarction.

Precautions

Monitor closely for widening of the QRS complex and third-degree block. The wider the QRS, the lower in the conduction system is the block, and further prolongation of the QRS may herald complete heart block. Since a temporary or permanent pacemaker is indicated for this rhythm, preparation for pacing would be prudent.

Treatment

Frequently, there will be need for temporary pacing while preparations are made for permanent pacemaker insertion. Atropine or isoproteronol may be required as temporizing measures; a pacemaker is the treatment of choice.

Third-degree (complete) AV block (Fig. 4.28)

Etiology

There is complete absence of conduction at the level of the AV node, bundle of His, or bundle branch level. If at the AV node, the block may be due to increased parasympathetic tone, drugs, or infarction/ischemia, but below the AV node, it is most often due to infarction or ischemia, and usually involves both right and left bundle branches [23]. If the block is at the AV node, a junctional pacemaker focus will usually be present, with a rate of 40–60/min, and the prognosis is more favorable. Infranodal third-degree block will (hopefully) result in a ventricular escape focus, but immediate pacing is still likely to be needed.

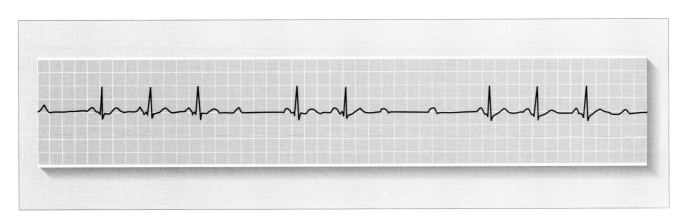

Fig. 4.27 Second-degree AV block, type II.

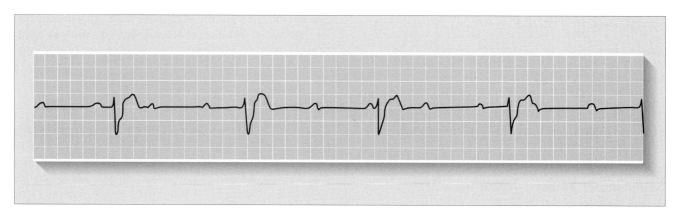

Fig. 4.28 Third-degree AV block.

Identifying characteristics

The atrial rate is faster than the ventricular rate. The rhythm is regular for both atrial and ventricular foci, but they are totally independent of each other. The P waves may be normal. The PR interval is random because of the lack of relationship between atrial and ventricular rhythms (there is no AV conduction). If the block is at the AV node, the QRS will be normal, indicating the presence of a junctional escape rhythm, usually at 40–60/min. For infranodal third-degree block, the QRS will be widened, particularly at the bundle branch level.

Risks

If the block is at the AV node and there is a junctional rhythm at a rate sufficient to maintain cardiac output, there may be adequate tissue perfusion. For infranodal complete heart block, there will likely be hemodynamic compromise. Even with a ventricular escape focus, this is not a stable rhythm, and there is a propensity to develop ventricular fibrillation or asystole.

Precautions

Monitor EKG for block at a lower level in the conduction system, ventricular fibrillation, or asystole. Provide oxygen. Begin preparations for pacemaker insertion.

Treatment

For block at the AV node with ventricular rate too slow to maintain adequate cardiac output, atropine is the drug of choice, with temporary pacemaker insertion if atropine fails. For infranodal block, a pacemaker is indicated. The patient's condition may require isoproteronol for chronotropic support prior to pacing.

PVC (Fig. 4.29)

Etiology

An irritable focus in the ventricle initiates an impulse before the next normally conducted beat. This may be seen in a variety of clinical situations, including hypoxia, acidosis,

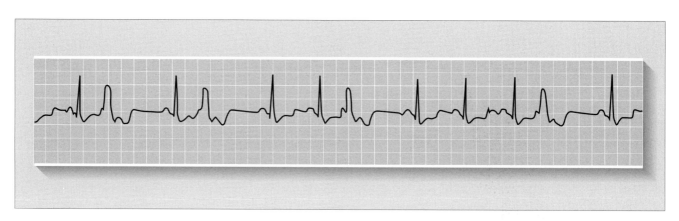

Fig. 4.29 Premature ventricular contraction.

bradycardia, electrolyte imbalance, drug toxicity, and myocardial infarction [23].

Identifying characteristics

The atrial and ventricular rates may be normal. The ventricular rhythm is irregular. P waves are not associated with the PVC complex unless there is retrograde atrial depolarization. The PR interval does not apply to the PVC. The QRS complex is wide and bizarre. Usually, there is a compensatory pause equal to two RR intervals following the normal beat prior to the PVC, because the sinus node impulse and PVC impulse tend to meet at the AV node, where neither can spread further because of the refractory period of the other [23,24]. Exceptions occur when the PVC falls between two normal sinus beats (interpolated PVC) resulting in "no pause", and when the PVC reaches the atria and depolarizes the AV node prior to its next spontaneous impulse, resulting in a "noncompensatory pause" of less than two RR intervals. The coupling interval (the time from the previous normal beat and the PVC) tends to be the constant for ventricular beats arising from the same ectopic focus, and their morphology is the same ("unifocal" PVCs). For ventricular beats arising from more than focus, or from the same focus and with varying conduction, the coupling interval and QRS morphology will vary (multifocal or multiformed PVCs). By definition, three or more PVCs in succession is termed ventricular tachycardia. PVCs occurring every other beat are termed "bigeminy", and every third beat "trigeminy".

Risk

Although it has been said that six or more PVCs per minute and PVCs falling on a T wave may be harbingers of ventricular tachycardia or fibrillation, the clinical setting in which the PVCs are occurring is probably a more important factor in risk assessment. PVCs of increasing frequency, and development of multifocal PVCs suggest increasing ventricular irrita-

bility, which in a clinical setting of acute myocardial infarction may have a different implication than in, e.g., a COPD patient with respiratory acidosis from carbon dioxide retention.

Precautions

Monitor for increasing frequency of PVCs, or multiformed PVCs. Depending on the clinical circumstances, consider preparing for lidocaine bolus and drip.

Treatment

Occasional PVCs in the asymptomatic patient without suspicion of heart disease do not require therapy. If the clinical situation indicates prompt treatment, IV lidocaine is the drug of choice, with procainamide for resistant cases [23,24].

Ventricular tachycardia (VT) (Fig. 4.30)

Etiology

A commonly cited cause of VT is a local focus of reentry, often due to a left ventricular scar from a previous infarction [45,46], which sets up a "circus movement" of electric current around the anatomic defect. This results in rhythmic impulse formation, conducted through the ventricles with variable effectiveness of contraction. Some VT will be slow enough to allow adequate time for ventricular filling, and if there is sufficiently organized ventricular mechanical activity, stroke volume may be enough to generate a pulse. More often, there is a precipitous fall in cardiac output [23]. VT is associated with multiple conditions, including CAD, dilated or hypertrophic cardiomyopathy, hypoxia, acidosis, and electrolyte imbalance. Nonsustained VT may occur in as many as 50% of all patients with congestive heart failure [47]. Despite its association with the above factors, the

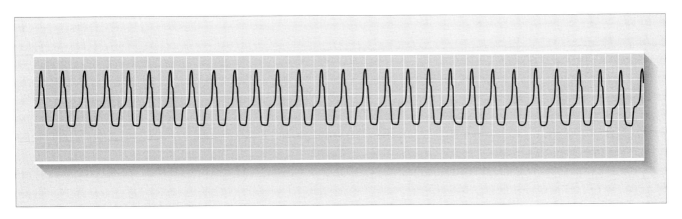

Fig. 4.30 Ventricular tachycardia.

prognosis for surviving cardiac arrest is greatest when the underlying mechanism is VT, and this is most commonly seen during in-hospital arrests [42].

Identifying characteristics

The rate is greater than 100 bpm, usually 120−220 bpm. The rhythm is regular. With ventricular rates slow enough, P waves may be visible, but because the AV node is being repeatedly depolarized by the ventricular impulses, there is complete AV dissociation. At faster rates, P waves are not visible. The PR interval does not apply. The QRS is wide and bizarre. There is no normal conduction, with an ectopic ventricular focus initiating impulse formation. Verapamil should *not* be administered as a diagnostic tool in wide complex tachycardia [45].

Risk

There are multiple risks associated with sustained VT. Even if the patient has a pulse and is hemodynamically stable, myocardial oxygen consumption is greatly increased and there is risk of deterioration to ventricular fibrillation (VF). If there is a pulse but insufficient cardiac output for tissue perfusion, cardiogenic shock will ensue. Pulseless VT, of course, is not a perfusing rhythm.

Precautions

If the patient is conscious and breathing, "cough version" may be employed if the onset of VT is witnessed. The patient is instructed to "cough hard and keep coughing!" [23]. Oxygen should be applied if the patient is breathing. Preparations for lidocaine administration and synchronized cardioversion or defibrillation should begin immediately.

Treatment

For hemodynamically stable VT with a palpable pulse, IV lidocaine is the drug of choice, followed by procainamide and bretylium. Patients who become hemodynamically unstable during the course of observation should receive synchronized cardioversion at 100−200 J. Pulseless VT is treated with defibrillation, using the same procedure as for VF.

Ventricular fibrillation (Fig. 4.31)

Etiology

There is a total lack of organized cardiac electric activity, with random, chaotic electric currents in the ventricles, and no ventricular contraction. As a result, there is *no cardiac output*. This is said to be the most common mechanism of cardiac arrest resulting from myocardial ischemia or infarction [24].

Identifying characteristics

The rate is too chaotic to count. There really is no rhythm, but it could be described as irregular (indeed random). There are, of course, no P waves, QRS complex, or T wave.

Risk

This is a *fatal rhythm*.

Precautions

Be sure it is VF and not artifact. If onset is witnessed on EKG, try cough version to gain a little time while the defibrillator is prepared and brought to the patient.

Treatment

Immediate defibrillation is the treatment of choice. CPR should be performed, but should not delay defibrillation. If the first series of shocks is unsuccessful, the patient is intubated and

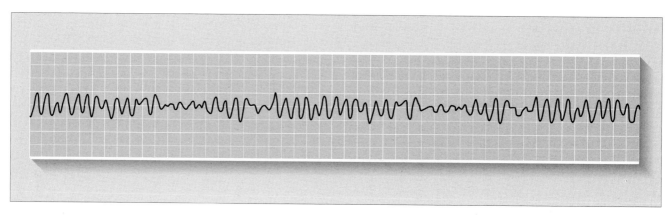

Fig. 4.31 Ventricular fibrillation.

IV access is established. Liberal use of epinephrine in conjunction with continued CPR [23,42,48] and repeated attempts at defibrillation are justified. Lidocaine may also be administered.

Defibrillation

Rapid defibrillation is the single most effective treatment for the patient in VF [23,24] and "the sooner a patient in ventricular fibrillation can be defibrillated, the better the chance for survival" [42]. This section is intended to review the basic principles and procedures relating to defibrillation. Basic life support (CPR) will not be covered. For a complete discussion, the practitioner is urged to complete an ACLS course (as provided by the American Heart Association). (See also references [23,24,42].)

With the introduction of automatic external defibrillators (Fig. 4.32), BLS-trained hospital staff are encouraged to provide early electric treatment of VF and pulseless VT, even before the code team arrives with ACLS capabilities [8–10,24]. As distinct from manual monitor defibrillators, which display the rhythm for the practitioner to interpret and act upon, these automated devices analyze the rhythm and advise "shock" or "no shock" depending upon the characteristics of the rhythm. It is up to the practitioner to determine unresponsiveness, lack of respirations, lack of pulse, and to apply the patches to the patient. The major advantage of this technology is the *rapid* availability of electric therapy to the patient in VF or pulseless VT, thus providing a "bridge" from CPR to formal ACLS therapy. Nonphysician BLS providers both in prehospital and in-hospital settings can readily be trained to operate this equipment, with resultant improved survival rates [24]. This technology is ideal for free-standing imaging centers, and would also be appropriate for hospital-based imaging departments with ACLS code-team back-up.

Successful defibrillation requires providing sufficient electric current passage through the myocardium to interrupt the arrhythmia, but not so much current as to cause morphologic damage [8]. The shocks should be given as soon as the defibrillator is available because of the decreasing chances of success with time, and because electric defibrillation is the treatment of choice in VF or pulseless VT [8,24]. With defibrillation, a substantial current of electric energy is passed through the heart in a very short period of time. The energy stored in the defibrillator and delivered to the patient is expressed as:

joules = watts × seconds.

Since it is the *current* of electric energy that depolarizes cardiac cells rather than the voltage, Ohm's law (energy equals current multiplied by resistance: $E = IR$) dictates that for a given voltage, resistance (in this case resistance of the chest) is the primary determinant of current applied to the myocardium. expressed as:

$$\text{current (amps)} = \frac{\text{potential (volts)}}{\text{resistance (ohms)}}.$$

Thus, the lower the transthoracic resistance (TTR), the greater the current delivered to the chest, and hence the myocardium. Grauer *et al.* [42] has reemphasized the importance of lowering the TTR in optimizing the chance of conversion and minimizing complications. Many factors influence TTR, including the chest wall configuration, paddle pressure applied to the chest wall, the skin/paddle interface, paddle size and placement, the total number of and interval between shocks, and phase of respiration. The practitioner can minimize TTR by the following.

1 Application of electrode gel or disposable electrode pads.
2 Correct paddle placement. "Sternum" paddle below the clavicle and just to the right of the sternum. "Apex" paddle lateral to the left nipple in the anterior axillary line.

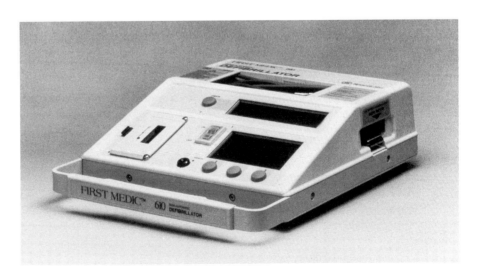

Fig. 4.32 Automatic external defibrillator. (Photograph courtesy of Spacelabs Medical, Redmond, Washington, USA.)

3 Firm (approximately 11 kg) paddle pressure against the chest.

4 Delivering the shock during exhalation (firm paddle pressure will aid forced exhalation).

TTR falls somewhat with successive shocks and with shorter interval between shocks, so if the initial attempt is unsuccessful, minimizing the time to deliver the next shock is important.

Duration of VF negatively influences success [24], placing a high premium on speed when attempting defibrillation, which is the single most important therapy that can be provided to the patient in VF or pulseless VT. The underlying health of the myocardium and the environment in which it is found also affect success. Previously healthy hearts respond to defibrillation better than diseased ones. Hypoxia, acidosis, electrolyte imbalance, hypothermia, and drug toxicity all render the fibrillating heart more resistant to therapy.

Manual defibrillator operation is somewhat variable, depending on the machine, but some generalizations are possible. Power switches to the monitor and defibrillator sections may be separate or combined. If the patient is not already on an EKG monitor, most defibrillators provide a "quick-look" feature that allows the paddles to act as EKG electrodes. Energy level is selected, and the capacitor is charged to that level. With the paddles in place as above, the usual technique employed is to require the practitioner to depress firing buttons simultaneously on both paddles. Most monitors/defibrillators label the controls for simplicity of operation (e.g., "one", "two", "three"), but the practitioner is urged to become familiar with the operation of the particular machine(s) that he or she may be called upon to use. Routine testing and documentation of the defibrillator at full output into a 50-Ω test load is recommended. In general, the procedure for manual defibrillation is the following.

1 Continue CPR only until the defibrillator is ready, i.e., do not delay defibrillation because of the need to perform CPR. CPR will need to be discontinued in order to confirm the rhythm without artifact from chest compressions.

2 Confirm that the rhythm is VF or pulseless VT, using either standard EKG leads, or "quick-look" paddles. Possible pitfalls include: motion artifact simulating VF, a lead off the patient, operator motion when using quick-look paddles, and selecting quick look when the standard limb leads are attached to the patient.

3 Apply conductive gel or disposable pads, confirm that defibrillator power is on, select energy, and charge the defibrillator.

4 Place the paddles as above, with a slight "twist" to distribute the conductive gel. Confirm that the rhythm is VF, and that all personnel are clear of the patient and anything that the patient touches.

5 Apply firm paddle pressure and depress both buttons simultaneously.

6 Check *rhythm and pulse* after each shock.

Synchronized cardioversion

The principle underlying synchronized cardioversion is to avoid delivering a shock during the "vulnerable period", roughly a 30-millisecond duration period just before the apex of the T wave, during which the heart is most susceptible to electrically induced VF. This is in distinction to defibrillation, which is timed only by the practitioner, and is therefore applied randomly with respect to the cardiac cycle. Synchronized cardioversion (sometimes called cardioversion) is accomplished by monitoring the patient in an EKG lead with a tall, upright R wave, which is sensed by the defibrillator when the appropriate controls are set. The machine then waits until it senses an R wave, and times the delivery of the shock so as to avoid the vulnerable period. It is most effective against arrhythmias of reentry origin, such as atrial flutter/fibrillation, PSVT, and ventricular tachycardia. The procedure is as follows.

1 Monitor the patient in a lead with a tall, upright R wave. (In VT with rates over 200 bpm and wide, bizarre QRS complexes, it may not be possible for the practitioner or the machine to tell the difference between the R and T waves. In this case, proceed with unsynchronized defibrillation.)

2 Activate the "synch" switch and confirm that the machine is sensing the R waves. Charge the defibrillator to the desired energy level.

3 Apply gel or disposable pads, place the paddles, and be sure all personnel are clear.

4 *Press and hold* the buttons on each paddle. Unlike defibrillation, the machine will not deliver the stored energy to the paddles until the R wave is sensed.

5 Check *rhythm and pulse* after each shock.

Precordial thump

This is a sharp, quick blow to the midsternum, delivered by the hypothenar eminence of the closed fist from a height of 20–30 cm above the chest. The concept is that a mechanical force applied to the myocardium will result in a depolarization of the order of 2–5 J, which may be enough to interrupt a local reentry pathway and terminate the rhythm [24]. *The precordial thump should not be used in VT with a pulse*, because this has caused VT to deteriorate to VF, asystole, or electromechanical dissociation (EMD) [8]. This maneuver, once advocated for the monitored onset of all VT and VF, can be viewed as having value primarily in a "no lose" situation. If a defibrillator is unavailable in a witnessed and monitored cardiac arrest, the patient will surely die if in VF or pulseless VT, and there is nothing to lose by trying the thump. If a manual or automatic defibrillator and trained personnel are immediately available, the time used to perform and evaluate the results of the thump may not be worth the potential risk of converting VT to VF. If there will be a delay of more than a few minutes in bringing the defibrillator to the patient, the thump may be used at the discretion of the practitioner [23]. Certainly if there is VT *with* a pulse, the thump should *not* be used.

Autonomic nervous system physiology

A complete discussion of the autonomic nervous system is well beyond the intent or scope of this chapter, but a brief review is appropriate before consideration of emergency medications. The sympathetic nervous system (SNS) and parasympathetic nervous system (PNS) comprise the autonomic nervous system, which is responsible for regulation of unconscious functions such as control of heart rate and blood pressure, intestinal motility, bladder control, and some hormonal activity (notably epinephrine release from the adrenal glands). Fibers of the preganglionic fibers of both the SNS and PNS, and the postganglionic fibers of the PNS mediate impulse formation by release of acetylcholine, and are thus termed *cholinergic*. Postganglionic fibers of the SNS are mediated by norepinephrine release, and are termed *adrenergic*.

A balance between PNS and SNS tone generally exists, and promotes homeostasis at rest. Generalized stimulation of the SNS results in the classic "fright and flight" response of tachycardia: raised blood pressure, pupillary dilatation, bronchial dilatation, anal sphincter contraction, and inhibition of intestinal peristalsis. This is accomplished through a combination of direct adrenergic innervation of target organs, and epinephrine release from the adrenal glands. As a rule, stimulation of the PNS has the opposite effect, sometimes termed "repose and repair". Thus, cholinergic stimulation results in slowing of the heart rate, a fall in blood pressure, and resumption of peristalsis.

The heart, as with many other organs, is innervated by both SNS and PNS fibers, whose end-point effects are mediated by acetylcholine and norepinephrine, respectively [23,24]. The vagus nerve comprises the direct PNS innervation of the heart, exerting its influence primarily on the SA node (slowed rate of spontaneous depolarization), and the AV node (prolonged AV conduction time). SNS innervation of the heart is mediated by adrenergic receptors located on cell surfaces, further divided into α_1-, α_2-, β_1-, and β_2-receptors.

α_1-Adrenergic receptors are postsynaptic, located predominantly on cellular surfaces of vascular smooth muscle. When stimulated, they produce vasoconstriction. α_2-Receptors, located on the presynaptic ends of the sympathetic neuron, inhibit further norepinephrine release when stimulated, thus functioning as an inhibitory feedback mechanism. For purposes of the following discussion, α-adrenergic stimulation will refer to α_1-receptors.

β_1-Adrenergic receptors are primarily located in the myocardium, and when stimulated, cause increased rate and strength of cardiac contraction (positive chronotropic and inotropic effects). β_2-Receptors are found on vascular smooth muscle where stimulation results in vasodilatation, and in bronchial smooth muscle where stimulation causes bronchodilatation. As mentioned above, homeostasis of cardiac function and blood pressure control depends on a balance between PNS and SNS stimulation. Excess PNS or PNS tone can "swing the pendulum" in one direction or another, as can exogenous adrenergic agents (Tables 4.5 & 4.6).

Emergency drugs

This section will present some basic pharmacology relating to commonly used drugs in the treatment of cardiac and contrast-related emergencies. Texts by Opie [17], Grauer and Cavallaro [23], Kofke and Levy [41], and Govoni and Hayes [49] are recommended for further reading. Unless otherwise specified, doses are for adults.

Table 4.5 Adrenergic receptors: location and effect

Designation	Location	Effect
α_1	Vascular smooth muscle	Vasoconstriction
α_2	Sympathetic neuron	Inhibits further norepinephrine release
β_1	Myocardium	Increased heart rate and strength of contraction
β_2	Vascular smooth muscle	Vasodilatation
	Bronchial smooth muscle	Bronchodilatation

Table 4.6 Adrenergic receptors: cardiovascular distribution and response

Site	Receptor type and relative predominance	Adrenergic response
Heart	β	Rate: increased Contractility: increased AV conduction: increased
Coronary arteries	$\beta > \alpha$	Dilatation > constriction
Peripheral arteries	$\alpha > \beta$	Constriction > dilatation

Adenosine

Actions/indications

Adenosine is a naturally occurring substance that binds to cardiac receptors in the SA and AV nodes and results in decreased heart rate, depressed conduction, and increased refractoriness of the AV node. It does not have significant effects on most accessory conduction pathways. It is very effective against reentry atrial, nodal arrhythmias, and AV reciprocating tachycardias, but is not effective against AF or atrial flutter, other than transiently to slow ventricular response due to AV block. It has an extremely short serum half-life of less than 5 seconds [8], which may allow the arrhythmia to recur, but also minimizes the duration of adverse effects [42]. Its primary utility lies in reliable and rapid termination of PSVT, although it may play a role in assisting diagnosis of some wide complex tachycardias by transiently increasing the degree of AV block, thereby unmasking underlying atrial activity [42,45].

Adverse effects

Dyspnea (it is a bronchoconstrictor), flushing, headache, and occasional angina are reported, but because the half-life is so short, these effects are transient, lasting less than 30–60 seconds [17]. Up to 50% of patients will have transient, usually asymptomatic, arrhythmias (PVCs, nonsustained VT, sinus pauses, and AV block) immediately following supraventricular tachycardia (SVT) termination [44].

Contraindications

Asthma, sick sinus syndrome, second- or third-degree AV block.

Dose

Initial dose: 6 mg IV bolus (1–3 seconds). Effect on the AV node is rapid. If unsuccessful within 1–2 minutes, repeat dose is 12 mg. If still unsuccessful, the 12-mg dose may be repeated in another 1–2 minutes, but if there is still no response, it is unlikely the drug will be effective [42].

Albuterol

Actions/indications

Albuterol is a synthetic β_2-selective agonist (with some β_1-activity) [17] whose primary usefulness in radiologic emergencies is for reversal of contrast-induced bronchospasm. It can be administered by metered dose inhaler, thus delivering drug directly to the target organ (β_2-receptors on bronchial smooth muscle).

Adverse effects

With excessive dosage, tachycardia may occur because of the β_1-component, but this is less of a problem than with aerosolized racemic epinephrine.

Contraindications

Hypertension, tachycardia.

Dose

One to two inhalations, repeated once in 1–2 minutes if needed. Maximum of four inhalations suggested. Observe for increased heart rate.

Atropine

Actions/indications

Atropine sulfate is a parasympathetic blocking agent, whose primary utility is in acceleration of symptomatic sinus bradycardia, with additional uses in second/third-degree AV block, slow idioventricular rhythm, and occasionally in asystole. It should not be given in asymptomatic bradycardia, unless perhaps the rate is less than 30 bpm, because of the potential risk of unmasking excessive underlying sympathetic tone [23,24].

Adverse effects

Pupillary dilatation, dry mouth, relatively unopposed sympathetic tone. The latter may be of import in acute myocardial infarction or myocardial ischemia, where tachycardia may increase myocardial oxygen demand beyond the ability of the coronary circulation.

Contraindications

Normal sinus rhythm or tachycardia. Use with caution in acute myocardial infarction or angina die to possibility of worsened ischemia with faster heart rate [8].

Dose

The usual dose is 0.5–1.0 mg IV every 5 minutes until the desired effect has been achieved, or a maximum dose of 3 mg (completely vagolytic in adults [8]). This may not be practical in the severely symptomatic patient, in whom more frequent or higher (1.0 mg) doses are required because of the urgency in reestablishing adequate tissue perfusion. Atropine can also be given per endotrachial tube (as can epinephrine or lidocaine), but the pharmacokinetics are not as favorable as with IV administration. Therefore, if given per endotracheal tube, it should be in 1.0-mg increments.

Bretylium

Bretylium prolongs the duration of cardiac cell action potential and refractory period. It is especially useful for reentrant arrhythmias with random conduction over multiple pathways, because it makes action potential duration more uniform throughout the myocardium [17,44]. Following an initial transient increase in blood pressure due to brief adrenergic stimulation, orthostatic hypotension is commonly seen. Primarily because of this, bretylium is not considered a first-line drug for VF or VT. In the acute setting, bretylium is used for refractory VT and VF, where it exerts an antifibrillatory effect that may facilitate subsequent electric defibrillation. There have also been reports of chemical defibrillation using bretylium after other methods have failed [44]. There may be a delayed onset of action from 2—10 minutes following bolus injection, so adequate circulation time should be allowed before concluding that no further defibrillation attempts are warranted [23,24]. Although the duration of action of a bolus dose is 2—6 hours, a lidocaine drip should probably be started once a perfusing rhythm has been established (see Lidocaine section, p. 81).

Adverse effects

Nausea and vomiting are common after IV injection. Postural hypotension is frequent, and may limit its use in hemodynamically stable VT. Bradycardia occurs, but is uncommon.

Contraindications

In a life-threatening situation, there are no absolute contraindications for use in ventricular arrhythmias [23]. Cautious use is advised in patients unable to increase their cardiac output in response to bretylium's expected hypotension (e.g., severe aortic stenosis, profound pulmonary hypertension, massive pulmonary embolism), digitalis toxicity, sinus bradycardia, and angina [17,44].

Dose

For refractory VF use 5—10 mg/kg IV bolus every 15—30 minutes, to a maximum of 30 mg/kg.

Digoxin

Actions/indications

Digoxin is one of the many foxglove derivatives that have found medicinal use, including increasing the force and velocity of myocardial contraction. It also prolongs the re-fractory period of the AV node, which is the basis for its use in slowing the ventricular response of SVT. In the emergency care setting, the indications for digoxin are limited to the latter [23], in part because of the relatively high incidence of digitalis toxicity, and because treatment of congestive failure with preload and afterload manipulation avoids the increased myocardial oxygen demand associated with the positive inotropic effects of digoxin.

Adverse effects

Digoxin has a low therapeutic index, with up to 20% of patients showing evidence of toxicity at some time [17]. There is large variation in response, a long half-life (1.5 days), and toxic manifestations may be life threatening. Noncardiac toxic symptoms are anorexia, nausea, vomiting, diarrhea, confusion, malaise, and visual disturbances. The cardiotoxic manifestations are more worrisome and include arrhythmias characterized by increased automaticity and conduction block: PACs, PVCs, AV block, SVT with or without 2:1 block, VT, and VF. The latter may be refractory to defibrillation. Factors that may potentiate digoxin toxicity are hypokalemia, hypercalcemia, hypomagnesemia, acidosis, renal insufficiency, quinidine therapy, and hypothyroidism [44]. Serum digoxin levels may be used as a gage of toxicity, with the usual therapeutic range 0.5—2.5 ng/ml [17]. Low levels with toxicity should prompt a search for the above potentiating factors.

Contraindications

Contraindications include established digitalis toxicity, significant AV block, hypertrophic obstructive cardiomyopathy, and Wolff—Parkinson—White (WPW) syndrome. Reduced dosage is suggested with hyperthyroidism, hypoxia, acute myocardial infarction, and electrolyte imbalance [17,23,44,49].

Dose

(For control of rapid ventricular response in SVT.)
● Loading dose: 0.25—0.50 mg IV.
● Incremental doses: 0.125—0.25 mg IV every 2—6 hours.
● End point: to desired ventricular rate, maximum of 0.75—1.0 mg, or signs of toxicity.

Dopamine

Actions/indications

Dopamine [17,23,24,44,49] is a catecholamine-like agent with varying effects dependent upon dose rate. At low infusion rates (1—2 µg/kg per min), so-called dopaminergic effects predominate, characterized by dilatation of renal and mesenteric vascular beds, but little effect on heart rate or blood pressure. At moderate (2–10 µg/kg per min) infusion rates, β-adrenergic effects are seen, resulting in increased cardiac output without much elevation of blood pressure. At the same time, renal blood flow is relatively preserved, up to about 7.5 µg/kg per min. At high infusion rates above 10 µg/kg per min, α-adrenergic effects predominate, and the drug behaves very much like epinephrine in this dose range. Thus, the benefit of preserved renal/mesenteric blood flow is lost, and peripheral vasoconstriction, raised blood pressure, and risk of tachyarrhythmias occur. Dopamine is used in cardiogenic and septic shock, bradycardia unresponsive to atropine, and electromechanical dissociation (EMD).

Adverse effects

As above, undesired elevation of blood pressure, PVCs, and various tachyarrhythmias may occur. If infused through a peripheral vein and extravasated, local tissue ischemia or necrosis may ensue, so whenever possible, administration through a central line is advised.

Contraindications

Ventricular arrhythmias and pheochromocytoma. MAO enzymatically inactivates norepinephrine, dopamine, and serotonin. MAOIs increase the concentration of catecholamines in the neuron and around the receptor, so the dose should be cut to 10% of what would normally be used [17,44].

Dose

Mix one ampule (200 mg) in 250 ml D5W and begin IV infusion at 1 µg/kg per min.

Titrate to desired clinical end point. Doses from 2 to 10 µg/kg per min generally have β-adrenergic effect, while at greater than 10 µg/min, α-adrenergic effects predominate [8].

Epinephrine

Actions/indications

Epinephrine is a potent endogenously occurring catecholamine with both α- and β-adrenergic effects [17,23,24,44]. At low concentrations, as may be seen with subcutaneous or slow IV infusion (1–2 µg/min), β-effects predominate, while at higher rates (2–10 µg/min), and bolus doses used in cardiac resuscitation, α-adrenergic effects predominate [50]. The α-effects are highly desirable in the treatment of the arrested heart, because of peripheral vasoconstriction, which raises blood pressure and relatively favors blood supply to the coronary and cerebral circulations [42,48]. Coronary blood flow is facilitated by the rise in aortic diastolic pressure which occurs with peripheral vasoconstriction. Cerebral circulation is favored because the external carotid (a peripheral branch) is selectively vasoconstricted, forcing blood flow into the internal carotid artery. The potent β-component results in a dramatic positive inotropic and chronotropic cardiac response. Because of shortened repolarization time and increased conduction velocities, epinephrine may theoretically facilitate defibrillation of VF. This may be evident as conversion of low-amplitude "fine" VF to higher amplitude "coarse" VF, which appears to be more susceptible to defibrillation [23,24]. It is used in EMD in an attempt to increase myocardial contractility and blood pressure [51–53]. In asystole, it may be able to generate some electric and mechanical activity [23,24]. As above, epinephrine is of great value in CPR because of preferential internal carotid perfusion.

Adverse effects

Epinephrine is a potent adrenergic agent and should be treated with respect in patients with established perfusing rhythms, in whom it will increase heart rate and blood pressure. This may result in severe hypertension, ventricular tachyarrhythmias, increased myocardial oxygen demand, angina, or left ventricular decompensation. Decreased renal blood flow may exacerbate renal injury in patients with preexisting renal insufficiency. If extravasated outside of a peripheral vein, local skin necrosis can occur.

Contraindications

VT, multiple PVCs, hypertension [17,23,24,44]. Use with caution in normotensive patients (e.g., anaphylaxis treatment) and in patients on tricyclic antidepressants and MAOIs.

Dose

Anaphylaxis

IV infusion of 0.1 mg (100 µg)/min [50] or 0.1–1.0 mg IV bolus. (Note adverse effects as above.)

Cardiac resuscitation

• IV bolus: 1.0 mg every 3–5 minutes as needed [8].
• IV infusion: mix 1 mg in 250 ml D5W, begin infusion at 1 µg/min.
• Endotracheal tube: 1.0 mg in 10 ml saline down endotracheal tube followed by several forceful insufflations.

Isoproteronol

Actions/indications

Isoproteronol is a synthetic catecholamine with β_1- and β_2-adrenergic effects. It is the most potent β-agonist available per microgram. At lower doses, its β_1-effects predominate, providing predominantly chronotropic effects. When higher doses are used, its β_2-effects become more predominant [23], and both positive cardiac inotropic effects and peripheral vasodilatation are seen. This may result in significantly increased cardiac output and demands on myocardial oxygen consumption. It is also a bronchodilator (β_2-component). Its primary utility in emergency cardiac care is for symptomatic bradycardia unresponsive to atropine and in high-degree AV block to increase the rate of idioventricular foci, and/or decrease the block as a temporizing measure prior to cardiac pacing. An exception to this is the patient who is so bradycardic that chest compression is required. In this circumstance, the lowered peripheral vascular resistance of isoproteronol is extremely detrimental, and epinephrine or high-dose dopamine would be a better choice [23]. Isoproteronol is *not* a pressor agent.

Adverse effects

Myocardial ischemia (especially with CAD) secondary to increased cardiac output and possible hypotension from peripheral vasodilatation. Sinus or ventricular tachyarrythmias are also seen.

Contraindications

Tachycardia, existing VA, angina. It should not be used in asystole, EMD, or VF [23].

Dose

Mix 1 mg in 250 ml D5W and begin infusion at 0.5 μg/min. Usual adult range is 0.5−20 μg/min.

Lidocaine

Actions/indications

Lidocaine [17,23,24,44,49] is a local anesthetic agent with very useful antiarrhythmic properties, largely confined to the ventricles, with very little antiarrhythmic effect on the atria or AV node. In toxic doses, however, it may depress automaticity of the sinus node. It preferentially decreases automaticity in ischemic ventricular tissue [54], and it is effective against orderly reentrant arrhythmias such as VT and bigeminy, by improving conduction time. For lidocaine to be optimally effective, hypokalemia must be corrected.

Lidocaine is cleared by the liver, so conditions that impair hepatic blood flow or function should be expected to raise lidocaine blood levels and raise the risk of toxicity. These would include hepatitis, congestive heart failure (pulmonary edema), shock, advanced age, and cimetidine [23]. In these patients, dosages should be reduced (approximately 50% usual dose). Indications for lidocaine in acute situations include suppression of frequent (> 6−8 bpm), multifocal, or ischemia-related PVCs, VT, and VF [23,24,44]. For recurrent VF after initially successful defibrillation, lidocaine may be given before additional defibrillation attempts, but other causes of recurrent or refractory VF such as hypoxia and acidosis should be sought and corrected.

Adverse effects

Adverse effects are uncommon with therapeutic levels, occurring usually as a manifestation of toxicity when therapeutic levels are exceeded. Inhibition of the sinus node with subsequent bradycardia and hypotension can occur, but the most common adverse reactions relate to the central nervous system. In rough order of increasing blood level, these include: numbness, dizziness, drowsiness, dysarthria, confusion, seizures, and respiratory arrest [23].

Contraindications

Bradycardia may be exacerbated, and escape beats (if present as a back-up mechanism) may be suppressed. Idioventricular rhythm may be converted to asystole, so lidocaine should never be given in third-degree AV block. As above, doses should be reduced in patients with reason to suspect decreased hepatic function, and there should be a higher index of suspicion of toxicity in these patients.

Dose

For PVC control and hemodynamically stable VT

- Loading dose: 1 mg/kg, repeated in 20 minutes if needed.
- Maintenance dose: 1−4 mg/min, titrate to effect.

Nonperfusing VT and VF

- Bolus of 1 mg/kg, repeated once in 2−5 minutes.
- Infusion at 1−4 mg/min, once a perfusing rhythm has been established.

Procainamide

Actions/indications

Procainamide [17,23,24,44,49] is a local anesthetic agent which acts by stabilizing cell membranes to decrease automaticity and conduction in both perfused and ischemic myocardium, as opposed to lidocaine, which preferentially influences ischemic regions. By decreasing conduction, it may convert regions of unidirectional block to bidirectional block, thereby interrupting reentrant arrhythmias. By inhibiting automaticity, it has utility against enhanced automaticity supraventricular arrhythmias. Although it has a wide spectrum of activity against atrial, AV nodal, and ventricular arrhythmias, its primary indication is for hemodynamically stable VT refractory to lidocaine.

Adverse effects

Hypotension secondary to vasodilatation is common, especially with dose rates above 25 mg/min [17]. AV block of varying degree may occur or progress. *Torsade de pointes* is an uncommon form of VT associated with a prolonged QT interval that may be caused or exacerbated by procainamide, quinidine, and other drugs [23]. Confusion and seizures can be seen with toxic doses.

Contraindications

Shock, heart block, and severe renal failure (renal clearance). Cimetidine inhibits renal clearance of procainamide, so dose should be reduced.

Dose

For hemodynamically stable VT refractory to lidocaine

- Loading: 10–50 mg/min to a total dose of 10–12 mg/kg [44] or until conversion of tachycardia, hypotension, or widening of the QRS by 50% occurs.
- Maintenance: 2–6 mg/min.

Propranolol

Actions/indications

Propranolol [17,23,24,44,49] is the prototype β-blocking agent, possessing both β_1- and β_2-antagonist effects. By blocking β_1-receptors, it slows heart rate, prolongs conduction, and decreases contractility. By blocking β_2-receptors, it tends to promote increased smooth muscle tone, which may lead to bronchospasm and cold extremities in susceptible patients. It is metabolized in the liver, so hepatic dysfunction or decreased hepatic blood flow (as can occur with cimetidine) may lead to toxicity. Although propranolol and other more selective β_1-blocking agents are in widespread use for treatment of hypertension, the indications for use in acute care situations are extremely limited. Propranolol is used in acute cardiac care situations as a third-line drug for control of SVT (especially AF and atrial flutter) refractory to digoxin

and verapamil, and occasionally for control of ventricular tachyarrhythmias.

Adverse effects

Bronchospasm and cold extremities may result from increased smooth muscle tone. Bradycardia, second- or third-degree AV block, and symptomatic hypotension may occur. With chronic use, central nervous system symptoms such as insomnia, fatigue, and confusion are reported.

Contraindications

Absolute contraindications include severe asthma, bronchospasm, symptomatic or severe bradycardia, second- or third-degree AV block, congestive heart failure, and severe peripheral vascular disease (rest pain, gangrene, threatened limb, accelerating claudication). Relative contraindications include treated congestive failure, recent IV verapamil, (synergistic effects of propranolol and verapamil may cause severe bradycardia or asystole), mild peripheral vascular disease, and hepatic dysfunction.

Dose

For control of rapid SVT unresponsive to digoxin and verapamil: 1 mg *slowly* over at least 5 minutes under constant monitoring. Repeat 1-mg increments as above to desired ventricular rate or maximum of 3–5 mg.

Verapamil

Actions/indications

Verapamil [17,23,24,44,49] is a calcium channel antagonist with wide therapeutic potential, including dramatically effective control of SVT. It inhibits the action potential in the upper and middle portions of the AV node (where depolarization is calcium mediated), and thus may inhibit the faster limb of reentry circuits responsible for perpetuation of a SVT. Additionally, it increases AV block and the relative refractory period of the AV node, accounting for its application in reduction of fast ventricular rates in atrial flutter and AF. Blood pressure is lowered secondary to peripheral vasodilatation due to vascular smooth muscle inhibition, and a direct negative cardiac inotropic effect. The expected tachycardia from the peripheral vasodilatation is generally counterbalanced by the negative chronotropic effect on the SA node, so that overall, there is little or variable effect on heart rate. Verapamil also has utility in therapy of MAT if correction of underlying hypoxia is unsuccessful.

Adverse effects

Headaches, facial flushing, dizziness, constipation, and ankle swelling are side-effects common to all calcium channel blockers. Hypotension, especially common in the elderly, is often seen, and may be controlled by slow incremental dosing or pretreatment with calcium chloride (see below). If given in the presence of preexisting AV block from disease or medication (e.g., β-blockade from propranolol), IV verapamil can severely slow the AV node and result in insufficient cardiac output. With sick sinus syndrome, asystole may follow IV injection.

Contraindications

IV verapamil is contraindicated in sick sinus syndrome, preexisting AV nodal disease (e.g., second- and third-degree AV block), digitalis toxicity, and quinidine therapy. It should not be given to patients with significant systolic hypotension, as its peripheral vasodilator effects may precipitate cardiovascular collapse [41]. In WPW syndrome with antegrade conduction through the bypass tract, it is theoretically possible for AF impulses to be conducted to the ventricles, precipitating VF; thus, IV verapamil should never be given to patients with WPW syndrome with AF or atrial flutter [41]. Despite this, verapamil can safely be used in the majority of narrow complex SVT. (See Adenosine section, p. 78.)

Dose

(Note: IV verapamil should only be given to monitored patients.)

For termination of reentrant SVT

- IV test dose of 1 mg, followed by 2.5–5.0 mg IV increments every 1–2 minutes until the tachycardia terminates, AV block develops, there is hypotension, or a total dose of 10–15 mg is given.
- Caution and/or decreased dosage is necessary in patients with left ventricular dysfunction or β-blocker therapy.

Note: hypotension may be treated with calcium infusion, or prevented by pretreatment with calcium chloride, 1 g IV over 5–10 minutes prior to IV verapamil. This appears to eliminate its hypotensive effect without diminishing its antiarrhythmic properties [55,56]. This may be especially appropriate in SVT with marginal (systolic blood pressure under 100 mmHg) blood pressure.

Resuscitation algorithms

The intention of this section is to review the steps outlined in the resuscitation algorithms presented in this chapter. *The practitioner desiring knowledge and skills in management of cardio-pulmonary emergencies is referred to Grauer and Cavalloro's text [23] and, for the most current information and concepts, is urged to complete the American Heart Association's ACLS course.* The problems to be covered are asystole, EMD, bradycardia, SVT, VT, VF, and contrast reaction. As with prehospital delivery of emergency medical services [5–7,23,24], the key to greater survival rates of in-hospital cardiopulmonary arrest and preservation of neurologic function lies in the "chain of survival" concept: prompt recognition of apnea and pulselessness, rapid activation of a system that provides immediate basic life support (CPR) and rapidly follows that with automatic external defibrillation (if available), and finally advanced life support (ACLS) techniques. In this regard, the radiology department can be thought of in terms of providing the primary recognition and early management of cardiopulmonary arrest, transitional care (including automatic external defibrillation) before the code team arrives, and institution of ACLS protocols. A systems approach is advocated, based on early recognition, prompt institution of therapy, communication with ACLS trained personnel, and integration of the emergency response of the radiology department into that of the hospital as a whole. Periodic drills, review sessions, equipment inventory/function checks, and BLS/ACLS certification are urged.

In general, the sequence of events begins with the "ABCs": airway, breathing, and circulation. The patient is assessed for unresponsiveness, and assistance is summoned. If not contraindicated, the head and neck are positioned to open the airway, and the adequacy of spontaneous respiratory efforts is assessed. If necessary, two quick breaths are given, and the carotid artery is checked for a pulse. If absent, CPR (preferably two person) is instituted and the code team summoned. Initial advanced life support measures are instituted as soon as qualified personnel and equipment are available.

Bradycardia (Fig. 4.33)

As a rule, bradycardias of multiple different etiologies lend themselves to algorithm discussion because of the similarities of treatment between sinus bradycardia, slow ventricular response due to AV block, and slow idioventricular rhythm. The key question to ask in any case of bradycardia is whether or not there is hemodynamic compromise (systolic blood pressure less than 90 mmHg, altered mental status, syncope, etc.). If not, observation and correction of the underlying cause (e.g., pain resulting in increased parasympathetic tone) is all that is necessary, unless the ventricular rate is less than 30 bpm, in which case atropine may well be considered because cardiac output is unlikely to be sufficient for long, and ventricular escape beats may occur.

If there is hemodynamic compromise, a volume infusion of 500 ml NS or LR can be started (unless contraindicated by CHF or pulmonary edema), and depending upon the urgency of the situation, 0.5–1.0 mg of atropine IV can be given

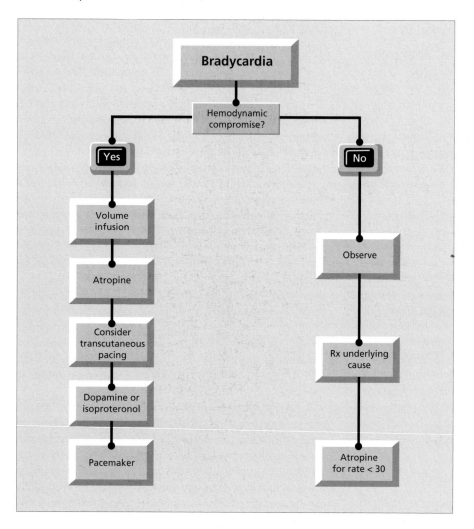

Fig. 4.33 Bradycardia treatment algorithm.

simultaneously, with repeated 0.5−1.0-mg increments to a total of 2.0−3.0 mg (completely vagolytic in most adults [23,24,50,57]. As with any case of hemodynamic compromise, oxygen should be given to maximize tissue oxygenation. If there is concern regarding volume excess, the infusion should be decreased as soon as a satisfactory rate is established. If the bradycardia is unresponsive to atropine, chronotropic dopamine or isoproteronol drips may be started and titrated to the desired ventricular rate [23,44]. As a last resort, a pacemaker may be required [23,58−60].

Asystole (Fig. 4.34)

Asystole occurring in a procedural setting may actually be profound bradycardia secondary to overwhelming parasympathetic tone [23], as distinguished from asystole occurring as a result of myocardial infarction. Obviously, the former has a much better prognosis, and although it is tempting to use atropine first because of this, epinephrine for asystole is a better initial choice because not only will it accelerate any potentially present sinus activity, it is the one

drug that preferentially preserves cerebral and coronary blood flow during cardiac arrest and CPR [42,48]. Since asystole is a "fatal rhythm", giving high doses of epinephrine is a "no-lose" situation. Frequent and liberal use of epinephrine is advocated [23,42], which can be given IV or via endotracheal tube every few minutes while CPR is in progress. Bicarbonate administration should ideally be guided by arterial blood gas determination. As with any cardiopulmonary emergency, detailed attention to the airway and adequacy of ventilation/oxygenation is of paramount importance, both to provide adequate tissue oxygenation and to facilitate respiratory correction of metabolic acidosis; both of which will improve the environment of the myocardium and favor successful conversion.

On occasion, "fine" VF may look like a flat-line EKG if the gain is set too low or the fibrillatory waves are perpendicular to the EKG lead being observed. Thus, it is necessary to confirm asystole in at least two leads (if using quick-look paddles, rotate paddle placement 90°) and to check that there is adequate gain on the monitor before concluding that there is no cardiac electric activity. Additionally, epinephrine

nodal conduction just long enough to interrupt a reentrant circuit that involves the AV node and, thus, terminate the tachycardia. Vagal maneuvers may also slow a SVT sufficiently to allow P waves to become visible, thus allowing greater diagnostic accuracy [23]. If vagal maneuvers are unsuccessful, adenosine is the first-line drug to be tried [16,41]. As discussed previously, it acts to interrupt atrial or AV nodal reentrant tachycardias by slowing AV conduction. It is given as a 6-mg IV bolus, followed in 1−2 minutes by 12-mg IV bolus if unsuccessful [17]. The 12-mg dose may be repeated in another 1−2 minutes if needed, but doses above this are unlikely to be successful [42]. If symptomatic SVT continues or recurs, IV verapamil is the next drug of choice, administered in 2.5−5.0-mg IV boluses every 1−2 minutes until the tachycardia is terminated, AV block ensues, hypotension occurs, or a total of 10−15 mg has been given [17,23]. As discussed previously, hypotension is a problem, which can be prevented or corrected with calcium administration [55,56].

WPW syndrome

Although a full discussion of accessory pathways and AV reciprocating tachycardias is well beyond the scope or intent of this chapter, a consideration of the WPW syndrome is appropriate at this point. For a full discussion, see references by Caruso [16], Grauer and Cavallora [23], Sager and Bhandari [41] and Arai and Kron [43] WPW is a form of preexcitation of the ventricles due to the presence of an accessory conduction pathway directly from the atrium to the ventricle, occurring with an estimated prevalence of 0.15%, although this may underestimate the true incidence. With normal sinus rhythm in WPW, the impulse reaches the ventricle sooner than expected, resulting in a PR interval that may be less than 0.12 seconds, and a "slurred" upstroke of the QRS (δ-wave) which represents the early depolarization of the ventricles. As a result, the QRS may be widened (>0.12 seconds). Two major arrhythmias are associated with WPW: AF and AV reciprocating tachycardia. Each will be considered as it relates to treatment of SVT.

AF may occur in 11.5−39% of WPW patients, although the exact mechanism for development of AF in these patients is unknown. If conduction is predominantly down the normal AV conduction system, the transmitted ventricular beats will have narrow QRS complexes, but every now and then a beat may be conducted by the accessory pathway, resulting in occasional wide QRS complexes. Thus, AF with a rapid response and occasional wide QRS complexes is suggestive of WPW. If conduction through the AV node is slowed by drugs such as verapamil or digoxin, the ventricular rate in WPW patients with AF may accelerate dramatically, or the rhythm may degenerate to VF. This may occur if the AF waves are conducted by the accessory pathway directly to the ventricle, or if an impulse is transmitted in the ventricle's

vulnerable period. Thus, a patient in AF with the WPW syndrome should not receive verapamil or digoxin. The goal of therapy in these patients should be to lengthen the antegrade refractory period by administration of procainamide. As with any other SVT, synchronized cardioversion is the treatment of choice should hemodynamic compromise (hypotension, angina, pulmonary edema, loss of consciousness, etc.) develop. If time and circumstances permit, sedation with midazolam or diazepam is advised.

Reciprocating AV tachycardia is possible in WPW because a circuit of conduction can occur involving the accessory pathway and the normal AV conduction system. A PAC or PVC, if timed just right, may be conducted up or down one path and not the other, thus comprising a unidirectional block and initiating a circus-movement tachycardia. The most common situation is for antegrade impulse conduction down the normal AV conduction system and up the accessory pathway (orthodromic SVT), and this may be the underlying mechanism in as much as 20% of all PSVT. Because the impulse enters the ventricles in a normal fashion, the QRS is narrow. Vagal stimulation, adenosine, and verapamil in orthodromic SVT may slow the antegrade limb of the reciprocating AV circuit enough to terminate the tachycardia.

In the minority of AV reciprocating tachycardia in WPW, there is antegrade conduction down the accessory pathway and retrograde up the normal AV conduction system (antidromic SVT). This results in a wide QRS because of the ventricular insertion point of the accessory pathway. With wide complex SVT, differentiation from VT may be difficult, and the best course of action is to presume that all wide complex tachycardias are VT until proven otherwise, and proceed accordingly. Fortunately, this does not involve the use of verapamil, because there is a high incidence of hemodynamic collapse, VF, and cardiac arrest when verapamil is given in VT. Additionally, procainamide and to a lesser extent lidocaine may terminate AV reciprocating tachycardia by blocking conduction in the accessory pathway, and both of these medications are included in the algorithm, although procainamide is used as a second-line drug (see VT section, below).

In summary, the majority of PSVT is due to reentrant mechanisms in the atria or AV node, and readily treated with sequential application of vagal stimulation, adenosine, and verapamil. Most WPW syndromes with reciprocating AV tachycardia respond to the same treatment. A regular wide complex tachycardia should be presumed to be VT until proven otherwise and treated as such, avoiding the use of verapamil.

VT (Fig. 4.37)

As with bradycardia and SVT, the management of sustained (>30 seconds) VT hinges on the clinical presentation. If there is no pulse, the situation is urgent because this is by

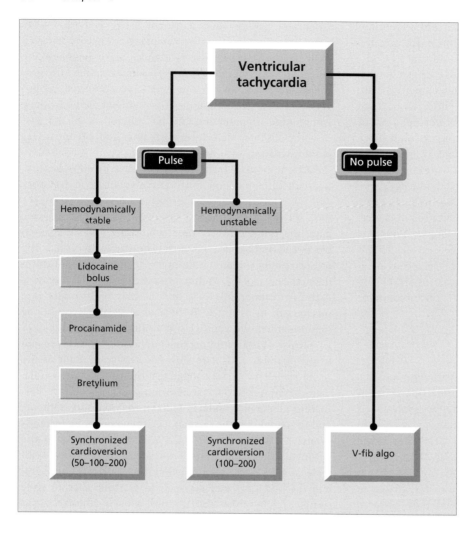

Fig. 4.37 VT treatment algorithm.

definition a nonperfusing rhythm. Pulseless VT is treated exactly the same as VF: immediate defibrillation starting at 200 J [23,24] (see VF section, below). As noted above, if there is uncertainty regarding whether or not the rhythm is SVT with aberrant conduction or VT, the patient should be treated for VT, as this is by far the most common cause of wide complex tachycardias, and is life threatening [45].

For VT with a pulse, the next question that must be answered is whether or not there is hemodynamic compromise. If so, or if during the course of pharmacologic treatment of hemodynamically stable VT the patient becomes unstable (angina, pulmonary edema, loss of consciousness, profound hypotension, etc.), then immediate synchronized cardioversion is the treatment of choice. Energy levels of 100–200 J are suggested for the first attempt, and if unsuccessful, 300–360 J for subsequent attempts [23,24,45]. (Sedation for the still conscious patient requiring emergency cardioversion is recommended [23,24].) As previously discussed, the rationale for synchronized cardioversion is to time the delivery of the shock so as to miss the vulnerable period

and hopefully avoid VF. Monitoring the patient in a lead with a tall, upright R wave is desirable in order for the defibrillator accurately to sense the R wave.

For hemodynamically stable VT, the initial drug of choice is lidocaine, particularly in a setting of myocardial ischemia, delivered as a bolus of 1 mg/kg, repeated in 5–20 minutes if required; a maintenance drip of 1–4 mg/min is recommended once the rhythm has been converted [17,23,24]. For patients with congestive heart failure or hepatic dysfunction, the infusion rate should be decreased by 50%. Procainamide is the next recommended drug, given as a slow injection of 10–12 mg/kg at a rate not to exceed 50 mg/min [44]. Widening of the QT interval, hypotension, and decreased left ventricular function are adverse effects. Once converted, a procainamide infusion at 1–4 mg/min may be started [23]. If refractory to procainamide, bretylium is the last routinely recommended drug, often reserved for resistant cases because of the common side-effects of hypotension and bradycardia. It is given as a 5–10-mg/kg bolus up to a total of 30 mg/kg [23], with hypotension seen as a major side-effect [17,23]. If all pharmacologic methods fail to control hemodynamically stable VT, then sedation and synchronized cardioversion can be attempted.

VF (Fig. 4.38)

The single most effective treatment for the patient in VF is early defibrillation [5–7,23,24]. As with the community emergency medical system (EMS) system, the greatest impact on patient outcome can be expected when there is a co-ordinated effort among the practitioners closest to the patient (in this case, radiology personnel), and those trained in automatic or manual defibrillation and ACLS techniques. To be optimally effective, the defibrillator and all associated oxygenation, ventilation, and suction apparatus, as well as resuscitative drugs need to be immediately available. Although intubation, IV access, and pharmacologic methods all are important, the initial focus should be on establishing the diagnosis of VF and *rapid* defibrillation. As discussed earlier, quick-look paddles may facilitate this process, as will training and familiarity with the equipment. CPR, of course, must continue until a perfusing rhythm is established or resuscitative attempts are abandoned. CPR should be interrupted as briefly as possible for defibrillation and intubation attemps.

The rationale underlying defibrillation starting at modest energy levels and progressing upward is that somewhat fewer complications (e.g., asystole, heart block) may occur at the lower energy levels, and it is possible that the rhythm may convert [23,42]. If unsuccessful, subsequent shocks at higher energies and at close intervals maximize the current delivered to the heart, presumably due in part to lowered transthoracic resistance with subsequent shocks [23,24]. Intubation and IV access have been previously discussed. It should be remembered that epinephrine and lidocaine may

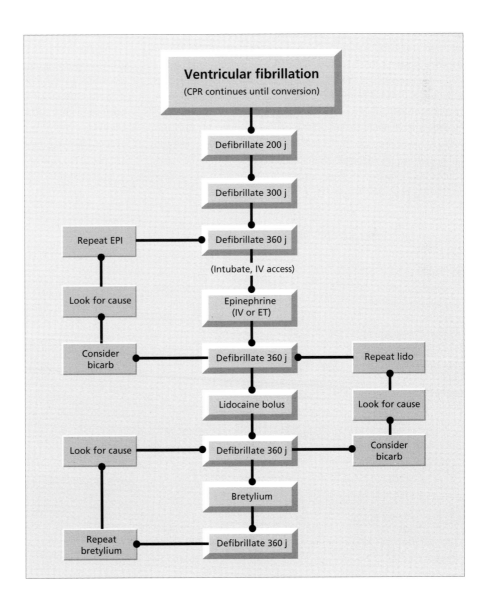

Fig. 4.38 VF treatment algorithm.

be given per endotracheal tube if IV access cannot be established. As with asystole and EMD, liberal and frequent use of epinephrine has been advocated because of its beneficial effects of preservation of coronary and cerebral blood flow, and positive inotropic and chronotropic cardiac effects [42]. One should allow sufficient time for the epinephrine to reach the central circulation while CPR is in progress before subsequent defibrillation attempts. Additional epinephrine may be given after lidocaine and bretylium if required. Likewise, there is no limit to the number of times defibrillation may be attempted [23].

If refractory to epinephrine and defibrillation, and hypoxia has been corrected, a lidocaine bolus of 1 mg/kg may be given, allowed to circulate with CPR, and defibrillation repeated. (It should be noted, however, that the use of lidocaine in refractory VF has recently been questioned, and further studies have been advocated [54,61]). The lidocaine bolus may be repeated in 2–5 minutes, but because hepatic blood flow by definition is decreased during CPR, lidocaine toxicity may occur somewhat sooner than with a perfusing rhythm. For this reason, it may be preferable to withhold the lidocaine infusion of 1–4 mg/min until the patient is converted out of VF, and there is a perfusing rhythm. If this is done, one should not forget to start the lidocaine drip once conversion has occurred [23,24].

Sodium bicarbonate may be considered if 5–10 minutes have elapsed, but ideally, bicarbonate administration should be governed by arterial blood gas determination [23,24]. Additionally, adequate ventilation should be able to counter much of the expected metabolic acidosis by respiratory correction.

Bretylium [17,23,44,49] may facilitate electrical conversion of VF, but its antifibrillatory effects may not be apparent for 10–15 minutes following administration, and thus it is not used as a first-line drug. The first dose of 5 mg/kg should be allowed to circulate for about 2 minutes before the next defibrillation attempt. The second dose of 10 mg/kg may be given after the next few unsuccessful defibrillation attempts, with repeated defibrillation after that. There is no theoretic limit to the number of times defibrillation can be performed [23].

Contrast reaction (Fig. 4.39)

This algorithm is included with arrhythmias only because of the potential for hypertension and tachyarrhythmias when epinephrine is used for treatment of anaphylaxis. A complete discussion of contrast-reaction treatment is covered elsewhere in this text (see Chapter 13). Flushing, nausea, and vomiting will not be discussed, as they are not considered life-threatening events, but they do constitute adverse drug reactions to the contrast media, and deserve due attention. As a rule, most contrast reactions are self-limited, and require not much more than close observation and reassurance. For example, hives need not be treated with antihistamines unless they are particularly widespread and symptomatic or are occurring in a sensitive location such as the eyelid.

Not infrequently, a contrast reaction will be manifest as

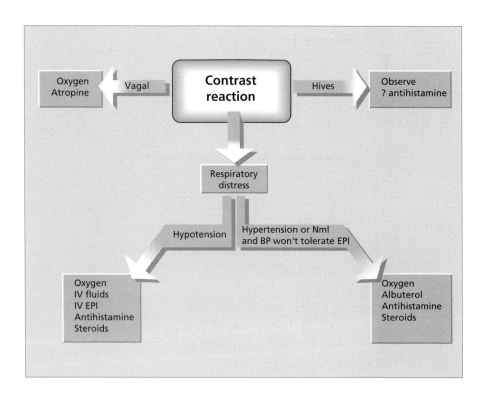

Fig. 4.39 Contrast-reaction treatment algorithm.

inappropriately increased parasympathetic tone. These vagal reactions are readily treated with Trendelenburg positioning, IV fluids, 0.5−1.0 mg IV atropine, and oxygen [50]. The same principles as outlined in the bradycardia algorithm may be used for treatment.

Many severe or life-threatening contrast reactions will have a component of respiratory distress, often secondary to bronchospasm or laryngeal edema. If associated with hypotension, then the mainstay of therapy is epinephrine, which should be administered IV in order to be sure that the dose has been delivered (peripheral vasoconstriction as a compensatory mechanism for anaphylactic shock may result in unpredictable subcutaneous absorption). Typical doses are 0.1−1.0 mg IV, depending upon the urgency of the situation and the patient's underlying cardiovascular status. Bush and colleagues [50,57] have pointed out that low-dose epinephrine in the range of 0.1 mg/min IV has the advantage of providing β_1- and β_2-adrenergic stimulation, while sparing the α-adrenergic effects at this dose level. van Sonnenberg *et al.* [12] have demonstrated the value of vigorous intravascular fluid replacement therapy, comprising 1−3 l of NS or LR at 200−300 ml/min. As discussed previously, this may be best accomplished through the use of a short, large bore peripheral IV cannula. Oxygen, of course, is desirable for any patient in respiratory or cardiovascular distress. Steroids may do little to alter the course of the acute reaction, but may offer some protection against recurrent reaction, and antihistamines (diphenhydramine and cimetidine) may decrease some histamine-mediated effects.

An occasionally encountered variation is the patient who develops respiratory distress and hypertension, or whose cardiovascular status is such that epinephrine would be poorly tolerated (e.g., angina, recent myocardial infarction, cardiomyopathy, etc.). Treatment in this circumstance is similar to hypotensive anaphylaxis, except that much more caution in regards to α-adrenergic receptors must be used. As advocated by Bush and colleagues [50,57], low-dose epinephrine may be used to maximize the β_1- and β_2-effects, or a selective β_1-agonist such as inhaled albuterol may be given.

Latex anaphylaxis

An infrequently seen but related problem is latex allergy. At the author's institution, we have seen four cases of potentially life-threatening anaphylaxis associated with inflation of latex rectal balloons used for barium enema examination. All were successfully treated with volume expansion, epinephrine, steroids, and support of blood pressure and oxygenation. Ownby *et al.* [62] reported six similar cases of immunoglobulin E (IgE)-mediated latex allergy, with classic signs and symptoms of anaphylaxis including facial erythema/edema, itching/burning eyes, urticaria, profound hypotension, and respiratory distress. There was one fatality.

Other reported cases of what appears to be IgE-mediated latex anaphylaxis include intraoperative exposure to rubber gloves, wearing of surgical or household latex gloves, rubber dams used in dental procedures, and use of latex gloves during vaginal examination [63−66]. Morales *et al.* [67] assume that the water-soluble allergen involved is hevein, a component of latex, and speculates that the recent (within the last decade) emergence of reported latex anaphylaxis may relate to changes in the latex manufacturing processes or other technical factors. The resuscitative approach to latex anaphylaxis is similar to that of contrast reaction, although it has been our experience (and by description, apparently that of Ownby *et al.* [62]) that these cases tend to be more severe than the "usual" contrast reaction. With the onset of profound hypotension and respiratory distress, immediate therapies include IV epinephrine, volume expansion, and support of ventilation/oxygenation. Steroids are also recommended, but may not play a role in immediate stabilization (see also p. 496).

Summary

As interventional radiologists accept a greater role in the management of increasingly complex clinical problems, there is a need for increased responsibility in the prevention and management of iatrogenic or spontaneously occurring emergencies. As the complexity and risk of interventional radiologic procedures increases, practitioners will need to hone skills to prevent, identify, and treat these complications. This chapter has summarized some aspects of preparing for, identifying, and dealing with adverse events occurring in association with interventional radiologic procedures. Preprocedural evaluation, patient preparation, intraprocedural care, monitoring, airway management, and arrhythmia recognition/management have been discussed. Application of these techniques will enhance the safe and effective application of image-guided interventions for the benefit of all our patients.

References

1 Health Care Financing Administration (HCFA). *Part-B Medicare Annualized Data (BMAD) file.* 1990.

2 Society of Cardiovascular and Interventional Radiology. *Standards of Practice.* Written Communication, April 1992.

3 Capek P, McLean GK, Berkowitz HD. Femoropopliteal angioplasty: factors influencing long term success. *Circulation* 1991; 83(2)(Suppl. I):1-70−1-80.

4 Hertzer NR. The natural history of peripheral vascular disease: implications for its management. *Circulation* 1991;83(2)(Suppl. I):1-12−1-19.

5 Montgomery WH. Prehospital cardiac arrest: the chain of survival concept. *Ann Acad Med* 1992;21(1):69−72.

6 Cummins RO *et al.* Improving survival from sudden cardiac arrest: the "chain of survival" concept. *Circulation* 1991;83(5): 1832−1847.

7 Hunt RC, McCabe JB, Hamilton GC, Krohmer JR. Influence of emergency medical services systems and prehospital defibrillation on survival of sudden cardiac death victims. *Am J Emerg Med* 1989;7:68−82.

8 Emergency Cardiac Care Committee and Subcommittees, American Heart Association. Guidelines for cardiopulmonary resuscitation and emergency cardiac care, I: introduction. *J Am Med Assoc* 1992;268:2171−2183.

9 Shuster M, Keller JL. Effect of fire department first-responder automated defibrillation. *Ann Emerg Med* 1993;22(4):721−727.

10 Schrading WA, Stein S, Eitel DR *et al.* An evaluation of automated defibrillation and manual defibrillation by emergency medical technicians in a rural setting. *Am J Emerg Med* 1993;11(2): 125−130.

11 Berkseth RO, Kjellstrand CM. Radiologic contrast-induced nephropathy. *Med Clin N Am* 1984;68(2):351−370.

12 van Sonnenberg E, Neff C, Pfister R. Life-threatening reactions to contrast media administration: comparison of pharmacologic and fluid therapy. *Radiology* 1987;162:15−19.

13 Becker DE. The respiratory effects of drugs used for conscious sedation and general anesthesia. *J Am Dent Assoc* 1989;119: 153−156.

14 Katayama H, Yamaguchi K, Kozuka T *et al.* Adverse reactions to ionic and nonionic contrast media. *Radiology* 1990;175(3): 621−628.

15 Lang DM, Alpern MB, Visintainer PF, Smith ST. Increased risk for anaphylactoid reaction from contrast media in patients on beta-adrenergic blockers or with asthma. *Ann Int Med* 1991;115: 270−276.

16 Caruso AC. Supraventricular tachycardia: changes in management. *Postgrad Med* 1991;90(2):000−000.

17 Opie LH. *Drugs for the Heart.* Philadelphia, PA: WB Saunders Company, 1991.

18 Hansten PD, Horn JR. *Drug Interactions and Updates.* Malvern, Pennsylvania: Lea and Febiger, 1990.

19 In: Young JR, Graor RA, Olin JW, Bartholomew JR, eds. *Peripheral Vascular Diseases.* Mosby Year Book, Inc., 1991.

20 Murphy TP, Dorfman GS, Becker J. Use of preprocedural tests by interventional radiologists. *Radiology* 1993;186:213−220.

21 Joint Commission on Accreditation of Healthcare Organizations. *Comprehensive Accreditation Manual for Hospitals.* Illinois: Joint Commission on Accreditation of Healthcare Organizations, 1994:134−137.

22 Trunkey DD, Collicot PE, Aprahamian C *et al. Advanced Trauma Life Support Course for Physicians.* Chicago: American College of Surgeons, 1984.

23 Grauer K, Cavallaro D. *ACLS, Certification Preparation and a Comprehensive Review,* 2nd edn. Missouri: St. Louis CV. Mosby Co., 1987.

24 ACLS Subcommittee, EEC Committee. *Textbook of Advanced Cardiac Life Support,* 2nd edn. Dallas: American Heart Association, 1990.

25 Stanley TE, Reves JG. Cardiovascular monitoring. In: Miller RD, ed. *Anesthesia,* 3rd edn. New York: Churchill Livingstone Inc., 1990.

26 Conroy JM, Rajogopolan PR, Baker JD 3rd, Bailey MK. A modification of the supraclavicular approach to the central circulation. *S Med J* 1990;83(10):1178−1181.

27 Sterner S, Plummer DW, Clinton J, Ruiz E. A comparison of the supraclavicular approach and the infraclavicular approach for subclavian vein catheterization. *Ann Emerg Med* 1986;15(4): 421−424.

28 Matthews NT, Worthley LG. Immediate problems associated with infraclavicular subclavian catheterization; a comparison between left and right sides. *Anaesth Intens Care* 1982;10(2): 113−115.

29 LaFreniere R. Indwelling subclavian catheters and a visit with the "pinched-off sign". *J Surg Oncol* 1991;47:261−264.

30 Zelcer J, White PF. Monitored anesthesia care. In: Miller RD, ed. *Anesthesia,* 3rd edn. New York: Churchill Livingstone Inc., 1990.

31 Alexander CM, Teller LE, Gross JB. Principles of pulse oximetry; theoretical and practical considerations. *Anesth Analg* 1989;68: 368−376.

32 Kelleher JF. Pulse oximetry. *J Clin Monit* 1989;5:37−62.

33 Freund PR, Overland PT, Cooper J *et al.* A prospective study of intraoperative pulse oximetry failure. *J Clin Monit* 1991;7(3): 253−258.

34 Severinghaus JW, Naifeh KH, Koh SO. Errors in 14 pulse oximeters during profound hypoxia. *J Clin Monit* 1989;5:72−81.

35 Barker SJ, Tremper KK. The effect of carbon monoxide inhalation on pulse oximetry and transcutaneous PO_2. *Anesthesiology* 1987; 66:667.

36 Boehmer RD. Continuous, real-time, non-invasive monitor of blood pressure: Penaz methodology applied to the finger. *J Clin Monit* 1987;3:282.

37 Davis RF. Clinical comparison of automated auscultatory and oscillometric and catheter−transducer measurements of arterial pressure. *J Clin Monit* 1985;1:114−119.

38 American Society of Anesthesiologists. *ASA Standards, Guidelines, and Statements.* Park Ridge, Illinois: American Society of Anesthesiologists, 1991.

39 Benumof JL. Respiratory physiology and respiratory function during anesthesia. In: Miller RD, ed. *Anesthesia,* 3rd edn. New York: Churchill Livingstone Inc., 1990:505−550.

40 Stone DJ, Thomas JG. Airway management. In: Miller RD, ed. *Anesthesia,* 3rd edn. New York: Churchill Livingstone Inc., 1990.

41 Sager PT, Bhandari AK. Narrow complex tachycardias, differential diagnosis and management. *Cardiol Clin* 1991;9:619−640.

42 Grauer K, Cavalloro D, Gums J. New developments in cardiopulmonary resuscitation. *Am Fam Physician* 1991;43(2):832−844.

43 Arai A, Kron J. Current management of the Wolff−Parkinson−White syndrome. *W J Med* 1990;152:383−391.

44 Larach DR, Kofke WA. Cardiovascular drugs. In: Kofke WA, Levy JH, eds. *Postoperative Critical Care Procedures of the Massachusetts General Hospital.* Boston: Little, Brown and Company, 1986:464−522.

45 Sager PT, Bhandari AK. Wide complex tachycardias; differential diagnosis and management. *Cardiol Clin* 1991;9(4):595−618.

46 Zaim S, Walter PF. Diagnosis and treatment of ventricular tachycardia. *Heart Dis Stroke* 1992;1(3):141−147.

47 Chakko S, de Marchena E, Kessler KM, Myerburg RJ. Ventricular arrhythmias in congestive heart failure. *Clin Cardiol* 1989;12: 525−530.

48 Waller DG, Robertson CE. Role of sympathomimetic amines during cardiopulmonary resuscitation. *Resuscitation* 1991;22: 181−190.

49 Govoni LE, Hayes JE. *Drugs and Nursing Implications.* Norwalk, California: Appleton and Lange, 1988.

50 Bush WH, Swanson DP. Acute reactions to intravascular contrast media: types, risk factors, recognition, and specific treatment. *Am J Roentgenol* 1991;157:1153−1161.

51 Kothari SS. Electromechanical dissociation: treatable causes of a

dire cardiac emergency. *Postgrad Med* 1991;90(7):75−78.

52 Cripps T, Camm J. The management of electromechanical dissociation. *Resuscitation* 1991;22:173−180.

53 Charlap S, Kahlam S, Lichstein E, Frishman W. Electromechanical dissociation: diagnosis, physiology, and management. *Am Heart J* 1989;118(2):355−360.

54 Wesley RC, Resh W, Zimmerman D. Reconsiderations of the routine and preferential use of lidocaine in the emergent treatment of ventricular arrhythmias. *Crit Care Med* 1991;19(11):1439−1444.

55 Haft JI, Habbab MA. Treatment of atrial arrhythmias: effectiveness of verapamil when preceded by calcium infusion. *Arch Int Med* 1986;146:1085.

56 Salerno DM, Dias VC, Kleiger RE *et al*. Intravenous verapamil for treatment of multifocal atrial tachycardia with and without calcium pretreatment. *Ann Int Med* 1987;107:623.

57 Bush WH. Treatment of systemic reactions to contrast media. *Urology* 1990;35(2):145−150.

58 Wood M, Ellenbogen KA. Bradyarrythmias, emergency pacing, and implantable defibrillation devices. *Crit Care Clin* 1989;5(3):551−568.

59 Kirschenbaum LP *et al*. Transthoracic pacing for the treatment of severe bradycardia during induction of anesthesia. *J Cardiothorac Anesth* 1989;3(3):329−332.

60 Fitzpatrick A, Sutton R. A guide to temporary pacing. *Br Med J* 1992;304:365−369.

61 Chamberlain DA. Lignocaine and bretylium as adjuncts to electrical defibrillation. *Resuscitation* 1991;22:153−157.

62 Ownby DR, Tomlanovich M, Sammons N, Mcgullough J. Anaphylaxis associated with latex allergy during barium enema examinations. *Am J Roentgenol* 1991;156:903−908.

63 Gerber AC, Jorg W, Zbinden S, Seger RA, Dangel PH. Severe intraoperative anaphylaxis to surgical gloves: latex allergy, and unfamiliar condition. *Anesthesiology* 1989;71:800−802.

64 Spaner D, Dolovich J, Tarlo S, Sussman G, Buttoo K. Hypersensitivity to natural latex. *J Allergy Clin Immunol* 1989;83:1135−1137.

65 Frosch PJ, Wahl R, Bahmer FA, Maasch HJ. Contact urticaria to rubber gloves is IgE-mediated. *Cont Derma* 1986;14:241−245.

66 Axelsson JGK, Johansson SGO, Wrangsjo K. IgE-mediated anaphylactoid reactions to rubber. *Allergy* 1987;42:46−50.

67 Morales C, Basomba A, Carreira J, Sastre A. Anaphylaxis produced by rubber glove contact. Case reports and immunological identification of the antigens involved. *Clin Exper Allergy* 1989;19:425−430.

CHAPTER 5

Infectious complications

Margaret E. Hansen

Introduction

Infectious complications are uncommon following radiologic procedures. As in surgery, most such infections probably result from environmental contamination, lapses in sterile technique, or microbial flora present within the patient. In recent years, however, health care workers (HCWs) and the public have become increasingly concerned about possible transmission of blood-borne pathogens in the health care setting. This chapter is intended to serve as an overview of these issues, to discuss precautions and regulations designed to reduce the risk of transmission of infectious agents during procedures, and to present recommendations in the event of an exposure.

Certain other situations, such as pregnant or immunocompromised patients, or HCWs, and the issue of antibiotic prophylaxis for radiologic procedures, merit special consideration as well, and will be discussed briefly.

Pertinent infectious agents

Infectious complications in radiology may result from virtually any infectious agent. Skin contaminants and flora of the gastrointestinal and upper respiratory tracts are common offenders, but other bacteria and classes of pathogens may also be responsible for infectious complications following radiologic procedures (Table 5.1), depending on the individual patient and the type of procedure being performed. This is particularly true in view of the increasing number of immunocompromised patients being treated in acute care settings, who may harbor unusual pathogens and are prone to opportunistic infections. A related and disturbing trend is the resurgence of tuberculosis as a significant — and increasingly widespread — pathogen [1,2]. Perhaps the most worrisome aspect of this phenomenon is the emergence of new strains of the tubercle bacillus, noted initially in urban hospitals in the eastern USA, which are resistant to standard multi-drug regimens [1,3]. These multi-drug resistant (MDR) strains are quite virulent, especially in immunocompromised individuals, in whom infection may rapidly lead to death.

Table 5.1 Major infectious agents of concern in radiologic procedures

Bacteria

Skin contaminants (*Staphylococcus epidermidis*, α-hemolytic streptococci)
Methicillin-resistant *S. aureus* (MRSA)
Mycobacteria (tuberculosis and atypicals, including drug-resistant strains)
Upper respiratory tract and gastrointestinal tract flora
  Escherichia coli, Bacteroides fragilis
  Enterococci, staphylococci
  Enterobacter, Clostridium, Pseudomonas spp.
  Haemophilus influenzae, Klebsiella pneumoniae
  Streptococcus pneumoniae, β-hemolytic streptococci

Viruses

Hepatitis B, hepatitis C
Human immunodeficiency virus (HIV)
Herpes varicella zoster
Cytomegalovirus (CMV)
Papillomavirus
Influenza
Mumps, measles, rubella

Parasites

Pneumocystis carinii
Toxoplasma gondii
Giardia lamblia
Entamoeba spp.

Fungi

Candida albicans
Aspergillus fumigatus
Mucor, Rhizopus spp.
Nocardia asteroides
Cryptococcus neoformans
Blastomyces dermatitidis
Histoplasma capsulatum
Coccidioides immitis

Several HCWs have contracted MDR tuberculosis, presumably from contact with infected patients [3].

Many other organisms have been reported to cause occupational infection in HCWs, although most are rare. Parenteral contact, through needlestick injury or contact with nonintact skin, is responsible in most cases. One of the most common of these is cutaneous infection with herpes simplex virus type 1 [4], but infection with cryptococcus, Rocky Mountain spotted fever, varicella zoster virus, *Staphylococcus aureus*, toxoplasma, malaria, papillomavirus, or syphilis has also occurred during patient care activities [5–10]. Infection with many other agents has been reported in laboratory workers or autopsy technicians as well [5]. While most of these cases are not directly relevant to the practice of radiology, they serve to indicate the range of occupational infection risk, and to emphasize the importance of safety awareness.

In addition to the above agents, blood-borne pathogens pose a potential threat to both patients and HCWs during invasive procedures. Major blood-borne agents of concern include human immunodeficiency virus (HIV) and the hepatitis viruses, which will be discussed in a later section. Other blood-borne organisms can also be transmitted during procedures, including syphilis, malaria, babesiosis, relapsing fever, brucellosis, leptospirosis, arboviral infections, viral hemorrhagic fever, Creutzfeldt–Jacob disease, and human T-lymphotropic virus type I (HTLV-I) [5,10]. Fortunately, most of these organisms are rare and infected individuals may not be infectious in all stages of a given disease.

Infectious complications of radiologic procedures

Potential infectious complications resulting from radiologic procedures range from relatively minor episodes, such as thrombophlebitis related to a peripheral intravenous line, to major and possibly life-threatening problems such as sepsis, prosthetic vascular graft infection, and endocarditis (Table 5.2). The distinction between minor and major infectious complications is somewhat arbitrary, as seemingly minor problems may be quite significant in some cases.

Study of postoperative infections has determined that in most cases the offending infectious agent is a contaminant from operating room personnel, spread by direct contact with hands or instruments, or derives from the patient's own flora [11]. Both *S. aureus* and *S. epidermidis* are commonly isolated from infected surgical wounds, and both are shed into the environment on skin scales by persons carrying these organisms [11–13]. Inanimate surfaces such as walls, floors, gurneys, and so on, play little part in surgical wound infection [11]. It is likely that the situation in radiology is similar. One difference is the possibility of

Table 5.2 Potential infectious complications of radiologic procedures

Minor complications
Folliculitis, localized skin infection
Superficial thrombophlebitis

Major complications
Line sepsis (intravenous or intraarterial lines/sheaths)
Prosthetic vascular graft infection
Native vessel infection/mycotic aneurysm formation
Endocarditis
Cholangitis
Urosepsis
Osteomyelitis; joint infection
Endometritis; salpingitis
Peritonitis
Empyema
Abscess
Meningitis

contamination through respiratory spread, as radiology personnel do not always wear face masks during procedures. However, the efficacy of face masks in preventing infection is not universally accepted [14].

Virtually any procedure performed in radiology can result in an infectious complication; fortunately, such complications are uncommon and, in general, are easily managed with appropriate therapy. A list of commonly performed radiologic procedures with potential infectious complications is given in Table 5.3. Although most are major invasive procedures, such as angiography and various nonvascular interventions, infectious complications can also occur after much less invasive procedures. Infection rates are highly dependent on procedure- and patient-related factors. Infection rates for selected procedures are listed in Table 5.4.

In addition to the risk of the patient suffering an infectious complication, some radiologic procedures pose a risk of infection to those performing them. Angiography and other invasive procedures, in which personnel may be exposed to blood, are obvious examples. Other procedures may not be considered to pose a risk at first glance, but do have theoretical potential for exposure to infectious agents. One such example is hysterosalpingography and Fallopian tube catheterization, in which personnel could be exposed to herpes simplex or papilloma viruses.

Infectious complications and intravascular contrast material

Many contrast media contain preservatives and therefore do not support bacterial growth. Some agents, however, such as those for intrathecal use, have no preservatives. One case of presumed septic shock after administration of iohexol has

been reported, which was probably related to improper handling of the contrast material [15].

Table 5.3 Procedures with risk of infectious complications or exposure

Vascular procedures
Angiography, venography, and related interventions
Lymphangiography

Nonvascular procedures
Abdomen and pelvis
   Percutaneous transhepatic cholangiography
   Percutaneous biliary drainage and related interventions
   Gastrointestinal tract intubation
   Abscess aspiration/drainage
   Lymphocele aspiration/drainage
   Percutaneous nephrostomy and related interventions
   Hysterosalpingography/Fallopian tube recanalization
   Peritoneal dialysis catheter repositioning
   Balloon dilatation of prostate
   Celiac plexus blockade
   Amniocentesis
   Paracentesis
   Pseudocyst drainage
Thorax
   Thoracentesis
   Chest tube placement
Miscellaneous
   Arthrography/joint aspiration
   Needle biopsy
   Intravenous administration of contrast or medications
   Lumbar puncture/myelography
   Phlebotomy
   Any procedure with potential exposure to body fluids

Table 5.4 Infection rates for selected radiologic procedures

Procedure	Infection rate (%)	Reference
Angiography	<1	[15–20]
Transjugular intrahepatic portosystemic shunt	2	[42–48]
Endovascular graft placement	0–15	[50–55]
Central/peripheral venous catheter placement	3–5	[63–66]
Venography	<1	[16]
Lymphangiography	10	[16, 68, 69]
Needle biopsy	<<1	[70–76]
Percutaneous abscess drainage	0.0–6.4	[79–85]
Pancreatic fluid collection drainage	3.7	[89–97]
Percutaneous transhepatic biliary drainage	20+	[107–112]
Gastrointestinal tract intubation	1–2	[113–123]
Peritoneal catheter placement/manipulation	1–2	[124–128,131]
Percutaneous nephrostomy	2.5	[132]
Fallopian tube catheterization	0	[142–144]
Needle biopsy of prostate	0	[145–147]
Thoracic interventions	<1	[149–162]
Arthrography/diskography	<1	[163–167]

Angiography (including cardiac catheterization)

Infectious complications occurring after angiography include infective endocarditis, fever or sepsis, mycotic aneurysm formation, local puncture site infection, and prosthetic vascular graft infection. The combined incidence of these complications is less than 1% [16–20].

Endocarditis has been reported after angiography in 0.003–0.02% of cases [16,17]. Causative organisms have included staphylococci and α-hemolytic streptococci. In some cases, endocarditis developed despite prophylactic administration of penicillin or other antibiotics prior to catheterization [17,21].

Transient bacteremia has been reported to occur in 0–18% of patients during angiography [22–25]. Cultures from catheters, guidewires, or blood obtained during angiography yielded positive results in 23% of patients in one study, with catheters being the most frequent source [22]. Organisms in some cases may have been contaminants, but in others pathogenic bacilli such as *Pseudomonas* and *Klebsiella* were found. Although single organisms were recovered in most cases, multiple organisms were found in five patients. However, no patient in this series developed sepsis, endocarditis, or puncture site infection. Eight of 23 patients with positive cultures had fever (35%), but 13 of 77 (17%) patients with negative cultures also had fever [22]. This series shows that it may be impossible to determine whether transient fever occurring after angiography represents an infectious complication or is due to other factors, such as pyrogens in contrast media or reactions to other drugs, as has been proposed in previous studies [16–19].

Infective arteritis developed in one of 12 367 patients in a cooperative study of cardiac catheterization, and was preceded by local infection at the cut-down site [17].

Local infections developed in 10 of 12 367 patients after cardiac catheterization (0.08%) [17]. *Escherichia coli* and staphylococci were the organisms most commonly isolated from these wounds, suggesting fecal contamination in some cases.

Both Gram-positive and Gram-negative organisms are commonly found in cases of prosthetic vascular graft infection [26–29], and mixed populations may also occur [26]. Graft infection is a grave problem, with high associated morbidity and mortality [26,29,30]. Any connection between preoperative arteriography and subsequent development of graft infection is therefore of great concern. Although angiography has a very low rate of infectious complications, some advocate prophylactic antibiotic administration before angiography in any patient who may soon thereafter undergo prosthetic graft placement [26,31]; others consider this unnecessary [27]. Landreneau and Raju [26], examining the influence of preoperative arteriography on graft infection, found that the incidence of postoperative groin infection was greater if the interval between angiography and surgery was more than 24 hours. This may be related to shaving the skin prior to angiography, as shaving of operation sites increases the infection rate of clean surgical wounds [32]. Shaving has been shown to produce small skin nicks [33] in which bacteria can grow, and a longer interval between angiography and surgery allows more bacterial growth to occur. This is consistent with surgical studies showing increased infection rates with longer intervals between shaving and surgery [32]. Landreneau and Raju [26] also found that 81% of wound complications occurred in the groin through which arteriography was performed, compared to 15% in the opposite groin, further supporting this relationship. Reduced infection rates when operative sites are not shaved [32,34] certainly cast doubt on the benefit of shaving the groin before angiography.

Transcatheter embolotherapy

Infections after transcatheter embolotherapy can occur as a result of contamination during the procedure or from bacterial seeding of devitalized tissue after embolization. It may be difficult to distinguish infection from the postembolization syndrome, which can cause fever, chills, leukocytosis, and other findings mimicking infection, and can be seen in 40% or more of patients following embolotherapy [35]. Difficulty is compounded by the fact that imaging studies, such as computed tomography or ultrasonography, are often not helpful, as gas may be seen in embolized solid organs without the presence of infection [36–40]. Prophylactic administration of antibiotics prior to high-risk embolization procedures, such as those involving the liver or spleen, can reduce the incidence of infectious complications after embolotherapy [35,41]. Soaking particulate emboli in antibiotic solution prior to injection may help as well [41].

Transjugular intrahepatic portosystemic shunt (TIPS)

TIPS is still a new procedure, with few reported infectious complications. In seven series totaling 243 patients, sepsis occurred in five cases (2%); the only organism specified in these reports was *S. epidermidis* [42–48]. Onset of sepsis was delayed (>30 days after the procedure) in one case [43], and may not have been procedure related. No other infectious complications have been described to date.

Endovascular graft placement

This too is a very new procedure, and is still considered investigational, although it is now being carried out in many centers around the world. Accordingly, there are few published data concerning the risk of infection associated with endovascular graft placement, although clearly this is a significant concern because of the high morbidity and mortality known to accompany infection of prosthetic grafts. Whether the angiography suite or the operating room is the most appropriate place for these procedures to be performed is controversial, and this is currently being addressed by the Society of Vascular Surgery and the Society of Cardiovascular and Interventional Radiology. If endovascular graft placement is to be undertaken in an angiography suite, the room should conform to the air-handling and traffic control requirements for operating rooms at that institution, and proper surgical scrub and attire are essential [49].

The incidence of wound or graft infection after endovascular graft placement appears to be relatively low. In two small series, local wound infection was reported in one of 27 patients (3.7%) [50] and one of 16 patients (6%) [51], respectively, but in several other series no infections were noted [52–54]. In a multicenter trial of an endovascular graft for treatment of abdominal aortic aneurysms in the USA, 15 wound infections occurred in the first 100 patients [55], one of which required local debridement, but no graft infections developed. Because most of these devices currently require an arterial cutdown for placement, prophylactic antibiotics should be given before the procedure, and meticulous aseptic technique must be used.

Indwelling arterial or venous catheters

Infection related to indwelling vascular catheters is most often due to *S. epidermidis*, a nearly universal skin contaminant, or *S. aureus*, although many other organisms have been associated with infusion-related bacteremia [56]. Cannula-related infections may derive from the patient's own flora or from bacteria on the hands of personnel handling or placing the cannula. The incidence of line-related complications, including infection and phlebitis, is related to the length of time the line has been present [56–58], although it is likely that contamination occurs at the time of insertion or shortly thereafter in most cases of infection [59]. Bacteremia due to peripheral intravenous (IV) catheters is rare unless they have been in place at least 48 hours; after 72 hours, it may occur in 2–5% of patients with plastic IV catheters [56]. The risk of infusion-related bacteremia can be reduced by limiting the duration of peripheral venous catheterization to 3 days and arterial catheterization to 4 days [60].

In patients in intensive care units, bacterial colonization has been reported in 4–10% of arterial catheters, 7–28% of central venous catheters, and 7–33% of pulmonary artery catheters [58,61]. Infection rates for peripherally inserted central catheters (PICC) appear to be lower than those for conventional central venous catheters [62].

Radiologic placement of long-term central venous catheters has an infection rate of 4.8%, identical to that of surgically placed catheters [63]. Infection rates are low even in patients who may be immunocompromised [64]. Venous

access ports implanted percutaneously in the arm have recently been described, with an infection rate of approximately 3% [65,66]. Length of central venous catheters does not affect infection risk, but operator inexperience may increase risk of infection [59]. Use of antibiotic ointment may reduce infection related to percutaneously placed catheters, but alters the microbial flora and may select for resistant organisms [67].

Venography and lymphangiography

Thrombophlebitis after extremity venography is not uncommon. Although generally ascribed to chemical irritation, infection may be responsible in some cases. Other infectious complications have been described in 0.02% of patients following peripheral venography [16].

Wound infection and delayed healing are seen in up to 10% of patients after lymphangiography [16,68,69], but involvement is most often superficial and limited to the skin incision site. Fever has been reported in up to 23% of patients [68,69], and may be due to a foreign body reaction to injected oil [68]. Serious infection, such as osteomyelitis, is extremely rare, occurring in only 0.01% of cases [16].

Needle biopsy

Percutaneous needle biopsy, whether with fine needle aspiration or core sampling techniques, has very low overall complication rates [70]. The most common complications are bleeding and other local problems, with infection being quite rare. In several large series [71–73], no infectious complications were encountered, although peritonitis has been reported following liver biopsy and after aspiration of an abdominal abscess [74,75]. One case of Gram-negative sepsis has also been reported after pancreatic aspiration [76].

Fever, with or without associated chills, has been reported in up to 15.5% of patients following transjugular liver biopsy [77,78]. Blood cultures, when obtained, were sterile in all cases. Fever after transjugular liver biopsy may be due to bacteria or pyrogens on the biopsy needle, and can be reduced by ultrasonic cleaning of the needle before sterilization [78] or use of disposable needles.

Percutaneous abscess drainage (PAD)

The incidence of infectious complications following PAD has decreased somewhat since early reports of this technique appeared [79,80]. In recent experience, the incidence of major and minor infectious complications after PAD has ranged from 0 to 6.4% [81–85], with no reported deaths from sepsis. This may be due to improvements in antibiotic therapy and equipment, but better understanding of patient management and catheter care is probably the most important factor [86,87]. It is now widely known that vigorous irrigation of an abscess cavity before all purulent material and debris has been evacuated can induce sepsis [86,88]. It is also recognized that inadequate drainage may contribute to death from sepsis [79,80], and that some abscesses require more than one catheter for successful drainage [86,87]. In addition, catheters must be of appropriate size for the viscosity of the abscess contents to permit effective drainage [86,88]. Finally, premature removal of drainage catheters can result in abscess recurrence and possible sepsis [86–88].

Pancreatic pseudocyst and abscess drainage

Infection following percutaneous drainage of pancreatic fluid collections occurred in 3.7% of combined cases from multiple series [89–97]. The reported infectious complications range from tract infection [92] or colonization of the fluid collection with nonpathogenic organisms [96], to infection of previously sterile collections [94–96] and empyema [93]. No cases of bacteremia or sepsis were noted in these series, which included 264 patients, despite the fact that many of the fluid collections were infected prior to catheter placement [89,92,93,96].

Lymphocele aspiration, drainage, and sclerosis

Aspiration, drainage, and sclerosis of lymphoceles is safe and effective, with few complications even in cases of infected fluid collections [98–100]. Infection is the most common complication, however, which is of concern because most patients with lymphoceles have renal transplants and are thus receiving immunosuppressive drugs. As with other abdominal and pelvic fluid collections, lymphoceles will become colonized after a few days of catheter drainage, but no serious infection results in most cases [99,100]. Repeated aspiration of a lymphocele, however, may result in sepsis and death, and should therefore be avoided [101].

Biliary tract procedures

Diagnostic and therapeutic procedures involving the gall bladder have a fairly low infection rate. Approximately 1% of patients develop bile peritonitis [102]. Cholangitis and sepsis are more common, occurring in up to 4% of patients after interventional gall bladder procedures [103–105].

Fever occurred in 1.7% of patients in one large series after percutaneous extraction of retained bile duct stones [106]. Cholangitis and local infection at the skin site each occurred in 3% of cases in a smaller series [105].

Infectious complications occur more frequently after percutaneous biliary drainage, probably because many of the patients undergoing this procedure are critically ill and may be immunosuppressed due to their underlying disease. Postprocedure bacteremia is more common in patients with

cholangitis at the time of drainage [107], and patients with malignant biliary obstruction are at greater risk of infectious complications than those with benign disease [108,109]. Cholangitis and/or sepsis has been reported in up to 54% of cancer patients undergoing biliary drainage, compared to 22% with benign disease [108]. Commonly isolated organisms include streptococci, *Klebsiella pneumoniae*, *E. coli*, *Enterobacter* spp., and *Pseudomonas aeruginosa* [108]. Nearly all bile will become infected after percutaneous drainage, and the mechanism of subsequent cholangitis and sepsis is not well understood. However, it is believed that reflux of bacteria from bowel into the biliary tree may be responsible. In addition, manipulation or injection of drainage tubes has been noted to precede most such episodes [108]. Transient fever is common after percutaneous biliary drainage, and subphrenic abscess has also been reported [110].

Placement of biliary endoprostheses has a fairly high rate of infectious complications as well; again, probably because of the patient population involved. Cholangitis, usually a delayed complication due to stent occlusion, can occur in up to 20% of patients after stent placement [111,112]. Abscess formation, bile peritonitis, and empyema have also been reported [111,112], but occur less often.

Gastrointestinal tract intubation

Infectious complications of percutaneous gastrostomy (PG) and gastroenterostomy (PGE) tube placement may be major, including peritonitis, sepsis, and death, or minor, such as superficial wound infection or transient postprocedure fever or leukocytosis [113]. The combined incidence of peritonitis in five large series of adult patients was 0.9%; sepsis occurred in 0.3% (with one death), and local wound infection in 1.8% [114–118]. Aspiration pneumonia occurred in one case (0.1%) [115]. Transient elevation of temperature or white blood cell count is not uncommon after PG or PGE placement, occurring in the majority of patients in one report [116]. In a series of pediatric patients, there were no cases of peritonitis or sepsis, but wound infection occurred in 12% [119]; these patients were immunosuppressed and were successfully treated with topical and oral antibiotics.

Although reported experience with percutaneous cecostomy tube placement is limited, no infectious complications of this procedure have been described [120–123].

Peritoneal catheter placement/manipulation

No infectious complications have been reported from manipulation of peritoneal dialysis catheters [124–126]. Strict attention to sterile technique is necessary during these procedures to minimize the risk of peritonitis. Recently, radiologic placement of peritoneal dialysis catheters has been reported in 32 patients, with acute peritonitis in one (2%)

and delayed peritonitis in three (6%), requiring catheter removal [127].

Paracentesis, whether diagnostic or therapeutic, also has a very low rate of infectious complications [128–131]. No infectious complications occurred in one series of 109 sonographically guided procedures [128]. There were two deaths from peritonitis in an earlier series of 100 procedures done without imaging guidance; one due to bowel perforation by the drainage catheter and the other to prolonged catheter placement (77 days) [129]. In a recent report describing percutaneous placement of intraperitoneal catheters for chemotherapy infusion and ascites drainage, peritonitis occurred after two of 134 procedures (1.5%) [131].

Percutaneous nephrostomy (PCN) and related procedures

Introduction of infection was the most common complication in a review of 1200 PCN placements, occurring in 2.5% of procedures [132]. If PCN placement is done for stone removal, infectious complications are more common, but most are minor. Percutaneous renal stone removal can result in sepsis if the urine or the stone is infected [133]. Transient fever occurred in 23% of patients in one large series, although significant infection was seen in only 0.8% [134]. In another series, infection occurred in 0.9% of patients [135]. Infection is very rare after simple antegrade pyelography, occurring in 0.4% in one large series [136]. The infection rate after Whitaker test performance is likewise quite low, reported to be 0.5% in the same series [136].

Infectious complications of ureteral stricture dilatation and stent placement are rare [137]. Patients may have transient fever after such procedures, but sepsis is uncommon if prophylactic antibiotics are used [137]. Stent obstruction and resultant fatal sepsis has been reported in patients with ileal urinary diversions [138]; presumably, mucus and urinary debris caused stent obstruction in these cases.

Infection has been reported after renal cyst puncture and aspiration, but is not a common complication, occurring in approximately 0.2% of cases [139]. Fever, chills, and leukocytosis were reported in 3% of patients in another series, in which cysts were injected with contrast material and/or sclerosing agents [140].

Transient fever and exacerbation of preexisting urosepsis have been reported after percutaneous drainage of renal and perinephric abscesses [141].

Hysterosalpingography (HSG) and related interventions

Complications of HSG and selective Fallopian tube catheterization are uncommon. Fallopian tube catheterization and dilatation has been performed in hundreds of patients without report of infectious complications [142]. Patients are treated with antibiotics before and after the procedure at most centers [142–144] (see Table 5.9, p. 112).

Transrectal ultrasound/biopsy of the prostate

Transrectal prostate ultrasound and biopsy no doubt has the potential to produce bacteremia in some patients. Because of the theoretical risk of fecal contamination, many centers administer prophylactic antibiotics (see Table 5.9, p. 112) to patients undergoing transrectal prostate biopsy [145]; some also advocate the use of cleansing enemas prior to the procedure [145]. In large series of diagnostic studies and transrectal biopsies [146–147], no infectious complications have been noted.

Transurethral balloon dilatation of the prostatic urethra

Few complications of this technique have been reported. Infection has been described in one case, in which a perineal abscess occurred after balloon dilatation [148]. This was the only significant complication in 150 cases performed at the reporting institution.

Thoracic interventions

Infection resulting from transthoracic needle biopsy of lung lesions is extremely rare [149–152]. In a series of 5300 biopsies in 2726 patients, there were two cases of empyema (0.04%), one case of spread of infection after puncture of a lung abscess (0.02%), and one case of superficial infection at the skin puncture site (0.02%) [152]. Even when performed to diagnose a suspected pulmonary infection or to identify the responsible organism, exacerbation or spread of infection has been reported in only one case [152].

Pleural interventions also have a very low rate of infectious complications. Infection due to image-guided pleural biopsy [153] or diagnostic aspiration of pleural fluid collections [154,155] has not been reported. Infection [156] and bacteremia [157] have occurred after placement of catheters for drainage of sterile or infected pleural fluid collections, but these are rare occurrences [154–160]. No cases of infection due to percutaneous placement of small chest tubes for treatment of pneumothorax have been described [161,162]. Transient fever after pleural sclerotherapy was noted in a case described by O'Moore *et al.* [154], and responded to antipyretics alone.

Musculoskeletal procedures

Infection resulting from arthrography is extremely rare, occurring in only one of 25 000 cases studied by Freiberger *et al.* [163]. The patient presented within 48 hours of the procedure with local pain and swelling, and the diagnosis was made by joint aspiration and culture, which revealed *S. aureus*. Arthrography or aspiration of infected joints did not result in any complications in this series.

Acute infection after diskography is also very rare, with a reported incidence ranging from 0.2 to 1.1% [164–166]. The risk of infection may be greater if meningitis is present at the time of disk puncture [165]. Chronic infection due to diskography may be difficult to document, but is probably rare as well.

The infection rate after automated percutaneous lumbar diskectomy reported in a review of experience with this technique in over 3600 patients is 0.2% [167], which compares favorably with other diskectomy methods.

Myelography

Infection after myelography is rare, probably occurring at a rate similar to those seen with diagnostic lumbar puncture or spinal anesthesia. In two large series of patients undergoing spinal anesthesia, subsequent bacterial meningitis occurred in one in 30 000 and one in 21 230 cases [168,169]. Inadequate skin preparation or contamination of instruments or injectables is probably responsible for most cases of postmyelography infection [170]. Some authors have also implicated lack of mask use during myelography [170–172], but others have questioned the value of masks in preventing infection [14]. Bacteremia at the time of lumbar puncture may predispose to subsequent meningitis [173]. Common organisms include *S. aureus*, *Pseudomonas* spp., enteric Gram-negative rods, and *Streptococcus* spp. [170–172,174]. Infection must be differentiated from chemical meningitis, which can occur even with nonionic contrast media [175] and can cause leukocytosis and elevated protein content in the cerebrospinal fluid (CSF) [170,171]. Fever and CSF leukocytosis are generally more pronounced in bacterial meningitis, and Gram stain of the CSF is positive in 70–80% of cases [170,171], but CSF culture is necessary to confirm the diagnosis, to identify the organism, and to determine appropriate therapy. In cases of suspected bacterial meningitis after myelography, parenteral antibiotic therapy should be started immediately [170]. If the CSF Gram stain reveals no bacteria, corticosteroids should also be given, to treat for possible chemical meningitis, until culture results are available [170, 171,175]. Lumbar puncture should be repeated if initial cultures are negative [175].

Contrast enemas

Bacteremia may occur in more than 20% of patients during contrast enemas [176,177]; its incidence is not affected by the presence or absence of intrinsic colonic disease [176]. Organisms isolated from blood cultures have included enterococci, *E. coli*, *K. pneumoniae*, *Proteus morganii*, *Bacteroides*, and other anaerobes [176,177]. Such bacteremia is generally

transient, self-limited, and without clinical sequelae, but fatal sepsis (due to *Clostridium perfringens* and *S. aureus*) has been reported in two immunocompromised patients after barium enema examinations [178,179].

Intervention in pediatric patients

A wide variety of interventional procedures have been performed on pediatric patients, with low rates of infectious complications comparable to those reported in adults [119, 130,180–184]. Certain procedures performed in children, such as splenic embolization, have a relatively high risk of infectious complications, but the risk is due to the procedure itself rather than the age of the patient.

Transmission of blood-borne pathogens during procedures

In recent years, concern has grown about possible transmission of blood-borne pathogens during medical procedures, whether from patients to HCWs, or from HCWS to patients. This has long been a recognized occupational risk in the health care field, but the advent of acquired immune deficiency syndrome (AIDS) has focused new attention on the issue of nosocomial infections.

Although concern has centered primarily on HIV, other blood-borne agents may be transmitted between patient and HCW and must also be considered. Chief among these are the hepatitis viruses, including hepatitis B virus (HBV), hepatitis C virus (HCV), and other strains [185]. It is estimated that 8700 HCWs acquire HBV infection occupationally each year; of these, approximately 10% become chronic carriers of the virus. Approximately 200 HCWs die each year of the illness or related complications [10]. In addition to the obvious health problems, medical personnel who become chronic carriers may transmit HBV to patients during invasive procedures. More than 20 clusters of such transmissions have been reported in the surgical and dental literature [10], and the risk of acquiring HBV infection after a single parenteral exposure to HBsAg-containing blood is between 7 and 30% [10].

The scope of occupational disease due to HCV is less well documented, but may be significant as well [185,186]. The first-generation HCV antibody test became available in May 1990, and is most sensitive in detecting chronic infection [185]. HCV is more likely than HBV to cause chronic infection, with up to 50% of patients becoming carriers of the virus [185]. Early seroprevalence investigations have found evidence of HCV exposure in 1–3% of HCWs, a rate similar to that found in the general population [185–189]. However, the first-generation HCV assay is not sensitive in either acute infection or resolved past HCV infection [185–190]. The second-generation antibody test is now available and detects anti-HCV in approximately 90% of infected individuals by 9 months after exposure [185,188]; in the remaining 10%, infection can be detected only by the use of the polymerase chain reaction or other research-based techniques [187]. Reports have documented HCV infection of HCWs resulting from needlestick injuries [184,190–192] and mucous membrane exposure [192,193]. The risk of HCV transmission after a needlestick injury with infected blood has been estimated at 2.7–4% [190], but was 6% in one recent study [192].

Although blood may be the most common vehicle for transmission of HIV or hepatitis strains in the health care setting, other body fluids can also be infectious. HIV may be present in semen, vaginal secretions, saliva, CSF, amniotic fluid, breast milk, and serous exudates [10]. HBV can also be found in most of these fluids [10]. Urine and feces, unless visibly contaminated with blood, do not contain significant quantities of either virus [10]. HCV is not found in as many body fluids as HBV or HIV: viral RNA has not been found in urine, feces, saliva, vaginal fluid, or semen from chronically infected patients, even when present in their blood [188].

HBV can survive on environmental surfaces up to 7 days at room temperature, but is killed by high-level disinfectants, such as bleach [10]. Low-level disinfectants, including quaternary ammonium compounds, do not kill the virus [10]. HIV is less hardy, surviving only briefly on environmental surfaces at room temperature. Like HBV, it is readily inactivated by dilute solutions of household bleach (sodium hypochlorite, 1:10–1:100) [10].

The risk of HIV transmission during radiologic procedures is unknown, but is probably lower than for surgical procedures. This is so because percutaneous injury occurs less often during invasive radiologic procedures than during surgery [194], and lower injury rates mean less risk for both patient and HCW. Surgical studies have found percutaneous injury rates ranging from 1.7 to 15.4% of operations, with most in the 3–6% range [195–199]. The injury rate in a recent study of invasive radiologic procedures, by comparison, was 0.6% of procedures [194]. In a survey of New York City surgeons, the median injury rate was two injuries/year [200], compared to a median of 0.3 injuries/year in a survey of interventional radiologists [201,202]. Another reason why radiologic procedures may pose less risk of physician to patient HIV transmission is that they do not generally involve work within open body cavities, thus reducing the chance of an injured HCW's blood coming into parenteral contact with the patient ("recontact"). Hansen *et al.* [201], in their survey, found that recontact occurred in only one of 527 procedure-related injuries that caused bleeding (0.2%) [201]. In contrast, recontact was observed after 29% of injuries to surgeons in a recent study by the Centers for Disease Control and Prevention (CDC) [198].

Patient to HCW transmission

Patient to HCW transmission of HIV has been serologically documented in 19 cases since 1983 [203]. In many additional cases, occupational exposure is considered the most likely means of transmission of the virus, although documentation is not conclusive [10,203].

Infection in most of these cases was the result of parenteral exposure from needlestick injuries [10]. In a few cases, contact of patient blood or body fluid with nonintact skin or mucous membrane surfaces was responsible for infection [10,204]. The risk of a HCW becoming infected after a single parenteral exposure to HIV-containing blood or body fluid depends most on the level of virus in the patient's blood [205], but other factors are probably involved.

HCW to patient transmission

Unlike patient to HCW transmission, transmission of HIV from HCW to patient has been documented in only a single cluster of five patients, all of whom were infected by a Florida dentist [206]. No other cases have been discovered in several investigations of HIV-infected practitioners [207–210]. It is generally agreed that the risk of HIV transmission is less than that of HBV transmission, but no data are available to determine the precise level of risk. The CDC and other investigators have estimated the risk of acquiring HIV infection after a single parenteral exposure at 0.4% [203, 211]. The risk of a surgeon transmitting the virus to a patient has been estimated to range from 1:28 000 to 1:500 000 if the surgeon is known to be HIV-positive [212,213]. However, such estimates are fraught with difficulty. Just as for patient to HCW transmission, the risk of an HIV-infected HCW transmitting the virus to a patient depends on many factors. These include the likelihood of the HCW being injured during a procedure, the likelihood of the HCW's blood contacting the patient as a result, the level of virus in the HCW's blood, and other factors [213].

At this time, there are no federal restrictions on the professional activities of HIV-infected HCWs, although recommendations issued by the CDC in 1991 include restrictions on performance of "exposure-prone" invasive procedures [214]. Invasive radiologic procedures, such as angiography, have not been considered in this context by CDC to date (D.M. Bell, personal communication). Several states have enacted legislation requiring HIV testing of HCWs, and practice restrictions for those testing positive. The remaining states were required to establish policy for HIV-infected HCWs by the end of 1992, according to a law passed by the USA Congress in October 1991. Legal and ethical issues surrounding the question of HIV-positive HCWs are, to say the least, complex and wide reaching [215–220]. Current recommendations by the American Medical Association (AMA) include voluntary HIV testing of HCWs who perform exposure-prone procedures and disclosure of HIV infection to local review panels; these panels would then establish practice restrictions on an individual basis [221].

Precautions

The risk of infectious complications during radiologic procedures is low, in part because of current understanding of modes of infectious transmission and near universal adherence to accepted principles of asepsis and sterile technique. Use of protective equipment, vaccination of HCWs, and observance of universal precautions during all invasive procedures can reduce the risk of disease transmission even further.

Safety guidelines and regulations

Use of universal precautions, or treating all blood/body fluid as if infectious, has been recommended by the CDC since 1987 [214,222]. Until recently, however, these recommendations did not have the force of law. With implementation of the new Occupational Safety and Health Administration (OSHA) blood-borne pathogen standard in 1992, use of universal precautions has become mandatory [10].

The OSHA blood-borne pathogen standard covers most HCWs, as well as many individuals in other occupations (Table 5.5). Its major elements (Table 5.6) include requirements for employers to provide protective equipment, training in infection control, free HBV vaccination, and postexposure prophylaxis and counseling to all employees at risk of occupational exposure to blood and/or body fluids. Engineering and work practice controls and housekeeping practices are also specified in the regulations (Table 5.6). Fines for noncompliance may be as high as $70 000. A concise introduction to the new standard may be found in a recently published summary [223].

The new OSHA standard clearly applies to invasive radiologic procedures such as angiography and various nonvascular interventions, including nephrostomy or biliary drainage tube placement, abscess drainage, biopsy, and so on. Applicability to other radiologic procedures, such as contrast enemas or cystography, is less clear. Urine and feces are not covered by the new regulations unless visibly contaminated with blood, or unless it is difficult or impossible to differentiate between them and other potentially infectious body fluids [10]. OSHA's Office of Compliance has issued a statement addressing radiology practice concerns, stressing that it is the responsibility of each employer to determine whether exposure to blood may be "reasonably anticipated" during a given procedure [224]. If so, employees involved in that procedure are covered by *all* provisions of the standard, including requirements for training in infection control, HBV vaccination, and availability and use of personal protective equipment. This is true whether exposure to blood occurs each time a procedure is performed or only seldom [224].

Elements of the standard pertaining to handling of soiled linens and infectious waste are also relevant to many areas

Table 5.5 OSHA blood-borne pathogen standard: coverage and definitions

Who is covered
- All workers in health care or other occupations who may be "reasonably anticipated" to be at risk for work-related exposure to infectious materials, except as below

Who is not covered
- Workers in medical facilities not subject to OSHA regulation (state, county, or municipal facilities in certain states)
- Medical, nursing, and allied health students, unless also employees
- Volunteers

Definition of infectious materials
- Blood and blood products
- Semen, vaginal secretions, CSF, synovial fluid, peritoneal fluid, pleural fluid, pericardial fluid, amniotic fluid, saliva in dental procedures, *any fluid visibly contaminated with blood, all fluids in cases where distinguishing between fluids is difficult or impossible*
- Unfixed tissues or organs from living or dead persons
- Cell, tissue, or organ cultures containing HIV or HBV
- Blood or other tissues from experimental animals infected with HIV or HBV

of radiology practice. Contaminated laundry must be placed and transported in color-coded or labeled containers; if wet, it must be placed in leakproof containers. Workers who handle contaminated linens are required to wear gloves (and other protective gear as needed) [10]. The OSHA standard requires that infectious waste be placed in leakproof, sealable containers which are labeled or color-coded; containers must be sealed prior to removal [10]. Disposal of infectious waste should be done in accordance with local regulations [224].

Safety devices

Concern about occupational exposure to blood-borne pathogens has led to a proliferation of products designed to improve procedure safety for HCWs. Newer personal protective equipment, such as fluid-impervious disposable gowns, gloves with longer cuffs, plastic face shields or shield–mask combinations (Figs 5.1 & 5.2) is relatively inexpensive and does not interfere with safe performance of procedures [225]. Devices have also been developed to reduce the risk of needlestick injuries, including improved sharps disposal containers (Fig. 5.3), special IV injection sets (Figs 5.4–6), needle holders for procedure trays (Figs 5.7 & 5.8) [226,227], and needle sheath guards (Figs 5.9 & 5.10). Still other devices have been designed to reduce operator exposure to blood and/or body fluid, including closed-system flush tubing (Fig. 5.11), "bloodless" puncture devices for angiography (Figs 5.12 & 5.13) [228], and closed abscess drainage

Table 5.6 OSHA blood-borne pathogen standard: major employer requirements

Exposure control plan
- Identify employees at risk for occupational exposure
- Detail how provisions of standard will be implemented
- Specify procedure for handling exposure incidents
- Be reviewed and updated at least once a year
- Be accessible to employees and to OSHA (written copy)

Personal protective equipment
- Includes gloves, gowns, masks/face shields, eye protection, shoe and hair covers, and other equipment as needed
- Use now mandatory, including gloves for phlebotomy
- Must be provided at no cost and in appropriate sizes
- Hypoallergenic or powder-free gloves or glove liners must be provided, at no charge, for employees allergic to standard gloves
- Must be clean, readily available, and in good repair; employer responsible for replacement/repair as needed

HBV/HIV protection and exposure
- Employees at risk an average of one or more times per month must be offered free HBV vaccination
- Employees declining vaccination must sign waiver
- Vaccination must be offered within 10 working days of initial assignment to area of risk
- Free booster doses of HBV vaccine must be provided as needed
- Free postexposure evaluation and follow-up must be provided for HBV and HIV exposures, including:
   antibody testing of employee and source
   counseling
   evaluation by physician or other health care provider
   postexposure prophylaxis

Training and record-keeping
- Training sessions must be provided for all employees at risk

- Content of training sessions stipulated in text of standard
- Training sessions must be repeated at least once a year
- Records of training must be kept for 3 years from training date
- Medical records must be kept for each at-risk employee for duration of employment + 30 years

Engineering and work practice controls
- Readily accessible hand-washing facilities must be provided
- Hands must be washed as soon as possible after removal of gloves or other protective equipment
- Skin must be washed with soap and water, and mucous membranes flushed with water, immediately after contact with potentially infectious material
- Personal protective equipment must be removed immediately upon leaving the work area
- Recapping of contaminated sharps by hand prohibited
- Use of food, drink, or cosmetics prohibited in areas of potential exposure; contact lens handling also prohibited
- Food or drink may not be kept in refrigerators or other areas where potentially infectious materials may be present

Housekeeping and labeling requirements
- Sharps disposal containers must be leakproof, puncture-resistant, closable, and as close as possible to area(s) where sharps are used
- Contaminated laundry must be placed in labeled or color-coded (red) bags; if wet, must be in leakproof bag
- Biohazard labels or red bags/containers must be used for all potentially infectious materials
- Specimens must be placed in labeled or color-coded (red), leakproof containers prior to handling, transport, shipping, or storage

---

systems [229]. Most have no adverse effect on procedure performance and are only slightly more expensive than standard products. The bloodless puncture systems, however, may impair tactile feel during guidewire introduction [225, 230], and should thus be used with caution to reduce risk of vessel injury.

Occult glove perforations occur during radiologic procedures, just as in surgery, and can result in exposure of procedure operators to blood or body fluid. The overall frequency of perforations was 10% in a recent study, with the vast majority of holes being unrecognized by the wearer [231]. The perforation rate increased significantly when gloves were worn 2 hours or longer, suggesting that gloves should be changed at or before 2 hours of wear even if no perforations are apparent. Double gloving is routine surgical practice at some institutions [195], but the value of this approach for radiologic procedures is unclear. Certainly, if an operator has cuts or other areas of nonintact skin on one or both hands, double gloving is advised. It may also be warranted if the procedure involves a high-risk patient, although selective double gloving violates the basic principle

of universal precautions, namely that *all* patients should be treated as though they are high risk.

Infection control practices

Despite the widespread availability of excellent protective equipment, adherence to universal precautions remains far from uniform in the current practice of radiology. For example, in a recent survey of interventional radiologists, it was found that only 20% of radiologists who do not wear corrective eyeglasses for procedures routinely wore eye protection, and only 32% routinely wore a face mask or shield, while performing invasive procedures [201,202]. In a study of blood contacts during invasive radiologic procedures, 10 of 14 cutaneous exposures (71%) could have been prevented by use of appropriate protective gear [194]. It is to be hoped that compliance with safety recommendations will improve in response to new OSHA regulations mandating use of protective equipment [10].

In addition to use of protective equipment, it is crucial to practice safe handling of sharp instruments. This includes

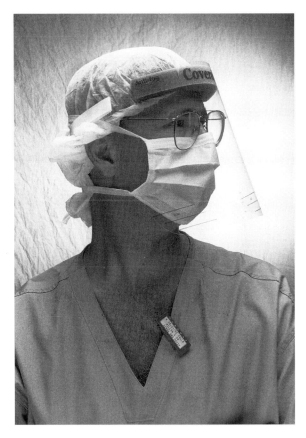

Fig. 5.1 Coverall[Tm] plastic shield (BFD Inc., Birmingham, AL; distributed by AliMed Inc., Dedham, MA) provides splash protection for eyes and face. Shield can be used over eyeglasses without fogging.

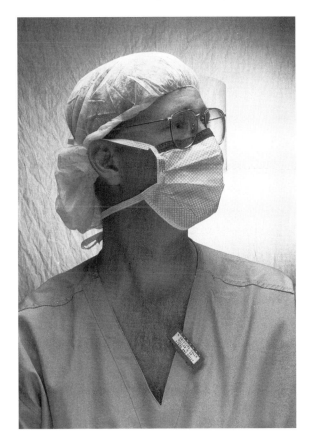

Fig. 5.2 Protector III[Tm] mask (Anago, Fort Worth, TX) combines a fluid-resistant face mask with a clear plastic shield to protect against splashes; shield has flaps for side protection as well.

not recapping used sharp instruments by hand (unless a one-handed method is used), disposing of used sharps properly, and not leaving exposed sharps on a procedure drape. It is also vital for members of a procedure team to communicate with each other when sharp instruments are being passed or put on a procedure tray, so that everyone is aware of the location of all sharps [225,232]. More than 25% of all injuries during invasive radiologic procedures could have been prevented by closer attention to safe handling of sharp instruments, according to the survey by Hansen *et al.* [201].

Although attention has been focused on blood-borne pathogens, other organisms are also of serious concern in many hospitals. Methicillin-resistant *S. aureus* (MRSA) and *Mycobacterium tuberculosis* (TB) are two such agents. MRSA may be found in the nares of HCWs, and is primarily spread by the hands of medical personnel [233]. Nasal carriage is important in only a minority of MRSA outbreaks, but may need to be treated during periods of high infection rates. Strict handwashing between patients is crucial in preventing MRSA transmission [233], but use of soap alone may not be adequate to eliminate bacterial colonization [234]. In

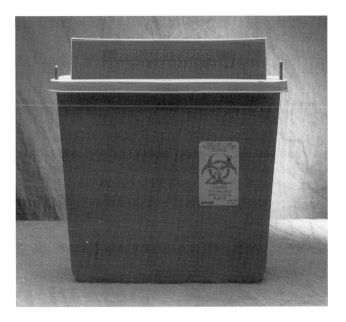

Fig. 5.3 Puncture-proof sharps disposal container (Sage Products Inc., Cary, IL) is constructed of rigid plastic; lid is spill-proof but allows easy placement of sharps into container.

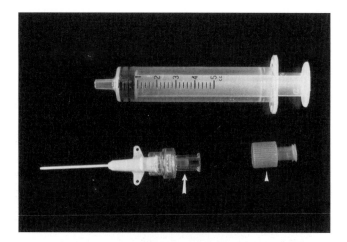

Fig. 5.4 SafSite™ (Burron Medical Inc., Bethlehem, PA) has luer lock fitting which attaches to IV cannula. One-way valve (arrow) is opened by inserting luer-slip syringe into fitting, which is covered with sterile cap (arrowhead) after use.

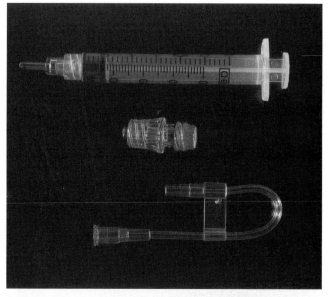

(a)

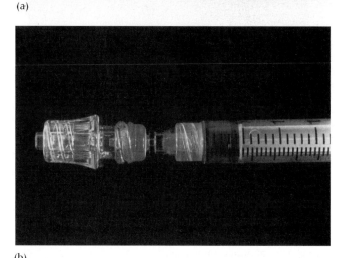

(b)

Fig. 5.5 (a) InterLink™ IV access system (Becton Dickinson, Franklin Lakes, NJ) has luer-lock adapter which connects to IV cannula directly or via luer-slip tubing. Syringe with blunt cannula is inserted through cap for access. Adapters are also available for drug vials. (b) Syringe inserted through cap.

addition, the use of gloves, masks, and gowns is recommended when caring for patients infected with MRSA [233].

TB is spread by droplet infection. Patients suspected of harboring this pathogen should be isolated in rooms that meet special criteria [235]. If undergoing procedures elsewhere, such as in the radiology department, they should wear masks or particulate respirators if possible. HCWs involved in the procedure should also wear particulate respirators. Respirators are preferred, because standard surgical masks do not filter out particles in the droplet size range (1–5 μm) and thus do not provide adequate protection [235]. A germicide or disinfectant is adequate for cleaning of procedure rooms after use for a known or suspected TB patient [235]. Reusable patient care equipment should be sterilized, except for items that come in contact only with intact skin. Such items do not transmit TB infection and need only be washed with detergent [235].

Vaccination

HCWs at risk for occupational exposure to blood and/or body fluids should be vaccinated against HBV. The currently available vaccine is a product of recombinant DNA technology and thus carries no risk of transmitting HIV or other pathogens [236]. Vaccination requires a series of three intramuscular injections, usually given over a 6-month period; response is confirmed by serologic testing. Booster doses of vaccine are not currently thought to be necessary as protection against infection appears to persist despite the decline in antibody levels with time [236]. It is not known whether HBV vaccine can cause harm to a fetus when given to a pregnant woman; vaccination during pregnancy should be avoided unless clearly indicated [236].

HCWs should also consider being vaccinated against rubella, tetanus, influenza, and measles. Although intense efforts are being made to develop a vaccine for HIV, none is currently available.

Prevention of intrauterine infection, which may cause serious fetal defects or death, is the major goal of rubella vaccination. Immunization is recommended during childhood for the general population. All medical personnel who do not have proof of immunity should be vaccinated, as transmission of rubella between HCWs and patients has occurred; HCWs may also infect coworkers, and patients may infect other patients as well [237]. Antibody titers may

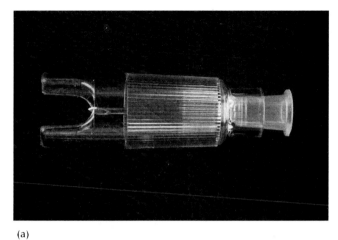

(a)

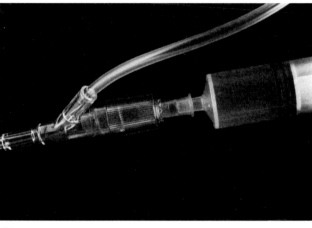

(b)

Fig. 5.6 (a) Safety-Gard™ IV needle (Becton Dickinson, Franklin Lakes, NJ) connects to heparin lock and Y site IV ports and can be used with any syringe or male luer fitting. Rigid shield extends beyond point of needle, providing passive needlestick protection. (b) Safety-Gard™ needle inserted into IV tubing Y site.

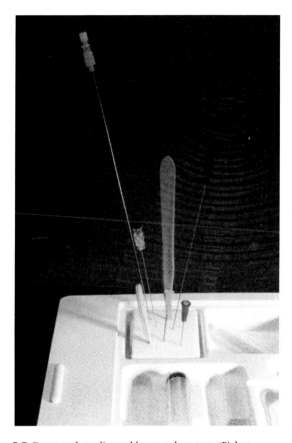

Fig. 5.7 Foam pad on disposable procedure tray (Picker International, Highland Heights, OH) keeps needles sterile and accessible on tray while protecting personnel.

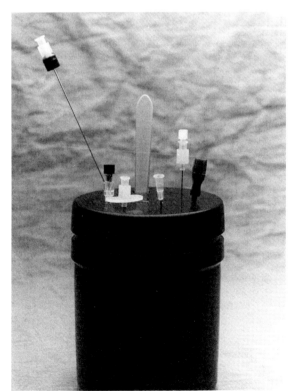

Fig. 5.8 Empty 105-mm film cannister (Kodak PFC film) with holes punched in lid can be sterilized and reused as a sharps holder for procedure trays. Needles of any length and scalpels can be accommodated; holes may be made in any size and shape.

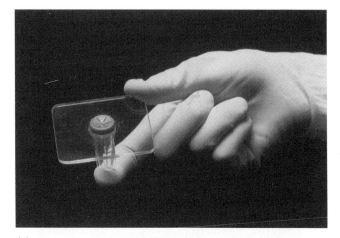

(a)

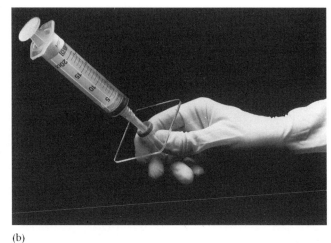

(b)

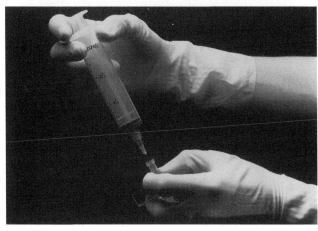

(c)

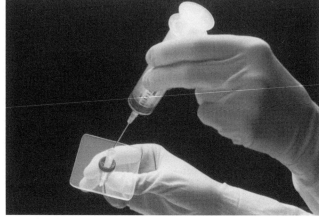

(d)

Fig. 5.9 Needle sheath guard (Hygenic Corp., Akron, OH; distributed by AliMed Inc., Dedham, MA). (a) Empty sheath holder. Unit can be washed and cold sterilized for reuse. (b) Sheathed needle is inserted into holder. (c) Sheath is held with one hand while needle is uncapped. (d) Needle is resheathed while holding guard with fingers behind protective flange.

decline below recommended levels years after vaccination, and repeat vaccination is then warranted. The rubella vaccine is a preparation of live, attenuated virus, and is given as a single subcutaneous injection. Rubella vaccine is contra-indicated during pregnancy, which should be avoided for 3 months after vaccination [237].

Tetanus vaccination is recommended for the population at large, with primary immunization during childhood and booster doses every 10 years [238]. Two formulations are available, both produced from formaldehyde-treated growth products of *Clostridium tetani*. The combination of tetanus and diphtheria toxoids (Td) is recommended for booster doses in adults [238], and is given as a single intramuscular injection.

The influenza vaccine consists of inactivated virus har-vested from infected chicken embryos, and is administered in a single intramuscular injection [239]. Influenza vaccines are formulated each year against the viral strains expected to be common in the subsequent year. Immunity lasts approximately 1 year, although variation is common. Influenza vaccination is recommended for HCWs, as they may transmit the virus to high-risk patients under their care [239].

Measles vaccine is a preparation of live, attenuated virus produced in chicken embryo cell culture [240], administered by subcutaneous injection. Vaccination with two doses given 1 month apart is recommended for medical personnel born in 1957 or later, who do not have documentation of immunity [240]. Measles vaccine is contraindicated during pregnancy, which should be avoided for 30 days after mono-valent measles vaccine, or 3 months if combined measles–rubella vaccine is given [240].

Recommendations in the event of exposure

Current recommendations in the event of parenteral (mucous membrane surfaces, percutaneous, or nonintact

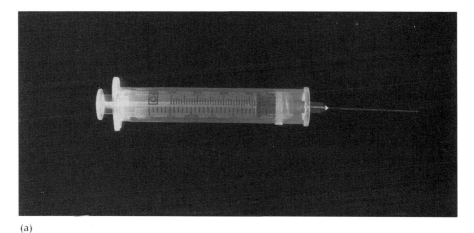

(a)

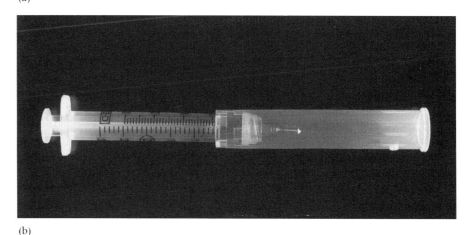

Fig. 5.10 (a) Safety-lok™ syringe (Becton Dickinson, Franklin Lakes, NJ) has plastic sleeve encasing barrel. Sleeve locks into open position for use. (b) After use, sleeve is pushed forward to cover exposed needle and clicked into position.

(b)

skin) exposure to blood or body fluid include testing of the source individual and the exposed individual for HIV and HBV as soon as possible after exposure occurs [10]. HCV testing has recently become available, but is not at present included in most postexposure recommendations. Other actions that should be taken depend on the results of the above tests.

If the source individual is HIV-positive, the exposed person should be counseled about receiving antiviral prophylaxis with zidovudine (AZT). AZT is a synthetic nucleoside, available in oral and IV forms, which is active against human retroviruses. Although it is widely used [241–243], the efficacy of zidovudine chemoprophylaxis has not been established and it is not currently considered the standard of care [188]. Nevertheless, many exposed individuals still choose to take it. As HIV infection may be established within hours of exposure, chemoprophylaxis should be started promptly — within 1 hour of exposure, if possible — if used [241]. Dosage regimens [241,242] are given in Table 5.7.

Counseling is an integral part of postexposure care, and should be provided by a health care professional experienced in this field. The exposed person should be retested for HIV at intervals of 3 and 6 months after exposure if the initial test

is negative, and should be advised to follow safe sexual practices during this period. Other precautions, such as not sharing toothbrushes, razors, or needles, should also be followed. In addition, the exposed individual should not donate blood, body organs, or sperm for 6 months following exposure. Preventing pregnancy for 6 months after exposure is probably advisable as well.

If the source individual has serologic evidence of HBV infectivity (HBsAg- or HBeAg-positive) and the exposed individual is not immune through vaccination or prior infection, the HBV vaccine series should be started within 7 days of exposure [244]. In addition, HBV immune globulin (HBIG) should be administered within 24 hours of exposure (Table 5.7). HBV vaccine and HBIG may inactivate each other if mixed in a syringe or injected in the same site [236]. HBIG is prepared from plasma that has been screened for HIV. No cases of HIV infection or AIDS due to HBIG administration have been reported [245]. Giving both the vaccine and HBIG is more effective in preventing infection than either agent given alone [188]. If the exposed individual has been vaccinated previously but not tested for immunity in the preceding 24 months, his or her anti-HBsAg level should be determined, because the duration of protection provided

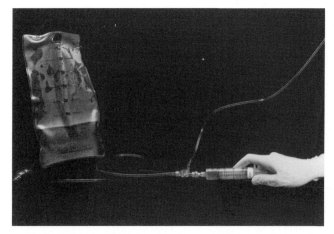

(a)

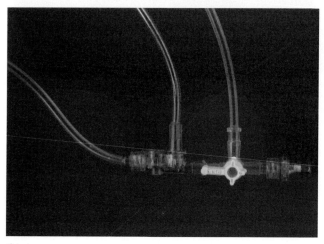

(b)

Fig. 5.11 (a) AngioFill[Tm] closed flush system (AngioDynamics, Glens Falls, NY) incorporates a check valve to allow refill and disposal of flush solution without need for a stopcock. Valve adapter prevents leakage when no syringe is attached. (b) Dual line version (AngioFill[Tm] II) has two fluid lines and a three-way stopcock to select active line.

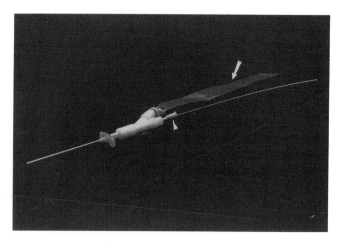

Fig. 5.12 Safe Stick[Tm] arterial puncture adapter (Cook Inc., Bloomington, IN) attaches to puncture needle; blood return from punctured artery fills plastic sleeve (arrow), and guidewire is introduced through side arm (arrowhead).

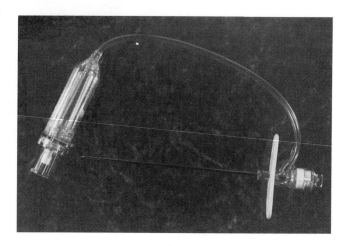

Fig. 5.13 Sos Pulse-Vu[Tm] puncture needle (AngioDynamics, Glens Falls, NY) is available in single- and double-wall designs. Blood flows from cannula to tubing, which has a one-way valve that allows injection of contrast but prevents egress of blood. The expanded portion of the tubing serves as a reservoir in which pulsations can be observed. Hemostatic valve on cannula prevents backflow but allows passage of guidewire.

by the vaccine is uncertain and titers fall gradually over several years [188]. Vaccine recipients whose anti-HBsAg titers are less than 10 mlU/ml should receive prophylaxis, as recommended by the Immunization Practices Advisory Committee [244]. Follow-up testing for infection or immunity should be performed at least 4–6 months after administration of HBIG [188]. Exposed individuals should be counseled about universal precautions and hygiene, but those who follow the recommended prophylaxis regimen pose a minimal risk to patients and household contacts, and there is no reason to restrict their patient-care activities during the interval between tests [188].

Recommendations for care after exposure to HCV include serologic testing acutely and again 6–9 months later [188], as well as counseling. If infection with HCV is diagnosed,

liver function testing should be performed so that appropriate treatment for hepatitis can be provided if necessary [188]. The use of immune globulin to prevent HCV infection after exposure is not recommended, because there is no evidence to support its efficacy [188]. Interferon alfa has been used in the treatment of chronic hepatitis C with some success [188], but currently has no role in prophylaxis. Because of the low risk of sexual transmission of HCV and the low risk of infection after exposure, no special precautions are essential during the 6- to 9-month interval between tests [188].

New OSHA rules, in addition to provisions designed to reduce exposure risks, also contain regulations on handling

Table 5.7 Recommendations in the event of exposure

OSHA regulations require
- Confidential medical evaluation and follow-up, to include:
  documentation of route and circumstances of exposure
  identification and documentation of source
  collection and testing of blood for HIV and HBV
  postexposure prophylaxis if medically indicated
  counseling
  evaluation of reported illnesses
- The written opinion of the health care provider performing the evaluation must be provided to the exposed individual within 15 days after evaluation is completed
- Medical records on exposed employees must be kept for the duration of employment + 30 years

Postexposure prophylaxis for HIV
- AZT (dosage regimens currently in use):
  200 mg p.o. q4h × 6 weeks (NIH)
  200 mg p.o. q4h (skip dose at 4 a.m.) × 4 weeks (SFGH)

Postexposure prophylaxis for HBV (exposed person not immune):
- HBV immune globulin (HBIG):
  one dose within 24 hours
- HBV vaccine series:
  first dose within 7 days

Postexposure prophylaxis for HCV:
- None currently recommended

q, every; NIH, National Institutes of Health; p.o., *per os* (oral administration); SFGH, San Francisco General Hospital.

of exposure incidents, including requirements for post-exposure treatment and record-keeping (Table 5.7) [10].

Special considerations

Situations that merit greater attention to infection control issues include pregnant patients/HCWs, immuno-compromised patients/HCWs, and patients who may need antibiotic prophylaxis prior to certain radiologic procedures.

Pregnancy

Concerns about pregnancy in the health care setting are primarily related to viral infections, especially rubella (German measles) and cytomegalovirus (CMV). Initial infection with these agents during pregnancy can result in serious harm to the fetus, including death. Pregnant HCWs (or those attempting to become pregnant) should not be exposed to patients with these viruses; similarly, HCWs with these infections should not care for patients who are or may be pregnant. HCWs who are not immune to rubella may transmit infection to patients and to coworkers, and immunization of all at-risk personnel should be performed [227].

Pregnant individuals are not more susceptible to HIV infection than other persons, and pregnant HCWs do not need to take any additional precautions when caring for HIV-infected patients [222]; however, strict adherence to universal precautions and other guidelines is advisable. Zidovudine chemoprophylaxis against HIV infection is not recommended for women who are pregnant or breastfeeding or for those of childbearing age who will not use contraception [188].

Immunocompromised patients/HCWs

Appropriate precautions should be taken by HCWs caring for patients who are immunocompromised, whether from AIDS, cancer, drug therapy, or other causes. Proper handwashing is the single most important precaution, and should be a standard part of radiology practice. Other precautions, such as gloves and face masks, may be needed depending on the type and severity of immunodeficiency.

Immunocompromised HCWs should discuss their job responsibilities with their personal physicians, and determine which activities are safe to perform and which, if any, should be avoided. HIV-positive HCWs, if otherwise healthy, may not be at significantly increased risk of acquiring infection from patients. However, medical judgment should be exercised in determining what job activities are safe for each worker. Because of their increased susceptibility to infection, it is probably prudent for HIV-positive HCWs not to be directly involved in caring for patients with TB.

Antibiotic prophylaxis

Antibiotic prophylaxis prior to certain invasive or surgical procedures is accepted practice for individuals with structural cardiac abnormalities. The revised American Heart Association (AHA) guidelines published in 1990 [246], however, no longer recommend prophylaxis for some procedures, such as gastrointestinal endoscopy or biopsy, for which it had previously been recommended [247]. The AHA guidelines do *not* recommend antibiotic prophylaxis for barium enema, cardiac catheterization, or angiography [246,247] but *do* recommend it for urethral dilatation, esophageal dilatation, urinary procedures if urinary tract infection is present, and biliary procedures. Recommended antibiotic regimens are included in the AHA guidelines [246]. In addition, recommendations for endocarditis prophylaxis, prophylaxis in surgery, and appropriate choice of antibacterial drugs are regularly updated in *The Medical Letter* [248–250]. A summary of prophylaxis regimens is given in Tables 5.8 and 5.9 [246–251].

Some feel that in addition to patients with cardiac lesions, those with prosthetic joints or other implanted orthopedic devices should receive antibiotic prophylaxis, but this is controversial. Antibiotic prophylaxis for patients in these groups may be warranted in the presence of factors that impair immune response, such as diabetes mellitus, cortico-

Table 5.8 Antibiotics for endocarditis prophylaxis

Oral/dental/upper respiratory tract procedures

Standard

Amoxicillin 3 g p.o. 1 hour before procedure, +1.5 g 6 hours after first dose (or 2 g IV or IM 30 minutes before procedure, +1 g IV/IM in 6 hours)

Penicillin allergy

Erythromycin ethylsuccinate 800 mg p.o. (or stearate, 1 g) 1 hour before procedure, +50% original dose in 6 hours
or
clindamycin 300 mg p.o. 1 hour before procedure, +150 mg p.o. in 6 hours (same doses can be given IV instead, with initial dose given 30 minutes before procedure)

Gastrointestinal/genitourinary procedures

Standard

Ampicillin 2 g IV/IM + gentamicin 1.5 mg/kg (maximum 80 mg) 30 minutes before procedure, + amoxicillin 1.5 g p.o. in 6 hours

Penicillin allergy

Vancomycin 1 g IV (given over 1 hour) + gentamicin as above

IM, intramuscularly; p.o., *per os* (orally).

Table 5.9 Antibiotic prophylaxis for radiologic procedures. These regimens are for *prophylaxis* only and are not intended for use in known/suspected infection. Drugs should be given just before the procedure unless otherwise stated

Procedure	Regimen
*Vascular procedures	
Standard	None
Graft puncture	Cefazolin 1 g IV or IM, or vancomycin 1 g IV
Lymphangiography	None
Needle biopsy (transcutaneous)	None
Biliary procedures	Cefazolin 1 g IV or IM
Gastrointestinal intubation	None
Drainage/aspiration of clear fluid collection (*not* suspected or known abscess)	None
Peritoneal catheter placement or manipulation	None
Genitourinary procedures	Cefazolin 1 g IV or IM
HSG	Doxycycline 100 mg p.o. b.i.d. × 5 days (start 2 days before procedure), *or* 200 mg p.o. × 1 just before procedure + 100 mg p.o. b.i.d. × 5 days thereafter
Transrectal prostate biopsy	Doxycycline 100 mg p.o. b.i.d. × 3 days (start 1 day before procedure)
Pulmonary/pleural interventions	None
Arthrography/diskography	None
Myelography	None

* Antibiotic prophylaxis is *not* indicated for routine vascular procedures, but may be used in patients with synthetic vascular grafts undergoing angiography, at the discretion of the radiologist and vascular surgeon involved.
b.i.d., twice a day; IM, intramuscularly; p.o., *per os* (orally).

steroid or other immunosuppressant therapy, and debilitating systemic diseases.

A related issue is whether patients with prosthetic vascular grafts should be given antibiotics prior to undergoing angiography or other invasive procedures. Antibiotic prophylaxis is clearly warranted before graft implantation surgery [252], but its value in patients with previously placed grafts undergoing angiography is less clear. Some believe that the risk of graft infection, while small, is sufficient to justify prophylaxis because of the high associated morbidity and mortality [30]. Others believe the risks of indiscriminate antibiotic use, including possible adverse reactions, organ damage, and selection of resistant organisms, outweigh the small risk of postprocedural infection in clean procedures [251–254]. Although experimental studies have shown newly implanted prosthetic grafts to be vulnerable to infection [255], clinical experience would seem to indicate a low risk of infection in patients with endothelialized grafts [256]. Because graft infection is uncommon, with an incidence of well under 2% [29], controlled studies to assess the value of antibiotics in this setting would be difficult to perform.

General principles of prophylactic antibiotic use are well understood. Timing of prophylactic antibiotic administration is most important, as antibiotics will have less effect if not given appropriately [251,253]. Adequate blood levels must be present during the entire period of risk, both at the beginning of a procedure and throughout its duration. A recent study of prophylactic antibiotic use in surgery [257], found maximum benefit of antibiotic prophylaxis when given no more than 1–2 hours before surgery. This study also found that prophylaxis was not correctly timed in about 40% of cases. Antibiotic doses should be repeated during long procedures, generally those lasting 3 hours or longer [254], so that blood levels are maintained. Continuation of prophylactic antibiotics after completion of the procedure has no proven benefit [251–254].

In deciding whether to give antibiotics prior to a particular radiologic procedure, it is necessary to evaluate the risk of infection associated with that procedure, as well as the status of the individual patient. Spies *et al.* [251] have classified radiologic procedures using an adaptation of the National Academy of Sciences/National Research Council classification of surgical wounds, which provides an excellent basis for risk assessment. Using this approach, procedures can be divided into clean, clean–contaminated, contaminated, or dirty. Vascular procedures are considered clean except for infusion therapy, which is clean–contaminated. Biliary procedures are best considered contaminated, due to the frequency of bacterial colonization of the biliary tree in patients undergoing invasive biliary procedures. In the genitourinary tract, procedures may be clean-contaminated, contaminated, or dirty. Aspiration and/or drainage of abdominal fluid collections, for the most part, are considered contaminated or dirty. Using this approach, antibiotics should be given prior to all procedures classified as contaminated or dirty [251]. Any procedure in which pus or other clinical evidence of infection is present is considered dirty.

Conclusions

The low rate of infectious complications in radiology is encouraging, but room for improvement remains, particularly in the area of infection control. Despite widely publicized recommendations by the CDC and other groups, use of universal precautions in current radiologic practice is far from uniform. Education and training of radiology personnel, both physicians and others, is needed to address this problem. Better understanding of infection risks and appropriate means of risk reduction will enhance procedure safety for HCWs and patients alike.

References

1 Goldsmith MF. Medical exorcism required as revitalized revenant of tuberculosis haunts and harries the land. *J Am Med Assoc* 1992;268:174–175.

2 Menzies D, Fanning A, Yuan L, Fitzgerald M. Tuberculosis among health care workers. *New Engl J Med* 1995;332:92–98.

3 Centers for Disease Control. Nosocomial transmission of multidrug resistant tuberculosis among HIV-infected persons — Florida and New York, 1988–1991. *MMWR* 91;40:585–591.

4 Hambrick GW, Cox RP, Senior JR. Primary herpes simplex infection of fingers of medical personnel. *Arch Dermatol* 1962;85:65–71.

5 Collins CH, Kennedy DA. Microbiological hazards of occupational needlestick and "sharps" injuries. *J Appl Bact* 1987;62:385–402.

6 Glaser JB, Garden A. Inoculation of cryptococcus without transmission of the acquired immunodeficiency syndrome. *New Engl J Med* 1985;313:266.

7 Sexton DJ, Gallis HA, McRae JR, Cate TR. Possible needle-associated Rocky Mountain spotted fever. *New Engl J Med* 1975;292:645.

8 Cannon NJ, Walker SP, Dismukes WE. Malaria acquired by accidental needle puncture. *J Am Med Assoc* 1972;222:1425.

9 Daniel Su WP, Muller SA. Herpes zoster: case report of possible accidental inoculation. *Arch Dermatol* 1976;112:1755–1756.

10 OSHA. Occupational exposure to bloodborne pathogens: final rule (29 CFR 1910.1030). *Fed Reg* 1991;56:64 003–64 182.

11 Ayliffe GAJ. Role of the environment of the operating suite in surgical wound infection. *Rev Infect Dis* 1991; 13(Suppl. 10):S800–S804.

12 Williams REO. Epidemiology of airborne staphylococcal infection. *Bact Rev* 1966;30:660–672.

13 Davies RR, Noble WC. Dispersal of bacteria on desquamated skin. *Lancet* 1962;2:1295–1297.

14 Behind the mask (editorial). *Lancet* 1981;1:197–198.

15 Pelz D, Fox AJ, Vinuela F. Clinical trial of iohexol vs. Conray-60 for cerebral angiography. *AJNR* 1984;5:565–568.

16 Hessel SJ, Adams DF, Abrams HL. Complications of angiography. *Radiology* 1981;138:273–281.

17 Swan HJC. Infectious, inflammatory, and allergic complications. *Circulation* 1968;37(Suppl. 3): 11 149–11 151.

18 Wennevold A, Christiansen I, Lindeneg O. Complications in 4413 catheterizations of the right side of the heart. *Am Heart J* 1965;69:173–180.

19 Bagger M, Biorck G, Bjork VO *et al.* On methods and complications in catheterization of heart and large vessels with and without contrast injection. *Am Heart J* 1957;54:766–777.

20 McAfee JG. A survey of complications of abdominal aortography. *Radiology* 1957;68:825–838.

21 Winchell P. Infectious endocarditis as a result of contamination during cardiac catheterization. *New Engl J Med* 1953;248:245–246.

22 Shawker TH, Kluge RM, Ayella RJ. Bacteremia associated with angiography. *J Am Med Assoc* 1974;229:1090–1092.

23 Kreidberg MB, Chernoff HL. Ineffectiveness of penicillin prophylaxis in cardiac catheterization. *J Pediatr* 1965;66:286–290.

24 Gould L, Lyon AF. Penicillin prophylaxis cardiac catheterization. *J Am Med Assoc* 1967;202:210–211.

25 Sande MA, Levinson ME, Lukas DS, Kaye D. Bacteremia associated with cardiac catheterizations. *New Engl J Med* 1969;281:1104–1106.

26 Landreneau MD, Raju S. Infections after elective bypass surgery for lower limb ischemia: the influence of preoperative transcutaneous arteriography. *Surgery* 1981;90:956–961.

27 Szilagyi DE, Smith RF, Elliott JP, Vrandecic MP. Infection in arterial reconstruction with synthetic grafts. *Ann Surg* 1972;176:321–333.

28 Conn JH, Hardy JD, Chavez CM, Fain WR. Infected arterial grafts: experience in 22 cases with emphasis on unusual bacteria and technics. *Ann Surg* 1970;171:704–714.

29 Fry WJ, Lindenauer SM. Infection complicating the use of plastic arterial implants. *Arch Surg* 1967;94:600–609.

30 Quinones-Baldrich WJ, Hernandez JJ, Moore WS. Long-term results following surgical management of aortic graft infection. *Arch Surg* 1991;126:507–511.

31 Hunter DW, Simmons RL, Hulbert JC. Antibiotics for radiologic interventional procedures. *Radiology* 1988;166:572–573.

32 Cruse PJE, Foord R. The epidemiology of wound infection: a 10-year prospective study of 62,939 wounds. *Surg Clin N Am* 1980;60:27–40.

33 Hamilton HW, Hamilton KR, Lone FJ. Preoperative hair removal. *Can J Surg* 1977;20:269–275.

34 Seropian R, Reynolds BM. Wound infections after preoperative depilatory versus razor preparation. *Am J Surg* 1971;121:251–254.

35 Hemingway AP, Allison DJ. Complications of embolization: analysis of 410 procedures. *Radiology* 1988;166:669–672.

36 Miller FJ Jr, Mineau DE. Transcatheter arterial embolization: major complications and their prevention. *Cardiovasc Intervent Radiol* 1983;6:141–149.

37 Rankin RN. Gas formation after renal tumor embolization without abscess: a benign occurrence. *Radiology* 1979;130:317–320.

38 Levy JM, Wasserman PI, Weiland DE. Nonsuppurative gas formation in the spleen after transcatheter splenic infarction.

Radiology 1981;139:375−376.

39 Siim E, Fleckenstein P. Gas formation following hepatic tumor embolisation. *Br J Radiol* 1982;55:926−928.

40 Hennessy OF, Allison DJ. Intra-hepatic gas following embolisation (letter). *Br J Radiol* 1983;56:348.

41 Spigos DG, Jonasson O, Mozes M, Capek V. Partial splenic embolization in the treatment of hypersplenism. *Am J Roentgenol* 1979;132:777−782.

42 LaBerge, JM, Gordon RL, Ring EJ. *Transjugular Intrahepatic Portosystemic Shunts with Use of the Wallstent Endoprosthesis: Midterm Results*. Washington DC: presented at 17th annual SCVIR meeting, April 4−9, 1992.

43 Zemel G, Becker GJ, Benenati JF, Katzen BT, Semba C, Julien W. *Transjugular Intrahepatic Portosystemic Shunts*. Washington DC: presented at 17 annual SCVIR meeting, April 4−9, 1992.

44 Hausegger KA, Lammer J, Flueckiger F, Klein GE, Aschauer M. *Transjugular Intrahepatic Portosystemic Shunt: First Clinical Experience*. Washington DC: presented at 17th annual SCVIR meeting, April 4−9, 1992.

45 Darcy MD, Picus D, Hicks ME *et al. Transjugular Intrahepatic Portosystemic Shunts with use of the Wallstent*. Washington DC: presented at 17th annual SCVIR meeting, April 4−9, 1992.

46 Maynar M, Cabrera J, Pulido-Duque JM *et al. Transjugular Intrahepatic Portosystemic Shunt*. Washington DC: presented at 17th annual SCVIR meeting, April 4−9, 1992.

47 Noeldge G, Rossle M, Perarneau JM, Richter GM, Palmaz JC, Wenz W. *Transjugular Intrahepatic Portosystemic Shunt: Follow-up to 42 Patients*. Washington DC: presented at 17th annual SCVIR meeting, April 4−9, 1992.

48 Mazer MJ, Moore DE, Layton B *et al. Tips on Transjugular Intrahepatic Portosystemic Shunts*. Washington DC: presented at 17th annual SCVIR meeting, April 4−9, 1992.

49 Katzen BT. *Performing Surgery in an Interventional Suite*. Miami, Florida: presented at 7th Annual International Symposium on Vascular Diagnosis and Intervention, January 21−25, 1995.

50 Chuter TAM. *Endovascular Bifurcated Graft Insertion for Aortic Aneurysm Repair*. Miami, Florida: presented at 7th Annual International Symposium on Vascular Diagnosis and Intervention, January 21−25, 1995.

51 Becker GJ. *Endoluminal Grafts: Miami Vascular Institute Experience*. Miami, Florida: presented at 7th Annual International Symposium on Vascular Diagnosis and Intervention, January 21−25, 1995.

52 Mialhe C. *Use of Covered Self-expanding Bifurcated Stent-Grafts for Abdominal Aortic Aneurysm*. Miami, Florida: presented at 7th Annual International Symposium on Vascular Diagnosis and Intervention, January 21−25, 1995.

53 Veith FJ. *Montefiore Experience with Endovascular Grafts for Repair of Aneurysmal, Occlusive and Traumatic Arterial Lesions*. Miami, Florida: presented at 7th Annual International Symposium on Vascular Diagnosis and Intervention, January 21−25, 1995.

54 Dake MD. *Transluminal Endovascular Stent-Grafts for the Management of Thoracic Aortic Aneurysms*. Miami, Florida: presented at 7th Annual International Symposium on Vascular Diagnosis and Intervention, January 21−25, 1995.

55 Katzen BT. *Preliminary Results of the EVT Endovascular Grafting System (EGS) versus Standard Surgery for the Treatment of Abdominal Aortic Aneurysms*. Miami, Florida: presented at 7th Annual International Symposium on Vascular Diagnosis and Intervention, January 21−25, 1995.

56 Maki DG. Nosocomial bacteremia: an epidemiologic overview. *Am J Med* 1981;70:719−732.

57 Bogen JE. Local complications in 167 patients with indwelling venous catheters. *Surg Gynecol Obstet* 1960;111:112−114.

58 Samsoondar W, Freeman JB, Coultish I, Oxley C. Colonization of intravascular catheters in the intensive care unit. *Am J Surg* 1985;149:730−732.

59 Bernard RW, Stahl WM, Chase RM Jr. Subclavian vein catheterizations: a prospective study. II: infectious complications. *Ann Surg* 1971;173:191−200.

60 Band JD, Maki DG. Infections caused by arterial catheters used for hemodynamic monitoring. *Am J Med* 1979;67:735−741.

61 Pinilla JC, Ross DF, Martin T, Crump H. Study of the incidence of intravascular catheter infection and associated septicemia in critically ill patients. *Crit Care Med* 1983;11:21−25.

62 Graham DR, Keldermans MM, Klemm LW, Semenza NJ, Shafer ML. Infectious complications among patients receiving home intravenous therapy with peripheral, central, or peripherally placed central venous catheters. *Am J Med* 1991;91(Suppl. 3B):95S−100S.

63 Taus LF, Deutsch LS, Miller DP, McKenzie RA, Brandon JC. Venous access: radiology versus surgery. *JVIR* 1992;3:33.

64 Dick L, Mauro MA, Jaques PF, Buckingham P. Radiologic insertion of Hickman catheters in HIV-positive patients: infectious complications. *JVIR* 1991;2:327−329.

65 Kahn ML, Barboza RB, Kling GA, Heisel JE. Percutaneous placement of the PAS-Port implantable venous access port: initial results. *JVIR* 1992;3:32.

66 Andrews JC, Ensminger WD, Walker-Andrews SC. Infusion port designed to be accessed with a Teflon angiocath: feasibility study. *JVIR* 1992;3:32.

67 Maki DG, Goldman DA, Rhame FS. Infection control in intravenous therapy. *Ann Intern Med* 1973;79:867−887.

68 Koehler PR, Wohl GT, Schaffer B *et al.* Lymphography: a survey of its recent status. *Am J Roentgenol* 1964;91:1216−1221.

69 Jackson RJA. Complications of lymphography. *Br Med J* 1966;1:1203−1205.

70 Gazelle GS, Haaga JR. Guided percutaneous biopsy of intra-abdominal lesions. *Am J Roentgenol* 1989;153:929−935.

71 Welch TJ, Sheedy PF, Johnson CD, Johnson CM, Stephens DH. CT-guided biopsy: prospective analysis of 1000 procedures. *Radiology* 1989;171:493−496.

72 Lees WR, Hall-Craggs MA, Manhire A. Five years' experience of fine-needle aspiration biopsy: 454 consecutive cases. *Clin Radiol* 1985;36:517−520.

73 Yankaskas BC, Staab EV, Craven MB, Blatt PM, Sokhandan M, Carney CN. Delayed complications from fine-needle biopsies of solid masses of the abdomen. *Invest Radiol* 1986;21:325−328.

74 Schulz TB. Fine-needle biopsy of the liver complicated with bile peritonitis. *Acta Med Scand* 1976;199:141−142.

75 Schnyder PA, Candardjis G, Anderegg A. Peritonitis after thin-needle aspiration biopsy of an abscess. *Am J Roentgenol* 1981;137:1271−1272.

76 Ferrucci JT Jr, Wittenberg J, Mueller PR *et al.* Diagnosis of abdominal malignancy by radiologic fine-needle aspiration biopsy. *Am J Roentgenol* 1980;134:323−330.

77 Gamble P, Colapinto RF, Stronell RD, Colman JC, Blendis L. Transjugular liver biopsy: a review of 461 biopsies. *Radiology* 1985;157:589−593.

78 Bull HJM, Gilmore IT, Bradley RD, Marigold JH, Thompson RPH. Experience with transjugular liver biopsy. *Gut* 1983;24:1057−1060.

79 Gerzof SG, Robbins AH, Johnson WC, Birkett DH, Nabseth DC. Percutaneous catheter drainage of abdominal abscesses: a five year experience. *New Engl J Med* 1981;305:653−657.

80 Haaga JR, Weinstein AJ. CT-guided percutaneous aspiration

and drainage of abscesses. *Am J Roentgenol* 1980;135:1187−1194.

81 vanSonnenberg E, Mueller PR, Ferrucci JT Jr. Percutaneous drainage of 250 abdominal abscesses and fluid collections. Part I: results, failures, and complications. *Radiology* 1984;151: 337−341.

82 Butch RJ, Mueller PR, Ferrucci JT Jr *et al*. Drainage of pelvic abscesses through the greater sciatic foramen. *Radiology* 1986; 158:487−491.

83 Mueller PR, Simeone JF, Butch RJ *et al*. Percutaneous drainage of subphrenic abscess: a review of 62 patients. *Am J Roentgenol* 1986;147:1237−1240.

84 Jeffrey RB Jr, Tolentino CS, Federle MP, Laing FC. Percutaneous drainage of periappendiceal abscesses: review of 20 patients. *Am J Roentgenol* 1987;149:59−62.

85 Mueller PR, White EM, Glass-Royal M *et al*. Infected abdominal tumors: percutaneous catheter drainage. *Radiology* 1989;173: 627−629.

86 vanSonnenberg E, D'Agostino HB, Casola G, Halasz NA, Sanchez RB, Goodacre BW. Percutaneous abscess drainage: current concepts. *Radiology* 1991;181:617−626.

87 Lang EK, Springer RM, Glorioso LW, Cammarata CA. Abdominal abscess drainage under radiologic guidance: causes of failure. *Radiology* 1986;159:329−336.

88 Mueller PR, vanSonnenberg E, Ferrucci JT Jr. Percutaneous drainage of 250 abdominal abscesses and fluid collections. Part II: current procedural concepts. *Radiology* 1984;151:343−347.

89 Karlson KB, Martin EC, Fankuchen EI, Mattern RF, Schultz RW, Casarella WJ. Percutaneous drainage of pancreatic pseudocysts and abscesses. *Radiology* 1982;142:619−624.

90 Kuligowska E, Olsen WL. Pancreatic pseudocysts drained through a percutaneous transgastric approach. *Radiology* 1985; 154:79−82.

91 Nunez D, Yrizarry JM, Russell E *et al*. Transgastric drainage of pancreatic fluid collections. *Am J Roentgenol* 1985;145: 815−818.

92 Torres WE, Evert MB, Baumgartner BR, Bernardino ME. Percutaneous aspiration and drainage of pancreatic pseudocysts. *Am J Roentgenol* 1986;147:1007−1009.

93 Freeny PC, Lewis GP, Traverso LW, Ryan JA. Infected pancreatic fluid collections: percutaneous catheter drainage. *Radiology* 1988;167:435−441.

94 Matzinger FRK, Ho C-S, Yee AC, Gray RR. Pancreatic pseudocysts drained through a percutaneous transgastric approach: further experience. *Radiology* 1988;167:431−434.

95 Sacks D, Robinson ML. Transgastric percutaneous drainage of pancreatic pseudocysts. *Am J Roentgenol* 1988;151:303−306.

96 vanSonnenberg E, Wittich GR, Casola G *et al*. Percutaneous drainage of infected and noninfected pancreatic pseudocysts: experience in 101 cases. *Radiology* 1989;170:757−761.

97 Grosso M, Gandini G, Cassinis MC, Regge D, Righi D, Rossi P. Percutaneous treatment (including pseudocystograstrostomy) of 74 pancreatic pseudocysts. *Radiology* 1989;173:493−497.

98 Gilliland JD, Spies JB, Brown SB, Yrizarry JM, Greenwood LH. Lymphoceles: percutaneous treatment with povidone-iodine sclerosis. *Radiology* 1989;171:227−229.

99 White M, Mueller PR, Ferrucci JT Jr *et al*. Percutaneous drainage of post-operative abdominal and pelvic lymphoceles. *Am J Roentgenol* 1985;145:1065−1069.

100 vanSonnenberg E, Mueller PR, Ferrucci JT Jr. Percutaneous drainage of 250 abdominal abscesses and fluid collections, I: results, failures, and complications. *Radiology* 1984;151:337−341.

101 Meyers AM, Levine E, Myburgh JA, Goudie E. Diagnosis and management of lymphoceles after renal transplantation. *Urology* 1977;X:497−502.

102 Teplick SK. Diagnostic and therapeutic interventional gallbladder procedures. *Am J Roentgenol* 1989;152:913−916.

103 Vogelzang RL, Nemcek AA. Percutaneous cholecystostomy: diagnostic and therapeutic efficacy. *Radiology* 1988;168:29−34.

104 vanSonnenberg E, Wittich GR, Casola G. Diagnostic and therapeutic percutaneous gallbladder procedures. *Radiology* 1986; 160:23−26.

105 Clouse ME, Stokes KR, Lee RGL, Falchuk KR. Bile duct stones: percutaneous transhepatic removal. *Radiology* 1986;160: 525−529.

106 Burhenne HJ. Percutaneous extraction of retained biliary tract stones: 661 patients. *Am J Roentgenol* 1980;134:888−898.

107 Lois JF, Gomes AS, Grace PA, Deutsch LS, Pitt HA. Risks of percutaneous transhepatic drainage in patients with cholangitis. *Am J Roentgenol* 1987;148:367−371.

108 Cohan RH, Illescas FF, Saeed M. Infectious complications of percutaneous biliary drainage. *Invest Radiol* 1986;21:705−709.

109 Yee ACN, Ho C-S. Complications of percutaneous biliary drainage: benign vs malignant disease. *Am J Roentgenol* 1987;148: 1207−1209.

110 Hamlin JA, Friedman M, Stein MG, Bray JF. Percutaneous biliary drainage: complications of 118 consecutive catheterizations. *Radiology* 1986;158:199−202.

111 Lammer J, Neumayer K. Biliary drainage endoprostheses: experience with 201 placements. *Radiology* 1986;159:625−629.

112 Mueller PR, Ferrucci JT Jr, Teplick SK *et al*. Biliary stent endoprostheses: analysis of complications in 113 patients. *Radiology* 1985;156:637−639.

113 Ho C-S, Yeung EY. Percutaneous gastrostomy and transgastric jejunostomy. *Am J Roentgenol* 1992;158:251−257.

114 vanSonnenberg E, Wittich GR, Cabrera OA *et al*. Percutaneous gastrostomy and gastroenterostomy: 2. Clinical experience. *Am J Roentgenol* 1986;146:581−586.

115 Halkier BK, Ho C-S, Yee ACN. Percutaneous feeding gastrostomy with the Seldinger technique: review of 252 patients. *Radiology* 1989;171:359−362.

116 O'Keeffe F, Carrasco CH, Charnsangavej C, Richli WR, Wallace S, Freedman RS. Percutaneous drainage and feeding gastrostomies in 100 patients. *Radiology* 1989;172:341−343.

117 Hicks ME, Surratt RS, Picus D, Marx MV, Lang EV. Fluoroscopically guided percutaneous gastrostomy and gastroenterostomy: analysis of 158 consecutive cases. *Am J Roentgenol* 1990;154:725−728.

118 Saini S, Mueller PR, Gaa J *et al*. Percutaneous gastrostomy with gastropexy: experience in 125 patients. *Am J Roentgenol* 1990; 154:1003−1006.

119 Towbin RB, Ball WS, Bissett GS III. Percutaneous gastrostomy and percutaneous gastrojejunostomy in children: antegrade approach. *Radiology* 1988;168:473−476.

120 Casola G, Withers C, van Sonnenberg E, Herba MJ, Saba RM, Brown RA. Percutaneous cecostomy for decompression of the massively distended cecum. *Radiology* 1986;158:793−794.

121 vanSonnenberg E, Varney RR, Casola G *et al*. Percutaneous cecostomy for Ogilvie syndrome: laboratory observations and clinical experience. *Radiology* 1990;175:679−682.

122 Morrison MC, Lee MJ, Stafford SA, Saini S, Mueller PR. Percutaneous cecostomy: controlled transperitoneal approach *Radiology* 1990;176:574−576.

123 Crass JR, Simmons RL, Frick MP, Maile CW. Percutaneous decompression of the colon using CT guidance in Ogilvie syndrome. *Am J Roentgenol* 1985;144:475−476.

124 Jaques P, Richey W, Mandel S. Tenckhoff peritoneal dialysis catheter: cannulography and manipulation. *Am J Roentgenol* 1980;135:83−86.

125 Davis R, Young J, Diamond D *et al.* Management of chronic peritoneal catheter malfunction. *Am J Nephrol* 1982;2:85−90.

126 Degesys GE, Miller GA, Ford KK *et al.* Tenckhoff peritoneal dialysis catheters: the use of fluoroscopy in management. *Radiology* 1985;154:819−820.

127 Stein M, Gray R, Jacobs I, Elliott D, Grossman H. Radiologic placement of peritoneal dialysis catheters: preliminary experience. *JVIR* 1992;3:33.

128 Ross GJ, Kessler HB, Clair MR, Gatenby RA, Hartz WH, Ross LV. Sonographically guided paracentesis for palliation of symptomatic malignant ascites. *Am J Roentgenol* 1989;153:1309−1311.

129 Appelqvist P, Silvo J, Salmela L, Kostiainen S. On the treatment and prognosis of malignant ascites: is the survival time determined when the abdominal paracentesis is needed? *J Surg Oncol* 1982;20:238−242.

130 Towbin RB, Strife JL. Percutaneous aspiration, drainage, and biopsies in children. *Radiology* 1985;157:81−85.

131 Kirk IR III, Carrasco CH, Richli WR, Lawrence DD, Charnsangavej C, Chuang VP. Percutaneous placement of intraperitoneal catheters under fluoroscopic guidance. *JVIR* 1992; 3:32.

132 Stables DP, Ginsberg NJ, Johnson ML. Percutaneous nephrostomy: a series and review of the literature. *Am J Roentgenol* 1978;130:75−82.

133 LeRoy AJ, Segura JW. Percutaneous removal of renal calculi. *Radiol Clin N Am* 1986;24:615−622.

134 Lee WJ, Smith AD, Cubelli V *et al.* Complications of percutaneous nephrolithotomy. *Am J Roentgenol* 1987;148:177−180.

135 Dunnick NR, Carson CC, Braun SD *et al.* Complications of percutaneous nephrostolithotomy. *Radiology* 1985;157:51−55.

136 Pfister RC, Newhouse JH, Yoder IC *et al.* Complications of pediatric percutaneous renal procedures: incidence and observations. *Urol Clin N Am* 1983;10:563−571.

137 Gordon RL, Banner MP, Pollack HM. Selected endourologic techniques. *Radiol Clin N Am* 1986;24:633−649.

138 Walther PJ, Robertson CN, Paulson DF. Lethal complications of standard self-retaining ureteral stents in patients with ileal conduit urinary diversion. *J Urol* 1985;133:851−853.

139 Lang EK. Renal cyst puncture and aspiration: a survey of complications. *Am J Roentgenol* 1977;128:723−727.

140 Branitz BH, Schlossberg IR, Freed SZ. Complications of renal cyst puncture. *Urology* 1976;VII:578−580.

141 Sacks D, Banner MP, Meranze SG, Burke DR, Robinson M, McLean GK. Renal and related retroperitoneal abscesses: percutaneous drainage. *Radiology* 1988;167:447−451.

142 Darcy MD, McClennan BL, Picus D, Hicks ME, Pineda J. Transcervical salpingosplasty: current techniques and results. *Urol Radiol* 1991;13:74−79.

143 Thurmond AS, Rosch J. Nonsurgical fallopian tube recanalization for treatment of infertility. *Radiology* 1990;174:371−374.

144 Lang EK, Dunaway HE Jr, Roniger WE. Selective osteal salpingography and transvaginal catheter dilatation in the diagnosis and treatment of fallopian tube obstruction. *Am J Roentgenol* 1990;154:735−740.

145 Rifkin MD, Dahnert W, Kurtz AB. State of the art: endorectal sonography of the prostate gland. *Am J Roentgenol* 1990;154:691−700.

146 Clements R, Griffiths GJ, Peeling WB. "State of the art" trans-

rectal ultrasound imaging in the assessment of prostatic disease. *Br J Radiol* 1991;64:193−200.

147 Bree R, Roberts J, Jafri S. Transrectal ultrasound guided biopsy of the prostate: techniques and results. *J Ultrasound Med* 1988; 7(Suppl.):S79.

148 Castaneda F, Hulbert JC, Letourneau JG, Hunter DW, Castaneda-Zuniga WR, Amplatz K. Perineal abscess after prostatic urethroplasty with balloon catheter: report of a case. *Radiology* 1990;174:49−50.

149 Westcott JL. Direct percutaneous needle aspiration of localized pulmonary lesions: results in 422 patients. *Radiology* 1980;137:31−35.

150 Perlmutt LM, Johnson WW, Dunnick NR. Percutaneous transthoracic needle aspiration: a review. *Am J Roentgenol* 1989;152:451−455.

151 Conces DJ Jr, Clark SA, Tarver RD, Schwenk GR. Transthoracic aspiration needle biopsy: value in the diagnosis of pulmonary infections. *Am J Roentgenol* 1989;152:31−34.

152 Sinner WN. Complications of percutaneous transthoracic needle aspiration biopsy. *Acta Radiol (Diag)* 1976;17:813−828.

153 Mueller PR, Saini S, Simeone JF *et al.* Image-guided pleural biopsies: indications, technique, and results in 23 patients. *Radiology* 1988;169:1−4.

154 O'Moore PV, Mueller PR, Simeone JF *et al.* Sonographic guidance in diagnostic and therapeutic interventions in the pleural space. *Am J Roentgenol* 1987;149:1−5.

155 Silverman SG, Saini S, Mueller PR. Pleural interventions: indications, techniques, and clinical applications. *Radiol Clin N Am* 1989;27:1257−1266.

156 Reinhold C, Illescas FF, Atri M, Bret PM. Treatment of pleural effusions and pneumothorax with catheters placed percutaneously under imaging guidance. *Am J Roentgenol* 1989; 152:1189−1191.

157 vanSonnenberg E, Nakamoto SK, Mueller PR *et al.* CT- and ultrasound-guided catheter drainage of empyemas after chest-tube failure. *Radiology* 1984;151:349−353.

158 Silverman SG, Mueller PR, Saini S *et al.* Thoracic empyema: management with image-guided catheter drainage. *Radiology* 1988;169:5−9.

159 Merriam MA, Cronan JJ, Dorfman GS, Lambiase RE, Haas RA. Radiographically guided percutaneous catheter drainage of pleural fluid collections. *Am J Roentgenol* 1988;151:1113−1116.

160 Westcott JL. Percutaneous catheter drainage of pleural effusion and empyema. *Am J Roentgenol* 1985;144:1189−1193.

161 Perlmutt LM, Braun SD, Newman GE *et al.* Transthoracic needle aspiration: use of a small chest tube to treat pneumothorax. *Am J Roentgenol* 1987;148:849−851.

162 Casola G, van Sonnenberg E, Keightley A, Ho M, Withers C, Lee AS. Pneumothorax: radiologic treatment with small catheters. *Radiology* 1988;166:89−91.

163 Freiberger RH, Kaye JJ, Spiller J. *Arthrography*. New York: Appleton-Century-Crofts, 1979:2.

164 Massie WK, Stevens DB. A critical evaluation of discography. *J Bone Joint Surg* 1967;49A:1243−1244.

165 Wiley JJ, Macnab I, Wortzman G. Lumbar discography and its clinical applications. *Can J Surg* 1968;11:280−289.

166 Gardner WJ, Wise RE, Hughes CR, O'Connell RB, Weiford EC. X-ray visualization of the intervertebral disk. *Arch Surg* 1952; 64:355−364.

167 Onik G, Helms CA. Automated percutaneous lumbar diskectomy. *Am J Roentgenol* 1991;156:531−538.

168 Bonica JJ. *Principles and Practice of Obstetric Analgesia and Anesthesia*. Philadelphia: FA Davis, 1967:726.

169 Arner O. Complications following spinal anesthesia: their significance and a technic to reduce their incidence. *Acta Chirug Scand* 1952;167(Suppl.):7–146.

170 Schlesinger JL, Salit IE, McCormack G. Streptococcal meningitis after myelography. *Arch Neurol* 1982;39:576–577.

171 Schelkun SR, Wagner KF, Blanks JA, Reinert CM. Bacterial meningitis following pantopaque myelography: a case report and literature review. *Orthopedics* 1985;8:73–76.

172 Rose HD. Pneumococcal meningitis following intrathecal injections. *Arch Neurol* 1966;14:597–600.

173 Fischer GW, Brenz RW, Alden ER, Beckwith JB. Lumbar punctures and meningitis. *Am J Dis Child* 1975;129:590–592.

174 Worthington M, Hills J, Tally F, Flynn R. Bacterial meningitis after myelography. *Surg Neurol* 1980;14:318–320.

175 Alexiou J, Deloffre D, Vandresse JH, Boucquey JP, Sintzoff S. Post-myelographic meningeal irritation with iohexol. *Neuroradiology* 1991;33:85–86.

176 LeFrock J, Ellis CA, Klainer AS, Weinstein L. Transient bacteremia associated with barium enemas. *Arch Intern Med* 1975;135:835–837.

177 Butt J, Hetges D, Pelican G et al. Bacteremia during barium enema study. *Am J Roentgenol* 1978;130:715–718.

178 Richman LS, Short WF, Cooper WM. Barium enema septicemia: occurrence in a patient with leukemia. *J Am Med Assoc* 1973;226:62–63.

179 Hammer JL. Septicemia following barium enema. *South Med J* 1977;70:1361–1363.

180 vanSonnenberg E, Wittich GR, Edwards DK et al. Percutaneous diagnostic and therapeutic interventional radiologic procedures in children: experience in 100 patients. *Radiology* 1987;162:601–605.

181 Ball WS Jr, Bissett GS III, Towbin RB. Percutaneous drainage of chest abscesses in children. *Radiology* 1989;171:431–434.

182 Lorenzo RL, Bradford BF, Black J, Smith CD. Lung abscess in children: diagnostic and therapeutic needle aspiration. *Radiology* 1985;157:79–80.

183 Hansen ME, Kadir S. Elective and emergency embolotherapy in children and adolescents: efficacy and safety. *Radiolöge* 1990;30:331–336.

184 Ball WS Jr, Towbin R, Strife JL, Spencer R. Interventional genitourinary radiology in children: a review of 61 procedures. *Am J Roentgenol* 1986;147:791–796.

185 Lettau LA. The A, B, C, D, and E of viral hepatitis: spelling out the risks for healthcare workers. *Infect Control Hosp Epidemiol* 1992;13:77–81.

186 Alter MJ. Hepatitis C: a sleeping giant? *Am J Med* 1991;91(Suppl. 3B):112S–115S.

187 Alter MJ. Occupational exposure to hepatitis C: a dilemma. *Infect Control Hosp Epidemiol* 1994;15:742–744.

188 Gerberding JL. Management of occupational exposures to blood-borne viruses. *N Engl J Med* 1995;332:444–451.

189 Cooper BW, Krusell A, Tilton RC, Goodwin R, Levitz RE. Seroprevalence of antibodies to hepatitis C virus in high-risk hospital personnel. *Infect Control Hosp Epidemiol* 1992;13:82–85.

190 Kiyosawa K, Sodeyama T, Tanaka E et al. Hepatitis C in hospital employees with needlestick injuries. *Ann Intern Med* 1991;115:367–369.

191 Marranconi F, Mecenero V, Pellizzer GP et al. HCV infection after accidental needlestick injury in health-care workers. *Infection* 1992;20:111.

192 Lanphear BP, Linnemann CJ Jr, Cannon CG, DeRonde MM, Pendy L, Kerley LM. Hepatitis C virus infection in healthcare workers: risk of exposure and infection. *Infect Control Hosp Epidemiol* 1994;15:745–750.

193 Sartori M, La Terra G, Aglietta M et al. Transmission of hepatitis C via blood splash into conjunctiva. *Scand J Infect Dis* 1993;25:270–271.

194 Hansen ME, Miller GL III, Redman HC, McIntire DD. Needlestick injuries and blood contacts during invasive radiologic procedures. *Am J Roentgenol* 1993;160:1119–1122.

195 Gerberding JL, Littell C, Tarkington A, Brown A, Schecter WP. Risk of exposure of surgical personnel to patients' blood during surgery at San Francisco General Hospital. *New Engl J Med* 1990;322:1788–1793.

196 Popejoy SL, Fry DE. Blood contact and exposure in the operating room. *Surg Gynecol Obstet* 1991;172:480–483.

197 Hussain SA, Latif ABA, Choudhary AAAA. Risk to surgeons: a survey of accidental injuries during operations. *Br J Surg* 1988;75:314–316.

198 Tokars JI, Bell DM, Culver DH et al. Percutaneous injuries during surgical procedures. *J Am Med Assoc* 1992;267:2899–2904.

199 Quebbeman EJ, Telford GL, Hubbard S et al. Risk of blood contamination and injury to operating room personnel. *Ann Surg* 1991;214:614–620.

200 Lowenfels AB, Wormser GP, Jain R. Frequency of puncture injuries in surgeons and estimated risk of HIV infection. *Arch Surg* 1989;124:1284–1286.

201 Hansen ME, Miller GL III, Redman HC, McIntire DD. HIV and interventional radiology: a national survey of physician attitudes and behaviors. *JVIR* 1993;4:229–236.

202 Hansen ME, McIntire DD, Miller GL III, Redman HC. Use of universal precautions in interventional radiology: results of a national survey. *Am J Infect Control* 1994;22:1–5.

203 Beekmann SE, Fahey BJ, Gerberding JL, Henderson DK. Risky business: using necessarily imprecise casualty counts to estimate occupational risks for HIV-1 infection. *Infect Control Hosp Epidemiol* 1990;11:371–379.

204 Centers for Disease Control. Update: human immunodeficiency virus infections in health-care workers exposed to blood of infected patients. *MMWR* 1987;36:285–289.

205 Mast St, Gerberding JL. Factors predicting infectivity following needlestick exposure to HIV: an *in vitro* model. *Clin Res* 1991;39:58A.

206 Centers for Disease Control. Update: transmission of HIV infection during an invasive dental procedure — Florida. *MMWR* 1991;40:21–27,33.

207 Sacks JJ. AIDS in a surgeon. *New Engl J Med* 1985;313:1017–1018.

208 Mishu B, Schaffner W, Horan JM, Wood LH, Hutcheson RH, McNabb PC. A surgeon with AIDS: lack of evidence of transmission to patients. *J Am Med Assoc* 1990;264:467–470.

209 Danila RN, MacDonald KL, Rhame FS et al. A look-back investigation of patients of an HIV-infected physician: public health implications. *New Engl J Med* 1991;325:1406–1411.

210 Centers for Disease Control. Update: investigations of patients who have been treated by HIV-infected health-care workers. *MMWR* 1992;41:344–346.

211 Henderson DK, Fahey BJ, Willy M et al. Risk for occupational transmission of human immunodeficiency virus type 1 (HIV-1) associated with clinical exposures: a prospective evaluation. *Ann Intern Med* 1990;113:740–746.

212 Lowenfels AB, Wormser G. Risk of transmission of HIV from surgeon to patient. *New Engl J Med* 1991;325–888–889.

213 Chamberland ME, Bell DM. HIV transmission from health care

worker to patient: what is the risk? *Ann Intern Med* 1992;116:871–872.

214 Centers for Disease Control. Recommendations for preventing transmission of human immunodeficiency virus and hepatitis B virus to patients during exposure-prone invasive procedures. *MMWR* 1991;40(RR-8):1–9.

215 O'Flaherty J. The AIDS patient: a historical perspective on the physician's obligation to treat. *Pharos* 1991;54(3):13–16.

216 Faria MA Jr. To treat or not — can a physician choose? A commentary. *Pharos* 1992;55(1):39–40.

217 Gostin L. HIV-infected physicians and the practice of seriously invasive procedures. *Hastings Cent Report* 1989;19(1):32–39.

218 Daniels N. HIV-infected professionals, patient rights, and the "switching dilemma." *J Am Med Assoc* 1992;267:1368–1371.

219 Lo B, Steinbrook R. Health care workers infected with the human immunodeficiency virus: the next steps. *J Am Med Assoc* 1992;267:1100–1105.

220 Association for practitioners in infection control; society of hospital epidemiologists of America. Position paper: the HIV-infected healthcare worker. *Infect Control Hosp Epidemiol* 1990;11:647–656.

221 *Delegates Report: 1991 Interim Meeting of the AMA House of Delegates.* Chicago, IL: American Medical Association; 1991.

222 Centers for Disease Control. Recommendations for prevention of HIV transmission in health-care settings. *MMWR* 1987;36(Suppl. 2S).

223 Decker MD. The OSHA bloodborne hazard standard. *Infect Control Hosp Epidemiol* 1992;13:407–417.

224 American College of Radiology. OSHA details application of bloodborne pathogen standard. *ACR Bull* 1992;48(8):3.

225 Wall SD, Olcott EW, Gerberding JL. AIDS risk and risk reduction in the radiology department. *Am J Roentgenol* 1991;157:911–917.

226 Mueller PR, Silverman SG, Tung G *et al.* New universal precautions aspiration tray. *Radiology* 1989;173:278–279.

227 van Sonnenberg E, Casola G. Maysey M. Simple apparatus to avoid inadvertent needle puncture. *Radiology* 1988;166:550.

228 Olsen WL, Jeffrey RB Jr, Tolentino CS. Closed system for arterial puncture in patients at risk for AIDS. *Radiology* 1988;166:551–552.

229 Palestrant AM, Esplin CA, Shaw GT. A closed irrigation and drainage system for use with percutaneous abscess drainage: technical note. *Cardiovasc Intervent Radiol* 1990;13:119–121.

230 Williams DM, Marx MV, Korobkin M. AIDS risk and risk reduction in the radiology department (commentary). *Am J Roentgenol* 1991;157:919–921.

231 Hansen ME, McIntire DD, Miller GL III. Occult glove perforations: frequency during interventional radiologic procedures. *Am J Roentgenol* 1992;159:131–135.

232 Bessinger CD. Preventing transmission of human immunodeficiency virus during operations. *Surg Gynecol Obstet* 1988;167:287–289.

233 Wenzel RP, Nettleman MD, Jones RN, Pfaller MA. Methicillin-resistant *Staphylococcus aureus*: implications for the 1990s and effective control measures. *Am J Med* 1991;91(Suppl. 3B):221S–227S.

234 Ehrenkranz NJ. Bland soap handwash or hand antisepsis? The pressing need for clarity. *Infect Control Hosp Epidemiol* 1992;13:299–301.

235 Centers for Disease Control. Guidelines for preventing the transmission of tuberculosis in health-care settings, with special focus on HIV-related issues. *MMWR* 1990;39(RR-17):1–29.

236 Hepatitis B virus vaccine inactivated. In: McEvoy GK, ed. *AHFS Drug Information.* Bethesda: American Society of Hospital Pharmacists, 1992;2026–2034.

237 Rubella virus vaccine live. In: McEvoy GK, ed. *AHFS Drug Information.* Bethesda: American Society of Hospital Pharmacists, 1992;2061–2065.

238 Tetanus toxoid, tetanus toxoid adsorbed. In: McEvoy GK, ed. *AHFS Drug Information.* Bethesda: American Society of Hospital Pharmacists, 1992;2012–2015.

239 Influenza virus vaccine. In: McEvoy GK, ed. *AHFS Drug Information.* Bethesda: American Society of Hospital Pharmacists, 1992;2034–2038.

240 Measles virus vaccine live. In: McEvoy GK, ed. *AHFS Drug Information.* Bethesda: American Society of Hospital Pharmacists, 1992;2038–2043.

241 Zidovudine. In: McEvoy GK, ed. *AHFS Drug Information.* Bethesda: American Society of Hospital Pharmacists, 1992;392–401.

242 Centers for Disease Control. Public Health Service statement on management of occupational exposure to human immunodeficiency virus, including considerations regarding zidovudine postexposure use. *MMWR* 1990;39(RR-1):1–14.

243 Henderson DK. Postexposure chemprophylaxis for occupational exposure to human immunodeficiency virus type 1: current status and prospects for the future. *Am J Med* 1991;91(Supp. 3B):312S–319S.

244 Centers for Disease Control. Protection against viral hepatitis: recommendations of the immunization practices advisory committee (ACIP). *MMWR* 1990;39(RR-2):1–26.

245 Hepatitis B immune globulin. In: McEvoy GK, ed. *AHFS Drug Information.* Bethesda: American Society of Hospital Pharmacists, 1992;1982–1988.

246 Dajani AS, Bisno AL, Chung KJ *et al.* Prevention of bacterial endocarditis: recommendations by the American Heart Association. *J Am Med Assoc* 1990;264:2919–2922.

247 Shulman ST, Amren DP, Bisno AL *et al.* Prevention of bacterial endocarditis: a statement for health professionals by the Committee on rheumatic fever and infective endocarditis of the Council on cardiovascular disease in the young. *Circulation* 1984;70:1123A–1127A.

248 Antimicrobial prophylaxis in surgery. *Med Letter* 1992;34:5–8.

249 The choice of antibacterial drugs. *Med Letter* 1992;34:49–56.

250 Prevention of bacterial endocarditis. *Med Letter* 1989;31:112.

251 Spies JB, Rosen RJ, Lebowitz AS. Antibiotic prophylaxis in vascular and interventional radiology: a rational approach. *Radiology* 1988;166:381–387.

252 Hopkins CC. Antibiotic prophylaxis in clean surgery: peripheral vascular surgery, noncardiovascular thoracic surgery, herniorrhaphy, and mastectomy. *Rev Infect Dis* 1991;13(Suppl. 10):S869–S873.

253 Bohnen JMA. Antimicrobial prophylaxis in general surgery. *Can J Surg* 1991;34:548–550.

254 Stone HH. Basic principles in the use of prophylactic antibiotics. *J Antimicro Chemother* 84;14(Suppl. B):33–37.

255 Moore WS, Rosson CT, Hall AD, Thomas AN. Transient bacteremia: a cause of infection in prosthetic vascular grafts. *Am J Surg* 1969;117:342–343.

256 Wade GL, Smith DC, Mohr LL. Follow-up of 50 consecutive angiograms obtained utilizing puncture of prosthetic vascular grafts. *Radiology* 1983;146:663–664.

257 Classen DC, Evans RS, Pestotnik SL, Horn SD, Menlove RL, Burke JP. The timing of prophylactic administration of antibiotics and the risk of surgical-wound infection. *New Engl J Med* 1992;326:281–286.

The pregnant and nursing patient

Robert A. Knuppel and Shyam B. Hatangadi

Introduction

The application of procedures using ionizing radiation and the current ubiquitous utilization of ultrasound in the pregnant patient has raised legitimate concerns regarding the detrimental effects of these imaging modalities. Radiologists are likely to encounter pregnant patients in three clinical situations.

1 A radiologic procedure may be requested by the obstetrician in the course of the management of a pregnancy.

2 A pregnant patient may present with medical or surgical problems unrelated to the pregnancy itself but which require diagnostic evaluation.

3 Patients not known to be pregnant may undergo a radiologic procedure only to discover the fact after the event.

In all these cases, the main concerns for both the parents as well as the treating physicians stem from the possible adverse effects that radiation may have on the unborn child.

Diagnostic examinations in the pregnant woman should be performed after careful consideration of the benefits conferred by their utilization, as opposed to the known risks. Unfortunately, when viewed in the context of possible damage to the fertile woman, her fetus, or future pregnancies, this trade-off is often unnecessarily perceived as a dilemma and nihilistic radiologic evaluation ensues. In addition, the profound anatomic and physiologic adaptations to pregnancy also affect radiologic appearances to a considerable degree. As a consequence, the radiologist must be familiar with these normal pregnancy induced changes in order correctly to interpret findings. The following discussion will address these issues. Attention will be focused on the true value of diagnostic/therapeutic radiologic procedures as compared to their potential for damage and an attempt will be made to provide pragmatic guidelines for the application of various imaging techniques in the management of the pregnant or nursing patient.

The developing fetus and newborn

Milestones

A knowledge of the important milestones of fetal development is critical to the ability to understand/interpret potentially teratogenic events, especially with regard to the role of radiation. The most commonly reported effects from *in utero* irradiation in humans are central nervous system defects, e.g., mental retardation, microcephaly, growth retardation, or the development of leukemia or other childhood malignancies [1−5]. A brief review of fetal development with special regard to the central nervous and hematopoietic systems is provided as a background for the discussion to follow. Table 6.1 demonstrates a profile of fetal organogenesis and maturation in relation to gestational age.

Gestation can be broadly stratified as follows: (i) preimplantation, which extends from fertilization until the embryo attaches to the uterine wall; (ii) organogenesis, which represents the period when the major organ systems develop; and (iii) the fetal period, during which continued growth and maturation of preformed structures take place. The preimplantation and organogenesis phase of development is called the embryonic period. In terms of gestational age, this period spans the first 8 weeks (postfertilization) of pregnancy, or 10 weeks from the first day of the last normal menstrual period (post-LNMP). For reasons of clarity and practical application, gestational age will hereafter refer to weeks post-LNMP.

Table 6.1 Embryonic development. (From Jones [6])

Age days	Length mm	Stage	Gross appearance	CNS	Eye	Ear	Face
4		III	Blastocyst				
7–12	0.1	V	Ectoderm Endoderm Yolk sac Amnionic sac				
19	1	IX	Heart Ant head fold Body stalk	Enlargement of anterior neural plate			
24	2	X early somites	Foregut Allantois	Partial fusion neural folds	Optic evagination	Otic placode	Mandible Hyoid arches
30	4	XII 21–29 somites		Closure neural tube Rhombencephalon, mesen., prosen. Ganglia V VII VIII X	Optic cup	Otic invagination	Fusion, mand. arches
34	7	XIV		Cerebellar plate Cervical and mesencephalic flexures	Lens invagination	Otic vesicle	Olfactory placodes
36	11	XVI		Dorsal pontine flexure Basal lamina Cerebral evagination Neural hypophysis	Lens detached Pigmented retina	Endolymphic sac Ext. auditory meatus Tubotympanic recess	Nasal swellings
44	17	XVIII		Olfactory evagination Cerebral hemisphere	Lens fibers Migration of retinal cells Hyaloid vessels		Choana, Prim. palate
52	23	XX		Optic nerve to brain	Corneal body Mesoderm No lumen in optic stalk		
56	26	XXII			Eyelids	Spiral cochlear duct Tragus	

Table 6.1 *Continued*

Extremities	Heart	Gut, abdomen	Lung	Urogenital	Other
					Early blastocyst with inner cell mass and cavitation (58 cells) lying free within the uterine cavity
		Yolk sac			Early amnion sac. Extraembryonic mesoblast, angioblast. Chorionic gonadotropin
	Merging mesoblast anterior to prechordal plate	Stomatodeum Cloaca		Allantois	Primitive streak Henson's node Notochord Prechordal plate Blood cells in yolk sac
	Single heart tube Propulsion	Foregut		Mesonephric ridge	Yolk sac larger than amnion sac
Arm bud	Ventric outpouching Gelatinous reticulum	Rupture stomatodeum Evagination of thyroid, liver and dorsal pancreas	Lung bud	Mesonephric duct enters cloaca	Rathke's pouch Migration of myotomes from somites
Leg bud	Auric. outpouching Septum primum	Pharyngeal pouches yield parathyroids, lat thyroid, thymus Stomach broadens	Bronchi	Ureteral evag. Urorect. sept Germ cells Gonadal ridge Coelom, Epithelium	
Hand plate. Mesench condens. Innervation	Fusion mid A-V canal Muscular vent sept.	Intestinal loop into yolk stalk Cecum Gall bladder Hepatic ducts Spleen	Main lobes	Paramesonephric duct Gonad ingrowth of coelomic epith.	Adrenal cortex (from coelomic epithelium) invaded by sympathetic cells = medulla Jugular lymph sacs
Finger rays. Elbow	Aorta Pulmonary artery Valves Membrane ventricular septum	Duodenal lumen obliterated Cecum rotates right Appendix		Fusion urorect. sept. Open urogen. memb. anus Epith. cords in testicle	Early muscle
Clearing, central cartilage	Septum secundum			S-shaped vesicles in nephron blastoma connect with collecting tubules from calyces	Superficial vascular plexus low on cranium
Shell, tubular bone				A few large glomeruli Short secretory tubules Tunica albuginea Testicle, interstitial cells	Superficial vascular plexus at vortex

While major organogenesis in the human is complete by 10 weeks (8 weeks postfertilization), it has been shown that the cerebral hemispheres undergo continued and rapid neuronal development from the tenth through the eighteenth weeks of life [7]. Indeed, the central nervous system as a whole continues to grow and develop throughout gestation into the first 2–3 years after birth [6]. Hematopoiesis in the embryo is first demonstrable in the yolk sac where the first stem-cell populations make their appearance at about 3–5 weeks. The main site of hematopoiesis then shifts, at approximately 12 weeks, probably by migration of stem cells to the liver, spleen, and finally to their definitive locations in the bone marrow. Current opinion favors the existence of different stem-cell lineages responsible for the generation of red and white blood cells [8,9].

Radiosensitivity of fetal/organ systems

Generally speaking, more radiation is required to destroy "mature" tissue, e.g., muscle, than is required to damage actively replicating, developing tissue, e.g., stem cells. For this reason, the fetus is thought to be more sensitive to radiation at certain points in gestation, i.e., the embryonic period than at others, i.e., the fetal period. Both animal as well as human studies have demonstrated a correlation between gestational age and radiation-induced damage [1,10] (Fig. 6.1). It appears that during the preimplantation (morula) stage of development, the embryo exhibits an "all or none" response to irradiation where the end result depends upon the number of fetal cells destroyed. The larger the number of

cells initially injured, the greater the likelihood of fetal demise. Conversely, the smaller the extent of damage, the greater the likelihood of the fetus emerging unscathed [1].

The incidence of malformations has not measurably increased after *in utero* irradiation [12]. This finding does not, however, discount the fact that genetic mutation may have occurred after *in utero* radiation exposure, but is not measurable. No increase in radiation-induced mutation in children of bomb survivors in Japan has been thus far confirmed [13]. Thus, previous fears regarding the possibility of hereditary damage caused by fetal gonad exposure may well be unfounded.

Experimentally, germ-cell sensitivity to mutation in the gonads of the embryo or fetus is not greater than that in the adult. As previously mentioned, the most commonly reported effects of high-dose *in utero* radiation exposure are microcephaly, mental retardation, growth retardation, leukemia, and other childhood cancers. Dekaban [1] studied 26 human conceptuses and constructed a timetable of pregnancy outcome following high-dose *in utero* radiation (> 2.5 Gy) to the human at various gestational ages (Table 6.2). The central nervous system and hematopoietic system appear to be the most sensitive organ systems. There is a general consensus that the most vulnerable periods extend through 4–16 weeks of gestation. It is, however, erroneous to believe that the last two trimesters are relatively "safe" periods for radiation exposure, as the fetus continues to grow and develop throughout pregnancy. While it is true that exposure during the organogenetic phase results in the most severe *in utero* growth retardation at term, irradiation later in pregnancy

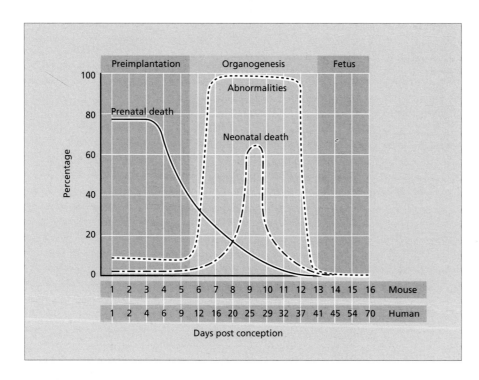

Fig. 6.1 Frequency of prenatal death, abnormalities, and neonatal death in murine embryos given a dose of 200 rad (2 Gy) at various times after fertilization. The lower scale consists of estimates of the equivalent stages for the human embryo. (From Hall [11].)

Table 6.2 Graphic summary of findings in 26 children who received irradiation during various stages of gestation. Observe that most abnormalities seem to occur following irradiation between 3 and 20 weeks, and that growth retardation is an almost universal finding. (From Dekaban [1])

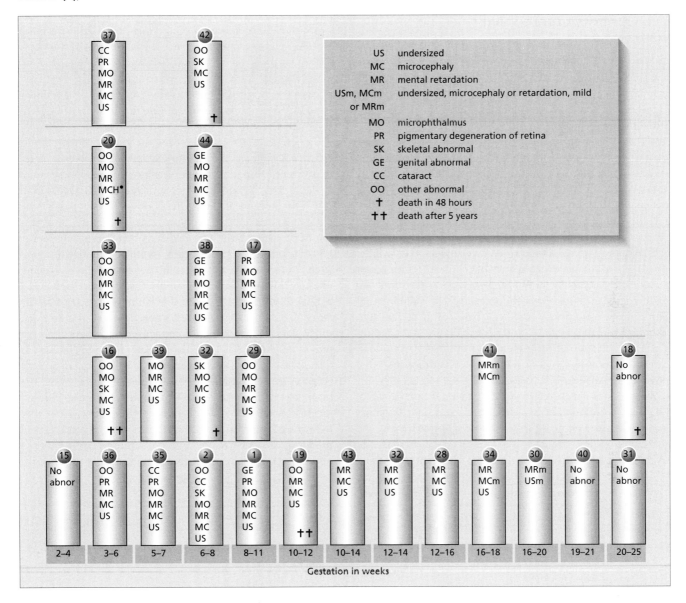

Table 6.3 Estimated dose to uterus from extraabdominal examinations (mrad/examination). (From Wagner *et al.* [15])

Examination	BRH $(1 \times 10^{-5}\,\mathrm{Gy})$	ICRP $(1 \times 10^{-5}\,\mathrm{Gy})$	UNSCEAR $(1 \times 10^{-5}\,\mathrm{Gy})$	Reported range $(1 \times 10^{-5}\,\mathrm{Gy})$
Dental		< 10	0.06	0.03−0.1
Head−cervical spine	< 0.5	< 10	< 10	< 0.5−3.0
Extremities	< 0.5	< 10	< 10	< 0.5−18.0
Shoulder	< 0.5	< 10		< 0.5−3.0
Thoracic spine	11	< 10		< 10−55
Chest (radiographic)	1		2	0.2−43
Chest (photofluorographic)	3	< 10	3	0.9−40
Mammography			< 10	
Femur (distal)		50	1	1−50

* BRH, Bureau of Radiological Health, 1976; ICRP, International Commission on Radiological Protection, 1970; UNSCEAR, United Nations Scientific Committee on the Effects of Atomic Radiation, 1972.

results in the largest degree of permanent growth retardation [14].

Teratogenicity of X-rays and contrast studies (see also Chapter 7)

The risks associated with radiation depend critically upon the gestational age and the amount of radiation delivered. It is important to remember that many radiographic examinations deliver very little radiation to the fetus. This is especially true of extraabdominal studies where the uterine doses are less than the dose of $5 \times 10^{-4} - 1 \times 10^{-3}$ Sv received from cosmic rays and other naturally occurring radioactive substances, e.g., carbon-14, during gestation [15] (Table 6.3). In contrast, examinations involving the lower abdomen such as pelvimetry or a lower abdominal series, deliver much more radiation to the fetus and may represent a greater threat (Table 6.4).

The amount of radiation delivered depends not only upon the dose and rate at which it is delivered, but also on other factors such as patient positioning, e.g., posterior–anterior or anterior–posterior views, the area exposed, and the proximity of the conceptus to the area exposed. In this regard, although the administered dose from various radiographic studies has been well documented, true intrauterine dose cannot be measured *in vivo*, but only in phantoms with the physical dimensions of a pregnant abdomen.

The dose is measured on the abdominal surface of a phantom corresponding to points on a pregnant woman. Inferences are then made about the intrauterine dose using scaling factors, and the calculated uterine dose approximated to the mean fetal dose. It is obvious that such estimations are greatly influenced by individual patient characteristics and can only remain a guide as to the true extent of exposure. Dosimetry for various radiographic studies can thus be easily calculated (Table 6.4). The ionizing effect of X-rays lasts only so long as exposure is maintained, following which the patient neither retains nor emits radiation.

Estimation of radiation dose received from radiopharmaceutical studies differs in an important aspect as radioactivity persists for a variable period following the study. In addition to administered isotope, background radiation contributes to the total exposure. Background radiation has been estimated to be less than 1×10^{-3} Gy over the course of pregnancy. Most of the exposure from nuclear medicine procedures are in the same order of magnitude as absorbed background radiation [16]. The radiation dose delivered to the fetus from radiopharmaceutical studies depends upon the type of study performed, the type of radiopharmaceutical used, the half-life of the agent, and whether or not the agent crosses the placenta (Table 6.5). In addition, pharmacokinetic properties such as distribution within the body and mode of excretion, impinge upon exposure to the fetus. For example, radioactive agents that are excreted via the kidneys may expose the fetus directly through the collection of radioactive urine in the bladder. There are limited data regarding placental transfer of radionuclides. Placental crossover for some agents such as free iodine-131 (^{131}I) and iron-59 (^{59}Fe) result in greater relative concentrations in the fetus as compared to the mother [15]. The gestational age of the fetus is also another factor to consider. For example, ^{131}I administered after 8-weeks gestation (i.e., following the onset of fetal thyroid function) can cause neonatal hypothyroidism [17]. Iodine is not concentrated by the fetal thyroid prior to 8 weeks of

Table 6.4 Estimated dose to uterus from abdominal examinations. (From Wagner *et al.* [15])

Examination	BRH (1×10^{-5} Gy)	ICRP (1×10^{-5} Gy)	UNSCEAR (1×10^{-5} Gy)	Reported range (1×10^{-5} Gy)
Upper gastrointestinal series	171	150		5–1230
Cholecystography				
Cholangiography	78	150	120	14–1600
Lumbar spine	990		560	27–3970
Lumbosacral spine		550	470	100–2440
Pelvis	290	340	320	55–2190
Hips and femur (proximal)	170	690	330	73–1370
Urography, intravenous or		960	810	70–5480
Retrograde pyelogram	810	1100	715	120–5480
Urethrocystography		2060		275–4110
Lower gastrointestinal tract (barium enema)	1240	1100	1200	28–12 600
Abdomen	300	690	290	25–1920
Abdomen (obstetric)		1370 fetal	410	150–2200
Pelvimetry		5480	850	220–5480
Hysterosalpingography		1650	1740	270–9180

BRH, Bureau of Radiological Health, 1976; ICRP, International Commission on Radiological Protection, 1970; UNSCEAR, United Nations Scientific Committee on the Effects of Atomic Radiation, 1972.

Table 6.5 Conceptus dose estimates from radiopharmaceuticals. (From Wagner *et al.* [15])

Radiopharmaceutical	Conception age (weeks)	Conceptus organ	Dose per unit of maternally administered activity (rad/mCi)	Isotope physical half-life
$^{99}Tc^m$-DTPA	1.5−6	Whole body	0.035	6.0 hours
$^{113}In^m$-DTPA	1.5−6	Whole body	0.035	2.8 days
$^{99}Tc^m$-gluconate	1.5−6	Whole body	0.034	
$^{99}Tc^m$-sodium pertechnetate	1.5−6	Whole body	0.027	
$^{99}Tc^m$-sodium pertechnetate	1.5−6	Whole body	0.037	
$^{99}Tc^m$-sodium pertechnetate	1.5−6	Whole body	0.039	6.0 hours
$^{99}Tc^m$-sodium pertechnetate	<8	Whole body	0.048−0.32	
$^{99}Tc^m$-polyphosphate	1.5−6	Whole body	0.025	
$^{99}Tc^m$-sulfur colloid	1.5−6	Whole body	0.007	
^{125}I-sodium iodide	1.5−6	Whole body	0.032	13.0 hours
^{131}I-sodium iodide	1.5−6	Whole body	0.10	
^{131}I-sodium iodide	1.5−6	Whole body	0.15	
^{131}I-sodium iodide	7−9	Whole body	0.88	
^{131}I-sodium iodide	11	Whole body	1.15	
^{131}I-sodium iodide	12−13	Whole body	1.58	8.1 days
^{131}I-sodium iodide	20	Whole body	3.00	
^{131}I-sodium iodide	11	Thyroid	715	
^{131}I-sodium iodide	12−13	Thyroid	1338	
^{131}I-sodium iodide	20	Thyroid	5900	
^{123}I-sodium rose bengal	1.5−6	Whole body	0.13	13.0 hours
^{131}I-sodium rose bengal	1.5−6	Whole body	0.68	8.1 days
^{67}Ga-citrate	1.5−6	Whole body	0.25	3.3 days
^{75}Se-methionine	1.5−6	Whole body	3.8	120.0 days
^{59}Fe-citrate	7−20	Whole body	38	
^{59}Fe-citrate	7−13	Liver	410	
^{59}Fe-citrate	20	Liver	330	45.0 days
^{59}Fe-citrate	11	Spleen	61.2	
^{59}Fe-citrate	12−13	Spleen	140	
^{59}Fe-citrate	20	Spleen	186	

^{59}Fe, iron-59; ^{67}Ga, gallium-67; $^{123/131}I$, iodine-123/131; $^{113}In^m$, indium-113 m; ^{75}Se, selenium-75; $^{99}Tc^m$, technetium-99m.

gestation. In a retrospective study of fetuses accidentally exposed to ^{131}I during the first or the first and second trimesters, six neonates out of 178 live births had hypothyroidism [17]. The use of radioactive iodine and, indeed, any contrast agent that contains iodine should be avoided during pregnancy, especially after the fetal thyroid achieves the capability to acquire iodine (see also p. 179).

The pattern of end-organ response also determines the result of irradiation *in utero*. For example, all available evidence indicates that radiation-induced carcinogenesis is a stochastic late effect. Stochastic implies an "all or nothing" effect. This means that the probability of the occurrence of leukemia itself is dose related, whereas the severity of leukemia is not. This would presumably hold for all organ systems that depend upon "stem cells" for differentiation. A number of studies have come out in support of the carcinogenic potential of prenatal irradiation [3,5,18,19]. Kneale and Stewart [18] postulate an increase by a factor of 1.5−2 over the natural incidence of childhood cancer with *in utero* doses of greater than 0.02 Gy. Hopton *et al.* [5] showed a positive

association with the incidence of leukemia/lymphoma diagnosed under 2 years of age. This association did not reach statistic significance at older ages. However, studies that question the role of radiation in the causation of childhood cancer also abound [20−22]. Yoshimoto *et al.* [20] in a study of cancer deaths and incidence in prenatally exposed children of bomb survivors showed no increase in childhood cancer. More recently, Mole [4] published the results of the largest ever case-control study on the risks of childhood cancer following prenatal exposure to diagnostic X-rays. The data refer to some 14 500 matched cancer case/control pairs culled from the records of the Oxford Survey of Childhood Cancer (OSCC). The period of examination spanned from 1940 to 1978. He found that radiography during the first trimester had a higher relative risk for malignant disease than during the third trimester, but postulated that increased radiation dose rather than intrinsic susceptibility was the reason. Although an association has been confirmed, whether or not the exposure to radiation *in utero* is genuinely a causal factor in childhood cancer remains a matter of debate.

A different situation is seen with central nervous system abnormalities. Data from the survivors of the Hiroshima and Nagasaki bombings reveal that during the most sensitive period of 8−15 weeks, the relationship between frequency of severe mental retardation and dose is apparently linear, without threshold, and has a risk coefficient of 40%/Sv [11,23]. However, there was no increased incidence of the above complications at doses less than 0.01 Sv. In 42 women who were exposed to 0.5 Gy or more after 17 weeks, only one infant was found to be mentally retarded [24]. Severe mental retardation was not observed at doses less than 0.5 Gy. Microcephaly often carries the implication of mental retardation, although this is not always the case [24]. At Hiroshima, microcephaly was most prevalent in fetuses exposed between 7 and 15 weeks. The minimum dose producing effect was found to be 0.1−0.19 Gy. Similar data from Nagasaki show that the threshold for microcephaly often exceeded 1.5 Gy. At maternal doses exceeding 1.5 Gy, microcephaly was often accompanied by mental retardation [24]. Growth retardation, microcephaly, and mental retardation are the predominant observable effects seen following direct exposures of greater than 0.5 Gy. Microcephaly may well be the most common malformation observed in humans exposed to high levels of radiation during pregnancy [14].

The difficulty in establishing a cause and effect attributable to imaging procedures in pregnancy derives from two confounding factors: (i) the high base rate of spontaneous abnormalities; and (ii) the myriad of other antenatal and postnatal factors, e.g., cigarette smoking, alcohol, and viral infections which may affect development. A determination of the true rate of fetal resorption/abortion induced by radiation during the preimplantation phase is confounded by the fact that up to 50% of confirmed pregnancies undergo spontaneous abortion; confirmed either clinicopathologically or biochemically.

It must be remembered that most of the evidence regarding the effects of ionizing radiation derive from studies performed on A-bomb survivors or from animal studies, and that conventional radiographic procedures deliver much smaller doses. All too often, the perceived risk from diagnostic radiation is evaluated without taking into account the considerable risks of normal pregnancy itself. Nevertheless, the clinician is faced with providing the patient with a cogent appraisal of the risks posed to her as well as to her unborn child. Assuming, on balance, that a risk does exist, a relative risk of 2 with regard to a background incidence of all childhood cancers of 1:1500, would translate to 2 additional cases per year or a percentage increase of 0.14% [18]. Considerations for the nursing mother may also be extrapolated from the above. Thus, in practical terms, with the possible exception of radioiodine studies, present estimates of the harmful effects of diagnostic radiologic procedures indicate that the benefit far outweights the risk.

It is important for the radiologist to be aware of the patient's pregnancy status before any type of X-ray is planned, both from the patient's as well as from a medicolegal standpoint. It allows the physician an opportunity to advise the patient of the risks involved and place them in perspective. More importantly, it allows the woman to make an informed choice. In emergency situations, the possibility of pregnancy must always be entertained. A pregnancy test must be obtained and if positive the parents accordingly counseled. The American College of Obstetricians and Gynecologists in conjunction with the American College of Radiology in 1977, issued a policy statement which affirmed that:

> Attempts to schedule abdominal X-ray examinations in relation to a woman's menstrual cycle are of little value. The developing ovum is at risk prior to ovulation as well as subsequently. Thus it is erroneous to assume that any time is "safer" for radiation exposure than another [25].

The official view of the American College of Radiology is that no single diagnostic procedure results in a radiation dose that threatens the well-being of the developing fetus or embryo [11]. The National Council of Radiation Protection and Measurements concluded that an exposure to the fetus of less than 0.05 Gy is associated with negligible risk, and studies suggest that the threshold for radiation effects may be 0.15−0.2 Gy [26]. Current recommendations set the annual public dose limit at 5 mSv and the occupational dose limit at 50 mSv.

Health care givers working in areas that would expose them to ionizing radiation are unlikely to absorb more than 1 mSv over the course of a pregnancy (9 months) if prescribed safe working practices are followed. The calculated risk of both hereditary effects as well as cancer to their child from this level of exposure would be 0.14% compared to a natural risk of roughly 4% [27]. The fatal cancer risk associated with 1-mSv exposure of the fetus is estimated to be 1:50 000. Nevertheless, the International Commission on Radiological Protection (IRCP) in 1992 has recommended that the dose limit during pregnancy be reduced to 2 mSv [28]. These recommendations have not, as yet, been accepted as general policy.

The only pregnancy specific indication for a radiographic procedure that entails direct irradiation of the fetus is pelvimetry. In this regard, computed tomography of the pelvis delivers much less radiation (4.4×10^{-4}−4.25×10^{-3} Gy) than conventional X-rays and should be employed wherever possible [29,30]. There is very little place for pelvimetry in the practice of modern obstetrics. Magnetic resonance imaging (MRI), at present, is not widely used for this purpose but represents an exciting alternate in terms of image quality as well as in being devoid of ionizing radiation.

Physiologic changes in pregnancy affecting radiologic appearances

Radiographic appearances can change drastically during

pregnancy primarily as a consequence of the profound changes that take place. These changes must be taken into account during the interpretation of radiologic findings.

In the nonpregnant woman, the uterus is a wholly pelvic structure weighing about 70 g. During the course of pregnancy, the uterus undergoes massive enlargement, finally achieving a 500–1000-fold greater capacity and weighing approximately 1 kg. In so doing, the uterus occupies an ever increasing proportion of the abdominal cavity, distorting the normal anatomic relations of other intraabdominal organs. For example, the cecum and the appendix are progressively pushed upwards and laterally by the enlarging uterus. Indeed, almost every organ system undergoes drastic anatomico-physiologic alterations in response to pregnancy.

Changes in the cardiovascular system can affect radiographic appearances to a large degree. Pregnancy induces a hyperdynamic state with a greatly exaggerated plasma volume, with an increase of up to 45% above nonpregnant levels. Total circulating erythrocyte volume also increases by roughly 33%. In response to the above, the heart enlarges with specific enlargement of the right atrium. There may be an "unfolding" of the aortic arch and prominence of the azygos vein system. In addition, the diaphragm is elevated progressively through pregnancy, resulting in the displacement of the heart to the left and upwards with some rotation along its long axis. It has also been noted that some degree of benign pericardial effusion may be noted in normally pregnant women [25].

Pregnancy also induces changes in the appearance of the thoracic cage. The level of the diaphragm rises about 4 cm, while the subcostal angle widens appreciably. The result is a 2–3-cm increase in the transverse diameter and a 6-cm increase in thoracic circumference [25].

Changes in the urinary system reflect both an increase in intrinsic renal function, e.g., glomerular filtration rate, renal plasma flow (RPF), and the effects of an enlarging uterus. The kidneys themselves enlarge during pregnancy. The most striking alterations, however, are seen in the collecting system. Varying degrees of pelvicalyceal and ureteral dilatation occur. Typically, the right side is more affected than the left. Elongation and lateral displacement of the ureter commonly accompany dilatation, thus giving the radiographic appearance of an enlarged collecting system with more or less acute angulations of the ureter along both its abdominal and pelvic course [25].

As mentioned previously, the stomach and intestines are displaced by the enlarging uterus. Gastric emptying time and intestinal transit time are prolonged [25].

Although impressive changes in liver function take place during pregnancy, the liver itself does not change appreciably in size or appearance. In summary, serum albumin concentration is reduced by about 25%, serum urea nitrogen is reduced, there is a mild elevation of liver enzymes, and excretion of sulfobromophthalein is delayed. Diminished

gall-bladder motility is found, and gall-bladder volume during resting conditions and following a test meal average twice the values found in the nonpregnant state [25]. In compensation to the growing uterus and its contents, increasing lumbar lordosis is also a feature of pregnancy. In addition, there is increased mobility of the sacroiliac, sacrococcygeal, and pubic joints [25].

After the second month of pregnancy, the breasts increase in size and assume a nodular consistency as result of alveolar hypertrophy. Thus, xeroradiography is not as helpful as a result of the parenchymal changes induced by the pregnant state, and due to the increased water density of the breasts, the discriminatory capacity of mammography tends to be reduced [31]. In general, for reasons of diagnostic accuracy, it is better to delay breast screening examinations until after 6 weeks postpartum.

The pituitary gland also enlarges to roughly 1.5 times the nonpregnant size. It is unusual, however, to find an increase in size sufficient to cause symptoms due to optic chiasm compression [25]. Microadenomas of the pituitary, however, may undergo rapid enlargement during gestation.

Notwithstanding concerns about the danger posed to the fetus from ionizing radiation during the present pregnancy, it will be useful to place the risk posed to the mother herself as well as any possible effects on any subsequent pregnancies in perspective. The main concerns in this area involve the carcinogenic potential of radiation and the mutagenic potential whereby a mutation caused in a germ cell will be expressed in some future generation. Although a wealth of information concerning these effects derived from animal experiments exists, the only data concerning the genetic effects of radiation in humans come from the children of the survivors of the attacks on Hiroshima and Nagasaki. There were only about 100 000 survivors. In terms of a genetic study, this number is relatively small. Several end points have been studied, and the doubling dose, i.e., the dose required to double the spontaneous mutation frequency, for some effects have been roughly estimated [32]. For example, the doubling dose for sex-linked chromosomal anomalies has been estimated at 2.52 Sv. No increase in radiation-induced mutation in children of bomb survivors in Japan has been thus far confirmed [13]. In 1982, the United Nations Scientific Committee on the Effects of Atomic Radiation (UNSCEAR) investigated the effect of radiation on genetic diseases with a multifactorial etiology. Although most authorities would concur that multifactorial diseases may be of great importance, it is unlikely that any meaningful estimates of the effect of radiation in their causation can be made.

There is also evidence to show that exposure to radiation can cause cancer in humans [11]. Most of these data have been derived from situations that involve high radiation exposure, e.g., radiotherapy. A major confounding factor is that these data must be extrapolated to the low-dose situation.

Also, the natural prevalence of cancer is affected by several factors such as race, age, sex, etc. All these must be taken into account when arriving at risk estimates. Table 6.6 summarizes a recent assessment of risks by the Biological Effects of Ionizing Radiation V and UNSCEAR committees for individuals exposed to 0.1 Sv [11]. The committees used a time-dependent, relative-risk model. The prevalence of cancer was found to vary both with age and interval since exposure, as well as the dose rate. It should be noted, however, that these risk estimates should be interpreted in the light of the knowledge that the natural prevalence of cancer and genetic disorders are themselves high. Any small increment in the prevalence or incidence due to radiation used for diagnostic purposes therefore will be very small and difficult to ascertain.

Forms of imaging not using ionizing radiation

Ultrasound

From its inception some 30 years ago, the use of ultrasound has achieved a preeminence among the various tools used to ascertain fetal well-being. As refinements in technique and equipment continue to take place, sonography above all other imaging modalities has the potential materially to improve pregnancy outcomes. It is estimated that in the USA, more than 50% of all pregnancies are examined ultrasonically. An additional factor is the remarkable safety record of ultrasound.

Ultrasound is in a class by itself because it utilizes purely acoustic "radiation". Sound waves emitted by the transducers represent mechanical compression waves that induce similar waves in their target tissue. Echoes are created at interfaces or boundaries of organs, tissues, fluids, or gases due to their differing acoustic properties. Ultrasound images are thus

maps of acoustic interfaces between different tissues determined by their reflective, absorptive, or conductive properties. In passing through tissue, the mechanical energy of the ultrasound wave is converted to other forms of energy. This transference of energy results in both thermal and nonthermal effects.

The nonthermal effects of ultrasound include the generation of "microstreams" or eddy currents near tissue boundaries. Microstreaming results in a number of effects such as applying twisting torques on macromolecules, e.g., deoxyribonucleic acid (DNA), or aggregative tendencies, e.g., human blood platelets, can be induced to clump *in vitro* by exposure from a fetal heart monitor. The interactions of ultrasound with micron-sized gas bubbles in tissue results in the phenomenon of *cavitation* [33]. Cavitation vastly enhances the nonthermal effects of ultrasound and can result in cell lysis. Apart from mechanical disruption, ultrasound-induced collapse of these gas bubbles have been noted to result in free radical and so-called sonochemical formation.

Thus, cells that survive the mechanical effects of cavitation may be subject to further attack from these agents. A possible mutagenic effect was demonstrated *in vitro* [34]. The exposure of Chinese hamster V79 cells in culture to 1 MHz continuous-wave ultrasound at spatial temporal peak averages (SPTA) at or greater than 35 W/cm^2, resulted in the induction of 6-thioguanine-resistant mutants. The frequency of mutation was 10% of that induced by X-rays at similar survival levels. Fortunately, at present, most of these findings have been confined to *in vitro* systems. Cavitation applies more to therapeutic ultrasound, e.g., lithotripsy, where a more continuous, less focused beam is used. The potential risks from the nonthermal effects of ultrasound in humans are at present unknown. To err on the side of caution this argues for the use of ultrasound only with the expectation of some medical benefit. With respect to this the American Institute of Ultrasound in Medicine (AIUM) in 1984 counseled the prudent use of ultrasound.

The thermal effects of ultrasound are a result of direct heating of the tissues by sound waves. Bone is the most sensitive tissue to this thermal effect and the heating rate of bone can be up to 50 times faster than in soft tissue. In the usual circumstance, exposed tissues are rapidly cooled by virtue of blood flow, and the excess heat is lost as a result of the normal thermoregulatory processes. Only at very high levels of exposure would these processes be unable to cope. In general a 1°C elevation in temperature is regarded as being safe [33].

The AIUM in its recommendations stated that mammalian bioeffects are not seen below a SPTA intensity of 100 mW/cm^2 [33]. SPTA values for conventional obstetric scans range from 0.1 to 200 mW/cm^2 [15]. Thus far, no untoward effects from the use of antenatal ultrasound have been reported. Epidemiologic studies of infants who were exposed to ultrasound *in utero* are continuing. Stark *et al.* [35] compared 425 children exposed to antenatal ultrasound to 381 matched

Table 6.6 Estimates of excess cancer mortality: lifetime risk per 100 000 individuals exposed to 0.1 Sv radiation. (From Hall [11])

| Type of cancer | BEIR V 1990 (USA population) | | UNSCEAR 1988 (Japanese population) |
	Male	Female	
Breast	—	70	60
Respiratory	190	150	151*
Digestive system	170	290	—
Stomach	—	—	126
Colon	—	—	79
Other solid tumors	300	220	194
Leukemia	110	80	100
Total	770	810	710

* Reported as deaths from lung cancer.
BEIR, Biological Effects of Ionizing Radiation.

controls. No biologically significant differences were found between the exposed and unexposed groups both in terms of neonatal course or on testing at 7–12 years of age. There was an apparently higher incidence of dyslexia among the exposed children (49:425 versus 26:381), but this did not reach statistic significance. Salvesen *et al.* [36] in a similar study found no statistically significant difference either in school performance or the incidence of dyslexia among a group of 309 exposed persons versus 294 matched controls. Although the results thus far indicate that exposure to ultrasound entails minimal or no risks, the general consensus is that further research on this topic is warranted [37]. At present, however, ultrasound appears to be the safest imaging modality available to obstetricians.

MRI

Similar to the ultrasound, MRI is an imaging modality that uses no ionizing radiation and can provide images in multiple planes. MRIs are related to the biochemical environment of the tissue in question and the response of individual molecules to strong externally applied magnetic fields [15]. In many ways a MRI reflects the functional integrity or developmental state of the areas being targeted [38]. For example, the maturing fetal lung accumulates increasing quantities of surfactant. This can be visualized by MRI through a secondary change in the properties of fetal lung water. MRI can thus potentially document the degree of lung maturation.

A number of effects resulting from the interaction of the electromagnetic fields used for MRI with the intrinsic magnetic moments of the molecules of the target tissue could theoretically cause damage to the developing fetus. Magnetic fields may affect the diffusion of charged ions across cell membranes or induce electric currents in tissues and, thus, affect normal neuronal or muscle function. Radiofrequencies (RFs) used in nuclear magnetic resonance (NMR) imaging, may result in tissue heating in a manner analogous to conventional microwave ovens. When rats and monkeys are subjected to RFs amounting to a mean specific absorption rate of more than 4 W/kg, a decrease in the animal's ability to perform tasks for which it had been trained has been noted [39]. Energy absorption rates in excess of 20 W/kg have been shown to cause anatomic deformities in the offspring of pregnant animals [39]. Most estimates of mean specific absorption rates during NMR average less than 0.1 W/kg. Men exposed to magnetic fields of up to 2 T, while adjusting large cyclotrons, have been noted to experience nausea, disorientation, and confusion. Such reports are, however, anecdotal and have not been reported in patients undergoing NMR imaging. No mutagenic effect has been noted in cultured mammalian cells or in human lymphocytes *in vitro* exposed to magnetic fields of up to 1 T [40,41]. Magnetic fields currently used in NMR range between 0.03 and 1.5 T [15]. No untoward effects in either isolated tissues or intact animals exposed to static magnetic fields at strengths approaching those used in NMR studies have been observed [39].

Because of the relatively long time needed to acquire MRI, the target tissue needs to be stationary over the period of time required for exposure. This is a drawback in terms of fetal imaging. Various methods to ensure fetal quiescence, e.g., maternal sedation, glucose loading, and paralyzing the fetus have been investigated but none have been entirely successful. MRI, in this regard, presents exciting possibilities but at present is used mainly as an experimental tool. Pelvimetry using MRI yields images comparable to those obtained from conventional X-rays or computed tomography scans [38].

In comparison to the studies examining the safety of ultrasound in obstetrics, relatively few investigations have looked into the teratogenic potential of NMR. Although at present this modality appears safe, current Food and Drug Administration (FDA) guidelines require labeling of MRI devices to the effect that the safety of MRI when used to image the fetus and infant has not been established yet [39], although it does not specifically contraindicate MRI. The National Radiological Protection Board in England in 1983 suggested that:

> Although there is no evidence to suggest that the embryo is sensitive to magnetic and radiofrequency at the intensities encountered in NMR imaging, it might be prudent to exclude pregnant women during the first trimester [39].

The board permits MRI in the second and third trimester, but only with the approval of the local medical ethics board. First-trimester MRI is allowed only if the patient has elected to terminate the pregnancy. Currently, the use of MRI during pregnancy in the USA is mainly restricted to research protocols approved by the local institutional review boards.

Summary

The teratogenic potential of various imaging modalities used in obstetrics has received valid attention in the world literature. Most data regarding the effects of ionizing radiation originate from animal studies or those performed on the survivors of the explosions at Hiroshima and Nagasaki. It is difficult to draw a parallel between these and conventional diagnostic X-rays. An association has been noted between prenatal irradiation and childhood cancers including leukemia. Whether X-rays are a causal factor is debatable. Central nervous system abnormalities and growth retardation as seen in bomb survivors are not seen at the doses administered during diagnostic radiology. Clinically, diagnostic X-rays in the first trimester that deliver less than 0.05 Gy to the fetus are not believed to be teratogenic. Concern about exposure between 0.05 and 0.1 Gy has been raised, but from a practical standpoint, serious risk to the fetus does not occur until the absorbed dose exceeds 0.1 Gy. Accumulated evidence suggests that overall, the risks are small. Nevertheless, a discriminatory approach on the part of the physician with careful weighing of the risk:benefit ratio is warranted. Pregnancy changes the radiologic appearance of normal tissue or organ systems. The radiologist must be familiar with these changes in order correctly to interpret findings. Ultrasound appears to be attended with minimal or no risks. Although MRI is generally considered safe during pregnancy, its wider use in obstetrics awaits a more thorough evaluation of the potential bioeffects.

References

1 Dekaban AS. Abnormalities in children exposed to X-radiation during various stages of gestation: tentative timetable of radiation injury to the human fetus. *J Nucl Med* 1968;9:471–477.

2 Mole RH. Consequences of prenatal radiation exposure for postnatal development. *Int J Radiat Biol* 1982;42:1–12.

3 Bithell JF, Stewart AM. Prenatal irradiation and childhood malignancy: a review of British data from the Oxford survey. *Br J Cancer* 1975;31:271–287.

4 Mole RH. Childhood cancer after prenatal exposure to diagnostic X-ray examinations in Britain. *Br J Cancer* 1990;62:152–168.

5 Hopton PA, Mckinney PA, Cartwright RA *et al.* X-rays in pregnancy and the risk of childhood cancer. *Lancet* 1985;ii:773.

6 Jones KL. *Smith's Recognizable Patterns of Human Malformation*, IVth edn. W.B. Saunders, 1988.

7 Dobbings J, Sands J. Qualitative growth and development of the human brain. *Arch Dis Child* 1973;48:757–767.

8 Kaufman MH. Critical role of the yolk sac in erythropoiesis and in the formation of the primordial germ cells in mammals. *Int J Radiat Biol* 1991;60:545–547.

9 O'Rahilly R, Muller F. *Human Embryology and Teratology*. Wiley Liss, 1992: 83.

10 Russell LB, Russell WL. An analysis of the changing radiation response of the developing mouse embryo. *J Cell Physiol* 1954;43 (Suppl. 1): 103–147.

11 Hall EJ. Scientific views of low-level radiation risks. *Radiographics* 1991;11:509–518.

12 Mole RH. Irradiation of the embryo and fetus. *Br J Radiol* 1987;60:17–31.

13 Sankaranarayan K. Invited review: prevalence of genetic risks of exposure to ionizing radiation. *Am J Hum Genet* 1988;42:651–662.

14 Brent RL. Teratology update: radiation teratogenesis. *Teratology* 1980;21:281–289.

15 Wagner LW, Lester RG, Saldana LR. *Exposure of the Pregnant Patient to Diagnostic Radiations: A Guide to Medical Management.* JB Lippincott, 1985:40.

16 Brent RL, Beckman DA, Jensh RP. In: Kriegel H, Schmal W, Gerler GB, Stieve FF, eds. *Radiation Risks to the Developing Nervous System.* New York: Gustav Fisher, 1986.

17 Stoffer SS, Hamburger JL. Inadvertant ^{131}I therapy for hypothyroidism in the first trimester. *J Nucl Med* 1976;17:146–149.

18 Kneale GW, Stewart AM. Mantel–Haenzel analysis of Oxford data. I. Independant effects of several birth factors including fetal irradiation. *J Natl Cancer Inst* 1976;56:879–883.

19 Harvey EB, Boice JD, Honeyman M, Flannery JT. Pre-natal X-ray exposure and childhood cancer in twins. *New Engl J Med* 1985;312:541–545.

20 Yoshimoto Y, Kato H, Schull WJ. Risk of cancer among children exposed *in-utero* to A-bomb radiation, 1950–84. *Lancet* 1988;ii:665–669.

21 Oppenheim BE, Greim ML, Meier P. The effects of diagnostic X-ray exposure on the human fetus: an examination of the evidence. *Radiology* 1975;114:529–534.

22 Jablon S, Kato H. Childhood cancer in relation to prenatal exposure to atomic bomb radiation. *Lancet,* 1970;Nov:1000–1003.

23 Otake M, Schull WJ. *In-utero* exposure to A-bomb radiation and mental retardation: a reassessment. *Br J Radiol* 1984;57:409–414.

24 Miller RW, Blot NJ. Small head size after atomic radiation. *Lancet* 1972;2:784–787.

25 Cunningham FG, MacDonald PC, Gant NF (eds). Maternal adaptations to pregnancy. In: *Williams Obstetrics*, XVIIIth edn. Norwalk, California: Appleton & Lange, 1989:129–162.

26 Brent RL. Ionizing radiation. *Contemp Ob/Gyn* 1987;30:20–29.

27 Given-Wilson R. Editorial. Pregnancy and work in diagnostic imaging. *Clin Radiol* 1993;47:75–76.

28 Clarke EA, Thompson WH, Notghi A, Harding LK. Radiation doses from nuclear medicine patients to an imaging technologist: relation to ICRP recommendations for pregnant workers. *Nucl Med Commun* 1992;13:795–798.

29 Adam Ph, Alberge Y, Castellano S, Kassab M, Escude B. Pelvimetry by digital radiography. *Clin Radiol* 1985;36:327–330.

30 Federle MP, Cohen HA, Rosenwein MF, Brant-Zawadzki MN, Cann CE. Pelvimetry by digital radiography: a low-dose examination. *Radiology* 1982;143:733–735.

31 Bland KI, Copeland III E.M (eds). The breast: comprehensive management of benign and malignant diseases. In: *The Breast.* Philadelphia: W.B. Saunders, 1991:1034–1045.

32 Neel JV, Schull WJ, Awa AA *et al.* The children of parents exposed to atomic bombs: estimates of genetic doubling doses of radiation for humans. *Am J Hum Genet* 1990;46:1053–1072.

33 Miller DL. Update on the safety of diagnostic ultrasonography. *J Clin Ultrasound* 1991;19:531–540.

34 Kaufman GE. Mutagenecity of ultrasound in cultured mammalian cells. *Ultrasound Med Biol* 1985;11:497–501.

35 Stark CR, Orleans M, Haverkamp AD, Murphy J. Short and long term risks after exposure to diagnostic ultrasound *in-utero*. *Obstet Gynecol* 1984;63:194–200.

36 Salvesen KA, Bakketeig LS, Eik-Nes SH, Undheim JO, Okland O. Routine ultrasonography *in utero* and school performance at age 8–9 years. *Lancet* 1992;339:85–89.

37 Enkin M, Kierse MJNC, Chalmers I *et al.* In: *A Guide to Effective Care in Pregnancy and Childbirth.* Oxford University Press, 1989.

38 Stark DD, Bradley WG. *Magnetic Resonance Imaging*, vol. I. St. Louis: CV Mosby, 1992:538.

39 The National Radiological Protection Board *ad hoc* Advisory Group on Nuclear Magnetic Resonance Clinical Imaging. Revised guidelines on acceptable limits of exposure during nuclear magnetic resonance clinical imaging. *Br J Radiol* 1983;56:974–977.

40 Cooke P, Morris PG. The effects of NMR exposure on living organisms. II. A genetic study on human lymphocytes. *Br J Radiol* 1981;56:622–625.

41 Schwartz JL, Crooks LE. NMR imaging produces no observable mutations or cytotoxicity in mammalian cells. *Am J Radiol* 1982;139:583–585.

42 Brent RL. Microwaves and ultrasound. *Contemp Ob/Gyn* 1987;30:19–25.

Part 2
Technical Considerations

CHAPTER 7

Radiation exposure in interventional radiology

M. Victoria Marx

Introduction

This chapter deals with the basic principles of radiation safety as they apply to the medical use of X-rays. Other types of radiations, such as γ-rays or high-energy particles are not included because they do not pertain to the practice of interventional radiology. It is assumed that the reader understands the basics of radiation physics and radiation biology. A brief review of radiation concepts and terminology is, however, in order because usage conventions may vary from one place to another.

Radiation exposure

The fundamental effect of radiation exposure on matter is the formation of ion pairs. The commonly used unit of radiation exposure is the röntgen (R), which is a measure of the number of ion pairs produced by X-rays in a standard volume of air. The SI unit correlating to the röntgen is coulomb per kilogram of air. One röntgen is equivalent to 2.6×10^{-4} C/kg.

With respect to the day to day practice of interventional radiology, röntgen determination is most important as a measure of the radiation output from the X-ray tube during fluoroscopy, and during the recording of permanent images (conventional filming, digital image acquisition, digital subtraction angiography, cineradiography, or videotape).

Radiation absorbed dose

Radiation exposure, or the interaction of radiation with air, does not reflect the energy deposited by the radiation in other substances (such as biologic tissue). This deposited energy is known as the absorbed dose of radiation. The absorbed dose of radiation is dependent not only on the energy and amount of the incident radiation, but also on the nature of the tissue being exposed. The commonly used unit of radiation absorbed dose per unit mass is the rad which is equal to 100 ergs/g. The corresponding SI unit is the gray (Gy), which is equivalent to 1 J/kg. One hundred rads is equivalent to 1 G (or 1 rad = 10 mGy).

With respect to the practice of interventional radiology, measurement of radiation absorbed dose is primarily of importance in determining patient dose. Retrospective estimation or calculation of patient dose may be indicated in some cases, such as when a patient is found, after the fact, to have been pregnant at the time of an interventional procedure.

Dose equivalent

The biologic effect of a given absorbed dose of radiation varies with the type of radiation. The biologic effect of radioactive particles (β-particles, α-particles, and neutrons) is greater than that of X-rays or γ-rays. Each type of radiation has been assigned a quality factor that is a numerical quantification of its relative biologic effectiveness. The quality factor for X-rays is 1. Dose equivalent is equal to the radiation absorbed dose multiplied by the appropriate quality factor for the type of radiation in question. The common unit of dose equivalent is the rem. The corresponding SI unit is the sievert (Sv). One hundred rems is equivalent to 1 Sv (or 1 rem = 10 mSv).

Radiation dose is expressed in terms of dose equivalent for purposes of personnel dosimetry. This common scale makes it possible to monitor and compare the occupational exposures of all radiation workers regardless of the type of radiation to which the workers are exposed. Therefore, film badge or thermoluminescent dosimeter readings are generally reported in terms of mrems or mSv.

Effective dose

The effective dose [1] is a concept that provides a way to relate partial body radiation dose to a uniform whole-body dose of equivalent overall risk. Sensitivity to radiation is greater for some tissues than for others. For example, the gonads, stomach, red bone marrow, and lung have higher radiosensitivity than do the thyroid gland, skin, and bone surfaces. The International Commission on Radiological Protection (ICRP) has assigned weighting factors to tissues that reflect their relative radiosensitivity [1]. The effective dose (E) is the sum of the dose equivalents (H_T) to each tissue (T), multiplied by their weighting factors (W_T) [1]:

$$E = \Sigma \ W_T \times H_T.$$

Although effective dose is not in common clinical use, it is an important concept for interventional radiology — both for patient care and for personnel monitoring. Neither the patient nor the interventionalist receives a uniform whole-body radiation dose during an interventional procedure. A patient's effective dose may be calculated, or at least estimated, from data recorded at the time of the procedure. The annual effective dose to personnel may be calculated or estimated from film badge readings, together with knowledge about the protective gear worn by each individual [2–5].

Radiation safety

The philosophic viewpoint

Ionizing radiation is a powerful tool. Its existence has permitted the development of both noninvasive means of medical diagnosis (diagnostic radiology) and minimally invasive diagnostic and therapeutic techniques (interventional radiology). There is, however, no free lunch. The use of ionizing radiation for medical purposes has its down side. X-rays cause intracellular ionization, the development of free radicals, and DNA damage. These events can lead to acute radiation injury such as hair loss and skin burns, as well as to the development of delayed sequelae such as cancer, genetic mutation, and degenerative problems including sterility and cataracts. In general, the ill-effects of radiation exposure are related to the radiation dose received, the dose rate, the time over which the total dose is received, the energy of the radiation, and the body part(s) and total volume of tissue exposed. There is no level of radiation dose that can be considered absolutely safe.

While the most dramatic instances of radiation injury relate to large-scale events, such as the Second World War atomic bombs and the explosion of the Chernobyl nuclear reactor, medical history contains many cases of radiation injury both to physicians and to patients. Early radiologists reported development of skin burns and skin cancers [6]. Studies have also shown an increased incidence of leukemia, aplastic anemia, lymphoma, liver cancer, and skin cancer among radiologists entering the field prior to 1940 [7].

With regard to patient exposure, widespread use of fluoroscopy to monitor tuberculosis treatments in the 1930s–1950s resulted in an increased incidence of breast cancer in the recipient population [8]. Increased numbers of cancers were also noted in populations receiving radiation therapy for the treatment of ankylosing spondylitis [9], postpartum mastitis [10], and enlargement of the thymus [11]. Use of radiation therapy for benign conditions has, therefore, been abandoned.

Because the medical community has learned from these experiences, and because an enormous number of technical developments have occurred that result in increased image quality at lower radiation exposures, diagnostic X-ray use is now considered to be "safe," i.e., when standard techniques are used, the health benefits of medical X-rays are assumed and the risk of measurable radiation-induced injury is considered to be negligible. Constant and meticulous attention to the issue of radiation safety on the part of the radiologic community, the health care system, and governments throughout the world have all contributed to this increased safety.

The issue of radiation safety in interventional radiology is of more than just academic interest or regulatory duty. The subspecialty of interventional radiology has a special responsibility with regard to the safe use of medical X-rays. Fluoroscopy is our primary imaging system: we use it to guide the performance of ever more complex and lengthy diagnostic and interventional procedures. Lengthy fluoroscopy times at typical radiation exposure rates of 1–5 R/min are a significant contribution to the overall radiation dose received by an individual patient. In addition, fluoroscopy is the largest source of occupational radiation exposure among medical workers [12,13]. Furthermore, recent anecdotal reports of acute radiation injuries to patients occurring as a consequence of lengthy interventional procedures have been brought to the attention of the USA Food and Drug Administration (FDA) [14]. The FDA's concern that such incidents be "nipped in the bud" has led to the publication of a formal FDA warning regarding the potential for X-ray-induced skin injuries during fluoroscopically guided procedures [15]. It is likely that the end result of this document will be the development of monitoring guidelines regarding permissable patient fluoroscopy dose and the institution of systems to monitor outcomes of patients whose skin doses exceed the level where skin injury may occur.

The interventional radiologist controlling the fluoroscopy foot pedal has an obligation to use this imaging tool judiciously, and to understand and use all available means to minimize patient and personnel exposure, while accomplishing the goals of the interventional procedure at hand. We must maintain a position of leadership within the medical community with regard to radiation safety issues to ensure the optimal care of our patients as well as to assure our continued participation in the formation of regulations regarding the use of medical X-rays.

The regulatory viewpoint

The potential for misuse of X-rays, and the need to develop guidelines for use, was recognized soon after their discovery in 1895. In the USA, this recognition led to the establishment of the National Council on Radiation Protection and Measurements (NCRP) in 1929, a nonprofit scientific organization which has operated under Congressional Charter since 1964. The NCRP is responsible for the development of recommendations concerning all uses of radiations, including medical X-rays. With respect to medical workers, the purpose of these recommendations and regulations is to ensure that radiation-related medical work, like other medical work, is a "safe" occupation, i.e., one that has less than 1:10 000 work related deaths per year [16]. These recommendations are the primary resource used by state regulatory agencies in establishing specific regulations relating to radiation safety.

Current NCRP recommendations are that yearly occupational total body radiation dose (effective dose equivalent) should not exceed 5 rem (50 mSv), and that cumulative lifetime occupational radiation dose should not exceed one's age in years multiplied by 1 rem (or age in years × 10 mSv) [16]. With regard to specific organ exposures, the lowest limit is set for the lens of the eye at 15 rem/year (150 mSv/year), while the yearly limit for extremity dose is 50 rem (500 mSv) [16]. Fetal exposure limits are 50 mrem/month (0.5 mSv/month).

In addition to setting occupational dose limits, the NCRP has articulated a philosophy stating that all occupational exposure to radiation should be kept at a level that is *as low as reasonably achievable (ALARA)* [13]. The goal of the ALARA philosophy is to encourage occupational practices and attitudes that will maintain actual occupational radiation exposure levels well below the limits noted above.

In Europe and other countries, the ICRP and the International Council on Radiation Protection and Units (ICRU) function in a manner similar to the NCRP. Although the recommendations regarding radiation safety of the ICRP, ICRU, and NCRP are not identical in all respects, they are similar. The most significant differences between ICRP and NCRP recommendations are that the ICRP has recently lowered its 5-year limit on occupationally received effective dose to 100 mSv (10 rem) [1].

Specific USA regulations regarding occupational exposure and personnel monitoring

In the USA, state regulatory agencies set rules in accordance with NCRP recommendations that all radiation workers must follow. All medical radiation workers must wear a dosimeter that is read at monthly intervals. For persons who routinely wear lead aprons, most states stipulate that the dosimeter should be worn at the collar level outside the lead apron [17]. For regulatory purposes, the dosimeter reading is assumed to be equal to the whole-body dose. Dosimeter readings must not exceed 400 mrem/month, 1250 mrem/quarter, or 5000 mrem/year. If an individual worker's doses exceed these limits, the institution's radiation safety officer must evaluate that person's radiation safety practices, indicate ways to lower the dose (which may include limiting clinical work time), and write a letter to the state regulatory agency explaining the cause of the excess exposure and what action has been taken.

Among all medical radiation workers, interventional radiologists (and cardiologists) are the most likely to approach or exceed regulatory dose limits due to the integral role played by fluoroscopy in the practice of these subspecialties. Because of this, personnel radiation monitoring practices in many interventional laboratories exceed state regulations. Personnel may wear multiple dosimeters: typical sites include the collar over the lead apron, at the waist under the lead apron, near the eyes, and on one or both hands. Data from multiple sites are quite helpful in evaluating the significance of an isolated high reading, i.e., relating that reading to one's effective dose [5].

Some interventionalists do not wear their dosimeters [4] and, therefore, do not comply with state regulations concerning personnel monitoring. The reasons for this behavior are not known with certainty but may include a belief that a point dosimeter reading does not accurately reflect the wearer's effective dose [5]. Incorporation of effective dose calculation into routine clinical practice is feasible [5] and has been recommended [4,16]. Compliance with state regulations is necessary for maintenance of radiation safety in the interventional laboratory.

Specific USA regulations regarding patient exposure

Medical radiation is the second largest source of radiation (behind natural background radiation) to the general public and is the largest source of artificial radiation exposure [18]. Despite this fact, there are no regulations concerning maximum radiation dose limits to patients. For each individual, it is assumed that the immediate benefit of the radiation exposure for medical purposes outweighs any potential associated risk to that person in the future. From a public health standpoint, medical radiation exposure is considered unlikely to harm the population as a whole because the group of persons receiving the most medical radiation is, on average, older and not as healthy. Therefore, on average, medically exposed persons are less likely to: (i) live long enough to develop a radiation-induced cancer; and (ii) reproduce and pass on genetic mutations to future generations.

The issue noted above regarding acute skin injury in association with lengthy fluoroscopically guided interventional procedures is a very serious one. As of September 9, 1994, the FDA had received, within a 1-year span, reports of serious skin injuries trackable to prolonged fluoroscopy with a single-beam entry site in 15 patients (T.B. Shope, personal communication, 1995). Currently, the procedures of highest risk are cardiac catheter radiofrequency ablations, neuroembolizations, and transjugular intrahepatic portosystemic shunting procedures. These procedures may be lifesaving for critically ill people but the aspect of possible skin injury must be factored into the risk:benefit ratio as clinical decisions are being made and as the consent process is carried out. No formal governmental quality assurance guidelines regarding this issue have, as of yet, been developed but they will undoubtedly appear.

The practical viewpoint

Strictly speaking, radiation safety in the interventional suite applies only to workers and not to patients. However, because patient exposures in the interventional laboratory can approach therapeutic levels [19], the ALARA philosophy [18] should be followed with respect to both patient and personnel exposure. Following this logic, the goal of the safety-conscious interventional radiologist should be to achieve a diagnostic and/or therapeutic goal with the lowest possible radiation dose to the patient and to all laboratory personnel.

A variety of factors affect the radiation dose received by these individuals, some of which, such as use of collimators, are under the control of the primary operator, and some of which, such as specific equipment features affecting dose, are not. All interventionalists must be familiar with the latter as well as the former in order to make optimal decisions at the time of equipment purchase.

In general, all factors that contribute to decreased patient dose also contribute to lowered operator dose. The majority of the following discussion emphasizes fluoroscopy because this is the primary source of radiation dose during lengthy interventional radiologic procedures.

The fundamental principles of radiation safety can be summarized in three words: *time*, *distance*, and *shielding*. Radiation output *rate* also affects radiation dose. Understanding these principles, learning to apply them to real life, and developing work habits that incorporate them is vital to the optimal and safe practice of interventional radiology.

Time of exposure

Radiation dose is directly proportional to the length of time of the radiation exposure. Therefore, during a fluoroscopically guided procedure, cutting the fluoroscopy time by 50% will decrease the radiation dose by a factor of two. Factors which can affect fluoroscopy time include the complexity of the task at hand, the experience level of the interventionalist, the quality of the imaging chain, and the availability of digital imaging options such as last image hold and roadmapping. Concern, or lack thereof, about radiation exposure on the part of the interventionalist may also result in behaviors that affect fluoroscopy usage.

The complexity of the fluoroscopically guided task is a primary determinant of fluoroscopy time. Nonselective angiography rarely requires more than 1 or 2 minutes of fluoroscopy, while superselective vascular embolization procedures may require fluoroscopy times of over 1 hour [20,21]. In the interventional suite, length of fluoroscopy "on-time" is rarely, if ever, viewed as a reason to terminate a procedure. Therefore, the concept of "cutting fluoroscopy time in half" to decrease operator and patient exposure is nice but not particularly practical.

No matter how complex the task, however, one work habit can decrease exposure time: *use fluoroscopy only when necessary* and *only for as long as is absolutely necessary*. Experience level obviously affects the speed and accuracy with which the operator interprets the fluoroscopic image and performs fluoroscopically guided maneuvers. Development of experience begins in residency, grows rapidly during fellowship, and continues throughout one's career. Longer procedure times and higher occupational exposures are an expected, and in general, accepted aspect of the training experience.

The length of fluoroscopy on-time necessary to complete a task is not completely under operator control. An imaging chain with suboptimal components can contribute to increased fluoroscopy time due to poor image quality. In addition, suboptimal function of the image intensifier can result in increased radiation dose because the equipment may compensate for decreased efficiency of X-ray detection by boosting X-ray tube output. It is the responsibility of the laboratory's assigned physicist to see that all equipment is in proper and optimal working order.

Two features available on all new computerized angiographic units can be used to decrease fluoroscopy time. *Last image hold*, where the fluoroscopic image is frozen on the television monitor after the operator lifts his/her foot from the pedal, allows the operator to ponder the image while making plans about what to do next without exposing anyone to radiation. *Roadmapping*, which allows the operator to superimpose a vascular tree opacified with contrast over a live fluoroscopic image of the same territory, increases the efficiency with which superselective vascular catheterizations and interventions can be performed.

Concern about radiation exposure is a very personal issue and is affected by one's personal perception of risk as well as the behavior and attitudes of one's teachers, role models, and work colleagues. Feedback about radiation time can be an effective tool in developing an appropriate level of concern about radiation exposure. Fluoroscopy time for each case should be recorded (timers are a standard feature on all angio/interventional equipment) for the benefit of the fluoroscopist as well as for the patient record, should retrospective estimation of dose be indicated. In addition, a pocket ionization chamber ("chirper") can provide instant feedback to the operator regarding occupational dose [22]. The chirping that occurs as often as 60 times/min in close proximity to the fluoroscopy beam, is so annoying that the wearer rapidly adopts behavior to decrease the rate of noise production — such as removing his/her foot from the fluoroscopy pedal when observation of the live image is not absolutely necessary for the forward progress of the case.

Rate of exposure

Radiation exposure rate during fluoroscopy usually varies between 1 and 5 R/min. Current federal regulations in the USA, limit tube output to 5 R/min during conventional fluoroscopy. Two relatively new equipment features can significantly affect this rate. *Pulsed progressive fluoroscopy,* where the X-ray beam is pulsed 30 times/min, can decrease patient dose by 30–50% compared to continuous fluoroscopy [21]. *High-level control (HLC) fluoroscopy,* on the other hand, can boost the radiation output to 20–120 R/min [19]. This feature can make some procedures possible, despite patient obesity, and when particularly tiny or relatively radiolucent objects must be visualized. HLC fluoroscopy should, however, be used judiciously because of the high dose rate which can approach therapeutic levels. In the USA, its use must be accompanied by a signal audible to the primary operator.

Because of increasing concern on the part of the FDA regarding X-ray exposure from fluoroscopy, USA regulations have recently changed. The dose limit for conventional fluoroscopy has been increased to 10 R/min, while HLC output is now limited to 20 R/min [14].

In the USA, there is no regulatory limit to radiation exposure during acquisition of permanent images. Exposure rates for image recording (conventional rapid-sequence filming or digital subtraction angiography) are much higher than those of fluoroscopy. Exposure time for each image is, however, much shorter — measured in milliseconds per image rather than minutes. Therefore, the relative contributions of filming and fluoroscopy to the overall patient dose will vary with the amount of fluoroscopy time and the number of filming runs. The job of the primary operator is to tailor the procedure in such a way that all necessary information is acquired in as efficient a manner as possible. Particular attention should be paid to filming rates and film sequence lengths during angiography: if the information can be recorded in 10 films, do not expose 20!

One final point about image recording should be made here. During conventional rapid-sequence angiographic filming, it is customary for all personnel to step out of the procedure room in order to decrease occupational radiation exposure. With the development of digital subtraction angiography, however, the primary operator frequently stays at the patient's side during image acquisition — either to inject the contrast manually or to continue with a complex intervention as soon as the images have been acquired [23]. New angiographic systems even include remote control devices for tableside control of image review, which, while convenient, further encourage the primary operator to remain in close proximity to the patient during digital image acquisition. Interventionalists who find it necessary to remain in the procedure room during digital subtraction runs, should step away from the patient during image acquisition and utilize supplemental shielding devices (see above).

Distance from the X-ray source

Because an X-ray beam diverges from its point source, the intensity of the beam decreases with distance from the source. Radiation dose decreases proportionally to the square of the distance from the radiation source (inverse square law). Therefore, doubling one's distance from the X-ray source will result in lowering one's dose by a factor of four. In the interventional suite, the physician in charge of the procedure receives the highest dose, while personnel who stand farther from the radiation source, such as technologists and circulating nurses, have lower exposures [24–26]. Anesthesia personnel may receive relatively high doses [27] because they stay with the patients throughout the procedures and prefer to sit, placing body parts not protected by a lead apron close to the point of maximum scatter radiation (Fig. 7.1).

In the interventional laboratory, where the majority of procedures are performed using C-arm or U-arm equipment, with the X-ray tube under the patient, there is little that can be done to increase the patient's distance from the X-ray source. The distance between the tube and the patient (or tabletop) is determined primarily by the geometry of the system and by the height of the primary operator, who must have the table positioned at a comfortable working height.

The primary source of radiation to the operator is the patient. Scatter radiation is most intense at table level where the primary beam first enters the patient. The distance between the operator and the part of the patient being

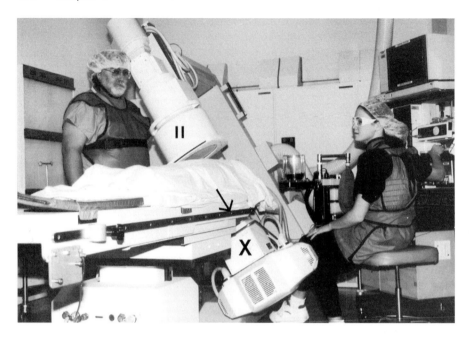

Fig. 7.1 Angiographic U-arm unit positioned with left posterior oblique geometry (X denotes X-ray tube). Physician stands to the patient's right while nurse anesthetist sits to the left. With this set-up, scatter radiation to the seated nurse is higher than to the physician. Point of maximum scatter is at tabletop level (arrow). The physician is protected from much of the scatter by the patient and the image intensifier (II) while the anesthetist is not.

exposed to radiation is determined primarily by the type of procedure being performed. The operator may be twice as far from the radiation source during a neuroembolization case than he/she would be during a percutaneous nephrostomy. For each type of procedure, the operator should learn not to stand any closer to the X-ray source than is necessary to perform the given task.

The above discussion assumes that the X-ray tube is located under the patient table (Fig. 7.2). Interventional radiologic procedures should never be performed using an X-ray unit with an over-the-table X-ray tube. Radiation dose to the operator's head, neck, and upper extremities is extremely high with this configuration because it includes backscatter of the primary beam as well as Compton scatter from the patient [28].

Tube angulation of a C- or U-arm unit can affect operator dose (Fig. 7.3). Scatter to the operator is increased when the tube is angled towards the working side of the table, and the image intensifier is angled away from the operator. Conversely, operator exposure is lowered when the X-ray tube is angled away from the working side of the table.

All ancillary personnel involved in interventional radiology cases, such as technologists, nurses, and anesthesia staff should be aware of the relationship between distance from the X-ray beam and radiation dose, and should develop work habits and personal shielding practices that incorporate this knowledge.

Shielding from the X-ray beam

Lead attenuates diagnostic X-rays very effectively. Therefore, lead shielding is a vital part of all radiation safety measures.

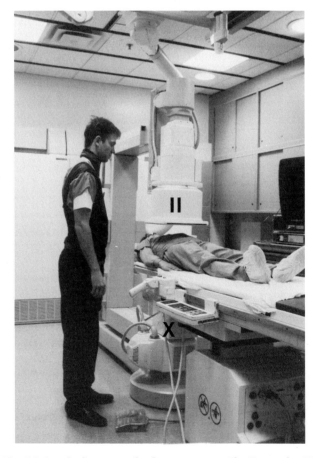

Fig. 7.2 Standard geometry for fluoroscopy use. The X-ray tube (X) is located beneath the table. The image intensifier (II) is over the patient. II should be as close as possible to the patient to minimize scatter radiation and to optimize image quality.

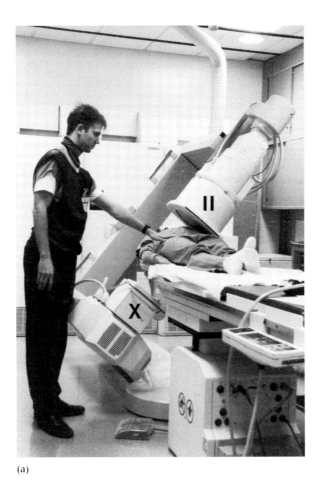

(a)

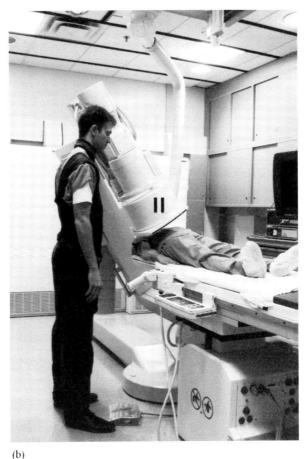

(b)

Fig. 7.3 Tube angulation with the operator at the right side of the supine patient. With right posterior oblique geometry (a), the scatter radiation to the operator is greater than with left posterior oblique geometry (b). When the tube is angled towards the operator, the operator receives backscatter from the primary beam as well as attenuated scatter from the patient. (a) Note particularly the proximity of the operator's left upper extremity to the X-ray tube as he or she touches the patient, and the direct line of sight between the operator's face and the X-ray tube. In (b), the operator is protected from primary beam backscatter by distance, the patient, and the image intensifier tower. X, X-ray tube; II, image intensifier.

Shielding devices include beam collimators, wearable items such as lead aprons, thyroid collars, leaded glasses, and mobile boom-mounted or floor-mounted leaded acrylic barriers.

Operator-controlled lead collimators are included in all angio/interventional X-ray units. Use of leaded collimators decreases radiation by decreasing the cross-sectional area of the beam emerging from the X-ray tube. Collimators contribute to radiation protection only if the interventionalist learns to use them and makes their use a habit. Fortunately, tight collimation to the area of interest has the added benefit of improving image quality by decreasing Compton scatter in the area. Therefore, the development of good habits regarding beam collimation comes easily to most practitioners.

Leaded aprons are mandatory for everyone who enters the angio/interventional room during a procedure. The lead apron covers all of the critical radiation-sensitive organs (intestine, lung, breast, and gonads) except for the lens of the eye and approximately 25% of the bone marrow [5]. Standard lead aprons provide 0.5 mm lead (Pb) equivalent thickness, which attenuates approximately 90% of the incident X-ray beam. A variety of styles are available. For angio/interventional personnel, wrap-around aprons are recommended — particularly for persons who are likely to have their backs to the X-ray source while the beam is on — such as technologists, nurses, and assistants to the primary operator. Wrap-around aprons are, however, heavy and the risk of radiation exposure must be weighed against the risk of chronic back problems when deciding what style of apron to adopt. Two part (skirt and vest) wrap-around aprons are available and divide the weight between the shoulders and hips quite effectively. Custom-fitted aprons are more expensive than "off-the-rack" styles, but can increase wearer comfort significantly. Full-time interventionalists find the investment in a custom-made apron extremely worthwhile.

Accessory items to the leaded apron include thyroid collars

and leaded glasses. The thyroid collar not only covers the thyroid gland, a moderately radiation-sensitive organ, but customizes the apron neck, covers a small amount of bone marrow, and provides a convenient location for clipping one's collar dosimeter. Their use is recommended for all interventional radiologists. Thyroid shielding is not necessary for ancillary personnel except perhaps for anesthesiology staff.

The lens of the eye is the most radiation-sensitive organ not covered by the lead apron. Cataracts can result from radiation doses of over 200–300 rad (2–3 Gy). The maximum permissible dose per year to the lens of the eye set by the NCRP is 150 mSv (15 rem) [16]. Busy interventionalists can approach that dose level [4,5]. In keeping with the principles of ALARA, therefore, leaded glasses are recommended for full-time interventionalists. Leaded glasses attenuate 90% of the scatter to the eyes and also shield the eyes from body fluids. As with thyroid shields, leaded glasses are not necessary for personnel who do not routinely stay in close proximity to the patient during the procedure.

Unfortunately, leaded glasses are heavy and can be quite burdensome to the nose during long cases. Therefore, many interventionalists do not use them. Investing in a pair of customized leaded glasses can increase comfort and therefore use of this shielding device. An alternative to leaded glasses is the boom-mounted leaded acrylic shield (see below). This item is harder to get used to, but does shield the entire head and neck from scatter radiation and body fluids.

Leaded surgical gloves have been developed. These items are of doubtful usefulness. They attenuate only 10–20% of the X-ray beam [29] and can decrease manual dexterity. The best way to protect one's hands is to avoid seeing them on the fluoroscopic image! Many tools designed to help the interventionalist keep his or her hands out of the beam have been developed.

Mobile leaded acrylic barriers are cumbersome to use for most people. They do, however, provide at least 0.5 mm Pb equivalent protection. Floor-mounted barriers that roll to the desired location on wheels are most useful when the primary operator must stand adjacent to the patient to inject contrast during permanent image recording (Fig. 7.4). They are also useful to give added protection to anesthesia staff who must stay at the patient's side.

Boom-mounted shields provide protection to the operator's head and neck (Fig. 7.5). They can be used throughout all fluoroscopically guided procedures because they do not interfere with arm and hand access to the patient. They have the added benefit of providing a fluid barrier to the face — not an inconsequential benefit in this day and age of concern about exposure to body fluids. Sterile transparent covers are available to drape these barriers so that they do not contaminate instruments. Unfortunately, this type of shielding frequently goes unused because it has been positioned in the room in an inconvenient spot, or because its design is not

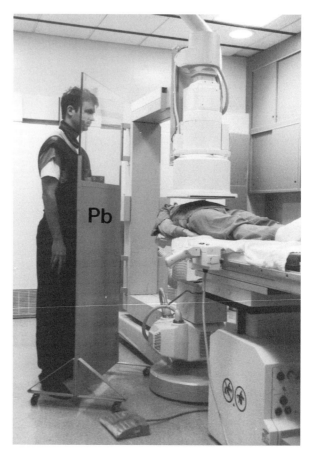

Fig. 7.4 This movable leaded shield (Pb) is appropriate for use by the operator when it is necessary to inject contrast by hand during filming. The top third of the protective barrier is translucent. This style of barrier is not appropriate for use at other times because it restricts access to the patient.

flexible enough. Careful planning during design of an angio suite is necessary to make use of this type of device practical.

Special considerations

The pregnant patient

Interventional radiologic procedures involving the use of X-rays should be avoided if the patient is pregnant. Fortunately, other imaging techniques such as external ultrasound or intravascular ultrasound can be used to guide some interventional procedures (such as percutaneous nephrostomy tube placement or inferior vena cava filter placement).

When the pregnant woman's life is at stake and the best therapeutic option for her is an X-ray guided procedure, it should be performed using the least amount of X-ray beam "on-time" possible. The uterus should be kept out of the primary beam if at all possible. Early involvement of a medical physicist is recommended in order most accurately

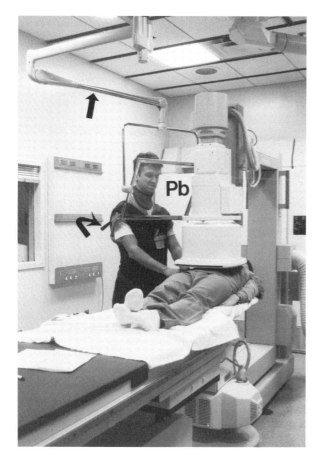

Fig. 7.5 Boom-mounted leaded acrylic shield provides supplemental radiation protection to the operator's head and neck without restricting access to the patient. Working behind a shield such as this also protects the face from splashing blood. The shield can be covered with a translucent self-adhesive sterile drape to avoid breaking sterile technique. Note that barriers such as this are only useful if they have a wide range of movement and are mounted in a convenient location in the ceiling. Arrow, articulated boom; curved arrow, operator handle; Pb, leaded barrier.

to determine the fetal dose. Concomitant involvement of a genetics counselor is also advisable to counsel the parents regarding the implications of the fetal exposure.

The pregnant worker

A pregnant member of the interventional radiology team must optimize her radiation safety practices for two reasons: (i) to minimize fetal dose; and (ii) to minimize her anxiety regarding fetal dose. Even for a busy interventional radiologist, it is possible to ensure that fetal dose remains well below the NCRP limit of 0.5 mSv/month [4].

The pregnant worker should wear a maternity apron that provides 1 mm Pb equivalent protection to the abdomen, and she should use behavior and shielding devices that will minimize her radiation exposure. Using a pocket ionization chamber ("chirper") can be quite useful by providing instant feedback to the pregnant worker about her radiation dose. She should wear an underapron dosimeter for documentation purposes, but this is not as useful as a chirper for educational purposes because it is read monthly and results can be quite delayed.

It is the pregnant worker's responsibility to notify her employer of her pregnancy. By USA federal law, she cannot be forced to discontinue her standard duties [30]. The implication of this law is that it is the responsibility of the employer to ensure that the working environment is safe. Adherence to optimal radiation safety practices by all members of the team is the key to ensuring this safety.

Conclusion

Interventional radiology is a specialty that provides vast benefit to patients. The potential for radiation-induced harm does, however, exist. Thorough education about radiation bioeffects and radiation safety is crucial to the safe practice of this specialty. Because our understanding of radiation continues to evolve, it is likely that radiation safety standards and practices will also change over time. It is each interventionalist's responsibility to adhere to optimal radiation safety practices throughout his or her career and to modify those practices as knowledge changes.

References

1 International Commission on Radiological Protection. 1990 recommendations of the International Commission on Radiological Protection. ICRP Publication 60. *Ann ICRP* 1991;21:1−25.
2 Faulkner K, Harrison RM. Estimation of effective dose equivalent to staff in diagnostic radiology. *Phys Med Biol* 1988;33:83−91.
3 Webster EW. EDE for exposure with protective aprons. *Health Phys* 1989; 56:568−569.
4 Marx MV, Niklason L, Mauger EA. Occupational radiation exposure to interventional radiologists: a prospective study. *J Vasc Intervent Radiol* 1992;3:597−606.
5 Niklason LT, Marx MV, Chan HP. Interventional radiologists: occupational radiation doses and risks. *Radiology* 1993;187:729−733.
6 Thomsen E. (Letters.) *Boston Med Surg J* December 10, 1896:610−611.
7 Matanoski GM, Sartwell P, Elliott E, Tonascia J, Sternberg A. Cancer risks in radiologists and radiation workers. In: Boice JD Jr, Fraumeni JF Jr, eds. *Radiation Carcinogenesis: Epidemiology and Biological Significance*. New York: Raven Press, 1984:83−96.
8 Boice JD, Monson RR. Breast cancer in women after repeated fluoroscopic examinations of the chest. *J Natl Cancer Inst* 1977; 59:823−832.
9 Court Brown WM, Doll R. Mortality from cancer and other causes after radiotherapy for ankylosing spondylitis. *Br Med J* 1965;2:1327−1332.
10 Shore RE, Hempelmann LH, Kowaluk E *et al.* Breast neoplasms in women treated with X-rays for acute post-partum mastitis. *J Natl Cancer Inst* 1977;59:813−822.

11 Hempelmann LH, Hall WJ, Phillips M *et al*. Neoplasms in persons treated with X-rays in infancy: fourth survey in 20 years. *J Natl Cancer Inst* 1975;55:519−530.

12 Hendee WR. Estimation of radiation risks: BEIR V and its significance for medicine. *J Am Med Assoc* 1992;268:620−624.

13 National Council on Radiation Protection and Measurements. *Implementation of the Principle of as Low as Reasonably Achievable (ALARA) for Medical and Dental Personnel*. NCRP Report No. 107. Bethesda, Md: National Council on Radiation Protection and Measurements, 1990.

14 Jacobson E. The FDA perspective on fluoroscopy. In: *Proceedings of the ACR/FDA Workshop on Fluoroscopy. Strategies for Improvement in Performance, Radiation Safety and Control*. Washington DC, October 16−17, 1992:2−3.

15 Food and Drug Administration. *Important Information for Physicians and Other Health Care Professionals: Avoidance of Serious X-ray-induced Injuries to Patients During Fluoroscopically-guided Procedures*. September 30, 1994.

16 National Council on Radiation Protection and Measurements. *Limitation of Exposure to Ionizing Radiation*. NCRP Report No. 116. Bethesda, Md: National Council on Radiation Protection and Measurements, 1993.

17 Bushong SC. Personnel monitoring in diagnostic radiology: revisited − again! *Health Phys* 1989;56:565−566.

18 National Council on Radiation Protection and Measurements. *Exposure of the US Population from Diagnostic Medical Radiation*. NCRP Report No. 100. Bethesda, Md: National Council on Radiation Protection and Measurements, 1989.

19 Payne JT. The ACR perspective on fluoroscopy. In: *Proceedings of the ACR/FDA Workshop on Fluoroscopy. Strategies for Improvement in Performance, Radiation Safety and Control*. Washington DC, October 16−17, 1992:1.

20 Brateman L, Marx MV. Fluoroscopic Radiation Safety. In: *Proceedings of the ACR/FDA Workshop on Fluoroscopy. Strategies for Improvement in Performance, Radiation Safety and Control*. Washington DC, October 16−17, 1992:33−35.

21 Gray JE. Fluoroscopic systems control, evaluation and performance. In: *Proceedings of the ACR/FDA Workshop on Fluoroscopy. Strategies for Improvement in Performance, Radiation Safety and Control*. Washington DC, October 16−17, 1992:14−15.

22 Hough DM, Brady A, Stevenson GW. Audible radiation monitors: the value in reducing radiation exposure to fluoroscopy personnel. *Am J Roentgenol* 1993;160:407−408.

23 Britton CA, Wholey MH. Radiation exposure of personnel during digital subtraction angiography. *Cardiovasc Intervent Radiol* 1988;11:108−110.

24 Renaud L. A 5-y follow-up of the radiation exposure to in-room personnel during cardiac catheterization. *Health Phys* 1992;62:10−15.

25 Jeans SP, Faulkner K, Love HG, Bardsley RA. An investigation of the radiation dose to staff during cardiac radiological studies. *Br J Radiol* 1985;58:419−428.

26 Bush WH, Jones D, Brannen GE. Radiation dose to personnel during percutaneous renal calculus removal. *Am J Roentgenol* 1985;145:1261−1264.

27 Berthelsen B, Cederblad A. Radiation doses to patients and personnel involved in embolization of intracerebral arterio-venous malformations. *Acta Radiol* 1991;32:492−497.

28 Boone JM, Levin DC. Radiation exposure to angiographers under different fluoroscopic imaging conditions. *Radiology* 1991;180:861−865.

29 Kelsy CA, Mettler FA. Flexible protective gloves: the emperor's new clothes? *Radiology* 1990;174:275−276.

30 *Federal Radiation Protection Guidance for Occupational Exposure*. Federal Register. Vol. 32, No. 17, p. 2822, January 27, 1987.

CHAPTER 8

Electric and mechanical hazards

Keith J. Strauss, Maria M. Damiano
and Ross S. Rulli

Introduction

Imaging and ancillary equipment used today in the health care field for diagnostic and/or interventional studies of patients, present numerous, potential electric and mechanical hazards to the patient, equipment operators, and other health care workers providing patient care. Numerous articles which define the scope of the electric hazards were written in the 1960s and early 1970s, when cardiologists and surgeons began applying electric currents directly to the heart, and other physicians, including radiologists and anesthesiologists increased their use of electric equipment in direct patient care [1–25]. Much less information has been written concerning the mechanical hazards [26,27].

This chapter lists the more common electric and mechanical hazards created by modern imaging and ancillary equipment used in radiology departments. The scope and causes of these hazards are discussed, followed by a listing of the programs necessary to minimize potential hazards and to eliminate accidents or injuries to patients and staff. (Practical information and examples are included.)

While the radiologist, cardiologist, surgeon, orthopedist, or other physician operating the equipment is responsible for the care and safety of their patients, these physicians must rely on others, e.g., equipment service vendors, third-party service groups, in-house biomedical engineering staffs, in-house X-ray engineering service personnel, and, at times, technologists/radiographers to provide appropriate, periodic inspections, maintenance, and/or repairs of equipment to eliminate or minimize the potential of hazards originating in the equipment. Fiscal pressures on health care providers today have caused some service providers to "cut corners" as opposed to improving their efficiency in order to lower service costs. The physician, or some other knowledgable individual within the institution, must periodically review the scope of services provided by their service personnel to ensure that patient and personnel safety are not being jeopardized.

Electric hazards

Electric shock is a direct potential hazard to patients and personnel when electric equipment is used. An additional indirect potential hazard may be created by distortion or alteration of displayed data from electronic monitoring equipment due to electromagnetic interference from low- or high-frequency electricity in the vicinity of the monitoring equipment.

Electric shock classifications

Electric current of sufficient intensity flowing through part of the body causes electric shock. Current is the flow of free electrons. In all electric circuits that conduct current from one location to another, the quantity of current flow (ampere) is determined by the size of the force pushing the electrons (volts) and the amount of resistance to the flow (ohms):

volt/ohm = amp.

An analogy is a water pipe. The quantity of water delivered per unit time (amp) is increased by an increase in water pressure (increased voltage), or by an increase in the diameter of the pipe (decreased ohms).

A person receives an electric shock if their hand touches a conductive surface, their foot touches another conductive surface, and a voltage is connected between the two points of contact (Fig. 8.1). This could happen if a person standing on a grounded conductive surface reached out and touched a piece of equipment with a voltage on its outer metal case. This voltage could be due to a failure within the equipment or due to a fault existing within the facility's electric system supplying the power to the piece of equipment. The patient's skin has a resistance to the electron flow of approximately 1000 Ω [29], which will reduce the amount of current flowing within the patient's body. But, the internal body tissues offer essentially no resistance to the current; the current seeks the shortest path through the body between the two points of contact with the conductive surfaces.

Two terms, recently deleted from some standards [29], but still found in common use to classify electric shock, are macroshock and microshock. *Macroshock* describes an electric shock that occurs when intact skin at the body surface contacts a conductive surface, and the current flow causes a sensation. The result may be a tingling sensation, involuntary muscle spasms, pain, convulsions, respiratory arrest, or ventricular fibrillation [30,31]. The actual result of the shock depends on the amount and frequency of the alternating voltage, the current, its duration, the conductivity of the skin, or the size and location of the electrodes that delivered the current to the body [29]. Table 8.1 lists the required levels of current at intact skin to experience macroshock sensations [31].

During interventional cases in which a conductor connected to an ancillary piece of equipment may be in direct contact with the heart, any shock (current flow) due to equipment failure would occur directly through the heart. Even a current of 100 μA [31] would cause ventricular fibrillation and would be potentially lethal. *Microshock* describes this small current, which is three orders of magnitude smaller than the macroshock level (Table 8.1) with the same biologic end point [31].

Source of electric hazards

A piece of electronic equipment is designed to contain the multitude of applied voltages and currents, associated with its normal operation, inside an outer case. The outer case should have no current flowing through it and should be at 0 V. This ideal is seldom achieved for two reasons. Insulating materials — materials with extremely large resistances to the flow of current — are used to isolate voltages and currents within the unit. However, since no material is a perfect insulator, very small currents conduct across the insulation and are present on the outer case of the instrument.

A second phenomenon — capacitive coupling — contributes additional stray currents to the outer metal case of equipment. The outer metal case is a conductor, capable of storing electrons or charges. The currents contained within the internal circuitry of the equipment create oscillating magnetic fields and electric potential fields. These fields can influence the free electrons on the outer metal case, despite no direct conductive connection between the fields and the case. This influence causes electrons to flow and be stored on the case. Due to its capacitive nature, as the number of

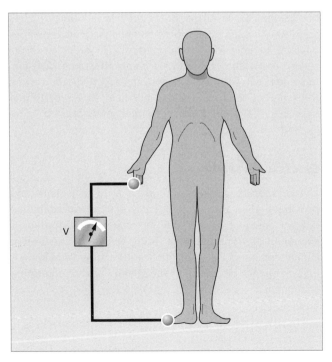

Fig. 8.1 Three conditions required to produce an electric shock: source of voltage connected to two different points of patient's body.

Table 8.1 Macroshock current thresholds at 60 Hz

Threshold (mA)	Sensation
1	Mild tingling sensation
5	Uncomfortable sensation
10	Muscle spasms
20	Pain, convulsions
100	Ventricular fibrillation

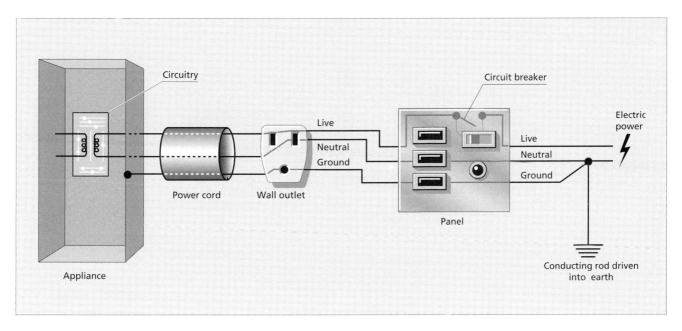

Fig. 8.2 Three-wire power source. The "hot" wire carries electric energy to the circuitry of the equipment. The neutral wire carries electric energy from circuitry of the equipment back to earth. The ground wire carries any fault or leakage currents on the external case of the equipment to earth.

stored charges increases, an increasing voltage is developed by the case. The outer case, which is no longer at 0 V, now is capable of being the force (Fig. 8.1) to cause an electric shock if an individual comes in contact with the outer case. *Leakage current* describes any current on the outer case of a piece of equipment due to imperfect insulation or capacitive coupling, which may be conveyed from the exposed surfaces of the equipment to anyone who comes in contact with the equipment.

Generic prevention of electric shock

Electric currents always flow over the path of least resistance, between the point of high electrical energy (voltage on the case of the instrument) to a point of zero electrical energy (the earth). The patient or personnel can be protected from shocks caused by electric equipment if the leakage current is given a pathway to earth with less resistance than the pathway provided by the patient's or worker's body. *Grounding* (called "earthing" in the UK) is the means of providing this low-resistance pathway to earth.

Figure 8.2 illustrates the principle of grounding. The power cord of the medical equipment contains three wires. The "hot" wire carries the electric energy (voltage and current) from the power company to the circuitry within the equipment. The neutral wire connects the internal circuitry of the equipment to the earth via a metal conductor driven into the ground. It carries the current from the circuitry within

the equipment back to ground potential. The third conductor directly connects the external chassis or external case of the equipment to earth. This third wire provides the necessary lower resistance pathway to earth than any grounded individual who might touch the metal case. This ground wire also conducts any other hazardous currents that may be created by faults or failures within the internal circuitry of the equipment to earth. Table 8.2 lists present maximum acceptable leakage current standards measured under different conditions established by the American National Standards Institute (ANSI) and Association for the Advancement of Medical Instrumentation (AAMI) [32–34].

Hard-wired imaging and ancillary equipment considerations

If tools are required to break the connection between the power cables of equipment and facility power, the equipment is *hard wired*. This type of connection is used for equipment that requires a large current or high-voltage power source. Table 8.2 lists three maximum allowed leakage currents for this equipment. The case to ground measurement (< 5000 μA) is performed when the equipment is initially installed with the ground cable removed. After installation the leakage current between any two components of the equipment which the patient or personnel could simultaneously touch, must be periodically measured. The acceptable value depends on the area in which the equipment is used. The maximum allowed leakage current in intensive care units must be more than a magnitude smaller than the leakage current in general care areas. The maximum leakage current values with ground connected are well below the threshold value for sensation in Table 8.1.

X-ray imaging equipment is a typical example of hard-

Table 8.2 Maximum leakage current limits

Equipment	Current (µA)
Hard-wired equipment	
Case to ground: ground removed	5000 [29]
Case to case after installation:	
critical care area	40 [29]
general care area	500
Portable equipment	
Case to ground: ground connected or removed	300
Patient lead to ground	
Nonisolated: ground connected or removed	100 (older equipment)
Isolated:	
ground connected	10
ground removed	50
Between patient leads (electrodes)	
Nonisolated: ground connected or removed	50 (older equipment)
Isolated:	
ground connected	10
ground removed	50
Isolation of patient leads (electrodes)	
Isolated: ground connected or removed	20

wired equipment found in health care facilities. In the USA, the necessary power wiring is typically provided by five cables. Three separate power "hot" wires or phases exist. The other two cables are the neutral wire and ground as discussed in Fig. 8.2. The voltage between each phase is typically 480 V; 277 V exist between each phase and the neutral cable connected to ground. Momentary maximum current draws during maximum-rated X-ray exposures range from 150–250 A. Special considerations that isolate the patients and operators from these high currents and voltages are discussed in the section on Facility considerations, p. 148.

The low level of leakage current between components (40 or 500 µA, depending on location; Table 8.2) is maintained only if each component of the equipment is connected to a low-resistance pathway to earth. Special attention over time is normally not required to maintain grounds of each fixed component. But, the hand or foot switches and other control devices attached to the unit by electric cords are frequently abused, which may jeopardize the connection of these components with earth. The cables and connections of these devices must be frequently checked for signs of wear. Most manufacturers of this equipment have reduced the risk of shock from these controls when the ground is violated by using only 12 or 24 V switching signals. These low-voltage signals control relays and switching devices controlling the circuits which carry the higher voltages and currents.

An X-ray machine may generate 60–150 kV to produce X-rays. These high voltages are delivered to the X-ray tube by flexible cables to allow movement of the X-ray tube relative to the remaining components of the machine. To reduce the required insulating materials in these cables, the transformer is designed to generate a maximum of 75 kV on each cable above and below ground. The three insulated wires carrying the three phases of high voltage are encased in an additional thick rubber insulator. Thick rubber is used further to insulate the current carrying wires. The thick rubber is surrounded by a heavy metal braid which is connected to ground. The braid is surrounded by an additional insulating sheath. These cables must be inspected periodically for cracks, punctures, or other signs of stress due to continual flexing or physical abuse of the cables. The equipment must be installed to prevent kinking, twisting, or sharp bends in the cables, which could lead to breakdown of the insulation or impair the conductive ability of the inner cables.

The high-voltage cables have special terminations to ensure integrity of the conductive pathways and isolation of the high voltage. The cable ends have connectors which are inserted into deep wells within the transformer or X-ray tube. The terminal connections are made at the bottom of each well. The wells in the transformer are filled with insulating oil; the wells in the X-ray tube are filled with insulating grease. Each is used to eliminate any atmospheric moisture which could cause arcing between the three conductors at the bottom of each well. The threaded retaining rings on each end of the cables must be securely fastened to its well to secure the mechanical connection and ensure the continuity of the braided metal of the cable with ground. The cables, retaining rings, and condition of the grease and oil in the wells must be inspected periodically to ensure electrical safety.

Portable imaging and ancillary equipment considerations

When the power cable of a piece of equipment contains a plug designed to be inserted into a power receptacle by the operator, the equipment or machine falls into the *mobile* or *portable* classification. Mobile X-ray machines, C-arm fluoroscopes, heat lamps, and any other electric devices with a power plug are examples. The "case to ground" maximum allowed leakage current in Table 8.2 applies to current flow from the outer case or chassis to ground of every portable piece of equipment, regardless of its age or application. The 300 μA is significantly lower than values required to produce a sensation from macroshock.

When equipment is designed to have electrodes attached to the patient's skin or inserted into the patient's body, maximum allowed leakage currents are much smaller, as listed in Table 8.2, due to the potential of microshock. The leads or electrodes contacting the patient must be electrically separated or isolated from the rest of the grounded circuitry in the unit to prevent any leakage currents reaching the patient. This is achieved by using optoisolators, which allow two different electric circuits with no conductive pathway between them to influence each other by nonconductive light beam connections. This design achieves the low leakage current values listed for the isolated equipment in Table 8.2. The maximum allowed leakage current rises for these units if the chassis ground is disconnected. The higher values in Table 8.2 for nonisolated equipment apply to older equipment manufactured before isolation circuit technology was developed.

The above criteria applies to electrocardiogram (EKG) monitoring equipment, defibrillator paddles, and the transducer of an ultrasound imager where an applicator comes in direct contact with the patient's skin. It also applies to contrast injection units. In this case, a nonconductive catheter is filled with a conductive contrast media which most likely will come in direct contact with the patient's heart [29]. The contrast media is completely isolated from the grounded internal electronic circuitry of the power injector by placing it in a plastic syringe, that is housed in the plastic chamber of the injector head, which incorporates a plastic piston for expelling the contrast media. The millions of ohms of resistance provided by the plastic effectively isolates the conductive fluid from the circuitry of the injector.

Mobile and portable equipment, or appliances, which come in direct contact with the patient, or are used in the patient vicinity must have a three-wire power cord with a grounding pin as discussed in Fig. 8.2. The resistance between the chassis or outer case of the equipment and the ground pin of the power cord must be less than or equal to 0.5 Ω

[29]. The power cord and plug, which are vital in maintaining the proper ground, probably receive more abuse than any other components of the equipment. The cord may be mechanically stressed or twisted by carts or other equipment wheeled over it. The plug is continually dropped, twisted, or forcefully jammed into power receptacles. Finally, a careless operator may remove the plug from its receptacle by yanking on the power cord [35].

For these reasons, heavy duty cords and plugs must be installed in the health care setting and must receive periodic inspections for wear and damage. The required gage of the conductors in the cord is determined by the length of the cord, the maximum voltage provided by the power source, and the maximum current draw during the operation of the equipment [29]. The plug must be durable enough to withstand the abuse commonly found in hospitals. "Hospital grade" plugs are not mandatory in the USA, today [29], since appropriate heavy duty plugs exist that are not rated as "hospital grade." These plugs, however, should not be confused with light duty or "household" grade plugs, which are not acceptable.

The three-conductor plug on the end of the power cord should only be installed by a properly trained individual. The ground pin on the plug is longer than the blades for the hot and neutral wires. This ensures that when the plug is inserted or removed from the power receptacle, the ground connection is made first and disconnected last. The ground wire within the plug should be at least 6.5 mm longer than the hot and neutral wires; the ground connection will be the last of the three connections to break if the strain relief of the plug fails and the cord is pulled out of the plug. The plug must be installed on the cord so that the internal wires within the plug are not stressed. The strain relief of the plug (mechanical clamp) must be snug, but not so tight that the insulation of the three wires within the cord is crimped.

In the USA, an exception is made with respect to the three-wire power cord. If the piece of equipment (e.g., portable mixer or other tool needed in the procedure room) is *double insulated*, it may be used in the vicinity of the patient with only a two-wire power cord, without a three-prong plug [29]. A double-insulated piece of equipment must contain deliberate design features to prevent the outer case from developing a voltage above ground potential. This criteria might be met by designing two independent layers of insulation. If the first layer breaks down, the second layer provides the necessary resistance to internal currents to prevent them from reaching the operator.

Pieces of office equipment or other common appliances (e.g., clocks, pencil sharpeners, typewriters, radios, etc.) may also find their way into the medical environment. Provided this equipment is not used "in the vicinity of the patient", codes in the USA allow the use of this type of equipment without double insulation, or without a three-conductor power cord with ground pin [29]. While the presence of this type of equipment at a nurse's station is allowed by national codes without a three-conductor cable, the practice may not be wise. Portable equipment typically migrates during its lifetime; someone unaware of the potential hazards of this equipment might move it into a procedure room or other patient vicinity.

Facility considerations

Proper grounding of both hard-wired and portable imaging and ancillary equipment in the procedure room cannot be overemphasized [36]. The integrity of this ground will always depend on the integrity of the conductive pathway from the procedure room back to a common metal rod driven into the earth (Fig. 8.2). The rod is made of conductive material; the soil into which the rod is driven may be treated chemically to improve the conduction. The size or gage of the ground conduit within the facility depends on the same factors mentioned previously for the portable power cord. In the case of X-ray imaging equipment, the potential current draw of $150-250$ A at 480 V requires heavy conduits. In new facilities in the USA [37,38], the resistance of the ground must be less than or equal to $0.1\,\Omega$ [29]. This maximum allowed resistance value increases to $0.2\,\Omega$ in existing facilities. The integrity of the facility's ground circuits must be checked by a properly trained individual prior to beginning the installation of new hard-wired imaging or ancillary equipment [38].

Two different problems can affect the integrity of the ground system. The first problem is *ground loops* within the facility's grounding system. A ground loop exists when a segment or leg of the facility's ground circuit has a different resistance than the rest of the grounding system, between true earth and the point of measurement. This resistance can be caused by corrosion of cabling or the loosening of connections over time. These changes can create a different voltage in a portion of the grounding system, which could lead to electric shock in the patient. The potential of ground loops is compounded when multiple power sources are used for equipment, e.g., a 480 V hard-wired piece of imaging equipment, and multiple 110 V pieces of monitoring and other ancillary equipment plugged into the power receptacles in the room on different circuits. All of these circuits must be checked periodically for the presence of ground loops.

The second problem arises if each individual component of a system of equipment (e.g., X-ray machine, etc.) is not properly connected to the facility's ground system. If not, each component or cabinet of the system can develop a voltage different from ground potential. Proper connection of hard-wired system components to the ground system is verified by measuring the leakage current between components or cabinets. This type of check should be performed annually after the integrity of the facility's grounding system is confirmed.

Circuit breakers must be provided on all incoming power sources to the procedure room. These terminate current flow when a fault occurs in the connected equipment. During some equipment failures, excessive amounts of current flow via the neutral wire or ground wire to earth. The excessive current draw causes the breaker switch to open and interrupt electric power to the equipment. The breaker should be installed in the circuit between the power source and the equipment to be protected, so that power is cut off only in the circuit in which the fault occurred. For example, if an imaging piece of equipment fails, the power should not be interrupted to other circuits in the procedure room which may be powering life-support equipment. If the circuit breaker is not located at the control desk of the equipment, a shunt trip, a switch that remotely trips the circuit breaker from the control desk in cases of emergency, should be installed in the circuit.

In addition to a circuit breaker, an electric circuit in a patient area may contain a *ground-fault circuit interrupter* [39]. This is a device installed in the circuit to interrupt the flow of electric energy to equipment if a fault current flows to ground that is significantly smaller than the size of current required to trip the circuit breaker. In patient care areas, ground-fault circuit interrupters are typically designed to trip at 6 mA [29].

The electric receptacles (sockets) in the room may receive considerable abuse. Only heavy duty, properly designed receptacles should be used in procedure rooms. If the receptacle appears to be damaged, or if the plug appears to fit loosely within the receptacle, the receptacle should be replaced immediately. These receptacles require periodic inspection and testing by properly trained personnel to ensure patient and personnel safety.

The interconnecting cables between components of imaging equipment, which carry large currents and voltages, must remain grounded and removed from the patient and operator. Each component of the imaging equipment must be directly connected to a common ground. The separation from patient and operator is achieved by placing the interconnecting cabling inside a metallic electric trough or conduit, which is also connected to ground. While the sections of metal trough are bolted together and should form a conductive path to ground, corrosion at the joints of the trough with time can jeopardize this continuity. Additional grounding wires should be added between each segment of the trough to ensure proper grounding.

The location, size, and shape of the electric trough can affect the performance and safety of the equipment over its lifetime. If the cross-sectional area of the trough crowds the required number of cables, the insulation on the individual cables can break down prematurely due to pressure and friction: this can lead to equipment malfunctions and potential electric hazards. The trough also should be located to minimize the effects of moisture and water over time.

Some types of floor trough are designed to be imbedded in

concrete floors with removable covers for access as shown in Fig. 8.3. This design is not recommended, as it can indirectly lead to equipment malfunctions and to electric hazards. The individual steel plates, which comprise the trough covers, must be sealed against liquids to prevent floor wax strippers and other fluids from leaking into the trough. In one case where the seals were faulty, less than 5 years after equipment installation, electric arcing occurred within the trough due to the breakdown of the insulation on the individual cables. This caused extensive equipment damage and created dangerous electric hazards to personnel and patient.

A better design for floor trough is shown in Fig. 8.4. The trough penetrates the floor and runs below the procedure room. The two-floor penetrations at each end of the trough can easily be sealed. The ends of the trough should extend about 5 cm above the finished floor to prevent flooding of the trough if water is spilled onto the floor. Since the cabling is pulled into the trough as opposed to being laid in place, large radius sweep bends should be used to change directions, as shown in Fig. 8.4, to prevent the excessive stress on the cables during pulling caused by right-angle bends. This design allows all cable installation from inside the procedure room, eliminates the cost of removable covers, and prevents fluids from entering the trough. This technique also eliminates floor discontinuities due to the trough, which are hard to keep clean and which can make it difficult to move carts, stretchers and other wheeled equipment about the procedure room.

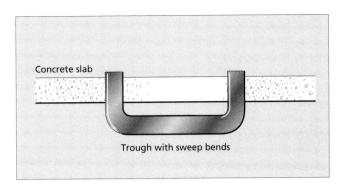

Fig. 8.4 Floor trough design that avoids potential hazards of trough design in Fig. 8.3. This design allows all cable installation from inside the procedure room, prevents fluid from entering the trough, and eliminates the unsightly, dirt-catching floor discontinuities created by removable covers illustrated in Fig. 8.3.

Electromagnetic interference (EMI): low- and high-frequency electricity

EMI is demonstrated by the distortion of displayed data or other electronic noise, from electronic equipment directly connected to only the facility power source and grounding system. If the magnitude of the interference is great enough to create incorrect data, the clinical management of the patient could be compromised. EMI is an indirect electric hazard to the patient in addition to electric shock [40,41].

If the objectionable noise is fed to the unit via the grounding system of the facility, one should first verify that no ground loops exist. If none exist, the interference can sometimes be eliminated by establishing a *quiet ground*. A quiet ground is a separate ground conductor which is directly connected to earth, independent of the portion of the facility grounding system responsible for the objectionable noise [29]. Since a quiet ground creates more than one connection to earth, one must carefully test the quiet ground relative to the facility ground to ensure the absence of ground loops. All the resistance and leakage current specifications previously stated must still be satisfied [29].

The interference may be due to high-tension power lines in the vicinity of the building, or to other power lines within the facility, that are carrying large currents. Interference can occur if the equipment is in the vicinity of heavy duty electric motors driving elevators, facility air conditioning systems, or other facility equipment with large current draws. Shielding of the affected instrument as discussed below may be necessary if the source of the interference cannot be eliminated. A new location for the equipment where the interference is absent is the simplest method of eliminating this hazard. For example, one should avoid locating an electrophysiology laboratory near large current devices in the facility. Unfortunately, clinical requirements frequently dictate the location of the affected equipment.

The above discussion assumes that the electric currents causing the EMI are of *low* frequency less than 100 000

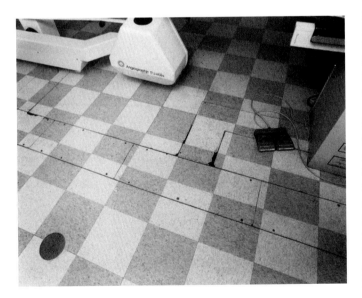

Fig. 8.3 Floor trough with removable covers at floor level, containing interconnecting cables between equipment components. If removable covers are not properly sealed, electric hazards can result.

cycles/s (100 kHz). High-frequency electricity — any current generated at frequencies exceeding 100 kHz — generates potential new electric and thermal hazards. Numerous examples of equipment using these frequencies now exist in the health care field. A few high-frequency converter X-ray generators in imaging equipment are now manufactured that produce wave forms at 100 kHz. Ultrasound imagers typically use 1−15 MHz transducers. Electrosurgery equipment, which uses heating effects of tissue to desiccate, fulgurate, coagulate, or cut tissues, operates in the 0.1−5.0 MHz region [29]. Depending on the stationary magnetic field strength of the magnetic resonance imager (MRI) unit, radiowaves in the 10−90 MHz region are produced. Radiofrequency (RF) diathermy units, which are used to provide a uniform heat distribution to tissue without damaging it, operate at approximately 25 MHz [29]. Microwave diathermy units operate at 2450 MHz [29].

As the frequency of the electric energy wave increases above 100 kHz, the current is no longer restricted to classical conductive pathways [29]. The high-frequency current can travel by radiation through space or other coupling mechanisms with the atmosphere, body tissues, or conductors found within equipment [29]. This can lead to RF interference (RFI), which can block the normal operation of a piece of monitoring equipment or cause thermal damage [29], in addition to the negative effects of EMI. Physiologic monitoring equipment, which today is based on digital circuitry, demonstrates significant sensitivity to RFI, sometimes demonstrated in nonobvious ways such as the production of erroneous data or random malfunctions [29].

RFI is only the beginning of the potential problems associated with the use of high-frequency powered equipment. A multitude of different types of burns can occur with electrosurgical equipment due to the difficulty in controlling heating of the tissues [29]. Explosions and fire can occur in the surgical suite, especially if flammable disinfectants, defatting agents, or cleaning agents are present. Hollow organs may contain methane which is an explosive gas [29]. Low-frequency electric shocks, as discussed previously, also remain as a potential hazard with high-frequency powered equipment.

The problems of RFI can be eliminated by shielding the source of the high-frequency electromagnetic energy, or by shielding the piece of equipment which is affected by the RF energy. The shield consists of a suitable conductor such as copper, which completely surrounds the equipment and is grounded at a single point. To avoid ground loops, any equipment within the conductive shield is attached to the same ground point. The shield is an effective barrier to electromagnetic energy attempting to escape or enter the enclosure. A common example of this shield technique in the health care field is MRI scanners. The image content of the MRI scan is contained in RF waves emitted from the body in the 50 MHz region. Since this is in the region of

frequency modulation radio broadcasts, the broadcast frequencies must be prevented from entering the procedure room; their presence would add noise to the MRI images. Conversely, these high-frequency waves generated by the MRI unit during scanning could potentially interfere with physiologic monitoring equipment outside the scanning room. Patient monitoring equipment is manufactured today with grounded internal conductive shielding to allow its use within MRI scanning rooms.

Mechanical hazards

Any equipment with moving parts or components some distance above the floor possess potential mechanical hazards to the patient and operator [28]. An example of this type of equipment is biplane special procedure X-ray imaging equipment shown in Fig. 8.5. The frontal imaging plane has significant mass (up to 680 kg) cantilevered off a base, which is bolted to the floor. The patient table has a floating top, capable of moving longitudinally up to 1.8 m, while supporting up to a 140−160-kg patient; the table and a 140-kg patient typically exceed 450 kg. The patient and tabletop are supported by a pedestal base, which is bolted to the floor. The lateral imaging plane is similar in weight to the frontal imaging plane; it is hung from overhead rails secured to the ceiling. Numerous television monitors are mounted on overhead suspension systems (combined weight up to 450 kg); the monitors are designed to move horizontally about the room on overhead rails. This suspension system may contain hydraulic supports which allow vertical adjustment of the monitors by the operator. Both imaging planes and the tabletop height are typically power driven. The

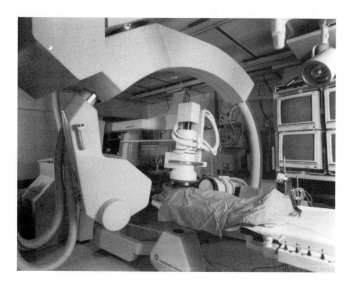

Fig. 8.5 Typical biplane special procedure X-ray imaging equipment, which surrounds the patient with suspended equipment components of significant mass and weight.

patient is positioned among all this equipment at the iso-center of the two imaging planes. This is a machine that presents a multitude of potential mechanical hazards to the patient and operator.

Gravity

If any individual component of the equipment shown in Fig. 8.5 fell from its suspended position, it would possess severe crushing force. This hazard must be minimized by designing redundant, secondary safety support mechanisms for protection if the primary support fails.

This secondary support may be of a different design. The joint, marked by the dark arrow in Fig. 8.6, of an overhead suspension system of a television monitor, receives considerable stress during routine use. It allows the monitor to swivel and rock while supporting the monitor's entire weight. One may not be able to inspect the internal components of this type of joint for signs of stress or weakness, which creates the potential of an undetected hazard. The joint illustrated is well designed and strong enough to support the monitor. This shaft should consist of more than a threaded bolt screwed into the cylindrical mount on top of the yoke of the unit. Manufacturers have addressed this type of hazard by

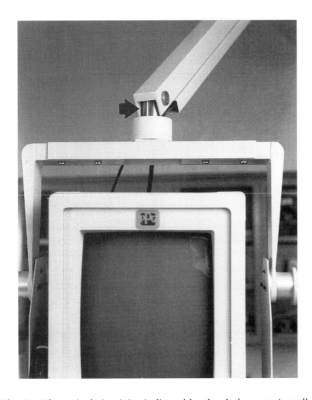

Fig. 8.6 The articulating joint indicated by the dark arrow is well designed to support the weight of the monitor while allowing it to swivel and rock. In the event of failure of this primary support, a secondary support mechanism should be provided.

connecting the two steel arms with a short steel cable, which would support the monitor if the joint broke. If accessible, the integrity of the cable and its connections to the two arms must be periodically inspected.

The secondary support may be of the same mechanical design as the primary. In this case, each individual support (e.g., steel cable, chain, bearing, etc.) must support all of the weight if its twin support fails. In this instance, each suspension system must be completely duplicated. It is not acceptable, e.g., for two cables to be secured with the same bolt at each end. The failure of one bolt would render both cables useless [27].

The extensive counterweights, which are required in most imaging equipment, add considerable moving mass to the system. A component of imaging equipment (overhead X-ray tube, wall bucky assembly, etc.) can be moved vertically upward by the operator without power assistance only if an equal weight is moving downward. Figure 8.7 illustrates a 90/90 tilting fluoroscopic table in its three orthogonal tilted positions. In each illustrated position, and each tilted position in between, when the image intensifier and carriage assembly are moved upward, an equal mass must be moving downward. This requires three different sets of counterweights attached to support rails that prevent swinging of the weights as the tilt of the table changes; each counterweight is connected to the carriage assembly by a steel cable and pulley system. Each cable, its attachment to the carriage assembly or counterweight, pulley, track, bearing, counterweight rubber bumper, etc., must be thoroughly inspected, cleaned, and/or lubricated periodically.

All bolts, lock washers, and nuts of equipment require careful attention. Vibration and jarring of fixed or portable equipment can loosen bolts and nuts over time. All of these items, especially if they secure weight, must be checked for tightness at least annually. The fasteners that secure the equipment to floor plates or overhead suspension systems connected to the facility, are typically checked by the equipment vendor or service engineer. The bolts or mechanical anchors used to secure overhead suspension systems or floor plates to facility structures must also be checked. (See "Facility considerations", p. 155.) In certain situations where vibrations or jarring may be present, bolts should be treated with a liquid which prevents loosening.

Overhead rails that support suspended equipment must be truly level. Any slope within the rails requires the operator to work against gravity as the equipment is moved uphill along the rails; this can lead to back strains and injuries. Sloping rails can cause unattended equipment to move down hill if the locks fail, which creates a potential collision hazard to patient or operator. Even if the rails are level, the potential for movement of the overhead tube crane exists if the locks fail due to the gravitational force exerted by the extended high-voltage cables within the large extended tube (indicated by the dark arrow in Fig. 8.8). This hazard can be

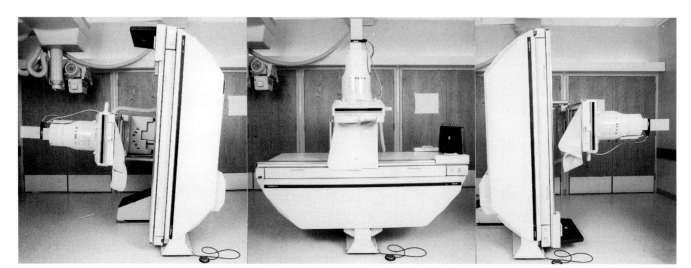

Fig. 8.7 A 90/90 tilting fluoroscopic table illustrated in its three orthogonal tilted positions. In all three illustrated positions, and each tilted position in between, three sets of counterweights are required to allow the operator freely to move the image intensifier and carriage through its three orthogonal motions.

eliminated by either installing a mechanical latch which secures the carriage in its parked position, or by relocating the location in the ceiling where the cables enter the room which reduces tension exerted by the cables. Finally, all horizontal rails must contain solid mechanical endstops to prevent overrun of the carriage beyond the rails. These

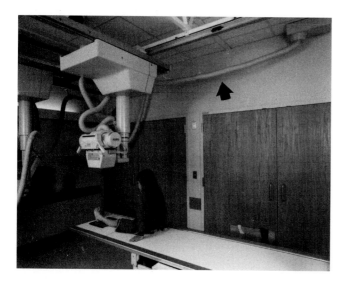

Fig. 8.8 The illustrated extended cable drape (dark arrow) exerts a force on the overhead tube crane assembly, which would cause the assembly to collide with the patient if the electromechanical locks failed. This hazard can be eliminated by installing a mechanical latch, which would secure the assembly in the event of power failure.

endstops must be inspected at least annually to ensure that they are not damaged or loose.

Power movements

Many of the required movements of complex imaging equipment are driven by electric motors. All of these motions require redundant safety features to prevent potential crushing hazards to the patient. A fault in any of the drive motors or their control circuitry (e.g., the patient table elevator drive) could crush the patient against other rigid components of the equipment. The manufacturer should provide an electric power emergency switch on each major component of the equipment. Since this may not be present or requires the operator quickly to recall its location in an emergency, the facility should provide an emergency shunt trip at the main control desk which allows the operator immediately to shut down all power to the equipment (Fig. 8.9).

The operator requires extensive training on the safe control of power movements of the equipment. The operator must be aware of the exact boundaries of all components of the piece of equipment he or she is moving to ensure that the equipment is not driven into the patient, other components of the machine, or other equipment in the vicinity of the machine. In many instances, the operator must split their attention between the safety of the patient and the safety of the equipment. The position of the equipment in Fig. 8.10 illustrates this need. The natural tendency is to concentrate on the patient and face of the image intensifier as one angulates the frontal plane in the caudal direction. But, this would cause the television camera of the frontal plane to collide with the stationary suspension system of the lateral plane. Whenever possible, stops or guards should be installed on the equipment to prevent these types of collisions. Figure 8.11 illustrates an elevating patient table with a cover, which will collide with a foot stool adjacent to its base when the table is driven downward. This hazard was effectively elim-

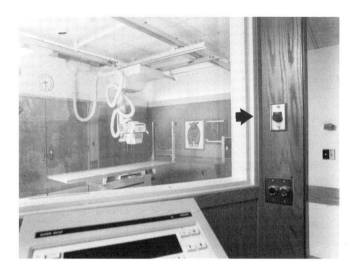

Fig. 8.9 Typical shunt trip, indicated by dark arrow, located at the main control desk of the equipment. This device allows the operator immediately to disconnect all electric power to the unit in case of emergency.

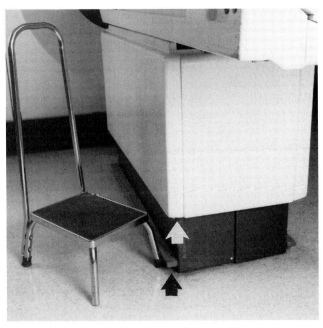

Fig. 8.11 The wooden rail at the base of the patient table (dark arrow), which was installed by the owner, prevents foot stools and other objects from being placed directly underneath the cover of the table (dark arrow), which could damage the equipment when the table is driven downward.

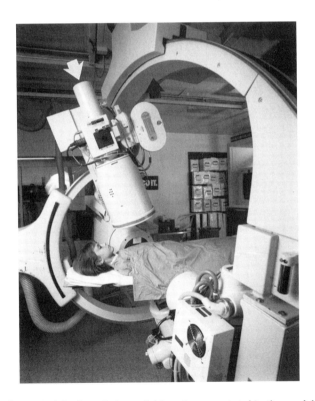

Fig. 8.10 If the frontal plane of this unit were rotated in the caudal direction, the television camera's cylindrical housing (white arrow) would collide with the stationary suspension system of the lateral plane (dark arrow). If mechanical stops that limit the source to image receptor distance in the frontal plane are not allowed by clinical requirements in the room, the operator must split their attention between the safety of the patient and the safety of the equipment.

inated by installing a wooden rail at the table base, which prevents foot stools from sitting directly under this cover.

Different types of electromechanical safety devices should be designed into the equipment. Each control of equipment movement must be of "deadman" design; when the control is released by the operator, the motion must immediately cease. The equipment should have either collision guards or slip clutches designed into their drive mechanisms to protect the patient in the event of a collision. The collision guards are typically mounted on springs and are the first surfaces that come in contact with the patient in the event of a collision. The guard moves and actuates a microswitch which shuts off the power to the drive motor. Slip clutches are mechanical couplings on drive motor shafts. When the equipment collides with the patient, the resistance to further movement causes the clutch to slip and prevent further advancement of the component.

All surfaces that are likely to come in contact with the patient due to collision should be smooth without sharp edges. When possible, these objects should be nonrigid, especially in the case of equipment designed with slip clutches. Figure 8.12 illustrates a flexible spacer mounted on the X-ray tube head, which is required by federal codes for radiation protection concerns [42]. The original spacer was constructed of rigid metal with hard edges. The redesigned spacer still satisfies federal codes, but flexes as required to prevent injury until slippage of the clutch occurs.

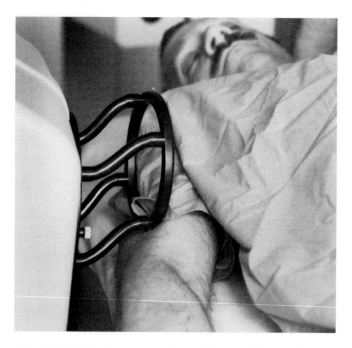

Fig. 8.12 The flexible, as opposed to a rigid spacer (illustrated in Fig. 8.11) on a lateral positioner with slip clutch design prevents the patient's arm from injury, by flexing until sufficient resistance to further movement causes the clutch to slip.

Both collision guards and slip clutches must be functionally tested periodically. Improperly adjusted slip clutches could cause injury from excessive force on the patient prior to slippage of the clutch. Collision guards require periodic cleaning and inspection for damage which could prevent them from moving freely on collision. Abrupt collisions have the potential of physically damaging the microswitch and rendering it inoperable.

All of the electromechanical safety devices designed into the equipment must be maintained in good operating conditions at all times. When these systems fail, a quick bypass allows the continued use of the room. This should *never* be allowed. Too often, the repair of the safety device is forgotten or significantly delayed because the room is completely functional. This practice courts potential disaster.

Cleaning and lubrication considerations

After each patient procedure, dirt, spilled contrast agents, and body fluids should be cleaned from all surfaces of the equipment accessible to the patient and other personnel. These agents may have the potential of spreading disease among patients and personnel, or can increase the risk of infection to the patient. Service personnel should clean and remove these agents from internal surfaces of the machine and from moving parts on a semiannual basis; any pathogens that are present could become air borne at a future time.

The build-up of these materials can create mechanical

hazards to the patient. Many imaging tabletops are designed to be rigidly held in place by energized electromagnets, or to float freely when the electromagnets are turned off. Any foreign materials can cause friction and prevent the table from floating when the electromagnets are released; this prevents the proper positioning of the patient. Conversely, the build-up may coat the electromagnet, reduce the holding force, and prevent the rigid locking of the tabletop when the electromagnets are energized.

Failure to remove spilled fluids and dirt from moving parts leads to excessive mechanical wear, increases the risk of premature failure, and can create mechanically hazardous situations due to poorly performing equipment. The dirt increases friction between moving parts. Stationary surfaces, like bearing races of overhead rails which must support the entire weight of the overhead tube assemblies, require special attention. When this track or the bearings are worn or pitted, more force must be exerted by the operator to move the overhead system which can lead to back strain or other injury of operators.

Lubrication is the second step after cleaning to eliminate unnecessary friction between moving parts. The types of lubricants recommended by the equipment manufacturer should be used. These lubricants vary depending on the application within the machine. If the manufacturer does not recommend lubrication, the cleaned surface should remain dry. A common error by service personnel is the lubrication of aluminum overhead rail surfaces. Manufacturers generally do not recommend this. Lubrication of aluminum rails causes the build-up of excessive grit and dirt, premature damage of the running surfaces, and poor mechanical performance of the bearings along these rails.

Heat considerations

The patient and operator must be protected from components of any imaging equipment that have the potential to overheat. The lamp that produces the light field of the collimator, used by the operator of X-ray equipment to position the patient, is typically contained under a cover at the surface of the collimator box. If the collimator lamp is left on for long durations of time, the temperature of this cover can cause skin burns. This hazard is eliminated by placing the lamp on a timing circuit which shuts the lamp off after a set period of time. This timer should be functionally tested periodically to ensure its correct operation.

The continual production of X-rays generates large quantities of heat within the X-ray tube. The insulating oil inside the tube housing must be allowed to expand into a bellows as it is heated. If the heat-loading ratings of the X-ray tube are exceeded, the oil may boil and generate excessive pressure within the tube. This may damage seals and spray boiling oil on the patient or operator. This hazard can be avoided by installing heat calculators or heat-sensing devices which prevent the continued production of X-rays when a heat-overload condition of the X-ray tube is approached. If the clinical application requires continual X-ray production, high heat capacity X-ray tubes with heat exchangers should be installed.

Facility considerations

Fixed equipment must be properly secured to the floor or ceiling of the facility. In the case of imaging equipment shown in Fig. 8.5, steel floor plates are typically provided by the manufacturer of the equipment. The manufacturer also specifies acceptable rigid structures which must be provided for attachment of any manufacturer supplied overhead rails or plates to which suspended equipment is mounted. In the case of suspended equipment, the manufacturer must specify static and momentary loads that will be exerted on the supporting structures as the suspended equipment is moved on its horizontal rails. The overhead supporting structures must be rigid enough to maintain true level as the equipment load shifts its location. These structures must provide enough mounting points with the manufacturer's rails to maintain true level along the rails. If any flexing occurs in the rails as the equipment is moved, the operator must strain against gravity.

Floor plates and overhead support structures attached to the equipment must be securely fastened to appropriate facility structures. Additional steel attached to the steel frame of the building may be necessary. If the floor deck without added steel can sufficiently bear the added weight, bored holes, which allow a steel plate to be secured on the opposite side of the deck, with bolts, lock washers, and nuts as illustrated in Fig. 8.13, provide one of the more secure attachments of floor plates. For overhead suspension systems, through bolts also are preferred as illustrated in Fig. 8.14.

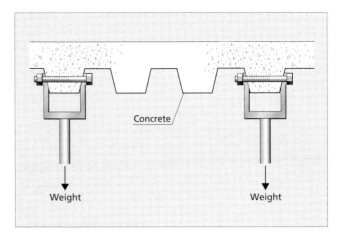

Fig. 8.14 Geometry of the preferred bolt-through scheme for overhead suspension systems.

If bolt-throughs are impossible, holes must be bored into the concrete and the threads of bolts must be tightened into anchors designed to grab the bolt threads and the cylindrical hole edges of the concrete. Structural engineers must ensure that the density and hardness of the cured concrete will resist breakdown and crumbling due to vibrations and other disturbances, which would loosen the anchor in the concrete. The long axis of the bolt and anchor should be perpendicular to the direction of force exerted by the secured equipment as illustrated in Fig. 8.15 (left). This orientation of the anchor and bolt will be more secure and less susceptible to failure than the parallel orientation illustrated in Fig. 8.15 (right).

Overhead tube cranes, floating tabletops, overhead monitor suspensions, or other equipment components may incorporate electromagnetic locks to prevent uncontrolled free-floating movements along their horizontal rails. Emergency

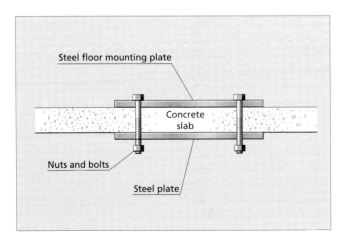

Fig. 8.13 Bolt-through scheme which attaches floor mounting plates securely to the floor deck by attaching a steel plate on the opposite side of the deck.

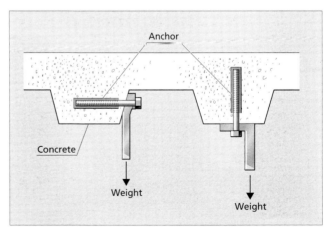

Fig. 8.15 If anchors must be used to secure overhead suspension systems, the long axis of the bolt should be perpendicular to the direction of force of gravity as shown on the left as opposed to parallel as shown on the right.

situations may occur (failure of the "deadman" fluoro-scopy pedal or uncontrollable power-driven motions) where the main circuit breaker must be opened. This also releases the electromechanical locks and causes free floating of the above components. This can cause collisions and potential injury to patients or personnel. These hazards can be avoided by supplying the electromagnetic locks with an independent source of electric power with independent circuit breakers [43]. If this is done, the electromagnetic locks must be connected to the common system ground to avoid the electric hazards associated with ground loops.

The procedure room should be free of obstructions to meet the needs of the equipment and operators in the room. Figure 8.16 illustrates a less than optimal special procedure room with a support column in the middle of the room. The column presents a collision hazard to the equipment. It may prevent the full range of movements designed into the machine which could potentially jeopardize patient care. The column may force personnel to perform their duties from less than optimal locations within the room. The column could make access to the patient much more difficult during emergency situations. Figure 8.17 illustrates equipment cables sprawling across the floor which should be in trough or conduit to avoid tripping hazards to personnel and to avoid cable damage, which could create electric hazards.

The size of the room along with adequate storage facilities are important considerations. If interventional procedures requiring anesthesia of the patient will be performed in the room, space requirements increase significantly due to the additional monitoring equipment and personnel that will be involved in the case. Adequate space must be provided

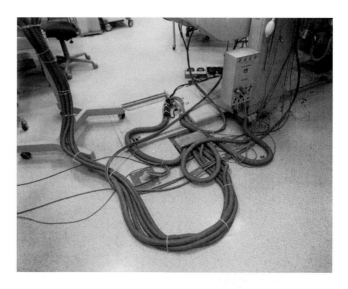

Fig. 8.17 Equipment cables sprawling across the floor create potential tripping hazards to personnel, and cable damage which could result in electric hazards.

around sterile tables to allow safe circulation of nonsterile personnel in the room without contamination of the sterile fields. Different intensities of lighting, each with independent rheostat controls should be available at different locations in the room. Storage of multiple catheters and supplies may be necessary. Figure 8.18 illustrates one solution. The catheters in their sterile packages are stored behind glass doors to minimize the build-up of dirt. The fluorescent light in these cabinets is turned on and off as the door to the closet is opened and closed, respectively. This provides the necessary light to select a catheter, but limits the amount of fluorescent light the catheter packaging is exposed to. Over time, the ultraviolet light emitted by the fluorescent fixtures can breakdown and damage any nylon, latex, or rubber materials contained within the packaging.

Discontinuities in floors can lead to premature failure of structural components of mobile X-ray equipment. If elevators do not stop level with the hallway floor, maintenance personnel should be contacted to make adjustments instead of risking damage to portable equipment. The skid plates that are commonly found on ramps (Fig. 8.19) can lead to premature failure of structural components of the vertical column of mobile X-ray units. As such equipment is driven over this uneven floor surface, an oscillating rocking of the unit occurs, causing premature breakage of support welds at the base of the steel support columns. If a choice exists, operators should avoid these types of floor surfaces when moving mobile X-ray equipment. The mobile X-ray equipment would be better served by a continuous skid pad as opposed to the typical alternating pattern of pad and linoleum flooring shown in Fig. 8.19.

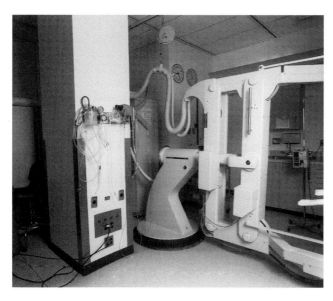

Fig. 8.16 The structural support column illustrated in this procedure room presents a collision hazard to the equipment and potential hazards to the patient and operators.

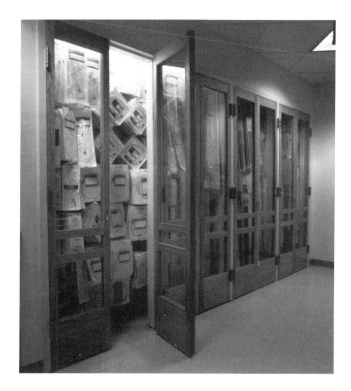

Fig. 8.18 Dirt and dust build-up on the sterile packages of catheters can be reduced by storage in enclosed closets or drawers. In this example, the fluorescent lights are automatically switched on only when the door is opened to identify a catheter.

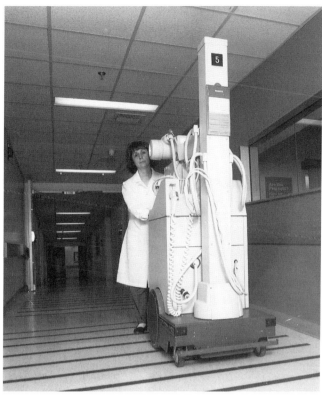

Fig. 8.19 Repetitive skid pads on ramps can create uneven floor surfaces which cause oscillating rocking of the mobile X-ray equipment as it is moved. Since this type of stress can potentially cause physical damage to this type of equipment, continuous as opposed to repetitive skid pads on ramps are preferred.

Methods to minimize hazards

Hazards associated with imaging or ancillary equipment are effectively minimized or eliminated by planning. Safety issues must be addressed during the planning of the facility that will house the equipment. Safety issues should be considered during the equipment selection process. The equipment must be installed properly and should be acceptance tested prior to first clinical use. Operator training before first clinical use and periodically during the equipment's lifetime is important. Finally, comprehensive, periodic, electric safety testing, mechanical inspections, and maintenance procedures must be performed to ensure continued safe use of the equipment and to extend the lifetime of the equipment [44]. Regardless of who has the responsibility within the institution to perform all of this work, someone within the user's department should periodically review, at least annually, all reports and documentation to ensure that the scope of the work performed is appropriate and that all required inspections, testing, and maintenance are completed according to recommended frequencies.

Facility planning

Potential safety issues must be addressed during the planning of the facility that will provide the working environment for the equipment. One must first identify the clinical needs of the patient, operator, and of the installed equipment [45]. This is achieved by asking questions of the physicians, technologists, and other users who will provide the clinical service. It is recommended that a medical physicist should review the range of features offered by the vendors of appropriate equipment on the market, by attending trade shows and reading the vendor's descriptive literature. The identified advantages and disadvantages of the range of equipment available should be discussed with clinical users. This allows tailoring of the purchased equipment to the specific clinical requirements and potential safety issues.

Facility planning and preparation has been discussed elsewhere [46–48]. Planning discussions should involve the clinical users, physicist, and design architect to ensure that the final attributes of the facility allow the operators and the equipment to function effectively, efficiently, and safely. The facility requirements should be communicated by the clinical users to the contracted facility planner, who generates facility site specifications and architectural drawings subject to the final review of the clinical users. The end user should control the facility's attributes, not the facility planner who may not understand the clinical requirements of the facility. This avoids problems such as improper floor trough as described in Fig. 8.3. The medical physicist must monitor each updated set of architectural drawings to ensure that all communications from the clinical users have been understood and included.

The specific facility requirements will be dictated by the type of equipment that will be installed and the clinical application of the equipment. One must consider proximity of the procedure room to other necessary support services (e.g., reception and waiting areas, patient toilets, dressing rooms, sedation and recovery areas, darkrooms, necessary emergency support services, other related clinical services, patient privacy, ambiance, etc.). The size of the procedure room must allow the maximum required number of operators and equipment to work effectively. The floor and ceiling decks must be capable of safely supporting the weight of installed equipment. The proper sized electric power supply and appropriately designed grounding system are imperative to providing an electrically safe environment. Special lighting may be dictated by the planned clinical work. Adequate storage for supplies and ancillary equipment must be provided. The heating, ventilation, and air conditioning systems (HVAC) for the facility must be given careful thought; heat gain to the room associated with modern imaging systems can be sizeable. If invasive procedures will be performed in the room, the air quality must be similar to that of an operating room. Adequate and appropriately designed storage space must be provided for ancillary equipment and supplies.

After the planning process is complete and construction has begun, an appropriate representative of the end users, such as a medical physicist or department manager, must monitor construction progress. This ensures that errors or oversights on the construction drawings and/or actual construction are corrected prior to facility completion. Corrections at this time are usually simpler and less costly, and minimize project completion delays.

Equipment acquisition

For years, complex equipment was purchased by hospitals by requesting quotations from a limited number of vendors. The vendor was selected based on price and the customer's previous experience with the vendors invited to provide quotations. This approach relied on the equipment vendor to specify the equipment with too little input from the clinical users. Equipment with too few or too many features typically was offered usually with little attention paid to the potential safety issues associated with the specific facility and its clinical application.

Better approaches to equipment acquisition have been developed [49–54], which return control of the process to the end user and ensure that safety concerns are addressed appropriately. One of these methods requires the end user to write a request for proposal (RFP). This invites vendors to respond to *user-defined* equipment requirements and purchase conditions. The vendor offers to sell the piece of equipment from their product line which best addresses the customer's clinical requirements and safety concerns. A customer team consisting of physicians, technologists, administrators, and physicist evaluate the RFP responses and objectively select the vendor. A purchase order is issued to the chosen vendor which incorporates all the purchase conditions defined in the RFP into the final purchase contract.

This evaluation team should consider the mechanical design and steps taken by each vendor with respect to mechanical safety issues. For example, some manufacturers "life test" their equipment. This consists of installing a new unit in the factory and operating all mechanical features continually until the machine has been subjected to a lifetime of motions. If any component fails during the process, it is redesigned, built, and the life test is repeated. As the president of one of these companies noted: "The equipment seldom fails in the way that mechanical design engineers would predict!"

The actual content of the RFP must be carefully written. The equipment specifications must be specific enough to define clearly the end user's clinical requirements, but general enough to foster competitive bidding among vendors [55]. If the specifications are narrowly written and appear to favor a specific vendor, other vendors will be discouraged from responding. The advantages to the customer of the competitive bidding process are lost.

Installation and acceptance testing

The final selection and purchase of equipment triggers the development of construction drawings by the chosen vendor. These should be carefully reviewed with the equipment vendor by the customer to ensure that all clinical objectives are addressed. These drawings are then reviewed with the architect. If the selected equipment places unique requirements on the facility which have not been previously addressed, the appropriate changes must be made on the construction drawings before actual construction begins.

Just prior to the installation of fixed, hard-wired equipment, the integrity of all grounds in the procedure room must be tested as outlined in the section "Periodic electrical safety testing and maintenance".

Test methods that the medical physicist can perform in the field designed to check the overall performance of installed equipment, should have been clearly defined in the RFP. Expected performance levels associated with these test methods should also be included in the RFP to define the objective criteria that will be used for acceptance of the installed equipment [55]. Vendors must be allowed to take exception to either the expected performance level or test method, provided an alternate method or performance level acceptable to both the customer and vendor can be identified. Since acceptance testing requires extensive operation of the equipment by the physicist, issues involving patient or operator electric or mechanical safety are typically identified and eliminated prior to first clinical use of the machine.

Personnel training

Initial and continuing education of all operators is necessary over the lifetime of equipment to ensure its continued safe operation. The radiologists, physicians, surgeons, anesthesiologists, technologists, nurses, and other ancillary personnel within the procedure room must follow some guidelines to eliminate electric hazards during procedures. Any control, foot or hand operated, attached to the equipment by a cord must be treated with care to maintain ground integrity of the control. The power cords and plugs of all portable equipment require the same attention. The plug should never be removed from the power receptacle by pulling on the power cord. Each electric circuit in hospitals that connects a number of power receptacles has either a 15 or 20 A capacity. The total current draw of all units plugged into one circuit must not exceed the rated capacity. Any receptacles that do not firmly hold an inserted plug or appear damaged should be reported immediately. The operators must know the exact location and effect of each circuit breaker or shunt trip in the room. A knowledge of which electric circuits in the room will be powered by the facility's emergency generators when commercial electric power is interrupted, is required. The operator must understand the emergency access controls on the equipment that allow immediate access to an arrested patient. A thorough knowledge of each positioning control of the equipment and the boundaries of each component of the equipment in the vicinity of, and remotely to, the patient as the machine moves through its entire range of motions is required [56].

Operators must avoid becoming conduits for leakage currents from powered equipment to the patient. Personnel should never touch the patient while in contact with the outer case of another piece of equipment. If the clinical procedure requires this type of contact, the operator can protect the patient by wearing rubber gloves, which provides an additional layer of insulation.

Operators must understand their responsibility immediately to report any situation that could create potential hazards. Attention to the condition of high-voltage cables and their retaining rings is necessary. Any apparent damage to electric facilities such as electric receptacles must not be ignored. Common appliances should not be indiscriminately moved into procedure rooms without first verifying that these appliances meet electric safety standards.

Throughout the lifetime of the equipment, accidents due to mechanical failure of the equipment can be avoided by an operator who listens carefully to the operational sounds emitted by the equipment during its normal operation. If the operator detects any unusual sounds of scraping, grinding, squeaking, chattering, etc., this may be a warning that a mechanical component within the system has either failed or is in need of maintenance. The operator should also pay attention to the appearance of the equipment, especially mobile X-ray units which suffer considerable physical abuse. Any unusual noise or change in operational sounds or problems noted visually should be reported immediately to service personnel prior to further incident.

The first clinical use of equipment will be more efficient and potentially safer for the patient, operator, and equipment if the physicians and technologists have an opportunity to operate the equipment repeatedly through all of its motions without a patient present. These practice sessions allow the operator to concentrate on equipment design, function, and built-in safety features. Better questions are asked of the equipment's applications specialist. Exercises with phantom patients enhance the operator's understanding. If abbreviated forms of these exercises are scheduled periodically during the lifetime of the equipment, supervisors have the opportunity to identify and eliminate staff member's bad habits before injuries to patients or staff, or damage to the equipment occurs. This practice also optimizes the utility and the performance of the equipment.

Complete service manuals and documentation are required on any equipment serviced by hospital personnel. If the equipment is complex and the manufacturer has developed training courses addressing service, hospital staff should attend. In the absence of formal courses, in-service lectures can sometimes be provided by the manufacturer's service organization on site if this service is negotiated as part of the purchase contract for the equipment. Service personnel who do not have adequate knowledge of the piece of equipment can inadvertently create electric or mechanical hazards which jeopardize the safety of the patients and personnel. Clearly, technologists, physicians, or other operators who are neither qualified as service personnel by training nor have the necessary knowledge concerning the mechanical and electric design of the equipment, have no business altering or attempting even simple repairs of the equipment unless these activities are under the direction of a qualified service person.

Periodic electric safety testing and maintenance

Both facility electric power systems and electric equipment require periodic inspections and maintenance to ensure their continued, safe operation [57]. Facility electric power systems (e.g., grounding systems, transformers, switch gear, emergency diesel generators, etc.) are either tested and inspected by personnel in the hospital maintenance department or these individuals are responsible to contract the work with outside vendors. Electric safety inspections and maintenance of ancillary equipment typically is completed by staff biomedical engineers. These same individuals may perform electric safety inspections of imaging equipment, but typically in the USA, the maintenance and repair of the imaging equipment are contracted to outside vendors.

The following facility components should be inspected and tested after completion of modifications or repairs, or at the recommended frequencies, whichever occurs first. Circuit breakers and associated shunt trips must be manually opened and closed annually [29]. It is strongly recommended, but not required, that periodically the circuit breaker should be electrically tested by placing a high value of current for a specified time across the circuit breaker [29]. Since this test procedure creates potential hazards, it should be performed only by qualified individuals at times when patients are not under examination in the procedure room.

Any ground-fault circuit interrupters installed in circuits must be tested annually [29]. This testing requires momentary application of the rated current of the interrupter between ground and the energized conductor of the circuit. While it is possible, depending on the test equipment and knowledge of the service personnel, to conduct this test safely while patient procedures are in progress, this testing should not be scheduled during patient examination if it can be avoided [29].

The integrity of all grounds must be tested at least annually [29]. The electric resistance between a grounding point of reference and the point in question (e.g., a receptacle in the room, the ground connection for a piece of hard-wired equipment, etc.) is measured to ensure that no ground loops exist. The ground of each power receptacle in the room must be checked since the operator may choose any of these power sources for ancillary equipment. The measured resistance shall not exceed 0.1 or 0.2 Ω in new or existing facilities, respectively.

Prior to checking the ground resistance of each receptacle in the room, its physical condition should be visually inspected. The presence of a ground should be verified. The polarity of the "hot" and neutral wires should be checked to ensure these wires are not reversed. The retention force exerted on the grounding pin of a plug by the receptacle must exceed 115 g [29]. Critical care areas may require testing of receptacles twice annually depending on use [29]. Prior to first clinical use of electric systems in new construction, or of altered systems in existing facilities, the appropriate testing must be completed [29].

The following parameters must be inspected and tested on each piece of portable equipment used in the procedure room in the vicinity of patients. This testing should be carried out after completion of modifications or repairs, or annually, whichever occurs first. The physical condition of the power cord, attached plug, and strain relief must be visually inspected [29]. This is followed by measuring the resistance (≤ 0.5 Ω) between the ground pin of the plug and any exposed conductive surface of the equipment. The cord should be flexed during the measurement at its connection to the strain relief of the plug [29]. After this measurement is complete, the plug is connected to a receptacle, the ground is removed, and two leakage current measurements are performed between the ground pin of the plug and any exposed conductive surface of the equipment; one with the power switch off and one with it on [29]. If the equipment contains leads, electrodes, or a transducer that will come in contact with the patient (e.g., EKG monitoring equipment, defibrillator, ultrasound imager, etc.) leakage current measurements must be completed between each lead and ground [29], and between each combination of two leads [29] when the power switch is on. Each of these leakage current measurements should be completed with the ground present and the ground removed. Finally, the isolation of the patient leads from the remaining circuitry of isolated equipment must be tested by attempting to drive a current through the leads back to ground.

Fixed, hard-wired equipment is inspected and tested differently than portable equipment since it is normally not possible to remove the ground of the equipment during required periodic testing. When the equipment is new, the equipment should be energized with the ground temporarily disconnected.

When the equipment is new, and at least annually thereafter, the continuity of each rack cabinet or case of the equipment system to ground is tested by measuring the resistance between one ground reference point selected in the procedure room and all the individual component cases of the system. Ideally, a ground buss should be used as the reference point, but in its absence the ground of a receptacle that has been previously checked may be used. The performance specification for facility grounds applies; the measured resistance between each component cabinet and the grounding point of reference should not exceed 0.1 Ω [29]. After this measurement is complete, the leakage current is measured between each component or accessible case of the equipment while the equipment is energized. Care must be exercised to attach the measurement leads of the test equipment on nonpainted conductive surfaces of each chassis.

The acceptable maximum leakage currents for isolated and nonisolated equipment, hard-wired or portable equipment under the test conditions described above are listed in Table 8.2. The instrumentation used for performing all of the above measurements must be tested for proper function at least annually and recalibrated [29]. The calibration must be traceable to standards maintained by the National Institute of Standards and Technology (NIST). The test equipment must have an input resistance of 1000 Ω [29]; this specification ensures that the leakage currents measured, model the leakage currents that would occur clinically if the patient or personnel formed the pathway to ground instead of the test instrument.

Periodic mechanical safety testing and maintenance

Comprehensive periodic mechanical safety testing and maintenance requires a thorough inspection of all mechanical systems for excessive wear and damage. This requires removal of system covers and some disassembly of the equipment depending on its design. This work is labor intensive even if completed properly by qualified personnel. The required duration of downtime is dependent on the design of the equipment; it ranges from 1 to a number of days, once or twice annually. Some components require cleaning and lubrication to prevent premature failure. The manufacturer's recommended type of lubrication and recommended frequencies should be rigorously followed. The individual performing the work should have information concerning the collective mechanical reliability, strengths, and weaknesses of a large number of installed machines to assist in identifying weaknesses before accidents occur. Typically, this work is performed by a service representative from the manufacturer. However, X-ray service personnel or staff in the hospital or health care facility who have received proper training and information from the manufacturer, can effectively perform this work.

Dirt, spilled contrast agents, and body fluids should be cleaned from all mechanical surfaces at least semiannually, using only the manufacturer's recommended cleaners and solvents. Other cleaners and solvents may damage these surfaces and lead to premature failure. Special attention must be paid to any lubricated surface where dirt and grit will be attracted and will lead to excessive mechanical wear of moving parts. After cleaning, manufacturer-recommended lubricants should be applied to appropriate surfaces.

After the completion of all recommended cleaning, but before the lubrication of recommended parts, one should complete a thorough mechanical inspection of all components. Wire rope or cable that suspends a system component or counterweights must be inspected for individual breaks in the steel strands. Manufacturers should specify the number of breaks per unit length of cable at which the cable should be replaced. The integrity of the attachments at the ends of the cables should be inspected, tightened, or repaired if necessary. If the manufacturer recommends the lubrication of the cable, the recommended lubricant should be applied.

All bearings should be checked for wear. The raceway or track on which the bearing travels should be replaced if it is damaged or exhibits wear. Each bearing should run down the center of its raceway. Throughout the entire range of motion of the component, the bearing should maintain consistent contact with its raceway as opposed to binding in some locations and lifting from the raceway in other locations.

Any brake systems in the system, mechanical or electromechanical, must be inspected for wear. Some machines have break systems that are designed to slip if excessive force is applied to the component to prevent damage to the equipment; service personnel must understand the design of the machine before appropriate adjustments can be made. The brake systems should be checked to ensure that no drag is present when the brake is fully released and the proper amount of tension is created when the brake is fully applied.

Chains must be carefully inspected. Some manufacturers recommend that chains be removed to allow proper inspection for cracked rollers in individual links or other signs of wear. Special attention must be given to sprockets and motors of drive mechanisms which support weight during the operation of the equipment. The tension of the chain should be carefully adjusted and the chain should be lubricated, both according to the manufacturer's recommendations. The chain tension should be checked with the drive mechanism in different positions to ensure uniform tension of the chain and the absence of misalignments or other problems within the drive mechanism.

All mechanical locks, stops, or joints must carefully be inspected for wear and to ensure that they are secure. Any stops at the ends of overhead rails that exhibit any damage or stress, which could jeopardize their strength, must be replaced. Plungers that are inserted and retracted into holes as part of center locks or source to image receptor distance locks on overhead rail systems, may become bent or worn with use which can prevent proper release or application of the lock. Joints of articulating arms on overhead suspension systems must be carefully inspected for wear or any other warning signs of imminent failure.

Counterweight systems within the machine require careful inspection. Wire rope integrity along the cable must be inspected followed by lubrication, if recommended; its attachment to the component and counterweight must be checked. Pulleys must be properly lubricated. The integrity of the attachment of the counterweight to its guide rail must be checked and lubricated if necessary. Any rubber bumpers attached to the counterweights or to the equipment must be inspected for wear and replaced if necessary.

All bolts and nuts in the system, especially those that are weight bearing (e.g., overhead rails, floor anchors, strain reliefs, tube holders, etc.) must be checked for tightness at least annually. These checks should be performed more frequently if the equipment is subject to vibration and jarring through normal use, e.g., mobile X-ray systems. These checks must include any bolts and nuts that secure floor-mounting plates or overhead suspension systems to the facility structures. Special attention must be paid to bolts that have been treated with a liquid to prevent loosening. If the bolt is turned while checking for tightness, the bold should be removed, cleaned, retreated, and secured.

Attention must be paid to high-tension cables and any other electric cables that are exposed within the procedure room. The integrity of any cable hangers must be checked. If these are designed to move on rails, all bearings and raceways must be checked. The exterior insulation of the cables must be checked for mechanical wear, cuts, or punctures, especially on mobile X-ray units. If initial signs of wear appear, the cable draping of the unit should be checked and altered, if necessary, to minimize continual wear of the cables.

A thorough functional check of every component within the equipment and facility support systems must be performed following cleaning, lubing, and maintenance. One should carefully listen for sounds of scraping, grinding, squeaks, chatter, etc., as each component is mechanically exercised. Counterweights within the system should be silent as they move. If counterbalancing or power-assist mechanisms are properly adjusted, the operator should not have to strain to cause a desired movement. Mechanical or electromagnetic locks should completely release and hold the component of the system according to the manufacturer's design. Drive motors should be tested by loading components to their maximum rated capacity and ensuring proper movement, e.g., elevating tables, etc. All collision guards must be functional and present only smooth surfaces to the patient. Systems with slip clutches should be tested with spring pulls to ensure that potentially harmful forces will not be exerted to the patient on collision. The functionality of all "emergency off" switches on components of the machine should be checked. Timers in collimators should be checked for proper function to avoid overheating of the collimator housing. Any heat calculator or sensor attached to the X-ray tube should be tested for proper function. The HVAC systems should be checked to ensure that proper maintenance is being performed. Any malfunctions in room lighting systems should be noted and repaired, or burned out lamps should be replaced. Finally, at least annually, the shunt trip and circuit breaker functionality should be checked.

Compliance issues

The Safe Medical Devices Act of 1990 (SMDA) became a law in the USA, effective from November 28, 1991 [58]. This law requires that hospitals or other health care facilities report information that reasonably suggests the probability that a piece of equipment or other medical device has caused or contributed to a death, serious injury, or serious illness. These reports must be submitted to the USA FDA and to the manufacturer of the involved equipment or other medical device [58,59]. The hospital must have written procedures documenting the training and education of employees concerning the obligations of this reporting. Documentation is also required that establishes an internal system within the hospital for identifying, communicating, and evaluating events which potentially should be reported.

For a health care organization to receive accreditation from the Joint Commission on the Accreditation of Health Organizations (JCAHO), comprehensive procedures and policies must be internally established within the institution, which ensure broad scope quality assurance with respect to patients and personnel. One component of this overall quality assurance program is the safety of all patients and personnel with respect to potential hazards created by imaging and ancillary equipment.

The SMDA and JCAHO compliance issues specifically regulate the clinical user. Federal regulations established in 1974 to regulate the manufacturer of X-ray equipment still exist [42]. The clinical user should remain abreast of changes to these regulations to monitor the equipment manufacturer's compliance [60].

Documentation

The results of all mechanical or electric safety testing during each piece of clinical equipment's entire life must be carefully and completely documented. This documentation or measured performance record is required to remain in compliance with JCAHO guidelines. The initial test results of optimally calibrated equipment immediately after installation are representative of the optimum performance level of the equipment. This provides an objective basis for initial acceptance of the equipment with respect to criteria established in the purchase contract. These original performance results provide a standard against which all subsequent performance evaluations can be compared. This equipment record may illustrate the slow development of a potential hazard over time and allow correction before a potential mechanical or electric hazard becomes an accident.

As described earlier in Personnel training, initial and continuing education of all operators to ensure the continued safe operation of equipment is an important factor in safety and patient care. Documentation of such training is also required to remain in compliance with JCAHO guidelines.

Summary

Optimal patient care under safe working conditions can be consistently provided when care is taken in proper planning of a facility, equipment selection and installation, proper maintenance programs are established and adhered to, and personnel are appropriately trained. Such routines as described throughout this chapter can be easily integrated into routine department operations. This results in a safe environment in which to provide patient care.

References

1 Albisser AM. Management of electrical hazards in hospitals. *Can Hosp* 1972;49:43.
2 Arbeit SR, Parker B, Rubin IL. Controlling the electrocution hazard in the hospital. *J Am Med Assoc* 1972;220:1581–1584.
3 Aronow S, Bruner JMR, Siegal EF, Sloss LJ. Ventricular fibril-

lation associated with an electrically operated bed. *New Engl J Med* 1969;281:31−32.

4 Atkin DH, Orkin LR. Electrocution in the operating room. *Anesthesiology* 1973;38:181−183.

5 Barry WF, Starmer CF, Whalen RE, McIntosh HD. Electric shock hazards in radiology departments. *Radiology* 1965;95(4): 976−980.

6 Bousvaros GA, Don C, Hopps JA. An electrical hazard of selective angiocardiography. *Can Med Assoc J* 1962;87:286−288.

7 Bruner JMR, Aronow S, Cavicchi RV. Electrical incidents in a large hospital: a 42-month register. *J Assoc Adv Med Instr* 1972;6: 222−230.

8 Bruner JMR. Hazards of electrical apparatus. *Anesthesiology* 1967; 28:396−425.

9 Burchell HB. Electrocution hazards in the hospital or laboratory. *Circulation* 1963;27:1015−1017.

10 Burchell HB, Sturm RE. Electroshock hazards. *Circulation* 1967; 35:227−228.

11 Camishion RC. Electrical hazards in the research laboratory. *J Surg Res* 1966;6:221−227.

12 Dobbie AK. Electricity in hospitals. *Bio-Med Engin* 1972;6: 12−20.

13 Friedlander GD. Electricity in hospitals, elimination of lethal hazards. *Inst Electrical Electronic Eng Spectrum* 1971;8:40−51.

14 Hopps JA. Electrical hazards in hospitals. *Med Biol Engin* 1971;9: 549−556.

15 Hopps JA, Roy OZ. Electrical hazards in cardiac diagnosis and treatment. *Med Electron Biol Engin* 1963;I:133−134.

16 Hopps JA. Shock hazards in operating rooms and patient-care areas. *Anesthesiology* 1969;31:142−155.

17 Leonard PF, Gould AB. Dynamics of electrical hazards of particular concern to operating-room personnel. *Surg Clin N Am* 1965; 45:817−828.

18 Mody SM, Richings M. Ventricular fibrillation resulting from electrocution during cardiac catheterization. *Lancet* 1962;2: 689−698.

19 Pengelly LD, Klassen GA. Myocardial electrodes and danger of ventricular fibrillation. *Lancet* 1961;i:1234.

20 Stanley PE. Hospital electrical safety and shielding. *J Assoc Adv Med Instr* 1967;2:8−12.

21 Starmer CF, Whalen RE. Current density and electrically induced ventricular fibrillation. *Med Instr* 1973;7:3−6.

22 Starmer CF, Whalen RE, McIntosh HD. Hazards of electric shock in cardiology. *Am J Cardiol* 1964;14:537−546.

23 Weinberg DI. Electrical safety in the operating room and at the bedside. In: Seigal BC, ed. *Engineering in the Practice of Medicine*. Baltimore: Williams & Wilkins, 1966.

24 Weinberg DI, Artley JL, Whalen RE, McIntosh MD. Electric shock hazards in cardiac catheterization. *Circul Res* 1962;11: 1004−1009.

25 Yarrow S. Electrical hazards associated with some new medical and surgical procedures. *N Z Med J* 1966;65:21−25.

26 Servomaa A. *Health Devices* 1989;18(1):53−54.

27 Higson GR. Electrical and mechanical hazards in the X-ray department. In: Ansell G, ed. *Complications in Diagnostic Radiology*, 1st edn. Oxford: Blackwell Scientific Publications, 1976: 452−469.

28 Servomaa A. *Health Devices* 1989;18(1):53−54.

29 Klein BR (ed.). *Health Care Facilities Handbook*, 3rd edn. Quincy, MA: National Fire Protection Association, 1992.

30 Dalziel CF. Electric shock hazard. *Inst Electrical Electronic Eng Spectrum* 1972;9:41−50.

31 Bruner JMR, Leonard PF. *Electricity, Safety, and the Patient*. Chicago and London: Yearbook Medical Publishers, 1989.

32 Safe Current Limits for Electromedical Apparatus (ANSI/AAMI ES1-1993). *Health Devices* 1993;22(8,9):413−415.

33 Staewen WS. Electrical safety reconsidered − the new AAMI electrical safety standard. *Biomed Instr Technol* 1994;March− April: 131−132.

34 Standards: what's new in NFPA 99 − 1993? *Health Devices* 1993; 22(8,9):413−415.

35 Bruner JMR. Common abuses and failures of electrical equipment. *Anesth Analg* 1972;51:810−820.

36 Albisser AM, Jackman WS, Pask BA. Isolated power is NOT the solution to electrical hazard problems. *Hosp Prog* 1971;52:52.

37 Albisser AM, Parson ID, Pask BA. A survey of the grounding systems in several large hospitals. *Med Instr* 1973;7:297−302.

38 Weinberg DI. Grounding for electrical safety. *Med Electron Biol Engin* 1964;2:435.

39 Dalziel CF. Transistorized ground fault interrupter reduces shock hazard. *Inst Electrical Electronic Eng Spectrum* 1970;7:55−62.

40 Guidance article: cellular telephones and radio transmitters − interference with clinical equipment. *Health Devices* 1993; 22(8,9):416−418.

41 Smyth NPD, Parsonnet V, Escher DJW, Furman S. The pacemaker patient and the electromagnetic environment. *J Am Med Assoc* 1974;227:1412.

42 Code of federal regulations. Title 21, Part 1020.32.f *Source to Skin Distance*. Washington: US Government Printing Office, 1984; 304−328.

43 Brateman L. Potential hazards from movable radiographic tables (letter to the editor). *Radiology* 1987;165(3):879.

44 Blinov NN, Danilenko TV, Leichenko AI, Leonov BI, Shengalia NA. Radiation methods and means for testing radiodiagnostic equipment. *Med Prog Technol* 1991;17:21−27.

45 Rossi RP. Identification of clinical needs (roentgenography). In: Hendee WR, ed. *The Selection and Performance Evaluation of Radiologic Equipment*. Baltimore: Williams & Wilkins, 1985: 9−12.

46 Roeck WW. X-ray room preparation: layout and design considerations. In: Siebert JA, Barnes GT, Gould RG, eds. *Specification, Acceptance Testing and Quality Control of Diagnostic X-ray Imaging Equipment*. New York: American Association of Physicists in Medicine, 1991: 1144−1177.

47 Hendee WR (ed.). *The Selection and Performance Evaluation of Radiologic Equipment*. Baltimore: Williams & Wilkins, 1985:88−97.

48 Rossi RP, Hendee WR. New equipment for room 2210: the critical path method. *Am J Roentgenol* 1980;134:1084−1088.

49 Gray JE, Morin RL. Purchasing medical imaging equipment. *Radiology* 1989;171:9−16.

50 Hendee WR, Rossi RP. Performance specifications for diagnostic radiologic equipment: a delicate interface between purchaser and supplier. *Proc Int Soc Optical Eng* 1975;70:238−241.

51 Hendee WR, Rossi RP. Performance specifications for diagnostic X-ray equipment. *Radiology* 1976;120:409−412.

52 Rossi RP, Hendee WR. The exchange of information between the purchaser and supplier of radiologic imaging equipment. *Proc Int Soc Optical Eng* 1977;127:167−171.

53 Rossi RP. Preparation of performance specifications (roentgenography). In: Hendee WR, ed. *The Selection and Performance Evaluation of Radiologic Equipment*. Baltimore: Williams & Wilkins, 1985: 41−46.

54 Stone T. Equipment acquisition procedures. *Proc Int Soc Optical Eng* 1977;127:167−171.

55 Strauss KJ, Rossi RP. Specification, acceptance testing, and quality control of mammography imaging equipment. In: Haus AG, Yaffe MJ, eds. *Syllabus: A Categorical Course in Physics: Technical Aspects of Breast Imaging.* Oakbrook: RSNA Publications, 1993: 213–240.

56 Damiano MM, Kandarpa K. Angiography: radiographic equipment and techniques. In: Kandarpa K, ed. *Handbook of Cardiovascular and Interventional Procedures.* Boston: Little Brown & Company, 1989: 167–175.

57 Duff WR, Maness JH. Technical note: safety testing of equipotential grounding systems. *J Assoc Adv Med Instr* 1971;5:355.

58 *Medical Device Reporting for User Facilities: Questions and Answers Based on the Tentative Final Rule.* US Department of Health and Human Services, FDA 92-4247, 1992: 1–44.

59 ECRI problem reporting system. *Health Devices* 1993;22(8,9): 421.

60 Kessler DA, Pape SM, Sundwall DN. The federal regulation of medical devices. *New Engl J Med* 1987;317:357–366.

CHAPTER 9

Diagnostic ultrasound

Hylton B. Meire

Introduction

One of the main reasons for the continuing rapid expansion in the clinical applications of diagnostic ultrasound is its freedom from the use of ionizing radiations. Many of the authors of early papers on the subject emphasized that the technique is painless, harmless, and noninvasive and that, where appropriate, it should be used in preference to alternate radiographic procedures.

In general, these views are still held, although many workers are now perhaps a little more cautious in emphasizing the complete freedom from hazard of diagnostic ultrasound. Although the general consensus of opinion is in favor of the absence of harmful biologic effects, a few papers have raised doubts that in some clinical situations and with certain types of equipment there are causes for concern. The field of biologic effects of ultrasound will be discussed in more detail later in this chapter.

There also has recently been an expansion in the application of ultrasound for the guidance of biopsy and aspiration techniques, both for diagnostic and therapeutic purposes. Clearly, these procedures are not devoid of complications and this subject is discussed at length in other chapters.

It is likely that the main source of hazard or complication to the patient from the use of ultrasound imaging, derives from its high reliance on operator expertise. Modern automatic realtime scanners are deceptively easy to use and the main hazard to the patient is likely to arise from an incorrect or inadequate diagnosis, possibly exacerbated by consequent incorrect medical or surgical treatment, or failure to treat an undiagnosed condition. Indeed, there is a rapidly rising number of medicolegal cases arising from missed or erroneous ultrasound diagnoses, especially in obstetrics.

Few attempts have been made to quantify the incidence or magnitude of patient hazard from this source, but the subject will be discussed in more depth and the results of a small trial will be presented later in this chapter.

There are now three reports of patients suffering harm as an indirect result of their ultrasound scans. One of these was a man who suffered a transient cerebral ischemic attack during a carotid Doppler examination [1]. This event was more likely to be attributable to the position of his neck than to the use of ultrasound. Another man suffered a pulmonary embolus during a Doppler examination of his thrombosed femoral vein [2]. The vein was being compressed by the ultrasound transducer at the time. Three patients have now been reported as suffering from water intoxication as a result of water ingestion prior to pelvic ultrasound scans, while suffering from the syndrome of inappropriate antidiuretic hormone secretion [3].

Contrast agents

A further departure from the otherwise noninvasive nature of ultrasound scanning has been the recent development of contrast agents, primarily to enhance the signal strengths reflected from within blood vessels. In their simplest form these comprise shaken saline or other inert fluids. However, these agents have a very short life and do not pass through the pulmonary bed and, thus, a variety of alternate agents have been investigated. Initially, animal experiments were undertaken with a range of supposedly inert particulate materials. These did not pass well through the pulmonary vascular bed and proved toxic if injected intraarterially [4]. Perfluorohydrocarbons were shown to be taken up by the liver and to increase its reflectivity. It was hoped that they would help in the diagnosis of malignant disease [5], but they had to be injected in very large doses to produce a detectable effect and have not proved acceptable for human use.

The most recent development has been the production of encapsulated gas bubbles. These comprise air, nitrogen, or carbon dioxide within a range of proprietary envelope materials, commonly polysaccharides or albumin, but also including polymers [6]. Some of these are capable of passing through the pulmonary and cardiac circulations after intravenous injection, and appear in low concentrations in the arterial tree. The large majority of the microspheres are, however, destroyed in the lungs or heart, but the envelope debris does not appear to result in any detectable adverse effects. However, there is some evidence from animal experiments that venous injection of albumin-coated microspheres is associated with a transient rise in pulmonary vascular resistance in the pig, although no effect has been detected in the monkey, rabbit, or dog [7,8]. At least one agent has used bovine albumin for its capsular material, and this has led to scares about possible transmission of bovine spongiform encephalopathy, while the use of human albumin has lead to concerns about transmission of a range of viral agents including hepatitis and human immunodeficiency virus (HIV). The clinical use of ultrasound contrast materials is still very limited and there are, as yet, no reported adverse incidents associated with their use, although it has been shown in the dog that intracoronary injection causes a transient impairment of myocardial contractility [9]. It has also been suggested that animals may produce antibodies to the human albumin component of these agents [10], but a search for antibodies in humans has produced negative results [11].

The move away from human albumin, or other biologic products, as envelope materials will obviate these anxieties.

Intracavitary scanners

Over the last 5 years, intracavitary ultrasound scanners have found increasing applications in many departments. These scanners comprise small transducers which can be passed into a range of body cavities. Those attached to gastroscopes have been shown to produce exquisitely detailed images of the pancreatic body and its duct system, and may have a role in the preoperative diagnosis of pancreatic disease. Dedicated rectal systems have been developed for imaging the prostate, and transvaginal scanning has become common place in gynecology and obstetrics. Minute catheter tip realtime transducers have been developed for intravascular imaging and are beginning to prove useful in the diagnosis and management of vascular disease.

The use of ultrasound in all these intracavitary imaging systems would not seem to make them more prone to complications or hazards than those normally associated with the analogous forms of endoscopy, although there is now a very acute awareness of the need to prevent crossinfection from patient to patient, especially with hepatitis and HIV. However, there are also theoretical hazards from the placement of electrically energized devices within the body cavities, but I have not been able to find any reported instances of patient electrocution from this source.

An additional family of scanners dedicated to intraoperative imaging have also appeared and, in general, they consist of small high-frequency sterilizable transducers which can be placed directly on such structures as the common bile duct, liver, or kidney during the search for calculi, to detect vessels or tumors within the liver, or to evaluate the adequacy of vascular anastomoses during arterial surgery. Once again, the complications associated with these dedicated systems are unlikely to be connected in any way with the utilization of ultrasound, although there may be a theoretical hazard from their use in an anesthetic-laden atmosphere. No instances of gas explosion caused by ultrasound scanners have been reported, to date, and there are no conspicuous examples of infection associated with peroperative scanning.

Effects of ultrasound on tissue

It has been known since the early years of this century that ultrasound can produce effects upon biologic systems. Experiments during the First World War succeeded in killing goldfish submitted to high-intensity ultrasound. A few years later it was shown that major lesions could be produced in the brains of cats subjected to high-intensity focused ultrasound, and experiments were undertaken to evaluate ultrasound as a potential alternate to radiotherapy for the destruction of localized neoplasms. More recently, ultrasound has gained wide clinical acceptance in physiotherapy departments and now virtually every professional sports organization has its own ultrasound therapy unit for treating the frequent soft tissue injuries associated with modern sports. There is good circumstantial evidence to show that the rate of resolution of soft tissue injuries is enhanced by treatment with therapeutic ultrasound, and similar results have been achieved in accelerating the healing of varicose ulcers, burns, and a range of other soft tissue conditions.

The mechanisms by which these beneficial effects are mediated are ill understood, although it seems likely that they are associated with a local heating effect and an increase in local blood flow. If we accept the existence of beneficial effects, then we must by inference accept the fact that ultrasound is capable of inducing changes in biologic systems, and it would not be surprising if some of these effects were harmful rather than beneficial.

Little scientific research seems to have been conducted into the harmful effects of therapy ultrasound, but, without revealing sources, I can report upon a well-proven clandestine use of an adverse biologic effect of therapy ultrasound in racing greyhounds. As with sportspersons, soft tissue injuries in greyhounds are often treated by therapy ultrasound. Certain greyhound owners have discovered that by mildly overtreating the rear limb muscles of their greyhounds they can marginally reduce the performance of these animals. It is possible, thereby, to influence the result of a race, and certain cartels of greyhound owners are known to be using this technique to enhance their winnings. One of the major advantages of this form of "nobbling" a greyhound is that it is short lived, reversible, and completely undetectable.

Having established that ultrasound is capable of producing effects on biologic systems, it becomes essential to assess the factors that determine the presence and degree of these bioeffects. Not surprisingly, the effects are directly related to the dose of ultrasound delivered to the target tissues. It is possible to demonstrate that increasing doses produce increasing bioeffects and that no effects are detectable at extremely low dose rates. There is some suggestion from the experimental evidence obtained to date that there appears to be a threshold level for dose below which no bioeffects have been observed [12] (Fig. 9.1), power levels well below 100 mW/cm^2 apparently being entirely safe, irrespective of the duration of the exposure.

The role of dosimetry is therefore of fundamental importance when we consider the potential bioeffects of ultrasound and the possibility of hazards to patients. Regrettably, ultrasound dosimetry is highly complicated and it is influenced by a wide variety of factors, many of which are unknown in clinical situations. Furthermore, the large majority of papers published on the findings of laboratory experiments into the bioeffects of ultrasound, incorporate poor dosimetry information which often completely negates their scientific value. As the question of dosimetry is so vital I will discuss it in some depth at this point.

Dosimetry

Diagnostic ultrasound is transmitted into patients either in very short pulses or as continuous ultrasound waves. Conventional imaging systems invariably employ pulsed ultrasound, whereas some Doppler systems, notably fetal heart detectors and simple peripheral vascular nonimaging systems, use continuous wave ultrasound. In the imaging systems the sound is transmitted from a small crystal and takes the form of a focused beam which passes down into the patient. The degree of focusing varies considerably between different types and makes of equipment and is now often under the influence of the scanner operator. The pulses of sound used for imaging have a duration of less than one-millionth of 1 second, and for Doppler scans are generally about 10 times this length. They are transmitted into the patient at a rate of 1000–10 000/s. In the interval between

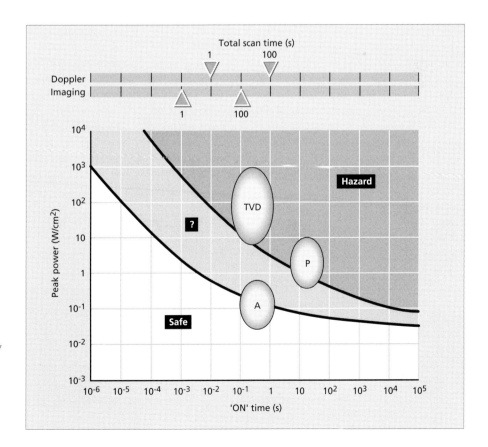

Fig. 9.1 Graph of ultrasound exposure power and time. When both time and power are low there is no evidence of adverse effects. As both increase the likelihood of effects increases. There is no evidence of effects, whatever the exposure time, if the power is below 100 mW/cm^2 (0.1 W/cm^2). The majority of extracorporeal scans lie in the region of "A" and are probably safe. Transvaginal Doppler (TVD) crosses the boundary into known adverse biologic effects. The exposure conditions for physiotherapy are indicated by "P."

pulses, the scanner merely "listens" for echoes returning to the surface from structures within the patient. As the sound passes through the patient the beam pattern is altered by refraction and, therefore, defocusing occurs with subsequent reduction in the power per unit area. At the same time, since biologic tissues are poor conductors of ultrasound, the beam is rapidly attenuated and may become undetectable before it reaches the distal tissues in the patient.

It can be appreciated, therefore, that in the average ultrasound imaging system the tissues beneath the ultrasound transducer are not being subjected to transmitted ultrasound for up to 99.9% of the duration of an ultrasound scan.

It is possible to measure ultrasound power in many different ways, including the instantaneous peak power during the height of a pulse (the temporal peak), the average power during the pulse (the pulse average), or as the time-averaged power over a period of several pulses (the temporal average). It is not yet clear from experimental results which of these is the most important for biologic effects. The matter is further complicated by changes in the pulse shape as it passes through the tissues. Most workers to date have assumed that the pulse shape does not alter and that the relationship between the above three values remains constant for a pulse as it traverses the tissues. This is now known to be false. As the pulse passes through the tissues the positive component of the pulse causes an increase in pressure in the tissues, producing tissue compression, and vice versa for the negative component (Fig. 9.2a). As the tissues are compressed the velocity of conduction of the ultrasound is marginally increased, and is reduced during the rarefaction phase. The effect of this is to cause the trailing edge of the positive pulse to catch up the leading edge (Fig. 9.2b), while the negative component becomes stretched out. After 5−6 cm of tissue path the positive component has become very short indeed (Fig. 9.2c) and is termed a "shock wave". The rate of change of energy in the pulse is now massively increased, as is the instantaneous peak power, although the total power content of the pulse (pulse average power) remains unchanged by

this process. These changes must inevitably have an adverse influence on the biologic effects of such a pulse and greatly complicate the already difficult problems of dosimetry.

The ultrasound beam is focused in order to improve image resolution and, as with sunlight focused through a lens, the focusing of ultrasound increases the power per unit area. In an average abdominal imaging system the transducer crystal has a diameter of roughly 20 mm and the beam width is reduced to approximately 3 mm in diameter at the focus. In the absence of attenuation, this results in the power per unit area at the focus being 44 times greater than at the transducer face. In order to take this into consideration it is essential in any experiment to take account of the focusing characteristics of the ultrasound beam and to specify precisely the point within the space beneath the transducer at which the ultrasound dose levels are assessed.

It is now general practice to consider the worst case, i.e., the peak power at the center of the focus (spatial peak). Fortunately, the majority of workers now confine their assessment to the spatial peak temporal average (SPTA) power, although there are occasions when the pulse average power (SPPA) may be more relevant. Neither of these values take into account any shock wave formation.

Power levels in diagnostic scanners

The reader would be forgiven for assuming that the majority of diagnostic ultrasound imaging systems have power levels that are broadly similar. In practice, this is far from the case. To date, most manufacturers have been reluctant to quote the power output characteristics of their equipment, but a number of independent laboratories have attempted to take measurements and their results are surprising. The SPTA levels of commercially available imaging equipment were found in 1985 to vary from 0.6 to 290 mW/cm^2 [13], and in the Doppler mode, powers of up to 825 mW/cm^2 were detected [14]. There has undoubtedly been a subsequent progressive increase in power outputs. Duck and colleagues

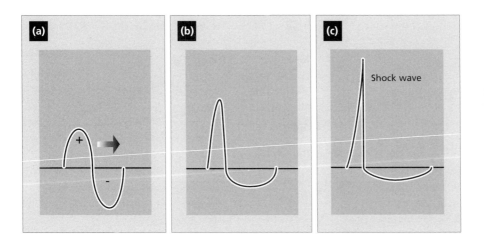

Fig. 9.2 The mechanism for "shock wave" production. (a) The positive and negative halves of the transmitted pulse are initially equal. (Arrow indicates direction of propagation of pulse.) (b) As the pulse passes through the tissues the positive half-cycle is foreshortened and the negative half-cycle is stretched. (c) At a tissue depth of 5−6 cm the positive half-cycle has been converted into a shock wave.

noted in 1991 that some diagnostic scanners now produce powers greater than those emitted by ultrasound therapy units [15,16].

There is no convincing evidence that the systems employing the higher power levels produce better images. More worrying are the power levels emitted by some equipment when used in the Doppler mode. In this mode there is almost invariably a marked increase in both the pulse length and the pulse power, giving rise to an increase in the total power output from 100 to 1000 times that used in imaging. In addition, there is a tendency for manufacturers to increase the power output of higher frequency transducers, to help compensate for the more rapid attenuation in the patient, and most array transducers have much higher outputs than single crystal devices. All these factors, combined with the short distance between the transducer and target tissue, may give rise to very high doses to the ovaries or conceptus during transvaginal Doppler studies (see Fig. 9.1). There are many commercially produced scanners, available in the early 1990s, which are capable of transmitting power levels of over $2000 \, mW/cm^2$ SPTA in the Doppler mode; occasional values of over $8000 \, mW/cm^2$ have been detected. Clearly, there is room for government legislation. Some countries (most notably the USA) are moving in this direction and the International Electrotechnical Commission is currently working on assessment of the thermal and mechanical effects of ultrasound radiation, with the intention of ultimately requiring all equipment manufacturers to incorporate in their scanners appropriate software to display the calculated thermal and mechanical indices on the screen of the scanner. The SPTA values for physiotherapy ultrasound equipment usually lie in the range of $100-1000 \, mW/cm^2$ (see Fig. 9.1). On the basis of this information it would seem very likely that certain diagnostic ultrasound systems are capable of producing biologic effects in some clinical situations.

Adverse biologic effects of ultrasound

To date, several thousand papers have been published reporting on clinical and laboratory experiments to assess the bioeffects of diagnostic ultrasound, and these have been reviewed at length elsewhere [17−20]. The vast majority of these have shown no adverse effects. In addition, several large clinical studies have reported on the follow-up findings in a range of populations exposed to ultrasound, usually during pregnancy [21−27]. Although the large majority of these have reported negative findings, there have been, and continue to be, occasional scares which often receive inappropriate and uninformed coverage in the popular press. At the time of writing this chapter two such papers are under discussion, one having reported an apparent increase in left handedness in children exposed to ultrasound *in utero* [28], and the other suggesting that frequent Doppler ultrasound in pregnancy is associated with reduced birth weight [29]. I

am sure that these studies will be repeated in the near future and it is highly likely that these findings will not be confirmed. When evaluating reports such as these it is important to be aware of both the scientific and statistical methods used in the studies. In the first study, a wide range of neurological signs were evaluated; the study was not designed specifically to investigate the effect of ultrasound on handedness. Similarly, in the second study, the project was not designed to test the effect of ultrasound on fetal weight. The fact that these observations have been made is almost certainly due to chance. Indeed, if one reads the original articles, the authors of the first actually state that their findings "may be due to chance" and the second accept that there is a possibility that "this finding was a chance effect". When analyzing data to assess the statistical significance of an observation we apply a test of probability. The accepted limit for probability is 95% confidence that the observation has not occurred by chance. The converse of this implies that out of every 20 random observations one will spuriously appear to be significant. Thus, if one takes any relatively large population and compares it with another for 20 different variables it is almost certain that one group will falsely appear to be significantly different from the other for one of the variables. If the test is repeated with two similar sized truly random groups, the apparent findings will be different. It is therefore very important that all studies which appear to show unexpected effects of ultrasound should be repeated, preferably with a study designed specifically to test for the effects on the specific variable. To date, no studies have shown any repeatable statistically significant adverse effects of ultrasound. This would suggest that if adverse effects do occur they are extremely mild, infrequent, or do not become manifest for a period of several years after the exposure.

By far the majority of published papers report the results of laboratory experiments. These are conducted either on intact small laboratory animals or on cell cultures or suspensions. Once again, the majority of investigators have reported negative findings, but there have been occasional apparently positive results. While many of these have not been reproducible there are a few which must now be taken seriously [30−35], and which I believe are very relevant to modern ultrasound scanning techniques. These experiments involved exposing pregnant mice to ultrasound at a range of different power levels. Some of these results are summarized in Table 9.1. It can be seen that when the SPTA was at or above $500 \, mW/cm^2$ there were reproducible effects. Experiments with SPTAs above $1000 \, mW/cm^2$ generally led to abortion of all fetuses.

The mechanisms by which these effects were mediated remain unproven, but it seems very likely that they were in part due to heating of the embryos, and the magnitude and reproducibility of the effects are roughly proportional to the heating effect. This hypothesis is supported by experiments which have shown that there is a significant increase in the

Table 9.1 Fetal anomaly induction in mice

Year	Power SPTA (mW/cm^2)	Reference
1971	40	Shoji *et al.* [30]
1977	<1000	Fry *et al.* [31]
1980	500	Stolzenberg *et al.* [32]
1981	500	Kimmel *et al.* [33]

fetal abnormality rate when pregnant rats and mice are heated by 2°C. If there temperatures are raised by more than 3°C all fetuses are killed.

A rather more worrying recent finding has been the production of pulmonary hemorrhage in primates who have been exposed to localized ultrasound exposure by a diagnostic imaging scanner [36]. Fortunately, the lung is not currently a target for ultrasound imaging, but the presence of air within the alveoli leads to deposition of most of the ultrasound energy into the lung when it does fall in the ultrasound beam. The mechanism for this effect is not yet clear but the effect appears real and is worrying. It may be thermal or mechanical in origin.

The heating effect of current ultrasound probes has thus been studied [37] and some alarming results have been seen (Table 9.2). It can be seen from this table that single crystal devices used for imaging only did not achieve any temperature rise, whereas all the array transducers heated during normal imaging. All transducers showed higher heating when used in the Doppler mode, and for one high-frequency phased array transducer this reached 50°C above room temperature. The temperature rises were roughly proportional to the probe frequency. There can be little doubt that this transducer is capable of producing power levels greater than that needed to induce adverse fetal effects in small mammals. When the results of the experiments on mice were published in the early 1980s little attention was paid to them as, at that time, all clinical scans were performed from the outside of the body and transducer output powers were very modest. In the intervening decade, output powers have increased, Doppler scanning is more frequent, and

Table 9.2 Transducer heating caused by ultrasound output levels. A summary of results from 30 transducers for a 5-minute temperature rise in air. (From Duck *et al.* [37])

Ultrasound probe	Minimum (°C)	Maximum (°C)
Imaging	0 (sc)	13.1 (pa)
Doppler	1.7 (sc)	52.2 (pa)
Color flow imaging		
2.5 MHz		1.6 (pa)
3.5 MHz		5.7 (pa)
7.0 MHz		7.0 (pa)

pa, Phased array transducer; sc, single crystal transducer.

intracorporeal scanning, especially transvaginal scanning, is bringing the transducer much closer to the potentially sensitive tissues.

It is always difficult to extrapolate the relevance of experimental laboratory findings to the application of ultrasound to the intact human. There must always be major uncertainties concerning the relative sensitivity of the tissues under consideration but, more importantly, the question of dosimetry arises once again. In laboratory experiments the transducer is likely to be held stationary over tissues or cells suspended in a nonattenuating medium. During clinical ultrasound scans the ultrasound beam is rapidly scanned through the field of view, and the field of view itself is moved rapidly around the patient's anatomy by the ultrasound operator, thus ensuring that the duration of exposure to any one tissue volume is extremely short. However, in Doppler studies the scanner is held stationary over the area of interest, both the pulse length and power are increased and the beam is no longer being scanned through the tissues.

Mechanisms of bioeffects

Four potential mechanisms have been identified by which these bioeffects may be mediated: heat, cavitation, streaming, and stress. The role of heating has been discussed above, the other mechanisms will be reviewed here and their relevance in the light of our expanding knowledge of ultrasound physics will be discussed.

Cavitation

Cavitation is a phenomenon in which small vapor-containing cavities are generated within fluid media under the influence of ultrasound energy. Several factors are thought to be necessary for the production of cavitation and, in general, this phenomenon has been observed only in free fluids under the influence of continuous-wave ultrasound at power levels greater than those used in most diagnostic systems. However, the longer and more powerful pulses used in Doppler scanning, possibly combined with the pulse distortion caused by shock wave generation, could theoretically give rise to conditions in which cavitation could occur by a process of "rectified diffusion". In this phenomenon, a small preexisting nidus in the tissue sucks in gas during the negative pressure phase of the passing pulse. If the positive phase is very brief, due to shock wave production, there is insufficient time for all the gas to escape before more is sucked in. The nidus thus gives rise to a rapidly expanding microbubble which, when it reaches a certain critical size, implodes with the very rapid release of huge amounts of energy. This rapid localized release of energy is very likely to cause tissue damage and there is some suggestion that the energy release might be of sufficient magnitude to induce free radicle production, analogous to that produced by ionizing radiations. This process can probably occur in biologic tissues at the higher range of power levels now found in some diagnostic equipment, and may be of potentially very grave importance as ultrasound has previously been thought to be free of the hazards associated with ionizing radiations.

Streaming

Streaming of fluids has been shown to occur in the presence of relatively high-power continuous-wave ultrasound and it can be used as a means of stirring liquids in industrial processes. It has been thought unlikely that streaming could be produced by diagnostic ultrasound imaging systems. However, it has now been shown that streaming can occur in free fluids within the body if the fluid contains reflective particles, although it remains unknown and doubtful if it occurs in intact cells. If streaming did occur within intact cells it could lead to disruption of the biochemical processes of the cell with consequent bioeffects.

Stress

As the ultrasound pulses pass through tissues, they are conducted from one point to another in the form of waves of mechanical compression and rarefaction of the tissues. The associated pressure changes are usually less than 2 MPa, and values of this magnitude are probably safe. It is, in fact, the peak negative pressure that is assumed to be of greatest importance, since it is this which is likely to "tear apart" structures and can lead to cavitation if the pulses are sufficiently long. Adverse effects can be shown if the peak negative pressure is greater than −4 MPa. The passage of these pressure waves through a medium induces mechanical stress which could, in theory, lead to disruption of cell membranes or intracellular structures, such as mitochondria or chromosomes. The likelihood of such damage occurring is increased if the instantaneous power, and rate of change of pressure, are increased due to shock wave formation. Such damage would be expected to lead to cell death, disordered biochemistry, or mutations in subsequent generations. Cell death and biochemical disturbance can be demonstrated only at power levels considerably higher than those used in diagnostic equipment, and no reproducible experiments demonstrating chromosomal damage have yet been published [38−40]. There have been a number of scares [41,42], notably the work published by MacIntosh and Davey in 1970 [43], but this work was later refuted by one of the original authors [44].

The role of the equipment operator

Ultrasound is a special investigation technique and, in common with other special radiologic techniques, requires particular experience and expertise from the operator. If the operator is not sufficiently skilled, an inadequate study may result in either a mistaken or missed diagnosis. The degree to which this occurs is extremely difficult to identify since any observer who was not present during an ultrasound examination is not in a position to criticize its quality. I have attempted on one occasion to assess operator adequacy in my own department.

A study was performed to evaluate the technical adequacy of measurements of the fetal abdominal circumference in late pregnancy. All scans were performed using a single manually operated static scanner and the images were recorded on large format video hard copy. At the end of the study period nearly 1000 images were analyzed retrospectively. The adequacy of each examination was assessed using a numerical score for four factors. These were: (i) the anatomic level at which the images had been obtained; (ii) evidence in the images of obliquity to the long axis of the fetus; (iii) evidence of movement of the fetus causing duplication of the outline; and (iv) the percentage of the outline of the fetal abdomen that was clearly definable in each image. Every image was scored by two assessors and neither was aware which operator had performed the examination. The total scores for each operator were then compiled and compared with the percentage of the departmental workload performed by that operator. The two operators who each performed more than 30% of the departmental workload achieved a satisfactory score in over 50% of their cases. Two other operators each performing less than 10% of the departmental workload achieved satisfactory scores in less than 10% of their cases. This study was able to confirm by numerical analysis the well-accepted observation that the technical competence of a person undertaking a special investigation is roughly proportional to the percentage of their time that they are able to devote to that technique.

A subsequent study on interobserver variability in the diagnosis of gallstones by ultrasound has shown similar findings [45]. In those departments where ultrasound examinations are performed by staff who are unable to devote more than about 20% of their time to this specialty, it is likely that the technical adequacy of many examinations is less than ideal.

Conclusion

The currently available evidence suggests that the hazards to a patient from ultrasound investigations are much more likely to be due to the inadequacies of the operator than the ultrasound energy dissipated within the patient. However, the development of transvaginal scanning, especially when combined with the Doppler technique, may be placing the developing ova and early conceptus at risk. Such scans should only be undertaken when there is a strong clinical indication and the as low as reasonably achievable (ALARA) principle should be applied to keep the power levels and exposure times as low as possible.

References

1 Dick MT, Cape CA. Complications of duplex carotid imaging. A case report. *Angiology* 1994;45(3):235−238.

2 Perlin SJ. Pulmonary embolism during compression US of the lower extremity. *Radiology* 1992;184(1):165−166.

3 Bhargava R, Lewandowski BJ. Water intoxication: a complication of pelvic US in a patient with syndrome of inappropriate antidiuretic hormone secretion. *Radiology* 1991;180(3):723−724.

4 Parker KJ, Tuthill TA, Lerner RM, Violante MR. A particulate contrast agent with potential for ultrasound imaging of liver. *Ultrasound Med Biol* 1987;13:555−566.

5 Mattrey RF, Stritch G, Shelton RE *et al.* Perfluorochemicals as ultrasound contrast agents for tumor imaging and hepatosplenography: preliminary clinical results. *Radiology* 1987;163:339−343.

6 Schneider M, Bussat P, Barrau MB *et al.* Polymeric microballoons as ultrasound contrast agents. Physical and ultrasonic properties compared with sonicated albumin. *Invest Radiol* 1992;27:134−139.

7 Ostensen J, Hede R, Myreng Y, Ege T, Holtz E. Intravenous injection of Albunex microspheres causes thromboxane mediated pulmonary hypertension in pigs, but not in monkeys or rabbits. *Acta Physiol Scand* 1992;144:307−315.

8 Walker R, Jeffrey BS, Wiencek BS *et al.* The influence of intravenous Albunex injections on pulmonary arterial pressure, gas exchange and left ventricular peak intensity. *J Am Soc Echocardiog* 1992;5:463−470.

9 Christiensen CW, Reeves WC, Holt GW. Intracoronary echocontrast agents: abnormalities in myocardial function in a normal and reduced coronary perfusion model in dogs. *Ultrasound Med Biol* 1988;14:199−211.

10 Walday P, Ostensen J, Holtz E. Human albumin base echocontrast agents-repeated use in animals may induce anaphylactic reactions. *Br J Radiol* 1994;67:112−113.

11 Christiansen C, Vebner AJ, Muan B *et al.* Lack of an immune response to Albunex, a new ultrasound contrast agent based on air-filled albumin microspheres. *Int Arch Allergy Immunol* 1994;104(4):372−378.

12 Wells PNT. Possibility of hazards in diagnosis. In: *Biomedical Ultrasonics*. London: Academic Press, 1977:466.

13 Duck FA, Starritt HC, Aindow JD, Perkins MA, Hawkins AJ. The output of pulse-echo ultrasound equipment: a survey of powers, pressures and intensities. *Br J Radiol* 1985;58:989−1001.

14 Evans DH, McDicken WN, Skidmore R, Woodcock JP. Safety considerations in Doppler ultrasound. In: Evans DH, *et al.* ed. *Doppler Ultrasound, Physics, Instrumentation and Clinical Applications.* Chichester: John Wiley & Sons, 1989:222.

15 Starritt HC, Duck FA. A comparison of ultrasound exposure in therapy and pulsed Doppler fields. *Br J Radiol* 1992;65:557−563.

16 Duck FA, Martin K. Trends in diagnostic ultrasound exposure. *Phys Med Biol* 1991;36:1423−1431.

17 Lele PP. Safety and potential hazards in the current applications of ultrasound in obstetrics and gynecology. *Ultrasound Med Biol* 1979;5:307−320.

18 Federal Drug Administration Report. *An Overview of Ultrasound Theory: Measurement, Medical Applications and Biological Effects.* New York: Bureau of Radiological Health, 1982.

19 World Health Organization. Ultrasound. In: Suess MJ, ed. *Nonionising Radiation Protection, WHO Regional Publications, European Series No 10.* Copenhagen: WHO, 1982.

20 Royal College of Obstetricians and Gynaecologists. *Report of the RCOG Working Party on Routine Ultrasound Examination in Pregnancy.* London: RCOG, 1984.

21 Hellman LM, Duffus GM, Donald I, Sunden B. Safety of diagnostic ultrasound in obstetrics. *Lancet* 1970;1:1133−1134.

22 Scheidt PD, Stanley F, Bryla DA. One year follow up of infants exposed to ultrasound *in utero*. *Am J Obstet Gynecol* 1978;131:743−748.

23 Wladimiroff JW, Larr J. Ultrasonic measurement of fetal body size: a randomized controlled trial. *Acta Obstet Gynaecol Scand* 1980;59:177−179.

24 Bennett MJ, Little D, Dewhurst J, Chamberlain G. Predictive value of ultrasound measurement in early pregnancy: a randomized controlled trial. *Br J Obstet Gynaecol* 1982;89:338−341.

25 Bakketeig LS, Eik-Nes SH, Jacobsen G *et al.* Randomized controlled trial of ultrasonographic screening in pregnancy. *Lancet* 1984;ii:207−210.

26 Eik-Nes SH, Okland O, Aure JC, Ulstein M. Ultrasound screening in pregnancy — randomized controlled trial. *Lancet* 1984;i:1347.

27 Stark CR, Orleans M, Haverkamp AD, Murphy J. Short and long term risks after exposure to diagnostic ultrasound *in-utero*. *Obstet Gynecol* 1984;63:194−200.

28 Salvesen KA, Vatten LJ, Eik-Nes SH, Hugdahl K, Bakketig LS. Routine ultrasonography *in utero* and subsequent handedness and neurological development. *Br Med J* 1993;307:159−164.

29 Newnham JP, Evans SF, Michael CA, Stanley FJ, Landau LI. Effects of frequent ultrasound during pregnancy: a randomised controlled trial. *Lancet* 1993;342:887−891.

30 Shoji R, Momma E, Shimizu T, Matsuda S. An experimental study of the effects of low intensity ultrasound on developing mouse embryos. *J Fac Sci Series 6* 1971;18:51−56.

31 Fry FJ, Erdmann WA, Johnson LK, Baird AI. Ultrasonic toxicity study. *Ultrasound Med Biol* 1978;3(4):351−366.

32 Stolzenberg SJ, Torbit CA, Edmonds PD, Taenzer JC. Effects of ultrasound on the mouse exposed at different stages of gestation: acute studies. *Radiat Environ Biophys* 1980;17:245−270.

33 Kimmel CA, Stratmeyer ME, Galloway WD, LaBorde JB, Brown N, Pinkavitch F. The embryotoxic effects of ultrasound exposure in pregnant ICR mice. *Teratology* 1983;27(2):245−251.

34 Hande MP, Devi PU. Effect of *in utero* exposure to diagnostic ultrasound on the postnatal survival and growth of mouse. *Teratology* 1993;48(5):405−411.

35 Carnes KI, Hess RA, Dunn F. Effects of *in utero* ultrasound exposure on the development of the fetal mouse testis. *Biol Reprod* 1991;45(3):432−439.

36 Tarantal AF, Canfield DR. Ultrasound-induced lung haemorrhage in the monkey. *Ultrasound Med Biol* 1994;20(1):65−72.

37 Duck FA, Starritt HC, ter Haar G, Lunt M. Surface heating of diagnostic ultrasound transducers. *Br J Radiol* 1989;62:1005−1013.

38 Warwick R, Pond JB, Woodward B, Connolly CC. Hazards of diagnostic ultrasonography — a study with mice. *IEEE Trans Sonics Ultrasonics* 1970;17(Suppl.):58−164.

39 Mannor SM, Serr DM, Tamari A, Meshorer A, Frei EN. The safety of ultrasound in fetal monitoring. *Am J Obstet Gynecol* 1972;113:653−661.

40 Akamatsu N. Ultrasound irradiation effects on preimplantation embryos. *Acta Obstet Gynecol (Japan)* 1981;33:369−378.

41 Kremkau FW, Witcofski RL. Mitotic reduction in rat liver exposed to ultrasound. *J Clin Ultrasound* 1974;2:123−126.

42 Liebeskind DE, Bases R, Mendez F, Elequin F, Koenigberg M. Sister chromatid exchanges in human lymphocytes after exposure to diagnostic ultrasound. *Science* 1979;205:1273−1275.

43 MacIntosh IJ, Davey DA. Chromosome aberrations induced by an ultrasonic fetal pulse detector. *Br Med J* 1970;4:92−93.

44 MacIntosh IJ, Brown RC, Coakley WT. Ultrasound and *"in-vitro"* chromosome aberrations. *Br J Radiol* 1975;48:230−232.

45 Allen-Mersh TG, Motson RW, Hately W. Does it matter who does ultrasound examination of the gall bladder? *Br Med J* 1985;291:389−390.

CHAPTER 10

Nuclear medicine

Colin R. Lazarus and Michael N. Maisey

The use of radioisotopes in medicine has proved to be a valuable and safe technique. The rapid progress of nuclear medicine has resulted, not only from developments in instrumentation and the wider use of computers, but also through the introduction of radioisotopes of short physical half-life attached to molecules of increasing complexity. The potential for complications occurring has increased in parallel with the developments in camera and computer technology, and the use of new radiopharmaceuticals. However, nuclear medicine has proved to be remarkably free of complications, but the potential user of the techniques should be aware of the possible complications that have arisen because these may affect the well-being of patients and the interpretation of images obtained from the patient study.

Adverse reactions to radiopharmaceuticals

The various interpretations of what constitutes an adverse reaction make the term difficult to define [1–3]. We will adopt the definition proposed by Cordova et al. [4], which comprises the important aspects of the various suggestions: "an unexpected reaction, or unusual and undesirable clinical manifestation to the vehicle, and not the radiation itself, of an administered radiopharmaceutical. The reaction does not result from an overdose, nor injury caused by poor injection technique."

The reactions themselves are of many kinds, but they can generally be grouped together as shown by the examples in Table 10.1.

The types of reactions usually reported are anaphylaxis, allergic, pyrogen, vasovagal, and a variety of miscellaneous

Table 10.1 Examples of reported clinical manifestations observed in adverse reactions to radiopharmaceuticals. (From Cordova et al. [4])

Clinical manifestation	Examples
Anaphylaxis/anaphylactoid (immediate reactions)	Nausea, vomiting Hypotension Incontinence Syncope Flushing Tachycardia
Allergic (delayed reactions)	Rash, urticaria, sometimes delayed Pruritus Flushing Dyspnea Nausea, vomiting Cyanosis Chest pain Sweating Palpitation Tachycardia
Pyrogen	Fever Headaches
Vasovagal	Faintness Blanching Sweating
Miscellaneous	Phlebitis Metallic taste Chills Cyanosis

reactions, such as phlebitis, metallic taste, and chills. The allergic reactions, such as rashes, urticaria, flushing, and dyspnea, were the most common, reported with the colloids and microspheres. Technetium-99m methylene diphosphonate ($^{99}Tc^m$-MDP) has been associated with rashes, often delayed by up to 4–24 hours after injection.

The reported incidence of adverse reactions to radiopharmaceuticals has remained low for many years. It is difficult to assess a true figure for incidence because the number of reports undoubtedly underestimates the true incidence. The majority of reactions are mild and transient, requiring little or no treatment. Serious reactions are occasionally reported such as cardiorespiratory arrest, tachycardia, dyspnea, and hypotension. On rare occasions fatalities have occurred. The various reporting systems acknowledge underreporting, particularly with mild reactions. It has been estimated [5] that the incidence probably lies between one and 20 reactions per 100 000 radiopharmaceutical administrations, which probably represents a reporting rate of less than 10% of all reactions.

Cordova *et al.* [4] have reviewed 277 adverse reactions reported to the USA Society of Nuclear Medicine (SNM) Adverse Reactions Registry, in an attempt to determine the probability that the reported clinical manifestations actually resulted from the administration of the radiopharmaceutical. Of the 277 reports, 17% were rated as definite, 40% as probable, 36% as possible, and 7% as unlikely. They have also characterized the reaction symptoms with each radiopharmaceutical. Keeling [6] has analyzed the adverse reactions in the UK from 1976 to mid-1992. In this period, there was a total of 330 reports of reactions to radiopharmaceuticals in the UK. Of these reports, 52 (16% of total reports) were reactions to the skeletal imaging agent $^{99}Tc^m$-MDP, and 44 reports (13%) to the renal imaging agent $^{99}Tc^m$-diethylenetriaminepentaacetic acid (DTPA). Earlier reports [4,7] showed that over the period 1978–1982, the radiopharmaceuticals accounting for most reactions were the colloids, 26% and 31% in the USA and UK, respectively. Preparations of human serum albumin such as $^{99}Tc^m$-macroaggregated albumin (MAA) and $^{99}Tc^m$-microspheres were the next highest group, with 13% in the UK series and 26% in that of the USA. The bone-imaging agents accounted for 27% of the earlier UK reports and 14.5% of the USA reactions. A summary of adverse reactions to radiopharmaceuticals in the UK from 1976 to mid-1992 is shown in Table 10.2. In this period, there were far fewer reports of reactions to colloids (10% compared to the earlier 31%), which probably reflects a decline in the usage of these materials. Reactions have also been reported to radiopharmaceuticals other than those labeled with $^{99}Tc^m$, e.g., iodine-131 (^{131}I) sodium iodide, gallium-67 (^{67}Ga) gallium citrate, indium-111 (^{111}In)-DTPA, and thallium-201 (^{201}Tl) thallous chloride. Table 10.3 shows examples of reported reactions to some radiopharmaceuticals.

The USA SNM has maintained a registry of adverse reactions since 1970. Similar reporting systems are also run in the UK and other European countries. These reports are collated and published annually in the *European Journal of Nuclear Medicine*. For the period 1980–1990, the European Association of Nuclear Medicine collated 349 reports of which 151 were allergic type reactions, 96 vasovagal, 15 local effects, and 77 other types. These reports are summarized in Table 10.4 for $^{99}Tc^m$-labeled radiopharmaceuticals, Table 10.5 for radioiodine radiopharmaceuticals, and Table 10.6 for a miscellaneous group. The reports came mainly from the UK (216 reports), Germany (35), Denmark (29), The Netherlands (34), and other European countries (46).

The SNM reported that there were 21 adverse reactions from an estimated 7 million radiopharmaceutical administrations in 1984, the last year for which results were published [8], emphasizing a consistent decline in reports over the previous 10 years. As with the European reports, the main reactions in 1984 were to $^{99}Tc^m$-MDP (seven reports) and $^{99}Tc^m$-DPTA (three reports). The other reported reactions were: $^{99}Tc^m$-human albumin microspheres (three reports); $^{99}Tc^m$-sulphur colloid (three reports); and one report each for $^{99}Tc^m$-dimercaptosuccinic acid (DMSA), $^{99}Tc^m$-glucoheptonate (GH), $^{99}Tc^m$-red blood cells, ^{131}I-sodium iodide, and nonradioactive pyrophosphate used for *in vivo* red blood cell labeling.

A more detailed account of adverse reactions to various radiopharmaceuticals is given in other reviews [6,9], where the pharmacologic mechanisms involved in reactions are discussed.

Where a reaction does occur, the patient's symptoms should be treated where necessary, and vital signs recorded.

Table 10.2 Some reported adverse reactions to radiopharmaceuticals in the UK from 1976 to mid-1992. (From Keeling [6])

Radiopharmaceutical	Number of reports	Percentage of total
$^{99}Tc^m$-MDP	52	16
$^{99}Tc^m$-Hydroxymethylene diphosphonate (HMDP)	16	5
$^{99}Tc^m$-MAA	23	7
$^{99}Tc^m$-Antimony colloid	16	5
$^{99}Tc^m$-Sulphur colloid	17	5
$^{99}Tc^m$-DTPA	44	13

Table 10.3 Some reported reactions to commonly used radiopharmaceuticals

Radiopharmaceutical	Reported reactions
$^{99}Tc^m$-Sulphur colloid	Nausea and vomiting, decreased blood pressure, incontinence, rash and urticaria, pruritus, dyspnea, cyanosis, dizziness, palpitations, pyrogen reactions
$^{99}Tc^m$-Tin colloid	Flushing, rash, dyspnea, nausea and vomiting, chest pain
$^{99}Tc^m$-Human albumin preparations	Flushing, nausea and vomiting, dyspnea, wheezing, rash, itching, cyanosis, chest pain, chills, sweating, tachycardia
$^{99}Tc^m$-MDP	Rash and itching (often late onset), flushing, headache, dyspnea, dizziness, nausea
$^{99}Tc^m$-Dimercaptosuccinic acid (DMSA)	Epigastric pain, flushing, nausea
$^{99}Tc^m$-DTPA	Dizziness, decreased blood pressure, blurred vision, weakness, low back pain
$^{99}Tc^m$-Gluceptate (GHA)	Nausea, dizziness, flushing, tachycardia
$^{99}Tc^m$-Mercaptoacetyl triglycine (MAG-3)	Rash, nausea, vomiting, faintness, sweating
$^{99}Tc^m$-Isonitriles	Vasovagal, metallic taste
$^{99}Tc^m$-Exametazime	Urticarial rash, vasovagal
$^{99}Tc^m$-Pertechnetate	Allergic, vasovagal, and others
^{123}I-Sodium iodide	Allergic, vasovagal, and others
^{123}I-Metaiodobenzylguanidine (MIBG)	Allergic, vasovagal, and others
^{131}I-Sodium iodide	Itching, urticaria, rash, swelling, nausea and vomiting, headache, hot and cold flushes
^{131}I-Orthoiodohippurate	Urticaria, decrease in blood pressure
^{131}I-MIBG	Allergic, vasovagal, and others
^{131}I-Norcholesterol	Allergic
^{67}Ga-Gallium citrate	Pruritus, skin rash, nausea, and vomiting
^{111}In-DTPA	Pyrogen reactions, aseptic meningitis
^{201}Tl-Thallous chloride	Pruritus, erythematous rash, flushing
^{51}Cr-Ethylenediaminetetraacetic acid (EDTA)	Allergic, local, and others
^{111}In-Oxine	Allergic, vasovagal, and local

Cr, chromium.

The suspect radiopharmaceutical should be removed from further use and an attempt made to establish the probability that the reaction is due to the radiopharmaceutical. Further steps should be taken depending on the progress of the reaction in the patient. The reaction should also be reported through the national reporting schemes.

Alterations in radiopharmaceutical biodistributions

The alteration of the biodistribution of a radiopharmaceutical by a pharmacologic or physiologic intervention, to provide further diagnostic information, is an integral part of many nuclear medicine procedures. For example, during a $^{99}Tc^m$-DTPA kidney study, the use of a diuretic, such as furosemide, can be used to differentiate between a physical and functional obstruction. The heart can be stressed by exercise and other physiologic methods, or by coronary dilatation using dipyridamole or adenosine. Dipyridamole may cause cardiovascular collapse [10] (see also pp. 41 & 78). During a

nuclear medicine procedure it is sometimes necessary to protect a critical organ from radiation, by either blocking the uptake of the radiopharmaceutical into that organ, or by increasing the rate of metabolism or excretion through the organ. Thus, the thyroid gland can be protected from radio-iodine, produced during the breakdown of administered radioiodinated material, by blocking the uptake with perchlorate. Laxatives can be used to promote the passage of ^{67}Ga through the intestines.

Many patients who present to the nuclear medicine department are on drugs that can alter the biodistribution of the administered radiopharmaceutical. The clinician should be aware of such unexpected alterations when making a diagnosis from an image; otherwise, it is possible to be misled into providing an inaccurate report. The administration of a second radiopharmaceutical can also lead to unusual biodistributions and erroneous interpretations.

Many of these drug-induced changes are now recognized and documented [9,11]. Alterations caused by procedures and agents other than drugs have also been reviewed [11].

Table 10.4 Summary of reports of adverse reactions to ^{99}Tc^m-labeled radiopharmaceuticals received by the European Association of Nuclear Medicine (1980–1990)

Radiopharmaceutical	Number of reports	Types of reaction	Number of patients requiring treatment
^{99}Tc^m-Albumin colloid	18	a,b,c	3
^{99}Tc^m-Antimony sulfide colloid	7	a,c	1
^{99}Tc^m-Tin colloid	7	a,c,d	2
^{99}Tc^m-Millimicrospheres	2	b	1
^{99}Tc^m-DTPA	51	a,b,d	7
^{99}Tc^m-Dimercaptosuccinic acid (DMSA)	2	a,d	2
^{99}Tc^m-Glucoheptonate (GH)	2	b	1
^{99}Tc^m-Mercaptoacetyltriglycine (MAG-3)	8	a,b	1
^{99}Tc^m-Sulfur colloid	6	a,b	2
^{99}Tc^m-Rhenium sulfide colloid	1	a	1
^{99}Tc^m-Methylenediphosphonate (MDP)	61	a,b,c,d	12
^{99}Tc^m-Hydroxymethylene diphosphonate (HMDP)	18	a,c,d	3
^{99}Tc^m-Pyrophosphate (PYP)	3	a,b,d	1
^{99}Tc^m-Exametazime	2	a,b	3
^{99}Tc^m-Isonitrile	4	b,d	—
^{99}Tc^m-MAA	21	a,b,c,d	7
^{99}Tc^m-Microspheres	6	a,b	3
^{99}Tc^m-Pertechnetate	5	a,b,d	—
^{99}Tc^m-Phytate	2	d	—
^{99}Tc^m-Plasmin	1	a	1
^{99}Tc^m-Red blood cells	11	a,b,d	1
^{99}Tc^m-Immunoglobulin	1	a	1
^{99}Tc^m-Diethyliodoaminodiacetic acid	1	a	1
^{99}Tc^m-Monoclonal antibodies	1	a	1

a, allergic; b, vasovagal; c, local effects; d, other effects.

Table 10.5 Summary of reports of adverse reactions to radioiodine-labeled radiopharmaceuticals received by the European Association of Nuclear Medicine (1980–1990)

Radiopharmaceutical	Number of reports	Types of reaction	Number of patients requiring treatment
^{123}I-Sodium iodide	4	a,b,d	1
^{123}I-Hippuran	4	a,b,c	2
^{123}I-Metaiodobenzylguanidine (MIBG)	17	a,b,d	1
^{123}I-Fatty acid	1	a	—
^{123}I-Isopropylamphetamine	1	d	—
^{125}I-Human serum albumin	2	d	—
^{131}I-Sodium iodide	6	a,d	2
^{131}I-Hippuran	6	a,b,d	2
^{131}I-MIBG	6	a,b,d	1
^{131}I-Norcholesterol	11	a	11
^{131}I-Monoclonal antibody	2	a	
^{131}I-Human serum albumin	3	b,d	1

a, allergic; b, vasovagal; c, local effects; d, other effects.

Contrast agents used in radiography can cause an alteration in biodistribution. Iodinated contrast agents can alter the uptake of radioiodine by the thyroid gland. This effect may last for weeks or months, and even years with contrast agents that are retained in the body. Radioopaque barium sulfate will absorb photons emitted from radionuclides giving the appearance of "cold" areas on an image. Some chemotherapeutic agents have been shown to have toxic effects resulting in abnormal localization of radiopharmaceuticals. Alterations in accumulation of ^{67}Ga in soft tissue

Table 10.6 Summary of reports of adverse reactions to miscellaneous radiopharmaceuticals received by the European Association of Nuclear Medicine (1980–1990)

Radiopharmaceutical	Number of reports	Types of reaction	Number of patients requiring treatment
[51]Cr-Ethylenediaminetetraacetic acid (EDTA)	4	a,c,d	—
[67]Ga-Gallium citrate	7	a,c,d	2
[75]Se-Selenocholesterol	4	a,c,d	4
[90]Y-Yttrium silicate	1	a	—
[111]In-Indium colloid	1	d	1
[111]In-Indium oxine	3	a,b,c	—
^{111}In-DTPA	1	d	—
[111]In-Monoclonal antibody	2	a,d	—
[111]In-Platelets	1	a	—
[113]In[m]-Indium chloride	1	b	—
[169]Yb-DTPA	3	d	3
[198]Au-Gold colloid	3	a	2
[201]Tl-Thallous chloride	6	a,c,d	4

a, allergic; b, vasovagal; c, local effects; d, other effect.
Au, gold; Cr, chromium; Se, selenium; Y, yttrium; Yb, ytterbium.

have been reported in some patients immediately after therapeutic irradiation [12]. The decreased detectability of some lesions with radioactive gallium has also been observed following irradiation [13]. Some bone-seeking ^{99}Tc^m-phosphate localization in soft tissue of the myocardium and breast has been reported following irradiation of the chest [14].

Care should be exercised in the interpretation of postoperative patients. Localization of radiopharmaceuticals has been observed in surgical scars [15,16], intramuscular injection sites [17], skin-pressure lesions, and broken ribs resulting from physiotherapy mimicking metastatic deposits.

Many drugs have been reported to cause an alteration in the distribution of radiopharmaceuticals. An excess breakthrough of aluminum ion in ^{99}Tc^m-generator eluates can cause flocculation of colloids resulting in the larger particles being trapped in the lungs [18].

Other causes of altered biodistributions of radiopharmaceuticals that have been reported include the effect of hemodialysis on a ^{67}Ga scan [17]. Problems associated with administration of a radioactive material can affect its biodistribution. Examples reported include the following.
1 Accidental intraarterial injection of ^{99}Tc^m-pyrophosphate [17].
2 The release of free ^{99}Tc^m from some ^{99}Tc^m-radiopharmaceuticals by iodinated antiseptic skin swabs.
3 The incorrect administration of radiocolloids can cause clumping of the particles and trapping in the lungs, e.g., clotting by mixing with blood in the syringe. This phenomenon has also been observed with ^{99}Tc^m-labeled lung imaging agents, such as microspheres and macroaggregates of human serum albumin.

4 Extravasation of a ^{99}Tc^m-bone agent has been noted at the site of injection together with uptake in an axillary lymph node [19].

It has been estimated that the rate of misadministrations of radiopharmaceuticals in the USA over a 10 year period, amounted to only one per 100 000 procedures performed, according to figures in the 1990 *Annual Report of the Nuclear Regulatory Commission* (NRC). This body defines a "misadministration" as any of the following events:
1 a radiopharmaceutical or radiation given to the wrong patient, or by a route of administration not intended by the prescribing physician, or from a sealed source other than the one intended;
2 a diagnostic dosage of a radiopharmaceutical more than 50% different from the prescribed dosage;
3 a therapeutic dosage of a radiopharmaceutical varying by more than 10% from the prescribed dosage, or different from the final prescribed total treatment dose from a sealed source by more than 10% [20].

Alterations of radiolabeling

Radiolabeling of red blood cells with ^{99}Tc^m is a common procedure in nuclear medicine. Many drugs have been reported to decrease the efficiency of radiolabeling, including antihypertensives [21] and drugs acting on the heart [22]. A similar effect has been observed when iodinated contrast-media administered to patients in the previous 24 hours were blamed for poor radiolabeling of their red blood cells. Interactions between radiopharmaceuticals causing unusual findings have also been noted. The use of *in vivo* red blood cell labeling was developed after it was observed that the stannous ions present in a $^{99}Tc^m$-bone-imaging radio-pharmaceutical caused a reduction of the $^{99}Tc^m$-pertechnetate ion, subsequently administered for a brain scan, resulting in the *in vivo* labeling of the patient's red blood cells [23].

It is apparent from the few examples described above that there are many potential traps, and images should be read bearing in mind the patient's drugs and other treatment as part of their history.

Drug-induced changes

Several authors [12,24–26] have reviewed drug-induced changes in the biodistribution of radiopharmaceuticals, and classified them in various ways. Some chemotherapeutic agents and antibiotics which have been reported to affect the biodistribution of radiopharmaceuticals are listed in Table 10.7 and Table 10.8, respectively. There is a large group of commonly prescribed drugs which have been implicated in the unusual handling in the body of radiopharmaceuticals (Table 10.9). Many drugs and chemicals have been reported to interfere with the uptake of ^{131}I-iodide into the thyroid gland [9], including iodine in Lugol's iodine, antitussives, iodine ointment, antithyroid drugs, perchlorate, sulfonamides, steroids, phenylbutazone, meprobamate, antihistamines, and some contrast-media. The alterations listed in Tables 10.7–10.9 can arise in a variety of ways. The distribution of the radiopharmaceutical can be altered as a result of the pharmacologic effects of the interfering drug or an *in vivo* physicochemical interaction between the radiopharmaceutical and patient medication. Some drugs will induce disease in body organs and systems, which can affect the transport of radiopharmaceuticals into that organ or system.

Table 10.8 Antibiotics reported to alter the biodistribution of radiopharmaceuticals

Antibiotic	Effect
Erythromycin	Increased uptake in the liver of $^{99}Tc^m$-diisopropyliminodiacetic acid (DISIDA) in hepatobiliary study
Gentamicin	Decreased glomerular filtration rate (GFR) with ^{51}Cr-ethylenediaminetetraacetic acid (EDTA)
Neomycin	Abnormal results for malabsorption of vitamin B_{12} ($^{57}Co/^{58}Co$) in Schilling test
Penicillin	Excretion of $^{99}Tc^m$-gluceptate (GHA) through biliary tract in renal study. Decrease in GFR with ^{51}Cr-EDTA
Sulfonamides	Abnormal uptake of ^{131}I-sodium iodide in thyroid gland
Sulfamethoxazole	Excretion of $^{99}Tc^m$-GHA through biliary tract in renal study

Cr, chromium; Co, cobalt.

Excretion of radioactivity in breast milk

A potential hazard with nursing mothers is the secretion into milk, and the subsequent ingestion by her infant, of radioactivity administered to the mother for a diagnostic or therapeutic purpose. There are few reports in the literature where this has actually occurred [27,28], but there are many reports that describe the measurement of levels of radioactivity in breast milk that has not been fed to the infant. A knowledge of the secretion of radioactivity into the milk is

Table 10.7 Some chemotherapeutic agents reported to affect the biodistribution of radiopharmaceuticals

Agent	Effect
Adriamycin	Uptake of $^{99}Tc^m$-pyrophosphate into damaged myocardium
Bleomycin	Uptake of ^{67}Ga into pulmonary lesions
Methotrexate	Increased uptake of $^{99}Tc^m$-pertechnetate in cerebral ventricles. Filling defects in liver with $^{99}Tc^m$-sulfur colloid due to hepatotoxicity
Cyclophosphamide	Abnormal uptake in blood pool, kidneys, and skeleton
Cyclophosphamide and doxorubicin	Intense renal uptake of $^{99}Tc^m$-pyrophosphate
Cisplatin	Abnormal uptake in kidneys of $^{99}Tc^m$-DMSA. Abnormal uptake in blood pool, kidney, and skeleton of ^{67}Ga-gallium citrate
Vincristine	Abnormal uptake. Increased blood pool and renal activity of ^{67}Ga-gallium citrate in tumor (abscess imaging)

Table 10.9 Examples of drugs implicated in altered radiopharmaceutical biodistribution

Drug	Effect	Drug	Effect
Aluminum hydroxide	Lung uptake of $^{99}Tc^m$-sulfur colloid. Altered biodistribution of $^{99}Tc^m$-EHDP. Liver and spleen uptake of $^{99}Tc^m$-pyrophosphate in myocardial imaging	Hydralazine	Poor labeling efficiency of red blood cells with $^{99}Tc^m$:-free pertechnetate
Analgesics (e.g., methadone, pethidine, morphine)	Delay in gastric emptying with $^{99}Tc^m$-pertechnetate	Iron salts	Abnormal uptake, accumulation of tracer at injection site of $^{99}Tc^m$-MDP/EHDP for bone imaging
Atropine	Delay in gastric emptying with $^{99}Tc^m$-pertechnetate in abdominal imaging	Metaclopramide	Increased uptake of ^{67}Ga-gallium citrate into breast
Chlorpromazine	Abnormal uptake of ^{67}Ga-gallium citrate in breast tumor imaging	Methyldopa	Increased uptake of ^{67}Ga-gallium citrate into breast. Poor labeling efficiency of red blood cells with $^{99}Tc^m$:-free pertechnetate
Contraceptives	Increased uptake into adrenals of ^{131}I-methylnorcholesterol in adrenal imaging. Filling defect due to medication-induced tumor in hepatic imaging with $^{99}Tc^m$-sulfur colloid	Nifedipine	Poor labeling efficiency of red blood cells with $^{99}Tc^m$:-free pertechnetate. Increased uptake of ^{131}I-metaiodobenzyl-guanidine (MIBG) into pheochromocytoma. Reduced skeletal uptake of $^{99}Tc^m$-MDP on bone imaging
Cortisone	Decrease in uptake of $^{99}Tc^m$-MDP in bone trauma. Reduced uptake of ^{111}In into white cells for abscess imaging	Nitrofurantoin	Abnormal or absence of $^{99}Tc^m$-HIDA in gall bladder in hepatobiliary image
Digoxin	Poor labeling of red blood cells with $^{99}Tc^m$:-free pertechnetate	Phenobarbitone	Enhanced biliary excretion of $^{99}Tc^m$-HIDA in hepatobiliary imaging
Fluphenazine	Increased uptake of ^{67}Ga-gallium citrate into breast in tumor imaging	Prazosin	Poor labeling efficiency of red blood cells with $^{99}Tc^m$:-free pertechnetate
Furosemide	Reduced uptake of ^{67}Ga-gallium citrate in tumor. Enhanced renal function with $^{99}Tc^m$-DTPA/DMSA in renal study giving misleading diagnosis	Paracetamol	Filling defects in liver due to hepatotoxicity in $^{99}Tc^m$-HIDA hepatic imaging
Haloperidol	Increased uptake of ^{67}Ga-gallium citrate into breast	Sodium bicarbonate	Decreased kidney uptake of $^{99}Tc^m$-DMSA in renal image
		Stilbestrol	Increased uptake of ^{67}Ga-gallium citrate into breast

important when considering the necessity of performing a radioisotope study on a nursing mother, or, if the necessity is established, advising the mother on how long she should stop breastfeeding her infant and use supplemental feeding. Difficulties are often met in making such a decision because the available data for guidance are often inaccurate. There are several factors that complicate the assessment of the levels of radioactivity secreted in breast milk, and the potential hazards to a suckling infant. The dose of the radionuclide and its effective half-life in the mother will determine the quantity of radioactivity secreted into the milk. This will be influenced further by the chemical form in which the radio-

activity is administered to the mother, the route of administration, and the metabolic fate of the radiopharmaceutical. The chemical form in which the radiopharmaceutical appears in the breast milk will influence its biodistribution in the infant, and the radiation dose to the infant will then depend on the frequency of breastfeeding and the volume of milk ingested at each feed.

There are many reports in the literature describing cases where radiopharmaceuticals have been administered to nursing mothers, and attempts have been made to assess the risk to the infant and make a recommendation. Much of the data in these reports have been presented in different ways, making it difficult to assess risks and recommendations from one report to another. However, recently, several publications have attempted to collate the literature reviews, assess the risks, and make recommendations on a more scientific basis. Lazarus and Edwards [29] have determined the concentrations of radioactivity in milk samples at the times at which maximum concentration is estimated to occur, and at a later time when the authors recommend that breastfeeding can recommence. They have assumed the chemical form of the radionuclide present in the milk to be the same as that administered to the mother, unless a different chemical form has been specified in the report. Romney *et al.* [30] have determined a formula to establish objective guidelines for the administration of radionuclides to nursing mothers. Mountford and Coakley [31] have attempted to calculate the fraction of the administered dose that is present in maternal milk feeds, and the total fractional radioactivity the infant would ingest in 1 day.

In the various reviews and guidelines that have been published, the authors have calculated the absorbed radiation doses to the infant critical organs and effective dose equivalents (EDEs). They have also estimated the radioactivity in maternal milk at which breastfeeding is considered safe to recommence. Lazarus and Edwards [29], in an attempt to provide a common basis for comparing the different radiopharmaceuticals, have calculated a risk factor based on the EDE to the infant per megabecquerel of radioactivity administered to the mother, assuming the resumption of breastfeeding at some stated time after the radioactivity was administered to the mother. The authors have also estimated the time delay to reduce the risk by a factor of 10. Romney *et al.* [30] have estimated maximum delays required before nursing can resume. Mountford and Coakley [31] have assigned radiopharmaceuticals to one of four categories:

1 interruption of feeding not essential;

2 interruption for a fixed period of time;

3 interruption until measurements indicate that breastfeeding can recommence;

4 complete cessation of breastfeeding.

In addition, they estimated the time delay after breastfeeding required to reduce the effective dose equivalent to the infant to below 1 mSv.

Some examples of the secretion of radioactivity into breast milk reported in the literature are given in Table 10.10. Mountford and Coakley [31] have calculated the EDE to a 4 kg infant per unit activity ingested for a range of radionuclides. While the EDE for ^{99}Tc^m-radiopharmaceuticals is low (0.28 mSv/MBq) and chromium-51 (^{51}Cr) (0.6 mSv/MBq), it is high for ^{131}I and ^{125}I (245 and 175 mSv/MBq, respectively). Other commonly used radionuclides have intermediate EDE values, e.g., ^{123}I, 2.3 mSv/MBq; ^{67}Ga, 3.4 mSv/MBq; and ^{111}In, 5.7 mSv/MBq. Their recommendations for interrupting breastfeeding are based on the period after administration of the radioactivity to the mother

required to reduce the EDE to the infant to below 1 mSv. For most commonly used ^{99}Tc^m-radiopharmaceuticals it is not necessary to interrupt feeding when the EDE to the infant is already below 1 mSv. However, with ^{99}Tc^m-pertechnetate and ^{99}Tc^m-red blood cells, they recommend an interruption in feeding until the EDE to the infant drops below 1 mSv, the level being determined by measurement of the radioactivity in the milk. An interruption of just 6 hours is necessary before breastfeeding can recommence after a maternal dose of ^{99}Tc^m-MAA. It is recommended that feeding should be stopped altogether after administration of some radiopharmaceuticals to the mother, where it takes several days for the infant's EDE to fall below 1 mSv, e.g., ^{67}Ga-gallium citrate, ^{131}I-iodide, and selenium-75 (^{75}Se)-selenomethionine.

The Administration of Radioactive Substances Advisory Committee (ARSAC) also gives guidance on diagnostic administrations to breastfeeding mothers [85]. Before administering a radiopharmaceutical to the mother, they suggest that consideration should be given: (i) as to whether the study could be delayed until after the mother has finished breastfeeding; and (ii) whether a more appropriate radiopharmaceutical could be used, e.g., the use of ^{99}Tc^m-DTPA or ^{99}Tc^m-glucoheptonate (GH) instead of ^{99}Tc^m-pertechnetate for brain imaging, and the use of ^{111}In-leukocytes instead of ^{67}Ga-gallium citrate for localization of infection. The recommendations on interruption of breastfeeding are similar to those of Mountford and Coakley [31], including the precaution to ensure that the radiation dose absorbed by the infant is below 1 mSv.

Radiopharmaceutical quality

Major requirements of a radiopharmaceutical needed to produce a successful patient study are that the radiopharmaceutical should be safe to administer to the patient, and it should be of a quality that is suitable for the performance of the test required. Consideration of safety includes the sterility and apyrogenicity of the injected material. Radiopharmaceuticals obtained from reputable commercial sources will have been tested before release to the user for sterility and freedom from pyrogens, and they can be used with confidence. It is advisable to use products that have been licensed for use by the appropriate national authorities. Fortunately, complications due to the presence of bacteria and pyrogens are now very rare with commercially supplied products. However, great care should be exercised in the preparation and use of radiopharmaceuticals manufactured or dispensed to "in-house" formulations. Complications arising from hazards associated with the radiations from the radiopharmaceutical will be dealt with later.

For a radiopharmaceutical to fulfil its function efficiently, it must localize in the organ to be imaged and not in other organs which may interfere with imaging or cause other

Table 10.10 Some examples of the secretion of radioactivity in breast milk

Radioisotope	Pharmaceutical	Reference
$^{99}Tc^m$	Pertechnetate	[27, 32–41]
	MAA	[41–48]
	Polyphosphate	[49]
	DTPA	[41, 46, 50]
	Ethylenediaminetetraacetic acid (EDTA)	[51]
	Macroaggregated ferrous hydroxide	[51]
	Glucoheptonate (GHA)	[40]
	Red blood cells (RBC)	[41, 47]
	Hexakismethoxyisobutylisonitrile (MIBI)	[52]
	Mercaptoacetyltriglycine (MAG-3)	[53]
	MDP	[41]
^{123}I	Iodide	[39, 54–58]
	Hippuran	[47, 59]
^{125}I	Fibrinogen	[60–62]
	Human serum albumin	[63]
	Hippuran	[41]
^{131}I	Iodide	[64–69]
	MAA	[51, 70]
	Hippuric acid	[41, 70–72]
	Insulin	[71]
	Human serum albumin	[70]
^{67}Ga	Gallium citrate	[28, 38, 73–76]
^{32}P	Sodium phosphate	[77]
	Chromic phosphate	[78, 79]
^{111}In	Leukocytes	[80–82]
$^{113}In^m$	Chelate complex	[83]
	Indium chloride	[38]
^{75}Se	Selenomethionine	[84]
^{51}Cr	EDTA	[41]

Cr, chromium; P, phosphorus; Se, selenium.

problems. Thus, localization in the liver of a portion of a kidney-imaging agent dose will interfere with a renal study because of the relative anatomic positions of the two organs. Another example can occur when the particles of a lung-imaging agent are too small and will pass through the lung capillary bed and localize in the liver and spleen: conversely, if the colloidal particles of a liver-imaging agent are too large they may be filtered from the bloodstream by the lung capillary bed.

There are several implications resulting from the use of poor quality radiopharmaceuticals. Radioactivity that is not bound to the pharmaceutical, or that has become unbound, will deliver an unnecessary radiation dose to the organ in which it inadvertently localizes. Unbound, or "free", technetium will be trapped in the thyroid, salivary glands, and the choroid plexus, and will also be secreted by the gastric mucosa into the lumen of the stomach. Similarly, radioiodine that is not bound to the pharmaceutical molecule will localize

in the thyroid and stomach, giving an appreciable radiation dose to these organs. It is advisable, therefore, to block the thyroid with nonradioactive iodine or perchlorate when radioiodine preparations are used. Even with such preparations of known high levels of radiolabeling, blocking should be performed because of the release of free radioiodine due to normal metabolism of the radioiodinated pharmaceutical.

Quality testing of radiopharmaceuticals

Certain tests for radiopharmaceutical quality are well within the scope of the department supplying radiopharmaceuticals, and some are so simple that they should be applied routinely to provide the assurance that they are satisfactory to administer. More than 85% of radiopharmaceuticals used today are labeled with $^{99}Tc^m$ which, due to its short physical half-life of 6 hours, is usually obtained from a commercially available generator sited within the user's facility. These generators, although tested by manufacturers before delivery, can be a source of problems, but these are rare with modern generators. On elution of a generator, it is advisable to perform a *molybdenum (Mo) breakthrough* assay to check for the presence of ^{99}Mo, the parent radionuclide from which ^{99}Tc^m is produced. The high-energy β-particles and γ-rays from ^{99}Mo, which has a physical half-life of 67 hours, can deliver an unacceptably high radiation dose to a patient if an eluate containing more than the pharmacopeial limit of 0.037 MBq of ^{99}Mo per 37 MBq of eluted radioactivity is used to prepare radiopharmaceuticals. Modern isotope calibrators, used for measuring radioactivity, can be supplied with a molybdenum breakthrough kit enabling the level of ^{99}Mo in the eluate to be assayed rapidly before use. Soluble aluminum ions, which can be produced under certain conditions within the chromatographic column of the generator, are another possible contaminant of the eluate. High levels of these ions can cause flocculation of colloidal particles which, if the problem is sufficiently bad, will localize in the lungs. The level of aluminum ion can be determined in several ways, but commercially available kits provide a rapid method of determining whether the eluate passes or fails the test.

A potentially more hazardous and difficult problem to cope with, is the presence of the radioisotope in chemical forms other than that intended. These radiopharmaceutical impurities will localize undesirably in other body organs. If this is sufficiently bad, an image obtained using such a preparation may be diagnostically unacceptable. A repetition of the study may be necessary, which entails a second dose of radioactivity. It will be necessary to wait a period of time, depending on the physical half-life of the radionuclide, before the second dose can be administered to allow the radioactivity from the first dose to decay to a sufficiently low level that will not interfere with subsequent imaging. This means a delay in diagnosis as well as an increase in the costs associated with the test. Incorrect data may be obtained from such a study leading to a missed diagnosis or false interpretation of the images obtained. For example, the presence of free ^{99}Tc^{m}O$_4$ in a preparation of the bone-imaging agent ^{99}Tc^m-MDP will be observed in the salivary and thyroid glands, and in the stomach. Insoluble forms of ^{99}Tc^m will localize in the liver and spleen. Rapid chromatographic tests are available for the examination of these preparations [86–91].

Some radiopharmaceuticals rely on, among other factors, the size of their radioactive particles for correct localization in the organ of interest, e.g., in the lungs and liver. Alterations in particle size can have a profound effect on the biodistribution of the radiopharmaceutical. It follows that careful attention must be paid in the formulation and preparation of the radiopharmaceuticals to ensure that the particle size distribution is correct. The relative distributions of radioactive colloidal particles in the liver, spleen, and bone marrow can be of diagnostic value in interpreting an image. If this distribution should vary as a result of incorrect particle size, rather than as a result of patient pathology or physiology, incorrect interpretation of the image may result. Variations in particle size of those diagnostic agents used for lymphoscintigraphy can have an effect on the flow of these particles through the lymphatic system. In addition to the previously mentioned potential problem of small particles for lung imaging passing through the lungs to the liver and the rest of the body, "clumping" of particles is also a potential problem. If several particles, each within the size range of 10–80 μm, stick together, then the effective size of the particle is drastically increased. This will result in localization of this particle, not in the lung capillary arterioles as required, but in the larger blood vessels of the lungs. If the problem is sufficiently bad, large "hot" spots can be seen in the lungs, and even outside the lungs in very severe cases. This problem can occur with some commercial lung preparations when the particles are mixed with blood in the syringe prior to injection. Care should be exercised in ensuring that this does not occur in the agent used by altering the injection technique if necessary. Particle size can be readily checked using a light microscope before administration of the preparation to the patient.

As with all preparations that are intended to be administered to patients by the parenteral route, they must be sterile and free from pyrogens. Sterilization of radiopharmaceuticals by virtue of their radiation does not occur. Consideration must be given to facilities, equipment, and techniques to ensure that the final preparation is sterile and free of pyrogens. One problem with radiopharmaceuticals is that, because of their short shelf-lives due to the short physical half-life of the radionuclides, the results of sterility tests and pyrogen tests cannot be obtained before the radiopharmaceutical is required for use. It is essential, therefore, that the facilities and techniques employed in preparative work ensure the maintenance of sterility and freedom from pyrogens in the final preparation. Some simple tests, and suggested frequency of testing, for ^{99}Tc^m-radiopharmaceuticals are shown in Table 10.11.

Guidance on facilities and techniques can be obtained from many sources. It is important, however, that the current rules and regulations in the user's own country are consulted. Lazarus [92,93] provides advice on facilities, preparation, handling, and control of radiopharmaceuticals.

Other problems in the use of radiopharmaceuticals can occur. The adsorption of ^{99}Tc^m-dimercaptosuccinic acid [94] and ^{99}Tc^m-colloids [95,96] onto the glass of injection vials has been reported. The adsorption of ^{99}Tc^m-MAA from one manufacturer was so high as to render the radiopharmaceutical useless [97]. Checks of compatibility between the vial, the vial closure, and the radiopharmaceutical are essential, especially when subdividing doses from the

Table 10.11 Some tests of quality of $^{99}Tc^m$-radiopharmaceuticals, their purpose, and suggested frequency of testing

Analytic test	Purpose of test	Suggested frequency
Radioactive concentration	To ensure correct dose of radioactivity	Every radiopharmaceutical prepared
Appearance	To ensure clarity and correct colour	Every radiopharmaceutical prepared
Freedom from particulate contamination	To ensure no foreign particles present, e.g., fragments of glass, fibers	Every radiopharmaceutical prepared
Radionuclide identity and purity, e.g., ^{99}Mo-breakthrough in eluate from $^{99}Tc^m$ generator	To ensure radioactivity is in the correct radionuclide form, thus reducing radiation burden to patient	First and last elution of radionuclide generator
Radiochemical purity	To ensure radioactivity is in the correct chemical form ensuring optimum dose of radioactivity in the target organ, and minimum amount of activity in nontarget organs, and as background	Beginning and towards the end of each batch of purchased kits. On all radiopharmaceuticals prepared using nonlicensed kits, or to "in-house" formulae
Particle size of colloids and aggregates	To ensure radioactivity is delivered to correct target organs, e.g., liver, lungs	Beginning and towards the end of every batch of kits purchased
Aluminum ion breakthrough	To ensure levels of aluminum ion in the eluate are not high enough to interfere with the formation of radiocolloids	On the first elution of each generator
pH	To ensure pH is in the correct range of pH 4.5−7.0	On the first elution of each generator
Sterility testing	To ensure sterile products	The remnants of the first vial of eluate from a generator, the final unmanipulated eluate, and the residues of at least three kits should be tested each week

manufacturer's vial into other vials for distribution to other nuclear medicine centers. It is sometimes necessary to dilute a radiopharmaceutical to obtain the desired radioactive concentration for a particular patient study. Breakdown of some radiopharmaceuticals can occur when they are diluted. Of six commercially available brands of $^{99}Tc^m$-DTPA, only two were stable on dilution and levels of free pertechnetate as high as 95% were measured [98]. The extraction of impurities from rubber syringe plungers by saline or water has been shown to occur, and localization of the resulting radiolabeled impurities in the kidney and hepatobiliary system has been demonstrated [99]. The implications of using a radiopharmaceutical of poor quality are shown in Table 10.12.

The use of commercially available "cold" kits for the preparation of $^{99}Tc^m$-labeled radiopharmaceuticals should

always be advocated. However, users should not assume that such preparations will always be perfect because problems can occur, and a policy of regular testing should be adopted. Where radiopharmaceuticals are prepared to in-house formulations, it is imperative that adequate "in

Table 10.12 Implications of the use of poor-quality radiopharmaceuticals

1 Unnecessary radiation with unintended organ localization
2 Possibility of patient infection and reaction to pyrogens
3 Missed or incorrect diagnosis
4 Delay in diagnosis if repetition of study is necessary
5 Undesirable effect on patient treatment of delay and repetition
6 Increased cost resulting from more radiopharmaceutical, and more camera, computer, technical, clinical, etc., time

process" testing and testing of the final preparation are carried out.

Hazards associated with the use of radiopharmaceuticals

In the previous sections, several complications that are encountered only sometimes with the use of radiopharmaceuticals in nuclear medicine have been described. A complication, however, associated with the use of all radiopharmaceuticals requires some attention, namely the problems associated with the *radiations* from the radionuclides themselves. It is not the intention here to discuss the effects of the radiations or dosimetry. It is worthwhile to review the various sources of radiation to which people can be exposed, in association with the nuclear medicine department and its procedures.

In contemplating the administration of a radiopharmaceutical to a patient, the harmful effects, both somatic and genetic, of radioactivity absorbed into the patient's tissues must be weighed against the benefits of the diagnostic procedure. Unlike an X-ray procedure where the radiation given to a patient lasts until the X-ray machine is switched off, the radiation from a radiopharmaceutical continues while the radionuclide is in the patient's body and/or the radioactivity has decayed. The effective half-life of a radionuclide is a reflection of the physical half-life of the radionuclide and the *biologic half-life* of the material within the body, and is represented by:

$$\frac{I}{t_{eff}^{1/2}} = \frac{I}{t_{biol}^{1/2}} + \frac{I}{t_{phys}^{1/2}}$$

where: $t_{eff}^{1/2}$ is the effective half-life; $t_{biol}^{1/2}$ is the biologic half-life; and $t_{phys}^{1/2}$ is the physical half-life.

The biologic half-life will depend not only on the formulation of the radiopharmaceutical, but also on the metabolic and physiologic processes that govern the way the radiopharmaceutical is handled in the body. Thus, e.g., $^{99}Tc^{m}$-DTPA will be rapidly cleared from the body by glomerular filtration, whereas $^{99}Tc^{m}$-red blood cells will remain within the vascular system until the red cells are destroyed; the radioactivity decaying long before this event occurs.

Once administered, a radiopharmaceutical will circulate within the blood or lymphatic system, pass through the gastrointestinal tract with some absorption, localize within an organ, and be excreted in the urine, feces, breath, or sweat. In following one or a combination of these processes, the radionuclide will irradiate not only the organ in which it is located, but all other organs and tissues within a distance, depending on the physical properties of the radionuclide. One can calculate, therefore, the radiation dose to the "target" organ, which is the organ under study, as well as the radiation dose to the whole body, radiation-sensitive tissues of the gonad and bone marrow, and other organs. Calcu-

lations of such doses have been performed for a range of radiopharmaceuticals, and are tabulated in the literature [100]. The radionuclide $^{99}Tc^{m}$ now accounts for the majority of imaging studies. The introduction into nuclear medicine of this, and other short-lived low-energy γ-emitting radionuclides, has resulted in a decrease in radiation doses to patients from diagnostic nuclear medicine procedures. However, radionuclides such as ^{111}In, ^{125}I or ^{201}Tl have significant Auger electron emissions and, because they enter the intracellular space, the microscopic distribution of radiation dose is a hazard that must be considered [101].

It must be borne in mind that once a radiopharmaceutical is administered to a patient, the patient is a radiation source for the duration of the radioactivity within the body. Furthermore, their urine and sometimes feces, breath, and sweat will be radioactive. Persons who come into contact with the patient, including nuclear medicine technicians, nurses, porters, secretaries, as well as ward nurses and staff, will be irradiated by the patient. In addition, the patient's own family and members of the general public are subject to radiations from the patient. Radiation-sensitive equipment may also be affected. Harding *et al.* [102] have measured the dose rates from 92 patients having nuclear medicine investigations over a period of 7 consecutive working days with a variety of commonly used radiopharmaceuticals labeled with $^{99}Tc^{m}$, ^{131}I, ^{67}Ga, ^{113}In^{m} and ^{201}Tl. They measured dose rates at 0.1 m, 0.5 m, and 1.0 m from the patients and calculated the values when the patient left the department, and the time-average dose rate over the next 8 hours. Their results showed, e.g., that the departure dose rate from an administered dose of 500 MBq of $^{99}Tc^{m}$ for bone imaging ranged from 96 μSv/h at a distance of 0.1 m from the patient, to 5.2 μSv/h at 1 m. The time-average dose rate for 8 hours for the same dose of radiopharmaceutical ranged from 63 μSv/h at 0.1 m to 3.4 μSv/h at 1 m. It can be shown from their results that a nurse working at 0.1 m from a patient for 20 minutes in a working day, would accumulate a dose of up to 60 μSv.

Contamination

Radiopharmaceuticals are normally prepared and administered as solutions or suspensions, and they are liable to be spilled. Precautions must be taken against such an event happening, and procedures adopted if contamination of skin, clothing, equipment, and environment occurs. With the increased use of radiopharmaceuticals, there is a move towards handling greater quantities of radioactivity in the preparation of radiopharmaceuticals. Facilities and techniques to cater for these functions are described in *National Codes of Practice*, and the reader is referred to these documents.

Miscellaneous factors complicating nuclear medicine procedures

An accurate diagnosis of a malfunctioning organ or diseased state depends very much on the use of radiopharmaceuticals of high quality. In addition, it depends on the optimum performance and correct use of the γ-camera and associated computer. Faults in the camera could result in images that can be misinterpreted by the unwary. In order to maintain imaging equipment operating at the peak of its performance, it is necessary to carry out regular maintenance. Servicing should be carried out by suitably qualified personnel, but there are other checks which can be performed at more frequent intervals by the nuclear medicine department staff.

Other imaging problems may occur due to artifacts arising from inadequate preparation of the patients. Metal objects left on the patient such as keys, coins in pockets, and metal belt buckles and buttons, will absorb photons and show as areas of decreased activity on images. The remedy is to remove the metal objects and repeat the imaging. Contamination of the patient's clothing, the imaging couch, and even the camera face with radioactive urine or saliva, will show up as areas of increased activity on an image. Decontamination will be necessary before repeating the image. The camera operator should be aware if a patient has a metal pacemaker, breast, or hip prosthesis, metal plates, or other objects that will absorb photons. The operator should also know if a patient has had a nuclear medicine scan recently because of the risk of any residual radioactivity from that scan interfering with the present study. For example, a bone scan performed within 24 hours of a liver–spleen scan will show the latter organs on a bone scan. Failure to block the choroid plexus with potassium perchlorate when performing a ^{99}Tc^m-pertechnetate brain scan will show the choroid plexus as a hot spot.

Incorrect use and administration of radiopharmaceuticals can sometimes produce misleading results. Infiltration of a part or whole of a dose can lead to breakdown of the radiopharmaceutical before it gets into the bloodstream, leading to alteration in biodistribution, as well as showing a hot spot at the injection site. Failure to shake a vial of MAA or microspheres before drawing a dose may result in too few particles being administered, giving an uneven lung scan. Patient positioning is very important. The patient's arm in a field of view will absorb photons and show an area of decreased uptake on a liver or lung scan. Similarly, breast artifacts on a liver scan can show as areas of decreased activity. Repositioning of the patient should remedy these problems. Images resulting from incorrect technical, pharmaceutical, and other faults are well presented in the literature [103].

It is important that the appearances on a patient image can be explained either as patient disease or as some form of imaging artifact. To achieve this, assurance is required that the radiopharmaceutical, γ-camera, and other instrumentation, and the imaging procedure are all controlled and satisfactory. Members of staff involved in obtaining and interpreting the images should be made aware of the conditions that can lead to pitfalls and how to cope with them. By doing this, not only will false-negative and false-positive image interpretations be avoided, but it will help to prevent the mismanagement of a patient that may occur as a result of something being reported on the image that may not be true.

References

1 Shani J, Atkins HL, Wolf W. Adverse reactions to radiopharmaceuticals. *Semin Nucl Med* 1976;6:305–328.

2 Williams ES. Adverse reactions to radiopharmaceuticals: a preliminary survey in the United Kingdom. *Br J Radiol* 1974;47: 54–59.

3 Atkins HL. Adverse reactions. In: Rhodes BA, ed. *Quality Control in Nuclear Medicine*. St Louis: Mosby, 1977:263–267.

4 Cordova MA, Hladik WB III, Rhodes BA. Validation and characterisation of adverse reactions to radiopharmaceuticals. *Noninvas Med Imag* 1984;1:17–24.

5 Keeling DH, Sampson CB. Adverse reactions to radiopharmaceuticals. United Kingdom 1977–1983. *Br J Radiol* 1984;57: 1091–1096.

6 Keeling DH. Adverse reactions and untoward events associated with use of pharmaceuticals. In: Sampson CB, ed. *Textbook of Radiopharmacy: Theory and Practice*, 2nd edn. New York and London: Gordon and Breach, 1994:285–298.

7 Keeling DH. Adverse reactions to radiopharmaceuticals. In: Kristensen K, Nørbygaard E, eds. *Safety and Efficacy of Radiopharmaceuticals*. Boston: Martinus Nijhoff, 1984:240–250.

8 Atkins HL. Reported adverse reactions to radiopharmaceuticals remain low in 1984. *J Nucl Med* 1986;27:327.

9 Sampson CB. Adverse reactions and drug interactions with radiopharmaceuticals. *Drug Safe* 1993;8(4):280–294.

10 Kahn D, Argenyi EA, Berbaum K, Rezai K. The incidence of serious hemodynamic changes in physically-limited patients following oral dipyridamole before thallium-201 scintigraphy. *Clin Nucl Med* 1990;15:678–682.

11 Sampson CB, Cox PH. Effect of patient medication and other factors on the biodistribution of radiopharmaceuticals. In: Sampson CB, ed. *Textbook of Radiopharmacy: Theory and Practice*, 2nd edn. New York and London: Gordon and Breach, 1994: 215–227.

12 Hladik WB, Nigg KK, Rhodes BA. Drug-induced changes in the biological distribution of radiopharmaceuticals. *Semin Nucl Med* 1982;12:184–210.

13 Bradley WP, Alderson PO, Eckelman WC *et al.* Decreased tumour uptake of gallium-67 in animals after whole-body irradiation. *J Nucl Med* 1978;19:204–209.

14 Soin JS, Cox JD, Youker JE *et al.* Cardiac localisation of Tc-99m-(Sn)-pyrophosphate following irradiation of the chest. *Radiology* 1977;124:165–168.

15 Jackson FI, Dierich HC, Lentle BC. Gallium-67-citrate scintiscanning in testicular neoplasm. *J Can Assoc Radiol* 1976;27: 84–88.

16 Poulose KP, Reba RC, Eckelman WC *et al.* Extraosseous localisation of 99mTc-pyrophosphate. *Br J Radiol* 1975;48:724–726.

17 Lentle BC, Scott JR, Noujaim AA, Jackson FI. Iatrogenic alterations in radionuclide biodistributions. *Semin Nucl Med* 1979;9: 131–143.

18 Haney TA, Ascania I, Gigliotti IA *et al.* Physical and biological preparation of a 99mTc-sulphur colloid preparation containing disodium edetate. *J Nucl Med* 1971;12:64–68.

19 Woldring MG. Drug radiopharmaceutical interactions and other possible modifications in radiopharmaceutical biodistribution. In: Kristensen K, Nørbygaard E, eds. *Safety and Efficacy of Radiopharmaceuticals.* Boston: Martinus Nijhoff, 1984:230–239.

20 News Briefs. Misadministration data released. *J Nucl Med* 1991; 32:34N.

21 Zimmer AM, Spies SM, Majewski W. Effect of drugs on *in vivo* RBC labelling: a proposed mechanism of inhibition. *Proceedings of Second International Symposium on Radiopharmacy.* Chicago, 1981.

22 Lee HB, Wexler JP. Pharmacologic alterations in Tc-99m binding by red blood cells. *J Nucl Med* 1983;24:894–897.

23 Ancri D, Lonchampt M-F, Basset J-Y. The effect of tin on the tissue distribution of 99mTc-sodium pertechnetate. *Radiology* 1977;124:445–450.

24 Sampson CB. Altered biodistribution of radiopharmaceuticals as a result of pharmacological or chemical interaction. In: Theobold AE, ed. *Radiopharmaceuticals and Radiopharmacy Practice.* London: Taylor and Francis, 1985:189–202.

25 Deckart H, Cox PH. *Principles of Radiopharmacology.* Jena: Gustav Fischer Verlag, 1986:224–239.

26 Cox PH. *Radiopharmacy and Radiopharmacology Yearbook 3.* London: Gordon and Breach Science Publishers, 1988:17–40.

27 Rumble WF, Aamodt RL, Jones AE, Henkin RI, Johnston GS. Accidental ingestion of Tc-99m in breast milk by a 10-week-old child. *J Nucl Med* 1978;19:913–915.

28 Rubow S, Klopper J, Scholtz P. Excretion of gallium 67 in human breast milk and its inadvertent ingestion by a 9-month-old child. *Eur J Nucl Med* 1991;18:829–833.

29 Lazarus CR, Edwards S. Radiopharmaceuticals. In: Bennett PN, ed. *Drugs and Human Lactation.* Amsterdam: Elsevier, 1988: 495–549.

30 Romney BM, Nickoloff EL, Esser PD, Alderson PO. Radionuclide administration to nursing mothers: mathematically derived guidelines. *Radiology* 1986;160:549–554.

31 Mountford PJ, Coakley AJ. A review of the secretion of radioactivity in human breast milk: data, quantitative analysis and recommendations. *Nucl Med Comm* 1989;10:15–27.

32 Ogunleye OT. Assessment of radiation dose to infants from breast milk following the administration of 99m-pertechnetate to nursing mothers. *Health Phys* 1983;45:149–151.

33 Pittart WB III, Bill K, Fletcher BD. Excretion of technetium in human milk. *J Paediatr* 1979;94:605–607.

34 Spencer RM, Cornelius EA, Kase NG. Breast secretion of 99mTc in the amenorrhea-galactorrhea syndrome. *J Nucl Med* 1970; 11:467.

35 Wyburn JR. Human breast milk excretion of radionuclides following administration of radiopharmaceuticals. *J Nucl Med* 1973;14:115–117.

36 Vagenakis AG, Abreau CM, Braverman LE. Duration of radioactivity in the milk of a nursing mother following ^{99m}Tc administration. *J Nucl Med* 1971;12:188.

37 Maisels MJ, Gilcher RO. Excretion of technetium in human milk. *Pediatr* 1983;71:841–842.

38 Hör G, Kriegel H, Heidenreich P, Schramm E. Investigations into the biological behaviour of radio-technetium, radio-indium and radio-gallium during lactation. *Int J Appl Radiat Isot* 1973; 24:525–529.

39 Hedrick WR, Di Simone RN, Keen RL. Radiation dosimetry from breast milk excretion of radioiodine and pertechnetate. *J Nucl Med* 1986;27:1569–1571.

40 Mountford PJ, Coakley AJ. Breast milk radioactivity following injection of $^{99}Tc^m$-pertechnetate and $^{99}Tc^m$-glucoheptonate. *Nucl Med Comm* 1987;8:839–845.

41 Ahlgren L, Ivarsson S, Johansson L, Mattson S, Nosslin B. Excretion of radionuclides in human breast milk after the administration of radiopharmaceuticals. *J Nucl Med* 1985;26: 1085–1090.

42 Berke RA, Hoops EC, Kereiakas JC, Saenger EL. Radiation dose to breast-feeding child after mother has $^{99}Tc^m$-MAA lung scan. *J Nucl Med* 1973;14:51–52.

43 Heaton B. The build up of technetium in breast milk following the administration of $^{99}Tc^mO_4$ labelled macroaggregated albumin. *Br J Radiol* 1979;52:149–150.

44 Tribukait B, Swedjemark GA. Secretion of $^{99}Tc^m$ in breast milk after intravenous injection of marked macroaggregated albumin. *Acta Radiol Oncol* 1978;17:279–382.

45 Pittard WB III, Merkatz R, Fletcher BD. Radioactive excretion in human milk following administration of technetium $^{99}Tc^m$ macroaggregated albumin. *Pediatr* 1982;70:231–234.

46 Mountford PJ, Hall FM, Wells CP, Coakley AJ. Breast milk radioactivity after $^{99}Tc^m$-DTPA aerosol/$^{99}Tc^m$ MAA lung study. *J Nucl Med* 1984;25:1108–1110.

47 Rose MR, Prescott MC, Herman KJ. Excretion of iodine-123-hippuran, technetium-99m-red blood cells, and technetium-99m-macroaggregated albumin into breast milk. *J Nucl Med* 1990;31:978–984.

48 Cranage R, Palmer M. Breast-milk radioactivity after $^{99}Tc^m$-MAA lung studies. *Eur J Nucl Med* 1985;11:257–259.

49 O'Connell MEA, Sutton H. Excretion of radioactivity in breast milk following $^{99}Tc^m$-Sn-polyphosphate. *Br J Radiol* 1976;49: 377–379.

50 Mountford PJ, Coakley AJ, Hall FM. Excretion of radioactivity in breast milk following injection of $^{99}Tc^m$-DTPA. *Nucl Med Comm* 1985;6:341–345.

51 Wyburn JR. Human breast milk excretion of radionuclides following administration of radiopharmaceuticals. *J Nucl Med* 1973;14:115–117.

52 Rubow SM, Ellmann A, Le Roux J, Klopper J. Excretion of technetium 99m hexakismethoxyisobutylisonitrile in milk. *Eur J Nucl Med* 1991;18:363–365.

53 Evans JL, Mountford PJ, Herring AN, Richardson MA. Secretion of radioactivity in breast milk following administration of $^{99}Tc^m$-MAG3. *Nucl Med Comm* 1993;14:108–111.

54 Lawes SC. ^{123}I excretion in breast milk — additional data. *Nucl Med Comm* 1992;13:570–573.

55 Blue PW, Dydek GJ, Ghaed N. Radiation dosimetry from breast milk excretion of iodine-123. *J Nucl Med* 1987;28:544.

56 Mountford PJ, Heap RB, Hamon M, Flat IR, Coakley AJ. Suppression by perchlorate of technetium-99m and iodine-123 secretion in milk of lactating goats. *J Nucl Med* 1987;28: 1187–1191.

57 Hedrick WR, Di Simone RN, Keon RL. Excretion of radioiodine in breast milk. *J Nucl Med* 1989;30:127–128.

58 Romney B, Nickoloff EL, Esser PD. Excretion of radioiodine in breast milk. *J Nucl Med* 1989;30:124–126.

59 Mountford PJ, Coakley AJ. Secretion of radioactivity in breast milk following administration of ^{123}I-hippuran. *Br J Radiol*

1989;62:388—389.

60 Palmer KE. Excretion of ^{125}I in breast milk following administration of labelled fibrinogen. *Br J Radiol* 1979;52:672—673.

61 Bowring CS, Ormsby PL, Keeling DH. Excretion of ^{125}I in breast milk following administration of labelled fibrinogen. *Br J Radiol* 1980;53:513.

62 Veall N, Smith T. Excretion of ^{125}I in breast milk following administration of labelled fibrinogen. *Br J Radiol* 1980;53:512—513.

63 Bland EP, Docker MF, Crawford JS, Farr RF. Radioactive iodine uptake by thyroid of breast-fed infants after maternal blood-volume measurements. *Lancet* 1969;ii:1039—1041.

64 Weaver JC, Kamm ML, Dobson RL. Excretion of radioiodine in human milk. *J Am Med Assoc* 1960;173:872—875.

65 Miller H, Weetch RS. The excretion of radioactive iodine in human milk. *Lancet* 1955;ii:1013.

66 Nurnberger CE, Lipscomb A. Transmission of radioiodine(^{131}I) to infants through human maternal milk. *J Am Med Assoc* 1952;150:1398—1400.

67 Honour AJ, Myant NB, Rowlands EN. Secretion of radioiodine in digestive juices and milk in man. *Clin Sci* 1952;11;447—462.

68 Dydek GJ, Blue PW. Human breast milk excretion of iodine-131 following diagnostic and therapeutic administration to a lactating patient with Graves' disease. *J Nucl Med* 1988;29:407—410.

69 Rubow S, Klopper J. Excretion of radioiodine in human milk following a therapeutic dose of I-131. *Eur J Nucl Med* 1988;14:632—633.

70 Karjalainen P, Penttilä IM, Pystynen P. The amount and form of radioactivity in human milk after lung scanning, renography and placental localisation by ^{131}I-labelled tracers. *Acta Obstet Gynaec Scand* 1971;50:357—361.

71 Hengst W. Uber die Ausscheidung von ^{131}I durch die Milch nach Radioisotopennephrographie (on the excretion of ^{131}I in milk after radioisotope renography). *Z Geburtschilfe Perinatol* 1967;166:284—290.

72 Schwartz K-D, Potschwadek B, Scholz B. Die Ausscheidung von ^{131}I in der Muttermilch bei der post partum durchgeführten Isotopennephrographie mit ^{131}I-Hippurat. *Radiobiol Radiother* 1968;9:259—262.

73 Tobin RE, Schneider PB. Uptake of ^{67}Ga in the lactating breast and its persistence in milk. Case Report. *J Nucl Med* 1976;17:1055—1056.

74 Larson SE, Schall GL. Gallium 67 concentration in human breast milk. *J Am Med Assoc* 1971;218:257.

75 Kriegel H. Biokinetics and metabolism of radio-gallium. *Nuklearmedizin* 1984;23:53—57.

76 Greener AW, Conte PJ, Steidley KD. Update on gallium-67 concentration in human breast milk. *J Nucl Med Technol* 1983;11:171—172.

77 Mountford PJ, Wells CP, Hall FM, Coakley AJ. Potential radiation dose to a breast-fed infant following administration of sodium ^{32}P-phosphate to the mother. *Nucl Med Comm* 1984;5:473—476.

78 Sharma SC, Osborne RP, Jose B, Carlson JA Jr. Dose estimation to the infant from breast milk following intraperitoneal administration of chromic phosphate ^{32}P for the treatment of early ovarian cancer. *Health Phys* 1984;47:452—454.

79 Carlson JA, Jose B, Sharma SC, Osborne RP. Radioactivity in breast milk after intraperitoneal chromic phosphate for the treatment of early ovarian cancer. *Am J Obstet Gynecol* 1983;147:840—841.

80 Butt D, Szaz KF. Indium-111 radioactivity in breast milk. *Br J Radiol* 1986;59:80—82.

81 Hesslewood SR, Thornback JR, Brameld JM. Indium-111 in breast milk following administration of indium-111-labelled leukocytes. *J Nucl Med* 1988;29:1301—1302.

82 Mountford PJ, Coakley AJ. Excretion of radioactivity in breast milk after an indium-111 leukocyte scan. *J Nucl Med* 1985;26:1096—1097.

83 Pullar M, Hartkamp A. Excretion of radioactivity in breast milk following administration of a 113m-ln-labelled chelate complex. *Br J Radiol* 1977;50:846.

84 Taylor DM, McCready VR, Cosgrove DO. The transfer of L-selenomethionine-^{75}Se to human milk and the potential dose to a breast-fed infant. *Nucl Med Comm* 1981;2:80—83.

85 Administration of Radioactive Substances Advisory Committee. *Notes for Guidance on the Administration of Radioactive Substances to Persons for Purposes of Diagnosis, Treatment or Research.* London: Department of Health, 1993; 37—40.

86 Zimmer AM, Pavel DG. Rapid miniaturized chromatographic quality-control procedures for Tc-99m radiopharmaceuticals. *J Nucl Med* 1977;18:1230—1233.

87 Frier M, Hesslewood SR (eds). *Quality Assurance of Radiopharmaceuticals. A Guide to Hospital Practice.* Nuclear Medicine Communications. Special Issue. London: Chapman and Hall, 1980.

88 Robbins PJ. *Chromatography of Technetium-99m Radiopharmaceuticals — a Practical Guide.* New York: The Society of Nuclear Medicine, 1984.

89 Coupal JJ, Shih W-J, Ryo UY. Airtight miniaturized chromatography: a safer method for radiopharmaceutical quality control. *J Nucl Med Technol* 1988;16:116—118.

90 Friede J, Dumesnil C, Caron C. Gamma camera and computer-assisted chromatography: a simple method. *J Nucl Med Technol* 1992;20:80—83.

91 Hayes AC. Effects of multiple factors on the stability of new technetium-99m labelled radiopharmaceuticals: MAG3, Cardiolite and Cardiotec. *J Nucl Med Technol* 1992;20:84—87.

92 Lazarus CR. Techniques for dispensing radiopharmaceuticals. In: Sampson CB, ed. *Textbook of Radiopharmacy: Theory and Practice*, 2nd edn. New York and London: Gordon and Breach, 1994;59—68.

93 Lazarus CR. Design of Hospital radiopharmacy laboratories. In: Sampson CB, ed. *Textbook of Radiopharmacy: Theory and Practice*, 2nd edn. New York and London: Gordon and Breach, 1994:51—58.

94 Millar AM. The adsorption of 99mTc-dimercaptosuccinic acid onto injection vials. *Nucl Med Comm* 1984;5:195—199.

95 Porter WC, Dworkin HJ, Gutkowski RF. Vial retention of technetium-99m sulphur colloid. *Am J Hosp Pharm* 1975;32:1141—1143.

96 Elliott AT, Murray T, Hilditch TE, Whateley TL. Investigation of factors affecting adhesion of ^{99}Tc^m labelled colloids to glass vials. *Nucl Med Comm* 1990;11:375—381.

97 Millar AM, Stewart E. The adsorption of 99mTc-radiopharmaceuticals on injection vials. *Nucl Med Comm* 1985;6:115—116.

98 Sampson CB, Keegan J. Stability of 99mTc-DTPA injection: effect of delay after preparation, dilution, generator oxidant, air and oxygen. *Nucl Med Comm* 1985;6:313—318.

99 Anderson ML, Garvie NW, Slater DM. Syringe extractables: effects on radiopharmaceuticals. In: Cox PH, Mather SJ, Sampson CB, Lazarus CR, eds. *Progress in Radiopharmacy.* Dordrecht: Martinus Nijhoff Publishers, 1986:509—511.

100 International Commission on Radiological Protection. *Radiation Dose to Patients from Radiopharmaceuticals*. Oxford: Pergamon Press, 1987.

101 Brill AB. Risk factors and dosimetry. In: Maisey MN, Britton KE, Gilday DL, eds. *Clinical Nuclear Medicine*, 2nd edn. London: Chapman and Hall, 1991;606−620.

102 Harding LK, Mostafa AB, Roden L, Williams N. Dose rates from patients having nuclear medicine investigations. *Nucl Med Comm* 1985;6;191−194.

103 Wells LD, Bernier DR. *Radionuclide Imaging Artifacts*. Chicago: Yearbook Medical Publishers, 1980.

Magnetic resonance imaging: bioeffects, safety, and patient management

Frank G. Shellock and Emanuel Kanal

Introduction

During the performance of magnetic resonance imaging (MRI), the patient is exposed to three different forms of electromagnetic radiation: (i) a static magnetic field; (ii) gradient magnetic fields; and (iii) radiofrequency (RF) electro-magnetic fields. Each of these may cause significant bioeffects if applied at sufficiently high exposure levels. Numerous investigations have been conducted to identify potential bioeffects of MRI [1−83]. Although none of these has deter-mined the presence of any significant or unexpected hazards [1−83], the data are not comprehensive enough to assume absolute safety. In addition, there are several areas of health concern for both the patient and health practitioner with respect to the use of clinical MRI.

The purpose of this chapter is to: (i) discuss the bioeffects of static, gradient, and RF electromagnetic fields with an emphasis on the data that pertains to MRI; (ii) describe and summarize the investigations that specifically apply to MRI; and (iii) provide an overview of other safety considerations and patient management aspects of this imaging technique.

Bioeffects of static magnetic fields

The literature on bioeffects of static magnetic fields is contra-dictory and often confusing. Unfortunately, there is a paucity

of data concerning the effects of high-intensity static magnetic fields on humans. Some of the original investigations on human subjects exposed to static magnetic fields were per-formed by Vyalov [84,85], who studied workers involved in the permanent magnet industry. These subjects were exposed to static magnetic fields ranging from 0.0015 to 0.35 T and reported feelings of headache, chest pain, fatigue, vertigo, loss of appetite, insomnia, itching, and other, more nonspecific ailments [84,85]. Exposure to additional potentially hazard-ous environmental working conditions (elevated room tem-perature, airborne metallic dust, chemicals, etc.) may have been partially responsible for the reported symptoms in these study subjects. Because this investigation lacked an appropriate control group, it is difficult to ascertain if there was a definite correlation between the exposure to the static magnetic field and the reported abnormalities. Subsequent studies performed with more scientific rigor have not sub-stantiated many of the above findings [86−89].

Temperature effects

There are conflicting statements in the literature regarding the effect of static magnetic fields on body and skin tempera-tures of mammals. Reports have indicated that static magnetic fields either increase or both increase and decrease tempera-ture, depending on the orientation of the organism in the static magnetic field [19,66]. Other articles state that static magnetic fields have no effect on skin and body temperatures of mammals [55,61,88,90].

None of the investigators that identified a static magnetic field effect on temperatures proposed a plausible mechanism for this response. In addition, studies that reported static magnetic field-induced skin and/or body temperature changes used either laboratory animals that are known to have labile temperatures, or instrumentation that may have been affected by the static magnetic fields [19,66].

Another investigation indicated that exposure to a 1.5 T static magnetic field does not alter skin and body temperatures in humans [90]. This study was performed using a special fluoroptic thermometry system demonstrated to be unperturbed by high-intensity static magnetic fields. Therefore, skin and body temperatures of human subjects are believed to be unaffected by exposure to static magnetic fields of up to 1.5 T [55,61].

Electric induction and cardiac effects

A magnetohydrodynamic effect may be observed during exposure to static magnetic fields and is caused by blood, a conductive fluid, flowing through a magnetic field. The result is an induced biopotential. This induced biopotential is exhibited by an augmentation of T-wave amplitude as well as by other, nonspecific waveform changes that are apparent on the electrocardiogram (EKG) and have been observed at static magnetic field strengths as low as 0.1 T [86,91,92]. The increase in T-wave amplitude is directly related to the intensity of the static magnetic field, such that at low static magnetic field strengths the effects are not as predominant as those at higher field strengths. The most marked effect on the T wave is felt to be caused when the blood flows through the thoracic aortic arch. This T-wave amplitude change can be significant enough falsely to trigger the RF excitation during a cardiac-gated MRI study.

Other potions of the EKG may also be altered by the static magnetic field, and this varies with the placement of the recording electrodes. Alternate lead positions can be used to attenuate the static magnetic field-induced EKG changes in order to facilitate cardiac gating studies [93]. Once the patient is no longer exposed to the static magnetic field, these EKG voltage abnormalities revert to normal.

Because there are no circulatory alterations that appear to coincide with these EKG changes, no biologic risks are believed to be associated with the magnetohydrodynamic effect that occurs in conjunction with static magnetic field strengths of up to 2.0 T [86,91,92].

Neurologic effects

Theoretically, electric impulse conduction in nerve tissue may be affected by exposure to static magnetic fields. How-

ever, this is another area in the biologic effects literature that contains contradictory information. Some studies have reported remarkable effects on both the function and structure of those portions of the central nervous system that were associated with exposure to static magnetic fields, whereas others have failed to show any significant changes [14,20, 34,68,69,76–79,94–99]. Further investigations of potential unwanted bioeffects are needed because of the relative lack of clinical studies in this field that are directly applicable to MRI. At the present time, exposure to static magnetic fields of up to 2.0 T does not appear significantly to influence bioelectric properties of neurons in humans [97–99].

In summary, there is no conclusive evidence of irreversible or hazardous biologic effects related to acute, short-term exposures of humans to static magnetic fields of strengths up to 2.0 T. However, as of 1991, there are at least four 4.0 T whole-body MRI scanners operating at various research sites around the world. A preliminary study has indicated that workers and volunteer subjects exposed to a 4.0 T MRI system have experienced vertigo, nausea, headaches, a metallic taste in their mouths, and magnetophosphenes (which are visual flashes) [50]. Therefore, considerable research is required to study the mechanisms responsible for these bioeffects and to determine possible means, if any, to counterbalance them.

Magnetic shielding and permanent magnet systems

Numerous MRI sites have been installed with magnetic shielding around the imaging magnet to limit the extent of the fringe static magnetic fields. Indeed, several vendors now provide systems in which the active or passive shielding is located within the casing or faceplate of the magnet. It might not be possible to recognize and differentiate shielded from unshielded systems on the basis of external appearance [99]. Furthermore, other systems are available in which the static magnetic field is provided by means of a permanent magnet in which fringe fields are tightly constrained by the design of the magnet. These designs offer the advantage of restricting the magnetic lines of force to areas deemed tolerable to the environments of the installed site [99].

While magnetic "shielding" seems to suggest a greater level of safety than that achieved with unrestricted systems, it is dangerous to treat such environments as magnetically safe [99]. For example, in the course of only a few inches or feet there may be a change from essential background field strength to a field strength of several hundred or even thousand gauss. This configuration would thus exert a force on the ferromagnetic object that is even greater than it would have been had there been a more gradual tapering of the fringe static magnetic fields. It is thus ironic that a shielded system might present an even greater hazard to the patient or health practitioner than a nonshielded system, because the former would provide less opportunity for a more gradual "warning" of attraction of an object inadvertently brought into this environment.

Similar statements might also be made about the permanent systems. In at least one episode an insulin-infusion pump on a patient was apparently permitted into the MRI system, because of a misconception about the safety of a low-field-strength permanent magnet system [99]. While the only injury in that episode was local bruising of the patient and damage to the pump (there were no long-term detrimental sequelae) such incidents illustrate the need for increased safety education and awareness among all MRI users.

Permanent magnet systems or systems with magnetic shielding are by no means immune to the considerations of the interactions of the static magnetic field with ferromagnetic objects. As noted above, it is entirely feasible that at certain locations relative to the magnet, a shielded system might actually exert a *greater* force on such ferromagnetic objects than in an otherwise identical nonshielded system [99].

Metal detectors and MRI

While only 4% of sites report the frequent use of metal detectors in a clinical setting [99], placement of significant emphasis on the abilities of metal detectors may be hazardous. Indeed, the use of a metal detector as the only means of detection of potentially hazardous ferromagnetic objects is inadequate for clearing patients into the imaging system. The ability of the metal detector actually to detect metal depends on several factors: (i) the size/mass of the metallic object; (ii) the sensitivity setting of the detector (this is generally user selectable); (iii) the proximity of the detector to the metallic object being sought; and (iv) the skill of the operator. Small or deeply embedded objects in biologically delicate locations (e.g., the eye) within the body might easily escape the detection of even a trained, expert examiner. Therefore, negative results from examination with a metal detector should never be construed as a definite clearance for MRI examinations. The results, rather, should at best be used in conjunction with patient history and other data to allow the patient to enter, or preclude the patient from entering, into the magnet room and undergoing a MRI examination. For all these reasons, we believe that metal detectors have no role in the safety evaluation of a patient about to undergo a MRI examination.

Cryogen and quench considerations of superconductive systems

Cryogen considerations

Hazards related to the use of cryogens in MRI magnets are often completely overlooked in safety discussions of MRI-related environments. This discussion, of course, applies only to superconductive magnet systems.

All superconductive MRI systems in clinical use today utilize liquid helium. Liquid helium, which maintains the magnet coils in their superconductive state, will achieve the gaseous state ("boil off") at approximately $-268.93°C$ (4.22 K) [99]. If the temperature within the cryostat precipitously rises, the helium will enter the gaseous state. In such a situation, the marked increase in volume of the gaseous versus the liquid cryogen (with gas—liquid volume ratios of 760:1 for helium and 695:1 for nitrogen) will dramatically increase the pressure within the cryostat [99]. A pressure-sensitive carbon "pop-off" valve will give way, sometimes with a rather loud popping noise, followed by the rapid (and loud) egress of gaseous helium as it escapes from the cryostat. In normal situations, this gas should be vented out of the imaging room and into the external atmosphere. It is possible, however, that during such venting some helium gas might accidentally be released into the ambient atmosphere of the imaging room.

Gaseous helium is considerably lighter than air. If any helium gas is inadvertently released into the imaging room, the dimensions of the room, its ventilation capacity, and the total amount of gas released will determine whether the helium gas will reach the patient or health practitioner who is in the lower part of the room [99]. Helium vapor looks like steam and is entirely odorless and tasteless, but it may be extremely cold. Asphyxiation and frostbite are possible if a person is exposed to helium vapor for a prolonged time. In a system quench, a considerable quantity of helium gas may be released into the imaging room. This might secondarily cause difficulty in opening the room door because of the pressure differential produced. In such a circumstance, the first response should be to evacuate the area until the offending helium vapor is adequately removed from the imaging room environment and safely redirected to an outside environment away from patients, pedestrians, or temperature-sensitive material [99].

Better cryostat design and insulation have allowed the use of only liquid helium in many of the newer superconducting magnets. However, there still are a great number of magnets in clinical use that utilize liquid nitrogen as well. Liquid nitrogen within the cryostat acts as a buffer between the liquid helium and the outside atmosphere, boiling off at 77.3 K. In the event of an accidental release of liquid nitrogen into the ambient atmosphere of the imaging room, there is a potential for frostbite, similar to that encountered with gaseous helium release. Gaseous nitrogen is roughly the same density as air and is certainly much less buoyant than gaseous helium.

In the event of an inadvertent venting of nitrogen gas into the imaging room the gas could easily settle near floor level; the amount of nitrogen gas within the room would continue to increase until venting ceased. The total concentration of nitrogen gas contained within the room would be determined on the basis of the total amount of gas released into the room, the dimensions of the room, and its ventilation capacity (the existence and size of other routes of egress, e.g., doors, windows, ventilation ducts, and fans). A pure nitrogen environment is exceptionally hazardous, and unconsciousness generally results as early as 5–10 seconds after exposure [99]. It is imperative that all patients and health personnel evacuate the area as soon as it is recognized that nitrogen gas is being released into the imaging room, and they should not return until appropriate corrective measures have been taken to clear the gas from the room [99].

Dewar (cryogen storage containers) storage should also be within a well-ventilated area, lest normal boil-off rates increase the concentration of inert gas within the storage room to a dangerous level (J.E. Gray, personal communication). At least one reported death has occurred in an industrial setting during the shipment of cryogens (J.E. Gray, personal communication), although to our knowledge no such fatality has occurred in the medical community. There is one report of a sudden loss of consciousness of unexplained cause by an otherwise healthy technologist (with no prior or subsequent similar episodes) passing through a cryogen storage area where multiple dewars were located (A. Aisen, personal communication). While there is no verification of ambient atmospheric oxygen concentration to confirm any relationship to the cryogens *per se*, the history is strongly suggestive of such a relationship.

Cryogens present a potential concern in clinical MRI despite an overwhelmingly safe record over the past 7 or more years of clinical service [99]. Proper handling and storage of cryogens, as well as the appropriate behavior in the presence of possible leaks, should be emphasized at each site. An oxygen monitor with an audible alarm, situated at an appropriate height within each imaging room, should be a mandatory minimum safety measure for all sites; automatic linking to, and activation of, an imaging room ventilation fan system when the oxygen monitor registers below 18 or 19% should be considered at each magnet installation [99].

Electric considerations of a quench

In addition to the potential for cryogen release, there is also a concern about the currents that may be induced in conductors (such as biologic tissues) near the rapidly changing magnetic field associated with a quench [99]. In one study, physiologic monitoring of a pig and monitoring of the environment were performed during an intentional quench from 1.76 T; there seemed to be no significant effect on the blood pressure, pulse, temperature, and electroencephalographic (EEG) and EKG measurements of the pig during or immediately following the quench [100]. While such a single observation does not prove safety for humans undergoing exposure to a quench, the data do suggest that the experience would indeed be similar, and that there would be no deleterious electric effects on humans undergoing a similar experience and exposure.

Bioeffects of gradient magnetic fields

MRI exposes the human body to rapid variations of magnetic fields due to the transient application of magnetic field gradients during the imaging sequence. Gradient or time-varying magnetic fields can induce electric fields and currents in conductive media (including biologic tissue) according to Faraday's law of induction. The potential for interaction between gradient magnetic fields and biologic tissue is inherently dependent on the fundamental field frequency, the maximum flux density, the average flux density, the presence of harmonic frequencies, the waveform characteristics of the signal, the polarity of the signal, the current distribution in the body, and the electric properties and sensitivity of the particular cell membrane [97–99].

For animals and human subjects, the induced current is proportional to the conductivity of the biologic tissue and the rate of change of the magnetic flux density [98,99,101, 102]. In theory, the largest current densities will be produced in peripheral tissues (i.e., at the greatest radius) and will linearly diminish towards the body's center [98,99,101,102]. The current density will be enhanced at higher frequencies and magnetic flux densities and will be further accentuated by a larger tissue radius with a greater tissue conductivity. Current paths are affected by differences in tissue types, such that tissues with low conductivity (e.g., adipose and bone) will change the pattern of the induced current.

Bioeffects of induced currents can be due either to the power deposited by the induced currents (thermal effects) or to direct effects of the current (nonthermal effects). Thermal effects due to switched gradients used in MRI are negligible and are not believed to be clinically significant [96,98,99].

Possible nonthermal effects of induced currents are stimulation of nerve or muscle cells, induction of ventricular fibrillation, increased brain mannitol space, epileptogenic potential, stimulation of visual flash sensations, and bone healing [98,99,101–104]. The threshold currents required for nerve stimulation and ventricular fibrillation are known to be much higher than the estimated current densities that will be induced under routine clinical MRI conditions [96–99,101]. To our knowledge there have been no reports of such effects during conventional clinical MRI at approved USA Food and Drugs Administration (FDA) levels.

The production of magnetophosphenes is considered to be one of the most sensitive physiologic responses to gradient magnetic fields [96–99]. Magnetophosphenes are supposedly caused by electric stimulation of the retina and are completely reversible with no associated health effects [96–99]. These have been elicited by current densities of roughly $17\,\mu A/cm^2$.

In contrast to this level, the currents that are required for the induction of nerve action potentials is roughly $3000\,\mu A/cm^2$, and those required for ventricular fibrillation induction of healthy cardiac tissue are calculated to be $100-1000\,\mu A/cm^2$ [96]. Although there have been no reported cases, to our knowledge, of magnetophosphenes for fields of 1.95 T or less, magnetophosphenes have been reported in volunteers working in and around a 4.0 T research system [50]. In addition, a metallic taste and symptoms of vertigo seem also to be reproducible and associated with rapid motion within the static magnetic field of these 4.0 T systems [50].

Time-varying extremely low-frequency magnetic fields have been demonstrated to be associated with multiple effects, including clustering and altered orientation of fibroblasts, as well as increased mitotic activity of fibroblast growth, altered deoxyribonucleic acid (DNA) synthesis, and reduced fentanyl-induced anesthesia [49,64,99]. Possible effects in multiple other organisms, including humans, have also been mentioned [99]. While, to our knowledge, no studies have conclusively demonstrated carcinogenic effects from exposure to time-varying magnetic fields of various intensities and durations, several reports suggest that an association between the two is still plausible [105-107].

The current recommendation issued by the USA FDA [108] for exposure to gradient magnetic fields during MRI, is that the rate of change should not be sufficient to cause peripheral nerve stimulation by an adequate margin of safety (at least a factor of three). In the event that significant electric currents are induced during MRI, it is predicted that cutaneous nerves or peripheral skeletal muscle will be stimulated and, thus, give ample warning before the occurrence of a more deleterious response, such as cardiac arrhythmia or fibrillation [96-99,101,102,108].

Although the current USA FDA guidelines are believed to provide a wide margin of safety with respect to exposure to gradient magnetic fields during MRI, it is imperative to realize that the newer echo-planar techniques that require more rapid and complex applications of gradient magnetic fields may easily exceed the recommended levels and must be thoroughly evaluated for potential health hazards. Preliminary studies performed in human subjects have demonstrated that induced eddy currents have resulted in peripheral nerve stimulation producing muscle twitches or contractions in synchrony with field pulses [12,15].

Bioeffects of RF electromagnetic fields

RF radiation is capable of generating heat in tissues as a result of resistive losses. Therefore, the main bioeffects associated with exposure to RF radiation are related to the thermogenic qualities of this electromagnetic field [96-99,108-116]. Exposure to RF radiation may also cause athermal, field-specific alterations in biologic systems that are produced without a significant increase in temperature [108-114]. This topic is somewhat controversial due to assertions concerning the role of electromagnetic fields in producing cancer and developmental abnormalities, along with the concomitant ramifications of such effects [108-114]. A report from the USA Environmental Protection Agency claimed that the existing evidence on this issue is sufficient to demonstrate a relationship between low-level electromagnetic field exposures and the development of cancer [107]. To date, there have been no specific studies performed to study potential athermal bioeffects of MRI. Those interested in a thorough review of this topic, particularly as it pertains to MRI, are referred to the extensive article written by Beers [113].

Regarding RF power deposition concerns, investigators have typically quantified exposure to RF radiation by means of determining the specific absorption rate (SAR) [108-112, 116-119]. SAR is the mass normalized rate at which RF power is coupled to biologic tissue and is indicated in units of watts per kilogram (W/kg). Measurements or estimates of SAR are not trivial, particularly in human subjects, and there are several methods of determining this parameter for RF energy dosimetry [108-112,119].

The SAR that is produced during MRI is a complex function of numerous variables including the frequency (which, in turn, is determined by the strength of the static magnetic field), type of RF pulse (i.e., 90 or 180 degrees), repetition time, pulse width, type of RF coil used, volume of tissue within the coil, resistivity of the tissue, configuration of the anatomic region imaged, as well as other factors [96-99]. The actual increase in tissue temperature caused by exposure to RF radiation is dependent on the subject's thermoregulatory system (e.g., skin blood flow, skin surface area, sweat rate, etc.) [97-99].

The efficiency and absorption pattern of RF energy are mainly determined by the physical dimensions of the tissue in relation to the incident wavelength [108-112]. Therefore, if the tissue size is large relative to the wavelength, energy is predominantly absorbed on the surface; if it is small relative to the wavelength, there is little absorption of RF power [108-112]. Because of the above relationship between RF energy and physical dimensions, studies designed to investigate the effects of exposure to RF radiation during MRI, that are intended to be applicable to the clinical setting, require tissue volumes and anatomic shapes comparable to that of human subjects. Of additional note is that there is no laboratory animal that sufficiently mimics or simulates the thermoregulatory system or responses of humans. For these reasons, results obtained in laboratory animal experiments cannot simply be "scaled" or extrapolated to human subjects [110-112,119].

Little quantitative data has been previously available on thermoregulatory responses of humans exposed to RF radiation prior to the studies performed with MRI. The few studies that existed did not directly apply to MRI because these investigations either examined thermal sensations or therapeutic applications of diathermy, usually involving only localized regions of the body [108−110,114].

Several studies of RF power absorption during MRI have been performed recently and have yielded useful information about tissue heating in human subjects [28,58−60,62,63,65]. During MRI, tissue heating results primarily from magnetic induction with a negligible contribution from the electric fields, so that ohmic heating occurs greatest at the surface of the body and approaches zero at the center of the body. Predictive calculations and measurements obtained in phantoms and human subjects exposed to MRI supports this pattern of temperature distribution [58−60,115,116].

Although one paper reported significant temperature rises in internal organs produced by MRI [65], this study was conducted on anesthetized dogs and is unlikely to be applicable to conscious adult human subjects because of factors related to the physical dimensions and dissimilar thermoregulatory systems of these two species. However, these data may have important implications for the use of MRI in pediatric patients since this patient population is typically sedated or anesthetized for MRI examinations.

An investigation using fluoroptic thermometry probes, which are unperturbed by electromagnetic fields [117], demonstrated that human subjects exposed to MRI at SAR levels up to 4.0 W/kg (i.e., 10 times higher than the level currently recommended by the USA FDA) have no statistically significant increases in body temperatures and elevations in skin temperatures are not believed to be clinically hazardous [62]. These results imply that the suggested exposure level of 0.4 W/kg for RF radiation during MRI is too conservative for individuals with normal thermoregulatory function [62]. Additional studies are needed, however, to assess physiologic responses of patients with conditions that may impair thermoregulatory function (e.g., elderly patients; patients with underlying health conditions such as fever, diabetes, cardiovascular disease, or obesity; and patients taking drugs that affect thermoregulation such as calcium blockers, β-blockers, diuretics, vasodilators, etc.), before subjecting them to MRI procedures that require high SARs.

Certain human organs that have reduced capabilities for heat dissipation, such as the testis and eye, are particularly sensitive to elevated temperatures. Therefore, these are primary sites of potential harmful effects if RF radiation exposures during MRI are excessive. Laboratory investigations have demonstrated detrimental effects on testicular function (i.e., a reduction or cessation of spermatogenesis, impaired sperm motility, degeneration of seminiferous tubules, etc.) caused by RF radiation-induced heating from exposures sufficient enough to raise scrotal and/or testicular tissue temperatures to 38−42°C [118].

Scrotal skin temperatures (i.e., an index of intratesticular temperature) were measured in volunteer subjects undergoing MRI at a whole-body averaged SAR of 1.1 W/kg [63].

The largest change in scrotal skin temperature was 2.1°C and the highest scrotal skin temperature recorded was 34.2°C [63]. These temperature changes were below the threshold known to impair testicular function. However, excessively heating the scrotum during MRI could exacerbate certain preexisting disorders associated with increased scrotal/testicular temperatures (e.g., acute febrile illnesses, varicocele, etc.) in patients who are already oligospermic, and could lead to possible temporary or permanent sterility [63]. Therefore, additional studies designed to investigate these issues are needed, particularly if patients are scanned at whole-body averaged SARs higher than those previously evaluated.

Dissipation of heat from the eye is a slow and inefficient process due to its relative lack of vascularization. Acute near-field exposures of RF radiation to the eyes or heads of laboratory animals have been demonstrated to be cataractogenic as a result of the thermal disruption of ocular tissues, if the exposure is of a sufficient intensity and duration [108,110]. An investigation conducted by Sacks *et al.* [53] revealed that there were no discernible effects on the eyes of rats produced by MRI at exposures that far exceeded typical clinical imaging levels. However, it may not be acceptable to extrapolate this data to human subjects, considering the coupling of RF radiation to the anatomy and tissue volume of the laboratory rat's eyes compared to those of humans.

Corneal temperatures have been measured in patients undergoing MRI of the brain using a send/receive head coil at local SARs up to 3.1 W/kg [59]. The largest corneal temperature change was 1.8°C and the highest temperature measured was 34.4°C. Since the temperature threshold for RF radiation-induced cataractogenesis in animal models has been demonstrated to be between 41 and 55°C for acute, near-field exposures, it does not appear that clinical MRI using a head coil has the potential to cause thermal damage in ocular tissue [59]. The effect of MRI at higher SARs and the long-term effects of MRI on ocular tissues remain to be determined.

Theoretically, RF radiation "hot spots" caused by an uneven distribution of RF power may arise whenever current concentrations are produced in association with restrictive conductive patterns. There has been the suggestion that RF radiation hot spots may generate thermal hot spots under certain conditions during MRI. Since RF radiation is mainly absorbed by peripheral tissues, thermography has been used to study the heating pattern associated with MRI at high whole-body SARs [57]. This study demonstrated no evidence of surface thermal hot spots related to MRI of human subjects. The thermoregulatory system apparently responds to the heat challenge by distributing the thermal load, producing a "smearing" effect of the surface temperatures. However, there is a possibility that internal thermal hot spots may develop from MRI [59].

USA FDA guidelines for MRI devices

On July 28, 1988, MRI diagnostic devices were reclassified from class III, in which premarket approval is required, to class II, which is regulated by performance standards, as long as the device(s) are within the "umbrella" of defined limits addressed below [120]. Subsequent to this reclassification, new devices had only to demonstrate that they were "substantially equivalent" to any class II device that was brought to market using the premarket notification process [510[k]], or, alternately, to any of the devices described by the 13 MRI system manufacturers that had petitioned the FDA for such a reclassification.

Four areas relating to MRI devices have been identified, for which safety guidelines have been issued by the FDA. These include the static magnetic field, the gradient magnetic fields, the RF power of the examination, and the acoustic considerations. Excerpts from the wording of the FDA Safety Parameter Action Levels are as follows [20].

Static magnetic field — Static magnetic field strengths not exceeding 2.0 T are below the level of concern for the static magnetic field. Should the static magnetic field strength exceed 2.0 T, additional evidence of safety must be provided by the sponsor.

Gradient magnetic field — Limit patient exposure to time-varying magnetic fields with strengths less than those required to produce peripheral nerve stimulation or other effects. There are three alternatives:

1 Demonstrate that the maximum dB/dt of the system is 6 T/sec or less.

2 Demonstrate that for axial gradients, dB/dt < 20 T/sec for p ≥ 120 msec, or dB/dt < (2,400/p) T/sec for 12 msec < p < 120 psec, or dB/dt < 200 T/sec for p ≤ 12 psec (p equals the width in microseconds of a rectangular pulse or the half period of a sinusoidal dB/dt pulse). For transverse gradients, dB/dt is considered to be below the level of concern when it is less than three times the above limits for axial gradients.

3 Demonstrate with valid scientific evidence that the rate of change of magnetic field for the system is not sufficient to cause peripheral nerve stimulation by an adequate margin of safety (at least a factor of three). The parameter dB/dt must be lower than that either of the two levels of concern by presentation of valid scientific measurement or calculational evidence sufficient to demonstrate that the time rate of magnetic field change (dB/dt) is of no concern.

RF power deposition — Options to control the risk of systemic thermal overload and local thermal injury caused by RF energy absorption are as follows:

1 If the specific absorption rate is 0.4 W/kg or less for the whole body and 8.0 W/kg or less spatial peak in any 1 gram of tissue, and if the specific absorption rate is 3.2 W/kg or less averaged over the head, then it is below the level of concern.

2 If exposure to RF magnetic fields is insufficient to produce a core temperature increase of 1 degree C and localized heating to no greater than 38 degrees C in the head, 39 degrees C in the trunk, and 40 degrees C in the extremities, then it is considered to be below the level of concern.

The parameter RF heating must be below either of the two levels of concern by presentation of valid scientific measurement or calculational evidence sufficient to demonstrate that RF heating effects are of no concern.

Acoustic noise levels — The acoustic noise levels associated with the device must be shown to be below the level of concern established by pertinent federal regulatory or other recognized standards-setting organizations. If the acoustic noise is not below the level of concern, the sponsor must recommend steps to reduce or alleviate the noise perceived by the patient [120].

MRI and acoustic noise

The acoustic noise produced during MRI represents a potential risk to patients. Acoustic noise is associated with the activation and deactivation of electrical current that induces vibrations of the gradient coils. This repetitive sound is enhanced by higher gradient duty cycles and sharper pulse transitions. Acoustic noise is thus likely to increase with decreases in section thicknesses, decreased fields of view, repetition times, and echo times.

Gradient magnetic field-related noise levels measured on several commercial MR scanners were in the range of 65–95 dB, which is considered to be within the recommended safety guidelines set forth by the USA FDA [120]. However, there have been reports that acoustic noise generated during MRI has caused patient annoyance, interference with oral communication, and reversible hearing loss in patients who did not wear ear protection [9,121]. A recent study of patients undergoing MR imaging without earplugs resulted in temporary hearing loss in 43% of the subjects [9]. Furthermore, the possibility exists that significant gradient coil-induced noise may produce permanent hearing impairment in certain patients who are particularly susceptible to the damaging effects of relatively loud noises [9,121].

The safest and least expensive means of preventing problems associated with acoustic noise during clinical MRI is to encourage the routine use of disposable earplugs [9,121]. The use of hearing protection has been demonstrated to avoid successfully the potential temporary hearing loss that can be associated with clinical MRI examinations [9,121]. MRI compatible headphones that significantly muffle acoustic noise are also commercially available.

An acceptable alternate strategy for reducing sound levels during MRI is to use an "antinoise" or destructive interference technique that not only effectively reduces noise, but also permits better patient communication [122]. This technique consists of a realtime Fourier analysis of the noise emitted from the MRI scanner [122]. A signal possessing the same physical characteristics, but opposite phase to the sound generated by the MRI scanner, is produced. The two opposite-phase signals are then combined resulting in a cancellation of the repetitive noise, while allowing other sounds such as music and voice to be transmitted to the patient [122]. A recent investigation demonstrated no significant degradation of image quality when MRI is performed with scanners that utilize this "antinoise" method [122]. While this technique has not yet found widespread clinical application, it has considerable potential for minimizing acoustic noise and its associated problems.

Investigations of MRI biologic effects

Investigations performed specifically to study the potential bioeffects of MRI are summarized in Table 11.1 [1–83]. The results of these MRI-related bioeffects studies have been predominantly negative, supporting the widely held view that there are no significant health risks associated with the use of this imaging modality. Experiments that yielded positive results either identified possible, nonspecific biologic responses, determined short-term biologic changes that were not considered to be deleterious, or found bioeffects that require further substantiation.

When perusing these studies, the reader should note that the dosimetric aspects of the exposure(s) to static, gradient, and/or RF electromagnetic fields were quite variable and include those that exceeded clinical exposures, simulated clinical exposures, or involved low-level chronic exposures. In certain cases, the effects of only one of the electromagnetic fields used for MRI was evaluated. Theoretically, there is a possibility that the combination of static, gradient, and RF electromagnetic fields may produce some unusual and/or unpredictable bioeffects that are unique to MRI.

"Window" effects are often present with respect to biologic changes that occur in response to electromagnetic radiation. Window effects are those biologic changes associated with a specific spectrum of electromagnetic radiation that are not observed at levels below or above this range [108,119]. Both field strength and frequency windows have been reported in the literature [108,119]. Virtually all of the experiments conducted to date on MRI biologic effects have been performed at specific windows and the results cannot be assumed to apply to all of the various field strengths or frequencies used for clinical MRI.

A variety of different biologic systems were also used for these experiments. As previously mentioned, since the coupling of electromagnetic radiation to biologic tissues is highly dependent on organism/subject size, anatomic factors, duration of exposure, the sensitivity of the involved tissues, and a myriad of other variables, studies performed on laboratory preparations may not be extrapolated or directly applicable to human subjects, or to the clinical use of MRI. Therefore, a cautionary approach to the interpretation of the results of these studies is advisable.

Table 11.1 Summary of MRI bioeffects studies

Study description	Results	Reference
2.0 T • Clinical imaging conditions • Rats • Studied effect of MRI on blood−brain barrier permeability	No MRI-induced difference was detected	Adzamil *et al.* [1]
1.5 T • Exposure to RF radiation in excess of clinical imaging conditions • Sheep • Studied RF radiation-induced heating	For exposure periods in excess of standard clinical imaging protocols, the temperature increase was insufficient to cause adverse thermal effects	Barber *et al.* [2]
0.5 and 1.5 T • Clinical imaging conditions • Human subjects • Studied effect of MRI on the EEG and evaluated neuropsychologic status	No measurable influence of MRI on cognitive functions	Bartels *et al.* [3]

Continued p. 198

Table 11.1 (*Continued*)

Study description	Results	Reference
0.04 T • Clinical imaging conditions • Human subjects • Studied effects of MRI on cognition	MRI did not cause any cognitive deterioration	Besson *et al.* [4]
1.6 T • Quenched magnet • Pig • Studied effect of quenching a magnet	Our findings, which in the circumstances of this experiment, suggested that the risks are small	Bore *et al.* [5]
MRI gradient-induced electric fields • Dogs • Studied bioeffects at high MRI gradient-induced fields	As the strength of MRI gradient-induced fields increases, biologic effects in order of increasing field and severity include stimulation of peripheral nerves, nerves of respiration, and finally, the heart	Bourland *et al.* [6]
0.38 T • Static magnetic field only • Deoxygenated erythrocytes • Studied orientation of sickle erythrocytes	Further studies are needed to assess possible hazards of MRI of sickle cell disease	Brody *et al.* [7]
0.35 and 1.5 T • Clinical imaging conditions • Human subjects with sickle cell disease • Studied effects of MRI on patients with sickle cell disease	No change in sickle cell blood flow during MRI *in vivo*	Brody *et al.* [8]
0.35 T • Clinical imaging conditions • Human subjects • Studied effects of noise during MRI on hearing	Noise generated by MRI may cause temporary hearing loss, and earplugs can prevent this	Brummet *et al.* [9]
• Varying gradient fields • Humans • Studied neural stimulation threshold with varying oscillations and gradient field strength	The threshold decreases with the number of oscillations and increases with frequency. The repeatable threshold of 63 T/s (1270 Hz) remains constant from 32 oscillations (25.6 ms) to 128 oscillations (102.4 ms)	Budinger *et al.* [10]
0.15 T • Simulated imaging conditions • HL60 promyelocytic cells • Studied effect of MRI on Ca^{2+}	Results demonstrate that time-varying magnetic fields associated with MRI procedures increase Ca^{2+}	Carson *et al.* [11]

Continued

Table 11.1 (*Continued*)

Study description	Results	Reference
Gradient magnetic fields up to 66 T/s in dogs and 61 T/s in humans • Dogs • Human subjects studied physiologic responses to large amplitude time-varying magnetic fields	Dogs — no motion, twitch, or EKG abnormalities Humans — brief minimal muscular twitches observed on various parts of the body due to magnetic stimulation	Cohen *et al.* [12]
0.5 and 1.0 T • Simulated imaging conditions • Cultured human blood cells • Studied effect of static magnetic fields and line-scan imaging on human blood cells	Neither treatment had any significant effect on any of the parameters measured	Cooke and Morris [13]
4.7 T • Exposures to static and RF electromagnetic fields only • Isolated rabbit hearts • Studied effects on cardiac excitability and vulnerability	No measurable effect on strength interval relationship or ventricular vulnerability	Doherty *et al.* [14]
Gradient magnetic fields only • Sinusoidal gradients at a frequency of 1.25 kHz with amplitudes up to 40 mT/min for a Z coil and 25 mT/min for an X coil • Human subjects studied physiologic effects, physiologic responses	Observed peripheral muscle stimulation, no extrasystoles or arrhythmias	Fischer [15]
0.3, 0.5, and 1.5 T • Simulated imaging conditions and static/RF and gradient fields separately • Rats • Studied blood–brain barrier permeability	Increased brain mannitol associated with gradient fluid flux may reflect increase blood–brain barrier permeability or blood volume in brain	Garber *et al.* [16]
2.2 to 2.7 T • Simulated imaging conditions • Mouse cells • Studied oncogenic and genotoxic effects of MRI	Data clearly mitigate against an association between exposure to MRI modalities and both carcinogenic and genotoxic effects	Geard *et al.* [17]
60 T/s • Gradient magnetic fields only • Human subjects • Studied effects of gradient magnetic fields on cardiac and respiratory function	No changes were observed	Gore *et al.* [18]
0.1 to 1.5 T • Static magnetic field only • Human subjects • Studied effects of static magnetic fields on temperature	Temperatures increased or decreased depending on field strength of magnet	Gremmel *et al.* [19]

Continued p. 200

Table 11.1 (*Continued*)

Study description	Results	Reference
2.11 T • Static magnetic field only • Isolated rat hearts • Studied effect of static magnetic field on cardiac muscle contraction	Static magnetic fields used in nuclear magnetic resonance imaging (NMRI) do not constitute any hazard in terms of cardiac contractility	Gulch and Lutz [20]
2.0 T • RF at 90 MHz • Simulated imaging conditions • Phantom • Capuchin monkey • Studied temperature changes in phantom and monkey brain during high RF power exposures	Blood flowing through the brain used the body as a heat sink	Hammer *et al.* [21]
0.35 T • Simulated imaging conditions • Mice • Studied teratogenic effects of MRI	Prolonged midgestional exposure failed to reveal any overt embryotoxicity or teratogenicity. Slight but significant reduction in fetal crown–rump length after prolonged exposure justifies further study of higher MRI energy levels	Heinrichs *et al.* [22]
1.5 T • Static magnetic field only • Human subjects • Studied effect of static magnetic field on somatosensory evoked potentials	Short-term exposure to 1.5 T static magnetic field does not effect somatosensory evoked potentials in human subjects	Hong and Shellock [23]
0.15 T • Simulated imaging conditions • Rats • Studied effects on cognitive processes	MRI procedure has no significant effect on spatial memory processes in rats	Innis *et al.* [24]
2.0 T • Static magnetic field only • Human subjects • Studied effect of static magnetic field on cardiac rhythm	Cardiac cycle length was significantly increased but this is probably harmless in normal subjects, safety in arrhythmic patients remains to be determined	Jehenson *et al.* [25]
1.5 T • Simulated imaging conditions • Frog embryo • Studied effect of MRI on embryogenesis	No adverse effects of MRI components on development of this vertebrate (*Xenopus laevis*)	Kay *et al.* [26]
2.3, 4.7 and 10 T • Static magnetic fields only • Physiologic solutions (2.3 and 4.7 T) and mathematic modeling (10 T)	A 10-T magnetic field changes vascular pressure in a model of the human vasculature by less than 0.2%	Keltner *et al.* [27]

Continued

Table 11.1 (*Continued*)

Study description	Results	Reference
• Studied hydrostatic pressure and electric potentials across vessels in presence of static magnetic fields		
1.5 T • Clinical imaging conditions • Human subjects • Studied physiologic changes during high field strength MRI	Temperature changes and other physiologic changes were small and of no clinical concern	Kido *et al.* [28]
1.5 T • Simulated imaging conditions • Rats • Studied effects of MRI on receptor-mediated activation of pineal gland indole biosynthesis	Strong magnetic fields and/or RF pulsing used in MRI inhibited β-adrenergic activation of the gland	LaPorte *et al.* [29]
3.5 to 12 kT/s • Gradient magnetic fields only • Mice • Studied effect of gradient magnetic fields on pregnancy and postnatal development	No significant difference between the litter numbers and growth rates of the exposed litters compared with controls	McRobbie and Foster [30]
• Various strong magnetic fields • Gradient magnetic fields only • Anesthetized rats • Studied cardiac response to gradient magnetic fields	The types of pulsed magnetic fields used in the present study did not affect the cardiac cycle of anesthetized rats	McRobbie and Foster [31]
1.89 T • Simulated imaging sequence • Rats • Studied taste aversion in rats to evaluate possible toxic effects of MRI	Rats exposed to MRI did not display any aversion to the saccharin solution	Messmer *et al.* [32]
1.89 T • Simulated imaging sequence • Mouse spleen cells • Studied possible interaction between ionizing radiation and MRI on damage to normal tissue	For the normal tissues studied, MRI neither increases radiation damage nor inhibits repair	Montour *et al.* [33]
0 to 2.0 T • Clinical imaging conditions • Human subjects • Studied the extent of changes of the brainstem evoked potentials with MRI	Routine MRI examinations do not produce pathologic changes in auditory evoked potentials	Muller *et al.* [34]
1.5 T • Simulated imaging conditions • Human subjects • Studied effect of MRI on somatosensory and brainstem auditory evoked potentials	It may be assumed that MRI causes no lasting changes	Niemann *et al.* [35]

Continued p. 202

Table 11.1 (*Continued*)

Study description	Results	Reference
0.75 T • Static magnetic field only • Hamster cells • Studied effect of static magnetic field on DNA synthesis and survival of mammalian cells irradiated with fast neutrons	Presence of the magnetic field either during or subsequent to fast-neutron irradiation does not effect the neutron-induced radiation damage or its repair	Ngo *et al.* [36]
1.89 T • Static magnetic field only • Mice • Studied effects of long-term exposure to a static magnetic field	No consistent differences found in gross and microscopic morphology, hematocrit and white blood cells, plasma creatine phosphokinase, lactic dehydrogenase, cholesterol, trigliceride, or protein concentrations in magnet groups compared to two control groups	Osbakken *et al.* [37]
0.15 T • Simulated imaging conditions • Rats • Studied effects of MRI on behavior of rats	Results fail to provide any evidence for short- or long-term behavioral changes in animals exposed to MRI	Ossenkopp *et al.* [38]
0.15 T • Simulated imaging conditions • Rats • Studied effect of MRI on murine opiate analgesia levels	MRI procedure alters both day and nighttime responses to morphine	Ossenkopp *et al.* [39]
1.0 T • Static magnetic field only • Mice • Studied effect of static magnetic field on *in vivo* bone growth	Results suggest that exposure to intense magnetic fields does not alter physiologic mechanisms of bone mineralization	Papatheofanis and Papatheofanis [40]
2.35 T • Static and gradient magnetic fields only • Nematodes • Studied toxic effects of static and gradient magnetic fields	Static magnetic fields have no effect on fitness of test animals. Time-varying magnetic fields cause inhibition of growth and maturation. Combination of pulsed magnetic field gradients in a static uniform magnetic field also has a detrimental effect on the fitness of the test animals	Peeling *et al.* [41]
2.35 T • Simulated imaging conditions • Mice • Studied the effect of MRI on tumor development	Immune response may be enhanced following MRI exposure, as indicated by the longer latency and smaller sizes of tumors in animals receiving MRI exposure	Prasad *et al.* [42]

Continued

Table 11.1 (*Continued*)

Study description	Results	Reference
4.5 T • Simulated imaging conditions • Mice • Studied the effects of high-field-strength MRI on mouse testes epididymes	Little, if any, damage to male reproductive tissues from high-intensity MRI exposure	Prasad *et al.* [43]
0.7 T • Simulated imaging conditions • Mouse bone marrow cells • Studied the cytogenic effects of MRI	NMR exposure causes no adverse cytogenic effects	Prasad *et al.* [44]
0.15 T • Simulated imaging conditions • Mice • Studied effects of MRI on immune system	MRI exposure has no adverse effect on the immune system, as evidenced by natural killer cell activity	Prasad *et al.* [45]
2.35 T • Simulated imaging conditions • Human peripheral blood mononuclear cells (PBMC) • Studied effect of MRI on natural killer cell toxicity of PBMC with and without interleukin 2	In neither case was cytotoxicity affected by prior exposure to MRI	Prasad *et al.* [46]
0.15 and 4.0 T • Simulated imaging conditions • Fertilized frog eggs studied effect of MRI on developing embryos	No adverse effect on early development	Prasad *et al.* [47]
0.7 T • Simulated imaging conditions • Frog spermatazoa, fertilized eggs, and embryos • Studied effects of MRI on development	NMR exposure, at the dose used does not cause detectable adverse effects in this amphibian	Prasad *et al.* [48]
0.15 T • Exposed separately to static, gradient, and RF electromagnetic fields • Mice • Studied separate effects of static, gradient, and RF electromagnetic fields on morphine-induced analgesia in mice	Time-varying, and to a lesser extent the RF, fields associated with the MRI procedure inhibit morphine-induced analgesia in mice	Prato *et al.* [49]
4.7 T • Clinical imaging conditions • Human subjects • Studied bioeffects of 4.7-T scanner	Mild vertigo, headaches, nausea, magnetophosphenes, metallic taste in mouth	Redington *et al.* [50]

Continued p. 204

Table 11.1 (*Continued*)

Study description	Results	Reference
0.04 T • Clinical imaging conditions • Human subjects • Follow-up study	Average follow-up time was 6 months. None of the 35 deaths recorded was unexpected. Using the magnetic field and RF levels currently in operation, we believe NMRI to be a safe, noninvasive method of whole-body imaging	Reid *et al.* [51]
4.0 T • RF at 8–170 MHz • No gradient magnetic fields • Human subjects • Studied response of human auditory system to RF pulses	In accordance with the used RF modulation envelope, three distinct chirps per sequence could be resolved. RF-induced auditory noise is usually completely masked by noise from simultaneously switched gradient fields	Roschmann *et al.* [52]
2.7 T • Simulated imaging conditions • Rats • Studied effects of MRI on ocular tissues	There were no discernable effects on the rat eye	Sacks *et al.* [53]
0.35 T • Simulated imaging conditions • Hamster ovary cells • Studied effects of MRI on observable mutations and cytotoxicity	NMRI caused no detectable genetic damage and does not affect cell viability	Schwartz and Crooks [54]
1.5 T • Static magnetic field only • Human subjects • Studied effect of static magnetic field on body temperature	No effect on body temperature of normal human subjects	Shellock *et al.* [55]
1.5 T • Clinical imaging conditions • Human subjects • Studied temperature, heart rate, and blood pressure changes associated with MRI	MRI not associated with any temperature or hemodynamic related deleterious effects	Shellock and Crues [56]
1.5 T • Clinical imaging conditions • Human subjects • Studied thermal effects of MRI of the spine	No surface "hot spots." Temperature effects were well-below known thresholds for adverse effects	Shellock *et al.* [57]
1.5 T • Clinical imaging conditions • Human subjects • Studied possible hypothalamic heating produced by MRI of the head	There was probably no direct hypothalamic heating produced by clinical MRI of the head	Shellock *et al.* [58]

Continued

Table 11.1 (*Continued*)

Study description	Results	Reference
1.5 T • Clinical imaging conditions • Human subjects • Studied effect of MRI on corneal temperatures	MRI causes relatively minor increases in corneal temperature that do not appear to pose any thermal hazard to ocular tissue	Shellock and Crues [59]
1.5 T • Clinical imaging conditions • Human subjects • Studied temperature changes associated with MRI of the brain	No significant increases in average body temperature. Observed elevations in skin temperatures were physiologically inconsequential	Shellock and Crues [60]
1.5 T • Static magnetic field only • Human subjects • Studied effects of static magnetic field on body and skin temperatures	There were no statistically significant changes in body or any of the skin temperatures recorded	Shellock et al. [61]
1.5 T • Clinical imaging conditions • Human subjects • Studied effect of MRI performed at high SAR levels	Recommended exposure to RF radiation during MRI of the body for patients with normal thermoregulatory function may be too conservative	Shellock et al. [62]
1.5 T • Clinical imaging conditions • Human subjects • Studied effect of MRI on scrotal skin temperature	Absolute temperature is below threshold known to affect testicular function	Shellock et al. [63]
0.15 T • Simulated imaging conditions • Anesthetized rats • Studied effect of MRI on blood−brain barrier permeability	These findings raise the possibility that exposure to clinical MRI procedures may also temporarily alter the central blood−brain permeabllity in human subjects	Shivers et al. [64]
1.5 T • Simulated imaging conditions • Anesthetized dogs • Studied effect of MRI performed at high SAR levels	These findings argue for continued caution in the design and operation of imagers capable of high specific absorption rates	Shuman et al. [65]
0.4 to 8.0 T • Static magnetic fields only • Mice • Studied effect of static magnetic field on temperature	Observed a field-induced increase in temperature	Sperber et al. [66]
0.4 to 1.0 T • Static magnetic field only • Human subjects • Studied the effects of static magnetic fields on tissue perfusion	Neither at the skin of the thumb nor at the forearm were the changes in local blood flow attributable to the magnetic fields applied	Stick et al. [67]

Continued p. 206

Table 11.1 (*Continued*)

Study description	Results	Reference
0.4 T • Static magnetic field only • Human subjects • Studied magnetic field-induced changes in auditory evoked potentials	Strong steady magnetic fields induce changes in human auditory evoked potentials	Stojan *et al.* [68]
0.15 T • Clinical imaging conditions • Human subjects • Studied effect of MRI on cognitive functions	No significant effect upon cognitive functions assessed	Sweetland *et al.* [69]
0.6 T/s • Gradient magnetic field only • Mice • Studied effect of gradient magnetic fields on the analgesic properties of specific opiate antagonists	Results indicate that the time-varying fields associated with MRI have significant inhibitory effects on analgesic effects of specific myopiate-directed ligands	Teskey *et al.* [70]
0.15 T • Simulated imaging conditions • Rats • Studied effects of MRI on survivability and long-term stress reactivity levels	Results fail to provide any evidence for changes in survivability and long-term reactivity levels in rats exposed to MRI	Teskey *et al.* [71]
0.01 and 1.0 T • Simulated imaging conditions and static magnetic field only • *Escherichia coli* • Studied effect of MRI and static magnetic field on various properties of *E. coli*	No mutations or lethal effects observed	Thomas and Morris [72]
1.5 T • Simulated imaging conditions • Mice • Studied the potential effects of MRI fields on eye development	These data suggest a potential for MRI teratogenicity in a strain of mouse predisposed to eye malformations	Tyndall and Sulik [73]
1.5 T • Simulated imaging conditions • C57BL/6J mouse • Studied combined effects of MRI and X-irradiation on the developing eye of the mouse	Results suggested that the MRI techniques employed for this investigation did not enhance teratogenicity of X-irradiation on eye malformations produced in the C57BL/6J mouse	Tyndall [74]
0.35 and 1.5 T • Clinical imaging conditions • Human subjects • Studied effects of MRI on temperature	No significant changes in central or peripheral temperatures resulting from the application of static or dynamic RF	Vogl *et al.* [75]

Continued

Table 11.1 (*Continued*)

Study description	Results	Reference
0.35 T • Static magnetic field only • Human subjects • Studied effect of static magnetic field on auditory evoked potentials	Magnetically induced shift may be explained by changes in electric capacities of the magnetically exposed biologic system	Von Klitzing [76]
0.2 T • Static magnetic field only • Human subjects • Studied effect of static magnetic field on power intensity of EEG	The increased control values following an inverted magnetic flux vector point to a reversible alteration of brain function induced by a static magnetic field	Von Klitzing [77]
0.2 T • Static magnetic field only • Human subjects studied • Studied encephalomagnetic fields during exposure to static magnetic field	Exposure to static magnetic fields as used in NMR equipment generates a new encephalomagnetic field in human brain	Von Klitzing [78]
1.5 and 4.0 T • Static magnetic fields only • Rats • Studied effect of magnetic field on behavior	At 4 T in 97% of the trials, the rats would not enter the magnet	Weiss *et al.* [79]
0.16 T • Static and gradient magnetic fields only • Anesthetized rats and guinea pigs • Studied effects of static and gradient magnetic fields on cardiac function of rats and guinea pigs	No change in blood pressure, heart rate, or EKG	Willis and Brooks [80]
0.3 T • Static magnetic field only • Mouse sperm cell • Studied effect of static magnetic field on spermatogenesis	Acute and subacute exposure to static magnetic fields associated with diagnostic MRI devices is unlikely to have any significant adverse effect on spermatogenesis	Withers *et al.* [81]
0.35 T • Simulated imaging conditions • Hamster ovary cells • Studied effect of MRI on DNA and chromosomes	The conditions used for NMRI do not cause genetic damage that is detectable by any of these methods	Wolff *et al.* [82]
• Varying gradient fields • Human subjects • Studied the effects of time-varying gradient fields on peripheral nerve stimulation using trapezoidal and sinusoidal pulse trains	The thresholds of trapezoidal pulses were higher than those of sinusoidal pulses by 11% and 30%, respectively, at equivalent power level	Yamagata *et al.* [83]

Electrically, magnetically, or mechanically activated implants and devices

The USA FDA requires labeling of MRI scanners to indicate that the device is contraindicated for patients who have electrically, magnetically, or mechanically activated implants, because electromagnetic fields produced by the MRI device may interfere with the operation of these devices [120]. Therefore, patients with internal cardiac pacemakers, implantable cardiac defibrillators, cochlear implants, neurostimulators, bone-growth stimulators, implantable electronic drug infusion pumps, and other similar devices that could be adversely affected by the electromagnetic fields used for MRI, should not be examined by this imaging technique [121,123–126]. Prior *ex vivo* testing of certain of these implants and devices may indicate that they are, in fact, MRI compatible.

The associated risks of scanning patients with cardiac pacemakers are related to the possibility of movement, reed switch closures or damage, programming changes, inhibition, or reversion to an asynchronous mode of operation, electromagnetic interference, and induced currents in lead wires [121,123,124,126]. At least one patient with a pacemaker has been scanned by MRI without incident [125]. A letter to the editor recently indicated that a patient who was not pacemaker dependent underwent MRI by having his pacemaker "disabled" during the procedure [125]. Although this patient sustained no apparent discomfort and the pacemaker was not damaged, it is unadvisable routinely to perform this type of maneuver on patients with pacemakers because of the potential to encounter the aforementioned hazards. Of note is the fact that there has been an MRI-related death of a patient with a pacemaker [99].

Of particular concern is the possibility that the pacemaker lead wire(s), or other similar intracardiac wire configuration, could act as an antenna in which the gradient and/or RF electromagnetic fields may induce sufficient current to cause fibrillation, a burn, or other potentially dangerous event [99,121,123,124,126]. Because of this theoretically deleterious and unpredicted effect, patients referred to MRI with residual external pacing wires, temporary pacing wires, Swan–Ganz thermodilution catheters, and/or any other type of internally or externally positioned conductive wire or similar device, should not undergo MRI because of the possible associated risks [99,120,127].

Some types of cochlear implants employ a relatively high-field-strength cobalt samarium magnet used in conjunction with an external magnet to align and retain a RF transmitter coil on the patient's head, while other types of cochlear implants are electronically activated [128]. Consequently, MRI is strictly contraindicated in patients with these implants because of the possibility of injuring the patient, and/or damaging or altering the operation of the cochlear implant.

Because there is a potential for demagnetizing implants that involve magnets (e.g., dental implants, magnetic sphincters, magnetic stoma plugs, magnetic ocular implants, and other similar devices) that may necessitate surgery to replace the damaged implant, these implants should be removed from the patient prior to MRI, if possible [128–130]. Otherwise, MRI should not be performed on a patient with a magnetically activated implant or device. A patient with any other similar electrically, magnetically, or mechanically activated implant or device should be excluded from examination by MRI unless the particular implant or device has been previously demonstrated to be unaffected by the magnetic and electromagnetic fields used for MRI [121].

Patients with metallic implants, materials, and foreign bodies

MRI is contraindicated for patients that have certain ferromagnetic implants, materials, or foreign bodies, primarily due to the possibility of movement or dislodgment of these objects [97–99]. Other problems may also occur when undergoing MRI, including the induction of electric current in the object, excessive heating of the object, and the misinterpretation of an artifact produced by the presence of the object as an abnormality [97,99,131–134]. These latter potentially hazardous situations, however, are encountered infrequently or are insignificant in comparison with movement or dislodgment of a ferromagnetic implant or foreign body by the magnetic fields of the MRI scanner.

Numerous investigations have evaluated the ferromagnetic qualities of a variety of metallic implants, materials, or foreign bodies by measuring deflection forces or movements associated with the static magnetic fields used by MRI [134–152]. These studies were conducted in order to determine the relative risk of performing MRI on a patient with a metallic object, with respect to whether or not the magnetic attraction was strong enough to produce movement or dislodgment.

A variety of factors require evaluation when establishing the relative risk of performing MRI in a patient with a ferromagnetic implant, material, device, or foreign body, such as: (i) the strength of the static and gradient magnetic fields; (ii) the relative degree of ferromagnetism of the object; (iii) the mass of the object; (iv) the geometry of the object; (v) the location and orientation of the object *in situ*; and (vi) the length of time the object has been in place [98,99]. Each of these should be considered before allowing a patient that has a ferromagnetic object to enter the electromagnetic environment of the MRI scanner.

To date, 261 different implants, materials, devices, or foreign bodies have been tested for ferromagnetism, including: 32 aneurysm and hemostatic clips; five carotid artery vascular clamps; 16 dental implants or materials; 29 heart valve prostheses; 14 intravascular coils, filters, and stents; 12 ocular implants; 15 orthopedic implants, materials, and devices; 56 otologic implants; 23 pellets, bullets, and shrapnel; nine penile implants or urinary sphincters; 33 vascular access ports; and 17 miscellaneous items [144]. Recently, a comprehensive summary of this information has been reported [144]. If a patient is identified as having an implant or foreign body during pre-MRI screening, this previously published compilation of implants, materials, or foreign bodies tested for ferromagnetism should be consulted in order to determine if the object is safe for MRI (i.e., there are no or only insignificant associated deflection forces associated with the object). Table 11.2 lists metallic implants, materials, and foreign bodies that are potential risks for patients undergoing MRI.

Aneurysm and hemostatic clips

Of the 32 different aneurysm ($n = 26$) and vascular clips ($n = 6$) studied and reported in the literature, 19 aneurysm clips and none of the vascular clips were found to be ferromagnetic. Therefore, only patients that definitely have non-ferromagnetic aneurysm clips should be exposed to the magnetic fields used for MRI, while any patient with one of the previously tested hemostatic clips may safely undergo MRI.

Table 11.2 Metallic implants, materials, and foreign bodies that are potential risks for patients undergoing MRI

Aneurysm clips
Drake (DR14, DR24), Edward Weck, Triangle Park, NJ
Drake (DR16), Edward Weck
Drake (301 SS), Edward Weck
Downs multipositional (17-7PH)
Heifetz (17-7PH), Edward Weck
Housepian
Kapp (405 SS), V. Mueller
Kapp curved (404 SS), V. Mueller
Kapp straight (404 SS), V. Mueller
Mayfield (301 SS), Codman, Randolph, MA
Mayfield (304 SS), Codman
McFadden (301 SS), Codman
Pivot (17-7PH), V. Mueller
Scoville (EN58J), Downs Surgical, Decatur, GA
Sundt-Kees (301-SS), Downs Surgical
Sundt-Kees Multi-Angle (17-7PH), Downs Surgical
Vari-Angle (17-7PH), Codman
Vari-Angle Micro (17-7PM SS), Codman
Vari-Angle Spring (17-7PM SS), Codman

Carotid artery vascular clamp
Poppen—Blaylock (SS), Codman

Dental devices and materials
Palladium clad magnet, Parkell Products, Farmindale, NY*
Titanium clad magnet, Parkell Products*
Stainless steel clad magnet, Parkell Products*

Intravascular coils, stents, and filters
Gianturco embolization coil, Cook, Bloomington, ID[†]
Gianturco bird nest IVC filter, Cook[†]
Gianturco zig-zag stent, Cook[†]
Gunther IVC filter, Cook[†]

New retrievable IVC filter, Thomas Jefferson University Philadelphia, PA[†]
Palmaz endovascular stent, Ethicon, Sommerville, NJ

Ocular implants
Fatio eyelid spring/wire*
Retinal tack (SS-martensitic), Western European

Otologic implants
Cochlear implant (3M/House)
Cochlear implant (3M/Vienna)
Cochlear implant, Nucleus Mini 22-channel, Cochlear, Englwood, CO
McGee piston stapes prosthesis (platinum/17Cr—4Ni SS), Richards Medical, Memphis, TN

Pellets, bullets, shrapnel, etc
BB's, Daisy
BB's Crosman
Bullet, 7.62×39 mm (copper, steel), Norinco
Bullet, 0.380 in (copper, nickel, lead), Geco
Bullet, 0.45 in (steel, lead), North America Ordinance
Bullet, 9 mm (copper, lead), Norma

Penile implants
Penile Implant, OmniPhase, Dacomed Corp., Minneapolis, MN*

Miscellaneous
Cerebral ventricular shunt tube, connector (type unknown)
Swan—Ganz Catheter, Thermodilution, American Edwards, Irvine, CA[‡]
Tissue expander with magnetic port, McGhan Medical, Santa Barbara, CA*

* The potential for these metallic implants or devices to produce significant injury to the patient is minimal. However, performing MRI in a patient with one of these devices may be uncomfortable for the individual and/or may result in damage to the implant.
† Ferromagnetic coils, filters, and stents typically become firmly incorporated into the vessel wall several weeks following placement and, therefore, it is unlikely that they will become dislodged by magnetic forces after a suitable period of time has passed.
‡ While there is no magnetic deflection associated with the Swan—Ganz thermodilution catheter, there has been a report of a catheter "melting" in a patient undergoing MRI. Therefore, this catheter is considered contraindicated for MRI.
The relative risks of performing MRI in patients with pellets, bullets, or shrapnel are related to whether or not the objects are positioned near a vital structure.
Manufacturer information is provided if indicated in previously published reference or if, otherwise, known.
SS, Stainless steel.

Carotid artery vascular clamps

Each of the five carotid artery vascular clamps evaluated for ferromagnetism exhibited deflection forces. However, only the Poppen−Blaylock clamp was considered to be contraindicated for patients undergoing MRI because of the significant ferromagnetism shown by this object. The other carotid artery vascular clamps are believed to be safe for MRI because of the minimal deflection forces relative to their use in an *in vivo* application (i.e., the deflection forces are insignificant and, therefore, there is little possibility of significant movement or dislodgment of the implant).

Dental devices and materials

Sixteen different dental devices and materials have been tested for ferromagnetism. Twelve of these demonstrated deflection forces, but only three of these pose a possible risk to patients undergoing MRI because they are magnetically activated devices.

Heart valves

Twenty-nine heart valve prostheses have been tested for ferromagnetism. Twenty-five of these displayed measurable deflection forces. However, the deflection forces were relatively insignificant compared with the force exerted by the beating heart. Therefore, patients with these heart valve prostheses may safely undergo MRI. The only possible exception is that MRI performed with a static magnetic field greater than 0.35 T may be potentially hazardous for a patient who has a Starr−Edwards Pre 6000 valve, if there is concern regarding the integrity of the annulus or the presence of valvular dehiscence.

Intravascular coils, filters, and stents

Five of the 14 different intravascular coils, filters, and stents tested were ferromagnetic [144,151]. These ferromagnetic devices are usually attached firmly into the vessel wall after approximately 4−6 weeks following introduction [151]. Therefore, it is unlikely that any of them would become dislodged by attraction from magnetic forces presently used for MRI. Patients with intravascular coils, filters, or stents in which there is a possibility that the device is not properly positioned or held firmly in place should not undergo MRI.

Ocular implants

Twelve different ocular implants have been evaluated for ferromagnetism. Of these, the Fatio eyelid spring and retinal tack made from martensitic stainless steel displayed measurable deflection forces. While it is unlikely that the associated deflection forces would cause movement or dislodgement of

these implants, it is possible that a patient with one of these implants would be uncomfortable or sustain a minor injury during MRI. Therefore, these two ocular implants are regarded as relative contraindications for MRI.

Orthopedic implants, materials, and devices

Fifteen orthopedic implants, materials, and devices tested for ferromagnetism have been demonstrated to be made from nonferromagnetic materials. Therefore, patients with these particular orthopedic implants, materials, and devices may be imaged safely by MRI.

Otologic implants

Three cochlear implants evaluated for ferromagnetism are considered to be contraindicated for MRI. Besides being attracted by static magnetic fields, these cochlear implants are also electronically and/or magnetically activated. Only one of the remaining tested otologic implants has associated deflection forces. This implant, the McGee stapedectomy piston prosthesis, composed of platinum and 17Cr−4Ni stainless steel, was made on a limited basis during mid-1987 and was recalled by the manufacturer. Patients with this otologic implant were issued warning cards that instructed them not to be examined by MRI.

Pellets, bullets, shrapnel, etc.

Most of the pellets and bullets previously tested for ferromagnetism are composed of nonferromagnetic materials [142,144]. Ammunition found to be ferromagnetic typically came from foreign countries and/or was used by the military. Shrapnel usually contains various amounts of steel and, therefore, presents a potential hazard for MRI. Furthermore, since pellets, bullets, and shrapnel may be contaminated with ferromagnetic materials, these objects represent relative contraindications for MRI. Patients with these foreign bodies should be regarded on an individual basis with respect to whether the object is positioned near a vital neural, vascular, or soft tissue structure. This may be assessed by taking a careful history and using plain film radiography to determine the location of the foreign body.

Penile implants and artificial sphincters

One of the nine penile implants tested for ferromagnetism displayed significant deflection forces. Although it is unlikely that this implant, the Dacomed Omniphase, would cause serious injury to a patient undergoing MRI, it would undoubtedly be uncomfortable for the patient. Therefore, this implant is regarded as a relative contraindication for MRI. Artificial sphincters that have been tested are made from nonferromagnetic materials. However, at least one artificial sphincter currently undergoing clinical trials has a magnetic component and, therefore, patients with this device should not undergo MRI.

Vascular access ports

Of the 33 different vascular access ports tested for ferromagnetism, two showed measurable deflection forces, but the forces were felt to be insignificant relative to the *in vivo* application of these implants [141]. Therefore, it is considered safe to perform MRI in a patient that may have one of these previously tested vascular access ports.

Miscellaneous

Various types of other metallic implants, materials, and foreign bodies have also been tested for ferromagnetism. Of these, the cerebral ventricular shunt tube connector (type unknown) and tissue expander, which is magnetically activated, exhibited deflection forces that may pose a risk to patients during MRI. An "O-ring" washer used as a vascular marker also showed ferromagnetism, but the deflection force was determined to be minimal relative to the *in vivo* use of this device.

Each of the contraceptive diaphragms tested for ferromagnetism displayed significant deflection forces. However, we have performed MRI on patients with these devices who did not complain of any sensation related to movement of these objects. Therefore, scanning patients with diaphragms is not believed to be considered to be physically hazardous to patients.

According to the "Policies, guidelines, and recommendations for MR imaging safety and patient management" information issued by the Society for Magnetic Resonance Imaging, Safety Committee [121], patients with electrically, magnetically, or mechanically activated, or electrically conductive devices should be excluded from MRI unless the particular device has been previously shown (i.e., usually by *ex vivo* testing procedures) to be unaffected by the electromagnetic fields used for clinical MRI, and there is no possibility of injuring the patient. During the screening process for MRI, patients with these objects should be identified before their examination and prior to being exposed to the electromagnetic fields used for this imaging technique. There are implants, materials, devices, or other foreign bodies that have yet to be evaluated for MRI compatibility which may be encountered in the clinical setting. Patients that have untested objects should not be allowed to undergo MRI.

Screening patients with metallic foreign bodies

Patients may present to MRI with a history of metallic foreign bodies such as slivers, bullets, shrapnel, or other types of metallic fragments. The relative risk of scanning these patients is dependent upon the ferromagnetic properties of the object, the geometry and dimensions of the object, and the strength of the static and gradient magnetic fields of the MRI scanner. Also important is the strength with which the object is fixed within the tissue and whether or not it is positioned in, or adjacent to, a potentially hazardous site of the body such as a vital neural, vascular, or soft tissue structure.

A patient who encounters the static magnetic field of an MRI scanner with an intraocular metallic foreign body is at particular risk for significant eye injury. The single reported case of a patient who experienced a vitreous hemorrhage resulting in blindness, underwent MRI on a 0.35 T scanner and had an occult intraocular metal fragment, that was 2.0×3.5 mm in size, dislodge during the procedure [153]. This incident emphasizes the importance of adequately screening patients with suspected intraocular metallic foreign bodies prior to MRI.

Research has demonstrated that small intraocular metallic fragments as small as $0.1 \times 0.1 \times 0.1$ mm in size are detected using standard plain-film radiographs [154]. Although thin slice (i.e., ≤ 3 mm) computed tomography (CT) has been demonstrated to detect metallic foreign bodies as small as approximately 0.15 mm, it is unlikely that a metallic fragment of this size would be dislodged during MRI, even with a static magnetic field up to 2.0 T [154]. Metallic fragments of various sizes and dimensions ranging from $0.1 \times 0.1 \times 0.1$ mm to $3.0 \times 1.0 \times 1.0$ mm in size have been examined to determine if they were moved or dislodged from the eyes of laboratory animals during exposure to a 2.0 T MRI system [154]. Only the largest fragment ($3.0 \times 1.0 \times 1.0$ mm) rotated, but did not cause any discernable damage to the ocular tissue [154]. Therefore, the use of plain-film radiography may be an acceptable technique for identifying or excluding an intraocular metallic foreign body that represents a potential hazard to the patient undergoing MRI [121]. Patients with a high suspicion of having an intraocular metallic foreign body (e.g., a metal worker exposed to metallic slivers with a history of an eye injury) should have plain-film radiographs of the orbits to rule out the presence of a metallic fragment prior to exposure to the static magnetic field. If a patient with a suspected ferromagnetic intraocular foreign body has no symptoms and plain-film series of the orbits does not demonstrate a radiopaque foreign body, the risk of performing MRI is minimal [121].

Using plain-film radiography to search for metallic foreign bodies is a sensitive and relatively inexpensive means of identifying patients who are unsuitable for MRI, and can also be utilized to screen out patients that may have metal fragments in other potentially hazardous sites of the body [121].

Each imaging site should establish a standardized policy

for screening patients with suspected foreign bodies. The policy should include guidelines as to which patients require work-up by radiographic procedures, the specific procedure to be performed (i.e., number and type of views, position of the anatomy, etc.), and each case should be considered on an individual basis. These precautions should be taken with regard to patients referred to MRI in any type of MRI scanner, regardless of the field strength, magnet type, and presence or absence of magnetic shielding [121].

Performing MRI during pregnancy

While MRI is not believed to be hazardous to the fetus, only a few investigations have examined the teratogenic potential of this imaging modality. By comparison, literally thousands of studies have been performed to examine the possible hazards of ultrasound during pregnancy, and controversy still exists concerning the safe use of this nonionizing radiation-imaging technique.

Most of the earliest studies conducted to determine possible unwanted bioeffects during pregnancy showed negative results [17,22,26,31,41,47,82]. More recently, one study examined the effects of MRI on mice exposed during mid-gestation [22]. No gross embryotoxic effects were observed. However, there was a reduction in crown–rump length [22]. In another study performed by Tyndall [73], exposure to the electromagnetic fields used for a simulated clinical MRI examination, caused eye malformations in a genetically prone mouse strain. Therefore, it appears that the electromagnetic fields used for MRI have the ability to produce developmental abnormalities.

A variety of mechanisms exist that could produce deleterious bioeffects with respect to the developing fetus and the use of electromagnetic fields during MRI [86,88,89,103, 108,109,118]. In addition, it is well known that cells undergoing division, as in the case of the developing fetus during the first trimester, are highly susceptible to damage from different types of physical agents. Therefore, because of the limited data available at the present time, a cautionary approach is recommended for the use of MRI in pregnant patients.

The current guidelines of the USA FDA requires labeling of MRI devices to indicate that the safety of MRI when used to image the fetus and the infant "has not been established" [155]. In Great Britain, the acceptable limits of exposure for clinical MRI recommended by the National Radiological Protection Board in 1983 specify that "it might be prudent to exclude pregnant women during the first 3 months of pregnancy" [155].

According to the Safety Committee of the Society for Magnetic Resonance Imaging [121], MRI is indicated for use in pregnant women if other nonionizing forms of diagnostic imaging are inadequate, or if the examination provides important information that would otherwise require exposure to ionizing radiation (i.e., X-ray, computed tomography, etc.). For pregnant patients, it is recommended to inform them that, to date, there has been no indication that the use of clinical MRI during pregnancy has produced deleterious effects. However, as noted by the FDA, the safety of MRI during pregnancy has not been proved [120].

Patients who are pregnant or suspect they are pregnant must be identified prior to undergoing MRI in order to assess the risks versus the benefits of the examination. Since there is a high spontaneous abortion rate in the general population during the first trimester of pregnancy (i.e., $> 30\%$), particular care should be exercised with the use of MRI during the first trimester because of associated potential medicolegal implications relative to spontaneous abortions.

MRI and claustrophobia, anxiety, and panic disorders

Claustrophobia and a variety of other psychologic reactions, including anxiety and panic disorders, may be encountered by as many as 5–10% of patients undergoing MRI. These sensations originate from several factors, including the restrictive dimensions of the interior of the scanner, the duration of the examination, the gradient-induced noises, the ambient conditions within the bore of the scanner, etc. [156–164].

Fortunately, adverse psychologic responses to MRI are usually transient. However, there has been a report of two patients with no prior history of claustrophobia who tolerated MRI with great difficulty and had persistent claustrophobia that required long-term psychiatric treatment [157]. Since adverse psychologic responses to MRI typically delay or require cancellation of the examination, several techniques have been developed and may be used to avert these problems [121,156–164]. These include the following.

1 Brief the patient concerning the specific aspects of the MRI examination, including the level of gradient-induced noise to expect, the internal dimensions of the scanner, and the length of the examination, etc.

2 Allow an appropriately screened relative or friend to remain with the patient during the procedure.

3 Use headphones with calming music to decrease the repetitive noise created by the gradient coils.

4 Maintain physical or verbal contact with the patient throughout the examination.

5 Place the patient in a prone position with the chin supported by a pillow. In this position, the patient is able to visualize the opening of the bore and thus alleviate the "closed-in" feeling. An alternate method to reduce claustrophobia is to place the subject feet-first instead of head-first into the scanner.

6 Use scanner-mounted mirrors, mirror or prism glasses within the scanner to allow the patient to see out of the scanner.

7 Use a large light at either end of the scanner to decrease the anxiety of being in a long, dark, enclosure.

8 Use a blindfold on the patient so that he/she is unaware of the close surroundings.

9 Use relaxation techniques such as controlled breathing and mental imagery [155]. Also, several case reports have shown hypnotherapy to be successful in reducing MRI-related claustrophobia and anxiety.

10 Use psychologic "desensitization" techniques prior to MRI scanning.

Several investigators have recently attempted to compare the effectiveness of some of the above-mentioned techniques in reducing MRI-induced anxiety and/or claustrophobia [158,159,162]. One such study demonstrated that providing detailed information about the MRI procedure in addition to "relaxation exercises" successfully reduced the anxiety level of a group of patients both before and during MRI. A similar anxiety reduction could not be shown in patients provided with only information or "stress-reduction" counseling. Relaxation methods have also been shown significantly to decrease anxiety during other medical procedures. Certain MRI system architectures employing a vertical magnetic field offer a more open design that might reduce the frequency of psychologic-related problems associated with MRI procedures.

Monitoring physiologic parameters during MRI

Because the typical MRI scanner is constructed such that the patient is placed inside a cylindrical structure, routine observations and vital signs monitoring is not a trivial task. Conventional monitoring equipment was not designed to operate in the MRI environment, where static, gradient, and RF electromagnetic fields can adversely affect the operation of these devices. Fortunately, MRI-compatible monitors have been developed and are commonly used in in-patient and out-patient MRI centers [165–173].

Physiologic monitoring is required for the safe utilization of MRI in patients who are sedated, anesthetized, comatose, critically ill, or unable to communicate with the MRI operator. All of the above categories of patients should be routinely monitored during MRI and, considering the current availability of MRI-compatible monitors, there is no reason to exclude these types of patients from MRI. Every physiologic parameter that can be obtained under normal circumstances in the intensive care unit or operating room can be monitored during MRI, including heart rate, systemic blood pressure, intracardiac pressure, end-tidal carbon dioxide, oxygen saturation, respiratory rate, skin blood flow, and temperature [166–173]. Table 11.3 lists examples of MRI-compatible monitors that have been successfully tested and operated at field strengths of up to 1.5 T. In addition, there are now MRI-compatible ventilators for patients who require ventilatory support.

Monitors that contain ferromagnetic components (i.e.,

Table 11.3 Examples of MRI-compatible monitors and respirators*

Device and manufacturer	Function
Omega 1400 In Vivo Laboratories, Inc. Orlando, FL	Blood pressure Heart rate
Fiber-Optic Pulse Oximeter Nonin Medical Plymouth, MN	Oxygen saturation Heart rate
525 Respiratory Rate Monitor Biochem International Waukesha, WI	Respiratory rate
MicroSpan Capnometer 8800 Biochem International Waukesha, WI	Respiratory rate End-tidal carbon dioxide
Aneuroid Chest Bellows Coulbourn Instruments Allentown, PA	Respiratory rate
Laserflow Blood Perfusion Monitor Vasomedics, Inc. St Paul, MN	Skin blood flow
Medpacific LD 5000 Laser–Doppler Perfusion Monitor Medpacific Corporation Seattle, WA	Skin blood flow
Fluoroptic Thermometry System Model 3000 Luxtron Santa Clara, CA	Temperature
Omni-Vent, Series D Columbia Medical Marketing Topeka, KS	Respirator
Ventilator, Model 225 Monaghan Medical Corporation Plattsburgh, PA	Respirator

* Note that these devices may require modifications to make them MRI-compatible and none of them should be positioned closer than 2.5 m from the entrance of the bore of a 1.5-T MRI scanner. Also, monitors with metallic cables, leads, or probes will cause mild to moderate imaging artifacts if placed near the imaging area of interest. Consult manufacturers to determine compatibility with specific MRI scanners and for additional safety information.

transformers, outer casings, etc.) can be strongly attracted by mid- and high-field MRI systems, posing a serious hazard to patients and possible damage to the MRI scanner. Since the intensity of standard static magnetic field falls off as the third power of the distance from the magnet, simply placing the monitor a suitable distance from the MRI scanner is sufficient to protect the operation of the device and to help prevent it from becoming a potential projectile [170,173]. If monitoring equipment is not placed in a permanently fixed position, instructions should be given to all appropriate personnel regarding the hazards of moving this equipment too close to the MRI scanner [170,173].

In addition to being influenced by the static magnetic field, monitors may be adversely affected by electromagnetic interference from the gradient, and RF pulses from the MRI scanner [170,173]. In these instances, increasing the length of the patient–monitor interface and positioning the equipment outside the RF-shielded room (e.g., the control room) will enable the monitor to operate properly. It is usually necessary to position all monitors with cathode ray tubes at a location in the magnetic fringe field such that the display is not "bent" or distorted.

Certain monitors emit spurious electromagnetic noise, which can result in moderate to severe imaging artifacts [170,173]. These monitors can be modified to work during MRI by adding RF-shielded cables, using fiberoptic transmission of the signals (which is becoming increasingly the method of choice in the MRI environment), or using special outer casing. Also, special filters may be added to the monitor to inhibit electromagnetic noise.

Of further concern is the fact that some monitoring equipment can be potentially harmful to patients if special precautions are not followed [170,173–176]. A primary source of adverse MRI scanner and physiologic monitor interactions has been the interface that is used between the patient and the equipment, because this usually requires a conductive cable or other device. The presence of a conductive material in the immediate MRI scanner area is a safety concern because of the potential for monitor-related burns. For example, there has been a report of an unfortunate accident involving an anesthetized patient who sustained a third-degree burn of the finger associated with using a pulse oximeter during MRI [175]. Investigation of this incident revealed that the cable leading from the pulse oximeter to the fingerprobe may have been looped during MRI and the gradient and/or RF magnetic fields induced sufficient current to exorbitantly heat the fingerprobe, resulting in the finger burn [175]. This problem may also occur with the use of EKG lead wires or any other cable that may be looped or form a conductive loop that contacts the patient.

Therefore, the following is recommended to prevent potential monitor-related accidents from occurring.
1 Monitoring equipment should only be utilized by trained personnel.
2 All cables and lead wires from monitoring devices that come into contact with the patient (e.g., the monitor–patient interface) should be positioned so that no conductive loops are formed.
3 Monitoring devices that do not appear to operate properly during MRI should be immediately removed from the patient and the magnetic environment.
The following is a brief description of some of the techniques of monitoring various physiologic parameters.

Monitoring blood pressure

Noninvasive blood-pressure monitors typically utilize the oscillometric technique for measuring blood pressure, using a pressure transducer connected to a pressure cuff via a pneumatically filled hose. Certain monitors (i.e., Omega 1400, In Vivo Research Laboratories Inc., Broken Arrow, OK) have adjustable audible and visual alarms as well as a strip-chart recorder.

Occasionally, the cuff inflation tends to disturb lightly sedated patients, especially pediatric patients, which may cause them to move and distort the MRI. For this reason, the noninvasive blood-pressure monitor may not represent the optimal instrument for obtaining vital signs in all patient groups. Direct pressure monitoring of systemic and/or intracardiac pressures, if necessary, can be accomplished using a fiberoptic pressure transducer made entirely of plastic.

Monitoring respiratory rate, oxygenation, and gas exchange

Monitoring of respiratory parameters during MRI of sedated or anesthetized patients is particularly important because the medications used for these procedures may produce complications of respiratory depression. Therefore, as a standard of care, a pulse oximeter, capnograph, or capnometer should always be used to monitor patients who are sedated or anesthetized during MRI.

The respiratory monitors utilized successfully on sedated pediatric or adult patients (i.e., the model 515 Respiration Monitor and model 8800 Capnometer, Biochem International, Waukesha, WI) are relatively inexpensive and can be modified for use during MRI by simply lengthening the plastic tubing interface to the patient so that the monitors can be placed at least 2.5 m from the unshielded MRI.

Pulse oximeters are used to record oxygen saturation and heart rate. Commercially available, modified pulse oximeters using hard-wire cables have been previously used to monitor sedated and anesthetized patients during the MRI study and the recovery period with moderate success. These pulse oximeters tend to work intermittently during MRI due to interference from the gradient and/or RF electromagnetic fields. In certain instances, patients have been burned, presumably as a result of excessive current being induced in inappropriately looped conductive cables attached to the patient probes of the pulse oximeters [174–176].

A newly developed portable fiberoptic pulse oximeter (Nonin Medical Inc., Plymouth, MN) has recently become available for use on patients during MRI [177]. Using fiberoptic technology to obtain and transmit physiologic signals from patients undergoing MRI has been demonstrated to be a technique that does not have any associated MRI-related electromagnetic interference. It is physically impossible for a patient to be burned using this fiberoptic monitor during

MRI because there are no conductive pathways formed by any metallic materials. A recent study conducted to evaluate this new fiberoptic pulse oximeter demonstrated acceptable performance during MRI using a 1.5 T/64 MHz MRI scanner, and a variety of conventional, as well as more sophisticated pulse sequences [177]. There were no interruptions in the operation of the fiberoptic pulse oximeter; heart and oxygen saturation were appropriately measured; and the monitor did not produce imaging artifacts during simulated clinical or actual clinical MRI procedures. To our knowledge, there is only one other commercially available fiberoptic pulse oximeter (In Vivo, Inc., Broken Arrow, OK). However, this is not a "stand-alone" unit, and requires extensive installation prior to operation in the MRI suite.

Monitoring cutaneous blood flow

Cutaneous blood flow can be monitored during MRI by means of the laser–Doppler velocimetry technique. This noninvasive measurement technique uses laser light that is delivered to and detected from the region of interest by flexible, graded-index fiberoptic light wires. The Doppler broadening of laser light scattered by moving red blood cells within the tissue is analyzed in realtime by an analog processor that is indicative of instantaneous blood velocity and the effective blood volume and flow. A small circular probe can be attached to any available skin surface of the patient. Areas with a relatively high cutaneous blood flow (such as the hand, finger, foot, toe, or ear) yield the best results.

Hard-copy tracings obtained by laser–Doppler velocimetry can be used to determine the patient's heart rate, respiratory rate, and cutaneous blood flow. An audible signal may be activated to permit the operator to hear blood-flow changes during monitoring. This technique of continuous physiologic monitoring is particularly useful when there is concern about disturbing a sedated patient, because it is easily tolerated.

Monitoring heart rate

Monitoring the EKG during MRI is typically required for: cardiac imaging; gating to reduce imaging artifacts from the physiologic motion of cerebral spinal fluid in the brain and spine; and for determining the patient's heart rate. Artifacts caused by the static, gradient, and RF electromagnetic fields may severely distort the morphology of the EKG, making determination of cardiac rhythm during MRI extremely difficult and unreliable. Although sophisticated filtering techniques can be used to attenuate the artifacts from the gradient and RF fields, the static magnetic field produces an augmentation of the T wave, as previously mentioned, and other nonspecific waveform changes that are in direct proportion to the strength of the field, which cannot be easily counterbalanced.

In some instances, static magnetic field-induced augmented T waves have a higher amplitude than the R waves, resulting in false triggering and an inaccurate determination of the beats per minute. EKG artifacts can be minimized during MRI by the following:

1 using special filters;
2 using EKG electrodes with minimal metal;
3 selecting lead wires with minimal metal;
4 twisting or braiding the lead wires;
5 using special lead placements [172].

The previously mentioned pulse oximeters may also be used accurately to record heart rate during MRI examinations. These devices have probes that may be attached to the finger, toe, or ear lobe of the patient.

Safety considerations of gadopentetate dimeglumine (Gd-DTPA)

At this time, Gd-DTPA (Magnevist, Berlex Laboratories, Wayne, NJ) is the only FDA-approved intravenous contrast agent available in the USA for use as an adjunct to MRI examinations in adults and children. Its safety has been well demonstrated and documented in several studies in the USA and abroad [99,178]. Studies of this agent in both adult and pediatric populations have demonstrated a high safety margin when compared, e.g., with iodinated contrast material. The median lethal dose of Gd-DTPA (in dogs, mice, and rabbits) is roughly 10 mmol/kg, roughly 100 times the diagnostic dose of 0.1 mmol/kg. Patient tolerance of this drug is also high: the total prevalence of adverse reactions of all types is approximately 2.3%.

Among the reactions noted to be temporally related to the administration of Gd-DTPA are headache, nausea, vomiting, local burning or cool sensation, and hives. There have also been reports of transient elevations in serum iron levels (15–30% of patients), which reverse within 24–48 hours [99,178]. There have been at least two reported cases of severe hypertension following the administration of this agent, these reactions may well have been drug related (P. Fedyshin, personal communication; Medical Affairs Department, Berlex Laboratories, Wayne, NJ, personal communication). Both reactions spontaneously resolved within 1 hour after onset, and both patients had previous histories of hypertension.

To our knowledge there have been six reported cases of fatalities at least temporally associated with the administration of Gd-DTPA. The actual relationship between the deaths and use of the drug is still unclear (Medical Affairs Department, Berlex Laboratories, personal communication). There have been rare reported incidents of anaphylactoid reactions associated with the injection, although the frequency of this appears to be less than 1 per 100 000 doses (Medical Affairs Department, Berlex Laboratories, personal communication).

The mild elevations in serum iron and bilirubin levels

suggest that mild hemolysis may be in some way associated with use of this drug. We stress, however, that this association is not definite or, if present, clearly understood, and there is no evidence of increased hemolysis when the agent is administered to patients with hemolytic anemia. It was theorized that secondary vascular occlusion and sickle crisis induction may occur in patients with sickle cell anemia, as sickled cells are known to align with external magnetic fields to which they are exposed [99]. Whether such forces are significant compared with normal physiologic forces on these cells in their intravascular course is unclear. We stress again that, to the best of our knowledge, there have been no reported incidents of sickle cell associated in any way (temporally or otherwise) with the intravenous administration of Gd-DTPA.

Although local irritative reactions can be expected from use of this hyperosmolar substance (at 1940 mosmol, it is roughly six to seven times the osmolarity of plasma), in some cases no severe adverse local reactions have occurred even when considerable quantities ($> 10\,nl$) of Gd-DTPA have extravasated; some of these cases have been at our own institution. There have been, however, several cases of erythema, swelling, and pain at the site of administration and proximally that were of delayed onset, typically appearing 1–4 days following the intravenous administration of Gd-DTPA [99]. The reaction typically progressed for several days, flattened out, and then resolved over several more days [179]. There has also been at least one incident in which a possible phlebitis was related (at least temporarily) to the intravenous administration of Gd-DTPA (Medical Affairs Department, Berlex Laboratories, personal communication). The mechanism(s) behind this is still unclear, although objective studies have demonstrated that tissue sloughing can occur as a result of extravasation of Gd-DTPA [99,178]. However, a theory that underlies potential safety considerations of this agent is as follows [180].

Initially, after intravenous administration of the agent, the intravascular copper and zinc (normally found in small amounts within the bloodstream), with their competing affinity for the DTPA chelate, will displace some of the gadolinium from the DTPA molecule, which will be released as free gadolinium ion (Gd^{3+}). Although this is a highly toxic substance, the total concentration of the released free Gd^{3+} is very low and is cleared very rapidly, allowing a very low concentration of the free ion to be maintained. As new physiologic sources of copper and zinc ions are "leaked" into the intravascular space in an attempt to reestablish concentration equilibrium, they too displace more Gd^{3+} from its chelate. This cycle continues until all the Gd-DTPA is cleared from the intravascular space. Because of this mechanism, however, the level of free Gd^{3+} may increase dangerously in patients with renal failure. Indeed, the safety of Gd-DTPA in patients with renal failure has not been clearly established, although results of at least one study suggest that it should be well tolerated. While it is theoretically possible that

decreasing the rate of clearance of the Gd-DTPA from the body might increase the concentration of free Gd^{3+} in the body, early data suggest that for a given level of renal function, administration of Gd-DTPA may be safer than administration of iodine-based contrast agents. Similarly, the safety of Gd-DTPA in patients with abnormally and considerably elevated levels of copper, such as patients with Wilson disease, or zinc has not been firmly established and will likely depend on such factors as the glomerular filtration rate and renal clearance rate, as well as the blood copper levels [180]. To our knowledge, to date there have been no studies that have demonstrated elevated free Gd^{3+} to clinically significant levels.

Gd-DTPA has been shown to cross the placenta and, indeed, appear within the fetal bladder during MRI. There are insufficient data presently available, however, to assess the safety of Gd-DTPA in pregnant women and, therefore, should be considered to be a contraindication. Gd-DTPA is also known to be excreted in the breast milk of nursing mothers [181].

Multiple new ionic and nonionic MRI contrast agents are now being developed and investigated. These agents are based on Gd^{3+} and other paramagnetic ions, the safety and efficacy of which are still being established.

References

1 Adzamil IK, Jolesz FA, Blau M. An assessment of blood–brain barrier integrity under MRI conditions: brain uptake of radiolabeled Gd-DTPA and In-DTPA-IgG. *J Nuc Med* 1989;30:839.

2 Barber BJ, Schaefer DJ, Gordon CJ, Zawieja DC, Hecker J. Thermal effects of MR imaging: worst-case studies in sheep. *Am J Roentgenol* 1990;155:1105–1110.

3 Bartels MV, Mann K, Matejcek M, Puttkammer M, Schroth G. Magnetresonanztomographie und Sicherheit: elektroenzephalographische und neuropsychologische Befunde vor und nach MR-Untersuchungen des Gehirns. *Fortschr Rontgenstr* 1986;145(4):383–385.

4 Besson J, Foreman EI, Eastwood LM, Smith FW, Ashcroft GW. Cognitive evaluation following NMR imaging of the brain. *J Neur Neurosurg Psych* 1984;47:314–316.

5 Bore PJ, Galloway GJ, Styles P, Radda GK, Flynn G, Pitts PR. Are quenches dangerous? *Mag Reson Imag* 1986;3:112–117.

6 Bourland JD, Nyenhuis JA, Mouchawar GA *et al.* Physiologic indicators of high MRI gradient-induced fields. In: *Book of Abstracts, Society of Magnetic Resonance in Medicine.* 1990:1276.

7 Brody AS, Sorette MP, Gooding CA *et al.* Induced alignment of flowing sickle erythrocytes in a magnetic field. A preliminary report. *Invest Radiol* 1985;20:560–566.

8 Brody AS, Embury SH, Mentzer WC, Winkler ML, Gooding CA. Preservation of sickle cell blood flow patterns during MR imaging. An *in vivo* study. *Am J Roentgenol* 1988;151:139–141.

9 Brummett RE, Talbot JM, Charuhas P. Potential hearing loss resulting from MR imaging. *Radiology* 1988;169:539–540.

10 Budinger TF, Fischer H, Hentschel D *et al.* Physiological effects of fast oscillating magnetic field gradients. *J Comp Ass Tomog* 1991;15:909–914.

11 Carson JJL, Prato FS, Drost DJ, Diesbourg LD, Dixon SJ. Time-varying fields increase cytosolic free Ca^{2+} in HL-60 cells. *Am J Physiol* 1990;259:C687–C692.

12 Cohen MS, Weisskoff R, Rzedzian R, Kantor H. Sensory stimulation by time-varying magnetic fields. *Mag Reson Med* 1990;14:409–414.

13 Cooke P, Morris PG. The effects of NMR exposure on living organisms. II. A genetic study of human lymphocytes. *Br J Radiol* 1981;54:622–625.

14 Doherty JU, Whitman GJR, Robinson MD *et al.* Changes in cardiac excitability and vulnerability in NMR fields. *Invest Radiol* 1985;20(2):129–135.

15 Fischer H. Physiological effects of fast oscillating magnetic field gradients. *Radiology* 1989;173:382.

16 Garber HJ, Oldendorf WH, Braun LD, Lufkin RB. MRI gradient fields increase brain mannitol space. *Mag Reson Imag* 1989;7:605–610.

17 Geard CR, Osmak RS, Hall EJ, Simon HE, Maudsley AA, Hilal SK. Magnetic resonance and ionizing radiation: a comparative evaluation *in vitro* of oncongenic and genotoxic potential. *Radiology* 1984;152:199–202.

18 Gore JC, McDonnell MJ, Pennock JM, Stanbrook HS. An assessment of the safety of rapidly changing magnetic fields in the rabbit: implications for NMR imaging. *Mag Reson Imag* 1982;1:191–195.

19 Gremmel H, Wendhausen H, Wunsch F. *Biologische Effekte statischef Magnetfelder bei NMR-Tomographie am Menschen.* Thesis, Radiologische Klinik, Christian-Albrechts-Universitat zu Kiel 1983.

20 Gulch RW, Lutz O. Influence of strong static magnetic fields on heart muscle contraction. *Phys Med Biol* 1986;31(7):763–769.

21 Hammer BE, Wadon C, Mirer SD, Ryan T. *In vivo* measurement of RF heating in Capuchin monkey brain. In: *Book of Abstracts, Society of Magnetic Resonance in Medicine.* 1991:1278.

22 Heinrichs WL, Fong P, Flannery M *et al.* Midgestational exposure of pregnant balb/c mice to magnetic resonance imaging. *Mag Reson Imag* 1988;6:305–313.

23 Hong C-Z, Shellock FG. Short-term exposure to a 1.5 Tesla static magnetic field does not effect somato-sensory evoked potentials in man. *Mag Reson Imag* 1990;8:65–69.

24 Innis NK, Ossenkopp KP, Prato FS, Sestini E. Behavioral effects of exposure to nuclear magnetic resonance imaging: II. Spatial memory tests. *Mag Reson Imag* 1986;4:281–284.

25 Jehenson P, Duboc D, Lavergne T *et al.* Change in human cardiac rhythm by a 2 Tesla static magnetic field. *Radiology* 1988;166:227–230.

26 Kay HH, Herfkens RJ, Kay BK. Effect of magnetic resonance imaging on Xenopus Laevis embryogenesis. *Mag Reson Imag* 1988;6:501–506.

27 Keltner JR, Roos MS, Brakeman PR, Budinger TF. Magnetohydrodynamics of blood flow. *Mag Reson Med* 1990;16:139–149.

28 Kido DK, Morris TW, Erickson JL, Plewes DB, Simon JH. Physiologic changes during high field strength MR imaging. *Am J Neuroradiol* 1987;8:263–266.

29 LaPorte R, Kus L, Wisniewski RA, Prechel MM, Azar-Kia B, McNulty JA. Magnetic resonance imaging (MRI) effects on rat pineal neuroendocrine function. *Brain Res* 1990;8:294–296.

30 McRobbie D, Foster MA. Cardiac response to pulsed magnetic fields with regard to safety in NMR imaging. *Phys Med Biol* 1985;30:695–702.

31 McRobbie D, Foster MA. Pulsed magnetic field exposure during pregnancy and implications for NMR foetal imaging: a study with mice. *Mag Reson Imag* 1985;3:231–234.

32 Messmer JM, Porter JH, Fatouros P, Prasad U, Weisberg M. Exposure to magnetic resonance imaging does not produce taste aversion in rats. *Physiol Behav* 1987;40:259–261.

33 Montour JL, Fatouros PP, Prasad UR. Effect of MR imaging on spleen colony formation following gamma radiation. *Radiology* 1988;168:259–260.

34 Muller S, Hotz M. Human brainstem auditory evoked potentials (BAEP) before and after MR examinations. *Mag Reson Med* 1990;16:476–480.

35 Niemann G, Schroth G, Klose U, Buettner UW. Influence of magnetic resonance imaging on somatosensory potential in man. *J Neurol* 1988;235:462–465.

36 Ngo FQH, Blue JW, Roberts WK. The effects of a static magnetic field on DNA synthesis and survival of mammalian cells irradiated with fast neutrons. *Mag Reson Med* 1987;5:307–317.

37 Osbakken M, Griffith J, Taczanowsky P. A gross morphologic, histologic, hematologic, and blood chemistry study of adult and neonatal mice chronically exposed to high magnetic fields. *Mag Reson Med* 1986;3:502–517.

38 Ossenkopp KP, Kavaliers M, Prato FS, Teskey GC, Sestini E, Hirst M. Exposure to nuclear magnetic imaging procedure attenuates morphine-induced analgesia in mice. *Life Sci* 1985;37:1507–1514.

39 Ossenkopp KP, Innis NK, Prato FS, Sestini E. Behavioral effects of exposure to nuclear magnetic resonance imaging: I. Open-field behavior and passive avoidance learning in rats. *Mag Reson Imag* 1986;4:275–280.

40 Papatheofanis FJ, Papatheofanis BJ. Short-term effect of exposure to intense magnetic fields on hematologic indices of bone metabolism. *Invest Radiol* 1989;24:221–223.

41 Peeling J, Lewis JS, Samoiloff MR, Bock E. Biological effects of magnetic fields on the nematode *Panagrellus redivivus*. *Mag Reson Imag* 1988;6:655–660.

42 Prasad N, Kosnik LT, Taber KH, Thornby JI. Delayed tumor onset following MR imaging exposure. In: *Book of Abstracts, Society of Magnetic Resonance in Medicine.* 1990:275.

43 Prasad N, Prasad R, Bushong SC, Ford JJ, Thornby JI. Effects of 4.5 T MRI exposure on mouse testes and epididymes. In: *Book of Abstracts, Society of Magnetic Resonance in Medicine.* 1990:606.

44 Prasad N, Bushong SC, Thornby JI, Bryan RN, Hazelwood RF, Harrell JE. Effect of nuclear resonance on chromosomes of mouse bone marrow cells. *Mag Reson Imag* 1984;2:37–39.

45 Prasad N, Lotzova E, Thornby JI, Madewell JE, Ford JJ, Bushong SC. Effects of MR imaging on murine natural killer cell cytotoxicity. *Am J Roentgenol* 1987;148:415–417.

46 Prasad N, Lotzova E, Thornby JI, Taber KH. The effect of 2.35-T MR imaging on natural killer cell cytotoxicity with and without interleukin-2. *Radiology* 1990;175:251–263.

47 Prasad N, Wright DA, Ford JJ, Thornby JI. Safety of 4-T MR imaging: a study of effects of developing frog embryos. *Radiology* 1990;174:251–253.

48 Prasad N, Wright DA, Forster JD. Effect of nuclear magnetic resonance on early stages of amphibian development. *Mag Reson Imag* 1982;1:35–38.

49 Prato FS, Ossenkopp KP, Kavaliers M, Sestini E, Teskey GC. Attenuation of morphine-induced analgesia in mice by exposure to magnetic resonance imaging: seperate effects of the static, radiofrequency and time-varying magnetic fields. *Mag Reson Imag* 1987;5:9–14.

50 Redington RW, Dumoulin CL, Schenck JF *et al.* MR imaging and

bio-effects in a whole body 4.0 Tesla imaging system. *Soc Mag Res Imag Book Abstr* 1988;1:20.

51 Reid A, Smith FW, Hutchison JMS. Nuclear magnetic resonance imaging and its safety implications: follow-up of 181 patients. *Br J Radiol* 1982;55:784–786.

52 Roschmann P. Human auditory system response to pulsed radiofrequency energy in RF coils for magnetic resonance at 2.4 to 170 MHz. *Mag Reson Med* 1991;21:197–215.

53 Sacks E, Worgul BV, Merriam GR, Hilal S. The effects of nuclear magnetic resonance imaging on ocular tissues. *Arch Ophthalmol* 1986;104:890–893.

54 Schwartz JL, Crooks LE. NMR imaging produces no observable mutations or cytotoxicity in mammalian cells. *Am J Roentgenol* 1982;139:583–585.

55 Shellock FG, Schaefer DJ, Gordon CJ. Effect of a 1.5 T static magnetic field on body temperature of man. *Mag Reson Med* 1986;3:644–647.

56 Shellock FG, Crues JV. Temperature, heart rate, and blood pressure changes associated with clinical MR imaging at 1.5 T. *Radiology* 1987;163:259–262.

57 Shellock FG, Schaefer DJ, Grundfest W, Crues JV. Thermal effects of high-field (1.5 Tesla) magnetic resonance imaging of the spine: clinical experience above a specific absorption rate of 0.4 W/kg. *Acta Radiol* 1986;369 (Suppl.):514–516.

58 Shellock FG, Gordon CJ, Schaefer DJ. Thermoregulatory responses to clinical magnetic resonance imaging of the head at 1.5 Tesla: lack of evidence for direct effects on the hypothalamus. *Acta Radiol* 1986;369 (Suppl.):512–513.

59 Shellock FG, Crues JV. Corneal temperature changes associated with high-field MR imaging using a head coil. *Radiology* 1986;167:809–811.

60 Shellock FG, Crues JV. Temperature changes caused by clinical MR imaging of the brain at 1.5 Tesla using a head coil. *Am J Neuroradiol* 1988;9:287–291.

61 Shellock FG, Schaefer DJ, Crues JV. Effect of a 1.5 Tesla static magnetic field on body and skin temperatures of man. *Mag Reson Med* 1989;11:371–375.

62 Shellock FG, Schaefer DJ, Crues JV. Alterations in body and skin temperatures caused by MR imaging: is the recommended exposure for radiofrequency radiation too conservative? *Br J Radiol* 1989;62:904–909.

63 Shellock FG, Rothman B, Sarti D. Heating of the scrotum by high-field-strength MR imaging. *Am J Roentgenol* 1990;154:1229–1232.

64 Shivers RR, Kavaliers M, Tesky CG, Prato FS, Pelletier RM. Magnetic resonance imaging temporarily alters blood–brain barrier permeability in the rat. *Neurosci Lett* 1987;76:25–31.

65 Shuman WP, Haynor DR, Guy AW, Wesbey GE, Schaefer DJ, Moss AA. Superficial and deep-tissue increases in anesthetized dogs during exposure to high specific absorption rates in a 1.5-T MR imager. *Radiology* 1988;167:551–554.

66 Sperber D, Oldenbourg R, Dransfeld K. Magnetic field induced temperature change in mice. *Naturwissenschaften* 1984;71:100–101.

67 Stick VC, Hinkelmann ZK, Eggert P, Wendhausen H. Beeinflussen starke statische Magnetfelder in der NMR-Tomographie die Gewebedurchblutung? (Strong static magnetic fields of NMR: do they affect tissue perfusion?) *Fortschr Rontgenstr* 1991;154(3):326–331.

68 Stojan L, Sperber D, Dransfeld K. Magnetic-field-induced changes in the human auditory evoked potentials. *Naturwissenschaften* 1988;75:622–623.

69 Sweetland J, Kertesz A, Prato FS, Nantau K. The effect of magnetic resonance imaging on human cognition. *Mag Reson Imag* 1987;5:129–135.

70 Teskey GC, Prato FS, Ossenkopp KP, Kavaliers M. Exposure to time varying magnetic fields associated with magnetic resonance imaging reduces fentanyl-induced analgesia in mice. *Bioelectromagnetics* 1988;9:167–174.

71 Tesky GC, Ossenkopp KP, Prato FS, Sestini E. Survivability and long-term stress reactivity levels following repeated exposure to nuclear magnetic resonance imaging procedures in rats. *Physiol Chem Phys Med NMR* 1987;19:43–49.

72 Thomas A, Morris PG. The effects of NMR exposure on living organisms. I. A microbial assay. *Br J Radiol* 1981;54:615–621.

73 Tyndall DA, Sulik KK. Effects of magnetic resonance imaging on eye development in the C57BL/6J mouse. *Teratology* 1991;43:263–275.

74 Tyndall DA. MRI effects on the teratogenicity of X-irradiation in the C57BL/6J mouse. *Mag Reson Imag* 1990;8:423–433.

75 Vogl T, Krimmel K, Fuchs A, Lissner J. Influence of magnetic resonance imaging on human body core and intravascular temperature. *Med Phys* 1988;15:562–566.

76 Von Klitzing L. Do static magnetic fields of NMR influence biological signals? *Clin Phys Physiol Meas (Bristol)* 1986;7(2):157–160.

77 Von Klitzing L. Static magnetic fields increase the power intensity of EEG of man. *Brain Res* 1989;483:201–203.

78 Von Klitzing L. A new encephalomagnetic effect in human brain generated by static magnetic fields. *Brain Res* 1991;540:295–296.

79 Weiss J, Herrick RC, Taber KH, Plisher GA. Bio-effects of high magnetic fields: a study using a simple animal model. *Mag Reson Imag* 1990;8(Suppl. 1):166.

80 Willis RJ, Brooks WM. Potential hazards of NMR imaging. No evidence of the possible effects of static and changing magnetic fields on cardiac function of the rat and guinea pig. *Mag Reson Imag* 1984;2:89–95.

81 Withers HR, Mason KA, Davis CA. MR effect on murine spermatogenesis. *Radiology* 1985;156:741–742.

82 Wolff S, Crooks LE, Brown P, Howard R, Painter RB. Tests for DNA and chromosomal damage induced by nuclear magnetic resonance imaging. *Radiology* 1980;136:707–710.

83 Yamagata H, Kuhara S, Eso Y, Sato K, Hiwake O, Ueno S. Evaluation of dB/dt thresholds for nerve stimulation elicited by trapezoidal and sinusoidal gradient fields in echo-planar imaging. In: *Book of Abstracts, Society of Magnetic Resonance in Medicine.* 1991:1277.

84 Vyalov AM. Magnetic fields as a factor in the industrial environment. *Vestn Akad Med Nauk* 1967;8:72–79.

85 Vyalov AM. Clinico-hygenic and experimental data on the effect of magnetic fields under industrial conditions. In: Kholodov Y, ed. *Influence of Magnetic Fields on Biological Objects.* Moscow: Translated by the Joint Publications Research Service JPRS-63-38, 1974:20–35.

86 Barnothy MF. *Biological Effects of Magnetic Fields*, Vols 1 & 2. New York: Plenum Press, 1964, 1969.

87 Persson BR, Stahlberg F. *Health and Safety of Clinical NMR Examinations.* Boca Raton, FL; CRC Press, Inc. 1989.

88 Tenforde TS. *Magnetic Field Effects on Biological Systems.* New York: Plenum Press, 1979.

89 Michaelson SM, Lin JV. *Biological Effects and Health Implications of Radiofrequency Radiation.* New York: Plenum Press, 1987.

90 Tenforde TS. Thermoregulation in rodents exposed to high-

intensity stationary magnetic fields. *Bioelectromagnetics* 1986;7: 341–346.

91 Beischer DE, Knepton J. Influence of strong magnetic fields on the electrocardiogram of squirrel monkey (*Saimiri sciures*). *Aerospace Med* 1964;35:939–944.

92 Tenforde TS, Gaffey CT, Moyer BR, Budinger TF. Cardiovascular alterations in Macaca monkeys exposed to stationary magnetic fields. Experimental observations and theoretical analysis. *Bioelectromagnetics* 1983;4:1–9.

93 Dimick RN, Hedlund LW, Herfkens RJ, Fram EK, Utz J. Optimizing electrocardiographic electrode placement for cardiac-gated magnetic resonance imaging. *Invest Radiol* 1987;22:17–22.

94 Abdullakhozhaeva MS, Razykov SR. Structural changes in central nervous system under the influence of a permanent magnetic field. *Bull Exper Biol Med* 1986;102:1585–1587.

95 Hong C-Z. Static magnetic field influence on human nerve function. *Arch Phys Med Rehab* 1987;68:162–164.

96 Budinger TF. Nuclear magnetic resonance (NMR) *in vivo* studies: known thresholds for health effects. *J Comp Ass Tomog* 1981;5:800–811.

97 Shellock FG, Crues JV. MRI: safety considerations in magnetic resonance imaging. *MRI Decis* 1988;2:25–30.

98 Shellock FG. Biological effects and safety aspects of magnetic resonance imaging. *Mag Reson Quart* 1989;5:243–261.

99 Kanal E, Talagala L, Shellock FG. Safety considerations in MR imaging. *Radiology* 1990;176:593–606.

100 Davis PL, Crooks L, Arakawa M, McRee R, Kaufman L, Margulis AR. Potential hazards in NMR imaging: heating effects of changing magnetic fields and RF fields on small metallic implants. *Am J Roentgenol* 1981;137:857–860.

101 Reilly JP. Peripheral nerve stimulation by induced electric currents: exposure to time-varying magnetic fields. *Med Biol Engin Comp* 1989;27:101–112.

102 Bernhardt J. The direct influence of electromagnetic fields on nerve and muscle and muscle cells of man within the frequency range of 1 Hz to 30 MHz. *Radiat Environ Phys* 1979;16:309–323.

103 Adey WR. Tissue interactions with nonionizing electromagnetic fields. *Physiol Rev* 1981;61:435–514.

104 Watson AB, Wright JS, Loughman J. Electrical thresholds for ventricular fibrillation in man. *Med J Aust* 1973;1:1179–1182.

105 Modan B. Exposure to electromagnetic fields and brain malignancy: a newly discovered menace? *Am J Indust Med* 1988;13:625–627.

106 Brown HD, Chattopadhyay SK. Electromagnetic-field exposure and cancer. *Canc Biochem Biophys* 1988;9:295–342.

107 Pool R. Electromagnetic fields: the biological evidence. *Science* 1990;249:1378–1381.

108 NCRP Report No. 86. Biological effects and exposure criteria for radiofrequency electromagnetic fields. *National Council on Radiation Protection and Measurements*. Bethesda: 1986.

109 Erwin DN. Mechanisms of biological effects of radiofrequency electromagnetic fields: an overview. *Aviat Space Environ Med* 1988;59(Suppl. 11):A21–A31.

110 Gordon CJ. Thermal physiology. In: *Biological Effects of Radiofrequency Radiation*. EPA-600/8-830-026A. Washington, DC: 4-1–4-28.

111 Gordon CJ. Normalizing the thermal effects of radiofrequency radiation: body mass versus total body surface area. *Bioelectromagnetics* 1987;8:111–118.

112 Gordon CJ. Effect of radiofrequency radiation exposure on thermoregulation. *ISI Atlas Sci Plants Anim* 1988;1:245–250.

113 Beers J. Biological effects of weak electromagnetic fields from 0 Hz to 200 MHz: a survey of the literature with special emphasis on possible magnetic resonance effects. *Mag Reson Imag* 1989;7:309–331.

114 Coulter JS, Osbourne SL. Short wave diathermy in heating of human tissues. *Arch Phys Ther* 1936;17:679–687.

115 Bottomley PA, Edelstein WA. Power disposition in whole body NMR imaging. *Med Phys* 1981;8:510–512.

116 Bottomley PA, Redington RW, Edelstein WA, Schenck JF. Estimating radiofrequency power disposition in body NMR imaging. *Mag Reson Med* 1985;2:336–349.

117 Wickersheim KA, Sun MH. Fluoroptic thermometry. *Med Electron* 1987;February:84–91.

118 Berman E. Reproductive effects. In: *Biological Effects of Radiofrequency Radiation*. EPA-600/8-83-026A. 1984.

119 Michaelson SM, Lin JC. *Biological Effects and Health Implications of Radiofrequency Radiation*. New York: Plenum Press, 1987.

120 FDA. Magnetic resonance diagnostic device; panel recommendation and report on petitions for MR reclassification. *Fed Reg* 1988;53:7575–7579.

121 Shellock FG, Kanal E. Policies, guidelines, and recommendations for MR imaging safety and patient management. *J Mag Reson Imag* 1991;1:97–101.

121 Hurwitz R, Lane SR, Bell RA, Brandt-Zawadzki MN. Acoustic analysis of gradient-coil noise in MR imaging. *Radiology* 1989;173:545–548.

122 Goldman AM, Grossman WE, Friedlander PC. Reduction of sound levels with antinoise in MR imaging. *Radiology* 1989;173:549–550.

123 Hayes DL, Holmes DR, Gray JE. Effect of a 1.5 Tesla nuclear magnetic resonance imaging scanner on implanted permanent pacemakers. *J Am Coll Cardiol* 1987;10:782–786.

124 Gangarosa RE, Minnis JE, Nobbe J, Praschan D, Genberg RW. Operational safety issues in MRI. *Mag Reson Imag* 1987;5:287–292.

125 Alagona P, Toole JC, Maniscalco BS, Glover MU, Abernathy GT, Prida XE. Nuclear magnetic resonance imaging in a patient with a DDD pacemaker. *Pacing Clin Electrophysiol* 1989;12:619.

126 Edelman RR, Shellock FG, Ahladis J. Practical MRI for the technologist and imaging specialist. In: Edelman RR, Hesselink J, eds. *Clinical Magnetic Resonance Imaging*. Saunders Co., 1990.

127 ECRI. *Health Devices Alert. A New MRI Complication?* 1988; May 27:1.

128 Dormer KJ, Richard GL, Hough JVD, Nordquist RE. The use of rare-earth magnet couplers in cochlear implants. *Laryngoscope* 1981;91:1812–1820.

129 Shellock F. *Ex vivo* assessment of deflection forces and artifacts associated with high-field MRI of "mini-magnet" dental prostheses. *Mag Reson Imag* 1989;7 (Suppl. 1):IT-03.

130 Liang MD, Narayanan K, Kanal E. Magnetic ports in tissue expanders: a caution for MRI. *Mag Reson Imag* 1989;7:541–542.

131 Lund G, Nelson JD, Wirtschafter JD, Williams PA. Tatooing of eyelids: magnetic imaging artifacts. *Ophthalm Surg* 1986;17:550–553.

132 Sacco JJ, Steiger DA, Bellon EM, Coleman PE, Haacke EM. Artifacts caused by cosmetics in MR imaging of the head. *Am J Roentgenol* 1987;148:1001–1004.

133 Jackson JG, Acker JD. Permanent eyeliner and MR imaging. *Am J Roentgenol* 1987;149:1080.

134 Pusey E, Lufkin RB, Brown RKJ *et al*. Magnetic resonance

imaging artifacts: mechanism and clinical significance. *Radiographics* 1986;6:891−911.

135 Buchli R, Boesiger P, Meier D. Heating effects of metallic implants by MRI examinations. *Mag Reson Med* 1988;7:255−261.

136 Shellock FG, Crues JV. High-field MR imaging of metallic biomedical implants: an *in vitro* evaluation of deflection forces and temperature changes induced in large prostheses. *Radiology* 1987;165:150.

137 Shellock FG, Crues JV. High-field MR imaging of metallic biomedical implants: an *ex vivo* evaluation of deflection forces. *Am J Roentgenol* 1988;151:389−392.

138 Dujovny M, Kossovsky N, Kossowsky R *et al.* Aneurysm clip motion during magnetic resonance imaging: *in vivo* experimental study with metallurgical factor analysis. *Neurosurgery* 1985;17:543−548.

139 Shellock FG, Schatz CJ, Shelton C, Brown B. *Ex vivo* evaluation of 9 different ocular and middle-ear implants exposed to a 1.5 Tesla MR scanner. *Radiology* 1990;177(P):271.

140 Shellock FG, Schatz CJ. High-field strength MRI and otologic implants. *Am J Neuroradiol* 1991;12:279−281.

141 Shellock FG, Meeks T. *Ex vivo* evaluation of ferromagnetism and artifacts for implantable vascular access ports exposed to a 1.5 T MR scanner. *J Mag Reson Imag* 1991;1:243.

142 Teitelbaum GP, Yee CA, Van Horn DD, Kim HS, Colletti PM. Metallic ballistic fragments: MR imaging safety and artifacts. *Radiology* 1990;175:855−859.

143 Shellock FG. MR imaging of metallic implants and materials: a compilation of the literature. *Am J Roentgenol* 1988;151:811−814.

144 Shellock FG, Curtis JS. MR imaging and biomedical implants, materials, and devices: an updated review. *Radiology* 1991;180:541−550.

145 Holtas S, Olsson M, Romner B, Larsson EM, Saveland H, Brandt L. Comparison of MR imaging and CT in patients with intracranial aneurysm clips. *Am J Neuroradiol* 1988;9:891−897.

146 Huttenbrink KB, Grobe-Nobis W. Experimentelle Untersuchungen und theoretische Betrachtungen uber das Verhalten von Stapes-metall-prosthesen im Magnetfeld eines Kernspintomographen. (Experiments and theoretical considerations on behaviour of metallic stapedectomy-prostheses in nuclear magnetic resonance imaging.) *Laryngol Rhinol Otol* 1987;66:127−130.

147 Becker R, Norfray JF, Teitelbaum GP *et al.* MR imaging in patients with intracranial aneurysm clips. *Am J Neuroradiol* 1988;9:885−889.

148 Randall PA, Kohman LJ, Scalzetti EM, Szeverenyi NM, Panicek DM. Magnetic resonance imaging of prosthetic cardiac valves *in vitro* and *in vivo*. *Am J Cardiol* 1988;62:973−976.

149 Romner B, Olsson M, Ljunggren B *et al.* Magnetic resonance imaging and aneurysm clips. *J Neurosurg* 1989;70:426−431.

150 Augustiny N, von Schulthess GK, Meier D, Bosiger P. MR imaging of large nonferromagnetic metallic implants at 1.5 T. *J Comp Ass Tomog* 1987;11:678−683.

151 Teitelbaum GP, Bradley WG, Klein BD. MR imaging artifacts ferromagnetism, and magnetic torque of intravascular filters, stents, and coils. *Radiology* 1988;166:657−664.

152 Yuh WTC, Hanigan MT, Nera JA *et al.* Extrusion of a magnetic eye implant after MR examination: a potential hazard to the enucleated eye. In: *Book of Abstracts, American Society of Neuroradiology.* 1991:97.

153 Kelly WM, Pagle PG, Pearson A, San Diego AG, Soloman MA.

154 Williams S, Char DH, Dillon WP, Lincoff N, Moseley M. Ferrous intraocular foreign bodies and magnetic resonance imaging. *Am J Ophthalmol* 1988;105:398−401.

155 McGuinness TP. Hypnosis in the treatment of phobias: a review of the literature. *Am J Clin Hyp* 1984;26:261−272.

156 Flaherty JA, Hoskinson K. Emotional distress during magnetic resonance imaging. *New Engl J Med* 1989;320:467−468.

157 Fishbain DA, Goldberg M, Labbe E, Zacher D, Steele-Rosomoff R, Rosomoff H. Long-term claustrophobia following magnetic resonance imaging. *Am J Psych* 1988;145:1038−1039.

158 Quirk ME, Letendre AJ, Ciottone RA, Lingley JF. Anxiety in patients undergoing MR imaging. *Radiology* 1989;170:463−466.

159 Quirk ME, Letendre AJ, Ciottone RA, Lingley JF. Evaluation of three psychological interventions to reduce anxiety during MR imaging. *Radiology* 1989;173:759−762.

160 Hricak H, Amparo EG. Body MRI: alleviation of claustrophobia by prone positioning. *Radiology* 1984;152:819.

161 Weinreb JC, Maravilla KR, Peshock R, Payne J. Magnetic resonance imaging: improving patient tolerance and safety. *Am J Roentgenol* 1984;143:1285−1287.

162 Klonoff EA, Janata JW, Kaufman B. The use of systematic desensitization to overcome resistance to magnetic resonance imaging (MRI) scanning. *J Behav Ther Exper Psych* 1986;17:189−192.

163 Granet RB, Gelber LJ. Claustrophobia during MR imaging. *New Jers Med* 1990;87(6):479−482.

164 Phelps LA. MRI and claustrophobia. *Am Fam Phys* 1990;42(4):930.

165 Karlik SJ, Heatherley T, Pavan F *et al.* Patient anesthesia and monitoring at a 1.5 T MRI installation. *Mag Reson Med* 1988;7:210−221.

166 Barnett GH, Ropper AH, Johnson KA. Physiological support and monitoring of critically ill patients during magnetic resonance imaging. *J Neurosurg* 1988;68:244−250.

167 Dunn V, Coffman CE, McGowan JE, Ehrhardt JC. Mechanical ventilation during magnetic resonance imaging. *Mag Reson Imag* 1985;3:169−172.

168 McArdle CB, Nicholas DA, Richardson CJ, Amparo EG. Monitoring of the neonate undergoing MR imaging: technical considerations. *Radiology* 1986;159:223−226.

169 Roth JL, Nugent M, Gray JE *et al.* Patient monitoring during magnetic resonance imaging. *Anesthesiology* 1985;62:80−83.

170 Shellock FG. Monitoring during MRI. An evaluation of the effect of high-field MRI on various patient monitors. *Med Electron* 1986;September:93−97.

171 Shellock FG. Monitoring sedated patients during MRI. *Radiology* 1990;177:586 (Letter).

172 Wendt RE, Rokey R, Vick GW, Johnston DL. Electrocardiographic gating and monitoring during NMR imaging. *Mag Reson Imag* 1988;6:89−95.

173 Holshouser BA, Hinshaw DB, Shellock FG. Sedation, anesthesia, and physiologic monitoring during MRI, American Roentgen Ray Society, Catagorical Course Syllabus. In: Hasso AN, Stark DD eds. *Spine and Body Magnetic Resonance Imaging.* May 1991.

174 Kanal E, Applegate GR. Thermal injuries/incidents associated with MR imaging devices in the US: a compilation and review of the presently available data. In: *Book of Abstracts, Society for Magnetic Resonance Imaging.* 1990:274.

175 Shellock FG, Slimp G. Severe burn of the finger caused by using a pulse oximeter during MRI. *Am J Roentgenol* 1989;153:

1105.

176 Kanal E, Shellock FG. Burns associated with clinical MR examinations. *Radiology* 1990;175:585.

177 Shellock FG, Myers SM, Kimble K. Monitoring heart rate and oxygen saturation during MRI with a fiber-optic pulse oximeter. *Am J Roentgenol.* (In press).

178 Goldstein HA, Kashanian FK, Blumetti RF, Holyoak WL, Hugo FP, Blumenfield DM. Safety assessment of gadopentetate dimeglumine in U.S. clinical trials. *Radiology* 1990;174:17−23.

179 Kanal E, Applegate GR, Gillen CP. Review of adverse reactions, including anaphylaxia, in 4260 intravenous bolus injections. *Radiology* 1990;177(P):159.

180 Haustein J, Endorf HP, Louton T. Renal tolerance of Gd-DTPA. a retrospective evaluation of 1,171 patients. *Mag Reson Imag* 1990;8(Suppl. 1):43.

181 Schmiedl U, Maravilla KR, Gerlach R, Dowling CA. Excretion of gadopentetate dimeglumine in human breast milk. *Am J Roentgenol* 1990;154:1305−1306.

CHAPTER 12

Lasers

Barry A. Sacks and Michael S. Feld

Introduction

This chapter concentrates on the complications of laser therapy, but to understand fully how and why these occur, it is important to discuss some basic technical and clinical concepts in laser therapy. This includes information about lasers, transmission of laser energy to the target site, the interaction of laser light and biologic tissue, and lastly, the concepts involved in designing a laser/catheter system. An understanding of this information will give the reader a better insight into laser applications and pitfalls of this form of therapy.

Established medical applications of lasers are in the fields of dermatology, ophthalmology, general surgery, gynecology, and to a lesser degree, urology, vascular surgery, and neurosurgery. In most of these applications, the laser light is delivered directly to the tissue target site, usually by an articulated arm. Because the laser delivery is simple, the choice of lasers is almost unlimited and can be decided depending on the required clinical effect. Endoscopic and angiographic applications require transmission of the laser light to a remote treatment site by *optical fibers*. This results in a number of limitations. In some instances, the most appropriate laser cannot be used because there are no suitable fibers to transmit that particular wavelength, the available fibers cannot transmit sufficient light for a therapeutic effect, or the suitable fibers may be either too inflexible or biologically incompatible. As a result, there are many trade-offs

when deciding to use the best combination of laser, dosimetry, and fibers for a specific indication.

Although there are a number of potential uses of laser therapy in interventional radiology, the largest experience is in the treatment of stenotic or occlusive atherosclerotic vascular disease. Most of this chapter will therefore be dedicated to vascular applications and their complications. The initial hope with laser angioplasty, or as we prefer, laser angiosurgery (LAS), was that it would solve a number of the inadequacies in percutaneous transluminal angioplasty (PTA) and atherectomy. Specifically, complete removal of the occlusive plaque and in an atraumatic way, giving a more predictable result and also reducing restenosis, as well as the ability to treat *diffuse* disease. Despite very optimistic initial results, it has been shown convincingly over the long term that laser treatment of atherosclerotic disease, at least as currently applied, offers very little real advantage over standard PTA.

The standard abbreviations for the units used throughout the text are defined in Table 12.1.

Lasers

The term laser stands for light amplification by stimulated emission of radiation. Regular white light from a light bulb is comprised of multiple wavelengths (all colors), dispersed in all different directions. Laser light, on the other hand, is pure, consisting of light waves of only one color or

Table 12.1 Units and definitions

Laser wavelength

Micron (μm)	10^{-6} m
Nanometer (nm)	10^{-9} m

Laser pulse duration

CW	Continuous
Millisecond (ms)	10^{-3} s
Microsecond (μs)	10^{-6} s
Nanosecond (ns)	10^{-9} s
Picosecond (ps)	10^{-12} s
Femtosecond (fs)	10^{-15} s

Laser energy parameters

Energy	Joule (J)
Fluence	J/mm^2
Power	Watt (W) (J/s)
Intensity (or irradiance)	W/mm^2

wavelength (monochromatic), all going in the same direction with a well-defined phase (coherent). Lasers have been developed to produce wavelengths throughout the electro-magnetic spectrum, from the far infrared (IR) to the ultra-violet (UV). The emitted laser light may be either continuous (CW) or pulsed. The pulses of pulsed lasers can vary in length from 0.25 seconds to as short as a few femtoseconds (10^{-15} seconds), and at variable repetition rates.

In its simplest form, a laser consists of a container with an amplifying medium placed between two mirrors aligned in parallel (optical resonator). The amplifying medium can be a gas, liquid, or solid. A laser can be viewed as an energy conversion device, in which the energy that activates the amplifying medium is converted into coherent light. Molecules within the amplifying medium are brought to an excited state, from which they can amplify light of a particular wavelength by a process known as stimulated emission. Photons of this wavelength traversing the amplifying medium grow in number, and after each pass the photons are reflected by the mirrors and undergo further amplification. The process is repeated many times, giving rise to a very large build-up of light. The parallel mirrors establish the direction-ality and collimation of the light waves. One of the mirrors is partially transmitting, typically 1%, allowing a beam of light to emerge for use.

Whereas most lasers generate light at a single, fixed wave-length, in others the emission wavelength can be varied or "tuned". The most important type of tunable laser for medical applications is the dye laser [1–3], in which a solution of dye is used as the amplifying medium. By inserting a rotatable prism (or other frequency selective filter) into the laser resonator, any desired output wavelength over a wide range of visible wavelengths can be selected.

Another important method of achieving different wave-lengths is nonlinear frequency mixing. As an example, infrared Nd:YAG laser light (wavelength 1.06 μm) can be "frequency doubled" in a mixing crystal to produce green light (530 nm), which is half the wavelength (twice the frequency) of the original light. Similarly, laser beams of two different frequencies can be "mixed" to produce light at the sum or difference frequency. Using these techniques, coherent radiation can be produced at virtually any desired wavelength in the UV, visible, or IR.

Laser–tissue interactions

Laser light is a source of energy delivered to a target, and the target for medical applications is biologic tissue. How the laser light interacts with the tissue depends on numerous variable factors, some related to laser parameters (wave-length, power, exposure time, CW, or pulsed), some to the tissue parameters (tissue composition, chromophores, calcification, vascularity), and others to the medium through which the light must travel in order to reach the tissue (air, saline, or blood). From all these variables, an enormous number of different combinations of therapeutic options are available. The challenge is to find the right combination of laser wavelength and dosage parameters to achieve the optimal required diagnostic or therapeutic effect.

The biochemical constituents in tissue that absorb light are called chromophores. The absorbed light excites chromo-phore molecules, changing their internal energy states in various ways. In most cases, this energy is converted to heat. This heating can raise the tissue temperature and, depending on the degree and rapidity, can change its phase (e.g., from solid to liquid, or liquid to vapor), and/or give rise to chemical decomposition. The heat will also diffuse to adjacent areas not directly illuminated by the laser light, causing indirect heating, usually at a lower temperature. Note that since light diffuses (scatters) much more rapidly than does heat, primary deposition of laser energy is nearly instan-taneous, whereas its subsequent thermal diffusion is rela-tively slow. Other types of laser–tissue phenomena include *shock wave formation*, which occurs when a large amount of energy is deposited very rapidly sending a mechanical wave through the tissue, and *ionization*, in which a very hot gaseous "plasma" (cloud of electrons) is formed and the plasma secondarily affects the tissue.

The power, diameter, and pulse duration of the laser beam determine which physical effects predominate. One can therefore tailor the laser–tissue interaction process to achieve the desired effect [4–19]. Laser light can be used to coagulate blood, incise, vaporize or fuse tissues, fragment calcifications, and rupture fibrous bands [10,20–30]. Each indication requires a different set of laser parameters, mode of delivery, and medium through which the laser light has to travel.

Understanding these basic laser–tissue interactions makes

it possible to adopt an educated approach to selection of the correct laser parameters and system components to accomplish the desired therapeutic result. The following section details the varying tissue responses to laser light, and the dangers both to the target and surrounding tissue. It also gives a slightly more detailed explanation of the different types of specific laser–tissue interactions.

Photocoagulation

Photocoagulation occurs when tissue is heated to a temperature high enough to cause denaturation of the structural proteins or damage to cell membranes or other small intracellular structures. This results in coagulative necrosis. This technique is used to coagulate tiny blood vessels to stop bleeding (cauterization). With rapid heating this usually occurs at about 60°C, but the exact same effect can be achieved by using lower temperatures for a longer time. CW Nd:YAG laser radiation at 1.06 μm is particularly well suited to this purpose. This near-infrared wavelength is weakly absorbed and penetrates deeply, heating a large volume of tissue.

Laser-induced photochemical changes

Laser light absorbed in tissue can excite chromophore molecules. Depending on the wavelength, intensity, and pulse duration of the light, this excitation can take many forms. Molecules raised to an excited state may become more reactive and combine chemically with other molecules. These chemical processes are well understood from studies in gaseous and other simple systems, but are not well established in the complex environment of biologic tissue. Processes sometimes attributed to laser photochemistry are often more likely due to thermal effects.

Shock fragmentation

Another process closely related to ablation is the fragmentation of mineralized deposits such as kidney and gallstones. In this case, a short pulse of laser light penetrates deeply into the stone, imparting shock waves. Where it is strongly and rapidly absorbed by small internal inhomogeneities, this can shatter the stone, and the resulting small fragments can more easily pass down the bile duct or ureter. Pulsed visible dye laser radiation is often used for this purpose. This process has been termed laser lithotripsy [31].

Plasma tissue removal

At sufficiently high laser intensities, the laser electric field becomes large enough substantially to accelerate electrons in the vaporized material. These then collide with tissue molecules, producing free electrons and ions. These charged particles are themselves accelerated by the laser field, resulting in further ionization. A dense hot plasma, composed of equal numbers of electrons and ions, develops. Plasma formation is usually accompanied by an audible "crack" and spark. The growing plasma strongly absorbs the laser light, producing temperatures as high as several thousand degrees centigrade. Such temperatures are sufficient to evaporate both calcified and soft components of tissue. Nanosecond pulses of Nd:YAG laser radiation at 1.06 μm produce ablation of this type.

Tissue ablation

Atraumatic removal — or more crudely put, tissue ablation — is the reaction desirable for the treatment of stenotic or occlusive vascular disease. This can be achieved in many different ways.

Hot tip tissue removal

Soft tissue can be removed by direct application of heat. A metal cap heated to several hundred degrees Celsius by laser light delivered through an optical fiber can evaporate the liquid component of soft tissue on contact. The energy is delivered by *thermal diffusion*, and the laser light plays no direct role in tissue removal. The device functions as a very sophisticated soldering tool. Thermal damage to adjacent tissue is substantial. Hot tip catheter devices with a blunt, heated metal probe at the distal end were the first to be used clinically to recanalize atherosclerotic vessels.

Laser–tissue ablation

This should be subdivided into ablation of "soft" and "hard" tissues. The latter refers to any tissue that contains either calcification or bone elements.

Soft tissues of the body contain a high percentage of water. They can be ablated by rapidly boiling the tissue water, thus evaporating it. The evaporation is so rapid, that microscopic tissue fragments are ejected at the same time. The energy required to heat and evaporate 1 mm^3 of soft tissue, assuming the tissue to be water, is about 2.5 J. (One joule is the power delivered by a 1-W laser beam in 1 second.)

Hard tissues such as bone and calcified plaque, on the other hand, are structurally different from soft tissue. Such tissues are composed of a distribution of small hard particles in a matrix of softer material [32]. For example, bone consists mainly of micron-sized microcrystalites of calcium hydroxyapatite embedded in collagen, with very little water present. The removal process and laser dosimetry parameters are therefore quite different. Different mechanisms have been proposed to explain how hard tissue is ablated. Some researchers have invoked photochemical decomposition and rapid breaking of structural bonds to account for the "cold" cutting and other features of excimer lasers [8–10,27,33–35]. Other studies suggest that the process is instead due to gas dynamic heating, in which the laser radiation rapidly vaporizes the soft component, and as this exits, it forcefully drags away the hard microparticles [28,32]. With appropriate laser parameters the particles generated in this blast can be very small, typically 1 μm or less in size, and unlikely to be an embolization threat to the distal tissue capillary bed.

Laser light is required for hard tissue ablation, because of the sufficiently high intensities required to evaporate the soft material rapidly enough to entrain the hard particles. Examples of lasers used to ablate hard tissue include the xenon fluoride excimer laser at a wavelength of 308 nm (UV), the pulsed dye laser at 480 nm (visible), and the hydrogen fluoride laser at 2.5 mm (IR).

Lasers, optics, and accessories

Optical fibers and catheters

As already suggested, optical fibers, which conduct light through circuitous pathways, are essential for transmission of the laser energy to the treatment site in both endoscopy and interventional radiology [4,7]. Because of the technical limitations, only certain wavelengths can be considered for optical fiber applications. These fibers also have to be able to withstand certain energy densities and peak powers. The fibers also have the physical characteristics that make them practical for clinical use. This includes flexibility, biological compatibility, safety, and nontoxic.

Fibers can be made of glass, quartz (actually fused silica), plastic, or other transparent materials. An optical fiber consists of a transmitting core surrounded by a thin layer of cladding material with a slightly lower refractive index, and is usually encased by a protective buffer coating. The fibers used in most medical applications have cores that are 100–400 μm in diameter. Light is coupled into the core by means of a lens.

Optical fibers are limited in their ability to carry pulsed laser light, and this is a hurdle for endoscopic and percutaneous applications. A light pulse will "break down" the fiber if its peak power exceeds a certain maximum value, or if too much energy is concentrated in too short a time. In addition, UV light can "solarize" an optical fiber, darkening it and limiting its useful life. Compromises must be made between what is ideal and what is feasible. Ideal fiber characteristics include safety, flexibility, reliability, transmission with negligible loss, and the ability to conduct light of adequate power and energy.

Computers and automatic mechanisms for controlling light

In complex laser delivery systems it is desirable to have the treatment parameters under computer control. This is especially true when multifiber catheters are used, and particularly when two or more functions (e.g., diagnosis and therapy) are combined in a single system. Hardware and software efficiently to run the various systems continues to be developed and improved.

Clinical applied systems

Because of the large number of variables and possible solutions, different investigators took very different approaches in applying laser therapy in the treatment of vascular disease (Fig. 12.1). The preceding discussion on the basic issues will help the reader to understand the thinking behind the development and application of the different clinical systems. The following is not only a summary of all the available systems, but also reflects the historic evolution of the clinical approaches. When a system was found to be lacking in certain qualities, e.g., the complication rate was too high, applications too limited, or the resultant recanalization inadequate, modifications were made to overcome these drawbacks. Rather than give a summary of every clinical study for each system, the clinical efficacy and results are given in Tables 12.2 & 12.3. This should allow a side by side comparison of the advantages and disadvantages of each, as well as indicate the particular problems specific to that system.

Bare fiber delivery devices

The first laser catheters used to treat atherosclerotic vascular disease employed an optical fiber introduced through a standard angiographic catheter at the time of diagnostic arteriography [36,37]. The catheter and fiber were positioned at the site of the obstruction, the laser fired, and the fiber alternately advanced and fired until the lesion was traversed. Unfortunately, clinical results were poor and the incidence of complications unacceptably high [36–41].

Adequate control of the light beam was difficult. As a result of this a number of complications were noted.
1 Too many perforations occurred as a result of either the misdirected beam burning through the vessel wall or the sharp inflexible fiber mechanically perforating it.
2 Coagulation of intervening blood between fiber and plaque produced microemboli.
3 The recanalized channel was very small, always requiring adjunctive PTA. The technique really did not offer any advantage over the sequence of passing a guidewire through the occlusion, particularly the new hydrophilically coated wires, or PTA.

The only well-documented clinical study using bare single-fiber delivery is that of Ginsberg *et al.* [36,37]. In that study, they modified the technique slightly to prevent perforation, advancing the catheter through the entire stenosis first (Dotter technique), positioning the optical fiber tip just

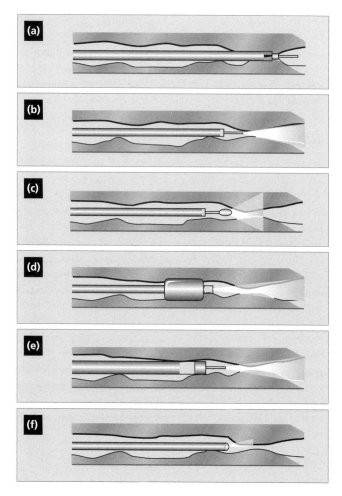

Fig. 12.1 Methods attempted to overcome the problems with bare fibers. (a, b) Initially, a catheter and fiber were advanced through the stenosis. With the fiber protruding beyond the catheter, the laser is fired on *withdrawal* through the stenosis. (c) The fiber can be modified by creating a ball tip. This has two functions: (i) to present a blunt end that is less traumatic; and (ii) to create a larger lumen both as a result of its increased tip size and devergence of the light. (d) Addition of a centering balloon allows clearing of the blood between the fiber and target and maintains the optical fiber axially within the lumen. (e) Angioscopic control theoretically affords laser therapy under direct vision. (f) Development of multifiber devices eliminates many of the problems associated with a single fiber.

beyond the catheter tip, and firing the laser during retrograde withdrawal of the entire unit through the stenotic or occlusive region. Despite initial enthusiasm with the first few cases, the study was abandoned after poor results in 16 patients.

Blunt tip catheters

Blunt tip catheters are single-fiber devices terminated at the distal end with an enlarged bulbous tip. The enlarged rounded tip served two purposes: better control (fewer perforations) as well as creation of a larger recanalized lumen. No substantial clinical experience was gained using these fibers.

Heated tip catheter

This approach used a laser source and a metal tipped optical fiber (Fig. 12.2). Instead of using the direct laser light to recanalize the vessel, a metal cap was firmly attached to the distal end of the fiber in a round blunted configuration. The laser beam, transmitted down the fiber, heated the metal cap to between 300 and 400°C. In other words, the laser was used as a very expensive energy source to create a hot poker. When the cap is brought in direct contact with the target tissue, the hot metal surface vaporizes the water within the tissue and partially decomposes the fibrous material (structural protein), shrinking it. The net effect is to debulk the tissue and enlarge the lumen. The recanalized lumen is substantially wider than that provided by a bare fiber alone.

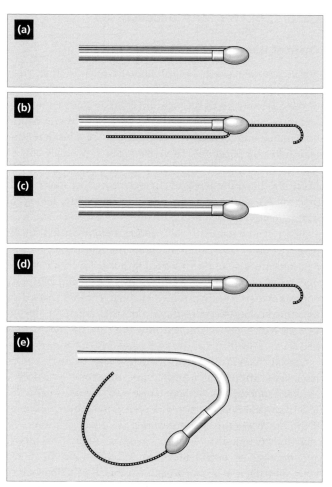

Fig. 12.2 Hot tip devices. (a) Standard Trimedyne laser probe. Metal cap at the end of an optical fiber. On the side is a safety wire to prevent loss of the metal cap. (b) Hot tip device with a guidewire. This addition was made to avoid possible perforation during advancement of the laser probe. (c) The Hybrid Trimedyne laser probe. This has a hole in the metal cap which allows transmission of a small amount of laser light through a sapphire shield. Thus, both the heated cap and direct laser light have an effect in recanalization.

The blunt shape of the metal tip also reduces, but does not eliminate, the likelihood of mechanical perforation. A metal tip catheter heated to 400°C cannot evaporate calcified plaque.

A modified version of this device, called the *Hybrid* catheter, is provided with a hole in the metal cap which allows about 20% of the laser light through directly to irradiate the target tissue [42]. However, with the latter design, direct contact or saline irrigation is required to remove blood from the field, particularly when argon ion laser light is used. A subsequent design has a small sapphire chip within the hole, between the fiber and the tissue.

Hot tip catheters were used to recanalize completely occluded arterial segments which could not be crossed with a standard guidewire. This was a major application in superficial femoral and popliteal arteries. It was only used occasionally below the knee or in the iliac system. Experience in the coronary and tibial vessels has shown mixed results, because thermal contact seems to induce considerable spasm in smaller vessels. In principle, in vessels 2−3 mm in diameter, the hot tip probe should have achieved an adequately recanalized lumen by itself, but in practice this was not always so. In larger vessels, the recanalized lumen was maximally 3 mm (limited by the size of the catheter that could be inserted through the percutaneous puncture hole). As a result, PTA was obligatory.

Several investigators have reported recanalization of occluded segments using the device, but without switching the laser on! Evidently, the rigid shaft and the "bullet" shape permit some completely occluded lesions to be crossed mechanically, equivalent to a "Dotterization" technique.

The energy source to heat the metal cap of a hot tip catheter need not be laser light. Electrical, chemical, and radiofrequency (RF) sources can all be used [43,44]. A RF probe, similar in configuration to the Trimedyne device — essentially an intravascular electrocautery device — was also evaluated. The cost would have been a fraction of the equivalent laser-heated system. The device failed to gain popularity.

Numerous clinical publications have described experience with the Trimedyne device in the superficial femoral artery (SFA)/popliteal region [18,45−63]. The results from many different investigators were comparable, independent of whether the probes were introduced surgically or percutaneously. In the vast majority of patients, the laser probe was used to create a pilot lumen, and subsequently PTA was performed. The hot tip catheter was used as "stand-alone" therapy in a few cases of distal popliteal and tibial disease. Using the Hybrid laser probe, Barbeau *et al.* [42] treated 51 lesions in 49 patients. The results were not significantly different from the standard hot tip studies.

Over 100 peripheral artery and numerous animal coronary laser thermal angioplasties were performed before the first patient with coronary artery disease was treated. The initial coronary artery studies were performed in two centers, one in England, the other in Boston, USA [59]. In the Boston study only high-grade stenoses were treated, but in England short occlusions were attempted. The first coronary laser probe was a modified 1.7-mm device and could only be used in straight sections of the coronary arteries. Subsequently, a more flexible heated tip "coil" catheter that could be advanced over a guidewire, allowed treatment of many more lesions. In a series by Linnemeier *et al.* [49], 29 coronary lesions were managed in 27 patients (12 native vessels and 17 saphenous vein grafts). Over-the-wire heated tip probes of varying sizes were used with either an argon or Nd·YAG laser source. In all but two lesions, subsequent PTA was performed.

Like the Trimedyne experience, data from clinical trials using the sapphire tip devices suggest primary results similar to that of conventional PTA. Adjunctive PTA is still necessary to create an adequately recanalized lumen.

Sapphire tip catheter

The design concept of the sapphire tip laser catheter, adapted from that of surgical laser systems, is similar to that of the hot tip catheters, but instead of a metal cap the distal tip is terminated in a sapphire bulb [26,64−66]. The sapphire tip also works as a direct contact device. Tissue is heated by two processes. First, the tip heats up considerably, providing appreciable thermal conduction to the tissue. In addition, laser light diffuses through the transparent tip, applying laser energy directly to the tissue. The laser source is usually CW light from a Nd:YAG laser ($1.06 \, \mu m$).

The configurations and heating characteristics of sapphire tip and hot tip devices are similar, and much of the discussion about the operating principles and performance of the hot tip devices also apply to sapphire tip catheters.

Sapphire tip devices are manufactured by Surgical Laser Technologies. Although used extensively in Europe, Food and Drugs Administration (FDA) trials in the USA were limited. The probe and disposables are considerably more expensive than the Trimedyne probes. Sapphire tip catheters are still in limited use in Europe. The largest reported multi-center study of 259 femoropopliteal occlusions [66], mean length 7.5 cm, demonstrated an 84% primary success rate. Long-term patency after 2 years was 74%. These results are impressive, and similar success has been confirmed by other workers (W. Arlart and L. Lorelius, personal communication).

Thermal PTA

Using this technique, laser energy was not used directly to recanalize vessels but rather to improve the results of conventional PTA and reduce the complications. The device is a modified angioplasty balloon catheter with a transparent balloon that both transmits laser light and can withstand

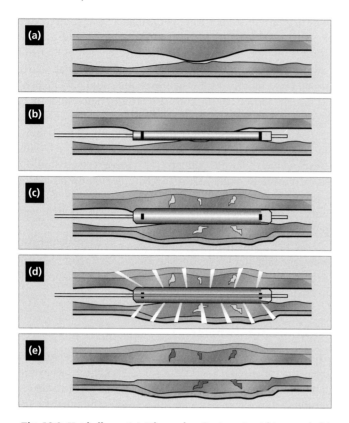

Fig. 12.3 Hot balloon. (a) Atherosclerotic stenosis within vessel. (b) Initial introduction of specialized angioplasty balloon. (c) Lesion dilated in standard fashion, with resultant disruption of the intima and the usual expected dissections. (d) Diffusing laser fiber illuminated with a Nd:YAG laser, causes heating of the vessel wall and fusing of the dissections to the media. (e) Following removal of the catheter, the lumen remains patent, preventing acute reclosure or thrombosis.

high temperatures (Fig. 12.3). Angioplasty was performed in the usual way and during balloon inflation a special 100-μm optical fiber with a helical diffusing tip was placed within the balloon. CWIR light from a Nd:YAG laser (1.06 μm) was transmitted through the walls of the balloon, radially heating the remodeled vessel wall [13,14,67].

The effects were threefold: (i) the dissected intimal flaps would be sealed against the media; (ii) the muscle wall itself would be altered; and (iii) any thrombus associated with the lesion would be dehydrated and remodeled. The sealed flaps would prevent dissection, avoiding potential acute closure. The heat was also intended to kill smooth muscle cells and completely denature the collagen in the artery wall, effectively producing a relatively rigid biologic stent. It was hoped that the effect of heating the vessel wall might also modify the cascade of events that result ultimately in intimal hyperplasia and restenosis.

The device was not difficult to manufacture and the technology straightforward to apply. The danger of damaging the artery wall during irradiation was less than for direct laser

ablation because the energy is diffused more evenly. Accurate temperature control was a concern as tissue temperature had to be maintained between 120 and 140°C. (The outer limits are 110−150°C.) Above this range, tissue damage and "hot tip" removal occurred. At lower temperatures, sealing was incomplete. Maintenance of a uniform temperature over the entire length of the balloon and throughout the thickness of the artery wall was difficult.

A published series of 55 patients [67] demonstrated excellent primary technical success (as would be expected in view of the similarity to conventional PTA). No deaths or major complications were attributable to the procedure. A slightly improved luminal diameter was achieved in this group, suggesting that the heat does improve the effectiveness of balloon dilatation. Among patients who were categorized as being of high risk for acute reclosure, either because of a prior such event or the appearance of the lesion, all were treated successfully. The experience is now much larger, with 350 patients having undergone laser balloon angioplasty (LBA), 130 of these in the high-risk category for acute reclosure (R. Spears, personal communication). The results have followed those of the initial experience, with very few minor complications.

The thermal PTA device, called the LBA catheter, was developed by USCI-Bard. The initial hopes for this approach were not realized and the long-term success rate was perhaps even worse than for standard angioplasty. Restenosis rates were extremely high, and as a consequence of this, the technique has been abandoned.

As with the electrically and RF-heated hot tip catheters, other methods of more cheaply heating balloons were explored. Note, however, that RF heating of the surface of a balloon is not identical to the radiant heating of LBA, in which the laser light penetrating the balloon material directly heats the tissue.

LASTAC system

The LASTAC system employed a single-fiber delivery catheter with a lens at its distal tip to diverge the laser beam. To prevent perforation, the fiber was centered within the vessel lumen by means of a modified angioplasty balloon. Another channel provided irrigation to remove blood from the segment between the fiber tip and atherosclerotic lesion. The LASTAC catheter system (developed by GV Medical, Minneapolis) was designed to treat totally occluded vessels [68−71]. The system used blue−green light from an 18 W CW argon ion laser.

The technique (Fig. 12.4) involved advancing the catheter to the site of the obstruction, inflating the centering balloon, and replacing the blood between the catheter tip and the lesion with saline solution. The fiber was introduced and positioned a fixed distance away from the lesion. The laser was fired, creating a channel in the occluded segment, and

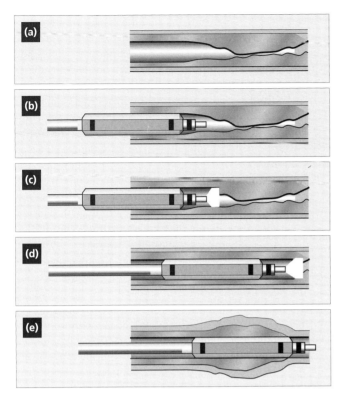

Fig. 12.4 LASTAC system. (a) Artery showing atherosclerotic stenosis. (b) LASTAC catheter advanced to lesion, balloon inflated, and blood evacuated with saline flush. (c) Argon ion laser light fired at stenosis through modified fiber. (d) After deflating the balloon, the catheter is advanced into the newly created channel and reinflated; in principle, angioplasting the segment. (e) Steps (b–d) repeated until the lesion has been completely traversed.

the catheter then advanced. This sequence was repeated until the obstruction was traversed. The recanalized lumen is approximately 1.5–2.0 mm in diameter. Each time the centering balloon was inflated, it also performed an angioplasty on the recanalized segment. In many cases, a standard high-pressure angioplasty balloon was used after removal of the laser catheter [68].

According to Foschi [69], argon ion laser irradiation facilitates guidewire entry through total occlusions which are otherwise refractory to guidewire alone. Clinical success occurred despite the fact that CW argon ion laser light cannot ablate calcified tissue. Perhaps the soft component of plaque was sufficiently vaporized to permit guidewire and balloon catheter passage mechanically to traverse the lesion and facilitate subsequent angioplasty.

Approximately 140 peripheral cases were performed in the USA, and over 300 worldwide. An overall primary success of 88% was reported. Although the CW argon should not affect calcified plaque, a number of calcified lesions were successfully treated. Nordstrom *et al.* [70–72] were the primary proponents of this technique and had the most clinical experience.

Medilase system

The Medilase system was a single fiber ablation catheter with angioscopic visualization to direct laser recanalization. A number of different catheter configurations were available, varying in size from 6 to 8 F. They all contained a fiber bundle for angioscopy, an occlusion balloon, and either three or four other lumens for irrigation and the laser ablation fiber. The catheters could be rotated to treat the entire cross-sectional area of the vessel lumen. Two separate lasers were used, a helium:neon laser for aiming and a pulsed flashlamp:pumped dye laser operating at 480 nm for ablation. No clinical data were collected to establish the effectiveness of this method.

The combination exemplified by this laser and catheter configuration may have many applications other than in the vascular system, e.g., in the management of ureteric and biliary calculi.

Multifiber laser catheters

A primary limitation of single-fiber ablation systems was the small size of the recanalized lumen, making it obligatory to use subsequent angioplasty. Multifiber laser catheters partially overcome this by using an array of fibers [73–75]. The combined effect of many fibers, each ablating a different portion of the lesion, will create a wider lumen, leaving less residual stenosis and improving the chances of longer term vessel patency. In actual practice, however, despite the larger lumen, there is almost always still a need for adjunctive angioplasty.

The distal end of a multifiber catheter is composed of an assembly of optical fibers, forming a smooth blunt tip, reducing the likelihood of mechanical perforation. The broad tip can be brought into direct contact with the lesion, displacing intervening blood. Direct contact permits the diameter of the light spots impinging on the tissue to be well defined, markedly improving the accuracy, specificity, predictability, and safety of tissue removal. Catheters with multiple small-core-diameter fibers provide flexibility as compared to a single, large diameter fiber with the same overall equivalent core area.

The following sections describe several multifiber systems using a variety of laser sources, catheter designs, and guidance techniques. All use pulsed laser light in the IR or UV range. These laser sources can ablate both calcified and noncalcified plaque without heating the vessel wall.

The recanalization procedure in all of these systems is much the same. If possible, the guidewire was advanced through the stenosis or occlusion and the laser catheter then brought into direct contact with the lesion. The laser was fired, removing the proximal end of the stenotic or occlusive lesion. The catheter was then advanced and the procedure repeated until the entire segment was recanalized. In peripheral vessels follow-up PTA was always performed, because even the largest multifiber catheters created a channel with a diameter in the range of 2.5−3.0 mm (the outer diameter of the device). The catheter diameter is limited by how safe and practical the size of the groin puncture should be. In a 5−6-mm SFA, a 2.5-mm channel would leave a 50% or greater stenosis, unequivocally requiring adjunctive PTA. In the larger iliac vessels, this would be an even more significant problem. On the other hand, in smaller vessels like the coronary or infrapopliteal arteries, laser recanalization potentially could be a "stand-alone" therapy because the size of these vessels matches the actual catheter diameter.

Most of the multifiber devices are advanced over a guidewire. Some have an additional method for guidance, namely spectroscopy.

Straightforward over-the-wire (OTW) systems

Excimer laser systems

These systems have been the most widely used clinically successful systems, and are still being used. Three systems have undergone percutaneous clinical trials in both peripheral and coronary vessels: two American (AIS and Spectranetics) and one European (Technolas). The laser catheters used range in diameter from 1.3 to over 2 mm and have similar designs. Each company manufactures catheters consisting of a ring of optical fibers surrounding a central guidewire lumen. One contains 12 200-μm core fibers and accepts an 0.018-in (0.46 mm) guidewire: another employs 14 200-μm core fibers and takes a 0.013-in (0.33 mm) guidewire; the third packs 41 100-μm core fibers in a ring. Other catheters of different diameters are also in use. Two companies also manufacture a 400-μm single-fiber device for establishing an initial pilot lumen in completely occluded vessels [76].

Grundfest, Litvak, and Forrester have a tremendous clinical experience with the AIS device (Fig. 12.5) [5,8−10,25,27,33, 34,43,50,76]. Their first study treated patients with femoro-popliteal stenoses and occlusions. For the occlusions, to create a pilot channel, a single-fiber catheter 400 μm in diameter was used to create a 1.2-mm channel, similar to the techniques already described, the only difference being the use of an excimer laser. For stenoses, a 1.4-mm diameter seven-fiber laser catheter was used over a guidewire. Primary technical success was approximately 85%, with almost all patients undergoing subsequent PTA to achieve adequate recanalization. Biamino [77] reported clinical results using the Technolas system in 208 patients with ileofemoral disease.

Early results in coronary arteries have been reported for several multifiber OTW systems [57,78−80]. A relatively large experience has been gathered. Litvak and Margolis

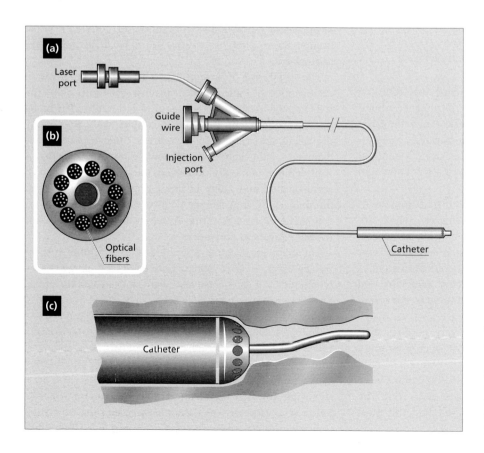

Fig. 12.5 AIS device. (a) A gross schematic view of the earlier AIS device. This is a multifiber device with a variety of outside diameters, fiber sizes, and number. Various ports allow contrast injection, a guidewire, and the laser light ablation. A number of subsequent improvements have been made. (b) The end-on view demonstrating the ring of fibers around a central guidewire lumen.

[81] summarized use of the AIS system in coronary arteries in 958 patients with 1151 lesions in the USA. (There have been additional cases in Europe.) Ghazzal *et al.* [82], in 1992, reported a series of 203 patients (220 lesions) treated with excimer laser systems, using 1.3-, 1.6-, and 2.0-mm diameter laser catheters. All residual stenoses greater than 40–50% underwent PTA.

Bittl [77] reported on the experience thus far with the Spectranetics excimer laser system. The multicenter experience with 284 patients and 314 lesions in coronary arteries was described. Stand-alone laser catheter therapy was performed in 14% of the cases treated.

Although unpublished, many more cases both in peripheral and coronary arteries have been performed using excimer systems (W. Grunfest, J. Isner, & G. Biamino, personal communication), in the range of thousands, but the results have really not changed. These have, however, only been performed in a few centers that have continued to try and advance the technology, resolve the pitfalls, or in the rare complicated case in which other technologies are unsuccessful.

IR delivery systems

A Ho/Tm:YAG multifiber OTW delivery system (Fig. 12.6) has been developed by Eclipse Surgical Technologies [78]. One catheter design is similar to the 1.6-mm UV laser catheters described above. In addition, Eclipse has developed a multifiber OTW catheter with a different configuration. A tapered tip projects beyond the ring of 26–37 100–150-mm fibers. By advancing this tip into the stenotic lesion, the catheter is centered and the fibers brought into direct contact with the plaque. Subsequent PTA is carried out in most cases. However, in some patients with coronary artery disease,

laser catheter recanalization alone is adequate. Catheter sizes vary from 1.5 to 2.0 mm in diameter.

Murphy-Chutorian [77] reported results with the Eclipse system in peripheral and coronary arteries. In peripheral vessels, 72 lesions were treated in 50 patients. In coronary arteries, 30 lesions were treated in 29 patients. Primary success of 80% was reported. Stand-alone laser catheter therapy was performed in 38% of the cases treated.

Spectroscopically guided systems

Spectral diagnosis is a promising technique for guiding LAS. As with intravascular ultrasound, information about tissue type, specifically normal arterial wall versus atherosclerotic plaque, can be gathered at the site of stenosis or obstruction and help make treatment decisions [83–86].

Spectroscopic information gathered by the catheter is analyzed by computer and a decision made whether or not to remove it. At present, laser-induced fluorescence (LIF) is the spectroscopic technique that is the most well developed for this purpose but near infrared raman spectroscopy may eventually surpass it [87,88]. It is performed by delivering a weak excitation laser light of an appropriate wavelength to the target tissue and collecting the return fluorescence. This is then analyzed by a spectrometer to provide diagnostic information. If the "feedback" signal indicates that the fiber is pointed at atherosclerotic plaque, a computer automatically triggers the decision to deliver an ablation dose of laser light; if not, the tissue is spared. The laser catheter is advanced after ablation, and the diagnosis/ablation sequence repeated until the lesion is crossed.

LIF guidance can, of course, be combined with OTW guidance to provide an extra margin of safety. On the other hand, if used without a guidewire, totally occluded vessels can also be treated.

MCM "smart" laser catheter

MCM Laboratories performed tests on a laser catheter with spectroscopic guidance. This catheter used a single 200-μm core silica fiber for both spectroscopy and ablation. Two different laser sources were used, a 325-nm He:Cd laser for spectroscopy and a 480-nm pulsed dye laser for ablation [1,2,89–91]. LIF return light from the fiber was spectrally analyzed and used to produce an electronic feedback signal for controlling the firing of the ablation laser.

The MCM system was a pioneering effort but had several difficulties in design. The use of 480-nm light for ablation is a poor choice for tissue removal, exfoliating surface material and producing fragments of debris (microemboli). In addition, light at this wavelength penetrates relatively deeply into tissue, and the resulting ablation craters are deeper than the thickness of tissue which can be analyzed by the shallower penetrating 325-nm diagnostic wavelength. In addition, the

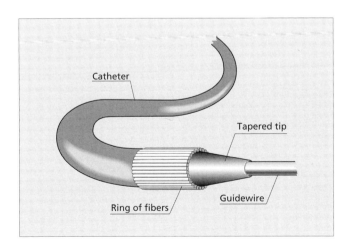

Fig. 12.6 The Eclipse system. This multifiber catheter has a ring of fibers surrounding the tapered tip. A central guidewire lumen is present.

MCM device collected diagnostic information from the entire catheter tip, thus averaging signals from both normal and diseased tissue. This provides faulty information for feedback control, which makes ablation decisions inaccurate.

Clinical results have been reported in 18 patients with femoropopliteal occlusions [2]. The National Institutes of Health (NIH) protocol used in this study required an initial attempt to pass the obstructed lesions with a conventional catheter and guidewire. This was possible in six patients. The remaining 12 patients qualified for treatment with the spectroscopically guided laser catheter. Primary recanalization and subsequent PTA was successful in 83 and 58% of the cases, respectively. PTA follow-up was always required to obtain adequate lumen size.

LAS system

Massachusetts Institute of Technology (MIT) and the Cleveland Clinic Foundation developed a multifiber laser catheter with spectroscopic guidance. This scheme, called the LAS system, incorporated features that ensure precise control of dose, as well as accurate aim [65,73–75,83,92–95]. The catheter had dual safety mechanisms, being advanced over a guidewire as well as having spectroscopic guidance capabilities.

Several variations of the catheter were produced, one having a 1.6-mm outer diameter, containing a single ring of 12 200-μm core diameter optical fibers, and a central lumen which accepts a 0.018-in (0.46 mm) standard guidewire. The fibers of the LAS catheter are enclosed in a transparent, protective "optical shield". By fixing the distance between the tips of the fibers and the shield, one can precisely select the diameter of the light spots on the output face of the shield, making it possible to determine dosimetry very accurately.

The same fibers are used for both spectroscopy and ablation. Spectral diagnosis is performed rapidly, one fiber at a time. LIF signals, produced using 1-ns pulses of 476-nm light from a nitrogen-pumped dye laser, are transmitted down the fibers, one by one. The return fluorescence signals are analyzed using an algorithm based on a model of tissue fluorescence in a turbid medium, which can differentiate normal tissue, calcified plaque, noncalcified plaque, and blood with greater than 90% accuracy [84]. A spectral image giving the distribution of these different tissue types at the catheter tip is formed. The fibers aimed at diseased tissue are automatically "armed" and, with the concurrence of the operator, the ablation laser is fired. Each fiber is separately controlled, and fibers are energized in contiguous groups. The ability selectively to activate only the desired fibers spares healthy tissue and blood, and offers the capability of treating eccentric lesions by firing only the fibers on the side containing the lesion.

The system used 355-nm ablation light from a frequency tripled solid-state Nd:YAG laser. The wavelength was chosen to fulfil two requirements: (i) it is short enough to provide shallow penetration of light into tissue, providing efficient ablation with clean cutting [32]; and (ii) it lies outside the UVB wavelength range, thus avoiding potential issues of mutagenicity [96]. In addition, the penetration depth at the diagnostic wavelength (476 nm) is three to four times larger than at the ablation wavelength, as required for proper feedback control.

An interesting technology was developed to provide pulses long enough to be transmitted through optical fibers at the desired energies [65].

Results

The results of the larger clinical series have been tabulated for easier comparison (Tables 12.2 & 12.3). A few general remarks are appropriate to understand the significance of the numbers, particularly as they look impressive. Most series have used the laser device to establish a channel through a stenosis or occlusion. If that is achieved, the procedure is considered a success. In the vast majority of

Table 12.2 Comparison of the new competitive technologies. (From Lau & Sigwart [81])

Clinical	DCA	TEC	Rotoblation	ELCA
Success (%)	85–95	90–98	85–95	85–99
Average	90	95	90	95
Diameter stenosis (%)				
Without PTCA	5–20	30–40	35–45	45–50
Adjunct PTCA required	Uncommon	32–85	30–40	40–78
(%)		60		60
Unfavorable lesions	Calcified, dissected diffuse, old SVG, complex, inexpert operator	Eccentric	NA	Ostial, chron occlus, dissection

DCA, directional coronary atherectomy; ELCA, excimer laser coronary angioplasty; NA, not available; SVG, saphenous vein graft; TEC, transluminal extraction-endarterectomy catheter.

Table 12.3 Results of large clinical trials

Number of lesions (patients)	Laser	Primary success (%)	Follow-up Patency (%)	Restenosis	Reference
1136 (967) C	308 XeCl	85	51	16.9%	Margolis [122]
55 (50) C	308 XeCl	75			Sanborn [98]
86 C	40 Ho:YAG	55		10.27	Geschwind [99]
	46 Excimer	71.7		7.24	
20 (203) C	Excimer	81.8			Ghazzal [82]
219 C	Hot tip	71	77 (1 year)		Sanborn [58]
64 C	32 Excimer	84	69 (1 year)		Huppert [66,123]
	32 Dye	78	63 (1 year)		
	32 PTCA	78	45 (1 year)		
	40 Nd:YAG	49	36 (1 year)		
	39 PTA	82	50 (1 year)		
167 (130) P	Hot tip	78–90			Leachman [124]
51 (49) P	Hybrid	81			Barbeau [42]
29 (27) C	Hot tip	83 (64% saphenous vein)	27		Linnemeier [49]
259 P	Sapphire tip	84			Lammer [66]
55 C	Laser-heated balloon				Spears [67]
68 P	LASTAC (argon)	87	75 (1 year)		Nordstrom [72]
37 (36) P		84			Foschi [69]
1151 (958) C	Excimer	92			Litvak (51%) [74]
314 (284) C	Excimer	70			Bittl (42%) [74]*
2 (50) P	Ho:YAG	80			Murphy-Chutorian [74]*
30 (29) C					
208 P	Excimer	100 (stenoses) 71 (occlusions)			Biamino [74]*

C, coronary; P, peripheral; PTCA, percutaneous transluminal coronal angioplasty.

* Spectranetics Corporation, personal communication.

cases, subsequent PTA is used, complicating evaluation. In fact, the laser has been used as the only method of recanalization in about 15% of some series.

It is important to understand that the recanalized lumen can only be as large as the outer diameter of the catheter. For practical reasons, this will always result in a recanalized channel that leaves a significant residual stenosis, particularly from the iliac to the popliteal. As a result, PTA is always necessary. Even in the infrapopliteal region and the coronary arteries, where complete recanalization with laser alone is possible, the restenosis rate is not better than plain old balloon angioplasty (POBA).

When both laser and PTA are used, is the procedure successful because of the laser device or the PTA? When there are follow-up complications, which is responsible? In many instances, the laser device was used only when conventional methods failed to traverse the lesion (in this situation the laser obviously offers something new), but in others the laser was used primarily. In many of these cases, it is entirely possible that a more standard approach may have worked. Although there are theoretical and sometimes even strong scientific reasons why one laser method is superior to others (multifiber versus single fiber, pulsed source versus CW), the reported results do not support any substantial advantage of one laser system or laser device over another.

One other important point should be made. In theory, the cases selected have been patients with more severe disease, less suited to PTA as a primary therapy. They would therefore not be expected to have as good an initial and long-term success as those who are well suited to PTA. Unfortunately, the patient selection process has not been uniform from series to series, making comparison of both method and results difficult. Definitions of a successful procedure vary. In some series, success was defined as the ability to achieve recanalization; in others, reduction in the stenosis by more than 20% for the laser alone, and a procedural success where the final stenosis reduction is more than 50% [82,97,98]. Others consider the complete procedure successful when the final residual stenosis is less than 30% [99].

Table 12.2 compares many of the new competitive technologies included in the article by Lau and Sigwart [81].

Table 12.3 demonstrates results from the larger series including the type of laser used, the primary success rate, follow-up data (where available), and the restenosis rate.

Complications

These comprise a combination of well-accepted complications that accompany all percutaneous intravascular interventions, as well as those that are more specific to the laser procedures themselves. When dealing with the specific laser complications, these can be divided into those that are general to all laser systems and those that may be specific to one particular system. The laser specific complications will be related to the laser itself (wavelength dependent, or related to CW versus pulsed delivery), or to the design of the laser catheter itself.

Overall complications can be divided into three categories.

1 *Acute* — related to the procedure itself. These include everything that can go wrong during the LAS procedure:

    (a) dissection, particularly in the total occlusions;

    (b) spasm and acute thrombosis;

    (c) perforation [100];

    (d) distal embolization;

    (e) groin hematomas;

    (f) limb loss.

2 *Subacute* — occurring immediately post procedure, to a few weeks or months later:

    (a) thrombosis;

    (b) embolization;

    (c) restenosis;

    (d) limb loss.

3 *Chronic* — occurring months later. There certainly can be overlap in the subacute and chronic categories:

    (a) restenosis;

    (b) aneurysm formation [101,102];

    (c) progression of disease.

Examples are shown in Fig. 12.7.

In dealing with the laser specific complications, a number of general points can be made. Because CW laser light is likely to be associated with more heat, the incidence of perforation, thromboembolic problems, spasm, and long-term aneurysm formation would be expected to be higher than with the pulsed systems. Dissection, although usually a technical complication, is more likely to be related to catheter design rather than the specific laser used. However, as expected, real results do not always follow the expected. What follows is a systematic reproduction of the literature, tabulating the specific incidence of complications for the different laser systems. Lau and Sigwart [81] compared the complication rate between the various methods of achieving vascular recanalization (Table 12.4). Complications from the larger series are shown in Table 12.5. The latest data from the Spectranetics excimer system are shown in Table 12.6.

Nonvascular applications for the radiologist

By and large, radiologists have not been active in development of nonvascular applications of laser therapy and diagnosis. Only a very few anecdotal reports have mentioned use by radiologists. Most of these indications are extensions of the use either by surgeons or endoscopist. Not enough is yet known about these applications really to comment on either their efficacy or the associated complications. For the sake of completeness the current status of the potential nonvascular applications is briefly discussed in the following sections.

Table 12.4 Comparison of complications. (From Lau & Sigwart [81])

Clinical	DCA	TEC	Rotoblation	ELCA
Complications (%) overall	2.3–18	2–5	3–5	5
Acute closure	1.0–3.7	1–3	6–10	2.7–7.0
Dissection	4.5	1.4	3–8	2–14
Spasm	2.5	NA	3–4	2–8
Thrombosis	NA	0.5	NA	2–6
AMI	4.8	—	6	2–3
Q wave	0.0–1.5	0.5	0.9	—
Non-Q wave	1.3–8.0	—	2.5–20.0	—
Emergency CABG	1.5–6.8	5.0–7.5	1–2	2.0–3.5
Embolization	1.0–6.9	1.4	10–20	1–2
Perforation	1–3	1–2	Rare	1.0–7.7
Death	0.0–0.6	1.5–2.0	Rare	0.3
Vascular repair	1.6–3.0	NA	NA	NA
Restenosis	30–50	40–45	30–50	30–60
Risk factors	>1 cm length, <3 mm diameter, SVG, restenosis, subint dissect, diffuse	NA	SVG, ostium prox LAD	SVG, Chronic occlus, post ELCA > 30%

AMI, acute myocardial infarction; CABG, coronary artery bypass graft; DCA, directional coronary atherectomy; ELCA, excimer laser coronary angioplasty; NA, not available; prox, proximal; SVG, saphenous vein graft; TEC, transluminal extraction-endarterectomy catheter.

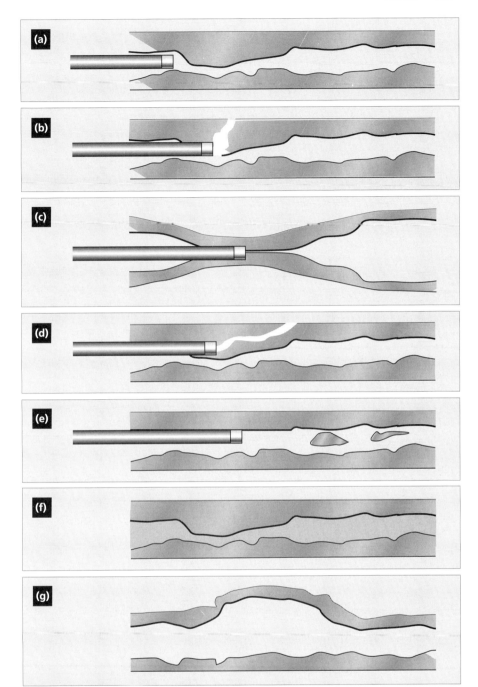

Fig. 12.7 Complications of LAS.
(a) Demonstrates the catheter in position
for laser therapy to a stenotic lesion.
(b) *Perforation* may occur as a result of
the laser beam penetrating through the
wall, or the catheter mechanically
traversing the wall. (c) *Spasm* may occur
as a result of the catheter mechanically
irritating the vessel wall, or as a
consequence of the laser ablation.
(d) *Dissection*, although often benign, can
result in acute closure of the arterial
lumen. (e) Ablated material may
embolize distally into the arterial capillary
bed. (f) *Thrombosis*, either during or
following therapy. (g) *Aneurysm*
formation occurs some time following
the procedure.

Lithotripsy [103–107]

(Urologic as well as biliary.) As discussed in the section
dealing with laser–tissue interactions, one of the mechanisms of pulsed laser light delivery, when applied to "solid"
(hard) tissue such as a renal or biliary calculus, is a shock
wave effect. This can result in fragmentation of a large stone
into multiple smaller fragments. This method of treatment is
therefore valuable in those instances where the stone is

either untreatable by standard extracaporial shock wave
lithotripsy (ESWL) or simple basket extraction.

Usually, a catheter is brought into contact with the stone
(via a nephrostomy, retrograde ureteral catheter, T-tube, or
transhepatic catheter). Even though this can be done with
simple fluoroscopic guidance, often direct visualization is
necessary (ureteroscopy, choledochoscopy, nephroscopy,
etc.). The fiber is then brought into contact with the stone
and laser energy applied. Usually, a tunable-dye laser is used

Table 12.5 Complications

Dissect.	Spasm	Thromb.	Perf.	Embol.	Em. op.	MI	Death	Hemat.	Ac. occl.	Reference
12.5	2	1.9	1.1	0.8	3.5	1.4	0		5.4	Margolis [122]
1.8	3.6	5.5	0	1.8	0	6.0	0		3.6	Sanborn [98]
										Geschwind [99]
7.5	10	15	2.5		0	0	0		7.5	(Ho)
28.3	13	6.5	2.5		0	0	0		17.1	(Exc)
16.4	1.4	4.5	1.4	1.8	2.4	0.5	0		4.5	Ghazzal [82]
2–14	2–8	2–6	1.0–7.7	1–2		2–3	0.3		2.7–7.0	Lau [125]
1.8		12	2.7					3.2		Sanborn [58]
40	0		5			8				Huppert [123]
										Lammer [126]
35		0.5		0						(Excim)
21.6		0.5		0.5						(Nd:YAG)
			10		1.1					Linnemeier [49]
		3.5	2.8					8.3		Nordstrom [72]
		Mechanical perf. 5.6								
22	6.1		2.4	2.3	3.1	3.3	0.7		6.1	Baumbach [128]
					0.6	4.6	1.0			Bittl [127]
4.5	3.5		1.4	2.4	2.1	0			0	Bittl [74]
1.8–40.0	0–13	1.9–15.0	0–10	0.0–2.7	0.0–3.5	0–6	0.0–0.3	3.2–8.3	2.7–17.0	Range

ac. occl., acute occlusion; dissect., dissection; em. op., emergency surgery; embol., embolization; hemat., groin hematoma; perf., perforation; thromb., thrombosis.

Table 12.6 Data from the Spectranetics excimer system. (From F. Stephenson, personal communication)

	Coronary	Peripheral	
	Overall $n = 695$ (%)	SCVIR Category 4 $n = 256$ (%)	Limb salavage $n = 164$ (%)
Clinical success	92.9	95 (fempop.) 92 (infrapop.)	94 (fempop.) 91 (infrapop.)
Major complications	5.2		
Dissection	4.9	0.4	0.6
Perforation	1.4	4.3	4.8
Acute reclosure	3.5	0	3.6
Embolization	2.7		
MI Q wave	0.85	0	0.6
Spasm		5.8	6.1
CABG	3.13		
Death	0.43		

CABG, coronary artery bypass graft; fempop., **femoropopliteal**; infrapop., infrapopliteal.

at 504 nm, with 1 µs pulses at 3–6 pulses/s (60 mJ/pulse). Following fragmentation, mechanical extraction or no further intervention may be instituted, depending on the specific clinical situation.

In terms of complications, these include perforation of the duct or ureter often due to mechanical injury. Perforation related to misdirected laser energy is very unusual.

Hemostasis [108]

As in the surgical management of acute bleeding, Nd:YAG laser light can be used to coagulate bleeding vessels. The major application for this is in endoscopic upper gastrointestinal bleeding. As with other indications, this function may also be accomplished using less sophisticated equipment.

Lasers as a diagnostic tool: spectroscopy [1,2,84−88,96,109−116]

Diagnostic application of laser light is an exciting new field. As already mentioned in the vascular section, LIF was used to differentiate between normal and atherosclerotic tissue. Several studies conducted on the colon, bladder and other organs have demonstrated that laser-induced fluorescence can be used to differentiate neoplastic (or potentially neoplastic) tissue from benign pathology [96,113−116]. Preliminary results have been promising and this field will almost certainly lead to new medical applications. The concept that can provide laser light histologic clues as to abnormalities of certain tissues has tremendous potential. It should be borne in mind that very few of the potential laser diagnostic approaches have even been investigated up to now.

Another spectroscopic technique, near infrared raman scattering, is also under study as a means of providing *in situ* analysis of the histological make-up of a suspected lesion in real time.

Tumor therapy [117−121]

In a manner similar to that used for other forms of tissue ablation, lasers have been used to debulk tumors, particularly those causing obstruction. Examples of this type of application include bronchoscopic ablation of obstructing endobronchial carcinomas, and endoscopic ablation of obstructing esophageal neoplasms. At this stage, the radiologists role is adjunctive; helping to guide the therapy, preprocedural planning, and postprocedural assessment of results. However, if the technique is found to have merit, there is no reason why a number of diseases should not be amenable to this approach by percutaneous means. This could include treatment of bile duct and ureteric obstructive lesions.

As already discussed, the interaction of laser light and tissue can be altered by the addition of extraneous chromophores, e.g., by giving a systemic medication. This enhanced reaction may take different forms, the most important of which is tissue destruction. This type of treatment is known as photodynamic therapy. Photochemical reactions resulting in tumor destruction have been shown to occur in patients who are first given hematoporphyrin derivative (HpD) and then exposed to 630-nm laser light. The HpD concentrates in all tissue, but clears from normal tissue much quicker, leaving higher concentrations within the tumor. Currently, however, despite clearing from normal tissue, enough remains to cause significant *photosensitivity* that lasts for a long time. Gatenby *et al.* [120] have attempted to overcome the problems with computed tomography-guided direct needle injection of HpD into the tumor. Three days later, the tumor is exposed to laser light (630 nm) via placement of a sheath in the lesion. In this way, the effect can be maximized and the side-effects minimized. Their results were a little disappointing, but they did demonstrate a variable reduction in tumor size, over a range of lesions in different locations. The complication rate was negligible, mostly pain related to the laser therapy. This form of treatment is promising and warrants further evaluation, especially if better and safer photosensitizers can be developed.

Conclusions

Laser technology has tremendous potential, not only in the vascular system but for a multitude of indications in other systems of the body. Applications in both diagnosis (spectroscopy) and therapy (ablation, fusion, coagulation, and fragmentation) are promising, and various combinations of the two appear likely.

As discussed earlier, achieving a particular biologic effect generally requires use of a specific wavelength, dosimetry, and delivery modality (CW versus pulsed). There is a vast selection of laser sources with different characteristics and, doubtless, as clinical opportunities are identified, many of these will be employed in specific applications in different medical specialties. Development of optical catheter systems to deliver the energy to remote sites, both endoscopically and percutaneously, also requires major refinement. Associated technology, including computer hardware and software, feedback sensing devices, and optical fiber development is evolving simultaneously, ultimately to be incorporated in the final systems.

LAS is probably the most complex and ambitious medical application of lasers to date. Laser catheter technology has rapidly evolved from bare fiber to heated tip and now to multifiber OTW delivery schemes; catheters incorporating feedback control are in their infancy. Laser use has shifted from CW sources (e.g., the argon ion laser) to the pulsed XeCl excimer gas laser, and now to pulsed solid-state lasers operating in the IR and UV spectral regions. In the coming years, one can expect to see continued innovations in laser catheter light delivery systems and continued major evolution of laser sources, the latter becoming smaller, cheaper, and easier to operate and maintain.

For the viability of intravascular laser therapy, a number of criteria will have to be met. The most important of these are: (i) providing the capability adequately to recanalize vessels of all sizes without needing adjunctive PTA; (ii) continuing to extend the range of vascular lesions amenable to laser therapy to include long segments of diffuse disease; and (iii) reducing the incidence of restenosis to below the level currently achieved by PTA. These are indeed challenging tasks, thus far unsuccessful.

In order to achieve a completely recanalized vessel lumen, particularly in larger vessels, a multifiber device is necessary. Recanalization is more easily achieved in the coronary arteries because of their smaller size by comparison with the iliac and proximal femoral arteries. At best, however, multifiber devices can produce channels which have the same diameter as the catheter. If the therapy is to be applied to larger vessels, methods must be developed for producing lumens significantly larger than the laser catheter's outer diameter.

Enthusiasm for vascular applications of lasers has significantly diminished in medical, industrial, and commercial circles. This is due, in part, to disappointment in the performance of hot tip laser catheters following the high level of expectations set up by premature publicity and excessive optimism in the media, coupled with the large capital investment required to develop and bring a laser treatment system into clinical fruition (research and development, clinical trials, and FDA approval). There is no doubt that the hot tip technology hurt the program to develop catheters for treatment of intravascular occlusions. Not only was that technique *not* laser therapy, but gave all laser therapy a bad reputation. Recent advances in mechanical atherectomy devices and stents have also diverted some of the initial interest in the laser-based technologies. However, it has to be admitted that even when the technology has been applied in the best of circumstances, to the most ideal lesions with good results, no real advantage over simple POBA has been demonstrated. Taking this into account and comparing the very large cost differential, it is not difficult to understand the waning interest. The most optimistic hope that the restenosis rate will be substantially reduced has not yet materialized.

Acknowledgments

We are grateful to all our colleagues of the Lester Wolfe Laser Angiosurgery Group at MIT and the Cleveland Clinic Foundation. Their years of devoted work have led to better understanding of the principles involved in application of this technology to medicine. Part of this work was carried out at the MIT Biomedical Research Center under an NIH grant.

References

1 Leon MB, Lu DY, Prevosti LG *et al.* Human arterial surface fluorescence: atherosclerosis plaque identification and effects of laser atheroma ablation. *J Am Coll Cardiol* 1988;12:94–102.

2 Leon MB, Almagor Y, Bartorelli AL *et al.* Fluorescence-guided laser assisted balloon angioplasty in patients with femoropopliteal occlusions. *Circulation* 1990;81:143–155.

3 Prince MR, Deutsch TF, Shapiro AH *et al.* Selective ablation of atheromas using a flashlamp-excited dye laser at 465 nm. *Proc Natl Acad Sci USA* 1986;83:7064–7068.

4 Eldar M, Battler A, Gal D *et al.* The effects of varying lengths and powers of CO_2 laser pulses transmitted through an optical fiber on atherosclerotic plaques. *Clin Cardiol* 1986;9:89–91.

5 Forrester JS, Litvack F, Grundfest WS *et al.* Vaporization of atheroma in man: the role of lasers in the era of balloon angioplasty. *Int J Cardiol* 1988;20:1–7.

6 Gerrity RG, Loop FD, Golding LAR, Ehrhart LA, Argenyi ZB. Arterial response to laser operation for removal of atherosclerotic plaques. *J Thorac Cardiovasc Surg* 1983;85:409–421.

7 Goth PR, Kramer JR, Kittrell C, Sacks BA, Feld MS. Optical fibers in medicine II. *Proc SPIE* 1987;713:58–63.

8 Grundfest WS, Litvack F, Doyle L *et al.* Comparison of *in vitro* and *in vivo* thermal effects of argon and excimer lasers for laser angioplasty. *Circulation* 1986;74(Suppl. 2):813(Abstract)

9 Grundfest WS, Litvack F, Forrester JS *et al.* Laser ablation of human atherosclerotic plaque without adjacent tissue injury. *J Am Coll Cardiol* 1985;5:929–933.

10 Litvack F, Grundfest WS, Goldenberg T *et al.* Pulsed laser angioplasty: wavelength power and energy dependencies relevant to clinical application. *Lasers Surg Med* 1988;8:60–65.

11 Selzer PM, Murphy-Chutorian D, Ginsburg R, Wexler L. Optimizing strategies for laser angioplasty. *Invest Radiol* 1985;20:860–866.

12 Shelton ME, Hoxworth B, Shelton JA, Virmani R, Friesinger GC. A new model to study quantitative effects of laser angioplasty on human atherosclerotic plaque. *J Am Coll Cardiol* 1986;7:909–915.

13 Spears JR. Percutaneous laser treatment of atherosclerosis: an overview of emerging techniques. *Cardiovasc Intervent Radiol* 1986;9:303–312.

14 Spears JR. Percutaneous transluminal coronary angioplasty restenosis: potential prevention with laser balloon angioplasty. *Am J Cardiol* 1987;60:61B–64B.

15 Spears JR, Serur J, Shropshire D, Paulin S. Fluorescence of experimental atheromatous plaques with hematoporphyrin derivative. *J Clin Invest* 1983;71:395–399.

16 Strikwerda S, Kramer JR, Partovi F, Feld MS. Considerations of dosimetry for laser-tissue ablation. In: Vogel JHK, King SB, eds. *Future Directions in Interventional Cardiology.* St. Louis: CV Mosby Co., 1989:54.

17 Strikwerda S, Partovi F, Cothren RM, Feld MS, Kramer JR. Ablation thresholds of atheromatous tissue for argon ion laser light exposures. *Lasers Life Sci* 1989;3:61–70.

18 Theis JH, Lee G, Chan MC *et al.* Effects of simultaneous viewing and vaporization of plaques using the steerable, laser-heated metal cap in the atherosclerotic monkey model. *Lasers Surg Med* 1987;7:414–420.

19 Welch AJ, Valvano JW, Pearce JA, Hayes LJ, Motamedi M. Effect of laser radiation on tissue during laser angioplasty. *Lasers Surg Med* 1985;5:251–264.

20 Abela GS, Conti CR. Laser revascularization: what are its prospects? *J Cardiovasc Med* 1983;September:977–984.

21 Abela GS. Laser recanalization: a basic and clinical perspective. *Thorac Cardiovasc Surg* 1988;36:137–141.

22 Abela GS, Normann S, Cohen D, Feldman RL, Geiser EA, Conti CR. Effects of carbon dioxide, Nd-YAG, and argon laser radiation on coronary atheromatous plaques. *Am J Cardiol* 1982;50:1199–1205.

23 Abela GS, Normann SJ, Cohen DM *et al.* Laser recanalization of occluded atherosclerotic arteries *in vivo* and *in vitro*. *Circulation* 1985;71:403–411.

24 Abela GS, Seeger JM, Barbieri E *et al.* Laser angioplasty with angioscopic guidance in humans. *J Am Coll Cardiol* 1986;8:184–192.

25 Adler L, Litvack F, Grundfest W *et al.* Excimer laser-balloon angioplasty treatment of peripheral vascular occlusions and stenoses. *Radiology* 1988;169(P):140(Abstract).

26 Cragg AH, Gardiner GA, Smith TP. Vascular applications of

laser. *Radiology* 1989;172:925−935.

27 Forrester JS, Litvack F, Grundfest W *et al.* The excimer laser: current knowledge and future prospects. *J Intervent Cardiol* 1988;1:75−80.

28 Izatt J, Sankey ND, Partovi F, Fitzmaurice M, Itzkan I, Feld MS. Ablation of calcific biological tissue using pulsed hydrogen fluoride laser radiation. *IQEE J Quant Elect* 1990;26:2261−2270.

29 Lee G, Ikeda RM, Stobbe D *et al.* Effects of laser irradiation on human thrombus: demonstration of a linear dissolution−dose relation between clot length and energy density. *Am J Cardiol* 1983;52:876−877.

30 Motarjeme A. Percutaneous laser angioplasty: a 2-year follow-up. *Radiology* 1988;169(P):140(Abstract).

31 Nishioka NS, Levins PC, Murray SC, Parish JA, Anderson RR. Fragmentation of biliary calculi with tunable dye lasers. *Gastroenterology* 1987;93:250−255.

32 Izatt JA, Albagli D, Itzkan I, Feld MS. Pulsed ablation of calcified tissue: physical mechanisms and fundamental parameters. In: Jacques SL, ed. *Laser−Tissue Interactions. Proc SPIE* 1990;1202:133−140.

33 Grundfest WS, Litvack F, Hickey A *et al.* The current status of angioscopy and laser angioplasty. *J Vasc Surg* 1987;5:667−672.

34 Grundfest WS, Litvack IF, Goldenberg T *et al.* Pulsed ultraviolet lasers and the potential for safe laser angioplasty. *Am J Surg* 1985;150:220−226.

35 Isner JM, Gal D, Steg G *et al.* Percutaneous, *in vivo* excimer laser angioplasty: results in two experimental animal models. *Lasers Surg Med* 1988;8:223−232.

36 Ginsburg R, Kim DS, Guthaner D, Toh J, Mitchell RS. Salvage of an ischemic limb by laser angioplasty: description of a new technique. *Clin Cardiol* 1984;7:54−58.

37 Ginsburg R, Wexler L, Mitchell RS, Profitt D. Percutaneous transluminal laser angioplasty for treatment of peripheral vascular disease: clinical experience with 16 patients. *Radiology* 1985;156:619−624.

38 Choy DS, Stertzer S, Rotterdam HZ, Sharrock N, Kaminow IP. Transluminal laser catheter angioplasty. *Am J Cardiol* 1982;50:1206−1208.

39 Choy DS, Stertzer SH, Rotterdam HZ, Bruno MS. Laser coronary angioplasty: experience with 9 cadaver hearts. *Am J Cardiol* 1982;50:1209−1211.

40 Choy DSJ, Stertzer SH, Marco P, Fournial G. Human coronary laser recanalization. *Clin Cardiol* 1984;7:377−381.

41 Choy DSJ, Stertzer SH, Myler RK, Marco J, Fournial G. Human coronary laser recanalization. *Clin Cardiol* 1984;7:377−381.

42 Barbeau G, Abela GS, Seeger JM. Laser recanalization: the hybrid probe. In: Sanborn TA, ed. *Laser Angiosurgery*. New York: Alan R. Liss Inc., 1989:47−58.

43 Litvack F, Warren W, Mohr F, Struhl B, Forrester J. Hot-tip angioplasty by a novel radiofrequency catheter. *Circulation* 1987;76(Suppl. 4):47(Abstract).

44 Lu DY, Leon MB, Bowman RL. A prototype catalytic thermal tip catheter: design parameters and *in vitro* tissue studies. *J Am Coll Cardiol* 1987;9:187A (Abstract).

45 Cumberland DC, Sanborn TA, Tayler DI *et al.* Percutaneous laser thermal angioplasty: initial clinical results with a laser probe in total peripheral artery occlusions. *Lancet* 1986;1:1457−1459.

46 Cumberland DC, Crew JR, Myler RK *et al.* Clinical laser angioplasty experience at Northern General Hospital and the San Francisco Heart Institute. In: Sanborn TA, ed. *Laser Angiosurgery*. New York: Alan R. Liss Inc., 1989:35−45.

47 Harrington ME, Schwartz ME, Sanborn TA *et al.* Expanded indications for laser assisted balloon angioplasty in peripheral arterial disease. *J Vasc Surg* 1990;11:146−155.

48 Lee G, Ikeda RM, Chan MC *et al.* Dissolution of human atherosclerotic disease by fiberoptic laser-heated metal cautery cap. *Am Heart J* 1984;107:777−778.

49 Linnemeier TJ, Rothbaum DA, Cumberland DC, Landin RJ, Hodes ZI, Ball MW. Percutaneous laser-assisted thermal coronary angioplasty in native coronary arteries and saphenous vein grafts: initial results and angiographic follow-up. *J Inv Cardiol* 1990;2:133−139.

50 Litvak F, Grundfest WS, Papaioannou T, Mohr FW, Jakubowski AT, Forrester JS. Role of laser and thermal ablation devices in the treatment of vascular disease. *Am J Cardiol* 1988;61:81G−86G.

51 McCowan TC, Ferris EJ, Barnes RW, Baker ML. Laser thermal angioplasty for the treatment of obstruction of the distal superficial femoral or popliteal arteries. *Am J Roentgenol* 1988;150:1169−1173.

52 Perler BA, Osterman FA, White RI Jr, Williams GM. Percutaneous laser probe femoropopliteal angioplasty: a preliminary experience. *J Vasc Surg* 1989;3:351−357.

53 Sanborn TA. Laser angioplasty: what has been learned from experimental studies and clinical trials? *Circulation* 1988;78:769−774.

54 Sanborn TA, Cumberland DC, Greenfield AJ, Welsh CL, Guben JK. Percutaneous laser thermal angioplasty: initial results and 1-year follow-up in 129 femoropopliteal lesions. *Radiology* 1988;168:121−125.

55 Sanborn TA, Faxon DP, Haudenschild CC *et al.* Experimental angioplasty: circumferential distribution of laser thermal energy with a laser probe. *J Am Coll Cardiol* 1985;5:934−938.

56 Sanborn TA, Haudenschild CC, Garber GR *et al.* Angiographic and histologic consequences of laser thermal angioplasty: comparison with balloon angioplasty. *Circulation* 1987;75:1281−1286.

57 Sanborn TA, Alexopoulos D, Marmur JD *et al.* Coronary excimer laser angioplasty: reduced complications and indium-111 platelet accumulation compared with thermal laser angioplasty. *J Am Coll Cardiol* 1990;16(2):502−506.

58 Sanborn TA. Initial multicenter training and experience with 1.5 and 2.0-mm peripheral laser probes. In: Sanborn TA, ed. *Laser Angiosurgery*. New York: Alan R. Liss Inc., 1989:29−34.

59 Sanborn TA. Percutaneous coronary laser thermal angioplasty. In: Sanborn TA, ed. *Laser Angiosurgery*. New York: Alan R. Liss Inc., 1989:101−110.

60 Tobis JM, Mallery JA, Macleay L *et al.* The mechanism of laser probe recanalization: thermal ablation vs. mechanical dissection. *Circulation* 1988;78(Suppl. 2):417 (Abstract).

61 Widlus DM, Osterman FA Jr. Evaluation and percutaneous management of atherosclerotic peripheral vascular disease. *J Am Med Assoc* 1989;261:3148−3154.

62 Wright JG, Belkin M, Greenfield AJ, Guben JK, Sanborn TA, Menzioan JO. Laser angioplasty for limb salvage: observation on early results. *J Vasc Surg* 1989;10:31−38.

63 Lammer J, Karnel F. Percutaneous transluminal laser angioplasty with contact probes. *Radiology* 1988;168:733−737.

64 Abela GS, Barbieri E, Khoury A, Roxey T, Conti CR. Coronary artery laser angioplasty without perforation using a sapphire lens tipped optical fiber. *J Am Coll Cardiol* 1987;9:222(Abstract).

65 Kramer JR, Feld MS, Loop FD *et al.* Laser angiosurgery: a biomedical system using photons to diagnose and treat athero-

sclerosis. In: Vogel JHK, King SB, eds. *Future Directions in Interventional Cardiology*, 2nd edn. St Louis: CV Mosby Co.

66 Lammer J, Pilger E, Karnel F *et al.* Austrian multicenter trial for laser angioplasty: 2-year results. *Radiology* 1988;169(P): 139(Abstract).

67 Spears JR, Reyes VP, Wynne J *et al.* Percutaneous coronary laser balloon angioplasty: initial results of a multicenter experience. *J Am Coll Cardiol* 1990;16(2):293–303.

68 Allen B, Loflin TG, Embry BM, Gaskin TA, Isobe JH, Martin RG. Occluded peripheral arteries: clinical utility of argon laser recanalization. *Radiology* 1990;176:543–547.

69 Foschi AE, Myers GE, Flamm MD. Laser-enhanced coronary angioplasty via direct argon laser exposures: early clinical results in totally occluded native arteries. *Circulation* 1989; 80(4):11–478.

70 Nordstrom LA, Castaneda-Zuniga WR, Lindeke CC, Rasmussen TM, Burnside DK. Laser angioplasty: controlled delivery of argon laser energy. *Radiology* 1988;167:463–465.

71 Nordstrom LA, Castaneda-Zuniga WR, Young EG, Von Seggern KB. Direct argon laser exposure for recanalization of peripheral arteries: early results. *Radiology* 1988;168:359–364.

72 Nordstrom LA. LASTAC clinical results: peripheral arteries. *Radiology* 1989;168:359–364.

73 Cothren RM, Hayes GB, Kramer JR, Sacks B, Kittrell C, Feld MS. A multifiber catheter with an optical shield for laser angiosurgery. *Lasers Life Sci* 1986;1:1–12.

74 Cothren RM, Kittrell C, Hayes GB *et al.* Controlled light delivery for laser angiosurgery. *IEEE J Quant Electron* 1986;22:4–7.

75 Cothren RM, Kramer JR, Hayes GB *et al.* Engineering of a multifiber catheter with an optical shield for laser angiosurgery. *IEEE Engin Med Biol Proc Ninth Ann Conf Boston MA* 1987:200.

76 Litvack F, Grundfest WS, Adler L *et al.* Percutaneous excimer laser and excimer-laser-assisted angioplasty of the lower extremities: results of initial clinical trial. *Radiology* 1989;172: 331–335.

77 Conference on the *Future Directions in Interventional Cardiology*, Santa Barbara, California, 1990.

78 Geschwind HJ, DuBois-Rande J-L, Murphy-Chutorian D, Tomaru T, Zelinsky R, Loisance D. Percutaneous coronary angioplasty with mid-infrared and a new multifiber catheter. *Lancet* 1990;336(8709):245–246.

79 Karsch KR, Haase KK, Voelker W, Baumbach A, Mauser M, Seipel L. Percutaneous coronary excimer laser angioplasty in patients with stable and unstable angina pectoris. Acute results and incidence of restenosis during a 6-month follow-up. *Circulation* 1990;81(6):1849–1859.

80 Karsch KR, Haase KK, Mauser M, Voelker W. Initial angiographic results in ablation of atherosclerotic plaque by percutaneous coronary excimer laser angioplasty without subsequent balloon dilatation. *Am J Cardiol* 1989;64(19):1253–1257.

81 Lau KW, Sigwart U. Novel coronary interventional devices: an update. *Am Heart J* 1992;123(2):497–506.

82 Ghazzal ZMB, Hearn JA, Litvak F *et al.* Morphological predictors of acute complications after percutaneous excimer laser coronary angioplasty. Results of a comprehensive angiographic analysis: importance of the eccentricity index. *Circulation* 1992; 86(3):820–827.

83 Kittrell C, Willett RL, de Los Santos-Pacheo C *et al.* Diagnosis of fibrous arterial atherosclerosis using fluorescence. *App Optics* 1985;24:2280–2281.

84 Richards-Kortum R, Rava R, Fitzmaurice M, Kramer JR, Feld MS. 476 nm excited laser-induced fluorescence (LIF) spectroscopy of human coronary artery: applications in cardiology. *Am Heart J* 1991;122:1141–1150.

85 Richards-Kortum R, Mehta A *et al.* Spectral diagnosis of atherosclerosis using an optical fiber laser catheter. *Am Heart J* 1989; 118:381–391.

86 Dasari RR, Feld MS. Spectroscopy. *Collier's Encyclopedia* 1993; 21:414–424.

87 Baraga JJ, Feld MS, Rava RP. In situ optical histochemistry of human artery using near infrared fourier transform raman spectroscopy. *Proc Nat Acad Sci* 1992;89:3473–3477.

88 Manoharan R, Wang Y, Feld MS. Histochemical analysis of biological tissues using raman spectroscopy. *Spectrochimica Acta* 1995 (in press).

89 Geschwind HJ, Boussignac G, Teisseire B, Benhaiem N, Bittoun R, Laurent D. Conditions for effective Nd-YAG laser angioplasty. *Br Heart J* 1984;52:484–489.

90 Geschwind HJ. Laser angioplasty: new modalities. *Ann Radiol* 1988;31:69–73.

91 Geschwind HJ, Teisseire B, Boussignac G, Vieilledent C. Laser angioplasty of arterial stenoses. *Cardiovasc Intervent Radiol* 1986; 9:313–317.

92 Cothren RM, Costello B, Hoyt C *et al.* Tissue removal using an 8F multifiber shielded laser angiosurgery catheter. *Lasers Life Sci* 1988;2:75–90.

93 Kjellstrom BT, Bylock AL, Bott-Silverman C *et al.* Removal of surgically induced fibrous arterial plaques by argon laser angiosurgery using a multifiber delivery system: an experimental study in the dog. *J Thorac Cardiovasc Surg* 1988;96:925–929.

94 Kramer JR, Bott-Silverman C, Ratliff NB *et al.* Removal of atherosclerotic plaque using multiple short exposures of argon ion laser light. *Am Heart J* 1987;113:1038–1040.

95 Kramer JR, Strikwerda S, Kittrell CK, Feld MS. Laser angiosurgery: a brief overview of tissue micromachining with spectral diagnostics. In: Bruschke AVG, Spaan JAE, Gittenberger AC, eds. *Coronary Circulation, From Basic Mechanisms to Clinical Implications*. Boston: Martinus Nijhoff, 1987:225.

96 Feld MS, Kramer JR. Mutagenicity and the XeCl Excimer laser: A relationship of consequence? *Am Heart J* 1991;122(6): 1803–1805.

97 Margolis JR, Mehta S. Excimer laser coronary angioplasty. *Am J Cardiol* 1992;69:3F–11F.

98 Sanborn TA, Torre SR, Sharma SK *et al.* Percutaneous coronary excimer laser-assisted balloon angioplasty: initial clinical and quantitative angiographic results in 50 patients. *J Am Coll Cardiol* 1991;17(1):94–99.

99 Geschwind HJ, Nakamura F, Kvasnicka J, Dubois-Randé JL. Excimer and holmium yttrium garnet laser coronary angioplasty. *Am Heart J* 1993;000:125–510.

100 Isner JM, Donaldson RF, Funai JT *et al.* Factors contributing to perforations resulting from laser coronary angioplasty: observations in an intact human postmortem preparation of intraoperative laser coronary angioplasty. *Circulation* 1985;72(Suppl. 2):191–199.

101 Preisack MB, Voelker W, Haase KK, Karsch KR. Case report: formation of vessel aneurysm after stand alone coronary excimer angioplasty. *Cathet Cardiovasc Diagn* 1992;27:122–124.

102 Nakamura F, Kvasnick J, Decoster HL, Geschwind HJ. Aneurysmal formation after successful pulsed laser coronary angioplasty. *Cathet Cardiovasc Diag* 1992;27:125–129.

103 Bogan ML, Hawes RH, Kopecky KK, Goulet RJ Jr. Percutaneous cholecystolithotomy with endoscopic lithotripsy by using a

pulsed-dye laser: preliminary experience. *Am J Roentgenol* 1990;155:781−784.

104 Faulkner DJ, Kozarek RA. Gallstones: fragmentation with a tunable dye laser and dissolution with methyl ter-butyl ether *in vitro. Radiology* 1989;170:185−189.

105 Hofmann R, Hartung R, Geissdorfer K *et al*. Laser induced shock wave lithotripsy: biological effects of nanosecond pulses. *J Urol* 1988;139:1077−1079.

106 Dawson SL, Mueller PR, Lee MJ, Saini S, Kelsey P, Nishioka NS. Treatment of bile duct stones by laser lithotripsy: results in 12 patients. *Am J Roentgenol* 1992;158:1007−1009.

107 Sullivan KL, Bagley DH, Gordon SJ *et al*. Transhepatic laser lithotripsy of choledocholithiasis: initial clinical experience. *JVIR* 1991;2:387−391.

108 O'Reilly GV, Forrest MD, Schoene WC, Clarke RH. Laser-induced thermal occlusion of berry aneurysms: initial experimental results. *Radiology* 1989;171:471−474.

109 Deckelbaum LI, Lam JK, Cabin HS, Clubb KS, Long MB. Discrimination of normal and atherosclerotic aorta by laser-induced fluorescence. *Laser Surg Med* 1987;7:330−335.

110 Fitzmaurice M, Bordagaray JO, Englemann GL *et al*. Argon ion laser-excited autofluorescence in normal and atherosclerotic aorta and coronary arteries: morphologic studies. *Am Heart J* 1989;118:1028−1038.

111 Hoyt CC, Richards-Kortum RR, Costello B *et al*. Remote biomedical spectroscopic imaging of human artery wall. *Lasers Surg Med* 1988;8:1−9.

112 Verbunt RJ, Cothren RM, Fitzmaurice M *et al*. Characterization of ultraviolet laser-induced autofluorescence of ceroid deposits and other structures in autofluoresclerotic plaques as a potential diagnostic for laser angiosurgery. *Circulation* (Submitted).

113 Itzkan I, Baraga JJ, Fitzmaurice M, Rava RP, Feld MS. Using laser spectroscopy to diagnose disease. In: *Proceedings of the International Conference on Lasers, 1992*. Mclean VA: SOQUE, 1993:780−786.

114 Cotheren RM, Sivak MV, Van Dam *et al*. Detection of dysplasia at colonoscopy using laser-induced fluorescence: a blinded study. *Gastrointest Endoscopy* 1996 (in press).

115 Cotheren RM, Arendt JT, Klein EA *et al*. *Lasers Surg Med* 1995 (submitted).

116 Ingrams DR, Roy K, Bottrill ID *et al*. Can laser-induced fluorescence detect early stage oral mucosa carcinoma. *Head Neck* 1995 (submitted).

117 Jaffe MH, Fleischer D, Zeman RK, Benjamin SB, Choyke PL, Clark LR. Esophageal malignancy: imaging results and complications of combined endoscopic−radiologic palliation. *Radiology* 1987;164:623−630.

118 Zwirewich CV, Muller NL, Lam SC T. Photodynamic laser therapy to alleviate complete bronchial obstruction: comparison of CT and bronchoscopy to predict outcome. *Am J Roentgenol* 1988;151:897−901.

119 Dachman AH, McGehee JA, Beam TE, Burris JA, Powell DA. US-guided percutaneous laser ablation of liver tissue in a chronic pig model. *Radiology* 1990;176:129−133.

120 Gatenby RA, Hartz WH, Engstrom PF *et al*. CT-guided therapy in resistant human tumors: phase 1 clinical trails. *Radiology* 1987;163:172−175.

121 Epstein BE, Lee D-J, Kashima H, Johns ME. Stage T1 glottic carcinoma: results of radiation therapy or laser excision. *Radiology* 1990;175:567−570.

122 Margolis JR, Litvak F, Krauthamer D, Trautwein R, Goldenberg T, Grunfest W. Coronary angioplasty with laser and high frequency energy. *Herz* 1990;15(4):223−232.

123 Huppert PE, Duda SH, Helber U, Karsck KR, Claussen CD. Comparison of pulsed laser-assisted angioplasty and balloon angioplasty in femoropopliteal artery occlusions. *Radiology* 1992;184:363−367.

124 Leachman DR. Techniques and experience in laser angioplasty at the Texas Heart Institute. In: Sanborn TA, ed. *Laser Angiosurgery*. New York: Alan R. Liss Inc., 59−76.

125 Lau KW, Sigwart U. Novel coronary interventional devices: an update. *Am Heart J* 1992;123(2):497−506.

126 Lammer J, Pilger E, Decrinis M, Quehenberger F, Klein GL. Stark G. Pulsed excimer laser versus continuous-wave Nd:YAG laser versus conventional angioplasty of peripheral arterial occlusions: prospective, controlled randomised trial. *Lancet* 1992;340:1183−1188.

127 Bittl JA, Sanborn TA, Tcheng JE, Siegel RM, Ellis SG. Clinical success, complications and restenosis rates with excimer laser coronary angioplasty. The Percutaneous Excimer Laser Coronary Angioplasty Registry. *Am J Cardiol* 1992;70(20):1533−1539.

128 Baumbach A, Bittl JA, Fleck E *et al*. Acute complications of excimer laser coronary angioplasty: a detailed analysis of multicenter results. *J Am Coll Cardiol* 1994;23(6):1305−1313.

Part 3
Intravascular Contrast Media

CHAPTER 13

Complications of intravascular iodinated contrast media

George Ansell

Pharmacology

Intravascular iodinated contrast media are a basic requirement for many imaging procedures. In comparison with other drugs, they have a relatively low toxicity but it is essential that all who use them should have a thorough understanding of the possible complications which may occur. The historic aspects and development of these media has been reviewed by Grainger [1] and Almen [2]. The general pharmacology and uses of radiologic contrast media have been discussed in some detail elsewhere [3] and the American College of Radiology has issued a guide on the use of iodinated contrast media [4]. Currently used radiologic contrast media are triiodinated derivatives of benzoic acid (Fig. 13.1). Cholegraphic media are discussed in Chapter 28, p. 497).

High-osmolar media

Conventional hyperosmolar ionic media, e.g., diatrizoate (Hypaque, Angiovist, Urografin, Renovist), iothalamate (Conray, Vascoray), metrizoate (Isopaque), and iodamide (Renovue, Uromiro) are monomeric salts with three atoms of iodine per molecule and two particles (ion and cation) in solution (ratio = 1.5). In terms of toxicity, on an equiosmolar basis, there are only slight differences between these negatively charged anions. Commercial preparations of contrast media [5] contain varying proportions of the positively charged cations sodium and methylglucamine; some media may also contain calcium and magnesium. Methylglucamine is heavier than sodium, therefore, for a given iodine content, the percentage value of contrast medium in solution (g/100 ml) is higher for methylglucamine media than for sodium media. In general, the osmolarity is related to the iodine concentrations of the media but there are slight variations with individual preparations [5] (Table 13.1).

Methylglucamine was originally introduced to increase the maximum concentration of contrast medium attainable in solution. In certain circumstances, methylglucamine decreases the local endothelial toxicity of contrast media. Prior to the introduction of lower osmolar media, this was mainly of value in the cerebral and coronary circulations, in peripheral angiography, and in venography. Methylglucamine may, however, have certain relatively minor disadvantages which are discussed elsewhere in this chapter (see pp. 247,249,268, 269).

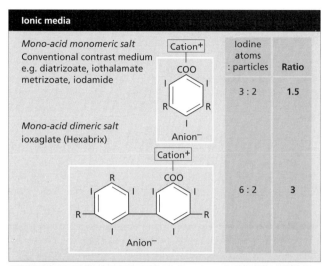

Ionic media

Mono-acid monomeric salt
Conventional contrast medium
e.g. diatrizoate, iothalamate
metrizoate, iodamide

Mono-acid dimeric salt
ioxaglate (Hexabrix)

	Iodine atoms : particles	Ratio
	3 : 2	1.5
	6 : 2	3

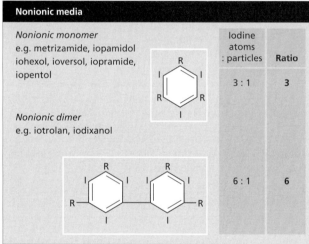

Nonionic media

Nonionic monomer
e.g. metrizamide, iopamidol
iohexol, ioversol, iopramide,
iopentol

Nonionic dimer
e.g. iotrolan, iodixanol

	Iodine atoms : particles	Ratio
	3 : 1	3
	6 : 1	6

Fig. 13.1 Structural formulae of contrast media. (Redrawn from Grainger [1].)

Lower osmolar media

A major factor in the toxicity of conventional contrast media is their hyperosmolarity (Table 13.1). Lower-osmolar *ratio-3* contrast media, with three atoms of iodine per particle in solution, are of two types. Sodium methylglucamine ioxaglate (Hexabrix) is an *ionic monoacid dimer*. This has six atoms of iodine per molecule with two particles in solution. The *nonionic monomers*, such as iopamidol and iohexol, have three atoms of iodine per molecule with one particle in solution. The *nonionic dimers* iotrolan and iodixanol have six atoms of iodine per molecule with one particle in solution (*ratio* = 6) (Fig. 13.1 & Table 13.1). At concentrations below 400 mgI/ml, the *nonionic dimers* are actually hypoosmolar with plasma: commercial preparations therefore contain small amounts of added saline to make them isoosmolar [6].

There has been increasing use of lower osmolar media. A recent review [7] indicated that these media are now exclusively used for intravascular purposes in Sweden, Norway,

Finland, and Japan. On the basis of 1990 and 1991 data, the lowest estimated use appeared to be in the Netherlands and France (20–30%), with intermediate use in other countries: Denmark, UK, USA, Spain (51–65%); Germany, Australia, Italy (75–80%). A recent survey in the UK reported the routine use of nonionic media in 78.8% of intravenous examinations [8].

Additives

Contrast media contain small quantities of the sequestrating agent ethylenediaminetetraacetic acid (EDTA) to stabilize them. This may be in the form of the disodium salt (Na_2EDTA) which causes calcium binding and may result in hypocalcemia, or as the calcium disodium salt ($Na_2CaEDTA$) which minimizes calcium binding. Small amounts of sodium citrate, which may be added as a buffer, may also cause calcium binding (see p. 250). EDTA is potentially allergenic [9].

Contaminants

Contrast media stored in natural-rubber-capped bottles may leach the rubber accelerator 2-mercaptobenzothiazole (MBT) from the rubber. MBT is a known allergen and has been suspected as a possible cause of a few contrast-media reactions. It has been suggested that such bottles should be stored upright. Likewise, prolonged contact of contrast media with rubber components of disposable syringes should be avoided [10]. Synthetic rubbers may overcome this problem.

When rubber-capped bottles are pierced by a needle, fragments of rubber may fall into the contrast medium. Likewise, when glass ampoules are broken open, fragments of glass may be sucked into the solution. After 30–60 seconds, larger particles sink to the bottom of the ampoule and may be avoided if the lower 3 mm of solution is not aspirated [11].

Lasser *et al.* [12] found evidence of an exogenous contact activator, causing accelerated complement activation by the contrast medium, in one out of four vials of nonionic medium. This increased activation was abolished by Millipore filtration, suggesting that particles in the particular vial may have acted as activating surfaces. "Punches" from rubber caps of various contrast-media vials, and also needles and catheters passed through contrast vial caps, likewise acted as exogenous contact activators. This might theoretically potentiate endogenous contact activation in a patient (12) (see p. 275). If this theory is correct, these findings might be relevant to some otherwise unexplained sporadic contrast-media reactions.

Contrast media may contain varying traces of nickel, probably derived from the vessels used during manufacture [13]. Nickel may cause a variety of hypersensitivity phenomena [9].

Table 13.1 Osmolarity and viscosity of representative contrast media. (From Fischer [5])

Generic name	Percentage in solution	Trade name	Iodine mg/ml	Osmolarity mosmol/kg	Viscosity	
					25°C	37°C
Diatrizoate sodium	50	Urovist	300	1550	3.2	2.4
Diatrizoate meglumine	65	Renovue	300	1558	8.7	5.7
Iothalamate sodium	54.3	Conray	325	1700	4.0	3.0
Iothalamate sodium	80	Angioconray	480	2400	14.0	9.0
Ioxaglate sodium meglumine	58.9	Hexabrix	320	600	15.7	7.5
Iohexol	64.7	Omnipaque	300	709	10.35	6.77
Iohexol	75.5	Omnipaque	350	862	18.5	11.15
Iopamidol	61	Isovue	300	616	8.8†	4.7
Iopamidol	76	Isovue	370	796	20.9†	9.4
Iodixanol*	55	Visipaque	270	290	11.3†	5.8
Iodixanol*	65.2	Visipaque	320	290	25.4†	11.4

* Manufacturers data
† Viscosity at 20°C.

Incompatibilities and interactions

Marshall *et al.* [14] showed that some conventional contrast media may be precipitated by antihistamines such as phenergan or diphenhydramine: they recommended that antihistamines and contrast media should not be mixed in the same syringe. Diatrizoate is also precipitated by amobarbital sodium used in the Wada test [15] and by protamine sulfate [16]. Ioxaglate (Hexabrix) is precipitated by papaverine, cimetidine [17,18], tolazoline, and diphenhydramine [19]. Nonionic media appear less reactive but immediate thrombosis has occurred following arteriography with papaverine and iopamidol [20].

Papaverine and iopamidol precipitate when mixed with plasma *in vitro*: heparin may increase the degree of precipitation [21]. Most of these incompatibilities appear to be due to pH changes. There was a possibility of contrast-medium precipitation by some batches of epinephrine with a low pH [22], but other studies did not find this [18,19].

In general, it is inadvisable to mix contrast media with drugs: precipitates may cause complement activation [23]. It is important to ensure that there are no incompatibilities: catheters should be flushed with saline between the administration of drugs and contrast media. Intraarterial injection of barbiturates or of many other emergency drugs may cause endarteritis and thrombosis [24]. In animal studies, administration of local anesthetics can double the intravenous toxicity of contrast media [25]. Likewise, strophanthin [26] and propranolol [27] may also increase the toxicity of diatrizoate. (See also drug interactions in the cardiovascular toxicity section, p. 251.)

Viscosity

The viscosities of representative contrast media are shown in Table 13.1. There is some variation between different compounds: in general, increase of iodine content increases viscosity. Sodium salts of the ionic monomers have the lowest viscosity. Methylglucamine increases viscosity, particularly in the low-osmolar ionic dimer ioxaglate. The nonionic monomers have a higher viscosity than the ionic monomers and viscosity increases still further in the nonionic dimers. Warming contrast media to 37°C reduces viscosity.

When contrast media are admixed with whole blood, there are changes in viscosity due to the effect of contrast media on red cells and plasma. Despite their higher viscosity, the nonionic contrast media appear to cause less rheologic change than the hyperosmolar media [28] (see also p. 261).

General aspects of toxicity

If large doses of ionic contrast media are administered intravenously to animals to determine the LD_{50} (i.e., the dose causing the death of 50% of the animals), a characteristic syndrome occurs [29]. As lethal dose levels are approached, the animals become apprehensive; vomiting, urination, and defecation occur, followed by muscle twitching and convulsions. At a later stage, capillary breakdown develops in the lungs causing pulmonary hemorrhage and right heart failure. The intravenous LD_{50} in mice for ionic monomers is of a magnitude of $5-10\,gI/kg$, whereas for the nonionic monomers it is $15-25\,gI/kg$. Thus, the tolerability of nonionic monomers is approximately three times higher than that of ionic monomers. The ionic dimer ioxaglate has an intermediate value [2]. The LD_{50} is mainly of value in comparing the toxicity of different contrast media, but it does not give a direct indication of the *safe* dose for clinical use in humans. In any large population sample, a dose—response curve would indicate that a few individuals would be unduly susceptible to a dose that is safe for the majority. At the other extreme of the curve, a few individuals would tolerate an even larger dose than the majority.

Intrinsic toxicity of contrast media is a function of *osmotoxicity* due to osmolarity, and *chemotoxicity* due to chemical structure. Osmotoxicity can be reduced by using ratio-3 or ratio-6 media. Chemotoxicity is related to the chemical structure of the compound and particularly to the presence of carboxyl (COO^-) radicals which are necessary for the solubility of ionic media. With nonionic media, there are no carboxyl radicals, solubility being achieved by multiple hydroxyl (^-OH) radicals which also lower chemotoxicity, particularly if they are evenly distributed around the molecule [1,2]. The *lipophilicity* of contrast media may also affect their toxicity; higher lipophilicity increases toxicity, especially in the central nervous system [6]. The carboxyl radical is particularly toxic in the central nervous system. Whereas the LD_{50} for *subarachnoid injection* of the nonionic monomers iohexol, iopamidol, or metrizamide is of a magnitude of $1000-2000\,mgI/kg$, for the ionic dimer ioxaglate and the ionic monomers diatrizoate, iothalamate and metrizoate which contain carboxyl radicals, the LD_{50} is below $200\,mgI/kg$ [2]. *The ionic media are therefore approximately 10 times more neurotoxic and should never be injected intrathecally. They are liable to cause myoclonic spasms, convulsions and other neurologic complications which are frequently fatal.* Although this has been widely recognized, intrathecal injection of ionic media continues to occur. Two recent papers [30,31] report 17 cases where ionic media were mistaken for nonionic media and inadvertently used for myelography: eight of these patients died. The USA Food and Drugs Administration (FDA) received 19 reports of mistaken intrathecal administration of ionic media in the 3 years up to 1993. The FDA has instructed manufacturers to place a boxed label on ionic media, warning against intrathecal use [32]. Ionic media may also be inadvertently injected into the subarachnoid space by other procedures such as discography [31], misplacement of an arteriography needle [33], or through an intrathecal catheter [34]: ionic contrast medium may be mistakenly injected into the cerebral ventricular system, or they may enter through a ventriculoperitoneal shunt following bladder rupture during cystography [35].

There may be an initial delay before neurotoxicity becomes evident. *Myoclonic spasms* and *convulsions* may be exacerbated by external stimuli. They may be controlled temporarily by intravenous diazepam, but general anesthesia with neuromuscular blocking agents may be required. Other complications include *rhabdomyolysis, fracture, hyperthermia,* and *acidosis*. Lavage of the subarachnoid space with isotonic saline may be life saving [33,34].

Vascular toxicity

Venous

Davies *et al.* [36] analyzed the incidence of *arm pain* immediately following intravenous urography. They found that pain at the injection site was usually due to a small subclinical perivenous injection, whereas pain extending up the arm was usually due to stasis of contrast medium in the vein. *Delayed arm pain* may occur several hours or days after the injection and is probably due to a toxic effect on the endothelium which may lead to *thrombophlebitis* [37]. Both immediate and delayed arm pain frequently occur with high concentrations of sodium, containing media such as Conray 420 (sodium iothalamate) and are less common with Conray 280 (methylglucamine iothalamate). Experimentally, minor endothelial changes appeared to be related to the concentration of sodium in the medium [38]. Using cultures of human endothelial cells from umbilical cord veins, Laerum [39] confirmed the toxic effects of conventional hyperosmolar media and the better tolerance of lower osmolar media, particularly nonionic media. With lower limb phlebography, there was significant reduction in thrombophlebitis with iopamidol, $300\,mgI/ml$, as compared with methylglucamine iothalamate, $280\,mgI/ml$ [40].

Arterial

It should be emphasized that the arterial system is less tolerant to irritant substances than the venous system. As mentioned above, some drugs which can be safely administered intravenously may cause endarteritis and thrombosis when administered intraarterially [24]. With contrast media, endothelial damage appears to be mainly related to hyperosmolarity, but other factors may also be involved [41]. Lower concentrations of contrast media should therefore be selected for arteriography: this may be less important with intraaortic injections provided that the catheter tip is correctly sited to allow mixing and dilution of the contrast medium. Digital subtraction procedures permit the use of even lower concentrations of contrast media.

Contrast media cause *vasodilatation*. This is partly due to the hyperosmolarity of the medium, but chemotoxicity is also an important factor; for example, acetrizoate had a more marked effect than an equiosmolar solution of diatrizoate. Methylglucamine salts appear to be less vasoactive in the peripheral vessels [42]. Such vasodilatation does not appear to be a histamine effect and it may be partially blocked by atropine [43]. It would be interesting to speculate on the possible involvement of nitric oxide in vasodilatation.

In peripheral arteriography, the injection of contrast media is painful and causes a sensation of heat. With lower osmolar media, there is considerable reduction in these symptoms [1], but some patients may experience pain with iohexol [44]. Ioxaglate appears to cause least pain [45]. *It is now generally agreed that lower osmolar media should be used for peripheral arteriography* [4,46]. Nonionic dimers, in particular, cause minimal discomfort and are valuable for arterial DSA.

Soft tissue toxicity

Extensive sloughing of the skin and muscles of the forearm occurred in a child receiving 20 ml Conray 325 into a vein on the dorsum of the hand [47], and in a debilitated patient following multiple punctures with injection of 60 ml Conray 420 through a Venflon catheter at the wrist [48]. Such cases are probably due to a combination of leakage with chemical cellulitis, venous thrombosis, and muscle compartment syndrome. Subcutaneous or intramuscular injection of ionic contrast medium in infants caused sloughing of the soft tissues in 14 cases [49]. A bullous eruption may rarely occur at the injection site as a reaction to contrast-medium extravasation in the soft tissues [50].

Experimental work in animals indicates that the severity of soft tissue damage is mainly dependent on the osmolarity of the contrast medium, but the contrast molecule itself also has an effect: with ionic media, methylglucamine salts cause more damage than sodium salts; *nonionic media cause least damage* [51,52].

Earlier experiments suggested that hyaluronidase aggravated muscle damage [49], but this remained unconfirmed and recent work has shown that *hyaluronidase significantly reduces skin toxicity* when injected immediately following contrast medium. Application of *cold* also significantly reduced skin toxicity whereas heat caused no improvement [53].

With rapid injection of large doses of contrast medium for computed tomography (CT), the risk of extravasation is increased. In a series of 20 950 contrast-enhanced CT studies using nonionic contrast media, extravasation was lowest with hand injection (0.1%). With power injection at 0.5 ml/s, the extravasation rate was 0.17%, while with power injection at 1.5 ml/s, the extravasation rate increased to 0.24% [54].

Extravasation may initially cause swelling, erythema, and/or pain. Surgical drainage has been used to treat large volume extravasation of ionic contrast media [55], but the necessity for this has been questioned [56]. With nonionic media, conservative treatment with elevation of the limb and careful observation usually resulted in resolution without sequelae [54,56]. In one case, however, accidental subfascial injection of nonionic contrast medium caused a compartment syndrome requiring fasciotomy [57]. Immediately after extravasation has been recognized, application of cold packs is rational, but ice should probably be avoided, or used with extreme care, due to the risk of cold burns. Systemic steroids with antibiotic cover may be useful to diminish the later chemical inflammatory reaction in the soft tissues [58,59]. Nonsteroidal anti-inflammatory drugs (NSAIDs) may also be considered, particularly if there is thrombophlebitis (see also p. 569).

An unusual local reaction occurred in an infant following accidental lymphatic injection of diatrizoate. There was soft tissue swelling with an inflammatory reaction and blistering of the skin. Contrast medium was shown in the blisters [60].

Overdose

Deaths due to cardiovascular failure with pulmonary edema and/or convulsions have, in the past, been reported in a number of infants due to accidental or mistaken administration of excessive doses of conventional ionic contrast media [61,62]. Pulmonary edema was also reported in a neonate receiving 4.7 ml/kg of Hypaque 50 [63]. These cases appeared to be mainly related to the hyperosmolar state induced.

More recently, gross overdosage occurred in a 7-year-old girl undergoing aortography for aortic coarctation: due to problems with the film changer, five injections of 68 ml Renografin 76 were administered in less than 20 minutes, giving a total dose of 340 ml (15.5 ml/kg). The patient developed status epilepticus followed by supraventricular tachycardia and died at 33 hours. CT showed persistent high concentrations of contrast medium in the brain: this was confirmed at autopsy and there was cerebral edema [64].

Adverse reactions

Adverse reactions to contrast media fall into two main categories.
1 *Direct effects on specific organs and systems* due to the demonstrable toxicologic properties of contrast media.
2 *Idiosyncratic reactions* due to abnormal reactivity of individual patients.
There may also be overlap between these two categories.

Toxic effects on organs and systems

Cardiovascular toxicity

In an analysis of 74 999 patients undergoing diagnostic cardiac catheterization during 1991, death was reported in 0.11% of cases, myocardial infarction (0.06%), neurologic complications (0.05%), arrhythmias (0.31%), contrast reactions (0.25%). In 17 073 coronary angioplasties, death occurred in 0.3% and myocardial infarction in 0.3% of cases. Nonionic media were used in 72% of cardiac catheterizations and in 77% of angioplasties [65].

Cardiovascular toxicity is likely to be more evident when contrast media are used for cardiac studies but this will be partially counterbalanced by the expertise and highly specialized treatment facilities immediately available during such studies (see Chapters 4, 16, 17, pp. 61, 328, 331).

Electrophysiologic changes

Intracoronary injection of contrast media may cause a variety of electrophysiologic changes, the most serious being *ventricular fibrillation, ventricular tachycardia,* or *asystole.* Other changes include sinus bradycardia, heart block, increase of the QT interval, QRS prolongation, ST depression with or without angina or increased T-wave amplitude. Changes are more marked after right coronary artery injection [66].

Early experiments indicated that pure *sodium* salts of contrast media increased cardiac toxicity and that methylglucamine appeared to have a protective effect [67]. Apparently as a result of this work, the manufacturers of Renografin 76 (sodium methylglucamine diatrizoate) altered the constitution of the contrast medium by removing almost all of its sodium content, but no announcement of the change was made. Radiologists using the altered contrast medium (subsequently redesignated Renografin M76), noticed an unexpected increase in the incidence of ventricular fibrillation in their patients during selective coronary arteriography. Subsequent animal experiments confirmed that this problem was apparently caused by prolongation of the depolarization time, and that this was reversed by the addition of small quantities of sodium [68–70].

Alterations in *plasma calcium* affect cardiac contractility and the fibrillation threshold. Renografin 76, which contains disodium edetate and trisodium edetate, causes significantly more *calcium binding* than Hypaque 76 which contains disodium calcium edetate. However, the diatrizoate ion itself, also produces significant calcium binding [71].

In a series of 2500 patients undergoing coronary angiography with Renografin 76, the overall incidence of ventricular fibrillation was 0.6%; the incidence being higher in patients with coronary artery bypass grafts (2.4%). In 2000 subsequent patients receiving Angiovist 370, which contains disodium calcium edetate, the overall incidence of ventricular fibrillation was only 0.1%. It was considered that this lower incidence of ventricular fibrillation was due to reduced calcium binding by Angiovist [72]. Blood ionized calcium in the coronary sinus is significantly depressed following coronary arteriography with Renografin 76: it has been suggested that if passage of contrast through the coronary circulation is

unduly prolonged, e.g., in patients with arteriosclerosis, this may lead to *electromechanical dissociation* [73]. Nonionic media do not bind calcium but they do contain disodium calcium edetate.

Nonionic media are associated with considerably less physiologic effects on the heart than ionic media [74]. It might therefore be expected that use of lower-osmolar media and particularly the nonionic media would reduce the incidence of adverse reactions in coronary arteriography, but the results of clinical trials have been somewhat inconsistent. In a large Norwegian series of 533 coronary angiograms performed with iohexol 350, Levorstad *et al.* [75] encountered only one case of ventricular fibrillation (0.019%). Surprisingly, in two randomized North American trials comparing ionic with nonionic media in a total of 1995 patients, no significant difference in the incidence of ventricular fibrillation was detected, but the numbers of patients involved were relatively small. There was, however, a significant decrease in the incidence of angina, bradycardia, and hypotension with nonionic media in both trials [76,77]. In a more recent cooperative randomized study of 1390 patients undergoing cardiac angiography, the incidence of severe cardiac events including ventricular fibrillation using a calcium-binding preparation of diatrizoate (Renografin 76TM) was more than twice that with iohexol (78).

In a comparison of ioxaglate and iopamidol for cardiac angiography in two randomized trials, *ioxaglate caused significantly more allergic reactions and nausea.* Ioxaglate also caused a significant increase in the QT interval which might predispose to ventricular fibrillation [79–81]. One patient receiving ioxaglate had severe bronchospasm and another had moderate bronchospasm. Patients with an allergic history appeared to be at greater risk with ioxaglate in comparison with iopamidol [80].

In the isolated rabbit heart, the addition of small amounts of sodium to nonionic media decreased still further the risk of ventricular fibrillation but may have a negative inotropic effect, reducing cardiac contractility. Small amounts of calcium counteract the negative inotropic effect of sodium, but excessive calcium may increase the risk of ventricular fibrillation. A careful balance is therefore required between sodium and calcium. Nonionic dimers, supplemented by low concentrations of electrolytes may prove advantageous in coronary arteriography despite their increased viscosity [74,82]. A small clinical study using the nonionic dimer iodixanol (320 mgI/ml) for cardioangiography has shown encouraging results [83].

Coronary artery spasm has rarely been reported during *anaphylactoid reactions* following coronary angiography with diatrizoate and ioxaglate, respectively [84,85]. In patients with a history of angina, cardiac *ischemic changes* have been reported following bolus injections of diatrizoate into the superior vena cava for *digital subtraction angiography,* and one patient in functional class IV failure developed ventricular fibrillation [86]. Transient ischemic ST changes were most common in patients with hypertension but also occurred in patients without previous heart disease [87].

Routine electrocardiogram (EKG) monitoring during excretion urography with ionic media showed unexpected cardiac arrhythmias, ischemic changes, tachycardia, and ectopic ventricular beats. Although these changes might occur in healthy patients, they were most common in patients with cardiac disease and in older patients. There was a direct relationship with the total dose of contrast medium and the rapidity of injection [88,89].

In a crossover study to assess the effect of stress, no significant EKG changes were noted during a preliminary injection of saline, but when the infusion was changed to diatrizoate, a number of asymptomatic heart rate changes and minor arrhythmias occurred [90]. However, in another similar study, a patient developed a severe vasovagal reaction with hypotension, transitory SA block, and nodal rhythm after a control injection of isotonic saline [91].

Vagal reactions

Reflex increase of vagal tone may cause depression of sinoatrial and atrioventricular nodal activity with inhibition of atrioventricular conduction resulting in bradycardia or even asystole. Peripheral vasodilatation also occurs and results in hypotension. Associated features include apprehension, sweating, nausea, vomiting, abdominal pain, diarrhea, and urinary incontinence [4,92–94] (see also pp. 270, 271, 281).

Hemodynamic effects

Bolus intravenous injections of hypertonic contrast medium cause withdrawal of water from the red cells, blood vessel endothelial cells, and tissues causing hypervolemia. Capillary permeability is increased and contrast molecules pass into the tissues causing increase in the lung water [95]. There may be a brief rise in systemic blood pressure followed by a more prolonged fall due to peripheral vasodilatation and depressed cardiac contractility. There is usually tachycardia but bradycardia may occur. Injection into the right heart or pulmonary arteries results in transitory pulmonary hypertension and systemic hypotension. Injection into the left ventricle or proximal aorta causes more profound hemodynamic changes with increase in stroke volume, heart rate, and cardiac output. There is also a rise in left and right atrial pressures, peak left ventricular pressure, and left ventricular end-diastolic pressure. There is a brief rise in systolic blood pressure followed by a more prolonged fall due to peripheral vasodilatation; venous pressure rises gradually [96].

Intracoronary injection of hypertonic medium, on the other hand, produces transitory direct depression of myocardial contractility causing a fall in left ventricular pressure which is not due to peripheral vasodilatation. This effect is greater in the ischemic state [97]. The depression of myocardial contractility results in decreased peripheral blood flow with increased peripheral resistance and increased venous pressure [98]. Intracoronary injection of the low-osmolar medium ioxaglate causes less decrease in cardiac contractility, while the nonionic monomers cause no myocardial depression and actually produce a slight positive inotropic effect [97].

Intravenous Renografin 76 caused large increases in coronary and femoral blood flow, while intravenous iohexol caused no significant change in coronary blood flow and a mild increase in femoral blood flow [99].

In patients with incipient cardiac failure, the injection of large doses of contrast medium, particularly hypertonic media, may cause pulmonary edema (see p. 269).

Drug interactions

Experimentally, there is a deleterious interaction between the calcium antagonist verapamil and Renografin 76 causing depression of atrioventricular conduction and myocardial performance during coronary arteriography, whereas iohexol has only a minimal interaction with verapamil [100]. In one patient, verapamil appeared to have a synergic effect in causing diastolic cardiac arrest [101]. The calcium antagonists nifedipine and diltiazem potentiated the hypotensive response following left ventriculography with diatrizoate, but this was not apparent with iopamidol [102]. β-Blockers depress cardiac contractility: they may potentiate hypotensive reactions and cause these to be resistant to therapy [103]. In animal experiments, the LD_{50} to diatrizoate was adversely affected by strophanthin [104] and by propranolol [105], but the clinical relevance has not been established.

Risk factors (Table 13.2)

Major risk factors include: severely ill patients with low-output left ventricular failure, recent myocardial infarction, severe coronary artery disease, coronary artery bypass grafts, and unstable angina [77]. Azotemia also appears to be a significant risk factor [78]. Nonionic media are generally preferable to ionic media and are more particularly indicated in selected higher risk patients undergoing cardiac angiography, but the possibility of an increased risk of thromboembolic complications cannot be excluded [106].

Table 13.2 Risk factors for cardiac toxicity. (From Barrett *et al.* [77])

Severely ill patients
Low output left ventricular failure
Recent myocardial infarction
Severe coronary artery disease
Coronary artery bypass graft
Unstable angina
Azotemia [78]

Nephrotoxicity

There is copious literature on renal toxicity, and in recent years there has been increasing recognition of the potential for contrast media to cause renal impairment. The earlier literature on this subject has been reviewed by Byrd and Sherman [107] and Mudge [108]. There have also been numerous recent reviews and, of these, a selection [109–123] is of interest for further reading.

Incidence

The overall reported incidence rates for contrast-media nephrotoxicity have varied from 0 to 22% [112,114]. In selected groups with particular risk factors, considerably higher incidence rates have been reported (see below). The divergence of findings depends partly on case mix, diagnostic criteria, and adequacy of follow-up. Unless patients are specifically monitored by serial measurements of serum creatinine (sCr), some cases of renal failure may be missed and the relation to contrast administration may be overlooked: for example, Van Zee *et al*. [124] initially encountered four patients with renal failure following urography. They then reviewed their hospital records over a 10-month period during which 2360 urograms were performed using 42.3 g iodine per examination. This brought to light 19 additional cases of previously unattributed renal failure in 395 patients with adequate records of sCr, giving an incidence rate of 4.9% or a minimum overall incidence rate of 0.8%, if it was assumed that there were no further cases that remained undetected. In another prospective study of 2216 hospital patients, there were 129 episodes of new renal insufficiency and 16 (12%) of these episodes were attributed to contrast media. This was the third most important cause of renal insufficiency in this study group and the most common cause of drug-induced nephrotoxicity [109].

Renal failure may be *oliguric* or *nonoliguric*. The serum creatinine may be raised in the first 24 hours after administration of contrast, but tends to peak between the third and seventh days. Contrast-induced renal failure is usually reversible over a period of 2 weeks, but in a few patients it may persist, requiring dialysis, or it may even be fatal [109,125].

Diagnostic criteria

The diagnostic criteria for contrast nephrotoxicity and renal failure have varied in different studies, ranging from an increase of sCr greater than 0.3 mg/dl above baseline to an increase of sCr greater than 1 mg/dl. Other studies have defined renal failure as an increase of sCr by 20–50% above baseline (Table 13.3).

Because of the relation between glomerular filtration rate (GFR) and the sCr level, halving the glomerular filtration in a patient with a baseline sCr 0.8 mg/dl will produce a rise in

Table 13.3 Diagnostic criteria for contrast nephropathy

Increase sCr above baseline	References
>1 mg/dl	109[†], 124, 126*, 127, 131*, 132*, 133*
>0.5 mg/dl	109*, 125, 128, 129*, 134*, 135[†], 136, 137, 133*
>0.3 mg/dl	131*, 138*, 132*
>50%	126*, 130*, 133*
>33%	129*
>25%	130*, 134*, 139, 140
>20%	131*, 138*, 132*

* Multiple criteria.
[†] Also ↑ sCr> × 2, dialysis, or sCr >4 mg/dl.

the sCr to only 1.6 mg/dl, whereas in a patient with a baseline sCr 4 mg/dl the same proportional reduction of GFR will increase the sCr to 8 mg/dl [114]. It should also be noted that the sCr may not rise above the normal range until the GFR falls below 30–50% of normal [115].

Older [141] drew attention to the predictive value of an abnormally *persistent or increasing nephrogram* following contrast administration: renal impairment (increase sCr > 0.6 mg/dl) developed in nine out 22 patients with such a nephrogram. D'Elia *et al*. [142] found that a persistent nephrogram had a sensitivity of 83% for nephrotoxicity, but that the predictive accuracy was only 19%. They recommended that in patients with preexisting azotemia, the sCr should be monitored at 24–48 hours after contrast administration with examination of the urinary sediment in selected patients. A persistent CT nephrogram 24 hours after contrast administration with a mean cortical density greater than 140 HU appeared to be an indicator of impending renal failure, while cortical density levels between 55 and 110 HU might indicate subclinical renal impairment [143]. With nonionic dimers· such as iodixanol, there may be a somewhat prolonged retention of the contrast medium in the kidney without renal failure [144].

Plasma contrast-medium concentrations can be rapidly measured by an X-ray fluorescent technique and clearance studies have been recommended as an early warning of potential nephrotoxicity in susceptible patients [145].

Risk factors (Table 13.4)

Renal insufficiency, diabetes

Most studies agree that the combination of preexisting renal insufficiency and insulin-dependent diabetes mellitus constitutes the most important risk factor for contrast nephropathy, although the numbers of cases reported in individual series

Table 13.4 Risk factors for contrast nephropathy

Renal insufficiency, diabetes
Previous contrast nephropathy
Dehydration
Dose, route of administration
Multiple contrast studies
Cardiovascular disease
Myelomatosis
Nephrotoxic drugs
Miscellaneous

are relatively few. In Van Zee's [124] series of high-dose pyelograms five out of 10 (50%) diabetics with sCr of 1.5–4.5 mg/dl and two out of two (100%) diabetics with sCr greater than 4.5 mg/dl developed contrast nephropathy (increase sCr greater than 1 mg/dl). In nondiabetics, the incidence of contrast nephropathy for sCr 1.5–4.5 mg/dl was 2/66 (3%) and for sCr greater than 4.5 mg/dl 5/16 (31%) [124]. Acute renal failure occurred in 12 out of 13 (92%) of patients with severe diabetic nephropathy undergoing coronary angiography [146]. In a prospective study of 378 nonrenal angiograms, patients with chronic azotemia had a 33% incidence of contrast nephropathy [142]. In a more recent prospective case-control study, administration of contrast to patients with preexisting renal insufficiency increased the risk of a mild nephropathy by a factor of 4.7 as compared with patients who did not receive contrast medium. The incidence of contrast nephropathy with preexisting renal insufficiency was 8.8% in diabetics and 4% in nondiabetics [130]. However, in three out of four (75%) diabetics, when sCr was greater than 2.25 mg/dl, the same group found a 25% increase of sCr with ionic media [134]. In diabetics without preexisting renal insufficiency, the risk of contrast nephropathy appears to be small. In another study [128], preexisting renal disease was considered to be the most important factor and a predictive model showed a sharp rise in the probability of contrast nephropathy when the baseline sCr exceeded 1.2 mg/dl.

Two studies, in particular, have questioned the clinical relevance of contrast nephropathy. In the first study, a retrospective analysis of 40 urograms from patients with moderate or severe renal failure, three patients had developed a transient rise in sCr without oliguria and in five patients, renal function was already deteriorating at the time of their urograms. The other patients showed no deterioration of renal function. There was, however, only one case of diabetic nephropathy in this series [147]. In another case-control study of patients undergoing CT with or without contrast medium, there did not appear to be an overall risk of renal impairment in patients receiving high-osmolar media, but an effect in particular subgroups could not be excluded in this study [148].

Vaamonde [149] was unable to produce renal failure with contrast medium in diabetic rats, but this experimental model does not mimic the chronic microvascular changes which may be an important contributing factor in the human disease.

Dehydration

Earlier studies suggested that fluid restriction and/or dehydration were major factors predisposing to contrast nephropathy [150–152] and the importance of adequate hydration is now widely recognized. However, in patients with substantial risk factors, avoidance of dehydration may not prevent contrast nephrotoxicity [153,154] and this may even occur in "hydrated" patients [126,128,154,155]. It should also be noted that vomiting, purgation, diarrhea, sodium restriction, and diuretics may all cause dehydration. Overhydration with isotonic saline has been recommended in patients with chronic renal failure, but this may cause a temporary increase in blood pressure and weight [156].

Dose, route of administration

Medullary necrosis or tubular changes occurred in seven out of 16 young infants who received more than 3 ml/kg ionic contrast medium for cardioangiography, and a follow-up study revealed a further eight infants who developed hematuria with a dose of 3–5 ml/kg. No hematuria occurred with doses below 3 ml/kg [157].

In a radionuclide study of renal function before and after arteriography, there appeared to be a direct relationship between the dose of contrast medium used and the degree of resulting transient renal dysfunction [158].

In two studies from the Mayo Clinic, patients with abnormal renal function showed a significantly higher incidence of contrast nephropathy with doses exceeding 125 ml (45 gI) of either ionic or nonionic contrast media [127,159]. Varying doses of contrast media have been identified as independent risk factors for contrast nephropathy in other studies, particularly when additional risk factors were also present [125, 126,146,153,160]. In one high-risk group of azotemic patients undergoing coronary angiography for pretransplant evaluation, a dose of more than 30 ml nonionic medium appeared to increase the risk of contrast nephropathy [139]. Other studies have not shown a significant effect of dose [128,134, 142], but methods of interpreting data may influence the findings [131]. *It seems probable that there is some dose relationship in causing nephrotoxicity, particularly in high-risk patients.*

Renal failure may occur after contrast administration by any route and has, e.g., been reported after cerebral angiography [161]. In one study, patients undergoing cardioangiography appeared to have a higher risk of nephrotoxicity when compared to those undergoing CT [relative risk = 3.44] [130]. Injection close to the renal arteries appears to increase nephrotoxicity [158] and conventional renal angiography was more likely to cause nephrotoxicity than renal angiography performed by intravenous digital vascular imaging using a similar dose of contrast medium [162]. One study found a higher risk of nephrotoxicity in abdominal aortography (15.8%) compared with arch aortography (4%) [126]. Contrast nephrotoxicity may be a problem with renal angiography during renal angioplasty: carbon dioxide has been suggested as an alternate contrast medium for this [163].

Multiple contrast studies in azotemic patients may increase the risk of renal failure [153,159,164]. Two separate episodes of renal failure with interstitial nephritis have occurred in a patient following ipodate and iothalamate [165]. A patient with a previous history of contrast nephropathy is likely to be at particular risk [154].

Cardiovascular factors

Congestive cardiac failure and low cardiac output were identified as risk factors for nephrotoxicity in three studies involving ionic media [126,135,159], but this did not appear to be a significant risk factor in patients receiving nonionic media [127,128]. Hypertension has been suggested as a possible risk factor [124,138], but this was not confirmed in other studies [128,159] and it may be an interrelated factor. One study suggested that a low mean arterial pressure may be a risk factor [160].

Myelomatosis

Myelomatosis has previously been regarded as a relative contraindication to contrast administration with a small risk of precipitating renal failure. In a recent review of 476 patients with myelomatosis who received contrast medium, the estimated risk of acute renal failure was 0.6–1.25%. It was concluded that contrast examinations may be performed if the clinical need arises and the patient is well hydrated [166]. Abdominal compression should be avoided. However, while the risk is relatively small, it should be noted that acute renal failure in myelomatosis is often fatal, in contradistinction to other types of contrast nephropathy. While the older contrast media such as diodone or acetrizoate, and also iodipamide, could precipitate Bence–Jones protein, this was considered to be unlikely with diatrizoate and iothalamate [167,168]. Nevertheless, renal failure has occurred in myelomatosis following use of diatrizoate [169]. Typically, acute renal failure in myelomatosis is associated with tubular damage and tubular blockage by casts. In an analysis of 14 cases of acute renal failure in myelomatosis, the most important etiologic factors were considered to be hypercalcemia, nephrotoxic antibiotics and volume depletion. Intravenous urography was performed in four cases, but was considered to be the primary cause of renal failure in only one case with dehydration as an associated factor [170]. However, it is arguable that urography may also have been involved in at least one of the other cases.

Hydration may not prevent renal failure. One patient with unsuspected myelomatosis who was azotemic and hyperuricemic developed acute oliguric renal failure within 24 hours of intravenous urography despite prior hydration and alkalization of the urine: he died 25 days later [155]. Reversible renal failure has also been reported in an unsuspected case of myelomatosis who had intravenous urography and renal angiography followed by surgery [171].

There appears to be a small but definite increased risk of acute renal failure when intravascular contrast media are administered in myelomatosis, particularly in patients with additional risk factors. It would still be prudent to avoid contrast media in myelomatosis unless there are compelling reasons for their use. While lower-osmolar media generally have somewhat reduced nephrotoxicity (see below), their effect in myelomatosis is as yet unknown. It should be noted that retrograde urography may also precipitate acute renal failure in myelomatosis [172].

Nephrotoxic drugs

There was a history of diuretic therapy in 68% of one series of contrast nephropathy [128] and other studies reported that furosemide was a significant risk factor [129,135]. Experimental work also suggests that furosemide and NSAIDs may be risk factors for contrast nephrotoxicity (see below). Antibiotic therapy may also be a factor in some cases of contrast nephrotoxicity [124,142,154,173]. Some cytotoxic and immunosuppressive drugs may be nephrotoxic and are potential risk factors for contrast nephropathy. Renal failure may also occur following cholangiography or after a combination of cholangiographic and other contrast media [165, 171,174–176]. A fatal case of renal failure with lactic acidosis has been reported following urography in a diabetic patient receiving metformin [177].

Other factors

Contrast nephropathy is approximately twice as frequent in males as in females [107,108]. A number of studies have found an increased risk of contrast nephropathy in the *older age groups* (60+ years) [107,113,126,128,138]. This may be related to the reduction of functioning nephrons which occurs in association with increasing age. However, some studies have not found age to be a significant factor [127, 130,135]. In a group of elderly patients, hyponatremia and hypoalbuminemia appeared to be risk factors [125]. One study indicated that atopy was a significant factor for contrast nephrotoxicity [135], but this has not been reported elsewhere. It appears rare for idiosyncratic reactions to progress to renal failure, but in at least one such case with "shock," the patient developed bilateral cortical necrosis [178].

Contrast media may cause hemolysis with *hemoglobinuria* resulting in renal failure [179] (see p. 262). This may also occur with *myoglobinuria* from rhabdomyolysis [180] (see

p. 262). Irreversible renal failure from *urate nephropathy* may occur from use of contrast medium in hyperuricemic children with *Burkitt's lymphoma* [181]. An experimental study suggested that intravascular ionic contrast media may precipitate renal failure in acute pancreatitis [182].

In patients with *renal transplants*, earlier studies suggested that allograft arteriography might contribute to, or elicit, acute rejection [183]: this was recorded in 50% of patients with markedly impaired renal function, but the risk appeared slight with normal renal function [184]. A later study suggested that the risk of renal damage was similar with or without contrast medium and related mainly to the level of plasma creatinine at the time of exposure [185]. Measurements of enzymuria in 26 renal transplant patients undergoing digital subtraction angiography with nonionic media, suggested that there was no appreciable nephrotoxicity [186]. Aortography in a patient with unilateral stenosis may deliver an increased dose of contrast medium to the contralateral kidney resulting in renal failure [187]. Similar considerations may apply with a unilateral kidney [113].

Cumulative effect

Variations in the findings from different studies are likely to be mainly due to differences in population samples, techniques, and methods of evaluation. This makes it difficult to produce a precise model for contrast nephrotoxicity, but consideration of the varying factors can usefully be employed in clinical decisions involving contrast administration. Moreover, risk factors have a cumulative effect: the more independent risk factors present, the greater the risk [125,131, 138]. Rarely, contrast nephropathy may occur without any significant preceding risk factor.

Pathogenesis

Hemodynamic factors

The pathogenesis of contrast nephropathy is still uncertain but it is believed to be multifactorial. There have been many attempts to investigate this problem using a variety of experimental approaches. Porter [188,189] has reviewed the hemodynamic effects of contrast injection into the renal arteries in dogs. This causes a well-recognized biphasic response with transitory vasodilatation, followed by a more prolonged vasoconstrictive stage and decrease in renal blood flow which is associated with a transient decrease in the filtration fraction. Experimentally, the decrease in renal blood flow produced by diatrizoate may be accompanied by a delayed patchy nephrogram which is dose related. This patchy contrast retention is associated with the presence of thrombi in the renal vascular bed. Iohexol and metrizamide cause only slight decrease in renal blood flow and do not cause patchy nephrograms [190]. The biphasic response is unique to the renal circulation and its degree is related to the

osmolarity of the injected contrast medium. The sensitivity of the renal vasculature is increased by sodium depletion in dehydrated dogs. Angiotensin II causes vasoconstriction of the efferent glomerular arterioles, but it also stimulates the secretion of vasodilator prostaglandins which counteract the constriction and restore renal autoregulation. It has been suggested that calcium or adenosine may interfere with the tubuloglomerular feedback mechanism since vasoconstriction can apparently be eliminated by calcium or by adenosine antagonists [189]. More recently, it has been suggested that contrast media may cause the release of endothelin, a renal vasoconstrictor, and that this may play a part in contrast nephrotoxicity [191,192]. The biphasic response is usually relatively brief and it is doubtful if it plays a major role in clinical contrast nephrotoxicity, but it may aggravate other nephrotoxic effects.

In patients with chronic renal failure, measurements of global renal blood flow showed no predictable relationship to the development of contrast nephropathy following coronary angiography, but these measurements could not exclude intrarenal alterations in blood supply [193]. In rats, *indomethacin*, which inhibits prostaglandin synthesis, causes a profound and selective reduction of renal medullary blood flow without alteration of global renal blood flow: this may predispose to acute and chronic hypoxic damage [194]. Heyman *et al.* [195] have produced acute renal failure in uninephrectomized rats preconditioned by *salt depletion* and *furosemide* injections, followed by the administration of *indomethacin and sodium iothalamate*. Regression analysis suggested a separate contribution for each of these treatments as a risk factor for the development of renal failure. The renal failure was associated with extensive vacuolar changes and necrosis in the proximal convoluted tubules. In some patients with chronic renal failure, Moreau *et al.* [196] found similar *tubular changes* in renal biopsies shortly after contrast administration, but these changes were not necessarily associated with declining renal function. Moreau attributed such changes to osmotic nephrosis. In the rat studies, however, electron microscopy did not support a diagnosis of osmotic nephrosis. The necrotic areas were radioopaque due to the presence of calcium and phosphorus, but there was no detectable iodine [195].

Vari *et al.* [197] produced reversible acute renal failure without histologic changes in salt-depleted rabbits given indomethacin and methylglucamine iothalamate. Pretreatment with DOCA and saline for 1 week prevented the renal failure, but acute infusion of saline or mannitol commencing 1 hour before contrast and indomethacin, did not prevent the renal failure. Neither indomethacin nor contrast medium alone caused renal failure, indicating the *cumulative* effect of multiple factors.

In vitro experiments suggest that contrast media have a direct toxic effect on renal proximal tubule cells and that this is aggravated by anoxia: iopamidol appeared to be less toxic than diatrizoate [198].

Renal hypoxia in rats, due to temporary bilateral renal occlusion, caused an increase in plasma urea at 24 hours. When contrast medium was administered prior to the arterial occlusion, there was potentiation of the renal injury. Somewhat surprisingly, there did not appear to be any significant difference in the degree of potentiation caused by either metrizoate, ioxaglate, iopamidol, or iohexol. It was suggested that the decreased cellular toxicity of the newer media might be counterbalanced by their increased concentration in tubular urine, due to the reduced diuresis associated with lower osmolar media [199].

If contrast medium is administered to kidney donors shortly before the harvesting of kidneys for transplantation, or to patients before operations involving a period of renal ischemia, the small residue of contrast medium may potentiate renal damage. It has been suggested that there should be an interval of at least 12 hours between such procedures, or longer if there is already renal impairment [200].

Proteinuria, enzymuria

Renal angiography may cause transient nonselective proteinuria [201,202]. The presence of large and medium weight proteins such as immunoglobulins and albumin in the urine is indicative of increased permeability of the glomerular filtering membrane. Low-molecular-weight proteins such as β_2-microglobulins, which are normally reabsorbed in the tubules, may show moderately increased excretion. This may be partly due to overload of the tubular reabsorption mechanism, but it may also be indicative of mild associated tubular damage. Isolated increase of β_2-microglobulin has been regarded as an early and sensitive sign of disturbed tubular function. Proteinuria following renal angiography usually appears to cause few significant changes in renal function, but massive albuminuria has rarely resulted in acute renal failure with coagulation of the proteins causing casts and tubular obstruction [203].

In dogs, nephroangiography with the nonionic medium iohexol caused considerably less albuminuria than diatrizoate, but with the older nonionic medium, metrizamide, there was no difference in the degree of albuminuria as compared with diatrizoate. This suggests that the glomerular effect is due to some *toxic factor* rather than to osmolarity alone [190]. In clinical renal angiography, ioxaglate and iohexol appear to cause less albuminuria than monomeric ionic media [204,205].

Enzymes derived from the tubular cells may be excreted in the urine and measurement of such *enzymuria* has been used as an early indication of tubular damage. These enzymes include *N*-acetyl-β-D glucosaminidase (NAG), alanine aminopeptidase (AA), alkaline phosphatase (ALP), retinol binding protein (RBP), and folate binding protein (FBP). Transient enzymuria has been reported following renal angiography

[202] and aortofemoral angiography [206]. It may also occur following intravenous contrast media [207,208]. The early effect of contrast media on urinary enzyme excretion may be partly due to increased diuresis, but the late effect at 24–48 hours cannot be explained by the osmotic load of the contrast medium [209]. Comparison of the effects of ionic and nonionic media on enzymuria show somewhat conflicting results. While some studies report that nonionic media cause no increase in enzymuria [206,210], others appear to show little difference in the effects of ionic and nonionic media [207,208] and one study reported that nonionic media caused a higher excretion of brush border antigen than ionic media [211].

Diatrizoate causes a small but significant decrease in the renal extraction of *p*-aminohippurate (EPAH): this seems to be due to a direct tubular depressant effect. Diatrizoate should therefore not be used for at least 30 minutes before estimation of EPAH [212].

Thomsen [115] suggests that the effects of contrast media in diseased kidneys may differ from that in normal kidneys. In rats with glycerol nephropathy due to rhabdomyolysis, diatrizoate caused more albuminuria than iohexol, but iohexol appeared to cause more prolonged enzymuria than diatrizoate in glycerol nephropathy and cyclosporine-A nephropathy. In doxorubicin nephrosis, both media caused a similar degree of prolonged enzymuria. Iohexol also appeared to cause a round cell response around the tubules in glycerol nephropathy [213]. In gentamycin nephropathy, tubular dysfunction and tubular necrosis was more marked after iohexol than after diatrizoate [214]. One study suggests that ioversol may be less nephrotoxic than either iothalamate, ioxaglate, or iohexol, but this requires further confirmation [191].

In CT studies, the nonionic dimer iodixanol appears to be retained in the kidneys for a longer period than iohexol [144]. Despite this slower excretion, a small clinical trial in patients with normal renal function suggests that iodixanol may possibly be less nephrotoxic than iohexol, but this requires further evaluation in higher risk patients [83]. Similarly, in the rat kidney, the reduced diuresis and high intratubular viscosity of the nonionic dimer iotrolan causes slow tubular flow with increase in intratubular pressure and prolonged depression of single nephron GFR [215].

Tamm—Horsfall protein (THP)

THP is a normal urinary mucoprotein which is present in the thick ascending limb of the loop of Henle [216]. Berdon *et al.* [217] described "flash filling" of the pelvicalyceal system followed by a nephrogram, and renal failure in dehydrated children and in adults with myeloma. They suggested that this might be due to gel precipitation of THP, causing tubular obstruction by casts: they stated that THP could be precipitated *in vitro* by urographic media [218].

Subsequent work failed to confirm precipitation of THP by ioxaglate, iothalamate, iohexol, or iopamidol, except at extreme acidity (pH = 1), but there was some precipitation by ioglycamate [219]. There was no increased excretion of THP during routine urography and no "aggregation" was found in the urine [220]. A more recent paper, however, reported that injection of 6 ml contrast medium into the renal arteries of dogs caused an increase in the urinary excretion of THP with hyaline and granular casts: this appeared to be, at least in part, mediated by oxygen free radicals [221]. The role played by THP in contrast nephropathy is uncertain. It would be interesting to speculate on the possibility that contrast-induced albuminuria might cause precipitation of THP.

Solutes

Fang *et al.* [222] reported a low fractional excretion of sodium associated with acute renal failure due to contrast media, but Schwab *et al.* [136] found that the fractional excretion of sodium was low in most patients after contrast administration, and that this did not appear to be related to nephrotoxicity. Contrast media are uricusuric agents but urate nephropathy is unlikely to be an important cause of contrast nephropathy [108]. Contrast media also increase the excretion of oxalates [223]. An antidiuretic hormone (ADH)-like effect, suggesting vasopressin release, has been reported after contrast administration, but it is uncertain if this is related to contrast nephropathy [116,223].

In a survey of delayed effects following examination with nonionic medium, an increase in *diuresis* for up to 4−7 days was reported in approximately 5% of patients [224]. A case of *nephrogenic diabetes insipidus* followed resolution of acute renal failure due to arteriography. Symptoms gradually improved over a period of 2−3 months [225].

Histology, immunology

Moreau *et al.* [196] found transitory changes resembling osmotic nephrosis in renal biopsies following contrast examinations in patients with chronic renal failure, but the changes were not necessarily associated with declining renal function. Medullary necrosis or tubular changes have occurred following high-dose cardioangiography in infants [157]. Acute tubular necrosis [173] and late tubular atrophy [187] have been reported in adults. In other cases, nonspecific changes due to chronic renal disease were found [154].

In two patients, there was eosinophilia with interstitial nephritis and it was suggested that this might be an immunologic reaction to contrast media [226,227]. In an isolated case report, a systemic idiosyncratic reaction was accompanied by acute renal failure and immunoglobulin M (IgM) antibodies were found to react with iothalamate, diatrizoate, acetrizoate, and iodipamide [228].

Prevention

Brezis and Epstein [114] have ably summarized the prevention of contrast nephropathy. In patients with no predisposing factors, the danger is slight. It is important, however, to identify higher risk groups such as patients with diabetic renal failure, severe cardiac disease with diminished renal blood flow, jaundice, preexisting azotemia, multiple myeloma, etc. The sicker the patient, the higher the risk. Contrast studies in such patients should be limited to those that are essential, weighing potential risks against expected benefits. Concomitant use of potentially nephrotoxic agents, especially NSAIDs should be avoided if at all possible. Optimum correction of morbid conditions should be attempted prior to contrast administration. Adequate hydration should be ensured. Where appropriate, slight volume expansion with half-isotonic saline can be used to induce a gentle diuresis (e.g., 75 ml/h) for several hours before and after administration of contrast medium. From a review of the literature, Rudnick *et al.* [229] conclude that there is insufficient evidence to support the use of mannitol for the prevention of contrast nephropathy. In the rat with contrast acute renal failure, Heymen *et al.* [230] found that furosemide had a potential protective effect but, from the data, saline with or without furosemide appeared more effective. Golman [231], moreover, found that furosemide potentiated renal failure due to temporary renal occlusion in the rat, and he advised against using furosemide as a protective agent. In a controlled study involving 60 patients with renal insufficiency undergoing arteriography, dopamine infusion (2.5 µg/kg per min) appeared to have a protective effect, but this requires further evaluation [232]. Neumayer *et al.* [233] claimed a beneficial effect from the calcium channel blocker, nitrendipine, but the protective effect of calcium channel blockers has not been confirmed [234] and there is a suggestion that they may even have a deleterious effect, particularly in patients receiving high-osmolar media or with diabetes [235,236]. This requires further study.

Experimental evidence suggested that lower-osmolar media had reduced nephrotoxicity, in so far as glomerular function was concerned, but tubular effects were equivocal (see above). Despite this, at least seven cases of acute renal failure have occurred in diabetic patients receiving the low-osmolar dimer ioxaglate [237,238]. A number of earlier randomized clinical trials comparing the nephrotoxicity of ionic and nonionic media showed either no significant difference in nephrotoxicity or only a trend to reduced nephrotoxicity with nonionic media [132,134,136,137,140,239,240]. However, there were relatively few high-risk patients in each of these studies for statistical significance to be achieved. In a larger more recent study, there was a relative increased nephrotoxicity risk of 5.2 for diatrizoate versus iohexol in patients with renal insufficiency [235]. The most convincing evidence comes from the preliminary results of the Iohexol

Co-operative Study. This was a multicenter randomized controlled trial in 1194 adult patients undergoing cardioangiography. In patients with preexisting renal insufficiency without diabetes, contrast nephropathy (increase sCr > 1 mg/dl) occurred in 7.4% of the diatrizoate group and in 4% of the iohexol group. For patients with renal insufficiency and diabetes, the incidence of contrast nephropathy was 27.3% with diatrizoate and 11.9% with iohexol ($P < 0.002$). In these patients, therefore, the incidence of contrast nephropathy was approximately halved with iohexol. In nonazotemic patients, there was no significant difference in nephrotoxicity between the media, namely: diabetics 0.7% and 0.6%, respectively, and nondiabetics, 0% for both media [133].

If the sCr in a patient increases by 1 mg/dl or more after contrast administration, this is likely to increase immediate treatment costs and may have an unknown effect on the future prognosis. This could provide an economic argument for using low-osmolar media in high-risk patients [122].

In general, low-osmolar nonionic media appear preferable for use in high-risk patients and for renal angiography. Whether there are any special conditions where this might not apply, e.g., possibly in gentamycin nephropathy [214] (see p. 256) remains to be evaluated. Absence of risk factors, however, does not preclude the development of contrast nephropathy, even with low-osmolar media. It would appear prudent to use the lowest dose of contrast medium that will provide the diagnostic information required. Management of contrast-induced acute renal failure is essentially similar to that arising from other causes. While contrast-induced renal failure is usually self-limiting, it may require dialysis and may rarely be fatal [109,125].

Miscellaneous

In patients with renal failure, heterotopic excretion of contrast medium may opacify the bowel or gall bladder [241,242]. Gall-bladder and colonic opacification may also occur with ioxaglate in the absence of renal failure [243].

Examination of the urine following contrast media may give misleading results. There is increase in specific gravity. There may be a false-positive test for protein when the sulphosalicylic acid or nitric acid ring test is used, but the bromophenyl dye test (Albutest) is not affected. There may also be a false black-copper reduction reaction when a Clinitest tablet is added to the urine, simulating alcaptonuria [244]. Ioxaglate causes a chalky precipitate with sulphosalicylic acid and a trace reaction with Albustix [245]. Diatrizoate crystalluria may be confused with other types of crystalluria in routine microscopy of the urine [246].

Methylglucamine may interfere with the periodate urinary estimation of metanephrins in pheochromocytoma and may produce a false low-level reading for catecholamines. At least 2 days should therefore elapse after a patient has received a methylglucamine-containing contrast medium before estimation of catecholamines [247].

Neurotoxicity (see also Chapters, 24 p. 437 and 25, p. 447)

Intraarterial administration

When contrast media are delivered directly to the cerebral circulation by the arterial route, alteration of the blood–brain barrier may occur and there may be associated neural toxicity. With conventional ionic contrast media, sodium salts have a higher neurotoxicity than methylglucamine salts. Neurotoxicity is predominantly related to the hyperosmolarity of these media and is reduced when lower-osmolar media are used [248].

With more recent studies of the blood–brain barrier in rabbits, using pertechnate-99m leakage as a measure of toxicity, the nonionic media iohexol, ioversol, iodixanol, and iotrolan showed a decreasing order of pertechnate leakage: equiosmolar mannitol showed no detectable leakage, indicating that even with the nonionic media there is some chemotoxic effect not related to osmolarity. These effects were, however, considerably less than those produced by conventional ionic media at similar iodine concentrations [249].

With conventional ionic contrast media, there may be focal electroencephalográm (EEG) changes and, if prolonged, these may be followed by evidence of neurologic involvement. There may also be reflex cardiovascular changes including bradycardia and hypotension, which may be followed by tachycardia and hypertension. Transient asystole may also occur [250]. Contrast-media complications of cerebral angiography are considered in greater detail in Chapter 24 (see p. 437).

Accidental diversion of concentrated ionic contrast medium to the spinal cord during aortography, bronchial arteriography, or parathyroid arteriography, has resulted in *paraplegia* and *tetraplegia*. In such cases, irrigation of the subarachnoid space with isotonic saline may be helpful [251]. *Transient cortical blindness* has occurred following left intercostal angiography to visualize a coronary artery graft, due to contrast medium entering the left vertebral artery [252,253], and similarly during coronary angioplasty [254]. Cortical blindness has also been reported after contrast medium in sickle cell disease [255] (see p. 261).

Intravenous administration

One of the major chemotoxic properties of contrast media is their convulsive effect. Large doses of ionic contrast media may cause *convulsions* in patients with a latent tendency to epilepsy [256]. Seizures may also occur in patients with cerebral tumors undergoing contrast-enhanced CT [257]. In these cases, seizures may even occur with lower doses of contrast medium [258]. There is an increased risk of such seizures in patients with a previous history of seizures, and in association with antineoplastic therapy. Diazepam (5 mg intravenously immediately before the contrast injection) is valuable in prophylaxis [259]. Fatal status epilepticus occurred following contrast CT in two patients with bilateral cerebral mass lesions [260] and in a patient with cerebral atrophy who had a previous history of seizures [261]. Severe neurotoxic reactions with two fatalities have also been reported in four children with supratentorial tumors undergoing contrast CT [262].

Skalpe [263] has reviewed the mechanisms of contrast enhancement of pathologic lesions in the brain. This can be associated with *disruption of the blood−brain barrier*, which allows extravasation of contrast medium into the extracellular space of the lesion. Nonionic media are less neurotoxic. In a series of 169 patients with brain metastases undergoing high-dose CT with iopamidol, there were no seizures even though no premedication against seizures was given [264].

Alteration of the blood−brain barrier may possibly also occur when there is *renal impairment*. Neurologic changes, including cortical blindness, occurred in an elderly patient 30 hours after aortography, renal angiography and renal angioplasty using a total dose of 4 ml/kg Hypaque 60. CT showed persisting opacification of the brain, and there were raised iodine levels in the plasma and cerebrospinal fluid [265].

It has been suggested that patients with *thrombocytopenic purpura* may have a greater risk of developing seizures during contrast examinations [593].

Stimulus-sensitive extensor spasms of the trunk and limbs occurred during CT in a patient with an arteriovenous malformation of the spinal cord [266]. Myoclonic spasms have also been reported following contrast administration in a patient with paraplegia [267].

In patients who develop an idiosyncratic reaction with *hypotensive collapse*, convulsions are likely to be due to cerebral anoxia and they may be a presenting feature of cardiac arrest.

Headache may occur in idiosyncratic reactions (see Table 13.8, p. 267). This is probably due to histamine release. (See also p. 273.)

Effects on muscle

Myopathies

A fatal case of contrast-induced *malignant hyperthermia* has been reported with muscle spasms, hyperventilation, tachycardia, hyperpyrexia, and acidosis. Adrenergic drugs are contraindicated in malignant hyperthermia which should be treated by a muscle relaxant such as dantrolene [268]. It is possible that some of the seven deaths associated with "fever"

in Lalli's analysis [269] may also have been due to malignant hyperthermia [270].

A transitory *acute myopathy* has been reported, commencing 1 hour after intravenous injection of iopamidol: there were severe muscle pains in both arms, pyrexia, and raised sCr phosphokinase (CPK). There was also an increase in serum urea and creatinine. Unfortunately, urinary myoglobin was not assessed. The condition resolved over a period of 3 days [271]. A similar case occurred following injection of diatrizoate in a patient with preexisting renal impairment. There was diffuse myalgia with proximal muscle weakness, raised CPK, myoglobinuria, and transient renal deterioration. *Rhabdomyolysis* was confirmed by muscle biopsy [180]. The author is aware of several additional anecdotal reports of transient severe muscle pains of a similar nature, but these were not investigated in detail.

Selective injection of large doses of the nonionic media, iohexol, iopramide, and iotrolan into the *external* carotid arteries in rabbits caused muscle twitching with electromyogram (EMG) changes localized to the arterial distribution. Mannitol caused similar but less marked changes. The twitching appeared to be due to a chemotoxic factor acting on the myoneural junction. Somewhat surprisingly, these effects did not occur with injection of the ionic medium methylglucamine iothalamate [272].

Tetany

Tetany may result from hyperventilation in an anxious patient, but occasionally they may occur following contrast administration in the absence of hyperventilation. The sequestrating agents EDTA and sodium citrate, which may be present in contrast media (see p. 246), may cause hypocalcemia which may produce a transitory increase in parathormone secretion [273,274]. The magnesium level may also be lowered [275]. The diatrizoate ion itself also binds to calcium, but the iopamidol molecule does not bind to calcium. Nevertheless, the nonionic media do contain EDTA [276]. It is possible that changes in calcium and magnesium levels may be a factor in causing tetany in predisposed individuals.

Rigors

Rigors may occur with high doses of contrast media. They appear to be more common with methylglucamine-containing media [277,278], but they may also occur with sodium media and with small doses. Rigors have sometimes been due to faulty batches of contrast medium containing pyrogens [256]. A contrast reaction with severe rigors possibly exacerbated adrenal deficiency in a patient with amyloidosis who was on steroid therapy after cardiac transplantation [279]. He responded to 15 mg of oral prednisolone (A.G. Mitchell, personal communication).

Myasthenic crisis

At least seven patients have developed an acute myasthenic crisis during contrast CT [280−283]. This usually presented with sudden respiratory distress or apnea requiring intubation. There was often prolonged deterioration of the myasthenic state. The majority of cases had received an ionic contrast medium but iopamidol was used in one patient [282]. Administration of diatrizoate to rabbits with experimental autoimmune myasthenia gravis produced significant but temporary impairment of muscle contraction response: this experimental neuromuscular blockade was partially reversed by calcium administration [283].

Hemic toxicity

Coagulation problems and thromboembolism

It has long been known that conventional contrast media may cause *hypocoagulability* to the blood with inhibition of clotting and impaired platelet aggregation [284,285]. They may also potentiate the anticoagulant action of heparin [286]. The low-osmolar ionic dimer ioxaglate has a similar degree of anticoagulant activity to diatrizoate, but the nonionic media have only relatively weak anticoagulant activity [287,288]. Robertson [289,290] drew attention to the occasional presence of clots when blood was drawn into syringes containing nonionic media: he also reviewed the FDA reports of possible thrombus formation and thromboembolism. Grollman *et al.* [291] reported thromboembolic complications in three out of 1380 coronary angiograms with iopamidol, whereas none had previously occurred in 6800 examinations using high-osmolar media. They emphasized the importance of avoiding aspiration of blood into the syringe. There has been considerable debate on the possibility that there may be an increased risk of thromboembolism with nonionic media, particularly in coronary angioplasty (PTCA). In a randomized double-blind study of 100 patients undergoing PTCA, Esplugas *et al.* [292] found evidence of thrombi in 2% of patients receiving ioxaglate and 22% of patients receiving iohexol. In a retrospective nonrandomized study of 124 PTCA patients, Gasperetti *et al.* [293] found new thrombus in 4% of patients with diatrizoate and 18% with iopamidol. In a randomized trial of 500 PTCA patients, Piessens *et al.* [294] reported 3.2% acute thrombotic events occurring during the procedure with ioxaglate, and 7.2% with iohexol. Although there was a somewhat higher incidence of pre-existing thrombi in the iohexol group, this was unlikely to account for the difference between the media. On the other hand, in a large prospective series of 8517 patients undergoing cardiac catheterization using iopamidol or iohexol, Davidson *et al.* [295] encountered thrombotic events in only 0.18% of patients. Thrombotic events tended to occur in clusters but no cause for this could be found.

Engelhart *et al.* [296] investigated the incidence of clotting when blood contaminated syringes containing contrast medium. The earliest clots detected were at 30 minutes: they estimated the probability of clot formation at 5 minutes to be 1.3% with iohexol and 1.9% with iopamidol, but their treatment of data has been challenged [297]. Clot formation was more frequent with nonionic media than with ionic media. The risk of clotting was appreciably greater in glass syringes, due to activation of the clotting mechanism by the glass wall of the syringe. Clotting was also more frequent in saline controls. With plastic syringes, the risk of clotting appears to be higher in styrene acrylonitrile syringes and least in polypropylene syringes [298].

Studies by Ing *et al.* [287], Kopko *et al.* [299], and Fareed *et al.* [288,300] provided evidence that blood contamination of iohexol or iopamidol might result in thrombin generation and inhibition of fibrin polymerization in a time-dependant manner: thrombin generation appeared to be somewhat less with ioversol. The absence of clots in such a mixture did not exclude the presence of thrombin and, if this material was reinjected into a patient, there was a theoretical risk of causing clotting, particularly if the procedure was prolonged [300]. Blood contamination of ioxaglate in syringes, on the other hand, did not appear to be associated with significant thrombin generation under normal circumstances.

Another study has suggested that the anticoagulant action of ionic contrast media may be partly due to inhibition of activation of coagulation-factor XII, and that nonionic media do not have this effect [301]. Both ionic and nonionic media may cause changes in fibrin assembly and structure, with production of thin fibrin fibrils that may be resistant to thrombolysis if thrombi are formed [302].

Electron microscopic studies showed some degree of clot formation on the inside wall of catheters following angiography when iopamidol was used, but no clots were found with use of ioxaglate [303]. *In vitro* studies showed similar findings [304].

It should be noted, however, that although ioxaglate appears to be associated with a lower incidence of thromboembolism, it has a higher incidence of systemic and possibly cardiac side-effects (see p. 250).

Grabowski *et al.* [305] have reviewed the question of thrombotic complications. They stated that "the predominant current view is that nonionic media are more permissive of thrombin generation rather than procoagulant." Clots arising in the syringe or catheter are only one aspect. Injury to the vascular endothelium by the catheter or contrast medium causing platelet aggregation adhesion and deposition may lead to peripheral thrombus formation. Nonionic media appear to cause less endothelial damage. With nonionic media, however, it is essential to ensure meticulous syringe and catheter techniques (see Chapter 14, p. 309 and Chapter 17, p. 338).

Heparin inhibits the generation of thrombin. Some of the

thromboembolic events reported may have been due to inadequate heparinization. Heparin resistance may occur and it has been suggested that heparin should be added to nonionic media before use [306], but others do not favor this approach [307]. Patients may also become sensitized to heparin and develop an antibody–antigen reaction with a resultant heparin–thrombin syndrome: this is usually mild but may rarely cause major thrombosis [308]. It has been recommended that in coronary angioplasty using nonionic media, the adequacy of systemic heparinization should be controlled by measurement of the activated clotting time, but two major thrombotic episodes have occurred despite this precaution [309].

A recent study suggests an additional possible mechanism for thrombotic events involving nonionic media. Iohexol and other nonionic substances were shown to produce profound degranulation of platelets *in vitro*. This was not related to thrombin generation and was not blocked by pretreatment with heparin or aspirin. Diatrizoate caused considerably less degranulation, while ioxaglate produced virtually no platelet degranulation [310].

Stormorken [311] provides a detailed review of the complex factors that control the hemostatic and thrombotic mechanisms that ensure the fragile homeostatic balance between hemorrhage and thrombosis. In general, the nonionic contrast media appear to produce fewer changes in this balance than the ionic media, but there is clearly need for further study on the thrombogenicity of contrast media.

It has been suggested that possible *risk factors* for thrombotic complications may include: antithrombin III deficiency, protein C or protein S deficiency, hyperfibrinogenemia, thrombocytosis, increased factor VIII levels, hemoconcentration, hyperviscosity syndrome, paraproteinemias, leukemias, hemolysis, hypercoagulable conditions, use of oral contraceptives, estrogen therapy, etc. [288]. Patients with homocystinuria have a particularly high risk of thrombotic complications following intravascular contrast medium. Hyperhomocysteinemia may be a possible risk factor for vascular disease [312].

A fatal reaction with massive intravascular thrombosis occurred in a patient with Waldenström's IgM paraproteinemia following injection of diatrizoate [313]. This appeared to be similar to a fatal case reported after the cholegraphic medium ioglycamate [314].

Thrombocytopenic purpura

Acute thrombocytopenic purpura has rarely occurred following the administration of contrast medium, and a sixth case has recently been reported [315]. The patient may present with chills and fever, and in one case there was hypotensive collapse [316]. Thrombocytopenia may recur on subsequent contrast administration [316]. Shojania [317] suggested an immunologic mechanism but this was not confirmed in the other cases. In one case, the findings were consistent with increased peripheral destruction of platelets [318]. These cases all involved the use of diatrizoate. To date, there do not appear to be any reported cases with nonionic media. Thrombocytopenia has also been reported with oral cholecystographic media (see p. 498).

Pancytopenia

An isolated case of pancytopenia has been reported [319]. The patient had three urographic examinations and a renal angiogram, each with diatrizoate, over a period of 15 days. One hour after angiography, there was a severe anaphylactic reaction and pyrexia. This was followed by a decrease in hematocrit, platelets, and leukocytes with a hypoplastic bone marrow. Four months later, the picture had returned to normal.

Sickling

There is a possibility that contrast media may occasionally cause sickle cell crises in patients homozygous for sickle cell hemoglobin (SSHb). Two such cases have been reported following cerebral angiography [320]. In a patient with sickle cell disease, multiple cerebral infarcts with cortical blindness occurred after angiocardiography with diatrizoate [255]. A fatality has been reported following selective coronary arteriography in a patient with unsuspected sickle cell disease: an immediate thrombus formed in the left coronary artery following the injection of 1 ml Renografin 76 [321]. Another patient with sickle cell disease developed severe hemolysis, thrombocytopenia, leukostasis, and pulmonary infiltrates, following left ventriculography and coronary angiography with meglumine diatrizoate [322].

The addition of diatrizoate to samples of SSHb blood *in vitro* caused sickling which was particularly marked when the concentration of diatrizoate exceeded 35%. In patients, the risk is probably greater during angiography when relatively high concentrations of contrast medium occur in the blood. On the other hand, with slower intravenous injections, admixture with blood will tend to decrease the concentration of contrast medium. Considering the widespread prevalence of sickle cell disease, surprisingly few incidents have been reported. Iopamidol causes significantly less sickling *in vitro* than conventional ionic contrast media [323]. *Preferential use of nonionic media has been advocated in sickle cell disease* [4]. *It is also preferable to dilute such media approximately 1:2 to render them approximately isosmolar with plasma* [324].

Other red cell changes

Aggregations of red cells may occur at the interface between blood and ionic or nonionic contrast-media. However, these aggregations are temporary: they disperse with shaking and do not recur. Likewise, they would be rapidly dispersed by the sheer rates which occur in the vascular system and they are now considered to be of little significance [325–327]. It was formerly believed that such aggregates and clumps of red cells might cause blockage of pulmonary capillaries with resultant exacerbation of pulmonary hypertension. This is no longer believed to be the explanation. However, hypertonic media do cause *increased rigidity* of the red cell wall, so that these cells become less deformable and less able to negotiate the capillaries, thereby causing blockage [328]. This effect also increases the microviscosity of the blood. Despite its lower osmolarity, metrizamide affects the red cell membrane and causes an increase in viscosity. Ioxaglate has only a minor influence on the red cell membrane and causes a much lower increase in microviscosity [329]. Ioxaglate does not appear to affect the filtrability of the blood, whereas iohexol causes some decrease in filtrability. This effect was somewhat more marked with iopamidol [330]. These *in vitro* studies suggest that there may be a chemical effect on the cell membrane in addition to the osmolar effect (see also p. 269). In pulmonary angiography, iohexol causes a lower increase in pulmonary artery pressure than diatrizoate [331].

Hemolysis

When red blood cells are mixed with hypertonic contrast media *in vitro*, there is initially a decrease in red cell diameter. As the concentration of contrast medium increases, the red cells begin to show an increase in diameter due to damage to the cell wall, and hemolysis may then occur [332]. Hemolysis and hemoglobinuria may result in renal failure [179,333]. Hemolysis does not occur with iohexol or ioxaglate: with these lower-osmolar media, the red cells may produce a transparent pink mixture which macroscopically resembles hemolysis, but when this is centrifuged, the intact red cells float on top and there is no evidence of hemolysis in the underlying contrast medium [325].

Eosinophilia

Transient eosinophilia may occur 24–72 hours after contrast administration and last for up to 6 days. This appears to be an incidental finding without clinical significance [334,335].

Chromosome changes

Several studies have reported increased chromosome aberrations and sister chromatid exchanges in lymphocytes up to 1 week after intravenous urography. The increase was more marked than would be expected from the radiation dose alone. It has been suggested that there might be photoelectric absorption of radiation by iodine atoms of the contrast medium in and around the lymphocytes. In one study, however, diatrizoate produced more changes than ioxaglate

even though the radiation doses were similar with both media: this suggests that a photoelectric effect was unlikely to be a major factor. There may therefore be a direct toxic mutagenic effect caused by contrast media or their impurities. The clinical implications of these findings are still uncertain [336–338].

Endocrine effects

Thyroid function

Several cases of thyrotoxicosis have been reported following the administration of contrast media to patients with previously nontoxic goitres [339]. In a recent case report, there was an acute exacerbation of preexisting thyrotoxic symptoms 5 hours after contrast CT and this progressed to a thyroid storm with proximal myopathy and loss of consciousness. There was elevation of T4, reverse T3 and thyroglobulin, but T3 was normal. Recovery occurred after intensive treatment with steroids and antithyroid drugs [340]. In another patient, severe thyrotoxicosis developed 20 days after celiac angiography [341]. In such patients with delayed onset, the relationship to contrast administration may be overlooked. In general, iodine-induced hyperthyroidism is associated with elevated free T4 and a suppressed thyroid-stimulating hormone (TSH) level [594].

Hyperthyroidism induced by contrast medium may sometimes be transitory. In one such case, the clinical signs and laboratory values returned to normal without specific treatment [342].

Small amounts of free iodide, sufficient to affect thyroid function, have been demonstrated in intravascular contrast media [343]. Systematic studies of thyroid function after contrast administration in patients with previously normal thyroid function have shown an increase in T3 and decrease in TSH at 6 weeks, with even more marked changes at 6 months [344]. Similar changes were noted at 28 days in 5.3% of patients after infusion urography in an area of endemic goitre [345].

Transient increase in thyrotrophic hormone secretion occurred in infants undergoing cardioangiography, suggesting a Wolf–Chaikoff effect on the thyroid gland due to transient *hypothyroidism* caused by free iodide. Interestingly, the effect was more marked after ioxaglate (31.4% of cases) than with iopamidol (19.4% of cases) [346].

Transient hypothyroidism has been reported in neonates following opacification of parenteral nutrition catheters with ioxaglate [595]. Contrast media may interfere with the accuracy of tests based on the binding capacity of thyroid hormones for up to 10 days after administration [347].

It has been suggested that patients at risk of developing hyperthyroidism might be treated with an oral dose of 1.2 g sodium perchlorate 30 minutes before and 6–8 hours after contrast exposure, temporarily to inhibit iodide uptake by the thyroid [348]. Since, however, symptoms of "iodism" may occur in the subsequent days after contrast administration (see p. 267), longer administration of perchlorate would appear to be more rational if indeed this therapy is considered for use in exceptional cases.

An unusual case of transitory swelling of the thyroid resembling an acute thyroiditis was associated with conjunctival injection and rhinorrhea [349]. Mild transitory thyroid enlargement has also been noted on the day following urography (G. Ansell, unpublished data).

Pancreas

Contrast media may cause release of vasoactive intestinal polypeptide (VIP) in vipoma of the pancreas (see p. 271).

Adrenal

Contrast media may precipitate a hypertensive crisis in patients with pheochromocytoma [350]. Preliminary results in an experimental study suggest that nonionic medium may be less likely to cause catecholamine release in pheochromocytoma [610]. Contrast reactions may possibly exacerbate adrenal deficiency (see pp. 259,267).

Idiosyncratic reactions

Classification and incidence

Idiosyncratic reactions can broadly be categorized into four grades of severity [256,351].
1 *Minor reactions.* These usually require no treatment.
2 *Intermediate reactions.* These usually require some form of treatment but there is no undue fear for the patient's safety and the response to treatment is usually rapid.
3 *Severe reactions.* There is often fear for the patient's life and intensive treatment is required in most cases.
4 *Fatal reactions.*
Different studies have used variations of this classification; for example, in some studies [352,353] the term "severe" is attributed to patients requiring hospitalization, but this begs the question as to how one classifies preexisting hospital in-patients.

Minor and intermediate reactions are not infrequent but severe and fatal reactions are relatively rare. A large series of cases is therefore required for analysis to be meaningful. This has usually been achieved by survey techniques. In the classical North American survey during 1942–1958, Pendergras *et al.* [354] found a mortality rate of 8.6 per million urograms (1:117 000). In that survey, the total number of urograms performed was estimated from manufacturers' data of contrast-media sales with appropriate allowances for breakage of ampoules, etc. This may have been a feasible approach at a time when the standard dose of contrast

medium was 20 ml per urogram! In later years, the wide variability of dosage rendered manufacturers' sales data unreliable as a basis for surveys. Between 1969 and 1981, the FDA received reports of 405 deaths due to contrast media and this was the second most common cause (3.8%) of reported deaths due to drugs [355].

In surveys, there may be problems with consistency of reporting and, in particular, underreporting may occur [351]. Additional difficulties are encountered when different surveys are compared, due to variations in classification criteria and contrast dose. Even in the combined survey by Shehadi and Toniolo [352], using the same criteria, Shehadi's mortality rate of 1:15 000 for North America and other countries was double that found by Toniolo in Italy. Representative rates for reactions to contrast media are shown in Table 13.5. The earlier surveys refer to conventional ionic contrast media. In the two nonrandomized studies comparing ionic and nonionic media, performed in Australasia [357] and Japan [353], the incidence rates for severe reactions varied, but in each study, there was an approximately five- to sixfold reduction using nonionic media. Wolf *et al.* [358] attempted a form of randomization in their North American study: this appeared to show an even greater reduction in reaction rates for nonionic media, but the numbers involved were small. In another study, the incidence rates for adverse reactions found in the iohexol preregistration trials were two to 10 times greater than those of subsequent reports in postmarketing surveillance. The relative risk for all reactions was three to six times higher for ionic media versus nonionic media and these odds ratios were similar in both pre- and postregistration studies [359].

The small numbers of deaths reported in surveys make it difficult to evaluate mortality rates. Hitherto, the generally accepted figure for conventional ionic media has been in the region of 1:40–45 000 [256,351] and the recent Australian study [357] gives a similar rate. Neither of the two deaths reported in the Japanese survey [353] was attributed to contrast media, but a mortality rate of even 1:169 000 for ionic media in this survey appears to be exceptionally low. The reason for this is unexplained but incomplete reporting might be a possibility. Some of the problems and inconsistencies of the Japanese survey have been discussed elsewhere [360,361]. There have been a number of published deaths using nonionic media [353,362–364,382,383] and a larger number of unpublished deaths with these media [605].

In the UK between 1984 and 1993, the Medicines Control Agency received reports of 16 deaths associated with the use of intravascular nonionic media (mean contrast dose 25.47 gI) and 12 deaths with ionic media (mean dose 22.24 gI). During this period, the estimated sales of nonionic media in the UK were equivalent to approximately 120 000 KgI and sales of ionic media were approximately 73 000 KgI (Fig. 13.2). Whilst there appeared to be a marginally higher risk factor in the nonionic group, there otherwise appeared to be a remarkable

Table 13.5 Reaction rates for intravenous ionic* and nonionic† contrast media

Reference	Number of examinations	Minor	Intermediate	Severe	Fatal
Shehadi (1980) N America [352]	146 904*	1:29	1:60	1:2800	1:15 000
Toniolo (1980) Italy [352]	67 129*	1:31	1:130	1:1200	1:34 000
Ansell *et al.* (1980) UK [351]	164 475*	1:15	1:76	1:4200	1:45 000
Hartman *et al.* (1982) Mayo Clinic [356]	300 000*				1:75 000
Palmer (1988) Australasia [357]	79 000* 30 000†	1:30 1:96	1:284 1:1010	1:1117 1:6056	1:40 000
Katayama *et al.* (1990) Japan [353]	169 284* 168 363†			1:394 1:2215	1:169 000 1:168 000
Wolf *et al.* (1991) USA [358]	6006* 8857†	1:35 1:227	1:86 1:738	1:316 1:8857	

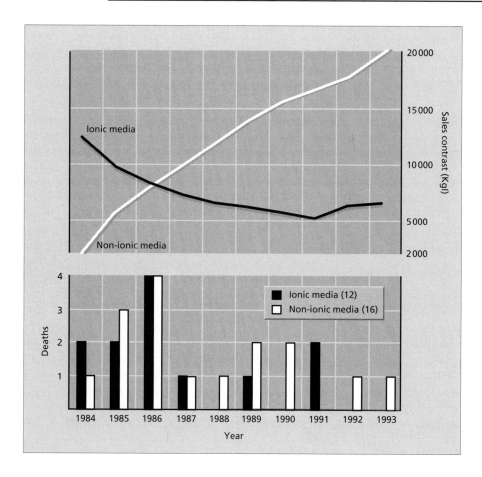

Fig. 13.2 Notified deaths in the United Kingdom and estimated sales of contrast media [365].

similarity in the numbers of notified deaths due to nonionic and ionic media, when these were related to contrast sales. These data should, however, be interpreted with considerable caution since it is probable that there was significant under-reporting of fatal reactions and it was impossible to determine if this applied equally to both types of media [365]. There appears to be a similar trend in the USA. Analysis of fatal contrast reactions reported to the FDA between 1978 and

1994 showed no decrease in reported annual deaths following the introduction of low-osmolar media in the USA in 1986, but limitation of data prevented correlation with risk factors, contrast sales and reporting trends [606].

It might be expected that the reduced incidence of severe reactions with nonionic media would also result in a lower mortality rate, but this is still speculative. Whichever contrast medium is used, it is important to have full facilities for emergency resuscitation and treatment.

Caro *et al.* [366] have undertaken a metaanalysis of contrast-media studies performed from 1980 onwards. They concluded that the incidence of severe reactions can be reduced by approximately 80% using low-osmolar media but, as yet, no alteration in the incidence of fatal reactions has been shown. It should be noted that this study was heavily weighted by the Japanese survey [353] and to a lesser extent by the Australasian survey [357]. Moreover, there was considerable nonuniformity of the other studies analyzed. The metaanalysis also failed to differentiate between ioxaglate and the nonionic low-osmolar media. Lawrence *et al.* [367] reported the findings of a large multidisciplinary working group who analyzed the published literature of severe and fatal reactions due to high- and low-osmolar contrast media. They drew attention to methodologic flaws in previous studies which made it difficult to determine accurate incidence rates, but they concluded that the risk of serious adverse reactions is very low with both high- and low-osmolar media. It might be noted in passing that even this high-powered evaluation could also be open to some criticism.

Time of onset of reactions

In the UK survey [58], approximately two-thirds of the severe and fatal reactions occurred in the first 5 minutes and 10% in the subsequent 10 minutes: 96% of these important reactions commenced in the first 20 minutes after injection. *This is the time when it is vital for the patient to be under constant observation* so that life-saving treatment can be commenced immediately. In Shehadi's series, 80% of the fatal reactions commenced in the first 5 minutes and the remaining 20% occurred between 5 and 15 minutes after the injection [355].

Occasionally, there may be *delayed hypotensive collapse* 1 or more hours after the injection [256]. A severe delayed reaction occurred several hours after injection of iohexol. At first, this was not recognized as a contrast-medium reaction. Symptoms were subsequently reproduced under controlled conditions [368]. Other types of delayed reactions are discussed on pp. 266—268, 270, 271, 274, 281.

Analysis of fatal reactions

Shehadi [355] analyzed the findings in 44 autopsies and noted edema of the upper respiratory tract in three cases

(6.8%), laryngeal edema in seven (15.9%), and pulmonary edema in 26 (59%). Lalli [269] analyzed manufacturers' data in 140 deaths following excretion urography in the USA and Canada and these are summarized in Table 13.6. The major factors in these deaths were cardiovascular or respiratory. Convulsions occurred in a few cases but it was uncertain whether these were toxic or secondary to anoxia. The mean age of these patients was 58 years. This corresponds with general experience in the various published series, where the great majority of urographic deaths occurred in patients *over the age of 50 years* [354,363]. In the UK survey [351], the mortality rate for the over-50 age-group doubled to approximately 1:20 000. In general, the cardiovascular system in older patients might be expected to be less resilient. An insult which in a younger patient might cause a moderate or severe reaction might prove fatal in an older patient. Older patients also appear to have an increased mortality rate with other drug reactions [369]. No age is completely immune to fatal reactions but they appear to be significantly less frequent in young adults [355]. In a subsequent analysis by Lalli involving manufacturers' data of 92 additional deaths following contrast media, it is surprising to find that only 16 patients had been subjected to autopsy [370]. A rare autopsy finding in a patient with idiopathic angioedema, who suffered a fatal contrast-medium reaction, showed occlusion of the trachea and bronchi by fluid-filled submucous blebs [349]. There is a scarcity of reliable information on the histology of fatal reactions. Findings have usually been nonspecific. In perhaps most cases, pathologists performing the autopsies have had no specialized experience in drug toxicology [371].

The first presentation of fatal reactions in Lalli's [269] series (Table 13.7) showed a wide range of symptoms and signs. Many of these were nonspecific as, e.g., nausea and vomiting. It should be noted that a reaction which initially appeared to be of minor importance might proceed to a fatality. This emphasizes the difficulty in recognizing the potentially fatal reaction and the importance of careful monitoring of even apparently trivial reactions. On the other hand, severe or fatal reactions may arise unexpectedly with startling suddenness (see also p. 266).

Table 13.6 Cause of death in 140 fatal urographic reactions (age = 6 weeks to 87 years; mean = 58 years. (From Lalli [269])

Cardiac	60
Pulmonary edema	20
Respiratory arrest	11
Cerebral or convulsions	10
Consumption coagulopathy	5
Bronchospasm	2
Laryngeal edema	2
Anaphylactic	1
Other	5
Unknown	24

Table 13.7 First sign in 140 fatal urographic reactions. (From Lalli [269])

Nausea and vomiting	20
Respiratory distress	20
Hypotension	13
Cardiac arrest or arrhythmia	10
Convulsions	8
Unconsciousness	8
Respiratory arrest	7
Apprehension	7

Other: rigors, erythema, peculiar sensation, sneezing, chest pain, attempt to sit up, arm pain, laryngeal edema, bronchospasm, rigidity, headache, diplopia, abdominal pain, urticaria, itching, hyperventilation

Analysis of nonfatal reactions

Whereas there is general agreement that the majority of fatal reactions occur in patients *over the age of 50 years* (see above), there is less certainty with regard to nonfatal reactions. Some studies have reported a higher incidence of severe reactions in the over-50 age-group [351,357,372]. This was not found in the Japanese survey [353], but grading criteria in this survey are unclear and show some discrepancies. Young infants may tolerate electrolyte imbalance badly, particularly with large doses of ionic contrast media. Severe delayed reactions occurred following excretion urography in two infants with congenital adrenal hyperplasia [373]. In the UK survey, the incidence rates for minor and intermediate urographic reactions peaked in the 20–29-year age-group and decreased with increasing age. The incidence rate for minor reactions also appeared to be slightly higher in female patients and there were more urographic examinations and reactions in females between the ages of 20 and 40 years, whereas after the age of 50 years, intravenous urograms were more frequently performed in males [351]. Lasser [374,375] subsequently also noted an increased incidence of reactions in women of childbearing years and in those receiving estrogen preparations: he suggested that this may be associated with their high estrogen state. Since minor and intermediate reactions constitute the overwhelming majority of reactions, it is possible that differences in sex distribution might account for the findings in some studies which claimed a lower incidence of reactions in the elderly compared with younger adults [353,376].

Clinical features of nonfatal reactions

The relative frequency of symptoms and signs reported in minor, moderate, and severe reactions in the UK survey of conventional ionic media are shown in Table 13.8 [58]. In individual cases, reactions often included more than one manifestation.

Trivial reactions

Trivial symptoms such as mild hot flush, metallic taste in the mouth, mild nausea, cough, sneezing, and tingling, occurred in most patients in one study [378]. Such trivial symptoms appeared to be related to dose and speed of injection [36]. Unpleasant perineal sensations may also occur such as burning, a feeling of wetness, or a desire to empty the bladder or rectum, sometimes accompanied by a spurious sensation of having done so. These perineal sensations appeared to be more common in women than in men [36,379].

Mucocutaneous reactions

Urticaria

Urticaria was the most common feature in intermediate reactions, occurring in approximately 50% of the cases, but it was reported in only 11.6% of severe reactions (Table 13.8). Lasser claims that in contrast reactions, urticaria is unique, in that its incidence is not increased in patients with a history of general allergy, or drug allergy, and that it is not prevented by corticosteroid pretreatment, except in patients with a previous history of allergy or a previous contrast reaction [374,375]. Urticaria may presage severe reactions.

Angioedema

Angioedema may occur in both intermediate and severe reactions. Commonly it affects the face. It has also been noted in the buccal mucosa [380] and in the bowel [381]. Angioedema is most hazardous when it affects the airways. It may cause a feeling of tightness in the throat. *Angioedema of the larynx may cause stridor with obstruction.* Angioedema may occasionally persist for up to 3 days. It may also present as a delayed reaction.

Necrotizing skin reactions

A small number of severe necrotizing skin reactions have been described, commencing up to several hours or days after contrast administration, often, but not exclusively, in patients with preexistent renal failure. The predominant feature appears to be a necrotizing vasculitis with widespread blistering and bullous changes [58]. There may also be multiorgan damage. *Patients with systemic lupus erythematosus (SLE) or those with a positive antinuclear factor due to hydrallazine appear to be at particular risk. Two patients developed fatal reactions with clinical features resembling Stevens–Johnson syndrome.* One of these patients had preexisting SLE and received iopamidol [382]. The other patient had a positive antinuclear factor due to hydralazine and received iohexol [383]. Nonfatal acute cutaneous vasculitis was precipitated by iopamidol in a patient who had an antinuclear factor due to hydralazine

Table 13.8 Clinical manifestations in nonfatal reactions [58]

Symptoms	451 minor reactions (%) (n)	335 intermediate reactions (%) (n)	43 severe reactions (%) (n)
Flushing	39.5 (178)	34.3 (115)	43.0 (10)
Pallor	2.2 (10)	8.0 (27)	30.0 (13)
Cyanosis		1.5 (5)	34.9 (15)
Urticaria	9.5 (43)	56.7 (190)	11.6 (5)
Conjunctival injection	0.9 (4)	8.2 (28)	18.6 (8)
Angioneurotic edema	0.2 (1)	9.3 (31)	16.3 (7)
Visual disturbance	0.2 (1)	2.7 (9)	2.3 (1)
Loss of consciousness		2.1 (7)	30.2 (13)
Convulsions		0.6 (2)	9.3 (4)
Tetani		1.5 (5)	
Headache	1.8 (8)	6.0 (20)	9.3 (4)
Faintness	6.9 (31)	11.3 (38)	37.2 (16)
Nausea	41.5 (187)	20.3 (68)	14.0 (6)
Retching	14.6 (66)	9.9 (33)	20.9 (9)
Vomiting	18.2 (82)	16.1 (54)	27.9 (12)
Abdominal pain	2.9 (13)	5.7 (19)	14.0 (6)
Diarrhea	0.2 (1)	0.3 (1)	
Sneezing	4.2 (19)	11.3 (38)	
Cough	1.8 (8)	11.6 (39)	9.3 (4)
Rhinorrhea	0.9 (4)	4.5 (15)	2.3 (1)
Bronchospasm	0.2 (1)	9.0 (30)	37.2 (16)
Laryngeal edema		3.6 (12)	14.0 (6)
Dyspnea	1.1 (5)	12.2 (41)	37.2 (16)
Circulatory collapse		4.5 (15)	62.8 (27)
Arrhythmia		0.9 (3)	4.7 (2)
EKG change			14.0 (6)
Pulmonary edema			9.3 (4)
Cardiac arrest			18.6 (8)
Arm pain	15.5 (70)	7.8 (26)	9.3 (4)
Chest pain	1.8 (8)	6.6 (22)	14.0 (6)
Rigors	1.3 (6)	6.0 (20)	4.7 (2)
Renal failure		0.4 (2)	2.3 (1)
Other	9.3 (42)	11.0 (37)	23.3 (10)

Numbers of manifestations in parentheses. Since reactions might consist of more than one manifestation, the totals for reactions are less than the sum of manifestations.

[384], and exacerbation of SLE has been reported following metrizamide myelography [385]. It is thought-provoking that all four of these cases had received *nonionic media*, but SLE and hydralazine therapy should probably be considered as contraindications to both ionic and nonionic media [384]. Two patients with endstage renal failure on peritoneal dialysis developed an *acute polyarthropathy* with severe constitutional illness 6 and 16 hours, respectively, after injection of iopamidol. One patient who had amyloidosis involving the adrenals also developed hypotension which responded promptly to hydrocortisone: there was no evidence of SLE [386].

A fatal case of *toxic epidermal necrolysis* occurred following urography with diatrizoate in a patient with malignant disease who had an earlier exposure to diatrizoate, suggesting the possibility of an immunologic mechanism [387]. There was also a history of malignant disease in two patients who developed nonfatal necrotizing vasculitis with purpuric rashes and acute nephritis [388]. These cases have occurred with both ionic and nonionic media. It seems possible that they represent some form of immunologic response to the iodine moiety resulting from deiodination and prolonged retention due to impaired renal excretion.

Typical *iododerma* with vegetative lesions occurred 3–4 days after high-dose urography in two patients with renal failure, and lasted up to 3 weeks [389,390]. In another patient with renal failure, an allergic vasculitis with bloody blisters, mild fever, and conjunctivitis was associated with salivary gland enlargement; the severity of symptoms correlated with serum iodine and sCr levels [391]. In a patient with seronegative rheumatoid arthritis and chronic renal failure requiring hemodialysis, venous shuntograms on two separate occasions caused iododerma and pulmonary infiltrates: biopsy of the skin lesions showed a *leukocytic vasculitis*

[392]. In another case of iododerma, the patient had an obscure pyrexial illness: the intravenous urogram was preceded by a lymphangiogram with lipiodol which may have been a sensitizing factor [393]. In most of these severe necrotizing lesions, there has therefore been some underlying disease which may have affected the immune system, and also the probability of prolonged exposure to iodide.

There have also been a number of isolated case reports of unusual dermatologic manifestations due to contrast media. In a case of *bullous lichen planus* a positive macrophage-migration inhibition factor to contrast medium was demonstrated *in vitro*, suggesting the possibility of an immunologic process [394]. In two patients, a localized transient fixed drug eruption occurred on several occasions following contrast examinations [596,597]. A patient who had a fixed drug eruption to aspirin subsequently developed a similar eruption with pyrexia following iohexol [396].

A *Koebner phenomenon* with skin lesions at the sites of previous scars may rarely occur following contrast administration [390,395]. An unusual reaction occurred following *lymphography* with *iodized* oil in a patient with carcinoma of the cervix. The patient developed *multicentric reticulohystiocytosis* with arthritis and skin papules: this was exacerbated on two occasions following *oral diatrizoate* [397].

Delayed onset and late phase reactions

Davies and colleagues [379,398] studied the incidence of delayed reactions in over 2000 patients and found an overall incidence of delayed skin rashes in 4.5% of patients. The rashes commenced within 3 days and lasted up to 8 days. They consisted of red blotches and lumps; itching was a prominent feature. Dry scaly skin occurred in two patients and mouth ulcers in seven patients. Recalculation of combined data from these two studies shows a significant difference in the incidence of rashes with different types of media, namely: sodium media = 3.3%; nonionic media = 5%; methylglucamine media = 7.5% (*P* = 0.006). It appears possible that the higher incidence of rashes with methylglucamine media may be related to the higher free iodide in such media [343]. Comparative chemical data are not available for measured free iodide contained in nonionic media, but the intermediate incidence of rashes suggests that they may possibly have a higher free iodide content than sodium media, or may be more prone to deiodination. Davies and colleagues also noted flu-like symptoms suggestive of iodism in 10% of patients, but some of these symptoms were nonspecific and it is not certain that they were all due to iodism. The overall incidence of delayed reactions was higher than that for immediate reactions [379,398,399,607].

In a large Japanese survey [399] of delayed symptoms in 2382 patients receiving nonionic media, the incidence of headaches was 2.6%, rashes 2.4%, and itching 1.7%. This survey only included symptoms up to 48 hours and some

delayed rashes may not have been included. In another large prospective Japanese survey [400], the incidence of delayed rashes was only 1.6%. However, only the "severest" symptom in each case was analyzed statistically in this study and, since arm pain and headache were more common, this may account for the relatively low incidence recorded for rashes.

A number of other delayed reactions and skin eruptions have been reported in the Japanese literature, the majority being due to iohexol or iopamidol [400–403]. In three cases, disseminated maculopapular eruptions developed 5–6 days after drip infusion pyelography with iohexol. Skin tests were apparently positive for iohexol and negative for other iodinated contrast media [404]. A late phase reaction with widespread erythema and edema appeared 6 hours after intravenous injection of the nonionic dimer iotrolan. An intradermal challenge of iotrolan provoked the same reaction in a previously affected area of skin but not in an unaffected area. Biopsy showed vascular and lymphatic dilatation and cellular infiltration. The white blood cell count showed marked decrease in granulocytes and marked increase in lymphocytes after the challenge. There was no crossreactivity with iohexol or iopamidol [405]. Another positive skin reaction has also been reported in a drug eruption due to iotrolan [406]. (In Japan and Germany during 1995, concern about a possible excess of troublesome delayed reactions following intravascular use of nonionic dimers resulted in precautionary temporary suspension of sales of iotrolan 280 [611].

Reports of severe drug eruptions have become more frequent since the introduction of nonionic media, but it is uncertain whether this is specifically related to the nature of nonionic media or whether it may be partly due to the more recent recognition of delayed reactions to contrast media and the increasing use of nonionic media, often in large doses. In a Japanese retrospective survey [407] using case records of 715 patients receiving ionic media and 902 patients receiving nonionic media for CT, the incidence of delayed reactions was 5% for methylglucamine ionic media and 4.9% following nonionic media. For other delayed reactions see pp. 265, 269–271, 274, 281.

Pulmonary reactions

Bronchospasm

Bronchospasm is an important feature. It occurred in 9% of intermediate reactions and 37% of severe reactions in the UK survey [58] (Table 13.8). Somewhat surprisingly, bronchospasm was not specifically evaluated in the Japanese survey where it was presumably included under the general category of dyspnea [353]. Laryngeal edema which occurred in 14% of severe reactions [58] may mimic bronchospasm. There was a preceding history of asthma or other allergy in 38% of reactions causing bronchospasm [58]. *Asthmatic patients form an unduly susceptible group* liable to severe reactions [351,408]. Severe bronchospasm may cause cyanosis: there may be accompanying hypotension or even cardiac arrest. As little as 0.5–1.0 ml of contrast may provoke a severe attack. However, only a small proportion of asthmatic patients actually develop an attack following contrast administration. In the Mayo Clinic series using methylglucamine diatrizoate, bronchospasm occurred in 6% of patients with a history of asthma and a severe attack occurred in one patient (0.7%) [378]. In the Japanese survey [353], the incidence of severe and very severe reactions in asthmatic patients was 1.88% with ionic media and 0.23% with nonionic media.

Patients receiving *β-adrenergic-blocking drugs* may also develop bronchospasm following contrast medium [409]. Moreover, β-blockers may increase the severity of a reaction and impair the response to treatment [408].

Methylglucamine is a potent histamine-releasing agent [410]. In individual cases, it appears that methylglucamine media may precipitate bronchospasm (G. Ansell, unpublished data). Bolus injection of large doses of ionic contrast medium frequently causes subclinical bronchospasm, as shown by measurement of peak expiratory flow. No difference was detected between sodium and methylglucamine media but the incidence was much reduced with iopamidol [411,412]. The significance of this type of subclinical bronchospasm requires further elucidation.

Nonionic media are now generally considered preferable in asthmatic patients but they should be combined with steroid prophylaxis (see p. 278). Severe bronchospasm occurred in a high-risk asthmatic patient receiving iopamidol without steroid premedication (see p. 279). Another severe reaction to iopamidol with hypotension and bronchospasm occurred during general anesthesia [413]. Bronchospasm also occurred in a fatal reaction to iohexol [362].

Pulmonary edema

Pulmonary edema was a frequent feature in fatal reactions [269,355] and occurred in some 9.3% of severe reactions to conventional contrast media [58] (Table 13.8, p. 267). The risk is greatest when large doses of hypertonic contrast media are given to patients with incipient cardiac failure [36,349,414]. With infusion urography, this may be partly due to the volume of fluid administered but the main factor is the high-osmotic load which causes withdrawal of fluids from the interstitial tissues into the cardiovascular compartments, with resulting hypervolemia. Pulmonary edema has also been reported after aortography [415] and following overdose of contrast media in infants [61,62].

Contrast media may also increase pulmonary capillary permeability. In rats, very large doses of diatrizoate produced transient pulmonary edema [416]. Iohexol caused negligible pulmonary edema whereas the low-osmolar dimer ioxaglate surprisingly produced a greater degree of pulmonary edema than diatrizoate. This suggests that there is also a chemotoxic effect on capillary permeability unrelated to osmolarity [417]. Pretreatment with methylprednisolone 24 and 0.5 hours before the injection of diatrizoate, significantly reduced the degree of this experimental pulmonary edema [418]. In patients with myocardial problems, nonionic media are preferable but pulmonary edema has occurred following a nonionic medium [419].

Noncardiogenic pulmonary edema

Noncardiogenic pulmonary edema has occurred during the course of acute anaphylactic reactions with hypotensive collapse. In these patients, central venous pulmonary artery and pulmonary artery wedge pressures excluded a congestive origin, while the colloid oncotic pressure and protein content of the pulmonary edema fluid resembled that of the plasma. This suggested that the pulmonary edema was due to increased capillary permeability, possibly as a result of an anaphylactoid phenomenon [420]: in one patient, there was also hypokalemia [421]. It is important to distinguish such cases from the congestive type, since they may *require fluid replacement*.

In a patient who had previously had clinical pulmonary edema following contrast medium, cardiac angiography for severe atypical chest pain was performed after premedication with prednisone and diphenhydramine, and again resulted in pulmonary edema. The pulmonary capillary wedge pressure was 2 mmHg indicating a noncardiogenic origin for the edema. There was no urticaria or angioedema [422]. Two atypical cases of pulmonary edema following contrast occurred in young adults. In one of these, there was initially generalized urticaria, and *delayed pulmonary edema* developed 2 hours later [423]. All of these patients had received conventional high-osmolar contrast media.

Four cases of noncardiogenic pulmonary edema have also been reported following the low-osmolar ionic dimer ioxaglate. In one patient, ioxaglate was injected intraarterially for mesenteric arteriography. Three of the patients had previous histories of myocardial infarction but there was no evidence of recent acute myocardial changes. One patient subsequently died. With a previous history of myocardial infarction, such patients may be misdiagnosed as cardiogenic pulmonary edema in the absence of hemodynamic measurements [424,425]. The experimental evidence suggesting increased toxicity of ioxaglate in pulmonary capillaries [417] (see above) may have some relevance in these cases.

Shock lung and adult respiratory distress syndrome (ARDS). Severe hypotensive reactions to contrast medium may be accompanied by a syndrome resembling shock lung with multiple pulmonary infiltrates [426]. An acute contrast reaction in a patient with urinary sepsis, commenced with dyspnea and progressed to an ARDS with disseminated intravascular coagulation [427].

Stevens—Johnson syndrome and iododerma. Pulmonary infiltrates may occur in the Stevens—Johnson syndrome [382,383] (see p. 266). They may also be present in association with iododerma [392] (see p. 267).

Eosinophilic pneumonia. A case of eosinophilic pneumonia with reticulonodular shadowing in the lung was attributed to cerebral angiography with iohexol, but the patient was an asthmatic [428].

Miscellaneous. Cough is usually a nonspecific symptom. While *dyspnea* can be an important symptom in major reactions, it may occasionally be present in minor and intermediate reactions without obvious significant cause. *Chest pain* may also be nonspecific.

Cardiovascular reactions

The direct effects of contrast media on the cardiovascular system are discussed above (see p. 249). However, cardiovascular manifestations are important in some idiosyncratic reactions and circulatory collapse was noted in some 60% of severe reactions (Table 13.8, p. 267).

Cardiac arrest

Sudden cardiac arrest occurred in approximately 20% of severe reactions (Table 13.8). With prompt and effective treatment, there is a reasonable chance of full recovery.

EKG changes

Arrhythmias and transitory *ischemic changes* may be present in severe reactions. These may initially be mistaken for myocardial infarction. Occasionally, however, hypotensive collapse may be associated with unequivocal evidence of *coronary infarction*, and it may be problematic to decide whether the coronary infarction occurred incidentally or if it resulted from a hypotensive reaction to contrast medium [256]. Tryptase levels may confirm an anaphylactoid reaction [429]. EKG changes are more likely to occur in older patients or in those with a previous history of heart disease, but *coronary artery spasm* has been demonstrated during an *anaphylactoid reaction* to contrast medium [84,85]. In some cases, arrhythmias including *ventricular fibrillation*, or ischemic changes, may have been due to *epinephrine* used to treat a reaction [256,430,431] (see also pp. 250, 285).

Hypotension

Hypotensive collapse is one of the most important features

of contrast-media reactions and it occurred in the majority of patients who experienced severe reactions. In this group, hypotension was usually profound, often associated with transitory loss of consciousness, and occasionally accompanied by incontinence. In the unconscious patient, there is a major risk of *airway obstruction* due to the tongue falling back, with resulting anoxia and cyanosis: this requires immediate attention. In reactions with hypotensive collapse, there was usually tachycardia with a thready pulse, but in approximately 25% of patients there was a vagal reaction with bradycardia usually responding to intravenous atropine [92—94] (see also p. 251).

Excluding vagal reactions, life-threatening hypotension occurred in 30 (0.05%) out of 60 000 contrast studies performed at the Massachusetts General Hospital between 1973 and 1983 [430]. With hypotensive collapse, the skin is often cold and clammy and there may occasionally be profuse perspiration. In some patients with severe hypotension, there was a diffuse erythematous rash preceded by nausea and vomiting [378]. *Syncope* may also occur due to fear or nausea, or it may occasionally result from decreased venous return to the heart following inferior vena caval obstruction due to abdominal compression. Minor degrees of hypotension usually require no treatment other than posture, reassurance, and observation.

Severe hypotension, however, may be associated with increased capillary permeability and loss of fluid into the tissues from the circulating blood, causing hypovolemia. Such cases usually respond best to fluid replacement [430]. Prolonged shock may be refractory until hypovolemia has been corrected [432]. A severe vasovagal reaction with hypotension, bradycardia, loss of consciousness, and convulsions resulted from the injection of 40 ml iohexol. This responded rapidly to intravenous fluids and atropine [433]. *Severe delayed hypotensive reactions* may rarely occur 1 or more hours after ionic media [256] or nonionic media [368].

Fischer *et al.* [434] monitored the blood pressure in 97 patients undergoing excretion urography and found six patients who became significantly hypotensive (mean blood pressure < 60 mmHg) without showing any obvious clinical manifestations other than slowing of the pulse in two cases. All six patients recovered spontaneously without sequelae and radiographs did not show any evidence of "shock kidneys". In the absence of routine monitoring, these cases would not have been detected after contrast administration: this suggests that significant subclinical hypotension may be more common than is generally realized. It is possible that in unfavorable circumstances, some similar cases may progress to an overt reaction and this may explain why some severe reactions arise suddenly without warning. It has been suggested that osmotic diuresis may be a cause of delayed hypotension [435].

Hypertension. While hypotension is usually the dominant

feature in the majority of severe contrast-media anaphylactoid reactions, it appears that rarely there may be a hypertensive response [436] (see also pp. 263, 276, 283, 285).

Gastrointestinal reactions

Nausea and vomiting. Nausea and vomiting are relatively nonspecific symptoms (Table 13.8), but vomiting can be distressing and it may even presage a fatal reaction [269]. In one patient, inhalation of vomit lead to death [349]. Rarely, the onset of vomiting may be delayed [256]. Ioxaglate has been associated with a higher incidence of vomiting and anaphylactoid effects, whereas nonionic media have a reduced incidence [80,437,438].

Delayed nausea and vomiting may be a feature of "recall reactions" when interleukin 2 (IL-2) causes sensitization to contrast media [439] (see p. 274).

In an anecdotal note, Nathan [440] suggests that vomiting may be caused by hypotension, and he claims that elevation of the limbs at the onset of nausea lowers the incidence of vomiting.

Diarrhea. Whereas diarrhea is not uncommon following cholegraphic media (see p. 499) it is relatively uncommon with the other intravascular media, but it may occur in vagal reactions. Sensitization with IL-2 can be associated with diarrhea (see p. 274).

Angioedema of the small bowel and ascites were noted during CT in a patient who developed cramping abdominal pain, abdominal distension, nausea, vomiting, and explosive diarrhea after receiving 50 ml meglumine diatrizoate-60 [381].

Another patient had severe continuous watery diarrhea and incontinence with a transitory hypotensive episode, shortly after injection of 100 ml diatrizoate-76. There was faint opacification of the small bowel on the 10 and 15 minute films and it was suggested that there might have been vicarious excretion of contrast medium [441].

In a patient with a *Vipoma of the pancreas* and hepatic secondaries, CT and angiography with diatrizoate caused release of VIP with a marked increase of watery diarrhea resulting in hypotension and temporary renal impairment. A cholecystogram with iopanoic acid also caused an increase in stool volume in the same patient and it was suggested that iodine may have augmented VIP-stimulated adenylcyclase activity [442].

An unexplained severe reaction to iopamidol commenced with abdominal cramping, vomiting, and diarrhea which was followed by hypotension, multisystem failure, and disseminated intravascular coagulation [443]. Circulatory collapse with prolonged unconsciousness may be followed on recovery by the passage of offensive blood-stained stools [349]. This may possibly be due to disseminated intravascular coagulation (see p. 276).

Salivary glands and pancreas

Parotid gland swelling (iodide mumps) was rarely reported with low doses of contrast media [444], but became more frequent with larger doses, particularly when there was prolonged retention of contrast medium due to renal failure [445]. This appears to be an idiosyncratic reaction and may occur in the same patient on repeated examinations. The parotid swelling usually occurs 3–4 days after contrast administration and may last for several days. In patients with renal failure, the swelling may persist for several weeks [391]. In uremic patients, the retained contrast medium is subject to deiodination *in vivo* [446]. There may be both organically bound iodine and inorganic iodide in the saliva [447]. Small but significant quantities of free iodide were found in commercial preparations of contrast media. The free iodide content of methylglucamine preparations (1.1–4.6 mg/100 ml) was higher than that in sodium-containing media (0.2–1.4 mg/100 ml) [343]. A case of iodide mumps has also been reported after iopamidol: it is stated that this medium may contain up to 4 mg free iodide/100 ml [448].

In an isolated case, parotid gland enlargement was associated with paralysis of the facial nerve, which developed over a period of 12 hours after the injection of 60 ml sodium diatrizoate-50. The parotid gland swelling responded to prednisone and diphenhydramine administered on the fourth day but the *facial palsy* persisted. Operative decompression of the facial nerve at 5 weeks revealed the presence of hemorrhage and edema and was followed by partial recovery and function [449]. Nerve involvement of this nature appears to be exceptional, but if a similar case should occur, it would be logical to commence steroid and possibly antihistamine therapy as early as possible. Iodide mumps and slight thyroid swelling occurred following cerebral angiography with iohexol in a patient with renal failure; diphenhydramine and cortisone were ineffective but improvement occurred after dialysis [450].

In a large follow-up survey of delayed reactions, symptoms suggestive of *parotitis* were noted in 0.87% of patients receiving sodium iothalamate and in 1.7% of patients receiving iopamidol. With the numbers involved, this difference lacked statistic significance but the trend is of interest [379].

Evanescent salivary gland enlargement has also been reported, commencing within a few minutes of injection of methylglucamine diatrizoate; the swelling subsided over a period of a few hours [451].

An unusually severe case of acute painful bilateral parotid enlargement with intense local erythema occurred 1 hour after intravenous ioxaglate; *acute anaphylactic shock* developed 10 minutes later. The shock responded rapidly to intravenous fluids and epinephrine, and this was followed by improvement of the parotid swelling. It is of interest that routine premedication with dexamethasone in this patient appeared ineffective [452].

In another patient, asymptomatic parotid gland enlargement occurred during a contrast CT examination. This was accompanied by marked global enlargement of the pancreas, shown on CT, and mild midback pain which rapidly subsided. Repeat CT at 4 hours showed that the pancreas had reverted to normal size; the parotid swelling had also subsided. St Amour *et al.* [453] suggested the term *pancreatic mumps* for this case, as part of the iodide mumps syndrome.

Abdominal pain

Severe abdominal pain may occur in anaphylactic reactions, presumably as a result of intestinal edema (see above) and/ or spasm. In one case, the pain was relieved by atropine (G. Ansell, unpublished data). Cramping abdominal pain was reported in several of the patients who developed severe hypotensive collapse with bradycardia due to *vagal overactivity* [92]. Hypotensive collapse might possibly induce abdominal angina in some patients, due to transitory visceral ischemia. In some patients, abdominal pain was associated with paresthesiae occurring elsewhere. Deficiency of C_1-esterase inhibitor is known to be a cause of attacks of abdominal pain [454]; this may possibly be a factor in rare cases.

Loin pain can occur during excretion urography due to the diuretic effect of contrast medium which may cause increased renal intracapsular pressure if there is partial obstruction, e.g., by a ureteric calculus. Severe abdominal pain due to pyelosinus extravasation into the perirenal space was at first mistaken for a contrast reaction [455]. Pancreatic pain is discussed above.

Risk factors for idiosyncratic reactions

History of previous reactions

In the UK Survey [351] (Table 13.9), patients with a history of a previous reaction to contrast media had an odds ratio of 10.9 for increased risk of a *severe reaction* occurring. In the Japanese survey [456], the odds ratio was 4.68. In cases where there had been a previous reaction to contrast medium, the risk of a recurrent reaction at a subsequent examination

was 35–40%, but even in these cases, repeat reactions were inconsistent and might be present on some occasions and not on others [351,378,457,458]. Shehadi [459] concluded that: "major life-threatening reactions do not tend to recur on reexamination." However, analysis of his data suggests that this conclusion is not valid [460]. It is also important to realize that reactions may occur *de novo* even though the patient has had previous uneventful examinations with contrast medium.

A severe reaction occurred in a radiographer who had apparently been sensitized by handling contrast media [256], and there is some evidence to suggest that *occupational exposure* to contrast media may induce hypersensitivity [461].

History of allergy

Asthma is the most important of the allergic predisposing factors for severe reactions. In the UK survey [351], the odds ratio for a severe reaction in patients with a history of asthma was 5.1 (Table 13.9). In the Japanese survey [456], the odds ratio was 10 and in a recent case-control study in the USA, the odds ratio was estimated at 4.5 [408]. In the Mayo Clinic series using sodium methylglucamine diatrizoate [378], approximately 6% of patients with a history of asthma developed an attack with contrast medium (see also p. 268).

A history of *urticaria* was more likely to be associated with an intermediate reaction. In the UK study [351], *eczema* had an odds ratio of 4.7 for severe reactions, but the small numbers were not statistically significant. Histories of *hay fever* or of adverse reactions to *drugs* including penicillin were moderate risk factors.

In the Mayo Clinic series [378], 6% of reactors gave a history of *food or seafood allergy* and 13% gave a history of allergy to *iodide*.

A fatal reaction occurred in a patient with *hereditary angioneurotic edema* and this should be regarded as a major risk factor [349].

Cardiac history

The effects of contrast media on the cardiovascular system

Table 13.9 Intravenous urograms: risk ratios related to clinical history. [(From Ansell *et al.* [351])

History	Minor reactions	Intermediate reactions	Severe reactions	Death
Allergy (all types)	1.6	2.6	3.9	
Hay fever	1.7	1.8	2.3	
Urticaria	1.5	4.8	2.0	
Asthma	1.2	2.7	5.1	
Previous reaction to contrast medium	6.9	8.7	10.9	
Previous reaction to other drugs	1.8	2	3.2	
Heart disease	1.1	0.9	4.5	8.5

have been discussed earlier (see p. 249), but a history of cardiac disease is also an important factor in severe idiosyncratic reactions. The majority of *cardiac arrests* in the UK survey occurred in patients with a history of cardiac disease. For *fatal reactions*, the odds ratio was 8.5 with an overall incidence of 1:9000. There was an increased risk of a severe reaction with all types of cardiac disease, particularly with congestive cardiac failure and coronary artery disease, but cardiac history did not appear to affect the incidence of minor or intermediate reactions. For patients with a history of *congestive cardiac failure* the mortality rate was 1:1600 [351]. In the Japanese survey, patients with cardiac disease had an odds ratio of 3 for severe reactions. In a theoretical model, combining the risk factors for "previous reactions, asthma, and cardiac disease" the calculated odds ratio for severe reactions was 120 [456].

Age (see pp. 265,266)

Dose

There is controversy concerning the effect of contrast medium dose on the incidence of reactions. On pharmacologic grounds, it would be reasonable to assume such a relationship, even though severe reactions may rarely occur after minute doses of contrast medium. In the UK survey, there was a very suggestive trend in that the incidence of *severe and fatal reactions* increased progressively from approximately 1:8000, with a dose below 20 g iodine, to 1:2000 when the dose exceeded 30 g iodine ($P < 0.05$) [58]. Similarly, Lasser *et al.* [372] found an approximate doubling of reactions requiring treatment for doses above 27 g iodine in comparison with doses below 15 g iodine. In the Japanese survey, however, the incidence of reactions was actually *lowest* in patients receiving more than 80 ml of contrast medium [353]: this appears inexplicable!

Injection rate

It is difficult to assess the influence of injection rate on reactions. Davies *et al.* [36] noticed an increased incidence of warmth after rapid injections, but otherwise the incidence of reactions did not appear to vary with injection speed. Jensen and Dorph [462] assessed the effects of injection rates in 334 patients using a relatively large dose of contrast medium (up to 120 ml Telebrix 380). Rapid injections within 10 seconds caused an increased sensation of warmth, metallic taste, and occipital headache, but these were mild. Otherwise, there was no increase in side-effects as compared with a slower injection over 2 minutes. However, they did not advocate rapid injection in patients with cardiac disease (patients with cardiac disease and other risk factors were excluded from this series). Lorenz *et al.* [23] have pointed out that drugs which cause histamine release are more likely to do so if

given by bolus injection rather than by a slow rate of injection. The sensation of warmth, metallic taste, and headache, noted by Jensen and Dorph, would be consistent with histamine release.

In animal experiments when large doses of contrast media were injected very rapidly, there was a considerable increase in toxicity. Whereas the LD_{50} of sodium diatrizoate by slow intravenous drip in the dog was 13 200 mg/kg, with rapid injection of 90% diatrizoate, the LD_{50} dropped to 2700 mg/kg. Death usually occurred rapidly and was associated with acute hypotension, marked EKG change, and hemorrhagic pulmonary edema [463]. Pfister and Hutter [89] showed that the incidence of abnormal EKG changes occurring during urography was related independently to the dose of contrast medium used and to the rapidity of injection. Therefore, it would appear that at least in the more susceptible older patients and in those with cardiac disease, a slower injection would be safer where this is consistent with the diagnostic requirement.

Route of administration

It is generally considered that adverse reactions occur more frequently following intravenous as compared with intra-arterial administration. In Dahlstrohm *et al.*'s series [464], the incidence following intravenous ionic media was approximately twice that of intraarterial administration. With iohexol, the incidence was lower and there was no difference between intravenous and intraarterial studies. Lasser [375] claims that the higher incidence of reactions following intravenous injections of ionic media relates mainly to gastrointestinal and skin symptoms. He suggests that this could be mainly due to mediators released from the first sweep of concentrated contrast medium through the lungs.

In a study of patients with previous histories of contrast-media reactions, there was no significant difference of recurrent reactions between intravenous and intraarterial examinations [465].

It should be recognized that in patients with a history of contrast-medium sensitivity, and in others, severe reactions may occur following arteriography [256,466] and more especially following left ventriculography or aortic-root injections [84,467−470].

β-Blockers

In patients under treatment with β-adrenergic blocking agents, there was an increased incidence of severe contrast-media reactions, including bronchospasm [409]. Severe hypotensive reactions may also occur [103]. In a case-control study, the odds ratio for increased risk of a significant reaction in patients receiving β-blockers was 3.43. These reactions may also be resistant to therapy and the odds ratio for such patients requiring hospitalization was 8.7 [408]. In one fatal reaction to iohexol, the patient was under treatment with a β-blocker for hypertension [471]. Greenberger [472] did not find β-blockers to be a problem, but his patients received prophylactic steroids and antihistamines (see p. 279).

The risk for increased severity of reactions in patients under treatment with β-blockers appears to involve both selective and nonselective agents. However, β-blocker therapy should *not* be withdrawn abruptly. An individual clinical assessment should be made in each patient. If a contrast examination is essential in a patient who also requires β-blockers, it would be logical to consider premedication with corticosteroids and use of a nonionic medium. Full facilities for resuscitation should, of course, be available (see also pp. 48, 49, 278, 282).

IL-2

IL-2 is an immune stimulant: 15−28% of patients who have received treatment with this substance may develop an unusual type of hypersensitivity: when they subsequently receive contrast media, even several weeks after treatment with IL-2, they develop a "recall reaction" resembling the toxic effects of IL-2. These reactions may occur 1−4 hours after contrast administration, and include diarrhea, fever, chills, nausea, vomiting, pruritus, skin rashes, wheezing, and edema. Severe reactions may cause *hypotension* and oliguria. This form of sensitization has occurred after intra-arterial or intravenous administration of IL-2, and is provoked by either intravenous or intraarterial administration of contrast media [439,473−475]. The reactions appear more likely to occur with ionic media. Reactions may occur up to 6 weeks after administration of IL-2, but they appear to be more common in the first 2 weeks. In earlier studies, corticosteroids and antihistamines appeared to be effective in treatment of these reactions, and when used prophylactically to premedicate sensitized patients. However, Shulman *et al.* [475] report a recurrent reaction despite steroid premedication and they advise against routine premedication with corticosteroids since this may block the IL-2 effector mechanism. They suggest that, instead, contrast media should be avoided in the first 2 weeks after IL-2, if possible. A reaction may, however, occur as long as 2 years after administration of IL-2 [598]. Local administration of IL-2 into the bladder, or by inhalation therapy, has also caused similar generalized sensitization reactions; these reactions included *pulmonary edema* and *hypertension* [476].

Ethnicity

In the UK survey, Indians appeared to have a significantly higher incidence of severe reactions than North Europeans or Africans, with an odds ratio of 8.1. The reason for this is uncertain but the role of ethnic factors merits further consideration in contrast-media studies [351].

Anxiety (see p. 277)

Miscellaneous

It is probable that patients in poor general condition may be unduly susceptible. Lasser *et al.* [477] suggested that a pre-existing clinical condition such as infection might prime the complement coagulation systems and interfere with the normal response of acute stress to contrast injection, thereby producing a more serious reaction [477,478]. In one study, the incidence of reactions in *trauma* patients was three times that in nontrauma patients [479]. Animal studies suggest that *dehydration* could be an adverse factor [480].

SLE and hydralazine therapy are major risk factors (see p. 266).

In a multivariate analysis, *diabetes* has been suggested as a risk factor for idiosyncratic reactions [481]. This is not generally agreed as being a risk factor, but it is conceivable that diabetic autonomic neuropathy might aggravate a reaction. Other individual case reports include *paraproteinemia* [313] and *malignancy* [387,388,482]. *Mastocytosis* is a theoretical risk [429,483]. Risk factors are summarized in Table 13.10.

Pathogenesis of idiosyncratic reactions

Although much effort and research have been devoted to the investigation of contrast media, the precise etiology of idiosyncratic reactions is still uncertain. The majority of these reactions appear to be pseudoallergic. It appears that a number of different factors may be involved in their causation, and some of these concepts will be discussed.

Table 13.10 Risk factors for severe idiosyncratic reactions

Major risk factors
Previous reaction to contrast medium
Asthma, allergy, iodism
Cardiac disease
Anxiety
β-Blockers
IL-2
Type contrast medium, dose
Age
SLE, hydralazine

Possible risk factors
General condition, dehydration, trauma, paraproteinemias, malignancy, mastocytosis, ethnicity, adrenal suppression, ?diabetes

Miscellaneous risk factors and complications
Convulsions, myasthenia gravis, sickle cell disease, homocystinuria, thromboembolism, thyrotoxicosis, pheochromocytoma, Vipoma

See also Tables 13.2, p. 251; 13.4, p. 253; and 13.9, p. 272.

Histamine liberation

Certain drugs can cause direct liberation of histamine from mast cells and other tissues without the intervention of an immunologic reaction. Mann [484] first drew attention to the resemblance of many features of contrast media reactions with those resulting from histamine liberation. She suggested that the susceptibility of atopic subjects to contrast-media reactions might be accounted for by the fact that the tissues in such patients contained a higher quantity of histamine than normal and that these subjects were more sensitive to the effects of histamine.

Histamine release may be associated with a wide range of symptoms and signs. These include flushing, hives, angioneurotic edema, pruritus, conjunctival injection, metallic taste, nausea, vomiting, cramps, diarrhea, sneezing, stuffy nose, tightness of the throat, tightness of the chest, coughing, dyspnea, bronchospasm, headache, tinnitus, tachycardia or bradycardia, hypotension, or hypertension. There may be complex cardiac changes with arrhythmias including ventricular fibrillation, coronary artery spasm, and cardiac arrest [23,483,485]. Histamine may cause vasodilatation, increased capillary permeability, pulmonary edema, and shock [486].

Contrast media and methylglucamine itself cause histamine release in animals and in humans [487,488]. Numerous studies have been performed on *in vitro* histamine release from animal mast cells, but it should be noted that mast cells are heterogeneous and results may vary depending on their site of origin and species. An *in vitro* study using leukocytes and platelets from healthy humans showed that contrast media liberated histamine from basophils and serotonin from platelets. Methylglucamine-containing media were more potent histamine-releasing agents than sodium media. In general, the higher-osmolar media caused greater histamine release than lower-osmolar media [489]. In patients, there did not appear to be any consistent correlation between elevated plasma levels of histamine and the occurrence of either contrast-media reactions or hemodynamic changes [488,490,491]. A later study using a sensitive method of estimating plasma histamine suggested that a peak plasma histamine level in excess of 1 μg/ml was more likely to be associated with adverse effects such as flushing, warmth, nausea, vomiting, rash, or urticaria, but there was a lack of uniformity, suggesting a possible variation in receptor sensitivity [492].

Histamine release may occur in many circumstances including trauma, pain, anesthesia, anoxia, ischemia, surgery, blood transfusion, and as a result of a wide variety of drugs [23]. In addition to, or in association with, histamine release, there are many mediators that theoretically might be involved in adverse reactions, including serotonin, bradykinin, prostaglandins, leukotrienes, and others. In considering the pathogenesis of an adverse reaction, histamine might be a causative factor, a contributory factor, a coincidental event, or a result of the adverse reactor itself. Lorenz *et al.* [493] devised a mathematical approach involving conditional probabilities and likelihood ratios. With this approach they showed that in the case of reactions to dextran, histamine appears to be a "contributory factor" leading to an increased probability of an adverse reaction: in cases in which the drug is given and histamine release is demonstrated, the incidence of adverse reactions is expected to be higher than in those cases in which the drug is given but no histamine release can be shown. Such histamine release does not always lead to an adverse reaction, e.g., because the release may be too small. Likewise, an adverse reaction to the drug is not always preceded by histamine release, e.g., because other mediators exist. Lorenz *et al.* suggest that there may be a similar relation between histamine release and contrast-media reactions. Bolus injections of contrast media might thus cause histamine release which might not necessarily cause a reaction apart from warmth, etc., but might be a contributory factor to more significant reactions.

Complement activation

Complement constitutes nearly 10% of the plasma globulins in humans and participates in many important biologic functions. The complement cascade may be activated by immunologic or nonimmunologic mechanisms with liberation of anaphylatoxins and various active mediators including histamine [494–496]. Lasser *et al.* [497,498] showed that contrast media may activate complement both *in vitro* and *in vivo*. High concentrations of contrast media may damage the endothelial lining of blood vessels, causing liberation of plasminogen activator and activation of factor XII, which is transformed into proteases and these then transform prekallikrein into kallikrein. Kallikrein potentiates the activation of factor XII and also hydrolyzes the high-molecular-weight kininogen, releasing the small peptide bradykinin, which is a considerably more potent mediator than histamine in producing the clinical features of anaphylaxis. Activation of the complement system is associated with reduction in the level of factor XII and depletion of control substances such as C_1-esterase inhibitor and hemolytic complement. In most patients, this process is stopped by inactivation and negative feedback, but occasionally the activation processes appear to go out of control. Lasser *et al.* found that in a group of contrast reactors, the average preinjection level of C_1-esterase inhibitor and hemolytic complement was lower than in a group of nonreactors, and they suggested that in some patients, preexisting subclinical activation may prime the patient for a reaction.

More recently, Lasser has demonstrated that a heparin-like substance, believed to be heparan sulfate, can act as an *endogenous contact activator*. It is present in increased concentration in the plasmas of some contrast medium reactor patients and in asthmatics; it probably originates in basophils and endothelial cells. The rate of activation is increased by zinc, and increased zinc levels were found in female asthmatic patients. Levels of this endogenous contact activator are increased by estrogen and generally decreased by pre-medication with corticosteroids. It is suggested that large granular lymphocytes, which are increased in patients with allergic asthma, may also be a potential source of heparan sulfate. The adherence of these cells to endothelium is in-creased by the presence of IL-2: this may be a factor in contrast-medium sensitization in patients receiving IL-2 (see p. 274). For more detailed discussion, the reader is referred to two recent reviews by Lasser *et al.* [374,499].

In a fatal contrast-medium reaction, autopsy showed the presence of leukostasis with aggregations of granulocytes impacted in the pulmonary arterioles and capillaries. It was suggested that this might have been due to complement activation [500]. Other authors [501−503] have confirmed the activation of complement by contrast media, but they were unable to demonstrate any significant correlation be-tween the various parameters and clinical contrast-media reactions. Dawson *et al.* [504] found that *in vitro*, diatrizoate, iopamidol, iohexol, and ioxaglate all activated complement with generation of C_{2a}-anaphylatoxin to a broadly similar extent. This does not appear to correlate with the established differences between the clinical toxicity of these media. Complement activation is an attractive hypothesis, but its role is still uncertain. In some patients, it may be a primary mechanism of a contrast reaction and in others, it may be a potentiating or an associated phenomenon.

Disseminated intravascular coagulation has been reported in association with a severe reaction accompanied by hypo-tensive collapse [505]. In another case, visceral angiography with iohexol, in a patient with immunologic disease and previous problems with diatrizoate, caused a severe delayed reaction with disseminated intravascular coagulation and *hypertension* [506].

Protein binding and enzyme inhibition

For many years, it has been known that contrast media may bind to plasma proteins [507,508]. The degree of protein binding appeared to correlate with the relative toxicity of various contrast media as shown by LD_{50} measurements, and it has been suggested that this may be partly due to the resulting alteration of proteins in cell membranes of blood vessel endothelium, or to alterations in the proteins of enzymes [509]. At relatively high concentrations of contrast media, there may be partial *in vitro* inhibition of various enzymes, such as acetylcholinesterase, lisozome, and alcohol dehydrogenase, and it was suggested that inhibition of acetyl-cholinesterase might produce various cholinergic side-effects such as diarrhea, vasodilatation, etc. [509,510]. However, addition of 1% albumin to the reaction mixture reverses the inhibition of acetylcholinesterase, suggesting that under physiologic conditions in the blood, it is unlikely that contrast media cause acetylcholinesterase inhibition [511]. On the available evidence at present, it appears unlikely that protein binding and enzyme inhibition play major direct roles in contrast-media reactions.

Allergic reactions?

For many years, it was initially assumed that contrast-media reactions were allergic in nature, but as early as 1955, Sandström [512] questioned this concept by showing that reactions might occur in patients who had not previously been exposed to contrast medium. Nevertheless, there have been a small number of reports where patients appear to have developed hypersensitivity to contrast media with in-creasingly severe reactions at subsequent reexposure [256, 458,466]. There are also a number of anecdotal reports suggesting that radiologists and radiographers may rarely become sensitized to contrast medium. In one study, 11 out of 17 nurses who were occupationally exposed to contrast media developed *positive lymphocyte transformation tests* and six of those with positive tests had a history of allergic symptoms on handling contrast media [461]. Wakkers-Garritsen [513] reported a reaction associated with a positive skin test to ioglycamate and a Prausnitz−Kustner reaction indicating the presence of IgE antibodies. Another case had an IgM antibody reacting to iothalamate, diatrizoate, acetri-zoate, and iodipamide [228]. In a recent report, a patient who had anaphylactic reactions with cardiac arrest following both ioxythalamate and diatrizoate had positive skin tests to diatrizoate, and positive basophil degranulation tests (HBDT) to diatrizoate and ioxythalamate. The degranulation test for ioxythalamate, repeated with heated serum, was negative, suggesting an IgE antibody. Skin and HBDT tests were negative for ioxaglate and iopamidol. Two subsequent examinations with iopamidol caused no reaction [514]. Several of the reactions associated with skin manifestations may possibly have an immunologic basis [394,404−406] (see p. 268). Theoretically, univalent radicles such as diatrizoate should not act as haptens, whereas divalent radicles might act as haptens (see below). This may be of particular relevance in the dimeric nonionic media and, indeed, positive skin tests to iotrolan have been reported in two cases [405,406].

Using radioimmunoassay techniques, Walker and Carr [515] were unable to demonstrate any evidence of specific antibodies of the IgG or IgE classes in the sera of 68 patients who had moderate or severe reactions to diatrizoate or ioglycamate. They acknowledge that this study could not definitely exclude antibodies of another class, e.g., IgM or IgA, but they consider that the majority of adverse reactions to contrast media are unlikely to be mediated by antibodies. Brasch [516] had earlier demonstrated elevated binding of diatrizoate to the serum globulin fraction in contrast-media reactors, but some nonreactors also had elevated binding.

Brasch suggested that patients who had not previously received contrast medium might develop cross-sensitivity to other halogenated benzene ring derivatives. In a guinea-pig animal model [516], anaphylaxis could be induced to a diatrizoate conjugate and to the divalent iodipamide, but not to the unconjugated monovalent diatrizoate. Lasser *et al.* [518] induced a hypersensitivity state in dogs by repeated injections of iothalamate, but no evidence of antibodies could be detected.

It appears probable that there may be an immunologic mechanism in at least a few contrast-media reactions. The possible immunogenicity of EDTA is discussed on p. 2.

Anxiety

Lalli [519] drew attention to the possible role of fear and anxiety in the causation of contrast-media reactions, and stressed the importance of a calm reassuring approach to the patient. He found that prior hypnotic relaxation significantly decreased the incidence of contrast-media reactions. In subsequent papers, he extended this hypothesis, suggesting that virtually all contrast-media reactions were explicable on a neurologic basis [269,520]. There is indeed evidence that anxiety may lower the ventricular fibrillation threshold [521], and cardiac arrest may even occur following routine venepuncture [522]. Patients who are unduly anxious may therefore be at increased risk of developing a reaction to contrast media. However, contrast-media reactions with severe hypotensive collapse have also been reported during general anesthesia [413,523,524]. This would indicate that fear could be only one of a number of factors involved in contrast-media reactions.

It would be ideal if an *in vitro* test could accurately predict individuals who would develop anaphylactoid reactions to contrast media. Claims have been made for a variety of such tests, including the lymphoblast transformation test [461,525,526], the basophil degranulation test [514,527, 599], prekallikrein–kallikrein conversion rate [528], zymosan activation of the complement cascade with measurement of C_{3a}, thromboxane B_2, and platelet factor IV [529]. However, as yet, *in vitro* tests remain unproven.

Prevention of reactions

Patient assessment

Prior to the administration of contrast media, it is important to assess the patient's history. Risk factors have been discussed earlier (see p. 272, and Tables 13.2, p. 251; 13.4, p. 253; 13.9, p. 272; and 13.10, p. 274). Patients with an allergic background may have an increased risk of developing a reaction to contrast medium, but in many severe and fatal reactions there may be no obvious preceding general history of allergy. However, patients with a history of *asthma, angioneurotic edema,* and particularly those with *previous reactions to contrast media* are exceptions in that they may be prone to develop quite severe or even fatal reactions (pp. 268, 272).

In those cases where a patient believes that he or she has previously had a reaction to contrast medium, careful enquiry by the radiologist will help to determine whether this was only a minor reaction such as nausea or flushing, in which case the examination can usually proceed as normal. If, however, there was a typical reaction to contrast medium, a decision has to be made whether the examination should be performed. If a patient has had a severe life-threatening reaction to contrast medium in the past, it would obviously be unwise to repeat the exposure unless there are imperative clinical reasons. With less severe reactions, the risk of recurrence with conventional ionic media appears to be 30–40% [256,378], and usually reactions that do occur are no more severe than on the previous occasion [378,457,459]. However, if there is a history of reactions on several occasions and if these were of increasing severity, this may indicate that the patient is developing a true hypersensitivity to the contrast medium [256,458].

If there has been a previous significant reaction to contrast medium or other serious risk factor, it will usually be appropriate to consult with the clinician to determine the importance of the proposed examination for the management of the patient's condition, and to explore whether the required information might be obtainable by alternate means. If the examination is considered essential, the examination may proceed with appropriate premedication and use of a non-ionic medium; there should be full provision to treat any emergency that might arise (p. 280).

Lalli [530] has described nine patients who previously suffered severe hypotensive reactions with unconsciousness following urography. In all of these patients, repeat urography, performed after adequate reassurance alone, caused no reaction. However, such bravura is not recommended.

It has been suggested that seeking "informed consent" might increase the risk of a reaction due to anxiety. A study of 1251 patients by Hopper *et al.* [531] indicated that the majority of patients attending an X-ray department already have an increased "anxiety score": explaining the possible risks of contrast media did not increase the score. It was therefore concluded that failure to obtain informed consent cannot be justified on this basis.

A vague history of "iodism" is another problem that occasionally arises. Questioning may reveal that there was nothing more than a skin burn resulting from tincture of iodine. In the Mayo Clinic series [378], patients with "iodism" appeared to have an increased liability to contrast-media reactions. Although the typical immediate contrast-medium reaction is not generally considered to be a manifestation of iodism, some of the delayed reactions may be of this nature (see pp. 267, 268). This may therefore be a problem if large doses are used, particularly in patients with renal failure.

Predictive testing

The technique of intravenous testing with 1 ml of contrast medium, followed by a pause of a few minutes before completing the injection, has generally fallen into disfavor. A patient may have no reaction to a small dose of contrast medium and yet develop a reaction to a larger dose [349]. Moreover, a test dose itself can cause death [457,532].

Shehadi [533] concluded that *pretesting* was of no significant value, but analysis of his data shows that in patients with a positive pretest, the incidence of subsequent reactions was approximately 12 times that in the series as a whole, and included two deaths — a mortality rate of 0.5%! In the recent large Japanese survey, the predictive value for a severe reaction to a full dose of ionic medium in patients with a positive pretest was 1.2% (sensitivity = 3.7%). With nonionic media the pretest showed no predictive value [534].

Yocumb *et al.* [465] introduced a more refined and safer pretesting procedure for use in patients with a previous history of anaphylactoid reactions to contrast media. Commencing with an intravenous injection of 0.1 ml of 1:10 000 dilution of contrast medium, subsequent injections of 0.1 ml of 1:1000, 1:100, and 1:10 dilutions are made at intervals of 15 minutes with subsequent injections of 0.1 ml, 1 ml, and 5 ml of full-strength contrast medium at similar intervals. If anaphylactoid symptoms occurred, the patient was treated with intravenous diphenhydramine and subcutaneous epinephrine: further pretesting was stopped and the pretest designated as positive. Two-thirds of the patients with a positive pretest developed reactions on subsequent re-exposure. This form of pretest may be useful in defining patients at particularly high risk of developing a repeat reaction. In such patients, the requirement for further contrast medium should be assessed: if this is clinically essential, appropriate prophylaxis should be used (see below). It is important to appreciate, however, that a negative pretest does *not* exclude the possibility of a reaction occurring.

In concurrence with Lasser [535], the author considers that it is a sensible precaution to wait a short period after injection of the first milliliter or so of contrast medium before proceeding with the full injection. If there is reason to fear a possible reaction, a slow rate of injection may allow the examination to be interrupted or abandoned at the earliest sign of trouble. This is a personal opinion and many radiologists consider that a rapid injection is acceptable [36, 462]. Fast injections may cause "histamine release" [23]. In patients with cardiovascular disease, and particularly in those with a history of coronary artery disease, a fast injection may predispose to arrhythmias [89]. A slower rate of injection is probably preferable in such patients if this is compatible with the diagnostic requirement.

A preliminary study in 100 patients suggested that reduction of the peak expiratory flow rate (PEFR), measured 10 minutes before contrast-medium administration, might

be a useful predictive test. Patients with a PEFR less than 400 l/min had a 3.8 times risk of reacting adversely to contrast medium [536].

Use of nonionic media

There is increasing use of nonionic contrast media. In a recent survey of 170 consultant radiologists in the UK, 78.8% routinely used nonionic media for intravenous examinations [8]. Where this is not the case, guidelines have been issued by the American College of Radiology [4] and the Royal College of Radiologists [324] to indicate those higher risk patients where it would be appropriate to select nonionic media for use. These include: patients with a history of previous significant reactions; asthmatics; atopic individuals; and those allergic to other drugs or agents; patients with known cardiac dysfunction; pulmonary hypertension or hemodynamic instability; high-dose procedures; renal impairment; elderly patients; patients with severe debilitation; circumstances where there is a risk of inhalation should vomiting occur, e.g., in CT; unduly anxious patients; and sickle cell disease (for the latter, the medium should preferably be diluted 1:2 to render it isosmolar).

In children, even minor reactions may affect image quality and upset the child emotionally and physically. Moreover, damage or pain due to extravasation may be a significant problem. This would justify the routine use of nonionic media in these young patients. In young infants, dosage should be calculated according to kilograms of body weight rather than by age, in order to avoid overdose [600].

Although use of nonionic contrast media is the most important factor in reducing the incidence of adverse reactions [353,357,358], such reactions may still occur and consideration should be given to premedication in high-risk patients.

Premedication (see also p. 565)

Corticosteroids

It has long been accepted that a combination of corticosteroid and antihistamine premedication can be of value in the prophylaxis of recurrent reactions to conventional ionic contrast media [608]. Animal experiments have shown that pretreatment with steroids over a period of 1–3 days has significant protective value against contrast-media reactions or toxicity, whereas the effect of a single intravenous injection of steroid before a challenging dose of contrast medium is variable and might even be detrimental [418,601]. Lasser suggested that the protective effect of steroid prophylaxis might be associated with elevation in the levels of C_1-esterase inhibitor, factor XII, and prekallikrein. He also found that administration of corticosteroids decreased the concentration of the endogenous contact activator heparan sulfate [374].

Corticosteroids cause transcription of ribonucleic acid (RNA) in the cell nucleus with coding for the production of regulatory peptides and proteins such as the protein kinases. One of the proteins, lipocortin, inhibits phospholipase A_2, the enzyme responsible for converting membrane phospholipids to arachidonic acid. It therefore reduces the synthesis of leukotrienes, prostaglandins, thromboxane, and platelet activating factor (PAF). This response occurs with very low drug concentrations several hours after drug administration. Corticosteroids may also have a bronchodilator action. The plasma half-life of prednisolone is approximately 2–3 hours [602].

In an important multicenter prospective randomized and blinded study of 6763 patients receiving conventional ionic media, Lasser *et al.* [377] investigated the value of corticosteroid premedication. In patients receiving a single dose of 32 mg methylprednisolone orally 2 hours before the examination, there was no significant difference from the controls. In patients receiving a two-dose oral regimen of 32 mg methylprednisolone 12 hours and 2 hours before contrast challenge, there was a significant reduction in the incidence of all grades of reaction ($P < 0.0001$): grade I reactions ($P = 0.001$), grade II reactions ($P = 0.06$), grade III reactions ($P = 0.04$). There was a greater reduction in the incidence of the more severe reactions, but in general the protective effect was similar in both high- and low-risk patients [372, 377]. Dawson and Sidhu [603] and others, have criticized the statistic methodology used in this study, but this criticism has been refuted by Lasser and Berry [604]. Dawson and Sidhu also question the added value of corticosteroid prophylaxis in high-risk patients when nonionic media are used, but their argument is not convincing. In their recent survey of 170 UK consultant radiologists, Seymour *et al.* [8] surprisingly found that only 55.3% used steroid prophylaxis in higher risk patients and that there was very considerable variation in the dosage regimens.

Lasser *et al.* [537] have now performed a carefully controlled prospective study in 1155 patients receiving *nonionic media*. In patients receiving a two-dose oral regimen of 32 mg of methylprednisolone (given 6–24 hours before, and again 2 hours before injection of contrast medium), there was a significant reduction in the incidence of grade I reactions compared with controls ($P = 0.004$). The incidence of reactions was also lower for grades II and III reactions, but the small numbers involved did not reach statistic significance. The problem in this study was the logistic difficulty of assembling a sufficient number of patients to achieve statistic significance in the less common grades II and III reactions. In the Japanese survey [534], no protective effect was found for corticosteroids, but it appears that these were given IV *immediately before* administration of contrast medium (H. Katayama, personal communication, quoted by Lasser), i.e., at a time when they might be expected to be ineffective [537].

In a series of 140 patients with a previous history of moderate or severe reactions to contrast media, Greenberger and Patterson [538] attained a rate of repeat reactions as low as 0.7% using a combination of nonionic media with a prophylactic regimen of prednisone 50 mg orally at 13, 7 and 1 hour, and diphenhydramine 50 mg orally 1 hour before repeat contrast examination. In a further 41 patients in whom there were no cardiac contraindications, ephedrine 25 mg orally was added to this regimen. In this three-drug regimen there were no reactions, but there may be other troublesome side-effects with ephedrine. Although this study was not randomized or blinded, the results are impressive and compare favorably with Wolf *et al.*'s [358] rate of 2.5% recurrent reactions in such patients for iohexol alone, or 5.5%, mainly minor, in Siegle *et al.*'s study [539].

Patients with asthma are at particular risk from contrast media (see pp. 268, 272). The value of corticosteroids in the prophylaxis and treatment of asthma is well-established clinically [602]. It is therefore entirely logical to combine corticosteroid prophylaxis with a nonionic medium when an examination is essential in such patients, but antihistamine may be less important.

Asthmatic patients who are currently under treatment with corticosteroids, or who have had corticosteroid therapy in the recent past, may have some degree of *adrenal suppression*. Consideration should be given to using a booster dose of steroids in these cases and in other patients who have received recent corticosteroid therapy. Some years ago, the author personally witnessed a case of severe bronchospasm with cardiovascular collapse following the administration of iopamidol without corticosteroid prophylaxis to an asthmatic patient. It subsequently emerged that steroid therapy had been discontinued 3–4 days before the examination (G. Ansell, unpublished data). In other conditions where the patient may have adrenal suppression from steroid therapy or hypoadrenal function, contrast media may precipitate severe reactions in the absence of appropriate prophylaxis [279,386,540] (see also pp. 259, 267).

In particularly high-risk patients, a 3–4 day prophylactic regimen with 32–50 mg of prednisone might be appropriate [540,541]. For emergency administration of radiocontrast medium in high-risk patients when time does not permit the normal premedication regimen, Greenberger recommends 200 mg hydrocortisone IV immediately, and every 4 hours, until the procedure is completed, with 50 mg diphenhydramine IV 1 hour before the procedure [542].

In the survey of Lasser *et al.* [537], exclusion criteria for routine corticosteroid prophylaxis included: diabetes mellitus, pregnant or nursing patients, active tuberculosis, systemic fungus disease or other infection, immune suppression, steroid psychosis, current peptic ulcer or diverticulitis, active leukemias or lymphoma which might be subject to breakdown. In children with lymphoreticular cancer, a single dose of corticosteroid may be sufficient to cause tumor lysis with severe metabolic disturbances and coagulopathy [543]. In myasthenia gravis, corticosteroid therapy may affect the dose of pyridostigmine required. Many of these contraindications are relatively theoretical for brief steroid use and the decision whether to undertake corticosteroid prophylaxis in high-risk patients with such conditions will depend on clinical assessment.

Providing that there are no clinical contraindications to corticosteroid prophylaxis, it is logical to combine this with use of nonionic media in those high-risk patients where the examination is essential [544,545]. Severe reactions may, however, still occur and full facilities must be available for treatment (see below). Prophylaxis of IL-2 recall reactions is discussed on p. 274.

Antihistamines

There does not appear to be any significant value in using intravenous H_1 antihistamines such as diphenhydramine, chlorpheniramine, or clemastin as a routine, prior to contrast examinations [36,546]. Intravenous antihistamines can produce undesirable and sometimes severe reactions with hypotension. Indeed, bolus injections of chlorpheniramine may cause histamine release [23,483]. Use of combined antihistamine corticosteroid prophylaxis is discussed above. In patients with uncomplicated hay fever, an oral preparation 1 hour before examination might be appropriate.

H_2 antihistamines also have significant antiallergic properties, and combined prophylaxis with H_1 and H_2 antihistamines has been advocated. Most of the studies have related to histamine release during surgical operations, hypovolemic shock, or from plasma expanders and blood transfusions where histamine release can cause serious consequences [23,483].

A randomized controlled trial of 800 routine intravenous urograms showed a significant reduction of urticaria and angioedema in patients receiving intravenous premedication with 0.03 mg/kg of the H_1 antagonist, clemastin, and 5 mg/ kg of the H_2 antagonist cimetidine given slowly 5 minutes before the examination [546]. Two other smaller trials have shown similar results, but the data appear to involve mainly minor reactions [547,548]. Greenberger and Patterson [549] found that the administration of cimetidine *increased* the incidence of reactions and he advised against its use for premedication. In another case report, premedication with clemastine, cimetidine, and prednisolone followed by iopamidol resulted in severe anaphylactoid shock [550]. Marshall and Lieberman [551] favor a pretreatment protocol using oral prednisone, intramuscular diphenhydramine, oral cimetidine, and oral ephedrine. Nevertheless, premedication with cimetidine must at present be regarded as controversial.

Aminocaproic acid

For many years, French radiologists placed great faith in a combination of 8 mg dexamethasone and 4 g ε-aminocaproic acid (EACA). This mixture was given to high-risk patients 5 minutes before the injection of contrast medium. It was claimed that this regimen prevented moderate and severe anaphylactoid shock reactions, but did not prevent other adverse effects such as cutaneous eruptions or vagal reactions [552]. Nevertheless, fatal reactions have occurred in patients pretreated with corticosteroids and EACA [553]. Aminocaproic acid was apparently suggested for such prophylactic use in 1965 on the simplistic theory that contrast-media reactions resulted from fibrinolysis: it was enthusiastically and dogmatically accepted without real validation. Coste *et al.* [554] reported a fatal case of massive intravascular coagulation during phlebography, which they attributed to EACA, and they suggested that use of EACA should be reconsidered. Soyer *et al.* [555] go further: they advise that premedication with antifibrinolytic drugs such as EACA should be prohibited.

EACA has an inhibitory effect on activation of complement by contrast media [556]. Side-effects that may occasionally occur with EACA include: nasal congestion, diarrhea, rash, transient hypotension, and transient delirious state [557]. In Europe, EACA has been replaced by tranexamic acid, which has similar actions but fewer side-effects. Tranexamic acid might possibly have a place for prophylaxis in those rare patients with *hereditary angioneurotic edema* when this is due to C_1-esterase deficiency [558].

Hyposensitization

Agardh *et al.* [559] described a program of hyposensitization used in 12 patients with a previous history of reactions to contrast media. Commencing with an intravenous injection of 1 ml of 1:100 dilution of contrast medium, 12 injections of gradually increasing doses were administered, spaced over a period of 3 days. This appeared effective if the repeat examination was performed within 5 days, but significant reactions occurred in two out of five patients who had examinations repeated after 5 days. It appears possible that this regimen involves tachyphylaxis and that the small doses of contrast medium may react with, and inactivate, those factors that might otherwise induce a reaction. This regimen may be considered in special cases of very high-risk patients in conjunction with other methods above.

Cromoglycate

There are theoretical reasons for believing that sodium cromoglycate (Intal) might be of prophylactic value in preventing contrast reactions, especially in asthmatics. In the UK survey there were 22 reports of moderate or severe reactions in patients with a history of asthma. None of these patients with reactions was receiving Intal, whereas the expected number should have been 1.3. The number of cases is too small to exclude a chance finding, but the trend is suggestive and it would be rational to consider the use of Intal in prophylaxis, especially in asthmatics [409].

Treatment of reactions (see also p. 567)

Since the mechanisms of contrast-media reactions are mainly still in doubt, treatment schemes are basically symptomatic and empirical. Several detailed programs for treatment of such emergencies have recently been published [4,560–563]. It is recommended that all those involved with the use of contrast media should read at least one of these publications. While they are broadly similar, there are some variations in emphasis and nuances: it would therefore be advantageous also to study the other programs if these are available. Each department should have a specific plan for treating reactions to contrast media: this should be updated as required and all personnel using contrast media should be skilled in basic resuscitation procedures [564,565]. *The most important factor in reducing mortality is the immediate availability and use of full facilities for resuscitation.* Provision should also be made for assessing and treating *delayed reactions* which may occur after a patient has left the X-ray department (see pp. 265, 266–268, 270, 271, 274).

General principles

It is prudent to administer contrast media through a needle or cannula that is securely taped: this should be left *in situ* as a means of access until it is considered safe to remove it. The patient should be under continuous observation for at least 20 minutes after contrast administration and there should be an alarm system to allow the technician or nurse to summon assistance without leaving the patient.

All reactions should be immediately assessed by the radiologist. If there is acute cardiac arrest, respiratory arrest, shock, or respiratory impairment, immediate vigorous treatment will obviously be required, and the crash team should be called. If the patient is unconscious, an adequate airway should be ensured with administration of oxygen: inhalation of vomit should be guarded against.

Minor and moderate reactions

It is neither desirable nor necessary to institute active drug treatment for each and every reaction. *Minor reactions* usually subside without treatment. Providing that the patient's general condition is satisfactory or improving, it is justifiable to spend a brief period in deciding whether the reaction is subsiding or whether active treatment is required. If drugs are required, they should generally be injected *slowly*, even in emergencies: appropriate dose corrections should be made for pediatric use.

Nausea and/or vomiting

These usually respond to slowing or interruption of the injection and reassurance. Inhalation of vomit should be prevented. Rarely, if vomiting is persistent, an antiemetic, e.g., metoclopramide may be required (see p. 27).

Urticaria

Mild scattered hives usually require no treatment but, if troublesome, an H_1 antihistamine may be given, orally, intramuscularly, or by *slow* intravenous injection. Prolonged or severe skin manifestations, particularly flushing or itching may sometimes be helped dramatically by combined H_1 and H_2 antihistamines (see below).

Treatment in severe reactions

Severe anaphylactoid reactions to contrast media may present with a variety of one or more clinical features including, bronchospasm, angioedema, laryngeal edema, severe hypotension, etc. Principles of treatment for these individual symptoms are briefly summarized in Table 13.11 (p. 283), which provides a rapid *aide memoire* for use in emergency. In all severe reactions 100% oxygen should be administered, but caution may be required in chronic obstructive airway disease with hypercapnia.

Hypotension

Simple syncope may respond to elevation of the legs which increases the return of blood to the heart. In more severe cases, there is usually tachycardia. Vasodilatation and increased capillary permeability may cause considerable fluid loss into the extravascular space. This requires replacement with rapid infusion of intravenous fluids. This is the most important therapeutic procedure and may frequently be effective without additional pharmacotherapy [430].

In anaphylactic and anaphylactoid cardiovascular collapse, plasma loss of up to 35% of blood volume may occur. Administration of fluid may be controlled by central venous pressure. Serial hemoglobin or hematocrit measurements are useful in estimating plasma loss. Up to 4 l of fluid or more may be required. Treatment may be commenced with crystalloids (e.g., isotonic saline) but hemoconcentration was less in patients receiving colloids. Epinephrine (see below) was an effective inotrope in most cases [566]. In a few cases, dopamine infusion may be required (see p. 38). In prolonged or refractory anaphylactoid hypotension, intravenous cimetidine (see below) may produce dramatic improvement. At least eight such cases have been reported [413,566–569].

Hypotension with bradycardia

Hypotension with bradycardia is usually of vagal origin [92–94,433]. In addition to fluid replacement as above, atropine 0.6–1 mg should be given by *slow* intravenous injection. This may be repeated at 5 minute intervals up to a total dose of 3 mg [4,560] (see also p. 38). In an athletic patient with a normally slow pulse rate, bradycardia in a reaction may be misleading [570].

Patients receiving *β-blockers* may develop *bradycardia* rather than tachycardia in hypotensive reactions. The reaction may be resistant to treatment with epinephrine but may respond to an infusion of *glucagon* [571]. Cimetidine should probably be avoided in such patients since it may decrease hepatic clearance of some β-blockers. (Ranitidine (p. 567) does not interfere with hepatic clearance.) In patients receiving β-blockers, a paradoxical effect may also occur whereby unopposed activation of α-receptors by epinephrine may result in coronary artery constriction, and may also cause *hypertension* [572] (see also pp. 48, 80).

Bronchospasm

Administer 100% oxygen. Bronchospasm may respond to deep inhalation of a β-agonist, e.g., albuterol — one or two puffs from a metered inhaler, preferably using a spacing device. If this is not practicable, albuterol may be given by injection (see p. 40). Epinephrine (see below) may be used as an alternative, particularly in progressive or severe bronchospasm. Intravenous steroids (see below) should be given as soon as possible on an empirical basis, particularly in asthmatics.

In resistant cases, combined H_1 and H_2 antihistamines may be considered as a second line of treatment (see below). Aminophylline may be effective in resistant bronchospasm but is now rarely used (see p. 37). In severe cases, positive pressure ventilation may be valuable.

Angioedema, laryngeal edema

Stridor due to laryngeal edema is unlikely to respond to β-agonists: epinephrine is preferable. An H_1 antihistamine, e.g., diphenhydramine or chlorpheniramine (see below) may be given as a *slow* intravenous injection. An H_2 blocker (e.g., cimetidine) may be considered as a second line of treatment (see below). Adequate oxygenation should be ensured. With severe laryngeal edema, intubation may be difficult or indeed dangerous in unskilled hands. Tracheotomy, laryngotomy, or minitracheotomy may be required. In emergency, oxygen may be administered via a large bore needle inserted through the cricothyroid membrane or upper trachea. Corticosteroid will usually be given empirically.

Pulmonary edema (see p. 269)

Administer oxygen and sit the patient upright if possible. Pulmonary edema is most commonly due to hypervolemia combined with congestive cardiac failure, particularly in patients with myocardial disease. Furosemide (20−40 mg) may be given by *slow* intravenous injection using a separate syringe, or by the intramuscular route. (Furosemide can produce bladder distension due to rapid diuresis: in unconscious patients catheterization is indicated.) Rotating venous tourniquets or, exceptionally, venesection may be useful. Use of morphine for left ventricular failure is discussed on p. 34. Possible use of aminophylline is discussed on p. 37.

Noncardiogenic pulmonary edema (see p. 269)

Initially, this may mistakenly be assumed to be cardiogenic in the absence of central venous pressure measurements. Administer oxygen. Increased capillary permeability may lead to *hypovolemia* which requires correction by intravenous infusion of colloids. Furosemide may be indicated to prevent fluid overload. Corticosteroid should be given in both cardiogenic and noncardiogenic pulmonary edema. Positive pressure ventilation may be helpful in selected cases.

Hypertension

Hypertensive crisis may occur in pheochromocytoma (see p. 263); following treatment of a reaction with epinephrine [573]; as a direct result of a contrast reaction (see p. 270); or following drug interactions between sympathomimetics with β-blockers, tricyclic antidepressants, or monoamine oxidase inhibitor agents (see pp. 48, 49).

For treatment with phentolamine or labetalol see pp. 41, 42.

Convulsions (see pp. 248, 249, 259)

Maintain airway; administer 100% oxygen. Anoxic convulsions resulting from cardiac arrest, hypotension, etc., usually respond to treatment of the primary cause.

More persistent convulsions, especially those due to chemotoxicity of contrast media, lidocaine, etc., likewise require 100% oxygen: in addition, diazepam (see p. 33) should be given by slow intravenous injection using the minimum dose to control convulsions. Assisted ventilation may be required. With more prolonged convulsions, consider intravenous phenytoin or general anesthesia.

Notes for **Table 13.1** (*opposite*)
√, Indicated;   ?, may be indicated;   ↑, increase;   ↓, decrease;   ×, contraindicated.
*, In patients receiving β-blockers, hypotensive reactions may present with a slow pulse and may be resistant to epinephrine (see p. 281).
†, Noncardiogenic pulmonary edema (low CVP): may require intravenous fluids.
‡, Convulsions due to anoxia usually respond to oxygen and treatment of cause.
§ See manufacturers' literature.
Do *not* mix antihistamine with hydrocortisone or other drugs in the same syringe.

Table 13.11 Symptomatic treatment for acute major contrast media reactions

Call crash team: *monitor:* pulse, EKG, blood pressure, oximetry, etc. airways (p. 54), ? suction

Reaction	Oxygen	Intravenous fluids	Corticosteroids	Salbutamol/ Albuterol	Adrenaline/ Epinephrine	H_1 antihistamines	Additional measures that may be required
Cardiac arrest	↑	✓	✓		✓		Thump, defibrillation, cardiopulmonary resuscitation, etc. (See Chapter 4, p. 47)
Arrhythmias	✓	✓	✓				See Chapter 4, p. 63, 83
Respiratory failure	↑	?	✓	?	?		Maintain airway, assisted ventilation (caution hypercapnia)
Unconscious	✓	?	✓		?		Maintain airway, check tongue, etc. Avoid: inhalation injury, etc. Treat as indicated ?Raise legs
Hypotension*	↑	↑	✓	?	✓		Raise legs. ?Dopamine (p. 38). ?H_1 (p. 35) and H_2 (p. 29)
Vagal reaction*	↑	↑	?	?	?		Raise legs. Atropine (p. 38)
Bronchospasm	↑	✓	✓	✓	✓	?	?Aminophylline (p. 37). ?H_1 (p. 35) and H_2 (p. 29). ?IPPV
Angioedema laryngeal edema	↑	✓	✓		✓	✓	Maintain airway (p. 54). ?Intubation. May require tracheotomy or alternative
Pulmonary edema†	↑	↓	✓				Sit up if possible. Furosemide (p. 43). ?Morphine (p. 34). ?Atropine (p. 38). ?Aminophylline (p. 37). ?Rotating tourniquets. ?Venesection. Maintain airway. ?IPPV. (?Catheterize bladder.)
Hypertension	✓	✓	?				?Phentolamine (p. 42). ?Labetalol (p. 41)
Toxic convulsions‡	↑	?	✓				Maintain airway. Avoid injuries. Diazepam (p. 33). Assisted ventilation. ?Phenytoin§ ?General anesthesia
Cerebral edema Coma	✓	↓	✓				?Mannitol§. ?Furosemide (p. 43). Consult neurologist
Myasthenic crisis	✓	?	✓				Edrophonium§. Maintain airway. ?Assisted ventilation
Hyperpyrexia	✓	↑	?	x	x		Avoid sympathomimetics. Consult anesthesiologist urgently. ?Dantrolene (p. 43)

For drug details see page 284.

✓, Indicated; ?, may be indicated; ↑, increase; ↓, decrease; x, contraindicated.

*, In patients receiving ß-blockers, hypotensive reactions may present with a slow pulse and may be resistant to epinephrine (see p. 281).

†, Noncardiogenic pulmonary edema (low CVP): may require intravenous fluids.

‡, Convulsions due to anoxia usually respond to oxygen and treatment of cause.

§ See manufacturers' literature.

Do *not* mix antihistamine with hydrocortisone or other drugs in the same syringe.

b

Blackwell Science

Table 13.11 Symptomatic treatment for acute major reactions

Call crash team: *monitor*: pulse, EKG, blood pressure, oximetry, etc. Airways (p. 54), ? suction

Reaction	Oxygen	Intravenous fluids	Corticosteroids	Albuterol	Epinephrine	H₁ antihistamines	Additional measures that may be required
Cardiac arrest	↑	√	√		√		Thump, defibrillation, cardiopulmonary resuscitation, etc. (See Chapter 4, p. 47)
Arrhythmias	√	√	√				See Chapter 4, p. 63, 83
Respiratory failure	↑	?	√	?	?		Maintain airway, assisted ventilation (caution hypercapnia)
Unconscious	√	?	√		?		Maintain airway, check tongue, etc. Avoid: inhalation injury, etc. Treat as indicated ?Raise legs
Hypotension*	↑	↑	√	?	√		Raise legs. ?Dopamine (p. 38). ?H₁ (p. 35) and H₂ (p. 29)
Vagal reaction*	↑	↑	?	?	?		Raise legs. Atropine (p. 38)
Bronchospasm	↑	√	√	√	√	?	?Aminophylline (p. 37). ?H₁ (p.35) and H₂ (p. 29). ?IPPV
Angioedema laryngeal edema	↑	√	√		√	√	Maintain airway (p. 54). ?Intubation. May require tracheotomy or alternative
Pulmonary edema†	↑	↓	√				Sit up if possible. Furosemide (p. 42). ?Morphine (p. 34). ?Atropine (p. 38). ?Aminophylline (p. 37). ?Rotating tourniquets. ?Venesection. Maintain airway. ?IPPV. (?Catheterize bladder.)
Hypertension	√	√	?				?Phentolamine (p. 42). ?Labetalol (p. 41)
Toxic convulsions‡	↑	?	√				Maintain airway. Avoid injuries. Diazepam (p. 33). Assisted ventilation. ?Phenytoin§ ?General anesthesia
Cerebral edema Coma	√	↓	√				?Mannitol§. ?Furosemide (p. 42). Consult neurologist
Myasthenic crisis	√	?	√				Edrophonium§. Maintain airway. ?Assisted ventilation
Hyperpyrexia	√	↑	?	×	×		Avoid sympathomimetics. Consult anesthesiologist urgently. ?Dantrolene (p. 43)

Cerebral edema

Give corticosteroid. Consider intravenous mannitol: this is contraindicated in overhydration and may aggravate congestive failure. Consult neurologist/neurosurgeon.

Myasthenic crisis (p. 260)

Intubation and assisted ventilation may be required in apnea. Edrophonium test distinguishes between myasthenic crisis and cholinergic crisis. Corticosteroids may affect the dose of pyridostigmine required in therapy of myasthenia.

Hyperpyrexia

Avoid sympathomimetic drugs. Administer oxygen. Consult anesthesiologist urgently. Consider dantrolene.

Selected drugs used in reactions (see also p. 44)

Corticosteroids (p. 36)

Corticosteroids should not be mixed in the same syringe with antihistamines due to risk of precipitation [560].

Corticosteroids are usually given empirically in severe contrast-media reactions. Their possible mode of action is discussed on p. 278. On the analogy of their effect in asthma and allergic reactions, they are likely to be of major value in severe contrast-media reactions, irrespective of the symptomatology. Indeed, in some fatal reactions, it is noteworthy that steroids had not been given [256].

Hydrocortisone sodium succinate (500 mg), or an alternative steroid preparation should be given by *slow* intravenous injection as soon as possible. In acute reactions, particularly in bronchospasm or in hypotensive shock, steroids may sometimes act very rapidly [386,560,574]. However, there may often be a delay of several hours before steroids are fully effective. It is therefore important to administer other symptomatic treatment. Following intravenous injection, blood levels of steroids decline after approximately 4 hours: additional booster doses may therefore be required to prevent a late relapse. Depending on the clinical circumstances, these may be given by the intravenous, intramuscular, or oral routes.

In very rare instances, intravenous hydrocortisone itself may cause severe allergic reactions, including rashes, bronchospasm, or even cardiac arrest. These appear to occur mainly but not exclusively in aspirin-sensitive asthmatics. Dexamethasone may be preferable in such patients. Some deaths have also been reported within 24 hours of an intravenous "pulse" of 1 g methylprednisolone [575,576]. The risk of tumor lysis in children with lymphoreticular cancer [543] has been mentioned earlier (see p. 279). In general, these very rare problems should not detract from the routine use of steroids in severe contrast-media reactions.

If, however, new symptoms or unexpected deterioration appear to be due to intravenous steroids, therapy should be reviewed and alternate antiallergic drugs should be considered.

Albuterol (Salbutanol)

See p. 40; see also section on bronchospasm above.

Epinephrine (Adrenaline) (p. 37)

Epinephrine is an important agent in the treatment of anaphylactic/anaphylactoid reactions and in the treatment of cardiac arrest. It has a physiologic antihistamine effect. It stimulates both α-adrenergic receptors causing primarily vasoconstriction and β-adrenergic receptors causing increase in the strength and rate of myocardial contraction. Stimulation of the β_2-adrenergic receptors results in smooth muscle relaxation, arteriolar vasodilatation, and, most importantly, bronchiolar relaxation. *Slow* administration of epinephrine causes predominant stimulation of the β-receptors, while fast administration causes predominant stimulation of the α-receptors [563].

In the early stage of anaphylaxis, when vasodilatation is present and if the peripheral circulation is satisfactory, epinephrine may be given subcutaneously. The standard dose is 0.3–0.5 mg (0.3–0.5 ml of 1:1000 solution) [577]. Others have suggested a lower initial dose of 0.1–0.3 mg for less severe reactions, repeated if necessary at 15 minute intervals up to a total dose of 1 mg, depending on the response [561]. Asthmatic patients who have received chronic treatment with sympathomimetics may become partially resistant and require higher doses. In severely shocked patients, absorption from the intramuscular route may be unpredictable. Absorption may be delayed and when the circulation subsequently improves following resuscitation, the sudden absorption of the epinephrine residue may then cause irreversible ventricular fibrillation [419].

In severe shock, the *intravenous route* may therefore be required, but epinephrine should be administered with extreme caution by this route, using a *diluted solution of 1:10 000*, preferably from a prepacked syringe. Initially, 1 ml (0.1 mg) of this diluted solution may be injected *slowly* over a period of 5–10 minutes, with further administration depending on the response.

Epinephrine may also be administered via the tracheal route where the rate of absorption through the highly vascular pulmonary alveoli may approach that of the intravenous route, but there may be some variability. For *intratracheal administration*, the epinephrine should preferably be *further diluted with saline to a concentration of 1:100 000* to provide a larger volume for injection, and the dose may be doubled (0.2 mg).

Epinephrine, particularly via the intravenous route, may cause serious *cardiac arrhythmias* [430] and may have been an etiologic factor in causing ventricular fibrillation in some fatal reactions [256]. The risks are higher in elderly patients, in those with cardiac disease, and in the presence of anoxia. However, severe *myocardial ischemia* and *hypertensive crisis* have also been reported in younger patients receiving intravenous epinephrine for anaphylactic shock [573,578]. *Drug interactions* may occur with β-blockers or antidepressants which may potentiate the pressor response of epinephrine (see Chapter 4, p. 49).

In the treatment of *cardiac arrest*, larger doses of epinephrine (0.5–1 mg) may be given intravenously [565] (see Chapter 4, p. 80).

H₁ antihistamines (p. 35)

H₁ antihistamines such as diphenhydramine (dose = 50 mg) or chlorpheniramine (dose = 10–20 mg) are mainly indicated for the treatment of urticaria or angioedema. They may be given either orally, intramuscularly, or, diluted, by *slow* intravenous injection. Rapid injection may cause histamine release [23]. Antihistamines should *not* be mixed with contrast media or other drugs in the same syringe. It is illogical to use H₁ antihistamines as a *routine* treatment for every type of reaction and they may on occasion cause hypotension [430].

H₂ antihistamines (p. 29)

There have been several reported cases of severe allergic reactions, including hypotensive shock, that failed to respond to standard therapy but which showed rapid improvement when the H₂ antihistamine cimetidine was given [566–569]. Likewise, a contrast reaction, causing extensive angioedema and early respiratory distress was unresponsive to diphenhydramine and steroids, but resolved with an infusion of cimetidine [579]. Rapid intravenous injection of cimetidine causes histamine release and cardiotoxic effects, but this does not occur with slow infusion [23]. Cimetidine (300 mg dissolved in 20 ml saline) is given as a *slow* intravenous infusion. Intravenous cimetidine should be preceded by an H₁ antihistamine. Cimetidine should preferably be reserved for treatment of reactions which have not responded to standard therapy (see also p. 280). Cimetidine may decrease the hepatic clearance of β-blockers and should be avoided in such patients (see above and p. 49).

Other drugs (see Chapter 3, p. 44)

Reactions in renal failure

Treatment of renal failure is outside the scope of this book. If a contrast-medium reaction persists in a patient with renal failure, dialysis may be required to remove the contrast medium [580].

Reactions following extravascular use of intravascular media

Typical idiosyncratic reactions varying from mild urticaria to anaphylactoid collapse may rarely occur when intravascular media are administered by other routes. The risk appears higher in patients with previous contrast reactions.

During retrograde pyelography using iodine-131 labeled diatrizoate, 12.5% of the medium was absorbed in a patient with pyelovenous intravasation, but in eight other patients absorption was less than 1% [581]. In micturating cystourethrography, the risk of a reaction may be increased by ureteric reflux [582,583], but in a child with a previous mild reaction to an IVU, micturating cystourethrography without reflux caused a severe allergic reaction with respiratory symptoms [584]. In another patient with a previous history of an IVU reaction, severe and prolonged hypotensive collapse occurred following antegrade pyelography through a nephrostomy tube into the ureter, using a nonionic medium under general anesthesia [585].

Severe contrast reactions have rarely been reported following endoscopic retrograde pancreatography [524,586], hysterosalpingography [587], or arthrography [609].

An anaphylactoid reaction occurred 2 hours after cervical myelography with metrizamide [588]. Exacerbation of SLE has also been reported following metrizamide myelography [385] (see also p. 267).

Oral iohexol caused diarrhea in 18 out of 40 patients. This did not appear to be an osmolar effect. There were three cases each of fever, nausea, and vomiting and one case of urticaria [589]. In another patient, oral iohexol caused a severe reaction with nausea, vomiting, abdominal cramps, hypotensive collapse, and slight dyspnea. The symptoms responded to treatment with intravenous hydrocortisone, chlorpheniramine, and plasma expanders [590].

Delayed cardiac tamponade developed 10 hours after accidental injection of iohexol into the pericardium during digital subtraction angiography [591].

Cross-sensitivity may occur with oily contrast media. A patient with a previous atypical reaction following contrast CT, and who ate seafood, developed profound hypotensive collapse 3 hours after lymphangiography with ethiodol, despite premedication with methylprednisolone [592].

Although reactions to extravascular administration of contrast media appear to be less frequent than after intravascular use, there should be appropriate provision for their prevention and treatment (see also p. 268).

References

1 Grainger RG. Intravascular contrast media — the past, the present and the future. *Br J Radiol* 1982;55:1–18.
2 Almen T. Contrast media: the relation of chemical structure, animal toxicity and adverse clinical effects. *Am J Cardiol* 1990; 66:2F–8F.

3 Swanson DP, Chilton HM, Thrall JH. *Pharmaceuticals in Medical Imaging*. Macmillan: New York, 1990.

4 American College of Radiology. *Manual On Iodinated Contrast Media* 1991.

5 Fischer HW. Catalog of intravascular contrast media. *Radiology* 1986;159:561−563.

6 Dawson P, Howell M. The non-ionic dimers: a new class of contrast agents. *Br J Radiol* 1986;59:987−991.

7 Thomsen HS, Dorph S. Review article. High-osmolar and low-osmolar contrast media. An update on frequency of adverse drug reactions. *Acta Radiol* 1993;34:205−209.

8 Seymour R, Halpin SF, Hardman JA, Coote JM, Ruttley MST, Roberts GM. Corticosteroid prophylaxis for patients with increased risk of adverse reactions to intravascular contrast agents: a survey of current practice in the UK. *Clin Radiol* 1994;49: 791−795.

9 Dukes MNG, ed. *Meyler's Side Effects of Drugs*, 12th edn. Elsevier: Amsterdam, 1992. (Edetic acid pp. 555−556; Nickel p. 531.)

10 Hamilton G. Contamination of contrast agent by MBT in rubber seals. *Canad Med Assoc J* 1987;136:1020−1021.

11 Winding O. Contaminants in contrast media and catheters. In: Ansell G, Wilkins RA, eds. *Complications in Diagnostic Imaging*, 2nd edn. Blackwell Scientific Publications: Oxford, 1987.

12 Lasser EC, Lyon SG, Petro Z. Iodinated agents — adverse effects and reaction mechanisms. Surfaces and sensitivity in contrast material reactions. *Invest Radiol* 1991;26:S20−S22.

13 Leach CA, Sunderman FW. Hypernickelemia following coronary arteriography caused by nickel in the radiographic contrast medium. *Ann Clin Lab Sci* 1987;17:137−144.

14 Marshall TR, Ling JT, Follis G, Russel M. Pharmacological incompatibility of contrast media with various drugs and agents. *Radiology* 1965;84:536−539.

15 Monsein LH, Miller TJ, Kuwahara SK, Sostre S, Debrun GM. Ionic iodinated contrast medium and amobarbital sodium mixtures: potential for precipitation. *Radiology* 1992;184:385−387.

16 Iannone LA. Protamine−renografin chemical embolus. *Am Heart J* 1975;90:678.

17 Pilla TJ, Beshany SE, Shields JB. Incompatibility of Hexabrix and papaverine. *Am J Roentgenol* 1986;146:1300−1301.

18 Shah SJ, Gerlock AJ. Incompatibility of Hexabrix and papaverine in peripheral arteriography. *Radiology* 1987;162:619−620.

19 Fischer HW. Incompatibilities between contrast media and pharmacologic agents. *Radiology* 1987;162:875.

20 Pallan TM, Wulkan IA, Abadir AR, Flores L, Chaudhry MR, Gintautas J. Incompatibility of Isovue 370 and papaverine in peripheral arteriography. *Radiology* 1993;187:257−259.

21 Finelli DA. Was heparin the culprit? and reply by Dr. Pallan. *Radiology* 1993;189:624−625.

22 Holman BL, Dewangee MK. Potential pH incompatibility of pharmacologic and isotopic adjuncts to arteriography. *Radiology* 1974;110:722−723.

23 Lorenz W, Ennis M, Doenicke A, Dick W. Perioperative uses of histamine antagonists. *J Clin Anesth* 1990;2:345−360.

24 Klatte EC, Brooks AL, Rhamy RK. Toxicity of intra-arterial barbiturates and tranquilising drugs. *Radiology* 1969;92:700−704.

25 Nilsson P, Almén T, Golman K *et al*. Addition of local anaesthetics to contrast media. II. Increase of acute mortality in mice with intravenous contrast administration. *Acta Radiol (Diagn)* 1988; 29:247−250.

26 Fischer HW, Morris TW, King AN, Harnish PP. Deleterious synergism of a cardiac glycoside and sodium diatrizoate. *Invest Radiol* 1978;13:340−346.

27 Virkkonen P, Luostarinen M, Johansson G. Diazepam, alpha and beta neurotransmission modifying drugs and contrast mortality in mice. *Acta Radiol (Diagn)* 1984;25:249−251.

28 Smedby O. Viscosity of some contemporary contrast media before and after mixing with whole blood. *Acta Radiol* 1992;33: 600−605.

29 Hoppe JO. Some pharmacological aspects of radiological compounds. *Ann NY Acad Sci* 1959;78:727−739.

30 Rosati G, Leto di Priolo S, Tirone P. Serious fatal complications after inadvertent administration of ionic water-soluble contrast media in myelography. *Eur J Radiol* 1992;15:95−100.

31 Bøhn HP, Reich L, Suljaga-Petchel K. Inadvertent intrathecal use of ionic contrast media for myelography. *AJNR* 1992;13: 1515−1519.

32 McClennan BL. Contrast media alert. *Radiology* 1993;189:35.

33 McCleery WNC, Lewtas NA. Subarachnoid injection of contrast medium. *Br J Radiol* 1966;39:112−114.

34 Tartiere J, Gerard J-L, Peny J *et al*. Acute treatment after accidental intrathecal injection of hypertonic contrast media. *Anesthesiology* 1989;71:169.

35 Dalkin B, Franco I, Reda EF, McLone D, Godine L, Kaplan WE. Contrast-induced central nervous system toxicity after radiographic evaluation of the lower urinary tract in myelodysplastic patients with ventriculoperitoneal shunts. *J Urol* 1992;148: 120−121.

36 Davies P, Roberts MB, Roylance J. Acute reactions to urographic contrast media. *Br Med J* 1975;2:434−437.

37 Panto PN, Davies P. Delayed reactions to urographic contrast media. *Br J Radiol* 1986;59:41−44.

38 Penry JB, Livingstone JB. A comparison of diagnostic effectiveness and vascular side-effects of various diatrizoate salts used for intravenous pyelography. *Clin Radiol* 1972;23:362−369.

39 Laerum F. Injurious effects of contrast media on human vascular endothelium. *Acta Radiol* 1983;366 (Suppl.):70.

40 Thomas ML, Keeling FP, Piaggio RB, Treweeke PS. Contrast agent induced thrombophlebitis following leg phlebography: iopamidol versus meglumine iothalamate. *Br J Radiol* 1984;57: 205−207.

41 Raininko R. Role of hypertoxicity in the endothelial injury caused by angiographic contrast media. *Acta Radiol (Diagn)* 1979;20:410−416.

42 Lindgren P. Hemodynamic responses to contrast media. *Invest Radiol* 1970;5:424−435.

43 Lasser EL. Hemodynamic responses to contrast media. *Invest Radiol* 1970;5:440−441.

44 Wolf GL. Adult peripheral angiography. Results from four North American randomised clinical trials of ionic media versus iohexol. *Acta Radiol* 1983;366 (Suppl.):166−170.

45 Murphy G, Campbell DR, Fraser DB. Pain in peripheral arteriography: an assessment of conventional versus ionic and non-ionic low osmolality contrast agents. *J Canad Assoc Radiol* 1988; 39:103−106.

46 Grainger R, Dawson P. *Guidelines For Use of Low Osmolar Intravascular Contrast Agents*. London: Royal College of Radiologists, 1991.

47 Leung PL, Cheng CY. Extensive local necrosis following the intravenous use of X-ray contrast medium in the upper extremity. *Br J Radiol* 1980;53:361−364.

48 Burd DAR, Santis G, Milward TM. Severe extravasation injury: an avoidable introgenic disaster? *Br Med J* 1985;290:1579−1580.

49 McAlister WH, Palmer K. The histologic effects of four commonly used media for excretory urography and an attempt to modify the response. *Radiology* 1971;99:511−516.

50 Kubota S, Tada S, *et al*. Skin injury due to iodinated contrast material: a side effect during intravenous urography. *Jap J Clin Urol* 1977;31.733.

51 Cohan RH, Leder RA, Bolick D *et al*. Extravascular extravasation of radiographic contrast media. Effects of conventional and low-osmolar agents in the rat thigh. *Invest Radiol* 1990;25:504−510.

52 Kim SH, Park JH, Kim YL, Kim C-W, Han MC. Experimental tissue damage after subcutaneous injection of water soluble contrast media. *Invest Radiol* 1990;25:678−685.

53 Elam EA, Door RT, Lagel KE, Pond GD. Cutaneous ulceration due to contrast extravasation. Experimental assessment of injury and potential antidotes. *Invest Radiol* 1991;26:13−16.

54 Sistrom CL, Gay SB, Peffley RN. Extravasation of iopamidol and iohexol during contrast-enhanced C.T.: report of 28 cases. *Radiology* 1991;180:707−710.

55 Loth TS, Jones DEC. Extravasations of radiographic contrast material in the upper extremity. *J Hand Surg (Am)* 1988;13:395−398.

56 Cohan RH, Dunnick NR, Leder RA, Baker ME. Extravasation of nonionic radiologic contrast media: efficiency of conservative treatment. *Radiology* 1990;176:65−67.

57 Memolo M, Dyer R, Zagonia RJ. Extravasation injury with non ionic material. *Am J Roentgenol* 1993;160:203.

58 Ansell G. Contrast media and urography. In: Ansell G, Wilkins RA, eds. *Complications in Diagnostic Imaging*, 2nd edn. Oxford: Blackwell Scientific Publications, 1987:1−36.

59 Zucherman SD, Jacobson G. Transtracheal bronchography. Complications of injection outside the trachea. *Am J Roentgenol* 1962;87:840−843.

60 Franken EA, Grosfield JL. Unusual local reaction to iodinated contrast media. *Radiology* 1975;116:629−630.

61 Ansell G. Fatal overdose of contrast medium in infants. *Br J Radiol* 1970;43:395−396.

62 McClennan BL, Kassner G, Becker JA. Overdose at excretory urography: toxic cause of death. *Radiology* 1972;105:383−386.

63 McAlister WH, Segel MJ, Shackelford GD. Pulmonary oedema following intravenous urography in a neonate. *Br J Radiol* 1979;52:410−411.

64 Junck L, Marshall WH. Fatal brain edema after contrast-agent overdose. *Am J Neuroradiol* 1986;7:522−525.

65 Johnson LW, Krone R. Cardiac catheterization 1991: a report of the society for cardiac angiography and interventions (S.C.A. & I.). *Cathet Cardiovasc Diagn* 1993;28:219−220.

66 Levin DC, Gardiner GA. Coronary arteriography. In: Braunwald E, ed. *Heart Disease. A Textbook of Cardiovascular Medicine*. Philadelphia: WB Saunders, 1992:238−239.

67 Gensini GG, Di Giorgi S. Myocardial toxicity of contrast agents used in angiography. *Radiology* 1964;82:24−34.

68 Snyder CF, Formanek A, Frech RS, Amplatz K. The role of sodium in promoting ventricular arrhythmia during selective coronary arteriography. *Am J Roentgenol* 1971;113:567−571.

69 Hildner CJ, Scherlag B, Samet P. Evaluation of Renografin M-76 as a contrast agent for angiocardiography. *Radiology* 1971;100:329−334.

70 Simon AL, Shabetai R, Lang JH, Lasser EC. The mechanism of production of ventricular fibrillation in coronary angiography. *Am J Roentgenol* 1972;114:810−816.

71 Morris TW, Sahler LG, Fischer HW. Calcium binding by radio-paque media. *Invest Radiol* 1982;17:501−505.

72 Murdock DK, Johnson SA, Loeb HS, Scanlon PJ. Ventricular fibrillation during coronary angiography: reduced incidence in man with contrast media lacking calcium binding additives. *Catheter Cardiovasc Diag* 1985;11:153−159.

73 Caulfield JB, Zir L, Harthorne JW. Blood calcium levels in the presence of angiographic contrast material. *Circulation* 1975;52:119−123.

74 Morris TW. The physiologic effects of nonionic contrast media on the heart. *Invest Radiol* 1993;28 (Suppl. 5):S44−546.

75 Levorstad K, Vatne K, Brodahl U, Laake B, Simonsen S, Aakhus T. Safety of the non-ionic contrast medium Omnipaque in coronary angiography. *Cardiovasc Intervent Radiol* 1989;12:98−100.

76 Steinberg EP, Moore RD, Powe NR *et al*. Safety and cost effectiveness of high-osmolality as compared with low-osmolality contrast material in patients undergoing cardiac angiography. *New Engl J Med* 1992;326:425−436.

77 Barrett BJ, Parfrey PS, Vavasour HM, O'Dea F, Kent RN, Stone E. A comparison of nonionic low-osmolality radiocontrast agents with ionic, high-osmolality agents during cardiac catheterisation. *New Engl J Med* 1992;326:431−436.

78 Hill JA, Winniford M, Cohen MB *et al*. for the Iohexol Cooperative Study. Multicenter trial of ionic versus nonionic media for cardiac angiography. *Am J Cardiol* 1993;72:770−775.

79 Klinke WP, Grace M, Miller R, Naqvi SZ, Roth D, Roy L. A multicenter randomized trial of ionic (ioxaglate) and nonionic (iopamidol) low-osmolality contrast agents in cardiac angiography. *Clin Cardiol* 1989;12:689−696.

80 Gertz EW, Wisneski JA, Miller R *et al*. Adverse reactions of low osmolality contrast media during cardiac angiography: a prospective randomized multicenter study. *JACC* 1992;19:899−906.

81 Lehman MH, Case RB. Reduced human ventricular fibrillation threshold associated with contrast-induced Q-T prolongation. *J Electrocard* 1983;16:105−110.

82 Bååth L, Besjacov J, Oksendal A. Sodium−calcium balance in nonionic contrast media. Effects on the risk of ventricular fibrillation in the isolated rabbit heart. *Invest Radiol* 1993;28:223−227.

83 Klow NE, Levorstad K, Berg J *et al*. Iodixanol in cardioangiography in patients with coronary artery disease. Tolerability, cardiac and renal effects. *Acta Radiol* 1993;34:72−77.

84 Druck MN, Johnstone DE, Staniloff H, McLaughlin PR. Coronary artery spasm as a manifestation of anaphylactoid reaction to iodinated contrast material. *Canad Med Assoc J* 1981;125:1133−1135.

85 Doyama K, Hirose K, Kosuga K *et al*. Coronary artery spasm induced by anaphylactoid reaction to a new low osmolar contrast medium. *Am Heart J* 1990;120:1453−1455.

86 Hesselink JR, Hayman LA, Chung KJ, McGinnis BD, Davis KR, Taveras JM. Myocardial ischemia during intravenous D.S.A. in patients with cardiac disease. *Radiology* 1984;153:577−582.

87 Neergaard K, Galloe AM, Dirksen KL, Andersen EB. Cardiac complications of intravenous digital subtraction angiography. *Eur J Radiol* 1989;9:105−107.

88 Stadalnik RC, Zakauddin V, Da Silva O *et al*. Electrocardiographic response to intravenous urography. Prospective evaluation of 275 patients. *Am J Roentgenol* 1977;129:825−830.

89 Pfister RC, Hutter AM. Cardiac alterations during intravenous urography. *Invest Radiol* 1980;15 (Suppl.):S239−S242.

90 Mindell JH, Gibson TC. ECG abnormalities during excretory

urography: the effect of stress. *Am J Roentgenol* 1988;150: 1327–1329.

91 Hald JK, Jakobsen JA, Andrew E, Stormorken H. Adverse reactions to contrast media: related to medium or procedure? Observations on a case. *Br J Radiol* 1988;61:337–338.

92 Andrews EJ. The vagus reaction as a possible cause of severe complications of radiological procedures. *Radiology* 1976;121: 1–4.

93 Stanley RJ, Pfister RC. Bradycardia and hypotension following use of intravenous contrast media. *Radiology* 1976;121:5–7.

94 Fischer HW, Colgan HJ. Opinion, contrast media reactions. *Radiology* 1976;121:223.

95 Morris TW. The cardiovascular effects of iodinated contrast media injections. *Invest Radiol* 1988;23 (Suppl. 1):S133–S136.

96 Fischer HW. Hemodynamic reactions to angiographic media. A survey and commentary. *Radiology* 1968;91:66–73.

97 Higgins CB. Overview of cardiovascular effects of contrast media. Comparison of ionic and nonionic media. *Invest Radiol* 1984;19 (Suppl.):S187–S190.

98 Kurnik PB, Tiefenbrun AJ, Ludbrook PA, Courtois MR. Peripheral hemodynamic effects of intraventricular and intracoronary contrast media in man. *Invest Radiol* 1985;20:203–211.

99 Higgins CB, Gerber KH, Mattrey RF, Slutsky RA. Evaluation of the hemodynamic effects of intravenous administration of ionic and nonionic contrast materials. *Radiology* 1982;142:681–686.

100 Higgins CB, Kuger M, Slutsky RA. Interactions between verapamil and contrast media in coronary arteriography: comparison of standard ionic and nonionic media. *Circulation* 1983;68: 628–635.

101 Gressier M, Beaune J, Amouroux C *et al.* Arrêt cardiaque prolongé en diastole au coup d'une coronarographie chez un patient atteint d'un angor de Prinzmétal traité par le vérapamil. *Nouv Presse Méd* 1980;9:1521.

102 Morris DL, Wisneski JA, Gertz EW, Wexman M, Axelrod R, Langberg JJ. Potentiation by nifedapine and diltiazem of the hypotensive response after contrast angiography. *J Am Coll Cardiol* 1985;6:785–791.

103 Hamilton G. Severe adverse reaction to urography in patients taking β-adrenergic blocking agents. *Can Med Assoc J* 1985;133: 122.

104 Fischer HW, Morris TW, King AN, Harnish PP. Deleterious synergism of a cardiac glycoside and sodium diatrizoate. *Invest Radiol* 1978;13:340–346.

105 Virkkunen P, Luostarinen M, Johansson G. Diazepam, alpha and beta neurotransmission modifying drugs and contrast media mortality in mice. *Acta Radiol (Diagn)* 1984;25:249–251.

106 Ritchie JL, Nissen SE, Douglas JS *et al.* ACC position statement. Use of nonionic or low osmolar contrast agents in cardiovascular procedures. *J Am Coll Cardiol* 1993;21:269–273.

107 Byrd L, Sherman RL. Radiocontrast induced acute renal failure. A clinical and pathophysiologic review. *Medicine* 1979;58:270–279.

108 Mudge GH. Nephrotoxicity of urographic radiocontrast drugs. *Kidney Internat* 1980;18:540–552.

109 Hou SH, Bushinsky DA, Wish JB, Cohen JJ, Harrington JT. Hospital-acquired renal insufficiency: a prospective study. *Am J Med* 1983;74:243–248.

110 Holtås S, Törnquist C. Renal complications of contrast media. In: Ansell G, Wilkins RA, eds. *Complications in Diagnostic Imaging*, 2nd edn. Oxford: Blackwell Scientific Publications, 1987:37–52.

111 Katzberg RW. Renal effects of contrast media. *Invest Radiol* 1988;23 (Suppl. 1):S157–S160.

112 Porter GA. Contrast-associated nephropathy. *Am J Cardiol* 1989; 64:22E–26E.

113 Berns S. Nephrotoxicity of contrast media. *Kidney Int* 1989;36: 730–740.

114 Brezis M, Epstein M. A closer look at radiocontrast-induced nephropathy. *New Engl J Med* 1989;320:179–181.

115 Thomsen HS. Contrast nephropathy. *Cur Opin Radiol* 1990;2: 793–802.

116 Dawson P, Trewhella M. Intravascular contrast agents and renal failure. *Clin Radiol* 1990;41:373–375.

117 Bettman MA. The evaluation of contrast-related renal failure. *Am J Roentgenol* 1991;157:66–68.

118 Nora NA, Krumlovsky FA. Use of iodinated contrast media in patients with chronic renal insufficiency and in end-stage renal disease. *Int J Artif Org* 1991;14:196–198.

119 Berns JS, Rudnick MR. Radiocontrast media; associated nephrotoxicity. *Kidney* 1992;24:1–6.

120 Spinler SA, Goldfarb S. Nephrotoxicity of contrast media following cardiac angiography: pathogenesis, clinical course, and preventive measures, including the role of low-osmolality contrast media. *Ann Pharmacother* 1992;26:56–64.

121 Goldfarb S, Spinler S, Berns JS, Rudnick MR. Low-osmolality contrast media and the risk of contrast-associated nephrotoxicity. *Invest Radiol* 1993;28 (Suppl. 5):S7–S10.

122 Goldfarb S, Spinler S, Berns JS, Rudnick MR. Low osmolarity contrast media and the risk of contrast-associated nephrotoxicity. *Invest Radiol* 1993;28 (Suppl. 5):S7–S10.

123 Porter GA. Contrast medium-associated nephropathy. Recognition and management. *Invest Radiol* 1993;28 (Suppl. 4):S11–S18.

124 Van Zee BE, Hoy WE, Talley TE, Jaenike JR. Renal injury associated with intravenous pyelography in non-diabetic and diabetic patients. *Ann Int Med* 1978;89:51–54.

125 Rich MW, Crecelius CA. Incidence, risk factors, and clinical course of acute renal insufficiency after cardiac catheterization in patients 70 years or older. *Arch Int Med* 1990;150:1237–1242.

126 Martin-Paredero V, Dixon SM, Baker JD *et al.* Risk of renal failure after major angiography. *Arch Surg* 1983;118: 1417–1420.

127 Taliercio CP, McCallister SH, Holmes DR, Ilstrup DM, Vliestra RE. Nephrotoxicity of nonionic contrast media after cardiac angiography. *Am J Cardiol* 1989;64:815–816.

128 Davidson CJ, Hlatky M, Morris KG *et al.* Cardiovascular and renal toxicity of a nonionic radiography contrast agent after cardiac catheterisation. A prospective trial. *Ann Int Med* 1989; 110:119–124.

129 Moore RD, Steinberg EP, Powe NR *et al.* Risk factors for contrast media-induced nephrotoxicity. *APC J Club* 1992; July/August:29.

130 Parfree PS, Griffiths SM, Barrett BJ *et al.* Contrast material-induced renal failure in patients with diabetes mellitus, renal insufficiency or both. A prospective controlled study. *New Engl J Med* 1989;320:143–149.

131 Lautin EM, Freeman NJ, Schoenfeld AH *et al.* Radiocontrast-associated renal dysfunction — incidence and risk factors. *Am J Roentgenol* 1989;157:49–58.

132 Lautin EM, Freeman NJ, Schoenfeld AH *et al.* Radiocontrast-associated renal dysfunction: a comparison of lower-osmolality and coventional high-osmolality contrast media. *Am J Roentgenol* 1991;157:59–65.

133 Wexler L, Cohen MB, Rudnick MR, Murphy MJ, Halpern EF. Multicenter trial of ionic and nonionic media: nephrotoxicity following cardiac angiography. *Radiol RSNA Ann Meet* 1991; Abstract:1159.

134 Barrett BJ, Parfrey PS, Vavasour HM *et al*. Contrast nephropathy in patients with impaired renal function: high versus low osmolar media. *Kidney Int* 1992;41:1274−1279.

135 Moore RD, Steinberg EP, Powe NR *et al*. Frequency and determinants of adverse reactions induced by high-osmolality contrast media. *Radiology* 1989;170:727−732.

136 Schwab SJ, Hlatky MA, Pieper KS *et al*. Contrast nephrotoxicity: a randomised controlled trial of a nonionic and an ionic radiographic contrast agent. *New Engl J Med* 1989;320:149−153.

137 Harding MB, Davidson CJ, Pieper KS *et al*. Comparison of cardiovascular and renal toxicity after cardiac catheterisation using a nonionic versus ionic radiographic contrast agent. *Am J Cardiol* 1991;68:1117−1119.

138 Cochrane ST, Wong WS, Roe DJ. Predicting angiography-induced acute renal functional impairment: clinical risk model. *Am J Roentgenol* 1983;141:1027−1033.

139 Manske CL, Sprafka JM, Strony JT, Wang Y. Contrast nephropathy in azotemic diabetic patients undergoing coronary angiography. *Am J Med* 1990;89:615−620.

140 Harris KG, Smith TP, Cragg AH, Lemke JH. Nephrotoxicity from contrast material in renal insufficiency: ionic versus nonionic agents. *Radiology* 1991;179:849−852.

141 Older RA, Korobkin M, Cleeve DM, Schaal R, Thompson W. Contrast-induced acute renal failure: persistent nephrogram as clue to early detection. *Am J Roentgenol* 1980;134:339−342.

142 D'Elia JA, Gleason RE, Alday M *et al*. Nephrotoxicity from angiographic contrast material. A prospective study. *Am J Med* 1982;72:719−725.

143 Love L, Lind JA, Olson MC. Persistent CT nephrogram: significance in the diagnosis of contrast nephropathy. *Radiology* 1989;172:125−129.

144 Jakobsen JÅ, Lundby B, Kristoffersen DT, Borch KW, Hald JK, Berg KJ. Evaluation of renal function with delayed CT after injection of nonionic monomeric and dimeric media in healthy volunteers. *Radiology* 1992;182:419−424.

145 Golman K, Almén T. Contrast media-induced nephrotoxicity. Survey and present state. *Invest Radiol* 1985;20 (Suppl. 1): S92−S97.

146 Weinrauch LA, Healy RW, Leland OS *et al*. Coronary angiography and acute renal failure in diabetic azotemic nephropathy. *Ann Int Med* 1977;86:56−69.

147 Webb JA, Reznek RH, Cattell WR, Fry IK. Renal function after high dose urography in patients with renal failure. *Br J Radiol* 1981;54:479−483.

148 Heller CA, Knapp J, Halliday J, O'Connell D, Heller RF. Failure to demonstrate contrast nephrotoxicity. *Med J Aust* 1991;54: 479−483.

149 Vaamonde CA, Bier RT, Papendick R *et al*. Acute and chronic renal effects of radiocontrast in diabetic rats. Role of anesthesia and risk factors. *Invest Radiol* 1989;24:206−218.

150 Bergman LA, Ellison MR, Dunea G. Acute renal failure after drug infusion pyelography. *New Engl J Med* 1968;279:1277.

151 Pillay VK, Robbins PC, Schwartz FD, Kark RM. Acute renal failure following intravenous urography in patients with long-standing diabetes mellitus and azotemia. *Radiology* 1970;95: 633−636.

152 Dudzinski PJ, Petrone AF, Persoff M, Callaghan EE. Acute renal failure following high dose excretory urography in dehy-drated patients. *J Urol* 1971;106:619−621.

153 Milman N, Gottlieb P. Renal function after high-dose urography in patients with chronic renal insufficiency. *Clin Nephrol* 1977; 7:250−254.

154 Feldman HA, Goldfarb S, McCurdy DK. Recurrent radiographic dye-induced acute renal failure. *J Am Med Assoc* 1974;229:72.

155 Shulman G. Bence Jones myelomatosis and intravenous pyelography. *S Afr Med J* 1977;51:574−576.

156 Teruel JL, Llorente MT, Herrero JA *et al*. Prevención de la nefrotoxicidad por contrastes yodados en pacientes con insuficiencia renal. *Med Clin (Barc)* 1988;91:281−282.

157 Gruskin AB, Oetliker OH, Wolfish NM, Gootman NL, Bernstein J, Edelman CM. Effect of angiography on renal function and histology in infants and piglets. *J Pediat* 1970;76:41−48.

158 Gates GF, Green GS. Transient reduction in renal function following arteriography: a radionuclide study. *J Urol* 1983;129: 1107−1110.

159 Taliercio CP, Vliestra RE, Fisher LD, Burnett JC. Risks for renal dysfunction with cardiac angiography. *Ann Int Med* 1986;104: 501−504.

160 Lang EK, Foreman JU, Schlegel JU, Leslie C, List A, McCormick P. The incidence of contrast medium induced acute tubular necrosis following arteriography. *Radiology* 1981;138:203−206.

161 Adornato B, Wienstock D. Acute renal failure, a complication of cerebral angiography. *Arch Neurol* 1976;33:687−688.

161 Krumlovsky FA, Simon N, Santhanam S. *et al*. Acute renal failure. Association with administration of radiographic contrast material. *J Am Med Assoc* 1978;239:125−127.

162 Khoury GA, Hopper JC, Varghese Z *et al*. Nephrotoxicity of ionic and non-ionic contrast material in digital vascular imaging and selective renal arteriography. *Br J Radiol* 1983;56:631−635.

163 Thompson K. Safety and efficiency of CO_2 as a contrast medium during renal artery angioplasty. *Andreas Gruntzig Soc Meet (Sydney)* 1994;6−13th February.

164 Barshay ME, Kaye JH, Goldman R, Coburn JW. Acute renal failure in diabetic patients after infusion pyelography. *Clin Nephrol* 1973;1:35−39.

165 Ihle BU, Byrnes CA, Simenhoff ML. Acute renal failure due to interstitial nephritis resulting from radio-contrast agents. *Aust NZ J Med* 1982;12:630−632.

166 McCarthy CS, Becker JA. Multiple myeloma and contrast media. *Radiology* 1992;183:519−521.

167 Lasser EC, Lang JH, Zawadzki ZA. Contrast media: myeloma precipitates in urography. *J Am Med Assoc* 1966;198:945−970.

168 Cwynarski MT, Saxton HM. Urography in myelomatosis. *Br Med J* 1969;1:486.

169 Myers GH, Witten DM. Acute renal failure after excretion urography in multiple myeloma. *Am J Roentgenol* 1971;113: 583−588.

170 De Fronzo RA, Humphrey RL, Wright JR, Cooke CR. Acute renal failure in multiple myeloma. *Medicine* 1975;54:209−223.

171 McEvoy J, McGeown MG, Kumar R. Renal failure after radiological contrast media. *Br Med J* 1970;4:717−718.

172 Brown M, Battle JD. The effect of urography on renal function in patients with myeloma. *Can Med Assoc J* 1964;91:786−790.

173 Gordon S, Barnes SJ. Acute renal failure after enhanced computer tomography. *Arch Int Med* 1983;143:1042−1043.

174 Mudge G. Cholecystography and renal failure. *Lancet* 1971;2: 872.

175 Harrow BR, Sloane JA. Acute renal failure following cholegraphy. A unique nephrographic effect. *Am J Med Sci* 1965;249:

26–35.

176 Blum M, Liron M, Aviram A. Acute renal failure following cholecystography. *Am J Proctol Gastroenterol Colon Rect Surg* 1984;August:11–14.

177 Jamet P, Lebas de Lacour JCl, Christoforov B, Stern M. Acidose lactique mortelle après urographie intraveineuse chez une diabétique recevant de la metformine. *Sem Hôp Paris* 1980;56: 473–474.

178 Przybylowski J, Buras B, Stefanowa-Urbaniak A, Snioch J. Bilateral necrosis of the renal cortex resulting from shock produced by intravenous contrast media. *Pol Tyg Lek* 1986;41: 373–375. (In Polish.)

179 Catterall JR, Ferguson RJ, Miller HC. Intravascular haemolysis with acute renal failure after angiocardiography. *Br Med J* 1981;282:779–780.

180 Carena J, Magnelli P, Puebla M, Smuckler C. Rabdomiolisis associada a medio de contraste iodado. *Medicina (Buenos Aires)* 1991;51:348–350.

181 Mandell GA, Swacus JR, Rosenstock J, Buck BE. Danger of urography in hyperuricaemic children with Burkitt's lymphoma. *J Can Assoc Radiol* 1983;34:273–277.

182 Schneider G, Marzi I, Kramann B. Effects of ionic and nonionic contrast media in renal function in acute hemorrhagic pancreatitis: an experimental study in rats. *RSNA Ann Meet* 1991; Abstract:843.

183 Heideman M, Claes G, Nilson AE. The risk of renal allograft rejection following angiography. *Transplantation* 1976;21:289–293.

184 Moreau JF, Kreis H, Barbanel C, Michel JR. Effects des produits de contraste iodés sur la fonction des reins transplantés. *Nouv Presse Med* 1975;4:2643–2646.

185 Peters C, Delmonico FL, Cosimi AB *et al.* Risks versus benefits of contrast medium exposure in renal allograft recipients. *Surg Gynec Obstet* 1983;156:467–472.

186 Hunter JV, Kind PRN. Non ionic contrast media: potential renal damage assessed with enzymuria. *Radiology* 1992;183: 101–104.

187 Stark FR, Coburn JW. Renal failure following methylglucamine diatrizoate (Renografin) aortography: report of a case with unilateral renal artery stenosis. *J Urol* 1966;96:848–851.

188 Porter GA. Effects of contrast agents on renal function. *Invest Radiol* 1993;28:S1–S5.

189 Porter GA. Experimental contrast-associated nephropathy and its clinical implications. *Am J Cardiol* 1990;66:18F–22F.

190 Törnquist C, Almén T, Golman K, Holtås S. Renal function following nephroangiography with metrizamide and iohexol. Effects on renal blood flow, glomerular permeability and filtration rate and diuresis in dogs. *Acta Radiol (Diagn)* 1985;26: 483–489.

191 Heyman SN, Clark BA, Cantley L *et al.* Effects of ioversol versus iothalamate on endothelin release and radiocontrast nephropathy. *Invest Radiol* 1993;28:313–318.

192 Morcos SK, Oldroyd S, Haylor SK. Role of endothelin in mediating the renal response to water-soluble contrast media. *RSNA Ann Meet* 1993;Abstract:507.

193 Weisberg LS, Kurnik PB, Kurnik BRC. Radiocontrast-induced nephropathy in humans: role of renal vasoconstriction. *Kidney Int* 1992;41:1408–1415.

194 Agmon Y, Brezis M. Nonsteroidal anti-inflammatory drugs (NSAIDs) induce outer medullary ischemia. *J Am Soc Nephrol* 1992;3:718.

195 Heyman SN, Brezis CA, Reubinoff CA *et al.* Acute renal failure with selective medullary injury in the rat. *J Clin Invest* 1988;82: 401–412.

196 Moreau JF, Droz D, Sabto J *et al.* Osmotic nephrosis induced by water-soluble tri-iodinated contrast media in man. A retrospective study of 47 cases. *Radiology* 1975;115:329–336.

197 Vari RC, Natarajan LA, Whitescarver SA, Jackson BA, Ott CE. Induction, prevention and mechanisms of contrast media-induced acute renal failure. *Kidney Int* 1988;33:699–707.

198 Humes HD, Cieslinski DA, Messana JM. Pathogenesis of radiocontrast-induced acute renal failure: comparative nephrotoxicity of diatrizoate and iopamidol. *Diagn Imag* 1987; 9 (Suppl.):12–18.

199 Cederholm C, Almén T, Bergquist D, Golman K, Takolander R. Acute renal failure in rats. Interaction between contrast media and temporary renal arterial occlusion. *Acta Radiol* 1989;30: 321–326.

200 Almén T, Bergquist D, Cederholm C *et al.* Interactive effects on renal function between renal ischemia and intravascular contrast media. *Invest Radiol* 1988;23 (Suppl. 1):S161–S163.

201 Tejler L, Almén T, Holtås S. Proteinuria following nephroangiography. I. Clinical experiences. *Acta Radiol (Diagn)* 1977;21: 634–647.

202 Nicot GS, Merle LJ, Charmes JP *et al.* Transient glomerular proteinuria, enzymuria, and nephrotoxic reaction induced by radiocontrast media. *J Am Med Assoc* 1984;252:2432–2434.

203 Tejler L, Ekberg M, Almén T, Holtås S. Proteinuria following renal arteriography. Report on two cases. *Acta Med Scand* 1977; 202:131–133.

204 Nillson PE, Holtås S, Tejler LT. Subjective responses and albuminuria induced during renal angiography in man. *Radiology* 1982;144:509–512.

205 Törnquist C, Holtås S. Renal angiography with iohexol and metrizoate. *Radiology* 1984;150:331–334.

206 Albrechtsson U, Hultberg B, Larusdottir H, Norgren L. Nephrotoxicity of ionic and non-ionic contrast media in aorto-femoral angiography. *Acta Radiol Diagn* 1985;26:615–618.

207 Bani E, Federighi F, Ghio R *et al.* The use of iohexol in pediatric urography: a comparison study with meglumine diatrizoate. *Int J Pediatr Nephrol* 1985;20:271.

208 Parvez Z, Ramamurthy S, Patel NB, Moncada R. Enzyme markers of contrast media-induced renal failure. *Invest Radiol* 1990;25:S133–S134.

209 Jakobsen JA, Nossen JØ, Jørgensen NP, Berg KJ. Renal tubular effects of diuretics and X-ray contrast media. A comparative study of equiosmolar doses in healthy volunteers. *Invest Radiol* 1993;28:319–324.

210 Skovgaard D, Holm J, Hemmingsen L, Skaarup P. Urinary protein excretion following intravenously administered ionic and non-ionic contrast media in man. *Acta Radiol* 1989;30: 517–519.

211 Rossi L, Spinetta G, Bergamaschi E *et al.* Nefrotossicita da mezzi di contraste ionici e non ionici in urografia. Valutazione con techniche immunoenzimatiche e anticorpi monoclonali. *Radiol Med* 1989;78:612–615.

212 Tidgren B, Golman K. Effect of diatrizoate on renal excretion of PAH in man. *Acta Radiol* 1989;30:521–524.

213 Thomsen HS. Contrast media- and pharmacologic-induced nephropathies. Effects of diatrizoate and iohexol on urine profiles in rats. *Invest Radiol* 1990;25:S129–S132.

214 Thomsen HS (quoted by Whalen E). Tenth meeting and postgraduate course of the Society of Uroradiology, September 1990. *Am J Roentgenol* 1991;156:190–191.

215 Ueda N, Nygren A, Hansell P, Erikson U. Influence of contrast media on single nephron glomerular filtration rate in rat kidney — a comparison between diatrizoate, iohexol, ioxaglate and iotrolan. *Acta Radiol* 1992;33:596−599.

216 Kumar S, Muchmore A. Tamm−Horsfall protein-uromodulin (1950−1990). *Kidney Int* 1990;37:1395−1401.

217 Berdon WE, Schwartz RH, Becker J, Baker DH. Tamm−Horsfall proteinuria. Its relationship to prolonged nephrogram in infants and children and to renal failure following intravenous urography in adults with multiple myeloma. *Radiology* 1969;92:714−722.

218 Schwartz RH, Berdon WE, Wagner J, Becker J, Baker DH. Tamm−Horsfall urinary mucoprotein precipitation by urographic contrast agents: *in vitro* studies. *Am J Roentgenol* 1970;108:698−701.

219 Dawson P, Freedman DB, Howell MJ, Hine AL. Contrast-medium-induced acute renal failure and Tamm−Horsfall proteinuria. *Br J Radiol* 1984;57:577−579.

220 Dawnay ABStJ, Thornley C, Nockler I, Webb JAW, Cattell WR. Tamm−Horsfall glycoprotein excretion and aggregation during intravenous urography. Relevance to acute renal failure. *Invest Radiol* 1985;20:53−57.

221 Bakris GL, Gaber AO, Jones JD. Oxygen free radical involvement in urinary Tamm−Horsfall protein excretion after intrarenal injection of contrast medium. *Radiology* 1990;175:57−60.

222 Fang LST, Sirota RA, Ebert TH, Lichtenstein S. Low fractional excretion of sodium with contrast media-induced acute renal failure. *Arch Int Med* 1980;140:531−533.

223 Gelman ML, Rowe JW, Coggins CH, Athanasoulis C. Effects of an angiographic contrast agent on renal function. *Cardiovasc Med* 1979;4:313−320.

224 Beyer-Enke SA, Zeitler E, Schneider R. Spätnebenwirkungen nach intravasaler Anwendung nichtionischer Röntgenkontrastmittel. *Radiologe* 1992;32:165−169.

225 Kovnat PJ, Lin KY, Popky G. Azotemia and nephrogenic diabetes insipidus after arteriography. *Radiology* 1973;108:541−542.

226 Borra S, Duguid W, Kaye M. Acute renal failure and nephrotic syndrome after angiocardiography with meglumine diatrizoate. *New Engl J Med* 1971;284:592−593.

227 Ihle BU, Byrnes CA, Simenhoff ML. Acute renal failure due to interstitial nephritis resulting from radio-contrast agents. *Aust NZ J Med* 1982;12:630−632.

228 Kleinknecht D, Deloux J, Homerg JC. Acute renal failure after intravenous urography: detection of antibodies against contrast media. *Clin Nephrol* 1974;2:116−119.

229 Rudnick MR, Goldfarb S, Murphy MJ. Mannitol and other prophylactic regimens in contrast media-induced acute renal failure. *Cor Art Dis* 1991;2:1047−1052.

230 Heymen SN, Brezis M, Greenfeld Z, Rosen S. Protective role of furosemide and saline in radiocontrast-induced acute renal failure in the rat. *Am J Kidney Dis* 1989;14:377−385.

231 Golman K, Cederholm C. Contrast medium-induced acute renal failure. Can it be prevented? *Invest Radiol* 1990;25:S127−S128.

232 Hans B, Hans SS, Mittal VK, Khan TA, Patel N, Dahn MS. Renal functional response to dopamine during and after arteriography in patients with chronic renal insufficiency. *Radiology* 1990;176:651−654.

233 Neumayer H-H, Junge W, Küfner A, Wenning A. Prevention of radiocontrast-media-induced nephrotoxicity by the calcium channel block nitrendipine: a prospective randomised clinical trial. *Nephrol Dial Transplant* 1989;4:1030−1036.

234 Cacoub P, Deray G, Baumelou A, Jacobs C. No evidence for protective effects of nifedipine against radiocontrast-induced acute renal failure. *Clin Nephrol* 1988;29:215−216.

235 Moore RD, Steinberg EP, Powe NR *et al*. Comparative frequency of and risk factors for nephrotoxicity in patients receiving high-versus low-osmolality contrast media. *Radiol RSNA Ann Meet* 1993;Abstract:1119

236 Olukotun Dr. Iodinated agent-pharmaconetics and renal function. Discussion. *Invest Radiol* 1991;26 (Suppl. 1):S89.

237 Aron NC, Feinfeld DA, Peters AT, Lynn RI. Acute renal failure associated with ioxaglate, a low-osmolality agent. *Am J Kidney Dis* 1989;8:189−193.

238 Spångberg-Viklund B, Nikonoff T, Lundberg M, Larsson R, Skau T, Nyberg T. Acute renal failure caused by low-osmolar radiographic contrast media in patients with diabetic nephropathy. *Scand J Urol Nephrol* 1989;23:315−317.

239 Denys BJ, Reddy PS, Uretsky BF. Nephrotoxicity of a nonionic (iopamidol) versus an ionic (diatrizoate) contrast agent in the patient after cardiac transplant with moderate cyclosporine-induced renal insufficiency. *Am J Cardiol* 1989;64:405−406.

240 Gomes AS, Lois JF, Baker JD, McGlade CT, Bunnell DH, Hartzman S. Acute renal dysfunction in high risk patients after angiography: comparison of ionic and nonionic contrast media. *Radiology* 1989;170:65−68.

241 Chamberlain MJ, Sherwood T. The extra-renal excretion of diatrizoate in renal failure. *Br J Radiol* 1966;39:765−770.

242 Segall HD. Gallbladder visualization following the injection of diatrizoate. *Am J Roentgenol* 1969;107:21−26.

243 Udeshi UL. Gall bladder and colonic opacification following parenteral ioxaglate. *Clin Radiol* 1985;36:497−498.

244 Lee S, Schoen I. Black-copper reduction reaction simulating alcaptonuria — occurrence after intravenous urography. *New Engl J Med* 1966;275:266−267.

245 Shanahan JC, Palmer C, Eggington J. Misleading urine tests after Hexabrix IVU. *Br J Radiol* 1985;58:389.

246 Ramsay AW, Spector M, Rodgers AL, Miller RL, Knapp DR. Crystalluria following excretory urography. *Br J Urol* 1982;54:341−345.

247 McPhaul M, Punzi HA, Sandi A, Borganelli M, Rude R, Kaplan NM. Snuff-induced hypertension in pheochromocytoma. *J Am Med Assoc* 1984;252:2860−2862.

248 Gonsette RE. Cerebral complications of angiography and computed tomography. In: Ansell G, Wilkins RA, eds. *Complications in Diagnostic Imaging* 2nd edn. Oxford: Blackwell Scientific Publications, 1987:103−113.

249 Evill CA, Wilson AJ, Sage MR. Chemotoxic effects of low-osmolar contrast media on the blood−brain barrier. *Invest Radiol* 1990;25:S82−S83.

250 Lundervold A, Engeset A. Cerebral angiography. In: Ansell G., ed. *Complications in Diagnostic Radiology*. Oxford: Blackwell Scientific Publications, 1976:151−182.

251 Mishkin MM, Baum S, Di Chiro G. Emergency treatment of angiography-induced paraplegia and tetraplegia. *New Engl J Med* 1973;288:1184−1185.

252 Henzlova MJ, Coghlan HC, Dean LS, Taylor JL. Cortical blindness after left internal mammary artery to left anterior descending coronary artery graft angiography. *Cathet Cardiovasc Diagn* 1988;15:37−39.

253 Parry R, Rees J, Wilde P. Transient cortical blindness after coronary angiography. *Br Heart J* 1993;70:563−564.

254 Bhola NR, Pagano TV, Delcore M, Knobel KR, Lee J. Cortical blindness after cardiac catheterization: effect of rechallenge

with dye. *Cathet Cardiovasc Diagn* 1993;28:149−151.

255 Banna M. Post-angiographic blindness in a patient with sickle cell disease. *Invest Radiol* 1992;27:179−181.

256 Ansell G. Adverse reactions to contrast agents. Scope of problem. *Invest Radiol* 1970;5:374−384.

257 Scott WR. Seizures a reaction to contrast media for computed tomography of the brain. *Radiology* 1980;137:359−361.

258 Pagani JJ, Hayman LA, Bigelo RH *et al*. Diazepam prophylaxis of contrast media induced seizures during computed tomography of patients with brain metastases. *Am J Neuroradiol* 1983;4:67−72.

259 Pagani JJ, Hayman LA, Bigelo RH *et al*. Prophylactic diazepam in prevention of contrast media induced seizures in glioma patients undergoing cerebral computed tomography. *Cancer* 1984;54:2200−2204.

260 Avrahami E, Weiss-Peretz J, Cohn DF. Epilepsy in patients with brain metastases triggered by intravenous contrast medium. *Clin Radiol* 1989;40:422−423.

261 Hyman N. Personal communication, 1987.

262 Haslam RHA, Cochrane DD, Amundson GM, Johns RD. Neurotoxic complications of contrast computed tomography in children. *J Pediatr* 1987;111:837−840.

263 Skalpe IO. Enhancement with water-soluble contrast media in computed tomography of the brain and abdomen. Survey and present state. *Acta Radiol* 1983;366 (Suppl.):72−75.

264 Leonardi M, Lavaroni A, Biasizzo E *et al*. High-dose contrast-enhanced computed tomography (CECT) with iopamidol in the detection of cerebral metastases. Tolerance of the contrast agent. *Neuroradiology* 1989;31:148−150.

265 Utz R, Ekholm SE, Isaac L *et al*. Local blood−brain barrier penetration following systemic contrast medium administration: a case report and an experimental study. *Acta Radiol* 1988;29:237−242.

266 Uhl GR, Martinez CR, Brooks BR. Spinal seizures following intravenous contrast in a patient with a cord AVM. *Ann Neurol* 1981;10:580−581.

267 Micheli F, Gatto E, Lehkuniec E. Myoclonus espinal secundario a la administracion endovenosa de contraste iodado. *Medicina (Buenos Aires)* 1991;51:548−550.

268 Mozley PD. Malignant hyperthermia following intravenous iodinated contrast media. Report of a fatal case. *Diagn Gynecol Obstet* 1981;3:81−85.

269 Lalli AF. Contrast media reactions: data analysis and hypothesis. *Radiology* 1980;134:1−12.

270 Lalli AF. Personal communication, 1986.

271 Stinchcombe SJ, Davies P. Acute toxic myopathy: a delayed adverse effect of intravenous urography with iopamidol 370. *Br J Radiol* 1989;62:949−950.

272 Whisson CC, Evill CA, Wilson AJ, Sage MR. Muscular and central nervous system side effects of intracarotid contrast media in rabbits. *Invest Radiol* 1990;25:S90−S91.

273 Mallette LE, Gomez LS. Systemic hypocalcemia after clinical injections of radiocontrast media: amelioration by omission of calcium chelating agents. *Radiology* 1983;147:677−679.

274 Berger RE, Gomez LS, Mallette LE. Acute hypocalcemic effects of clinical contrast media injections. *Am J Roentgenol* 1982;138:283−288.

275 Kutt H, Milhorat TH, McDowell E. The effect of iodinised contrast media upon blood proteins, electrolytes and red cells. *Neurology* 1963;13:492−499.

276 Morris S, Sahler LG, Fischer HW. Calcium binding by radiopaque media. *Invest Radiol* 1982;17:501−505.

277 Doyle FH, Sherwood T, Steiner RE *et al*. Large dose urography. Is there an optimum dose? *Lancet* 1967;ii:964−966.

278 Smith MJG, Kendall BE, Tomlinson S. Adverse reactions to high doses of methylglucamine based contrast media. *Br J Radiol* 1974;47:566−569.

279 Hall R, Hawkins PN, Scott J *et al*. Grand rounds − Hammersmith Hospital cardiac transplantation for AL amyloidosis. Good quality of life is possible for several years. *Br Med J* 1994;309:1135−1137.

280 Chagnac Y, Hadani M, Goldhammer Y. Myasthenic crisis after intravenous administration of iodinated contrast agent. *Neurology* 1985;35:1219−1220.

281 Van den Bergh P, Kelly JJ Jr, Carter B, Munsat TL. Intravascular contrast media and neuromuscular junction disorders. *Ann Neurol* 1986;19:206−207.

282 Anzola GP, Capra R, Magoni M, Vignolo LA. Myasthenic crisis during intravenous iodinated contrast medium injection. *Ital J Neurol Sci* 1986;7:273.

283 Eliashiv S, Wirguin I, Brenner T, Argov Z. Aggravation of human and experimental myasthenia gravis by contrast media. *Neurology* 1990;40:1623−1625.

284 Stein HL, Hilgartner MW. Alteration of coagulation mechanism of blood by contrast media. *Am J Roentgenol* 1968;104:458−463.

285 Parvez Z, Moncada R, Fareed J, Messmore L. Antiplatelet action of intravascular contrast media. Implications in diagnostic procedures. *Invest Radiol* 1984;19:208−211.

286 Parvez R, Moncada R, Messmore HL, Fareed J. Ionic and nonionic contrast media interaction with anticoagulant drugs. *Acta Radiol (Diagn)* 1982;23:401−404.

287 Ing JJ, Smith DC, Bull BS. Differing mechanisms of clotting inhibition by ionic and nonionic contrast agents. *Radiology* 1989;172:345−348.

288 Fareed J, Walenga JM, Saravia GE, Moncada RM. Thrombogenic potential of nonionic contrast media? *Radiology* 1990;174:321−325.

289 Robertson HJF. Blood clot formation in angiographic syringes containing nonionic media. *Radiology* 1987;162:621−622.

290 Robertson HJF. Nonionic contrast media in radiology: procedural considerations. *Invest Radiol* 1988;23 (Suppl. 2):S374−S377.

291 Grollman JH, Liu CK, Astone RA, Lurie MD. Thromboembolic complications in coronary angiography associated with the use of non-ionic contrast medium. *Cathet Cardiovasc Diagn* 1988;14:159−164.

292 Esplugas E, Cequier A, Jara F. *et al*. Risk of thrombosis during coronary angioplasty with low osmolality contrast media. *Am J Cardiol* 1991;68:1020−1024.

293 Gasperetti CM, Feldman MD, Burwell LR *et al*. Influence of contrast media on thrombus formation during coronary angioplasty. *J Am Coll Cardiol* 1991;18:443−450.

294 Piessens JH, Stammen F, Vrolix MC *et al*. Effects of an ionic versus a nonionic low osmolar contrast agent on the thrombotic complications of coronary angioplasty. *Cath Cardiovasc Diagn* 1993;28:99−105.

295 Davidson CJ, Mark DB, Pieper KS *et al*. Thrombotic and cardiovascular complications related to non-ionic media during cardiac catheterisation: analysis of 8517 patients. *Am J Cardiol* 1990;65:1481−1484.

296 Engelhart JA, Smith DC, Mawney MD, Westengard JC, Bull BS. A technique for estimating the probability of clots in blood/contrast agent mixtures. *Invest Radiol* 1988;23:923−927.

297 Grabowski EF. Reviewer's comments. *Invest Radiol* 1989;24: 940–941.

298 Dawson P, McCarthy P, Allison DJ, Garvey B, Bradshaw A. Non-ionic contrast agents, red cell aggregation and coagulation. *Br J Radiol* 1988;61:963–965.

299 Kopko PM, Smith DC, Bull BS. Thrombin generation in non-clottable mixtures of blood and nonionic contrast agents. *Radiology* 1990;174:459–461.

300 Fareed J *et al.* Reply to correspondence. *Radiology* 1990;177: 283–284.

301 Laurie AJ, Lyon SG, Lasser EC. The effects of contrast media on coagulation factor XII. *Invest Radiol* 1991;26:S23–S25.

302 Granger CB, Gabriel DA, Reece NS *et al.* Fibrin modification by ionic and nonionic contrast media during cardiac catheterization. *Am J Cardiol* 1992;69:821–823.

303 Casalani E. Role of low-osmolality contrast media in thromboembolic complications: scanning electromicroscopy study. *Radiology* 1992;183:741–744.

304 Himi Z, Takemoto A, Himi S *et al.* Hematologic effects of iodinated media. Anticoagulant effect of ionic and nonionic contrast media. Scanning electron microscopic study on clot formation. *Invest Radiol* 1991;26:S92–S95.

305 Grabowski EF, Head C, Michelson AD. Nonionic contrast media, procoagulants or clotting innocents? *Invest Radiol* 1993;28 (Suppl. 5):S21–S24.

306 Grollman JH. Thrombogenic potential of nonionic media? — correspondence. *Radiology* 1990;177:282.

307 Dawson P, Grabowski EF. The clotting issue: etiological factors in thromboembolism. II. Clinical considerations. Discussion. *Invest Radiol* 1993;28 (Suppl. 5):S38.

308 Stormorken H. Nonionic contrast media in radiology. Procedural considerations. Discussion. *Invest Radiol* 1988;23 (Suppl. 2): S376–S377.

309 Doorey AJ, Stillabower ME, Gale N, Goldenberg EM. Catastrophic thrombus development despite systemic heparinization during coronary angioplasty: possible relationship to nonionic contrast. *Clin Cardiol* 1992;15:117–120.

310 Chronos NAF, Goodall AH, Wilson DJ, Sigwart U, Buller NP. Profound platelet degranulation is an important side effect of some types of contrast media used in interventional cardiology. *Circulation* 1993;88:2035–2044.

311 Stormorken H. Effects of contrast media on the hemostatic and thrombotic mechanisms. *Invest Radiol* 1988;23 (Suppl. 2): S318–S325.

312 Clarke R, Daly L, Robinson K *et al.* Hyperhomocystenemia: an independent risk factor for vascular disease. *New Engl J Med* 1991;324;1149–1155.

313 Burchardt CP, Fenker H, Schoop HJ, Tödlicher Kontrastmittelzwischenfall bei unberandertem morbus Waldenström. *Dtsch Med Wschr* 1981;106:1223–1225.

314 Bauer K, Tragl KH, Baur G *et al.* Intravasale Denaturierung von Plasma–Proteinen bei einer IgM Paraproteinämie ausgelost durch ein intravenös verabreichtes lebergangiges Röntgenkontrastmittel. *Wien Klin Wschr* 1974;86:766–769.

315 Kudoh Y, Kijima T, Imura O. Acute thrombocytopenic purpura after intravenous infusion of radiographic contrast medium. *Jap J Nephrol* 1991;33:61–64.

316 Lacey J, Brober-Sorcinelli KE, Farber LR, Glickman MG. Acute thrombocytopenia. *Am J Roentgenol* 1986;146:1298–1299.

317 Shojania AM. Immune-mediated thrombocytopenia due to an iodinated contrast medium (diatrizoate). *Can Med Assoc J* 1985; 133:123.

318 Chang JC, Lee D, Gross HM. Acute thrombocytopenia after IV administration of a radiographic contrast medium. *Am J Roentgenol* 1989;152:947–949.

319 Stemerman M, Goldstein ML, Schulman PL. Pancytopenia associated with diatrizoate. *NY St J Med* 1971;71:1220–1222.

320 Richards D, Nulsen FE. Angiographic media and the sickling phenomenon. *Surg Forum* 1971;22:403–404.

321 McNair JD. Selective coronary angiography. Report of a fatality in a patient with sickle cell haemoglobin. *Calif Med* 1972;117: 71–75.

322 Rao AK, Thompson R, Durlacher L, James F. Angiographic contrast agent-induced acute hemolysis in a patient with hemoglobin SC Disease. *Arch Intern Med* 1985;145:759–760.

323 Rao VM, Rao AK, Steiner RM *et al.* The effect of ionic and non-ionic contrast media on the sickling phenomenon. *Radiology* 1982;144:291–293.

324 Grainger R, Dawson P. Guidelines for use of low osmolar intravascular contrast media. *Fac Clin Radiol Roy Coll Radiol Lond*, 1991.

325 Aspelin P, Schmid-Schönbein H, Mallotta H. Do nonionic contrast media increase red cell aggregation and clot formation? *Invest Radiol* 1988;23 (Suppl. 2):S326–S333.

326 Aspelin P. Do nonionic contrast media increase red cell aggregation and clot formation? *Invest Radiol* 1990;25:S119–S120.

327 Kallio T, Alanen A, Kormano M. Red blood cell aggregability and contrast media. Recent results of quantitative dynamic ultrasonic analysis. *Invest Radiol* 1990;25:S121–S122.

328 Aspelin P, Schmid-Schönbein H. Effect of ionic and non-ionic contrast media on red cell aggregation in vitro. *Acta Radiol (Diagn)* 1978;19:767–784.

329 Staubli M, Braunschweig J, Tillman U. Changes in the rheological properties of the blood as induced by sodium/meglumine diatrizoate and metrizamide. *Acta Radiol (Diagn)* 1982;23:71–78.

330 Le Mignon MM, Ducret MN, Bonnemain B, Donadieu AM. Effect of contrast media on whole blood filtrability. An *in vitro* comparative study of iohexol, iopamidol and ioxaglate on rat blood. *Acta Radiol* 1988;29:593–597.

331 Tajima H, Kumazaki T, Tajima N, Ebata K. Effect of iohexol and diatrizoate on pulmonary arterial pressure following pulmonary angiography. A clinical comparison in man. *Acta Radiol* 1988; 29:487.

332 Bernstein EF. Discussion. Symposium on contrast medium toxicity. *Invest Radiol* 1970;5:416–422.

333 Cohen LS, Kokko JP, Williams WH. Hemolysis and hemoglobinuria following angiocardiography. *Radiology* 1962;92: 329–332.

334 Vincent ME, Gerzof SG, Robbins AH. Benign transient eosinophilia following intravenous urography. *J Am Med Assoc* 1977; 237:2629.

335 Plăvsić, B, Zumanić I, Rotvić I. Eosinophilia caused by iodinated radiographic media. *Clin Radiol* 1983;34:636–642.

336 Cochran CT, Khodadoust A, Norman A. Cytogenic effects of contrast material in patient undergoing excretion urography. *Radiology* 1980;136:43–46.

337 Matsubara S, Suzuki S, Suzuki H *et al.* Effect of contrast medium on radiation induced chromosome aberrations. *Radiology* 1982;144:295–301.

338 Nuñez MA, Sinués B. Cytogenic effects of diatrizoate and ioxaglate on patients undergoing excretory urography. *Invest Radiol* 1990;25:692–697.

339 Blum W, Weinberg U, Shenkman L, Hollander CS. Hyperthyroidism after iodinated contrast medium. *New Engl J Med*

1974;291:24−25,682−683.

340 Shimura H, Takazawa K, Endo T, Tawata M, Onaya T. T$_4$-thyroid storm after CT scan with iodinated contrast medium. *J Endocrinol Invest* 1990;13:73−76.

341 Sereno L, Massini R, Di Ciommo V. Hyperthyroidism after iodinated contrast media. Discussion of a clinical case. *Policlin Sez Med* 1979;86:366−369.

342 Shetty SP, Murthy GG, Shreeve WW, Nwaz AM, Ryder SW. Hyperthyroidism after pyelography. *New Engl J Med* 1974;261: 682.

343 Coel MN, Talner LB, Lang JH. Mechanism of radioactive iodine uptake depression following intravenous urography. *Br J Radiol* 1975;48:146−147.

344 Breuel H-P, Breuel Ch, Emrich P *et al.* Changes in thyroid function after application of iodinated media to normal subjects. *Med Klin* 1979;74:1492−1496.

345 Steidle B, Grehn S, Seif FJ. Iodine-induced hyperthyroidism due to contrast media. *Dtsch Med Wschr* 1979;104:1435−1438.

346 Von Rohner G, Rautenberg HW, Höpfner B. Transiente Hypothyreose bei Säuglingen nach Röntgenkontrastmitteln. *Röntgenpraxis* 1983;36:301−304.

347 Beyer HK, Schultze B. Einflussnahme von Röntgenkontrastmitteln auf Schildrasenhonen-parameter als Saforteffet. *Nuklearmedizin* 1985;24:122−126.

348 Westhoff-Bleck M, Bleck JS, Jost S. The adverse effects of angiographic radiocontrast media. *Drug Safety* 1991;6:28−36.

349 Ansell G. A national survey of radiological complications: interim report. *Clin Radiol* 1968;19:175−191.

350 Gold RE, Wisinger BM, Geraci AR, Heinz LM. Hypertensive crisis as a result of adrenal venography in a patient with pheochromocytoma. *Radiology* 1972;102:579−580.

351 Ansell G, Tweedie MCK, West CR, Evans DAP, Couch L. The current status of reactions to intravenous contrast media. *Invest Radiol* 1980;15 (Suppl.):S32−S39.

352 Shehadi WH, Toniolo G. Adverse reactions to contrast media. A report from the Committee on Safety of Contrast Media of the International Society of Radiology. *Radiology* 1980;137:299−302.

353 Katayama H, Yamaguchi K, Kozuka T, Takashima T, Seez P, Matsuura K. Adverse reactions to ionic and non-ionic media. A report from the Japanese Committee on the Safety of Contrast Media. *Radiology* 1990;175:621−628.

354 Pendergras HP, Tondreau L, Pendergras EP *et al.* Reactions associated with intravenous urography: historical and statistical review. *Radiology* 1958;71:1−12.

355 Shehadi WH. Death following intravascular administration of contrast media. *Acta Radiol (Diagn)* 1985;26:457−461.

356 Hartman GW, Hattery RR, Witten DM, Williamson B. Mortality during excretory urography: Mayo Clinic experience. *Am J Roentgenol* 1982;139:919−922.

357 Palmer FG. The R.A.C.R. Survey of intravenous contrast media reactions: final report. *Australas Radiol* 1988;32:426−428.

358 Wolf GL, Mishkin MM, Roux SG *et al.* Ionic contrast agents, ionic agents combined with steroids, and nonionic agents. *Invest Radiol* 1991;26:404−410.

359 Andrew E, Haider T. Incidence of roentgen contrast medium reactions after intravenous injection in pre-registration trials and post-marketing surveillances. *Acta Radiol* 1993;34:210−213.

360 Bettman MA. Ionic versus nonionic contrast media: are all the answers in? *Radiology* 1990;175:616−618.

361 Gerstman SB. Epidemiologic critique of the report on adverse reactions to ionic and nonionic contrast media by the Japanese Committee on the Safety of Contrast Media. *Radiology* 1991; 178:787−790.

362 Curry NS, Schabel SI, Reiheld CT, Henry WD, Savoca WJ. Fatal reactions to intravenous nonionic contrast material. *Radiology* 1991;178:361−362.

363 Cashman JD, McCredie J, Henry DA. Intravenous contrast media: use and associated mortality. *Med J Aust* 1991;155: 618−623.

364 Pozzato C, Marozzi F, Brenna F, Gattoni F. Un caso di morte consequente all somministrazione endovenoza di mezzo di contrasto organiodato a basa osmolalita. *Radiol Med* 1990;80: 107−108.

365 Ansell G. Fatal reactions to ionic and non-ionic contrast media. Birmingham: Röntgen Centenary Congress, 1995.

366 Caro JJ, Trinade E, McGregor M. The risk of death and of severe nonfatal reactions with high- vs. low-osmolarity contrast media: a meta-analysis. *Am J Roentgenol* 1991;156:825−836.

367 Lawrence V, Matthai W, Hartmair S. Comparative safety of high-osmolality and low-osmolality radiographic contrast agents. Report of a multidisciplinary working group. *Invest Radiol* 1992; 27:2−28.

368 Bolz K-D, Bolle R, Due J, Østerud B. Severe contrast medium reaction after iohexol (omnipaque) with *in vivo* proven monocyte stimulation. *Tidsskr Nor Laegeforen* 1986;106:2493,2559.

369 CSM update. Blood dyscrasias. *Br Med J* 1985;291:1269.

370 Lalli AF. Contrast media deaths. *Australas Radiol* 1984;28:133−135.

371 Ansell G. Epidemiology of adverse reactions to intravascular iodinated contrast media. *Toxicol Lett* 1992;64/65:717−723.

372 Lasser EC, Berry CC, Talner LB *et al.* Protective effects of corticosteroids in contrast material anaphylaxis. *Invest Radiol* 1988;23 (Suppl.):S193−S194.

373 Silverman SH, Nyhan WL. Shock following intravenous pyelography in patients with congenital adrenal hyperplasia. *J Pediatr* 1976;88:269−270.

374 Lasser EC. Sex, surfaces, sulfation and sensitivity. *Invest Radiol* 1991;26:S16−S19.

375 Lasser EC. Contrast reactions: eked data from contrast reactions − surveys. *Invest Radiol* 1990;25:S14−S15.

376 Macht SC, Williams RM, Lawrence PS. Study of 3 contrast agents in 2,234 intravenous pyelographs. *Am J Roentgenol* 1966;98:79−87.

377 Lasser EC, Berry CC, Talner LB *et al.* Pretreatment with corticosteroids to alleviate reactions to intravenous contrast material. *New Engl J Med* 1987;317:845−849.

378 Witten DM, Hirsch FD, Hartman GW. Acute reactions to urographic contrast medium. Incidence, clinical characteristics and relationships to hypersensitivity states. *Am J Roentgenol* 1973; 119:832−840.

379 McCullough M, Davies P, Richardson R. A large trial of intravenous Conray 325 and Niopam 300 to assess immediate and delayed reactions. *Br J Radiol* 1988;62:260−265.

380 Tuck JS, Martin DF. Reactions to intravenous contrast media. *Br J Radiol* 1990;63:230−231.

381 Polger M, Kuhlman JE, Hansen FC, Fishman EK. Computed tomography of angioedema of small bowel due to reaction to radiographic contrast medium. *J Comput Assist Tomogr* 1988;12: 1044−1046.

382 Savill JS, Barrie R, Ghosh S *et al.* Fatal Stevens−Johnson syndrome following urography with iopamidol in systemic lupus erythematosus. *Postgrad Med J* 1988;64:392−394.

383 Goodfellow T, Haldstock GE, Brunton FJ, Bamforth J. Fatal

acute vasculitis after high-dose urography with iohexol. *Br J Radiol* 1986;59:620−621.

384 Reynolds NJ, Wallington TB, Burton JL. Hydrallazine predisposes to acute cutaneous vasculitis following urography with iopamidol. *Br J Dermatol* 1993;129:82−85.

385 Gelmers HJ. Exacerbation of systemic lupus erythematosus, aseptic meningitis and acute mental symptoms following metrizamide lumbar myelography. *Neuroradiology* 1984;26:65−66.

386 Donnelly PK, Williams B, Watkin EM. Polyarthropathy — a delayed reaction to low osmolality angiographic contrast medium in patients with end stage renal disease. *Eur Radiol* 1993;17:130−132.

387 Kaftori JK, Abraham Ż, Gilhar A. Toxic epidermal necrolysis after excretory pyelography. Immunologic-mediated contrast medium reaction? *Int J Dermatol* 1988;27:346−347.

388 Kerdel FA, Fraker DL, Haynes HA. Necrotising vasculitis from radiographic contrast media. *J Am Acad Dermatol* 1984;10:25−29.

389 Heydenrich G, Olhom Larsen P. Iododerma after high-dose urography in an oliguric patient. *Br J Dermatol* 1977;97:567−569.

390 Lauret Ph, Godin M, Bravard P. Vegetating iodides after an intravenous pyelogram. *Dermatologica* 1985;171:463−468.

391 Reutter FW, Eugster C. Akuter Iodismus mit Sialadenitis allergischer Vaskulitis und Konjuctivitis nach Verabreichung jodhaltiger Kontrastmittel. *Schweitz Med Wochenschr* 1985;115:1646−1651.

392 Vaillant L, Pengloan J, Blanchier D, De Muret A, Lorette G. Iododerma and acute respiratory distress with leukocytic vasculitis following the intravenous injection of contrast medium. *Clin Exp Dermatol* 1990;15:232−233.

393 Sparrow GI, Rhodes GP. Iododerma due to radiographic contrast medium. *J Roy Soc Med* 1979;72:60−61.

394 Grunwald MH, Halevi S, Livini E, Feuerman E. Bullous lichen planus after intravenous pyelography. *J Am Acad Dermatol* 1985;13:512−513.

395 Shah AM, Hutchison SJ. Case report: the Koebnor phenomenon — an unusual localization of a contrast reaction. *Clin Radiol* 1990;42:136−137.

396 Borofsky HB, Barnard CM, Lang EV. Fixed bullous drug eruption due to iohexol. *Adv X-Ray Contr* 1993;1:58−60.

397 Bork K, Hoede E. Paraneoplastische multizentrische Reticulohistiozytose: durch jodhaltige Röntgen-kontrastmittel ausgelöst und provozierbar. *Z Hautkr* 1985;60:729.

398 Panto PN, Davies P. Delayed reactions to urographic media. *Br J Radiol* 1986;59:41−44.

399 Yoshikawa H. Late adverse reactions to non-ionic contrast media. *Radiology* 1992;183:737−740.

400 Higashi TS, Takizawa K, Nagashima J *et al*. Prospective two-phase study of delayed symptoms after intravenous injection of low-osmolality contrast media. *Invest Radiol* 1991;26:S37−S39.

401 Mineyama H, Katayama Y, Go H. Delayed reactions to non-ionic contrast media. *West Jap Urol* 1989;51:2022−2026.

402 Hidano A. Drug eruption. *J Tokyo Wom Coll* 1991;61:172−177.

403 Akiyama M, Iijima M, Fujisawa R. Clinical analysis of drug eruption due to iohexol (omnipaque). *Jap J Dermatol* 1990;100:1057−1060.

404 Asano S, Ikeda M, Ichikawa E *et al*. Drug eruption due to iohexol (Omnipaque). *Rinsho-Hoshasen* 1990;35:533−536.

405 Kanzaki T, Sakagami H. Late phase allergic reaction to a CT contrast medium (Iotrolan). *J Dermatol* 1991;18:528−531.

406 Mitsuya K, Akai Y, Masuda R, Hamabuchi M. A case of drug eruption due to Iotrolan (isovist 300). *Skin-Res* 1993;35:257−260.

407 Yamaguchi K, Takanashi I, Kanauchi T, Hoshi T. Retrospective survey of delayed adverse reactions to ionic and non-ionic contrast media. *RSNA Ann Meet (Chicago)* 1991;Abstract:Paper 97.

408 Lang DM, Alpern MB, Visintainer PF, Smith ST. Increased risk for anaphylactoid reaction from contrast media in patients on β-adrenergic blockers or with asthma. *Ann Int Med* 1991;115:270−276.

409 Ansell G, Tweedie MCK, West CR, Evans DAP. Risk factors for adverse reactions in intravenous urography. In: Amiel M, ed. *Contrast Media in Radiology*. Berlin: Springer-Verlag, 1982:7−10.

410 Lasser EC, Walters AJ, Lang J. An experimental basis for histamine release in contrast media reactions. *Radiology* 1971;110:49−59.

411 Littner MR, Ulreich S, Putman CE *et al*. Bronchospasm during excretory urography: lack of specificity for the methylglucamine cation. *Am J Roentgenol* 1981;137:477−481.

412 Dawson P, Pitfield J, Britton J. Contrast media and bronchospasm: a study with iopamidol. *Clin Radiol* 1983;34:227−230.

413 Jantzen J-PAH, Wangeman B, Wisser G. Adverse reactions to non-ionic iodinated contrast media do occur during general anesthesia. *Anesthesiology* 1989;70:561.

414 Cameron JD. Pulmonary edema following drip-infusion urography. Case report. *Radiology* 1974;111:89−90.

415 Malins AF. Pulmonary oedema after radiological investigation of peripheral vascular disease. Adverse reactions to contrast media. *Lancet* 1978;1:413−415.

416 Måre K, Violante M. Pulmonary edema induced by high intravenous doses of diatrizoate in the rat. *Acta Radiol Diagn* 1983;24:419−424.

417 Måre K, Violante M, Zack A. Contrast media induced pulmonary edema. Comparison of ionic and non-ionic agents in an animal model. *Invest Radiol* 1984;19:566−569.

418 Måre K, Violante M, Zack A. Pulmonary edema following high intravenous doses of diatrizoate in the rat. Effects of corticosteroid pretreatment. *Acta Radiol Diagn* 1985;26:477−482.

419 Dawson P. Personal communication, 1983.

420 Chamberlin WH, Stockman GD, Wray NP. Shock and non cardiogenic pulmonary edema following meglumine diatrizoate for intravenous pyelography. *Am J Med* 1979;67:684−686.

421 Soloman DR. Anaphylactoid reaction and non-cardiac pulmonary edema following intravenous contrast injection. *Am J Emerg Med* 1986;4:146−149.

422 Borish L, Matlof SM, Findlay SR. Radiographic contrast media-induced non cardiogenic pulmonary edema: case report and review of the literature. *J Allergy Clin Immunol* 1984;74:104−107.

423 Greganti MA, Flowers WM Jr. Acute pulmonary edema after the intravenous administration of contrast media. *Radiology* 1979;132:583−585.

424 Delacour JL, Floriot C, Wagschal G *et al*. Non-cardiac pulmonary edema following intravenous contrast injection. *Intens Care Med* 1988;15:49−50.

425 Bouachour G, Varache N, Szapiro N *et al*. Noncardiogenic pulmonary edema resulting from intravascular administration of contrast material. *Am J Roentgenol* 1991;157:255−256.

426 Eddie RR, Burtis BB. Lung injury in anaphylactic shock. *Chest* 1973;63:636−638.

427 Bisbe E, Escolano F, Diez A, Castaño J. Distrés respiratorio del adulto y coagulación intravascular diseminada tras la admistración de contraste yodado. *Rev Esp Anestesiol Reanim* 1990;37:156−159.

428 Jennings CA, Deveikis J, Azumi N, Yeager H. Eosinophilic pneumonia associated with reaction to a radiographic contrast medium. *South Med J* 1991;84:92−94.

429 Schwartz LB, Metcalfe DD, Miller JS, Earle H, Sullivan T. Tryptase levels as an indicator of mast cell activation in systemic anaphylaxis and mastocytosis. *New Engl J Med* 1987;316:1622−1626.

430 Van Sonnenberg E, Neff CC, Pfister RC. Life-threatening hypotensive reactions to contrast media administration: comparison of pharmacologic and fluid therapy. *Radiology* 1987;162:15−19.

431 Horak A, Raine R, Opie LH, Lloyd EA. Severe myocardial ichaemia induced by intravenous adrenaline. *Br Med J* 1983;286:519.

432 Delorme P, Letendre J. Prolonged shock after intravenous pyelography. *Radiology* 1972;151:31−33.

433 Poulsen J, Rasmussen F, Georgsen J. Hypotensive shock associated with bradycardia after intravenous injection of contrast medium. *Radiology* 1987;164:275−276.

434 Fischer HW, Katzberg RW, Morris TW, Spataro RF. Systemic response to excretory urography. *Radiology* 1984;151:31−33.

435 Benotti JR. The comparative effects of ionic versus nonionic agents in cardiac catheterisation. *Invest Radiol* 1988;2 (Suppl. 2):S366−S373.

436 Madowitz JS, Schweiger MJ. Severe anaphylactoid reaction to radiographic contrast media. Recurrence despite premedication with diphenhydramine and prednisone. *J Am Med Assoc* 1979;241:2813−2815.

437 Manhire AR, Dawson P, Dennet R. Contrast agent-induced emesis. *Clin Radiol* 1984;35:369−370.

438 Vacek JL, Gersema L, Woods M, Bower C, Beauchamp GD. Frequencies of reactions to iohexol versus ioxaglate. *Am J Cardiol* 1990;66:1277−1278.

439 Fishman JE, Abere DR, Moldawer NP, Belldegrun A, Figlin RA. Atypical contrast reactions associated with systemic interleukin-2 therapy. *Am J Roentgenol* 1991;156:833−834.

440 Nathan MH. Prevention of vomiting induced by IV contrast media. *Am J Roentgenol* 1991;156:633.

441 Cho S-R. Personal communication, 1988.

442 Weinstein GS, O'Doriso TM, Joehl RJ *et al*. Exacerbation of diarrhoea after iodinated contrast agent in a patient with a VIPoma. *Digest Dis Sci* 1985;30:588−592.

443 Lucas LM, Colley CA, Gordon GH. Case report: multisystem failure following intravenous iopamidol. *Clin Radiol* 1992;45:276−277.

444 Sussman RM, Miller J. Iodide mumps after intravenous urography. *New Engl J Med* 1956;255:433−434.

445 Nakadar AS, Harris-Jones JM. Sialadenitis after intravenous urography. *Br Med J* 1971;3:351−352.

446 Talner LB, Coel MN, Lang JH. Salivary secretion of iodine after urography. *Radiology* 1973;106:262−268.

447 Talner LB, Lang JH, Brasch RC, Lasser EC. Elevated salivary iodide and salivary gland enlargement due to iodinated contrast media. *Am J Roentgenol* 1971;112:380−382.

448 Wylie EJ, Mitchell DB. Case report: iodide mumps following intravenous urography with iopamidol. *Clin Radiol* 1991;43:135−136.

449 Koch RL, Byl FM, Firpo JJ. Parotid swelling with facial paralysis: a complication of intravenous urography. *Radiology* 1969;92:1043−1044.

450 Berman HL, Delaney V. Iodide mumps due to low-osmolality contrast material. *Am J Roentgenol* 1992;159:1099−1100.

451 Navani S, Taylor CE, Kaufman SA, Parle RH. Evanescent enlargement of salivary glands following tri-iodinated contrast media. *Br J Radiol* 1972;45:19−20.

452 Melki Ph, Mugel Th, Cléro B, Belin X, Moreau J-F. Parotidite aigue bilatérale. Prodrome isolé d'un choc anaphylactoide après injection de produit de contraste iodé. *J Radiol* 1993;74:51−54.

453 St Amour TE, McLennan BC, Glazer HS. Pancreatic mumps: a transient reaction to IV contrast media (Case report). *Am J Roentgenol* 1986;147:188−189.

454 Marenah CB, Quiney JR. C1 esterase inhibitor deficiency as a cause of abdominal pain. *Br Med J* 1983;286:786−787.

455 Collins CD, King DM, Gleeson JA. Bilateral pyelosinus extravasation secondary to probable radiation induced fibrosis. *Br J Urol* 1993;72:385−386.

456 Katayama H, Yamaguchi K, Takashima T *et al*. Full scale investigation into adverse reaction in Japan: risk factor analysis. *Invest Radiol* 1991;26:S33−S36.

457 Fischer HW, Doust VL. An evaluation of pre-testing in the problem of serious and fatal reactions to excretory urography. *Radiology* 1972;103:497−501.

458 Rapoport S, Bookstein JJ, Higgins CB *et al*. Experience with metrizamide in patients with previous severe anaphylactoid reactions to ionic contrast agents. *Radiology* 1982;143:321−325.

459 Shehadi WH. Contrast media adverse reactions: occurrence, recurrence and distribution patterns. *Radiology* 1982;143:11−17.

460 Barker KH, McClennan BL, Miller JP. Adverse reactions to contrast material. *Radiology* 1983;149:325.

461 Stejskal V, Nilson R, Grepe A. Immunologic basis for adverse reactions to radiographic contrast media. *Acta Radiol* 1990;31:605−612.

462 Jensen N, Dorph S. Adverse reactions to urographic contrast medium. Rapid versus slow injection. *Br J Radiol* 1980;53:659−661.

463 Bernstein EF, Palmer JD, Aaberg TA, Davis RL. Studies on the toxicology of Hypaque-90 per cent following rapid venous injection. *Radiology* 1961;76:88−95.

464 Dahlstrom K, Shaw DD, Claus W *et al*. Summary of U.S. and European intravascular experience with iohexol based on the clinical trial program. *Invest Radiol* 1985;20 (Suppl.):S117−S121.

465 Yocumb MW, Heller AM, Abels RI. Efficiency of pretesting and antihistamine prophylaxis in radiocontrast media-sensitive patients. *J Allergy Clin Immunol* 1978;62:309−313.

466 Cho KJ, Thornbury JR. Severe reaction to contrast material by three consecutive routes: intravenous, subcutaneous and intra-arterial. *Am J Roentgenol* 1978;131:509−510.

467 Seymour J. Severe laryngeal oedema during injection of metrizoate (Triosil). Survival after emergency laryngostomy. *Br Heart J* 1969;31:529−530.

468 Obeid AI, Johnson L, Potts J *et al*. Fluid therapy in severe systemic reaction to radiographic dye. *Ann Int Med* 1975;83:317−320.

469 Slack JD, Slack LA, Orr C. Recurrent severe reaction to iodinated contrast medium during cardiac catheterisation. *Heart Lung* 1982;11:348−352.

470 Mohan JC, Reddy DS, Bhatia ML. Anaphylactoid reaction to angiographic contrast media: recurrence despite pretreatment with corticosteroids. *Cathet Cardiovasc Diagn* 1984;10:465−469.

471 Pozzato C, Marozzi F, Brenna F, Gattoni F. Un cazo di morte conseguente alla somministrazione endovenosa di mezzo di contrasto organiodato a bassa osmolalita. *Radiol Med* 1990;80: 107−108.

472 Greenberger PA, Patterson R, Tapio CM. Prophylaxis against repeated radiocontrast media reactions in 857 cases: adverse experience with cimetidine and safety of β-adrenergic antagonists. *Arch Intern Med* 1985;145:2197−2200.

473 Zukiwski AA, David CL, Coan J *et al*. Increased incidence of hypersensitivity to iodine-containing radiographic contrast media after interleukin-2 administration. *Cancer* 1990;65: 1521−1524.

474 Abi-Aad A, Figlin RA, Belldegrun A, de Kernion JB. Metastatic renal cell cancer and interleukin-2 toxicity induced by contrast agent injection. *J Immunother* 1991;10:292−295.

475 Shulman KL, Benyunes MC, Winter TC, Fefer A. Adverse reactions to intravenous contrast media in patients treated with interleukin-2. *J Immunother* 1993;13:208−212.

476 Heinzer H, Huland E, Huland H. Adverse reaction to contrast material in a patient treated with local interleukin-2. *Am J Roentgenol* 1992;158:1407.

477 Lasser EC, Lang JH, Hamblin AE *et al*. Activation systems in contrast idiosyncrasy. *Invest Radiol* 1980;15 (Suppl.):S2−S5.

478 Lasser EC, Lang JH, Lyon SG, Hamblin AE. Changes in complement and coagulation factors in a patient suffering a severe anaphylactoid reaction to injected contrast material: some considerations of pathogenesis. *Invest Radiol* 1980;15 (Suppl.): S6−S12.

479 Brinkmann H, Gunther M. Increased incidence of contrast medium reactions in children undergoing urography after accidents. *Klin Pädiat* 1984;196:100−102.

480 Katzberg RW, Morris TW, Schulman G *et al*. Reactions to intravenous contrast media. Part 1: severe and fatal cardiovascular reactions in a canine dehydration model. *Radiology* 1983;147:327−330.

481 Moore RD, Steinberg EP, Powe NR *et al*. Frequency and determinants of adverse reactions induced by high-osmolality contrast media. *Radiology* 1989;170:727−732.

482 Duda D, Lorenz W, Menke H *et al*. Histamine release during induction of anaesthesia in patients undergoing general surgery: incidence and clinically severe cases. *Agents Act Spec Confer Iss* 1992;C149−C154.

483 Lorenz W, Dietz W, Ennis B, Doenicke A. Histamine in anaesthesia and surgery; causality analysis. In: Uvnas B, ed. *Handbook of Experimental Pharmacology*. Berlin: Springer-Verlag, 1991: 385−439.

484 Mann RM. The pharmacology of contrast media. *Proc Roy Soc Med* 1961;54:473−475.

485 Wolf AA, Levi R. Histamine and cardiac arrhythmias. *Circul Res* 1986;58:1−16.

486 Martindale. *The Extra Pharmacopoea*, 29th edn. London: Pharmaceutical Press, 1989:941.

487 Lasser EC, Walters A, Lang JH. An experimental basis for histamine release in contrast media reactions. *Radiology* 1974; 110:49−50.

488 Brasch RC, Rockoff SD, Kuhn C, Chraplyvy M. Contrast media as histamine liberators. II. Histamine release into venous plasma during intravenous urography in man. *Invest Radiol* 1970;5: 510−513.

489 Assem ESK, Bray K, Dawson P. The release of histamine from human basophils by radiological contrast agents. *Br J Radiol* 1983;56:647−652.

490 Rockoff SD, Aker CT. Contrast media as histamine liberators. IV. Arterial plasma histamine and haemodynamic responses following angio-cardiography in man with 75% Hypaque. *Invest Radiol* 1972;7:403−406.

491 Cogen FL, Norman ME, Dunsky E, Hirshfield J, Zweiman B. Histamine release and complement changes following injection of contrast media in humans. *J Allergy Clin Immunol* 1979;64: 299−303.

492 Robertson PW, Frewin DB, Robertson AR, Mahar LJ, Jonsson JR. Plasma histamine levels following administration of radiographic contrast media. *Br J Radiol* 1985;58:1047−1051.

493 Lorenz W, Röhner HD, Doenicke HD, Omann CH. Histamine release in anaesthesia and surgery: a new method to evaluate its clinical significance with several types of causal relationship. *Clin Anaesthesiol* 1984;2:403−426.

494 Watkins J, Salom V (eds). *Trauma, Stress and Immunity in Anaesthesia and Surgery*. London:Butterworth, 1982.

495 Westaby S, Dawson P, Turner MW, Pridie RB. Angiography and complement activation. Evidence for generation of C2a anaphylatoxin by intravascular contrast agents. *Cardiovasc Res* 1985;19:85−88.

496 Lieberman P. Review article. Anaphylactoid reactions to radiocontrast material. *Ann Allergy* 1991;67:91−100.

497 Lasser EC, Lang JH, Hamblin AE *et al*. Activation systems in contrast idiosyncrasy. *Invest Radiol* 1980;15 (Suppl.):S2−S5.

498 Lasser EC, Lang JH, Lyon SG, Hamblin AE. Changes in complement and coagulation factors in a patient suffering a severe anaphylactoid reaction to injected contrast material: some considerations of pathogenesis. *Invest Radiol* 1980;15 (Suppl.): S6−S12.

499 Lasser EC. Sulfated surfaces in sensitivity: an "on−off" switch for anaphylaxis? *Med Hypoth* 1991;34:13−19.

500 Schneiderman H, Hammerschmidt DE, McCall A, Jacob HS. Fatal complement-induced leukostasis after diatrizoate injection. *J Am Med Assoc* 1983;250:2340−2342.

501 Arroyave CM, Schatz M, Simon RA. Activation of the complement system by radiographic contrast media in vivo and in vitro. *J Allergy Clin Immunol* 1979;63:276−280.

502 Simon RA, Schatz M, Stevenson DD *et al*. Radiographic contrast media infusion. Measurement of histamine, complement, and fibrin split products in correlation with clinical parameters. *J Allergy Clin Immunol* 1979;68:281−288.

503 Gonsette RE, Delmotte P. *In vivo* activation of serum complement by contrast media: a clinical study. *Invest Radiol* 1980; 15:S26−S28.

504 Dawson P, Turner MW, Bradshaw AW, Westaby S. Complement activation and generation of C2a anaphylatoxin by radiological contrast agents. *Br J Radiol* 1983;56:447−448.

505 Zeman RK. Disseminated intravascular coagulation following intravenous pyelography. *Invest Radiol* 1977;12:203.

506 Skjennald A, Heldas J, Høiseth A. Comparison of iohexol and meglumine−Na−Ca metrizoate. *Acta Radiol* 1983;366 (Suppl.): 158.

507 Lasser EC, Farr RJ, Fujimagara T, Tripp WM. Significance of protein-binding of contrast media in roentgen diagnosis. *Am J Roentgenol* 1962;87:338−360.

508 Kutt H, Milhorat TH, McDowall F. The effect of iodinised contrast media upon blood proteins, electrolytes and red cells. *Neurology* 1963;13:492−499.

509 Lasser EC. Metabolic basis of contrast media toxicity states. *Am J Roentgenol* 1971;113:415−422.

510 Howell MJ, Dawson P. Contrast agents and enzyme inhibition.

II. Mechanisms. *Br J Radiol* 1985;58:845−848.

511 Tamura A, Suzuki T, Yamasaki T, Morita R, Sato T, Tatsuzo F. Effect of radiological iodinated contrast media on acetylcholinesterase activity. *Br J Radiol* 1991;64:768−770.

512 Sandström C. Secondary reactions from contrast media and the allergy concept. *Acta Radiol* 1955;44:233−242.

513 Wakkers-Garritsen BG, Houwerzigl LJ, Nater JP, Walkers PJM. IgE-mediated adverse reaction to a radiographic contrast medium. *Ann Allergy* 1976;36:122−126.

514 Kanny G, Maria Y, Mentre B, Moneret-Vautrin DA. Case Report: recurrent anaphylactic shock to radiographic contrast media. Evidence supporting an exceptional IgE-mediated reaction. *Allergy Immunol* 1993;25:425−430.

515 Walker AC, Carr DH. Reactions to radiographic control media: an attempt to detect specific anti-contrast medium antibodies in the sera of reactor patients. *Br J Radiol* 1986;59:531−536.

516 Brasch RC. Evidence supporting an antibody mediation of contrast media reactions. *Invest Radiol* 1980;15 (Suppl.):S29−S31, S46−S48.

517 Brasch RC, Kay J, Mark S, Nitecki D. Allergy to radiographic contrast media: accumulated evidence for antibody-mediated human toxicity and a new animal model. In: Amriel M, ed. *Contrast Media in Radiology*. Berlin: Springer-Verlag, 1982: 16−19.

518 Lasser EC, Sovak M, Lang JH. Development of contrast media idiosyncrasy in the dog. *Radiology* 1976;191:91−95.

519 Lalli AF. Urographic contrast media reactions and anxiety. *Radiology* 1974;112:267−271.

520 Lalli AF, Greenstreet R. Reactions to contrast media: testing the CNS hypothesis. *Radiology* 1981;138:47−49.

521 Lown B, Verrier RL, Rabinowitz SH. Neural and psychologic mechanisms and the problems of sudden cardiac death. *Am J Cardiol* 1977;39:890−902.

522 Tizes R. Cardiac arrest following routine venepuncture. *J Am Med Assoc* 1976;236:1846.

523 Gottlieb A, Lalli AF. Hypotension following contrast media injection during general anesthesia. *Anesth Analg* 1982;61: 387−389.

524 Gmelin E, Kramann B, Weiss H-D. Kontrastmittel-zwischenfall bei einer endoskopischen retrograden Cholangio-pancreatikographie. *Munch Med Wschr* 1977;119:1439.

525 Halpern B, Ky NT, Amache N. "*In vitro*" lymphoblast transformation test (L.T.T.) as a tool for the study of drug hypersensitivity. *Proc Eur Soc Study Drug Tox* 1969;10:27−35.

526 McClennan BL, Periman PO, Rockoff SD. Positive immunological responses to contrast media. *Invest Radiol* 1976;11:240.

527 Camussi G, Stratta P, Bosio D, Rotunno M, Dogliani M, Vercellone A. Ipersensibilita ai mezzi di contrasto iodati in corso di urografia. Importanza pratica del test di degranulazione del basofili. *Min Nefr* 1979;26:299−303.

528 Lasser EC, Lang JH, Lyon SG *et al.* Prekalikrein−kallikrein conversion rate as a predictor of contrast material catastrophies. *Radiology* 1981;140:11−15.

529 Eaton SM, Hagan JJ, Tsay HM *et al.* A predictive test for adverse reactions to contrast media. Preliminary results. *Invest Radiol* 1988;23 (Suppl. 1):S206−S208.

530 Lalli AF. Urography, shock reaction and repeated urography (editorial). *Am J Roentgenol* 1975;125:264−268.

531 Hopper KD, Houts PS, Tenhave TR *et al.* The effect of informed consent on the level of anxiety in patients given IV contrast material. *Am J Roentgenol* 1994;162:531−535.

532 Lalli AF. Contrast media reactions: data analysis and hypothesis. *Radiology* 1980;131:1−12.

533 Shehadi WH. Adverse reactions to intravenously administered contrast media. A comprehensive study based on a prospective survey. *Am J Roentgenol* 1975;125:264−268.

534 Yamaguchi K, Katayama H, Takashima T, Kozuka T, Seez P, Matsuura K. Prediction of severe adverse reactions to ionic and nonionic contrast media in Japan: evaluation of pretesting. A report from the Japanese Committee on the Safety of Contrast Media. *Radiology* 1991;178:363−367.

535 Elliot LS. Adverse reactions to contrast media: an interview with Elliott Charles Lasser, M.D. *Appl Radiol* 1980;9:63−66.

536 Bertrand PH, Rouleau PH, Alison D, Chastin I. Use of peak expiratory flow rate to identify patients with increased risk of contrast medium reaction. Results of preliminary study. *Invest Radiol* 1988;23 (Suppl. 1):S203−S205.

537 Lasser EC, Berry CC, Mishkin MM, Williamson B, Zheutlin N, Silverman JM. Pretreatment with corticosteroids to prevent adverse reactions to nonionic contrast media. *Am J Roentgenol* 1994;162:523−526.

538 Greenberger PA, Patterson R. The prevention of immediate generalized reactions to radiocontrast media in high-risk patients. *J Allergy Clin Immunol* 1991;87:867−872.

539 Siegle RL, Halvorsen RA, Dillon J, Morris LG, Halpern E. The use of iohexol in patients with previous reactions to ionic contrast material. A multicenter clinical trial. *Invest Radiol* 1991;26:411−416.

540 Greenberger PA, Gutt L, Meyers SL. An immediate generalized reaction to iopamidol. *Arch Int Med* 1987;147:2208−2209.

541 Lasser EC. Pretreatment with corticosteroids to prevent reactions to IV contrast material: overview and implications. *Am J Roentgenol* 1988;150:257−259.

542 Greenberger PA, Halwig M, Patterson R, Wallemark CB. Emergency administration of radiocontrast media in high-risk patients. *J Allergy Clin Immunol* 1986;77:630−634.

543 Fineman SL, Healy MV, Parker BR. Corticosteroid pre-treatment for potential contrast reaction in children with lymphoreticular cancer. A word of caution. *Am J Roentgenol* 1990;155:357−358.

544 Ansell G. Corticosteroid prophylaxis for contrast media reactors. *Clin Radiol* 1994;49:508.

545 Dunnick NR, Cohan RH. Cost, corticosteroids, and contrast media. *Am J Roentgenol* 1994;162:527−529.

546 Ring J, Rothenberger K-H, Clauss W. Prevention of anaphylactoid reactions after radiographic contrast media infusion by combined histamine H_1- and H_2-receptor antagonists: results of a prospective controlled trial. *Int Archs Allergy Appl Immunol* 1985;78:9−14.

547 Tauber R, Reiman J, Kersting H, Schmidt U. Pramedication mit H_1- and H_2-Rezeptorantagonisten vor Applikation von Röntgenkontrastmitteln. *Munch Med Wschr* 1985;27:1052−1054.

548 Beyer HK, Kukulies R, Schmitt WGH, Schultze B. Nebeneffekte und Komplikationen nach Röntgenkontrastmittelgabe − Riskoverminderung und Prävention. *Röntgenpraxis* 1987;40:459−465.

549 Greenberger PA, Patterson R. Adverse reaction to radiocontrast media. *Prog Cardiovasc Dis* 1988;31:239−248.

550 Böckmann S, Bodman KF, Schuster HP. Anaphylaktischer shock nach Röntgenkontrastmittel trotz Prämedikation mit Ausbildung eines akuten Myokardinfarktes. *Intensivmed Notfallmed* 1989;26:385.

551 Marshall GD, Lieberman PL. Comparison of three pretreatment protocols to prevent anaphylactoid reactions to radiocontrast media. *Ann Allergy* 1991;67:70−74.

552 Michel JR. Prevention of shocks induced by intravenous urography. In: Amiel M, ed. *Contrast Media in Radiology.* Berlin: Springer-Verlag, 1982:11−13.

553 Pinet A, Lyonnet D, Maillet P, Groleau JM. Adverse reactions to intravenous contrast media in urography. Results of a National Survey. In: Amiel M, ed. *Contrast Media in Radiology.* Berlin: Springer-Verlag, 1982:14−15.

554 Coste F, Tremolières F, Bousquet M et al. Coagulation intravasculaire massive fatal au coup d'une phlébographie. Responsabilité de l'acide epsilon aminocaproique? *Presse Médicale* 1985;14:832−834.

555 Soyer Ph, Levesque M, Rouleau P. Prevention of adverse reactions to intravascular contrast media. *Internat J Risk Safety Med* 1991;2:21−27.

556 Neoh SH, Sage MR, Wilis RB et al. The *in vitro* activation of complement by radiologic contrast materials and its inhibition with ε-aminocaproic acid. *Invest Radiol* 1981;16:235−239.

557 Wysenbeck AJ, Sella A, Vardi M, Yeshurun D. Acute delirious state after ε-aminocaproic acid. *Lancet* 1978;1:221.

558 Scheffer AL, Fearon DT, Austen KF. Tranexamic acid: preoperative prophylactic therapy for patients with hereditary angioneurotic oedema. *J Allergy Clin Immunol* 1977;60:38−40.

559 Agardh C-D, Amer C-D, Ekhom S, Boijsen E. Desensitisation as a means of preventing untoward reactions to ionic media. *Acta Radiol (Diagn)* 1983;24:235−239.

560 Faculty of Clinical Radiology *Guidelines for the Management of Reactions to Intravenous Contrast Media.* London: The Royal College of Radiologists, 1993:1−6.

561 Cohan RH, Dunnick NR, Bashore TM. Treatment of reactions to radiographic contrast material. *Am J Roentgenol* 1988;151:263−270.

562 Bush WH, Swanson DP. Acute reactions to intravascular contrast media: types, risk factors, recognition, and specific treatment. *Am J Roentgenol* 1991;157:1153−1161.

563 Bush WH, McClennan BL, Swanson DP. Contrast media reactions: prediction, prevention and treatment. *Postgrad Radiol* 1993;13:137−147.

564 European Resuscitation Council Basic Life Support Working Group. Guidelines for basic life support. *Br Med J* 1993;306:1587−1589.

565 European Resuscitation Council Working Party. Adult advanced cardiac life support: the European Resuscitation Council guidelines 1992 (abridged). *Br Med J* 1993;306:1589−1593.

566 Fisher MMcD. Clinical observations on the pathophysiology and treatment of anaphylactic cardiovascular collapse. *Anaesth Intens Care* 1986;14:17−21.

567 Mayumi H, Kimura S, Asano M, Shimokawa T, Au-Yong T-F, Yayama T. Intravenous cimetidine as an effective treatment for systemic anaphylaxis and acute allergic skin reactions. *Ann Allergy* 1987;58:447−450.

568 Kambam R, Merrill WH, Smith BE. Histamine$_2$ receptor blocker in the treatment of protamine related anaphylactoid reactions: two case reports. *Can J Anaesth* 1989;36:463−465.

569 Yarborough JA, Moffitt JE, Brown DA, Stafford CT. Cimetidine in the treatment of refractory anaphylaxis. *Ann Allergy* 1989;63:235−237.

570 Shellock FG, Hahn NP, Mink JH, Itskovich E. Adverse reaction to intravenous gadoteridol. *Radiology* 1993;189:151−152.

571 Zaloga GP, Delacey W, Holmboe E, Chernow B. Glucagon reversal of hypotension in a case of anaphylactoid shock. *Ann Intern Med* 1986;105:65−66.

572 Toogood JH. Editorial. Risk of anaphylaxis in patients receiving beta-blocker drugs. *J Allergy Clin Immunol* 1988;81:1−5.

573 Barach EM, Nowak RM, Lee G, Tomlanovich MC. Epinephrine for treatment of anaphylactic shock. *J Am Med Assoc* 1984;251:2118−2123.

574 Dawson P. Personal communication, 1995.

575 Heyns W. Corticotrophins and corticosteroids. In: Dukes MNG, ed. *Side Effects of Drugs Annual 5.* Amsterdam: Excerpta Medica, 1981:354.

576 Heyns W. Corticosteroids and corticotrophins. In: Dukes MNG, ed. *Side Effects of Drugs Annual 7.* Amsterdam: Exerpta Medica, 1983:379.

577 Fisher M. Treating anaphylaxis with sympathomimetic drugs. In severe anaphylaxis, adrenalin by any route is better than none. *Br Med J* 1992;305:1107−1108.

578 Horak A, Raine R, Opie LH, Lloyd EA. Severe myocardial ischaemia induced by intravenous adrenaline. *Br Med J* 1983;286:519.

579 Myers GE, Bloom FL. Cimetidine (Tagamet) combined with steroids and H$_1$ antihistamines for the prevention of serious radiographic contrast material reactions. *Cathet Cardiovasc Diagn* 1981;7:65−69.

580 Saxton HM. Review article: urography. *Br J Radiol* 1969;42:321−346.

581 Lytton B, Brooks MB, Spencer RP. Absorption of contrast material from urinary tract during retrograde pyelography. *J Urol* 1968;100:779−782.

582 McAlister WH, Cacciarelli A, Shackelford GD. Complications associated with cystography in children. *Radiology* 1974;111:167−172.

583 Weese DL, Greenberg HM, Zimmern PE. Contrast media reactions during voiding cystourethrography or retrograde pyelography. *Urology* 1993;41:81−84.

584 Bettenay F, de Campo J. Allergic reaction following micturating cysto-urethrography. *Urol Radiol* 1989;11:167−168.

585 Gaiser RR, Chua E. Anaphylactic/anaphylactoid reaction to contrast dye administration in the ureter. *J Clin Anesthes* 1993;5:510−512.

586 Lorenz R. Allergic reaction to contrast medium after endoscopic retrograde pancreatography. *Endoscopy* 1990;22:196.

587 Elias JA. Systemic reaction to radiocontrast media during hysterosalpinography. *J Allergy Clin Immunol* 1980;66:242.

588 Gelmers HJ. Adverse side effects of metrizamide in myelography. *Neuroradiology* 1979;18:119−123.

589 Cohen MD, Towbin R, Baker S et al. Comparison of iohexol with barium in gastrointestinal studies in infants and children. *Am J Roentgenol* 1991;156:345−350.

590 Glover JR, Thomas BM. Case report: severe adverse reaction to oral iohexol. *Clin Radiol* 1991;44:137−138.

591 Gallant MJ, Studley JGN. Case report: delayed cardiac tamponade following accidental injection of non-ionic contrast medium into the pericardium. *Clin Radiol* 1990;41:139−140.

592 Lossef SV, Barth KH. Severe delayed hypotensive reaction after ethiodol lymphangiography despite premedication. *Am J Roentgenol* 1993;161:417−418.

593 Benear JB, Vannatta JB, Hosty TA, Hughes WL. Contrast-induced seizure associated with thrombocytopenic purpura. *Arch Intern Med* 1985;145:363−364.

594 Stokigt JR. Hyperthyroxinemia secondary to drugs and acute illness. *Endocrinologist* 1993;3:67−73.

595 Girouk JD, Sizun J, Rubio S et al. Hypothyroide transitoire après opacification iodées des cathéters epicutanéocaves au réanimation néonatale. *Arch Fr Pediatr* 1993;50:273.

596 Benson PM, Giblin WJ, Douglas DM. Transient, nonpigmenting fixed drug eruption caused by radiopaque contrast media. *J Am Acad Dermatol* 1990;23:379−381.

597 Good AE, Novak E, Sonda LP. Fixed eruption and fever after urography. *South Med J* 1980;73:948−949.

598 Choyke PL, Miller DL, Lotze MT *et al*. Delayed reactions to contrast media after interleukin-2 immunotherapy. *Radiology* 1992;183:111−114.

599 Assem ESK. Diagnostic and predictive test procedures in patients with life-threatening anaphylactic and anaphylactoid drug reactions. *Allergol Immunopathol* 1984;12:61−70.

600 Cohen MD. A review of the toxicity of nonionic contrast agents in children. *Invest Radiol* 1993;S87−S93.

601 Lasser EC, Lang J, Sovak M *et al*. Steroids. Theoretical and experimental basis for utilisation in prevention of contrast media reactions. *Radiology* 1977;125:1−9.

602 Tattersfield A. Asthma. Management and treatment. In: Brewis RAL, Gibson GJ, Geddes DM, eds *Respiratory Medicine*. London: Bailliere Tindall, 1990:644−673.

603 Dawson P, Sidhu PS. Is there a role for corticosteroid prophylaxis in patients at increased risk of adverse reactions to intravascular contrast agents. *Clin Radiol* 1993;48:225−226.

604 Lasser EC, Berry CC. Corticosteroid prophylaxis in patients at increased risk of adverse reactions to intravascular contrast agents. *Clin Radiol* 1994;49:582−584.

605 Whalen E. Tenth meeting and postgraduate course of the Society of Uroradiology, September 1990. *Am J Roentgenol* 1991;156:189−195.

606 Spring DB, Bettmann MA. Contrast material-related deaths spontaneously reported to the US Food and Drug Administration 1978−1994: changes with the advent of low osmolar contrast agents. *Radiology* 1995;197 (Suppl. RSNA Scientific Program Abstract 1348):346−347.

607 Mikkonen R, Kontkanen T, Kivisaare L. Acute and late reactions to low-osmolal contrast media. *Acta Radiol* 1995;36:72−76.

608 Zweiman B, Mishkin MM, Hildrith EA. An approach to the performance of contrast studies in contrast-material reactive persons. *Ann Intern Med* 1975;83:159−162.

609 Newberg AH, Munn CS, Robbins AH. Complications of arthrography. *Radiology* 1985;155:605−606.

610 Peppercorn PD, Kaltas G, Reznek RH *et al*. Does intravenous injection of nonionic contrast medium result in elevation of catecholamine levels in patients with pheochromocytoma? *Radiology* 1995;197 (Suppl. RSNA Scientific Program Abstract 1800):422−423.

611 Niendorf HP. Delayed allergy-like reactions to X-ray contrast media. Problem statement exemplified with iotrolan (Isovist) 280. *European Radiology Supplement* 1996 (in press).

Part 4
Organ Systems

Complications of diagnostic angiography

Charles E. Ray, Jr and John A. Kaufman

Introduction

Angiography has been performed as a diagnostic tool for more than 90 years. As with any invasive procedure, there have been many complications described with diagnostic angiography. Since Seldinger [1] wrote his landmark article in 1953 describing a percutaneous technique using guidewires, there have been numerous publications describing complications related to guidewires and catheters as well as those related to arterial punctures and contrast media. In addition, utilization of interventional procedures such as angioplasty, stent placements, and thrombolytic therapy carry additional unique risks.

There have been many previous studies describing complications of diagnostic angiography. In 1963, Lang [2] surveyed radiologists, vascular surgeons, and urologists in a retrospective review of 11 402 patients who underwent percutaneous angiography using the Seldinger technique. In this study, the incidence of fatal complications was 0.06% and the incidence of serious nonfatal complications was 0.71%. A prospective study undertaken by Sigstedt and Lunderquist [3] of 1217 patients undergoing peripheral angiography, demonstrated a serious complication rate of 0.14% at the puncture site and thromboembolic complications occurring in an additional 0.74% of the patients. In a separate study, prospective data collected on 2475 consecutive patients undergoing cerebral angiography demonstrated nonneurologic complications in 7.3% of patients; however, many of these incidents were minor, with complications requiring further intervention occurring in only 0.7% of all patients [4].

Due to the invasive nature of diagnostic angiography, a certain risk is assumed by both the physician and patient regarding the possibility of an adverse outcome. The majority of complications may be considered minor, e.g., not requiring further intervention, such as small thromboemboli or groin site hematomas. Threshold level guidelines for complication rates for diagnostic peripheral angiography have been compiled by the Quality Assurance program of the Society of Cardiovascular and Interventional Radiology (SCVIR) (Table 14.1) [5]. The majority of published literature addressing complication rates, and in particular those quoted in recent studies, suggest that most rates fall well below the guidelines set by the SCVIR.

This chapter describes complications related to diagnostic peripheral angiography including those occurring secondary to arterial puncture, complications related to guidewires and catheters, and systemic complications. Complications arising from coronary and pulmonary angiography, as well as those related to contrast exposure and peripheral vascular intervention are discussed elsewhere (Chapters 16 & 17) and will not be reviewed here.

Table 14.1 Threshold level guidelines for complication rates for diagnostic peripheral angiography

Indicators (complications)	Threshold (%)
Puncture site	
Hematoma requiring transfusion, surgery, or delayed discharge	<3.0
Occlusion	<0.5
Pseudoaneurysm	<0.5
Arteriovenous fistula	<0.1
Contrast extravasation	<1.0
Nonpuncture site	
Distal emboli	<0.5
Dissection or occlusion of selected vessel	<2.0

Complications

Puncture site

The most frequently encountered complications occur at the arterial puncture site. Common complications include hematoma formation, pseudoaneurysms (PSA), arteriovenous fistulae (AVF), and occlusion of the artery at or near the puncture site. The incidence of complications varies with regard to the site of entry, with axillary, brachial, and translumbar approaches generally demonstrating higher complication rates than femoral artery punctures.

Femoral artery punctures

Complications arising from femoral artery punctures may be seen with punctures occurring anywhere along the length of the common femoral artery. In addition, however, specific complications may arise from punctures occurring either above or below the common femoral artery segment. Punctures occurring too high result in cannulation of the external iliac artery above the inguinal ligament, precluding adequate manual compression and tamponade of the artery post-procedure, placing the patient at risk for intraperitoneal hemorrhage [6]. Punctures performed too low are associated with an increased incidence of both AVF and PSA formation.

PSA formation is a complication directly related to the arterial puncture site. PSAs result from persistent arterial flow into an adjacent hematoma and occur most frequently following inadequate hemostasis after removal of the catheter. Since hematoma formation is a prerequisite for development of a PSA, adequate hemostasis precludes development of such a complication. In the event of development of a hematoma, our practice is to apply aggressive diffuse manual compression in order to disperse the hematoma which may decrease the likelihood of PSA.

Recent literature suggests that a significant percentage of PSAs caused by femoral artery catheterization will require intervention. In one recent study, at least one-third of PSAs required surgical repair [7]. The same study indicated that asymptomatic AVF do not require intervention and can be safely followed clinically.

Puncture of the arterial system below the common femoral artery bifurcation is associated with an increased incidence of PSA. In a review of 6200 femoral arteriograms, Rapoport *et al.* [8] demonstrated PSA complications in six cases, all of which occurred secondary to puncture below the femoral bifurcation. Many of the older studies in the literature do not report PSA complications or, if described, suggest a lower incidence of PSA than the more current studies. In 1963, Lang [2] reviewed over 11 000 angiograms and reported three cases of PSA that underwent surgical repair. In contrast, a study by McCann *et al.* [9] in 1991 demonstrated 150 of 16 350 patients who underwent cardiac catheterization

required surgical repair of PSA at the puncture site. This represents a greater than 30-fold increase in the percentage of patients requiring surgical repair of a PSA. The apparent increase in PSA complications is difficult to explain, but may in part be secondary to the increased size of sheaths used in radiologic or cardiologic interventions, as well as intra-procedural/postprocedural anticoagulation.

AVF formation is more likely to occur with punctures at or below the level of the bifurcation of the common femoral artery, largely due to the anatomic relationship of the femoral artery to the adjacent vein (Fig. 14.1). In the normal anatomic setting, the common femoral artery and vein lie adjacent to one another in a side by side fashion, while below the bifurcation the vein more commonly lies deep to the superficial femoral artery [10] (Fig. 14.2). Therefore, by using the standard double-wall technique there is an increased incidence of simultaneous artery and vein puncture when the puncture is centered too low, concomitantly increasing the likelihood of AVF formation.

Kim and Orron [11] retrospectively reviewed nearly 1000 femoral arteriograms and demonstrated that in 95% of the

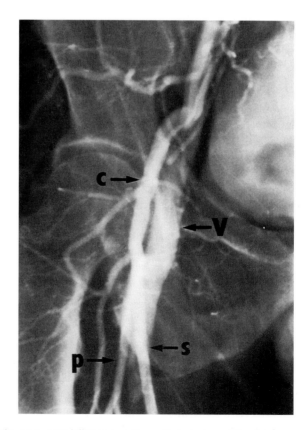

Fig. 14.1 AVF following cardiac catheterization. AP pelvic angiography performed after cardiac catheterization from a right femoral approach demonstrating visualization of the femoral vein (V) during the midarterial phase of an aortic injection. c, common femoral artery; p, profunda femoral artery; s, superficial femoral artery.

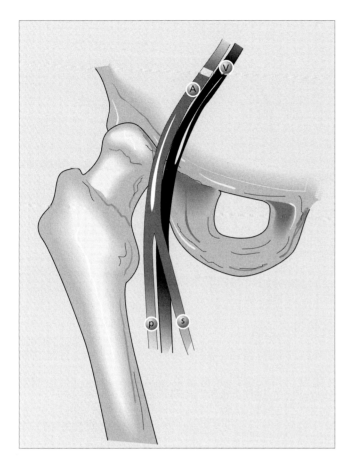

Fig. 14.2 Anatomy of vascular structures below the inguinal ligament. At the level of the femoral head, the common femoral artery (A) and femoral vein (V) lie adjacent to one another. After the common femoral artery bifurcation, however, the superficial femoral artery (s) lies superficial to the femoral vein. p, profunda femoral artery.

cases, the common femoral artery bifurcation was located within 3 cm below and 2 cm above the inferior border of the femoral head. Therefore, puncture of the femoral artery at or above the level of the midfemoral head significantly decreases the likelihood of puncturing either the femoral vein or the superficial or profunda femoris arteries, and therefore would result in a decrease in the incidence of both PSA and AVFs.

Hematomas at the puncture site account for the majority of complications encountered in diagnostic angiography. The incidence of large hematomas from diagnostic angiography ranges from 1.5 to 4.0% [2,3] and account for up to 40% of all reported complications [2]. The incidence of clinically insignificant hematomas, defined in one study as those measuring less than 5 cm in diameter, can occur in as many as 15–20% of patients [12]. Perhaps the best measure of significance of hematomas is the necessity of further therapy such as blood transfusion or surgical evacuation. The incidence of such complications ranges from 0.26 to 1.5%, as

demonstrated in previous studies [2,13]. More recent studies suggest an increased incidence of hematomas requiring intervention in patients undergoing peripheral interventions or cardiac catheterization when compared with those patients undergoing diagnostic peripheral angiography [14]. Trerotola *et al.* [6] described 21 patients with significant postcatheterization bleeding with positive findings on computed tomography (CT) scan; all but one of these patients underwent cardiac or peripheral intervention, with the remaining patient undergoing a venous study. A complicating factor in patients undergoing percutaneous intervention is the frequent concurrent use of heparin and thrombolytic agents. Other studies have also suggested a correlation with catheter size and complication rates, such as PSA formation [8]; however, a recent study by Cragg *et al.* [12] demonstrated no difference in large hematoma formation following catheterization with 7-F catheters when compared with 5-F catheters.

Bleeding complications are particularly important when associated with a high puncture site, especially those cephalad to the inguinal ligament [15]. The etiology of hemorrhage from a high puncture site is inadequate tamponade of the external iliac artery after catheter removal, and significant blood loss into the retroperitoneum can occur. Hemorrhage can dissect from the femoral sheath into the prevesical space of Retzius which may contain up to 2.5 l of fluid without a palpable mass [16]. Further accumulation can result in extension into the rectus sheath and retroperitoneum.

Puncture of the femoral artery below the inguinal ligament greatly decreases the likelihood of hematoma extension into the retroperitoneum. In an anatomic study of the inguinal ligament in cadavers, Rupp *et al.* [17] demonstrated that punctures centered over the midportion of the femoral head would essentially preclude punctures of the external iliac artery. As stated previously, similar puncture sites would alleviate complications of AVF and PSA due to puncture of the vessels caudad to the common femoral artery bifurcation. Therefore, it is our routine to fluoroscope the groin prior to all punctures and puncture the common femoral artery at the level of the midfemoral head.

The incidence of hematoma formation is increased in certain patient populations. In particular, obese patients are prone to hematoma formation regardless of other variables [12]. Due to the variation in anatomic location of the inguinal crease, especially in obese patients, it is imperative in this patient population that fluoroscopic guidance be used prior to arterial puncture [18]. Other clinical factors, such as coagulopathy and the inability of a patient fully to cooperate during or after angiography, are further predisposing conditions to the formation of groin site hematomas [19].

In addition to clinical factors, technical factors represent a role in the formation of puncture site hematomas. As noted previously, recent data suggest that catheter size is not a significant factor in hematoma formation [12]. The use of angiographic needles with or without a stylet does not appear to make a significant difference on the pathologic changes one sees in the artery postpuncture [20]. Additionally, use of mechanical implements to tamponade the artery postprocedure have been described, both to stop bleeding primarily [21] or to decrease the risk of recurrent or late bleeding [22,23]. Some success has been seen with both of these mechanical aides.

Femoral punctures of synthetic vascular grafts may be performed safely. Studies in the literature demonstrate no increased incidence of clinically significant hematomas, PSA, distal thromboembolic events, or graft infections [24–26]. Overdilatation of the puncture site does not increase the incidence of significant puncture site complications in these patients [26]. Previously demonstrated complications from puncture of femoral grafts have included catheter separation on withdrawal [27]. However, with advances in wire and catheter technology this complication is less common.

Other puncture sites

Common puncture sites other than the femoral artery include axillary and brachial arteries, with translumbar approaches reserved for select cases. Although some authors have suggested an increased incidence of puncture site complications related to sites other than the femoral artery [13], the SCVIR guidelines outlining thresholds for complications do not specifically address the puncture site but rather suggest a complication rate threshold for all puncture sites combined (see Table 14.1).

Axillary puncture

Axillary punctures are most frequently used as an alternate approach in the setting of occluded femoral or iliac arteries. Occasionally, in the setting of patent iliofemoral segments, a combination of the patient's pathology and technical factors may indicate the need for an approach cephalad to the site of pathology. Examples of this include selective catheterization of visceral arteries in patients with severely ectatic or aneurysmal abdominal aortas, or patients with groin infections.

Factors that must be considered before attempting axillary punctures include ability of the patient to cooperate, results of coagulation studies, previous axillary intervention such as operative dissection, osseous abnormalities precluding positioning of the arm in adequate position during and following the procedure (e.g., severe arthritis), and whether or not the patient is normotensive.

The axillary artery extends between the lateral border of the first rib and the inferior margin of the teres major muscle (Fig. 14.3). The origins of the subscapular and humeral circumflex arteries indicate the transition from axillary to brachial artery. Care should be taken during axillary punctures regarding the proximity of the brachial plexus, and any

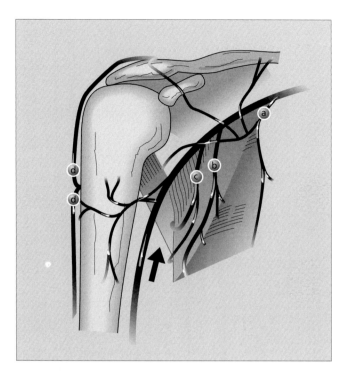

Fig. 14.3 Vascular anatomy of the axilla. The axillary artery forms the brachial artery at the inferior margin of the teres major muscle (arrow). Branches of the axillary artery include the thoracoacromial trunk (a), lateral thoracic artery (b), subscapular artery (c), and circumflex humeral artery (d).

neurologic complaints (paresthesias, numbness, electric sensations) during or following the puncture should alert the operator to possible complications involving the brachial plexus. Additionally, the axillary artery is more mobile than the femoral artery, making control of the artery difficult during the puncture as well as during compression.

The axillary artery is palpated with the patient's hand positioned underneath the head with the arm abducted to approximately 135°. Fluoroscopic guidance allows marking of the skin superficial to the artery as it courses over the humeral head. The puncture is made 1–2 cm lateral to the tendon of the pectoralis major muscle. Although termed axillary punctures, this site actually results in very high brachial artery punctures since the puncture site is distal to the lateral margin of the teres major muscle (Fig. 14.4).

Puncture of the artery at the described location should be adhered to closely. Punctures centered too high have an increased incidence of hemorrhage due to relative incompressibility of the artery, because of mobility of the artery in the axilla and relative lack of osseous structures against which to apply compression. Additionally, the axilla represents a large potential space, allowing accumulation of large amounts of blood before becoming clinically obvious. Neurologic complications may also be encountered with punctures centered too high due to the anatomic position of with catheter sizes ranging from 5-F to 8-F; hematoma formation occurred in 26 patients (8.1%), the majority of which did not require further intervention.

A serious complication of axillary punctures is neurologic deficit due to injury to the brachial plexus. Signs or symptoms related to the brachial plexus occurs in approximately 1.0% of axillary punctures [29,30]. Brachial plexus injuries may result from compression by a large axillary hematoma or PSA, as well as direct nerve injury during the puncture. Smith *et al.* [29] described the medial brachial fascial (MBF) compartment syndrome, believed to be due to hematoma formation within the thick and nonpliable MBF. The brachial fascia surrounds the arm from the clavicle to the elbow and lies superficial to the axillary sheath at the level of the brachial plexus. The musculocutaneous and radial nerves exit the MBF proximal to the usual puncture site of the axillary artery, while the ulnar and median nerves remain within the MBF to the level of the distal humerus and elbow, respectively. In the described syndrome, there is early involvement of the median and ulnar nerve distributions secondary to compression by the hematoma within the confines of the relatively inelastic MBF, with relative sparing of the remainder of the brachial plexus until the hematoma expands.

Neurologic complications involving the brachial plexus may also be seen with axillary punctures due to direct damage to the nerves during the needle insertion. This may be compounded in proximal punctures due to an increased number of brachial plexus fibers over the axillary artery when compared with the high brachial artery [28].

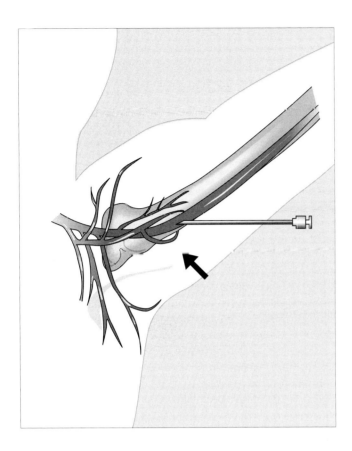

Fig. 14.4 Position of the arm and puncture site location for an axillary puncture. The correct site for axillary puncture is the proximal brachial artery, approximately 2 cm distal to the origin of the circumflex humeral artery (arrow).

the median nerve, which lies just ventral to the distal axillary artery [28,29]. Low puncture sites carry certain risks as well, including spasm or occlusion, which are in part due to the decreased size of the artery punctured. Very low puncture sites, such as the midbrachial artery, are discussed below.

The incidence of complications from axillary punctures varies according to the author. Hessel *et al.* [13] demonstrated an overall puncture site complication rate of 1.7% for transaxillary diagnostic angiography, compared to a rate of 0.47% for femoral punctures. In this study, hematomas and arterial obstruction each accounted for over 40% of the axillary site complications (0.68% and 0.74% of all axillary punctures, respectively), with PSA formation accounting for the majority of the remaining complications. In a review of complications of 1762 consecutive axillary punctures, largely for cardiac arteriography, Molnar and Paul [30] demonstrated hematoma formation in 1.2% and PSA formation in 0.2%. Antonovic *et al.* [31] described hematoma formation in 9.5% of axillary puncture sites, but only 1.0% required surgical intervention. In this study, hematoma formation was not related to catheter size but did increase in incidence with greater numbers of catheter exchanges. In 1989, Smith *et al.* [29] retrospectively reviewed 320 axillary catheterizations

Brachial artery punctures

Brachial artery punctures may be used for peripheral, neurologic, and coronary angiography and have become more commonplace with the advent of smaller catheter and guidewire systems. The brachial approach gives the angiographer a viable alternate in patients in whom femoral or axillary arteriography are not feasible, and is used more frequently today than the translumbar approach.

The brachial artery may be punctured anywhere along its course. The antecubital fossa is most frequently used during cutdown procedures for coronary angiography, while most radiologists prefer a more proximal puncture site for percutaneous techniques. Some authors advocate the use of introducer sheaths and have shown a decreased incidence of major complications when sheaths are used [32]. Complications such as hematomas are seen in the setting of brachial artery punctures; however, due to the anatomic location of the brachial artery, hemostasis should be somewhat easier to obtain. Multiple studies have indicated, however, that hematomas form at the puncture site in 1.8–9.5% of patients [32–36]; hematomas requiring surgical intervention are far less common, occurring in less than

0.25% of patients in all studies but one [33–36], which demonstrated one of 27 patients requiring evacuation of a hematoma (3.7%) [32]. PSA formation is also a known complication of brachial artery punctures but occurs only rarely [33].

Complications that are specific to brachial artery punctures include obturation and spasm. Compared to the femoral artery, the brachial artery is relatively small in diameter at the puncture site. Even small diameter catheter systems may cause a significant impediment to flow, and the larger systems used in interventional procedures carry a significant risk for arterial occlusion. Thrombosis of the brachial artery at the puncture site is most likely influenced by the small diameter and spastic properties of the brachial artery. The incidence of this complication is 0.15–8.0% [28,32,34,35]. The likelihood of arterial thrombosis may be decreased with the use of small sized catheters; Morin *et al.* [36] performed 71 brachial artery punctures with 4-F catheters and had no complications of brachial artery thrombosis. While thrombosis is a serious complication, surgical correction is generally not difficult and usually consists of arteriotomy and thrombectomy performed under local anesthesia. Due to the ease and rapidity of the surgical approach, few angiographers will consider thrombolysis in the setting of acute thrombosis at the puncture site. Finally, another factor complicating brachial punctures is the irritability of the brachial artery and its predisposition for spasm. While the pathologic basis for this is uncertain, some angiographers empirically use vasodilators to decrease the likelihood of spasm and subsequent thrombosis.

Translumbar aortic punctures

Translumbar aortography (TLA) has largely been supplanted by other vascular access routes as a diagnostic tool. In certain select cases, however, TLA may still be performed as a relatively safe angiographic approach. Although the inherent complication rate is generally higher, and many recently trained angiographers have little experience with TLA technique, the risks associated with not performing the procedure must be compared to the risk of TLA itself. Often, in the setting of "no peripheral access", the primary question may be answered by other imaging modalities such as CT, ultrasound US, magnetic resonance imaging (MRI), or magnetic resonance angiography (MRA). The noninvasive imaging modalities are fraught with their own drawbacks and artifacts, however, and contrast angiography may still be necessary, in which case TLA may prove to be the only viable access route.

In the past, the translumbar approach was typically used for aortic and lower extremity angiography. However, with the advent of smaller catheters and torque control wires and catheters the translumbar approach can be used for selective work as well [37].

Complications encountered with TLA are similar to those seen with other puncture sites. Hematoma formation is the most frequent complication encountered with the TLA technique, due to the inability to apply compression postprocedure. Many authors have described bleeding as a common complication but usually of no clinical significance [2,37–41]. Lang [2] reviewed 3240 cases of TLA and described small retroperitoneal hematomas in 34 patients (1.1%) as evidenced by changes visualized on follow-up intravenous urograms. Serious retroperitoneal hemorrhage or dissecting aneurysm occurred in only four patients (0.1%). Hessel *et al.* [13] found a hemorrhagic complication rate of 0.53% in reviewing 4118 cases. Many authors have described higher rates of retroperitoneal hemorrhage. For instance, Dorph and Folke [42] demonstrated retroperitoneal hematomas in 10% of cases. Another study, in which all patients underwent operation following TLA, demonstrated retroperitoneal hemorrhage in 12.1% of patients [40]. Bakal *et al.* [41] showed a 6% or greater drop in hematocrit in 15% of patients. Studies in which post-TLA CT scanning is routinely performed have demonstrated very high rates of periaortic hemorrhage, ranging from 71 to 87% [38,39].

Intramural or perivascular extravasation during contrast injection may also occur with TLA. Rates of such a complication range from 2 to 13% [42,43]. Most patients have few symptoms other than pain at the injection site, and sequelae from contrast extravasation are rare.

Case reports of other complications arising from TLA have been described, including vertebral osteomyelitis [44], puncture of the left ventricle [45], hemothorax, and pulmonary infarction [46].

Catheters and guidewires

Complications related to catheter and guidewire manipulation have evolved over time and are related to both the changes in catheter and wire technology as well as the common use of various contrast agents and heparin. Complications related to intravascular heparin administration will be discussed later in this chapter. The use of nonionic contrast agents has an association with increased thrombogenicity [47]; however, adverse outcomes associated with contrast agents are discussed in other chapters and will not be reviewed here (see Chapter 13). Rather, complications related solely to guidewire and catheter manipulation or to properties of the materials themselves will be discussed.

Dissection

Perhaps the most feared and serious complication associated with catheter and wire manipulation is dissection (Fig. 14.5). Dissection of the artery during manipulations is difficult to quantitate, particularly since it is frequently associated with other complications such as subintimal injection of contrast

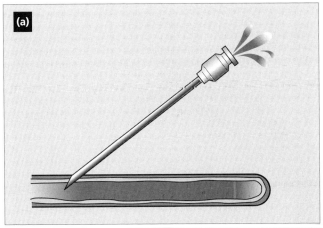

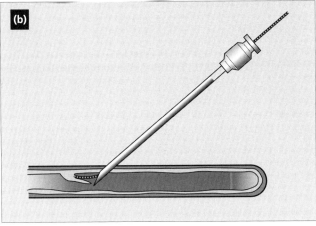

Fig. 14.5 Arterial dissection during guidewire introduction. (a) Placement of a single wall needle within the arterial wall with only a portion of the needle in the vessel lumen. (b) Advancement of a guidewire through the media of the vessel, raising a dissection flap.

or thrombosis of the artery. Few review articles separate arterial dissection as an individual complication. However, one article demonstrated 30 deaths in 118 591 angiograms (0.03%) from aortic dissection and aneurysm rupture combined [13].

Dissections may be recognized by subintimal injections of contrast material (Figs 14.6 & 14.7). This may be seen following placement of a catheter over a guidewire which has dissected into an intramural position. Repositioning of straight or curved catheters without the use of a guidewire can also cause intramural injection due to undermining of a plaque, and blunt dissection of the arterial wall by the unprotected catheter end. Catheters without side holes are more likely to cause intramural injection due to the jet phenomenon (see below). Intramural injections are more significant with larger volume injections due to a more extensive dissection, and if large enough may lead to occlusion of the artery [11].

Certain technical factors are associated with an increased risk of arterial dissection. One such factor is the use of a single-wall needle with a long bevel, which allows pulsatile return when only a portion of the needle is within the arterial lumen and predisposes to guidewire dissection [11] (Figs 14.5 & 14.8).

Thromboembolic events

A second serious complication arising from catheter and guidewire manipulation is arterial thrombosis (Fig 14.9). The majority of arterial occlusions secondary to thrombus occur at the puncture site, most likely due to stripping of pericatheter thrombus or fibrin sheath upon removal of the catheter or wire. Thromboembolic events may also originate from the more distal catheter–wire system. They may occur secondary to thrombus forming on the catheter or guidewire, or plaque or cholesterol embolized during manipulation of the catheter.

Material from which the catheters and wires are made may make the system more or less prone to thrombus formation. Catheters made from Teflon are the most likely to form thrombus, while those made from polyethylene are the least thrombogenic [48]. The porous surface of Teflon seems to be a factor in thrombus formation, and the surface irregularities seen with polyurethane make it more prone to form thrombus than polyethylene materials [49]. Similarly, Teflon-coated guidewires are more thrombogenic than their stainless steel counterparts [48]. Regardless of the wire material, a wet gauze pad should be used to wipe the wire after use rather than a dry swab since the latter are prone to subsequent cotton fiber embolization, due to contamination of both the irrigation fluid and the guidewire itself [50].

The number of side holes in a catheter may also play a role in thrombus formation. Although clotting may be prevented in end-hole catheters with low-pressure continuous flushing [51], preferential flow into the proximal side holes of multiple side-hole catheters has been documented when a low-pressure flushing system is used. This increases the risk of thrombus formation in the distal side holes and end holes [48] (Fig. 14.10). For this reason, many angiographers prefer the manual double-flush technique when working with multihole catheters.

Catheter size does not appear to have a significant role in thrombus formation. While some authors suggest that the increased surface area of larger catheters increases the chance of thrombus formation, the same investigators demonstrated no difference in thrombus formation when comparing catheters sized 6–9-F [52]. Other investigators have suggested that catheter diameter is a less important variable than the number of side holes; Dawson and Strickland [48] indicated that distal side holes and end holes of smaller catheters require more pressure to flush than larger catheters and, hence, are more prone to thrombus formation.

All other variables aside, many authors have suggested

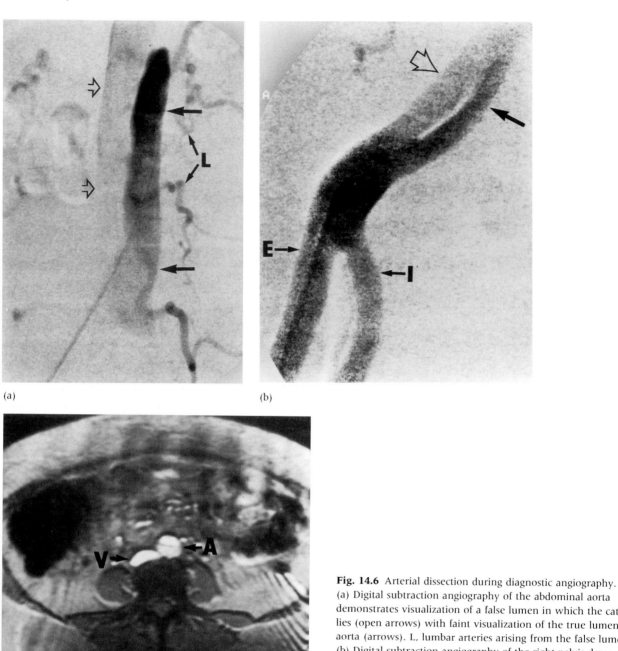

(a)

(b)

(c)

Fig. 14.6 Arterial dissection during diagnostic angiography. (a) Digital subtraction angiography of the abdominal aorta demonstrates visualization of a false lumen in which the catheter lies (open arrows) with faint visualization of the true lumen of the aorta (arrows). L, lumbar arteries arising from the false lumen. (b) Digital subtraction angiography of the right pelvis demonstrates visualization of both the true (arrow) and false (open arrow) lumens. E, external iliac artery; I, internal iliac artery. (c) Axial GRE MRI image of the lower abdominal aorta clearly demonstrating the intimal flap within the aorta (A). V, inferior vena cava.

that the single most important factor in the risk for thromboembolic events is the experience of the angiographer. Judkins and Gander [53] demonstrated a 10-fold increase in the rate of thromboembolic events during coronary angiography when the procedures were performed at an institution performing less than 100 angiograms/year when compared with institutions doing more than 400/year. Other authors reached the same conclusion regarding angiographic tech-

nique as being the dominant factor in precluding thromboembolic events [48,54].

The intraprocedural use of heparin is highly variable. The complications of heparin administration, such as bleeding at or distal to the puncture site, must be weighed against the advantages of the anticoagulant properties of heparin. Miller [55] surveyed all members and fellows of the SCVIR, regarding the use of heparin during angiography and received

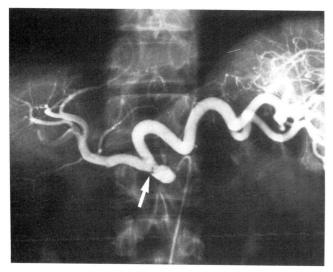

(a)

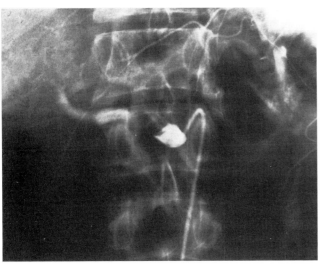

(b)

Fig. 14.7 Subintimal injection of contrast. (a) Early arterial phase angiogram during a celiac angiogram demonstrating irregularity of the celiac axis with an intraluminal filling defect (arrow). (b) Late arterial phase angiogram from the same injection demonstrating persistent contrast stain in the proximal celiac artery corresponding to the area of irregularity noted during the early arterial phase.

Fig. 14.9 Catheter-induced thromboembolism. (a) Angiogram centered over the pelvis during an aortic injection demonstrates a normal appearing ileocolic branch of the superior mesenteric artery (arrows). G, aortobifemoral bypass graft. (b) Angiogram performed in a slightly different projection following selection of the superior mesenteric artery now demonstrates a well-defined intraluminal filling defect within the ileocolic branch (arrow), indicating a catheter-induced thromboembolism.

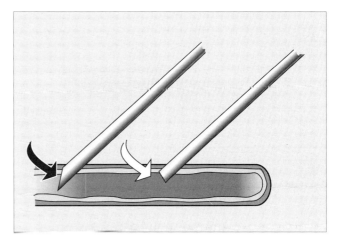

Fig. 14.8 Single-wall needle versus double-wall arterial needle. Placement of the bevel of the single-wall needle into the vessel wall may allow pulsatile return of blood flow simulating complete entry into the vessel lumen (arrow). Conversely, following removal of the inner stylet, pulsatile return from a double-wall needle indicates adequate and safe placement of the arterial needle (open arrow).

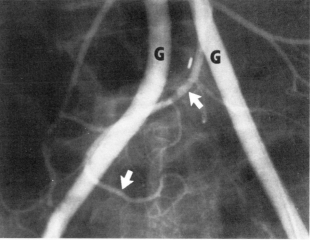

(a)

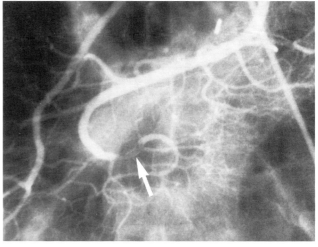

(b)

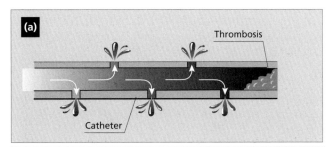

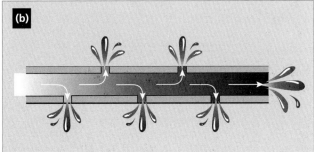

Fig. 14.10 Thrombus formation at the distal end of a multihole catheter. (a) Low-pressure flushing technique flushes only the proximal side holes and allows thrombus to form at the distal end of the catheter (arrow). (b) Flushing technique using higher pressure ensures adequate flushing of both proximal and distal holes.

a broad spectrum of answers to his questionnaire. Indeed, less than 20% of respondents formed their policy towards heparin based on literature review, while one respondent admitted to "paranoia" as his or her sole reason for systemic heparinization!

Wallace *et al.* [56] routinely used both systemic (mean 3000 IU) and flush solution heparin (2 IU/ml saline) in 525 patients and demonstrated no thrombotic complications and no bleeding complications requiring intervention other than administration of protamine sulfate. Additionally, angiograms performed at the puncture site just prior to removal of the catheter demonstrated pericatheter thrombus in two of 78 patients (2.6%), compared with a 50% incidence quoted in nonheparinized patients [52]. In the same paper, the authors also showed that heparin given only in the flush solution resulted in a peak elevation of activated clotting time (ACT) and activated partial thromboplastin time (PTT) at the time of catheter removal, while systemic heparinization resulted in a peak ACT at 10 minutes and peak PTT at 30 minutes following bolus administration of systemic heparin.

Anderson *et al.* [57] compared systemic heparinization, heparin-coated guidewires, and both versus no anticoagulation in an experimental canine model. All forms of anticoagulation were superior to the control group. Coated wires combined with systemic heparinization demonstrated a complete absence of fibrin accumulation and fewer platelets adhering and aggregating to the guidewires than either wire coating or systemic heparinization in isolation.

Antonovic *et al.* [58] examined 400 patients prospectively by comparing systemic heparinization (45 IU/kg body weight) with flush system heparin (2 IU/ml). They demonstrated a decrease in the number of nonocclusive thrombi at the entry site in the systemically heparinized patients; however, there was also a significant increase in the number of cases of delayed bleeding in the systemically heparinized group. The authors recommended systemic heparinization with control of bleeding complications by the use of protamine sulfate as needed.

In a study of interventional neuroradiology patients, Debrun *et al.* [59] compared systemic heparin versus flush solution heparin. Both groups received either 1−2 g of aspirin prior to the procedure, or 1 g of acetylsalicylate was added to the flush solution. In the group receiving systemic heparinization, bolus administrations were given at regular intervals to keep the PTT levels above 110 seconds. The results from this study demonstrated no thromboembolic complications in the 57 patients receiving systemic heparin and aspirin, while four thromboembolic complications occurred in the 25 control patients. The authors recommended routine use of systemic heparin and aspirin for all diagnostic and interventional neuroradiologic procedures.

Heparin-coated catheters have been shown to have a decreased incidence of cell aggregations, thrombus, or fibrin formation when compared to noncoated catheters [57,60, 61]. However, the heparin coating of the catheter quickly dissolves, and many angiographers do not consider the extra cost of heparinized catheters worthwhile in the clinical setting [48].

Cholesterol embolization is a frequently serious but very rare complication, most typically associated with prolonged catheter or guidewire manipulation in a heavily diseased aorta [62]. Small cholesterol emboli are dislodged from aortic plaques and embed in the microvasculature of the kidneys, toes, or other organs. Emboli to the kidney invoke a foreign body reaction causing delayed renal failure 1−2 weeks following the angiogram [63]. Involvement of the foot may range from livedo reticularis or blue toe syndrome to dry gangrene [63]. Although a rare clinical entity, pathologic studies suggest that clinically silent cholesterol embolization occurs far more frequently than previously suspected [64]. Very rarely, cholesterol emboli may occur in routine angiography with minimal catheter manipulations [65].

Miscellaneous catheter and guidewire complications

Inadvertent selective injection of smaller arteries may be caused by a number of factors. Multiple side-hole catheters are less likely to cause selective injection due to a portion of the side holes frequently being outside the selected vessel. End-hole catheters, however, are more dangerous in terms of inadvertent selective injection because the entire contrast bolus will be deposited into the selected vessel at higher rates than usually used in such vessels. Additionally, if catheters are injected at flow rates above those recommended, whipping or uncoiling of the catheter may occur, increasing the risk of inadvertent selective injection. This may also rarely occur with flow rates below the maximum recommended rates (Fig. 14.11).

The angiographic jet phenomenon is defined as endothelial injury caused during contrast injection by the force of the injected contrast. Vascular injury can range from endothelial contusion and subendothelial hemorrhage, to gross dissection of the vessel. If radiographic evidence suggesting injury is seen, i.e., contrast staining, severe injury to the vessel has occurred [66]. The jet phenomenon is particularly prone to occur when end-hole catheters are used, since the entire force of the injection is directed largely in one vector. Multiple hole catheters decrease the jet phenomenon; however, high flow multihole catheters demonstrate preferential flow through the endhole and distal side holes when high flow rates are used. One study suggested the use of catheters with larger proximal side holes when compared with the distal holes, allowing nearly constant velocity throughout the length of the catheter, and decreasing the jet phenomenon through the end hole [67].

Occasionally, a catheter may become knotted during manipulation; this is most likely to occur during the reformation of reverse curve catheters such as a Simmons catheter [68]. Multiple techniques have been described to unknot catheters, which may be as simple as advancement

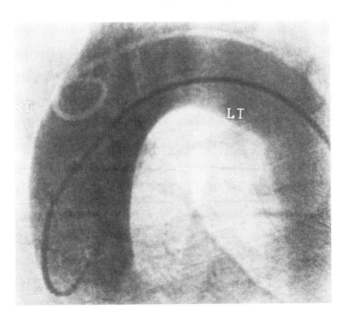

Fig. 14.11 Unwinding of pigtail catheter during contrast injection. Magnified view of digital subtraction angiogram during aortic arch injection demonstrating the original position of the pigtail catheter prior to injection (white) and uncoiling of the catheter during injection of 25 ml/s of contrast (Hypaque-76) (black). This catheter is rated by the manufacturer for injection rates up to 29 ml/s.

of the stiff end of a guidewire or may require more advanced techniques such as utilization of tip-deflecting wires or snares [11,68]. If the knot is small enough, the hub of the catheter may be removed and a large vascular introducer sheath placed over the catheter, through which the knotted catheter may be withdrawn. Surgical removal after withdrawal of the catheter to the groin may be the only means of retrieval in some cases.

Systemic complications

Systemic complications from diagnostic angiography may arise from multiple causes such as contrast exposure, anesthesia, adverse reactions to pharmacologic adjuncts, or inadequate aseptic technique. In addition, bleeding complications may arise from the systemic effects of heparin or thrombolytic therapy.

The incidence of bacteremia during angiography ranges from 0 to 23%, however, the incidence of clinically significant infection is negligible [69–71]. Studies in which blood draws were performed from a site other than the angiography catheter, demonstrate a low incidence of bacteremia [70], while studies in which blood cultures were drawn from the catheter itself tend to show growth of Grampositive organisms of low virulence frequently found on the skin surface [69,71]. The onset of postprocedural fever is not associated with bacteremia, but rather may be due to pyrogen on the catheters, sensitivity to catheter materials, or inflammation at the site of catheter introduction [69]. Prophylactic antibiotics seem to have little if any protective effect against bacteremia or postprocedure fever [69,72]. Local infections at the puncture site have been reported, such as septic arthritis of the hip following femoral artery puncture [73], and retroperitoneal abscess [42], and vertebral osteomyelitis following TLA [74].

Adverse reactions from pharmacologic agents used in diagnostic angiography may also occur. Intraarterial nitroglycerine, used as a short-acting vasodilator, may cause hypotension due to the systemic effects of vasodilatation. Intraarterial lidocaine, used during extremity angiography in conjunction with ionic contrast material to decrease the amount of pain felt during injection, may cause arrhythmias. Lidocaine should not be injected intraarterially if there is the possibility of retrograde flow into the cerebral circulation due to placement of a catheter too proximally during upper extremity angiography. Lidocaine injected into the cerebral circulation has been associated with transient tinnitus and seizures [75]. Other pharmacologic agents used in angiography, such as benzodiazepines and narcotics given for conscious sedation, carry certain risks which must always be weighed against the advantages of giving such drugs.

General anesthesia is not commonly used for standard diagnostic angiography but may prove helpful in select cases. In a study comparing local, spinal, and general anesthesia in 12 313 procedures, McAfee [76] demonstrated a higher neurologic complication rate with both general and spinal anesthesia compared to local anesthesia only. The overall complication rate was lowest with locally anesthetized patients (0.65%) and highest in patients undergoing spinal anesthesia (2.06%).

Outpatient angiography

With increased emphasis on decreasing the cost of health care, many investigations have been undertaken evaluating diagnostic angiography performed on an outpatient basis. Most of the studies on this subject were performed in the mid-1980s, and although acceptance of outpatient procedures by radiologists has been relatively slow, many angiographers will perform select procedures on an outpatient basis.

Adams and Roub [77] performed diagnostic angiography and interventional procedures on 195 patients as outpatients. Of these patients, 163 had diagnostic angiography, with only two outpatients having vascular intervention (PTA). While the majority of the patients in this study underwent angiography by a femoral artery approach, some patients did undergo axillary punctures. All patients received only oral sedation and were observed for 3–4 hours following the procedure; catheter sizes ranged from 5 to 7-F. The results of the study demonstrated no significant difference in complications with examinations performed on outpatients compared with inpatients. In particular, there were no complications with the outpatient population that were not appreciated during the observation period, i.e., inpatients who had already left the hospital. The total potential savings in this study was $28 930.

A separate retrospective study was performed on 2029 outpatients with a control group of 3864 inpatients over an 11-year period [78]. A 3-hour observation period followed the procedure, and no mention was made of sedation. Catheters ranged from 5 to 8-F, with an emphasis on the smaller sized catheters. The results of this study demonstrated 39 major complications, only six (0.30%) of which were seen in the outpatient group. One patient after arriving home was referred to an emergency room for an expanding hematoma; the other five complications were recognized during the observation period. Estimated cost savings from this study was $702 000 over the 11-year period.

A prospective study on 100 patients undergoing peripheral or neurologic diagnostic angiography demonstrated similar results [79]. Catheter sizes ranged from 5 to 8-F, and patients were observed for 4 hours following the procedure; there was no mention in this study of the sedation given. Again, there were no reported complications following the procedure that were not noticed in the observation period, and 94 of the 100 patients went home after the observation period as planned.

Rogers and Moothart [80] reviewed a total of 95 patients undergoing peripheral, visceral, and cerebral arteriograms, many of whom were given intravenous sedation (diazepam and/or meperidine) and intravenous heparin. Once again, there was no increase in the complication rate with procedures performed on an outpatient basis, and intravenous sedation was not proven to be a liability with the exception of increasing the observation time to 4–6 hours.

Transbrachial arteriography performed on outpatients has also been shown to be a safe procedure, particularly with the utilization of smaller (4-F) catheters. Gritter *et al.* [81] retrospectively reviewed 660 patients who underwent transbrachial arteriography using 4-F catheters, demonstrating complications requiring surgery in only two (0.3%) patients. Delayed or minor complications were observed in an additional 137 patients; however, more than 50% of these were simple ecchymoses [81].

Pediatric angiography

While any of the complications previously described with adult patients may occur in the pediatric population, the small size of the artery in infants and children predisposes this group of patients to more thromboembolic events and vascular spasm.

Thrombosis at the puncture site occurs with much greater frequency in children than in adult patients. One series demonstrated partial or complete arterial occlusion in nine of 50 patients, with the vast majority occurring in patients aged less than 8 years [82].

Arterial spasm is also more likely to occur in the pediatric population than with adult patients. Due to decreased flow and vascular stasis, arterial spasm may be a predisposing factor in arterial thrombosis. The incidence of arterial spasm ranges from 18 to 62%, with the majority of spasm causing no clinically significant sequelae [83–85]. Franken *et al.* [85] demonstrated that the primary cause of arterial spasm is the size of the catheter relative to the artery. Therefore, as expected, spasm was seen most frequently in the neonate and in older children when larger catheter sizes were used. With the advent of high flow smaller diameter catheters, both arterial spasm and thrombosis should decrease in incidence.

Conclusion

Diagnostic angiography is by definition an invasive procedure, and as such will always entail some risk. Despite the recent progress in noninvasive imaging modalities, diagnostic angiography continues to have an important role in the evaluation and management of patients with vascular disorders. The overall safety of angiography has improved steadily with the development of specialized technology and postgraduate training. Meticulous attention to technique during angiographic procedures will continue to minimize the incidence and severity of complications for our patients.

Acknowledgment

The authors wish to thank Stacy Erickson, BS, for the illustrations included in this chapter.

References

1 Seldinger SI. Catheter replacement of the needle in percutaneous arteriography. A new technique. *Acta Radiol* 1953;39:368−376.

2 Lang EK. A survey of the complications of percutaneous retrograde arteriography: Seldinger technic. *Radiology* 1963;81:257−263.

3 Sigstedt B, Lunderquist A. Complications of angiographic examinations. *Am J Roentgenol* 1978;130:455−460.

4 Waugh JR, Sacharias N. Arteriographic complications in the DSA era. *Radiology* 1992;182:243−246.

5 Spies JB, Bakal CW, Burke DR *et al.* Standard for diagnostic arteriography in adults. *J Vasc Intervent Radiol* 1993;4:385−395.

6 Trerotola SO, Kuhlman JE, Fishman EK. Bleeding complications of femoral catheterization: CT evaluation. *Radiology* 1990;174:37−40.

7 Kent KC, McArdle CR, Kennedy B *et al.* A prospective study of the clinical outcome of femoral pseudoaneurysms and arteriovenous fistulas induced by arterial puncture. *J Vasc Surg* 1993;17:125−131.

8 Rapoport S, Sniderman KW, Morse SS *et al.* Pseudoaneurysm: a complication of faulty technique in femoral arterial puncture. *Radiology* 1985;154:529−530.

9 McCann RL, Schwartz LB, Peiper KS. Vascular complications of cardiac catheterization. *J Vasc Surg* 1991;14:375−381.

10 Baum PA, Matsumoto AH, Teitelbaum GP *et al.* Anatomic relationship between the common femoral artery and vein: CT evaluation and clinical significance. *Radiology* 1989;173:775−777.

11 Kim D, Orron DE. Techniques and complications of angiography. In: Kim D, Orron DE, eds. *Peripheral Vascular Imaging and Intervention.* St Louis: Mosby Year Book, 1992:83−109.

12 Cragg AH, Nakagawa N, Smith TP *et al.* Hematoma formation after diagnostic angiography: effect of catheter size. *J Vasc Intervent Radiol* 1991;2:231−233.

13 Hessel SJ, Adams DF, Abrams HL. Complications of angiography. *Radiology* 1981;138:273−281.

14 Fraedrich G, Beck A, Bonzel T, Schlosser V. Acute surgical intervention for complications of percutaneous transluminal angioplasty. *Eur J Vasc Surg* 1987;1:197−203.

15 Kaufman JL. Pelvic hemorrhage after percutaneous femoral angiography. *Am J Roentgenol* 1984;143:335−336.

16 Auh YH, Rubenstein WA, Schneider M *et al.* Extraperitoneal paravesical spaces: CT delineation with US correlation. *Radiology* 1986;159:319−328.

17 Rupp SB, Vogelzang RL, Nemcek AA *et al.* Relationship of the inguinal ligament to pelvic radiographic landmarks: anatomic correlation and its role in femoral arteriography. *J Vasc Intervent Radiol* 1993;4:409−413.

18 Lechner G, Jantsch H, Waneck R *et al.* The relationship between the common femoral artery, the inguinal crease, and the inguinal ligament: a guide to accurate angiographic puncture. *Cardiovasc Intervent Radiol* 1988;11:165−169.

19 Quint LE, Holland D, Korobkin M *et al.* Role of femoral vessel catheterization and altered hemostasis in the development of extraperitoneal hematomas: CT study in 44 patients. *Am J Roentgenol* 1993;160:855−858.

20 Frood LR, Smith DC, Pappas JM *et al.* Use of angiographic needles with or without stylets: pathologic assessment of vessel walls after puncture. *J Vasc Intervent Radiol* 1991;2:269−272.

21 Semler HJ. Transfemoral catheterization: mechanical versus manual control of bleeding. *Radiology* 1985;154:234−235.

22 Christenson R, Staab EV, Burko H *et al.* Pressure dressings and postarteriographic care of the femoral puncture site. *Radiology* 1976;119:97−99.

23 Colapinto RF, Harty PW. Femoral artery compression device for outpatient angiography. *Radiology* 1988;166:890−891.

24 Eisenberg RL, Mani RL, McDonald EJ. The complication rate of catheter angiography by direct puncture through aorto-femoral bypass grafts. *Am J Roentgenol* 1976;126:814−816.

25 Smith DC, Grable GS, Shipp DJ. Safe and effective catheter angiography through prosthetic vascular grafts. *Radiology* 1981;138:487−488.

26 Wade GL, Smith DC, Mohr LL. Follow-up of 50 consecutive angiograms obtained utilizing puncture of prosthetic vascular grafts. *Radiology* 1983;146:663−664.

27 Weinshelbaum A, Carson SN. Separation of angiographic catheter during arteriography through vascular graft. *Am J Roentgenol* 1980;134:583−584.

28 Lipchik EO, Sugimoto H. Percutaneous brachial artery catheterization. *Radiology* 1986;160:842−843.

29 Smith DC, Mitchell DA, Peterson GW *et al.* Medial brachial fascial compartment syndrome: anatomic basis of neuropathy after transaxillary arteriography. *Radiology* 1989;173:149−154.

30 Molnar W, Paul DJ. Complications of axillary arteriotomies: an analysis of 1762 consecutive studies. *Radiology* 1972;104:269−276.

31 Antonovic R, Rosch J, Dotter CT. Complications of percutaneous transaxillary catheterization for arteriography and selective chemotherapy. *Am J Roentgenol* 1976;126:386−393.

32 Watkinson AF, Hartnell GG. Complications of direct brachial artery puncture for arteriography: a comparison of techniques. *Clin Radiol* 1991;44:189−191.

33 Gaines PA, Reidy JF. Percutaneous high brachial aortography: a safe alternative to the translumbar approach. *Clin Radiol* 1986;37:595−597.

34 Gritter KJ, Laidlaw WW, Peterson NT. Complications of outpatient transbrachial intraarterial digital subtraction angiography: work in progress. *Radiology* 1987;162:125−127.

35 Barnett FJ, Lecky DM, Freiman DB *et al.* Cerebrovascular disease: outpatient evaluation with selective carotid DSA performed via a transbrachial approach. *Radiology* 1989;170:535−539.

36 Morin ME, Willens BA, Kuss PA. Carotid artery: percutaneous transbrachial selective arteriography with a 4-F catheter. *Radiology* 1989;171:868−870.

37 Maxwell SL, Kwon OJ, Millan VG. Translumbar carotid arteriography. *Radiology* 1983;148:851−852.

38 Bergman AB, Neiman HL. Computed tomography in the detection of retroperitoneal hemorrhage after translumbar aortography. *Am J Roentgenol* 1978;131:831−833.

39 Chuang VP, Fried AM, Chun-Quan C. Computed tomographic evaluation of para-aortic hematoma following translumbar aortography. *Radiology* 1979;130:711−712.

40 Gmelin E, Rinast E. Translumbar catheter angiography with a needle-sheath system. *Radiology* 1988;166:888−889.

41 Bakal CW, Friedland RJ, Sprayregen S *et al.* Translumbar arch aortography: a retrospective controlled study of usefulness, technique, and safety. *Radiology* 1991;178:225–228.

42 Dorph S, Folke K. Complications in translumbar aortography: a comparison of direct needle puncture and aortic catheterisation. *Acta Radiol (Diagn)* 1972;12:750–756.

43 Taheri SA, Sheehan FR. Translumbar aortography as an outpatient procedure. *Am J Roentgenol* 1981;137:1287.

44 Szilogyi ED, Smith RF, Elliott JP *et al.* Translumbar aortography. *Arch Surg* 1977;112:399.

45 Haut G, Amplatz K. Complication rates of transfemoral and transaortic catheterization. *Surgery* 1968;63:594–596.

46 Poulias GE, Stergiou LE. Pulmonary infarction and haemothorax as a post-translumbar aortography sequel. *Br J Radiol* 1968;41:866–869.

47 Grollman JH, Liu CK, Astone RA *et al.* Thromboembolic complications in coronary angiography associated with the use of nonionic contrast medium. *Cathet Cardiovasc Diagn* 1988;14:159–164.

48 Dawson P, Strickland NH. Thromboembolic phenomena in clinical angiography: role of materials and technique. *J Vasc Intervent Radiol* 1991;2:125–132.

49 Thomson HK, Kjeldsen K, Hansen JF. Thrombogenic properties of arterial catheters: a scanning electron microscopic examination of the surface structure. *Cathet Cardiovasc Diagn* 1977;3:351–358.

50 Kay JM, Wilkins RA. Cotton fibre embolism during angiography. *Clin Radiol* 1969;20:410–413.

51 Dahlborn M, Cronestrand R, Klintmal G *et al.* Blood inflow and coagulation in vascular catheters: comparison of the effects of polysaccharide solutions, saline and contrast medium. *Acta Radiol (Diagn) (Stockh)* 1980;21:715–720.

52 Formanek G, Frech RS, Amplatz K. Arterial thrombus formation during percutaneous catheterization. *Circulation* 1970;41:830.

53 Judkins MP, Gander MP. Complications of coronary arteriography. *Circulation* 1974;49:599–602.

54 Davis K, Kennedy JW, Kemp MG *et al.* Complications of coronary arteriography from the collaborative study of coronary artery surgery (CASS). *Circulation* 1979;59:1105–1112.

55 Miller DL. Heparin in angiography: current patterns of use. *Radiology* 1989;172:1007–1011.

56 Wallace S, Medellin H, De Jongh D. Systemic heparinization for angiography. *Am J Roentgenol* 1972;116:204–206.

57 Anderson JH, Gianturco C, Wallace S *et al.* Anticoagulation techniques for angiography: an experimental study. *Radiology* 1974;111:573–576.

58 Antonovic R, Rosch J, Dotter C. The value of systemic arterial heparinization in transfemoral angiography: a prospective study. *Am J Roentgenol* 1976;127:223–225.

59 Debrun GM, Vinuela FV, Fox AJ. Aspirin and systemic heparinization in diagnostic and interventional neuroradiology. *Am J Roentgenol* 1982;139:139–142.

60 Kido DK, Paulin S, Aienghat JA. Thrombogenicity of heparin and non-heparin coated catheters: clinical trial. *Am J Roentgenol* 1982;139:957–961.

61 Amplatz K. A simple non-thrombogenic coating. *Invest Radiol* 1971;4:280–288.

62 Gaines PA. Cholesterol embolization after angiography. *Lancet* 1988;19:643.

63 Knutson DW, Abt AB. Pathophysiology, pathology, and clinical features of renovascular hypertension. In: Strandness DE, van

Brede A, eds. *Vascular Diseases: Surgical and Interventional Therapy.* New York: Churchill Livingstone, 1994:684.

64 Ramirez G, O'Neill WM, Lambert R *et al.* Cholesterol embolisation, a complication of angiography. *Arch Int Med* 1978;138:1430–1432.

65 Henderson MJ, Manhire AR. Case report: cholesterol embolization following angiography. *Clin Radiol* 1990;42:281–282.

66 Lipton MJ, Abbott JA, Kosek JC. Cardiovascular trauma from angiographic jets; validation of a theoretic concept in dogs. *Radiology* 1978;129:363–370.

67 Hansen EC, Hawkins MC, Hawkins IF *et al.* New high-flow "cloud" catheter for safer delivery of contrast material. *Radiology* 1989;173:461–464.

68 Gerlock AJ, Mirfakhraee M. *Essentials of Diagnostic and Interventional Angiographic Techniques.* Philadelphia: WB Saunders, 1985.

69 Clark H. An evaluation of antibiotic prophylaxis in cardiac catheterization. *Am Heart J* 1969;77:767–771.

70 Sande MA, Levinson ME, Lukas DS *et al.* Bacteremia associated with cardiac catheterization. *New Engl J Med* 1969;13:1104–1106.

71 Shawker TH, Kluge RM, Ayella RJ. Bacteremia associated with angiography. *J Am Med Assoc* 1974;229:1090–1092.

72 Kriedberg MB, Chernoff HL. Ineffectiveness of penicillin prophylaxis in cardiac catheterization. *J Pediat* 1965;66:286–290.

73 Resnick CS, Sawyer RW, Tisnado J. Septic arthritis of the hip: a rare complication of angiography. *J Can Assoc Radiol* 1987;38:229.

74 Schwartz H, Berkow AE, Love L. Vertebral osteomyelitis following translumbar aortography. *Angiology* 1977;28:487.

75 Chuang VP, Widrich WC. Complications from intraarterial lidocaine in upper extremity arteriography. *Am J Roentgenol* 1978;131:906.

76 McAfee JG. A survey of complications of abdominal aortography. *Radiology* 1957;68:825–838.

77 Adams PS, Roub LW. Outpatient angiography and interventional radiology: safety and cost benefits. *Radiology* 1984;151:81–82.

78 Wolfel DA, Lovett BP, Ortenburger AI *et al.* Outpatient arteriography: its safety and cost effectiveness. *Radiology* 1984;153:363–364.

79 Saint-Georges G, Aube M. Safety of outpatient angiography: a prospective study. *Am J Roentgenol* 1985;144:235–236.

80 Rogers WF, Moothart RW. Outpatient arteriography and cardiac catheterization: effective alternatives to inpatient procedures. *Am J Roentgenol* 1985;144:233–234.

81 Gritter KJ, Laidlaw WW, Peterson NT. Complications of outpatient transbrachial intraarterial digital subtraction angiography: work in progress. *Radiology* 1987;162:125–127.

82 Mortensson W. Angiography of the femoral artery following percutaneous catheterization in infants and children. *Acta Radiol (Diagn)* 1976;17:581–593.

83 Rubenson A, Jacobsson B, Sorensen SE. Treatment and sequelae of angiographic complications in children. *J Pediat Surg* 1979;14:154–157.

84 Jacobsson B, Curtin H, Rubenson A *et al.* Complications of angiography in children and means of prevention. *Acta Radiol (Diagn)* 1980;21:257–261.

85 Franken EA, Girod D, Sequeira FW *et al.* Femoral artery spasm in children: catheter size is the principal cause. *Am J Roentgenol* 1982;138:295–298.

CHAPTER 15

Complications of venography

Max P. Rosen and Ducksoo Kim

Introduction

Ascending lower extremity venography was once the only modality available to diagnose deep vein thrombosis (DVT). The standard for performing ascending venography of the lower extremity has been described by Rabinov and Paulin [1]. With the development of high-resolution realtime ultrasound (US) equipment, compression US has become the primary modality to diagnose lower extremity DVT. Cronan and Dorfman [2] initially reported compression US to be 89% sensitive and 100% specific in diagnosing acute femoral or popliteal vein DVT. However, compression US is less accurate in diagnosing calf vein DVT [3], and often unable reliably to differentiate acute from chronic DVT [4]. It is in these two situations (diagnosis of calf vein DVT and recurrent DVT), that ascending venography plays a current role.

With the advent of compression US and other noninvasive tests, the number of venographies performed at most institutions has dramatically decreased in recent years. As the frequency of this procedure has diminished, practicing radiologists may become less proficient at performing peripheral venography. A new generation of radiology residents is emerging which has had limited experience with this technique. This diminished familiarity can be compensated for by a heightened awareness of early signs of an impending severe complication as well as an understanding of the measures that can be taken to reduce the overall incidence of mild adverse reactions.

Descending lower extremity venography is performed for evaluation of patients with varicose veins and chronic venous insufficiency. The complications of this procedure differ from those associated with ascending venography and will be discussed separately.

Ascending venography

Complications associated with peripheral venography can be divided into two categories: (i) adverse reactions related to the systemic effects of contrast medium; and (ii) the local complications specifically associated with peripheral venography. The systemic complications associated with contrast-medium administration are discussed in detail (see Chapter 13). Local complications include pain, contrast extravasation, postvenography syndrome, postvenographic DVT, tissue necrosis, and pulmonary embolism (PE).

Numerous variables have been associated with a modification of the incidence of local complications. These factors include the osmolarity and sodium content of the contrast agent, the use of ionic or nonionic contrast, and the duration of contact of the contrast agent with the venous endothelium.

Pain

In 1977, Bettmann and Paulin [5] compared the incidence and intensity of pain associated with venography performed with Renografin 60 (8% sodium diatrizoate, 52% meglumine diatrizoate) (Squib, New Brunswick, NJ) and Renografin 60 diluted to 75% concentration with 5% dextrose−water. There was a statistically significant reduction in moderate or marked pain associated with the dilute Renografin (59−30%), without any change in diagnostic accuracy. In a subsequent study, Bettmann and Robbins [6] reported a decrease in patient's assessment of pain during lower extremity venography when the nonionic iopamidol was used when compared to the ionic iothalamate meglumine. Forty-four per cent of patients experienced discomfort during the study when iothalamate was used (38% mild, 4% moderate, and 2% severe), whereas 18% experienced discomfort with

317

iopamidol (all mild). The iodine content of both these agents is essentially equivalent (200 mg/ml iopamidol, 202 mg/ml iothalamate meglumine). A similar reduction of pain has been reported by Thomas and Briggs [7] when iopamidol 61 (Bracco, Industria Chimica, SpA, Milan, Italy) was compared with Conray 60.

Reduction in pain and cramping associated with peripheral venography has been accomplished by addition of Xylocaine to the contrast medium. Silverbach [8] performed venographies using 75% strength Conray 60 and compared the pain experienced when 10 or 20 mg Xylocaine was added to each 100 ml of contrast. Thirteen per cent of patients who received the 20 mg Xylocaine reported pain, compared with 30% of patients who received the 10 mg mixture. Admixture of local anesthetics may increase the systemic toxicity of contrast media [9].

An additional contributor to pain associated with venography is the sodium content of the contrast. Four of 14 patients (30%) receiving meglumine diatrizoate (Hypaque 60) reported pain, compared to 14 of 17 patients (82%) receiving sodium diatrizoate (Hypaque 50). Of the four patients who received Hypaque 60 and experienced pain, three patients reported mild and one patient reported moderate pain. Of the 14 patients who received Hypaque 50 and experienced pain, six reported mild, six reported moderate, and two reported severe pain [10].

Postvenography syndrome

Delayed side-effects of venography consist of pain, warmth, erythema, and swelling, often several centimeters cephalad of the venopuncture site. The onset of this reaction usually begins between 2 and 12 hours after the study, and is usually maximal at 12–24 hours and then gradually subsides over several days [11,12]. Occasionally, these findings are associated with malaise and fever. Although the physiologic and morphologic nature of this reaction is not clear, its inflammatory character is probably related to a direct toxic effect on the endothelium and a more generalized, systemic effect related to the hypertonicity of the contrast [5]. A reduction of these symptoms has been associated with dilute contrast, nonionic contrast, and low-osmolar contrast.

When full strength Renografin 60 was compared to 75% strength Renografin, Bettmann and Paulin [5] reported a decrease in the incidence of postvenography syndrome from 24 to 7.5%. In both groups, the incidence of postvenography syndrome was higher in patients who had a negative study than in patients in whom a DVT was documented. The reason for this observation is unclear. Possibly, the reduced incidence of postvenography syndrome in the patients with DVT is related to the effect of heparin, which the DVT patients received.

Arndt et al. [13] investigated the incidence of postvenography thrombophlebitis in patients who received heparin flush prior to and after venography was performed with Reno M-60. The flush consisted of 250 ml of 5% dextrose in water containing 1000 U of heparin, which was attached to the indwelling venography cannula. The infusion was begun prior to contrast injection with the patient partially upright, and continued with the patient supine after completion of the venogram. The incidence of postvenography thrombophlebitis was 4.37% in patients who did not receive the heparin flush, compared to 1.97% in patients who did receive the heparin flush.

A similar reduction in postvenography thrombophlebitis has been reported by Coel and Dodge [14] by performing the venography in a supine position. In this study, 95 ml of 76% meglumine diatrizoate (Renografin M-76, Squibb) was injected at a rate of 1–2 ml/s. Immediately after injection, the contrast media was flushed form the veins with 250–500 ml 5% dextrose in water. Using this technique, the incidence of postvenography thrombophlebitis was 1.5%. This rate is significantly lower than that reported by Bettmann and Paulin [5] (even though full-strength Reno M-76 was used instead of 75% strength Reno 60), and is lower than that reported by Arndt et al. [13] using full-strength Reno 60 but followed by heparinized flush. The reduction in postvenography thrombophlebitis is thought to be related to a decrease in the time that the contrast medium is in contact with the endothelium when compared to the semiupright positioning described by Rabinov and Paulin [1]. The lower sodium content of Renografin M-76 (0.04 mEq/ml) compared to 75% strength Renografin 60 (0.16 mEq/ml) used by Bettmann and Paulin [5] may also contribute to the diminished adverse effects reported using the supine technique.

A decrease in postvenography phlebitis has also been observed when nonionic is compared to ionic contrast. Thomas and Briggs [7] reported delayed foot and/or leg swelling in 11 out of 46 (24%) patients imaged with iopamidol (nonionic) compared to 22 out of 46 (48%) patients imaged with Conray 60 (ionic). Delayed foot swelling was noted in 4% of patients in the nonionic group, compared to 30% in the ionic group. The reduction in these symptoms is most likely related to the decreased osmolarity of iopamidol (0.574 osmol/kg H_2O) compared to Conray 60 (1.485 osmol/kg H_2O). In Western Europe, lower-osmolar media have been used, almost exclusively, for lower limb venography, over a period of several years.

Postvenographic DVT

An example of postvenographic DVT is shown in Fig. 15.1. Several studies have investigated the incidence of postvenographic DVT using the iodine-125 (^{125}I) fibrinogen uptake test. This test has been shown to be highly sensitive, but not very specific for diagnosing DVT. The ^{125}I fibrinogen test is unable to distinguish superficial from DVT. The diagnostic accuracy of the test in detecting clinically significant

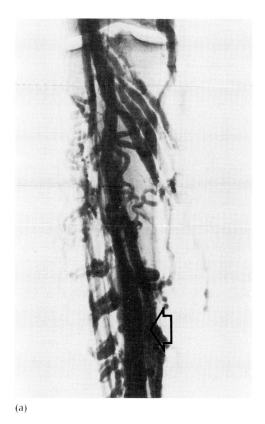

(a)

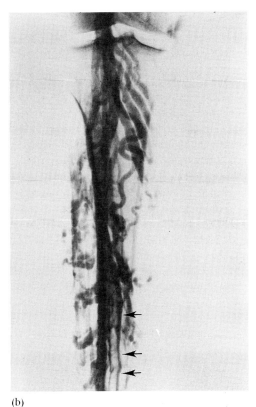

(b)

Fig. 15.1 Postvenogram DVT. A 50-year-old man presented with calf pain and swelling following a transcontinental flight. A venogram was performed (a) which failed to demonstrate any evidence of DVT. The peroneal veins are well visualized (open arrow). The patient returned 3 days later with persistent complaints. A repeat venogram (b) demonstrated new thrombus in the peroneal veins (straight arrows).

DVT is further limited by its sensitivity to intravascular fibrin deposition without gross thrombosis, extravascular, or intramural deposition of fibrin in a hematoma or inflammatory reaction, or the detection of thrombus which can not be visualized radiographically [15]. While the incidence of DVT will be less than the incidence of positive ^{125}I scans, a comparison of the positive scan rate for various contrast agents serves as a useful barometer for comparing the relative incidence of postvenographic DVT associated with these contrast agents.

Reduced concentrations of ionic contrast, nonionic contrast, and low-osmolar contrast have all been associated with a reduction in the incidence of positive ^{125}I fibrinogen uptake tests following venography. The incidence of positive ^{125}I scans for various contrast agents is given in Table 15.1. As this table indicates, reducing the concentration of ionic contrast (Renografin) from 60 to 45% significantly reduces the incidence of positive ^{125}I uptake. There is no significant difference in the incidence of positive scans between Renografin 45 (ionic), Conray 43 (ionic), and nonionic

iopamidol. The use of low-osmolar Hexabrix results in a further reduction in the incidence of positive scans.

A 13.3% incidence of positive ^{125}I scans has been reported by Minar *et al.* [17] using the ionic contrast methylglucamine iodamide (Uromiro 300; 300 mg I/ml, 65%, 1590 mosmol/kg H_2O). This has been achieved by immediately flushing the veins with 100 ml of physiologic saline containing 10 000 IU of heparin. This concentration of heparin is 10 times greater than that used by Arndt *et al.* [13] and yields a positive scan rate similar to that achieved with either ionic contrast of lower concentration, nonionic, or low-osmolar contrast.

Table 15.1 The incidence of positive ^{125}I scans for various contrast agents

Contrast	Positive ^{125}I uptake (%)	Reference
Renografin 60 (ionic)	39	[6]
Renografin 45 (ionic)	9	[6]
Conray 43 (ionic)	10	[6]
Iopamidol (nonionic, low osmolar)	10	[6]
Hexabrix (ionic, low osmolar)	3.3	[16]
Uromiro (ionic, followed by heparin flush)	13.3	[17]

Contrast extravasation

Extravasation of contrast medium at the puncture site is a common complication (Fig. 15.2) which can cause a chemical cellulitis accompanied by acute pain, swelling, and skin changes such as bullae. Soft tissue or skin necrosis, sloughing, and gangrene may rarely follow, particularly if the circulation is impaired [18]. Extravasation of contrast at the venopuncture site can be minimized by frequent fluoroscopy of the site during contrast injection. If any extravasation is noted the injection should be immediately terminated. Any complaints of pain at the venopuncture site or generalized foot discomfort should be evaluated immediately by the radiologist. An increased risk of contrast extravasation is associated with: (i) injections over the dorsum of the foot or ankle; (ii) multiple punctures of the same vein; (iii) prolonged placement of a tourniquet; (iv) injection peripheral to a tourniquet [19]; (v) injection through metal needles (as compared to plastic sheaths); and (vi) excessively forcible injections.

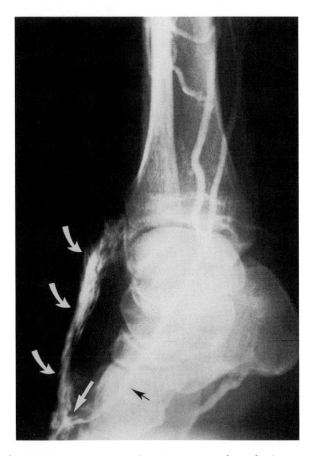

Fig. 15.2 Contrast extravasation. Venogram performed using a 19-gage butterfly needle inserted in an antegrade fashion. The tip of the needle (straight white arrow) has become dislodged from the vein (straight black arrow) resulting in extravasation of contrast material into the soft tissues of the dorsum of the foot (curved arrows).

If contrast extravasation has occurred, recommended treatment includes massage to dissipate the contrast medium, application of warm compress, foot elevation to accelerate absorption of extravascular contrast medium, and occasionally, immobilization [12]. Some authors advocate injection of hyaluronidase into the area of extravasation [20], in order to break down the affected connective tissue and promote absorption of the extravasated contrast. However, in another study [21], injection of hyaluronidase has been found markedly to increase the amount of inflammation, necrosis, and scarring. Currently, the local administration of hyaluronidase for the treatment of contrast extravasation remains controversial. The efficacy of other interventions such as administration of local steroids, or infiltration with procaine, isoproterenol, or propranolol have not been proven. Full demarcation of the injured site may take several days [21]. Once an ulcer appears, early and aggressive surgical debridement has been shown to relieve pain and functional impairment and to promote healing. Split-thickness skin grafts or skin and/or muscle flaps may eventually be necessary [21]. Water-soluble contrast medium of larger volume, higher osmolarity, higher iodine content, and meglumine salts rather than sodium salts have been shown to cause more severe tissue damage [22]. The risk of tissue damage is decreased with lower osmolar media [18] (see also pp. 249, 569).

PE

Although PE is a very rare complication of lower extremity venography (Fig. 15.3), it has been reported [23–25]. It is therefore important to avoid any active or passive maneuvers that might dislodge fresh thrombi, such as muscle exercise, massaging or milking the calf or thigh muscles, or direct groin compression prior to obtaining films of the extremity, iliac veins, and inferior vena cava [26]. If DVT is seen on the film, the patient should not actively contract his/her calf during the heparinized flush nor should the leg be massaged.

Descending venography

Descending venography is performed for evaluation of patients with primary varicose veins or chronic venous insufficiency, and for determination of the site of incompetence of venous valves of the lower limb [27,28]. The common femoral vein is catheterized using a 4 or 5-F catheter. With the table elevated 45–60°, contrast medium is slowly injected into the iliac or femoral vein under fluoroscopic observation. During normal respiration, spot films are obtained over the iliofemoral region, thigh, and leg. Complications involving descending venography are usually related to femoral vein puncture, including hematoma, thrombosis of the femoral vein, and arteriovenous fistula formation. Hematoma at the groin is uncommon and is usually small and self-limited. Femoral vein thrombosis can

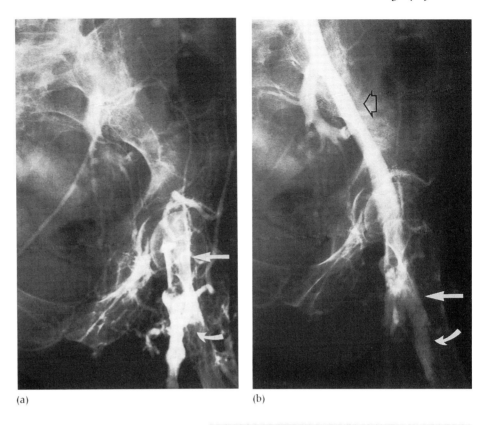

(a)　　　　　　　　　　　(b)

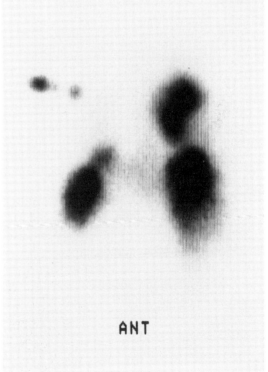

Fig. 15.3 Femoral vein DVT causing PE during venography. Two films of the femoral region performed 25-seconds apart during an ascending venogram. (a) This demonstrates extensive DVT in the common femoral (straight arrow) and superficial femoral (curved arrow) veins. The external iliac vein is not filled. A second film exposed 25-seconds later (b), demonstrates almost complete filling of the superficial femoral (curved arrow), common femoral (straight arrow), and external iliac veins (open arrow). Immediately following the second film, the patient sustained a complete cardiopulmonary arrest. A perfusion scan (c) showed multiple, bilateral perfusion defects consistent with PE. (From Montgomery [23].)

(c)

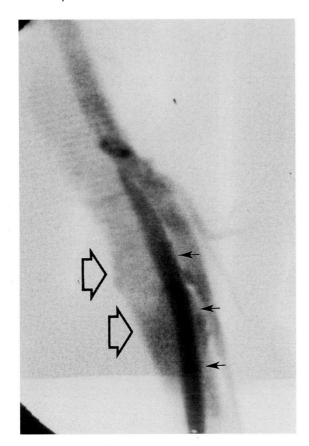

Fig. 15.4 Arteriovenous fistula following descending venogram. Arteriogram performed from a contralateral femoral artery approach. The common femoral vein (open arrows) is opacified at the same time as the superficial femoral artery (straight arrows) indicating the presence of an arteriovenous fistula.

occur, but is also uncommon. Arteriovenous fistula can occur (Fig. 15.4) as in other venous catheterizations, especially with lower puncture of the femoral vein [29–31].

Conclusion

Complications of ascending lower extremity venography include complications related to the systemic effects of contrast medium, the local effects of the contrast medium on the venous endothelium, and complications associated with extravasation of contrast medium into the soft tissues of the foot. The use of low-osmolar, nonionic, or dilute ionic contrast can reduce the incidence of many of these complications. Complications associated with descending lower extremity venography are usually related to the femoral vein puncture. The incidence of most of these complications can be reduced by paying strict attention to any complaints of pain or discomfort reported by the patient during the venogram.

References

1 Rabinov K, Paulin S. Roentgen diagnosis of venous thrombosis in the leg. *Arch Surg* 1972;104:134–144.

2 Cronan JJ, Dorfman GS, Scola FH, Schepps B, Alexander J. Deep venous thrombosis: US assessment using vein compression. *Radiology* 1987;162:191–194.

3 Rose SC, Zwiebel WJ, Nelson B *et al.* Symptomatic lower extremity deep venous thrombosis: accuracy, limitations, and role of color duplex flow imaging in diagnosis. *Radiology* 1990;175:639–644.

4 Cronan JJ, Leen V. Recurrent deep venous thrombosis: limitations of US. *Radiology* 1989;170:739–742.

5 Bettmann MA, Paulin S. Leg phlebography: the incidence, nature and modification of undesirable side effects. *Radiology* 1977;122:101–104.

6 Bettmann MA, Robbins A, Braun SD, Wetzner S, Dunnick NR, Finkelstein J. Contrast venography of the leg: diagnostic efficacy, tolerance, and complication rates with ionic and nonionic contrast media. *Radiology* 1987;165:113–116.

7 Thomas ML, Briggs GM. Comparison of triiodoisophthaldiamide with meglumine iothalamate in phlebography of the leg. *Am J Roentgenol* 1982;138:725–727.

8 Silverbach S. The use of Xylocaine to diminish leg cramps in venography. *Radiology* 1979;133:788–789.

9 Nilsson P, Ahmén T, Golman K *et al.* Addition of local anesthetics to contrast media. II. Increase of acute mortality in mice with intravenous contrast administration. *Acta Radiol (Diagn)* 1988;29:247–250.

10 Sommer FG, Laglia A, Goldberg RT. Pain accompanying leg venography: a comparison of sodium and methylglucamine diatrizoates. *Radiology* 1979;133:790–791.

11 Thomas ML. Phlebography. *Arch Surg* 1972;104:145.

12 Kim D, Orron DE, Porter DH. *Venographic Anatomy, Technique and Interpretation. Peripheral Vascular Imaging and Intervention.* St Louis: Mosby-Year Book, Inc, 1992.

13 Arndt RD, Grolman JH, Gomes AS, Bos CJ. The heparin flush: an aid in preventing post-venography thrombophlebitis. *Radiology* 1979;130:249–250.

14 Coel MN, Dodge W. Complication rate with supine phlebography. *Am J Roentgenol* 1978;131:821–822.

15 Bettmann MA, Saltzman EW, Rosenthal D *et al.* Reduction of thrombosis complicating phlebography. *Am J Roentgenol* 1990;134:1169–1172.

16 Thomas ML, Briggs GM, Kuan BB. Contrast agent-induced thrombophlebitis following leg phlebography: meglumine ioxaglate versus meglumine iothalamate. *Radiology* 1983;147:399–400.

17 Minar E, Ehringer H, Sommer G, Marosi L, Czembirek H. Prevention of postvenographic thrombosis by heparin flush: fibrin uptake measurements. *Am J Roentgenol* 1984;143:629–632.

18 Thomas ML. Phlebography. In: Ansell G, Wilkins RA, eds. *Complications in Diagnostic Imaging,* 2nd edn. Oxford: Blackwell Scientific Publications Ltd., 1987:288–299.

19 Coulthard A. Gangrene of the foot following peripheral phlebography [letter; comment]. *J Roy Coll Surg Edin* 1992;37:137.

20 Spigos DG, Thane TT, Capek V. Skin necrosis following extravasation during peripheral phlebography. *Radiology* 1977;123:605–606.

21 Cohan RH, Dunnick NR, Bashore TM. Treatment of reaction to radiographic contrast material. *Am J Roentgenol* 1988;151: 263−270.

22 Kim SH, Pary JH, Kim YI, Kim CW, Han MC. Experimental tissue damage after subcutaneous injection of water soluble contrast media. *Invest Radiol* 1990;25:678−685.

23 Montgomery S. Pulmonary embolism during venography: report of a rare complication. *Cardiovasc Intervent Radiol* 1989;12: 196−198.

24 Zeitler E, Milbert L, Richter EI *et al*. Special complications in leg phlebography. *ROFO Fortschr Geb Rontgenstr Nuklearmed* 1983; 138:670−677.

25 Werner HL, Clemson J, Browse NL *et al*. Hazards and complications in roentgenological venous diagnosis. *Fortschr Roentgenstr* 1962;96:655−665.

26 Thomas ML. *Phlebography of the Lower Limb*. Edinburgh: Churchill Livingstone, 1982.

27 Kistner RL, Ferris EB, Randhawa G, Kamida C. A method of performing descending venography. *J Vasc Surg* 1986;4: 464−468.

28 Morano JU, Raju S. Chronic venous insufficiency: assessment with descending venography. *Radiology* 1990;174:441 444.

29 Grassi CJ, Bettmann MA, Rogoff P *et al*. Femoral arteriovenous fistula after placement of a Kimray-Greenfield filter. *Am J Roentgenol* 1988;151:682.

30 Heystraten FMJ, Fast JH. Ateriovenous fistula as a complication of the Seldinger procedure of the femoral artery and vein. *Diagn Imaging* 1983;52:197−201.

31 Altin RS, Flicker S, Naideck HJ. Pseudoaneurysm and arteriovenous fistula after femoral artery catheterization: associated with low femoral puncture. *Am J Roentgenol* 1989;152:629−631.

CHAPTER 16

Complications of pulmonary angiography

Maurice John Raphael

Definition

Pulmonary angiography may be defined as the opacification of the pulmonary arteries, capillaries, and veins with radiopaque contrast medium and their visualization by plane radiographic techniques as opposed to the cross-sectional imaging techniques of computed tomography (CT) scanning. The subject and its history have been well reviewed by Goodman [1]. The most common indication for the performance of pulmonary angiography appears to be for the visualization of the pulmonary arteries for suspected pulmonary thromboembolic disease [2]. As the largest series of pulmonary angiograms concern pulmonary thromboembolic disease [3,4], it seems reasonable to consider the complications that might be encountered in this area in considerable detail, and to consider the other applications, for which, in general, there is no particular hazard, afterwards.

Thromboembolic disease [5]

Three clinical syndromes are recognized:
1 acute massive pulmonary embolism;
2 subacute pulmonary embolism;
3 chronic thromboembolic large vessel pulmonary hypertension.
Isotope lung scanning has a differing role in each of these three conditions.

Acute massive pulmonary embolism

The patient usually has an appropriate clinical history of previous surgery, immobility, or oral contraception. Evidence of deep vein venous thrombosis in the legs will often be lacking. Presentation is usually with circulatory collapse which may be severe or fatal, although often with premonitory emboli. The cause is usually embolization of large thrombus, originating from the larger veins of the thigh or more proximal veins of the pelvis or abdomen. When the diagnosis is suspected, it is usually quicker to mobilize the X-ray department for pulmonary angiography, which will give a decisive answer, rather than attempting to obtain an isotope scan, particularly if the episode occurs out of working hours.

Subacute pulmonary embolism

The progressive arrival of smaller emboli in the lungs may produce attacks of shortness of breath, chest pain, and even hemoptysis with no diagnostic physical signs. There may be no useful history or evidence of deep venous thrombosis. The isotope lung scan is less helpful than might be thought as the majority of patients have chronic lung disease or are smokers and have frequent perfusion abnormalities. It is in this group that the most careful pulmonary angiography must be performed.

Chronic thromboembolic pulmonary hypertension

These patients present with shortness of breath and have the physical signs of pulmonary hypertension. All such patients should have a perfusion lung scan. This will be normal in those patients with small vessel disease who are treated medically, but the perfusion lung scan will show gross abnormalities of perfusion in those patients with large vessel abnormalities who may be amenable to surgical thrombo-endarterectomy [6]. Such patients should proceed to pulmonary angiography for surgical evaluation. In this group, pulmonary angiography may be technically difficult as there is often tricuspid incompetence and a large right atrium, and also dangerous because of the severe pulmonary arterial hypertension and the hemodynamic effects of the contrast medium.

Angiographic technique

Angiography is indicated when the isotope study, if available, is nondiagnostic [7]. A normal isotope scan virtually excludes the diagnosis of pulmonary embolism [8], a "high probability scan" will detect 90% of patients with pulmonary embolism. Between 40 and 70% of scans will be nondiagnostic and may need to proceed to pulmonary angiography. A variety of imaging techniques have been applied. Large-film format using a film changer seems to be the most popular [3,4] (but, Bell and Simon [9] noted that of 176 supposedly positive angiograms submitted for study, a panel found no evidence of pulmonary embolism in five, and disagreed in 11, giving a significant error rate for the basic examination). Cine-filming and photospot techniques [2] have been advocated either as the primary imaging technique, or as a supplement to large films.

Digital subtraction (DSA) [10] is not considered sufficiently accurate to diagnose small emboli. Recently, direct digital imaging has become available and I feel that this will become the definitive investigation. Magnification angiography, up to three times, using a fine focal-spot tube, has been advocated for detecting very small pulmonary emboli [11]. Elegant pictures are produced, but the majority of workers do not find it necessary to utilize magnification techniques to diagnose or exclude pulmonary emboli. Careful selective angiography [12], guided by isotope scanning, will usually suffice to detect any clinically significant pulmonary emboli.

With wedged pulmonary angiography, very small vessels, almost down to pulmonary arterioles, may be resolved and the pulmonary veins opacified [13]. The technique has little role in the investigation of pulmonary thromboembolic disease, and has been less helpful than hoped in the study of pulmonary vascular disease secondary to heart disease. The danger of overinjection rupturing vessels has also to be considered [13].

In congenital heart disease, when congenital or acquired pulmonary atresia prevents direct access to the pulmonary arteries, they may be opacified by retrograde injection of contrast through catheters wedged in the pulmonary veins [14].

Pulmonary angiography

Pulmonary angiography, as currently performed, requires:
1 the introduction of a catheter into the systemic venous circulation;
2 its passage through the heart to the pulmonary arteries — venous or right atrial injections, as well as not permitting hemodynamic measurements, produce inadequate studies [15];
3 the injection of radiopaque contrast medium.
Complications may relate to each of these three phases of the procedure (Table 16.1).

Venous access

Currently [4], percutaneous catheterization of the femoral vein is the preferred route of venous access. The standard technique may be used for open-ended catheters, or a venous sheath may be used for blocked-end catheter access. Relative contraindications to the use of the femoral vein are the presence of groin scars following surgery, iliac vein occlusion, or thrombus in the iliac vein or inferior vena cava [2]. On puncturing the femoral vein it is wise to make a test injection of contrast medium and confirm that the iliac veins are clear, and after introducing the catheter, make a further test injection to make sure the vena cava is clear [17]. There does not appear to be any significant risk of detachment of thrombus and subsequent embolization if the femoral vein approach is utilized. The percutaneous technique can also be used on antecubital veins with the availability of 5-F or smaller catheters. The lypophilic wires, now available, reduce the incidence of venospasm and also allow the utilization of laterally running veins, as with these wires it is almost invariable to reach the heart via the cephalic vein. The majority of older work utilized the vein of the elbow, which was dissected out and the catheter introduced by venotomy, the vein being tied afterwards [18]. To some degree, the choice of venous access is governed by the inclination of the operator, but if the patient has a large right atrium, an arm approach, and even preferably from the left arm, gives a better natural curve to the pulmonary artery and might be considered. Major hemorrhage as a complication of venous access is excessively rare, occurring in only one anticoagulated patient of 1111 patients who had pulmonary angiography [4]. Phlebitis appears even rarer. Problems with puncturing the femoral artery inadvertently while attempting to puncture the femoral vein are not recorded, even in the patients that are anticoagulated. In only three of 1114 patients did venous access fail [4].

Complications of right heart catheterization

Although this area is covered in other parts of this book, it is

Table 16.1 Complications of pulmonary angiography

Number of patients	Deaths	Respiratory distress	Arrhythmias	Angina	Contrast reaction	Cardiac perforations	Bleeding	Miscellaneous	Reference
1350	3	CPR catheter induced 5	11 severe		11	14*	3	14†	Mills *et al.* [3]
1434‡	2§	10 / 5 CPR	15 severe	3	Unknown				Perlmutt *et al.* [16]
1114¶	5**	8 / 4 CPR	6	2 CCU	16	0	2††	19‡‡	Stein *et al.* [4]

* One aspirated.

† No sequelae.

‡ Includes 388 patients with severe pulmonary hypertension.

§ All patients had severe pulmonary hypertension. Death followed the contrast injection.

¶ Includes three patients without venous access and eight patients in whom pulmonary angiography was not successful.

** Two patients died before angiography, and in three the authors felt that the cause of death was the severity of the underlying disease rather than the procedure.

†† Required transfusion.

‡‡ Includes 13 patients who developed renal impairment, of whom three required dialysis, four patients developed pulmonary congestion, and two hypotension, all managed conservatively.

CCU, required transfer to coronary care unit; CPR, required cardiopulmonary resuscitation.

appropriate to make some reference to it in this section. Complications to be anticipated are the production of cardiac arrhythmias as the catheter passes through the heart, and perforation of the heart [3]. Ventricular ectopic beats, as the catheter passes through the tricuspid valve and into the right ventricle, are rarely sufficiently sustained to lead to hemodynamic deterioration and can usually be controlled by repositioning the catheter. Catheter manipulations within the right atrium may precipitate atrial fibrillation [15]. If this does not revert immediately, it may require active management. Passage through the right ventricle may initiate ventricular tachycardia or fibrillation, particularly in patients with a compromised circulation, and clearly requires defibrillation. In the urokinase–pulmonary embolism trial (U–PET) [18] study there were five episodes of ventricular arrhythmias which required treatment in 310 angiograms, but no deaths or residual disability.

Perforation of the heart by the catheter, either during manipulation through the heart, or by catheter recoil during powered contrast injection, has been identified as a not infrequent complication of the procedure. Cardiac perforation was identified as a complication of pulmonary angiography; once in 310 cases [18] in 1973, and in 1% of studies [3] in 1980, but with no clinical sequelae noted. The one death in 176 patients noted by Bell and Simon [9] occurred in a patient with cardiomyopathy who died of probable tamponade 3 days after perforation. The complication of perforation prompted the abandonment of standard curve open-ended catheters by Mills *et al.* [3] who confined the use of the NIH (blocked end, side holes only) catheter to the arm approach, and preferred a Grollman [19] catheter from the

femoral vein. Use of the Grollman catheter or a standard pigtail catheter [20], while it may lower the risk of myocardial perforation as compared to a standard curved catheter, may still precipitate serious arrhythmias, and limits the degree of selectivity of the pulmonary angiogram to simple right and left pulmonary artery injections. This would be clearly adequate for massive central pulmonary embolism, but is quite unsatisfactory for the selective pulmonary angiography needed to pursue equivocal lung scans [21]. Perforation should clearly be avoided, or identified promptly, if thrombolytic therapy is to follow angiography [22].

When cardiac perforation leads to tamponade, there is deterioration in the patient's condition with the development of chest pain and (further ?) shortness of breath. The physical signs are: (i) a falling systemic blood pressure; (ii) a rising pulse rate; and (iii) a rising systemic venous pressure. Pulsus paradoxus, a fall in blood pressure during inspiration, may be present. Fluoroscopy may reveal the pericardial collection if there is sufficient epicardial fat to outline the heart beating within the fluid-filled pericardium. If the right atrial wall is displaced away from the pericardium by blood, the position of the catheter, or a right atrial contrast injection may be helpful, but can be confusing if contrast is inadvertently injected into either of the great veins and streaming makes the soft tissue gap appear large. Even echocardiography may mislead unless a comprehensive evaluation is done, as serious pericardial hematomas may be localized to only part of the pericardium. Urgent aspiration may be required, preferably by fluoroscopic and ultrasound control with the exploring needle attached to an electrocardiography (EKG) display (see also pp. 286, 339).

Rather limited pulmonary angiography may now be performed using a flow-guided float catheter, such as the Berman, which has an inflatable balloon at its tip with a lumen suitable for angiography, although at low flow rates.

Contrast injection

The contrast injection in pulmonary angiography may present a number of serious problems. The hemodynamic effects of radiopaque contrast medium of both the traditional high-osmolar contrast agents and the new nonionic low-osmolar agents are similar but markedly lesser in the latter group [23]. Contrast injection into the pulmonary artery produces, in general, a rise in pulmonary artery pressure for which no proper explanation is available, although promotion of rouleaux formation [24], aggregation of red cells [25], or even disaggregation [26], or an increase in red cell rigidity [27] may produce a transient increase in resistance to flow through the pulmonary circulation. Of the available contrast agents, the ionic but low-osmolar preparations produce the least effect on blood viscosity experimentally [28], but the clinical significance of such observations is unclear. When injected into one pulmonary artery in patients with basically normal pulmonary circulations, nonionic contrast media produced significantly less rise in both systolic and diastolic pulmonary artery pressures, and quicker recovery times than ionic agents [29] (see also p. 261).

Following arrival in the systemic circulation, passage of contrast into the coronary arteries [24] produces an impairment of contractility and may also produce bradycardia. Arrival in the peripheral arterioles produces vasodilatation, and this combined with the impairment of myocardial contractility leads to a fall in systemic blood pressure. After an interval, contrast-induced hemodilution leads to an increase in cardiac output. Pulmonary arteriography is associated with a transient rise in pulmonary artery pressure and a significant fall in systemic blood pressure.

The three deaths out of 1350 pulmonary angiograms noted by Mills *et al.* [3] all had severe pulmonary hypertension, and all died following a marked fall in systemic blood pressure associated with bradycardia following contrast injection. Perlmutt *et al.* [16] noted that 388 of 1434 patients having pulmonary angiography had significant pulmonary hypertension, and 82 had right ventricular dysfunction as indicated by right ventricular end-diastolic pressure of 20 mmHg or greater. Two deaths occurred in patients with severe pulmonary hypertension and moderate right ventricular dysfunction. This paper seemed to reinforce the suggestion that pulmonary arteriography carried a significantly higher risk of death in patients with significant pulmonary hypertension and right ventricular dysfunction, than in those without. The levels of pulmonary arterial hypertension considered in this paper were more those that occur in chronic pulmonary hypertension than the rises seen in

acute pulmonary embolism, but the case mix is not specified. Caldini *et al.* [30] in 1959 recorded a death during pulmonary angiography and, in reviewing the literature, noted that death appeared much more common when right heart catheterization was carried out in the presence of pulmonary hypertension, than in its absence, and may occur even before contrast was injected. Snider *et al.* [31] reporting a death in 1973, speculated on the mechanism of death following contrast injection in the presence of pulmonary hypertension. Keane *et al.* [32] called attention to the dangers of performing cardiac catheterization and pulmonary angiography in children with primary pulmonary vascular obstruction and concluded that it was: "an unusually hazardous, often fatal, undertaking". It might thus be concluded that pulmonary arteriography is more hazardous in chronic pulmonary hypertension when the pressure is markedly raised, than in acute pulmonary hypertension, secondary to acute massive pulmonary embolism. In contrast to these gloomy reports, Nicod *et al.* [33] reviewed the safety of angiography in 67 consecutive patients with moderate to severe primary pulmonary hypertension, or hypertension secondary to chronic thromboembolic occlusions of the pulmonary arteries. They encountered no deaths, major rhythm disturbances, or systemic hypotension requiring therapy. They concluded that pulmonary angiography could be done safely despite the presence of severe pulmonary hypertension and right ventricular failure.

Contrast injections may also damage the lung directly when the catheter tip of a nonpigtail catheter is too distal during power injection. The whole injected segment may show an intense persisting contrast blush, associated with coughing, but this rarely proceeds to lung infarction, usually clearing over minutes. It can be difficult, using standard catheters, to position the tip to avoid recoil, even with blocked-end catheters, from left or right pulmonary arteries into the main, or even the right ventricle. If the catheter is too far in, there is a risk of lung damage; if not far enough, the risk of recoil and poor pictures, or even right ventricular damage.

Mortality

Stein *et al.* [4] encountered five deaths in 1111 patients with angiography performed or attempted for acute pulmonary embolism. They doubted whether three of the five deaths could be attributed to the catheterization procedure or pulmonary angiography in the presence of severe underlying cardiac or respiratory disease. They attributed most of their deaths and major complications to the severity of the underlying disease and indeed commented that only four of 11 patients with major complications actually had pulmonary embolism. Moses *et al.* [34] noted two deaths shortly after injection in patients with greater than 95% vascular bed obstruction out of their 298 patients with pulmonary embolism, and related mortality to the severity of vascular obstruction. Although it is clear that in the majority of patients with severe pulmonary hypertension pulmonary angiography may be performed safely, it is also clear that in a number of the reported deaths it is the injection of the contrast medium that precipitates the fatal event, and this is initiated by a fall in systemic blood pressure.

The mechanism of death is not agreed, although most authors have noted a rise in pulmonary artery pressure after contrast injection. It may be, however, that as patients with severe pulmonary hypertension cannot easily increase their cardiac output, the fall in blood pressure due to systemic vasodilatation as the contrast arrives in the systemic circulation can not be compensated for by an increase in cardiac output. This would impair coronary perfusion and depress ventricular contractility, leading to a further fall in blood pressure and a vicious circle of falling blood pressure and falling cardiac output results. It would thus seem prudent to be prepared to keep the blood pressure up if it should fall following the contrast injection. I prefer to monitor the systemic blood pressure closely rather than the pulmonary artery pressure, to have an intravenous infusion running, and to have the correct pressor agent, phenylephrine, readily available. This is the correct agent on theoretical grounds but there is no published information on its efficacy. On theoretical grounds the use of the low-osmolar or nonionic contrast agents might not only improve patient comfort but also improve safety. No large series has compared the safety of the two groups of agents in a control trial, but Saeed *et al.* [35] noted that patient comfort was greater and coughing less with a nonionic contrast agent. They discovered no significant hemodynamic differences between ionic and nonionic agents in a relatively small group comparing the two.

Contrast reactions

Mills *et al.* [3] noted 11 contrast reactions in their 1350 pulmonary angiograms. Eleven of these were urticaria, two were laryngeal edema, one transient hypertension, and one asthma. There were no sequelae to these contrast reactions. Stein *et al.* [4] had 16 examples of urticaria, itching, or periorbital edema in their 1111 patients, but curiously enough only one example of nausea and vomiting. Thus, allergic contrast reactions in pulmonary angiography appear infrequent and relatively easily managed by straightforward measures. In patients with a known sensitivity to contrast media, I would use a nonionic or low-osmolar preparation and also pretreat with steroids [36] (see also p. 263).

Renal function

Curiously enough, only Stein *et al.* [4] make specific comment on the problem of renal impairment induced by the contrast material, particularly in elderly patients. Their study, using ionic high-osmolar contrast agents, shows 10 out of 1111 patients developed some evidence of renal impairment, including three requiring dialysis, although all reverted to their previous status.

Miscellaneous

Stein *et al.* [4] had four patients with sufficiently severe respiratory distress to require cardiopulmonary resuscitation or intubation, two patients with pulmonary congestion responding to drugs, and two with hypotension responding to drugs and fluid. Two developed angina requiring monitoring. There were nine hematomas that did not require transfusion and two that did. Six patients developed an arrhythmia that reverted spontaneously or responded promptly to drug treatment.

Comment

As might be expected, the mortality and morbidity of pulmonary angiography depend far more on the cases being investigated than on the procedure itself. Mortality and morbidity will be high in the very elderly and in the very ill, even if the illness is not due to pulmonary arterial disease. Mortality and morbidity will be higher in patients with severe pulmonary vascular disease, whether it be acute massive pulmonary embolism with clinical shock or chronic severe pulmonary vascular disease with severe pulmonary hypertension and right ventricular impairment. Taken overall, the procedure carries about a 0.5% mortality on best current figures: nonfatal complications of varying severity probably occur in 10 times that number at around 5%.

Similar risks are probably present during the injection of contrast medium into the pulmonary arteries in patients with pulmonary hypertension secondary to congenital heart disease, particularly those with the Eisenmenger reaction to a high-pressure left to right shunt. It seems likely that the mechanism is similar to that provoking death in patients with acquired pulmonary hypertension on the basis of thromboembolic disease.

In theory, the use of low-osmolar or nonionic contrast agents should not only improve patient comfort and reduce coughing but should also reduce mortality and morbidity in pulmonary hypertension. Cumberland [37] felt that the use of a low-osmolar agent in a patient with pulmonary hypertension secondary to congenital heart disease led to a much lower rise in pulmonary artery pressure than a high-osmolar ionic agent, and advised its use in patients with severe pulmonary hypertension, but there are no controlled trials to confirm this.

Other indications for pulmonary angiography

Acquired lesions

Pulmonary angiography may also be used for a variety of primarily vascular abnormalities of the pulmonary circulation such as pulmonary arteriovenous fistulae [38] and aneurysms [39]. Of lung lesions, sequestrated segment and its more complex variant, the Scimitar syndrome [40], might be encountered. Pulmonary angiography is rarely indicated in the investigation of pulmonary tumors, either to show intrinsic circulation, obstruction of pulmonary vessels, or bleed. In many of these lesions, pulmonary angiography is performed prior to a potentially hazardous intervention [41].

Lesions usually associated with congenital heart disease

Peripheral pulmonary artery stenoses, congenital absences of one pulmonary artery, and pulmonary arterial communication to the right atrium, together with the even more complex malformations associated with congenital pulmonary atresia [42], are usually considered in the remit of the pediatric cardiologist rather than the general radiologist.

References

1 Goodman PC. Pulmonary angiography. *Clin Chest Med* 1984;5: 465−477.
2 Gomes AS. Pulmonary angiography. In: Marcus ML, Schelbert HR, Skorton DJ, Wolf GL, eds. *Cardiac Imaging. A Companion to Braunwald's Heart Disease.* Philadelphia: WB Saunders, 1991: 149−161.
3 Mills ST, Jackson DC, Older RA, Heaston DK, Moore AV. The incidence, etiologies and avoidance of complications of pulmonary angiography in a large series. *Radiology* 1980;136:295−299.
4 Stein PD, Athanasoulis C, Alavi A *et al.* Complications and validity of pulmonary angiography in acute pulmonary embolism. *Circulation* 1992;85:462−468.
5 Raphael MJ. Pulmonary angiography. *Br J Hosp Med* 1970;3: 377−389.
6 Auger WR, Fedullo PF, Moser KM, Buchbinder M, Petersion KL. Chronic major vessel thromboembolic pulmonary artery obstruction appearance at angiography. *Radiology* 1992;182:393−398.
7 Morrell NW, Seed WA. Diagnosing pulmonary embolism. Editorial. *Br Med J* 1992;304:1126−1127.
8 Kipper MS, Moser KM, Kortman KE, Ashburn WL. Long-term follow-up of patients with suspected pulmonary embolism and a normal lung scan perfusion scans in embolic suspects. *Chest* 1982;82:411−415.
9 Bell WR, Simon TL. A comparative analysis of pulmonary perfusion scans with pulmonary angiograms. *Am Heart J* 1976;92: 700−706.
10 Musset D, Rosso J, Petitpretz P *et al.* Acute pulmonary embolism: diagnostic value of digital subtraction angiography. *Radiology* 1988;166:455−459.
11 Greenspan RH, Simon AL, Ricketts HJ, Rojas RH, Watson JC. *In vivo* magnification angiography. *Invest Radiol* 1967;2:419.
12 Bookstein JJ. Segmental arteriography in pulmonary embolism. *Radiology* 1969;93:1007−1012.
13 Raphael MJ. *Flow patterns in the pulmonary veins of man: studied by the technique of wedged pulmonary angiography.* MD thesis, University of Cambridge, 1971.
14 Nihil MR, Mullins CE, McNamara DG. Visualisation of pulmonary arteries in pseudotruncus by pulmonary vein wedge angiography. *Circulation* 1978;58:140.
15 Dalen JE, Brooks HL, Johnson LW, Meister SG, Szucs MM, Dexter L. Pulmonary angiography in acute pulmonary embolism: indications, techniques, and results in 367 patients. *Am Heart J* 1971;81:175−185.
16 Perlmutt LM, Braum SD, Newman GE, Oke EJ, Dunnick NR. Pulmonary arteriography in the high risk patient. *Radiology* 1987;162:187−189.
17 Alderson PO, Martin EC. Pulmonary embolism: diagnosis with multiple imaging modalities. *Radiology* 1987;164:297−312.
18 U-PET. Urokinase−Pulmonary Embolism Trial. *Circulation* 1973; 47 (Suppl. 2):38−45.
19 Grollman JH, Gyepes MT, Helmer E. Transfemoral selective bilateral pulmonary arteriography with a pulmonary-artery-seeking catheter. *Radiology* 1970;96:202−204.
20 Green GS. Use of the pigtail catheter for pulmonary angiography. *Radiology* 1980;136:744.
21 Novelline RA, Balterowich AH, Athanasoulis CA, Waltman AC, Greenfield AJ, McKusick KA. The clinical course of patients with suspected pulmonary embolism and a negative pulmonary arteriogram. *Radiology* 1978;126:561−567.
22 Meyerovitz MF. How to maximize the safety of coronary and pulmonary angiography in patients receiving thrombolytic therapy. *Chest* 1990;97:132S−135S.
23 Raphael MJ, Donaldson RB. *Contrast Media.* Edinburgh: Churchill Livingstone, 1988:97−103.
24 Fischer HW. Hemodynamic reactions to angiographic media: a survey and commentary. *Radiology* 1968;91:66−73.
25 Read R, Meyer M. The role of red cell agglutination in arteriographic complications. *Surg Forum* 1959;10:472.
26 Aspelin P, Schmid-Schonbein H. Effect of ionic and non-ionic contrast media on red cell aggregation *in vitro. Acta Radiol Diagn* 1978;19:766−784.
27 Dawson P, Harrison MJG, Weisblatt E. Effect of contrast media on red cell filtrability and morphology. *Br J Radiol* 1983;56: 707−710.
28 Strickland NH, Rampling MW, Dawson P, Martin G. Contrast media-induced effects on blood rheology and their importance in angiography. *Clin Radiol* 1992;45:240−242.
29 Tajima H, Kumazaki T, Tajima N, Ebata K. Effect of iohexol and diatrizoate on pulmonary arterial pressure following pulmonary angiography. *Acta Radiol Scand Diagn* 1988;29:487−490.
30 Caldini P, Gensini GG, Hoffman MS. Primary pulmonary hypertension with death during right heart catheterisation. *Am J Cardiol* 1959;4:519−527.
31 Snider GL, Ferris E, Gaensler EA *et al.* Primary pulmonary hypertension: a fatality during pulmonary angiography. *Chest* 1973;64:628−635.
32 Keane JF, Fyler DC, Nadas AS. Hazards of cardiac catheterisation in children with primary pulmonary vascular obstruction. *Am Heart J* 1978;96:556−558.
33 Nicod P, Peterson K, Levine M *et al.* Pulmonary angiography in

severe chronic pulmonary hypertension. *Ann Int Med* 1987;107: 565–568.

34 Moses DC, Silver TM, Bookstein JJ. The complementary roles of chest radiography, lung scanning and selective pulmonary angiography in the diagnosis of pulmonary embolism. *Circulation* 1974;69:179–188.

35 Saeed M, Braun SD, Cohan RH *et al.* Pulmonary angiography with Iopamidol: patient comfort, image quality and hemodynamics. *Radiology* 1987;165:345–349.

36 Reidy JF. Reactions to contrast media and steroid pretreatment. *Br Med J* 1988;296:809–810.

37 Cumberland DC. Hexabrix — a new contrast in angiocardiography. *Br Heart J* 1981;45:698–702.

38 Dines DE, Arms RA, Bernatz PE, Gomes MR. Pulmonary arteriovenous fistulas. *Mayo Clin Proc* 1974;49:460–465.

39 Guttentag AR, Shepard JO, McLoud TC. Catheter-induced pulmonary artery pseudoaneurysm: the halo sign on CT. *Am J Roentgenol* 1992;158:637.

40 Folger GM. The scimitar syndrome. *Angiology* 1976;27:373–407.

41 Remy-Jardin M, Wattinne L, Remy J. Transcatheter occlusion of pulmonary arterial circulation and collateral supply: failures, incidents and complications. *Radiology* 1991;180:699–705.

42 Rees S. Arterial connection of the lung: the inaugural Keith Jefferson Lecture. *Clin Radiol* 1981;32:1–15.

Complications of diagnostic and interventional angiocardiography

Michael S.T. Ruttley

Introduction

Cardiac catheterization allows the study of cardiopulmonary disease by physiologic measurement (manometry, oximetry) and angiocardiography. Angiocardiography may be defined as the radiographic demonstration of the heart, great vessels, or coronary arteries opacified by radiologic contrast media.

History

The development of these diagnostic procedures was based on the first passage of a catheter (ureteric!) from an arm vein to the right atrium (his own!) by Forssman in 1929 [1]. Two years later, Moniz et al. [2] injected sodium iodide through such cardiac catheters to obtain radiographs of the opacified pulmonary arteries — "angiopneumography" — in patients. Safer contrast media became available and, in the late 1930s, Castellanos et al. [3] used peripheral venous injections with appropriately timed penetrated chest radiographs to demonstrate heart chambers in children with congenital heart disease. Robb and Steinberg [4] extended this technique to adults, and it was not until 1947 that Chavez et al. [5], claiming that better images could be obtained from intracardiac injections, publicized a return to cardiac catheterization for angiocardiography. Their catheter entry was by jugular venous cut-down, and access to arteries or veins by surgical exposure was favored by cardiologists for many years, even after Seldinger's [6] 1953 description of the now ubiquitous percutaneous needle technique.

Advances in imaging saw the replacement of direct radiography, and the many devices for rapid film changing, by cinefluoroscopy, a "movie" technique more appropriate to the beating heart. This was soon supplemented by videotape

recording for immediate playback of the ever-improving fluoroscopic images. Recognition of the value of radiographic projections additional to those in the transverse plane for coronary arteriography in the 1970s [7] led to the manufacture of the X-ray tube — image intensifier C-arm or U-arm mountings capable of movement around the patient, removing the inglorious and potentially dangerous need to shove and turn patients, with catheters in place, for oblique projections. The numerous projections now so readily available are increasingly being obtained by digital imaging in "filmless" cardiac catheter laboratories. Storage of the huge amount of digital information from an angiocardiogram is still a major technical problem, presently dealt with by analog video archiving in most institutions.

These improvements in imaging have undoubtedly contributed to the safety of cardiac catheterization and new or replacement installations are usually of the latest technology, with economic arguments confined to the need for a single or biplane facility. Advances in the chemistry of contrast media have also made considerable contributions to safety in angiocardiography, but use of the latest and safest media is usually qualified by economic constraints in even the richest countries [8].

The techniques of diagnostic cardiac catheterization were already being applied to endovascular treatment by the late 1960s, and examples of such interventions from that decade are Rashkind's balloon atrial septostomy [9] and Portsmann et al.'s percutaneous closure of the patent ductus arteriosus [10]. Dotter and Judkins [11] had introduced percutaneous transluminal angioplasty (PTA) for peripheral vascular disease in 1964, and 10 years later PTA was revolutionized by the Gruntzig balloon catheter [12]. PTA was no longer confined to vessels near to and in line with the catheter entry site, and in 1977 Dotter's prediction that angioplasty would be applied to the coronary arteries was realized: in that year Gruntzig successfully performed the first percutaneous transluminal coronary angioplasty (PTCA) in a patient with intractable angina due to a left anterior descending coronary artery stenosis [13].

PTCA was rapidly embraced and developed by cardiologists; it is now the most widely practised cardiovascular catheter intervention and is accepted by most as a major advance in the treatment of ischemic heart disease. Its acceptance has had a "knock-on" effect in popularizing PTA at other sites and has provided a commercial stimulus for improvements in catheter, guidewire, and balloon technology to the considerable benefit of all interventions. There has been an explosive growth in interventional catheterizations since 1977 and in cardiology they now include balloon valvotomy, closure of intracardiac as well as great vessel shunts, and embolotherapy of arteriovenous malformations. PTCA continues to dominate — 1300 procedures/ 1 000 000 population were estimated for the USA and 168/ 1 000 000 for the UK in 1991 [14] — and while balloon technology is still the mainstay, attempts to deal with complications, improve the restenosis rate, and widen the scope of application have led to a succession of laser, radiofrequency, mechanical, and ultrasound devices, all looking for their niche in the catheter treatment of coronary atherosclerosis.

The radiologist and cardiac catheterization

Radiologists have been of considerable importance in the growth of cardiac angiography and intervention, as the eponyms of the most widely used coronary diagnostic and PTCA guiding catheters (Judkins, Amplatz) show. A 1983 USA InterSociety Commission for Heart Disease Resources report on cardiac catheterization facilities accorded equal status to operators whose basic training was: ". . . in internal medicine, pediatrics or radiology with special training in cardiac radiology" [15]. Radiologists continue to introduce interventional techniques for development in conjunction with cardiology colleagues, but their day to day involvement in cardiac catheterization is probably on the wane. Cardiac radiologists perform a proportion of the diagnostic and interventional cardiac catheterizations in most UK cardiac centers [16], but this is idiosyncratic in global terms — a 1990 survey with 117 responses from predominantly USA cardiac catheterization laboratories [17], found that radiologists were responsible for catheterization in only 2% of the laboratories and had little input, even for reporting, in the remainder. Authoritative statements on training included in reports on PTCA from the American College of Cardiology/American Heart Association [18] and from the International Society and Federation of Cardiology/World Health Organization [19] make no mention of radiologists, referring only to cardiologist trainers and trainees. Guidelines on PTCA train-

ing from the Council of the British Cardiovascular Intervention Society (a society that welcomes radiologists among its members) are very specific regarding the level of general medical and cardiologic experience required of trainees, and indicate that these mean:

> that angioplasty trainees will usually be junior cardiologists. Radiologists who intend to pursue careers in interventional catheterisation must have received training in, and be able to manage competently, the recognised cardiological complications of PTCA [20].

No responsible physician would wish to undertake such potentially life-threatening procedures unless able to comply with this prescription, but there is some doubt that even suitably trained radiologists are acceptable as independent operators [21].

Whatever the future holds for radiologists in this area of catheter work, there would be general agreement that while angiocardiography may be appropriately performed by a single trained operator, interventional procedures usually demand a team approach and the variety of 'ologist leading in a given case is of less importance than their level of competence. This must at least match published guidelines and include the knowledge and ability to instigate correct management for recognized complications.

Involvement of radiologists in cardiac catheterization is not confined to the procedure itself and increasingly includes the assessment, and in some instances treatment, of its peripheral vascular complications by noninvasive imaging or angiography.

Complications

Death, myocardial infarction, and stroke

These are the most severe complications of cardiac catheterization. They are interrelated and will be the end result of one or more of the adverse events to be considered later. Their incidence varies with the complexity and length of the procedure, and the status of the patient: most at risk are the severely diseased, infants, and the aged.

The first major survey of cardiac catheterization was conducted in 16 USA centers in 1963–1964 [22]. Total mortality was 0.45% with a figure of 0.14% when neonates and infants under 2 years of age were excluded. The relevance of these overall figures to current practice is limited, not least because only 26% of the patients had coronary arteriography. The increasing role of coronary arteriography in later years is evident from a 1977–1982 Veterans Administration cooperative study of catheter complications [23] in males with valvular heart disease: coronary arteriography was performed in 92% of the 1559 preoperative catheter assessments. Mortality was 0.13%, nonfatal myocardial infarction (MI) 0.19%, and stroke 0.26%.

The Society for Cardiac Angiography and Interventions (SCAI) reported a mortality of 0.11% among 59 792 patients who underwent diagnostic catheterization in 63 laboratories in 1990 [24]; the figures for MI and cerebrovascular accident (CVA) were 0.05% and 0.07%, respectively. The mortality for PTCA in the same report was 0.32% among 12 011 patients; MI occurred in 0.61% and CVA in 0.05%. There was a mortality of 4.6% among 87 various valvuloplasty procedures.

An audit of British figures for 1991 showed a mortality of 0.11% for diagnostic studies, and 0.23% for PTCA in 16 participating centers [25].

Voluntary involvement of laboratories in multicenter and continuing surveys probably introduces a bias towards best practice, but they are the most comprehensive studies currently available.

Coronary arteriography was performed in 94% of the patients undergoing diagnostic catheterization in the SCAI study [24], and the complications of adult angiocardiography today are essentially those of coronary arteriography and its usual accompaniment, left ventriculography. In 1973, Adams *et al.* [26], reported a USA nationwide survey of selective coronary arteriography, with responses from 173 of 373 institutions. Death, MI, or cerebral embolus occurred in 1.3% of patients. An overall mortality rate of 0.45% was significantly increased in institutions with low case loads and significantly greater for transfemoral than for transbrachial catheterization; the same pattern was true for MI and cerebral embolus.

The unacceptable and the inevitable

One of the disturbing facts in the Adams *et al.* [26] survey was that particular hospitals with low case loads reported mortalities between 5.2 and 7.7%, "... hardly acceptable for a diagnostic study." Judkins and Gander [27] were uncompromising in an editorial response, deploring "cookbook, self-taught angiographers" and demanding proper training and maintenance of skills. They suggested that:

> ... laboratories with a death rate of over 0.1% should give serious thought and study to methods of reducing their total serious complication rate. Laboratories with death rates over 0.3% should terminate coronary arteriography ....

Bourassa and Noble [28] in a review of 5250 patients examined at their institution between 1970 and 1974 with catheters similar to those of Judkins, reported a mortality rate of 0.23% and felt a lower figure was not attainable in similar case mixes (left main coronary disease, a major risk factor, was present in all their deaths) without more aggressive supportive measures.

Prospective data of 7553 consecutive patients undergoing coronary arteriography in 13 institutions as part of the Collaborative Study on Coronary Artery Surgery (CASS) showed an overall mortality of 0.2% in highly reputable centers in 1975–1976 [29]. This figure was for the period of catheterization and the following 48 hours; the 24-hour

figure was 0.11%. A similar 0.12% mortality was reported from the Beth Israel Hospital a decade later [30], and we have already noted 0.11% mortalities in more recent surveys [24,25]. No doubt these were despite the "serious thought and study" advocated by Judkins and Gander [27].

No mortality can really be described as acceptable in a diagnostic study, but it appears that annual rates around 0.1% are currently inevitable. Individual subsets of patients will have greater or lesser rates depending on the presence and severity of cardiac disease (a significant number of patients with chest pain and normal coronary arteries feature in coronary arteriography practice), and of other risk factors which will be considered later.

Routes and risks

Transbrachial coronary arteriography equated with the Sones and Shirey technique [31] in the era surveyed by Adams *et al.* [26]. The Sones catheter is passed from a brachial artery cut-down and requires skilled manipulation selectively to intubate each coronary orifice. Percutaneous transfemoral coronary arteriography was introduced by Ricketts and Abrams in 1962 [32]; improved (and very different) preformed catheter designs for the technique were added by Judkins [33] and by Amplatz *et al.* [34] in 1967. The Judkins preformed catheters home in to the coronary ostia with disconcerting ease in most cases and the discrepancy between the safety of the femoral and brachial techniques revealed by the Adams survey could have been in part due to this very ease, which opened coronary arteriography to the relatively unskilled: "... with little experience in transfemoral catheterisation techniques, and in dealing with cardiac complications ..." [26]. Another possible explanation was the greater potential for catheter-related thromboembolism with the femoral technique, in which differently shaped catheters for each coronary artery and a catheter for left ventriculography are introduced and exchanged over a guidewire; the single Sones catheter is used without such a potentially thrombogenic leading wire. Anticoagulation was cited as a possible remedy; Judkins and Gander [27] pointed out that heparinization was an integral part of a brachial cut-down and recommended its adoption in all coronary arteriography.

Arguments for and against the two main techniques of coronary arteriography were pursued with almost religious fervor in the 1970s, but by acolytes not the masters. The latter stressed the excellence of both and the need for proficiency in one or the other [27]. Enthusiasts of the percutaneous femoral route stressed its ease and speed; safety and immediate sutural hemostasis were emphasized for the brachial cut-down in this period between the Adams *et al.* [26] and CASS [29] reports.

These reports showed interesting and contrasting differences between the two approaches. In the earlier survey, brachial and femoral representation was roughly equal whereas in the later CASS, femoral procedures outnumbered brachials by about 5:1 (neither survey was random but they were large and probably reflected the USA practice of their times). Adams *et al.* [26] found that the femoral approach was associated with a significantly higher mortality than the brachial [0.78% versus 0.13%), but this was reversed in the CASS (0.14% versus 0.51%).

Adams *et al.* [26] pointed out that the difference in major complication rates was only marginal when the two institutes with the highest case load of each technique were compared; similarly, in the CASS the increased risk of death with the brachial approach did not apply in laboratories using it for 80% or more of procedures. It should also be noted that the mortality for transbrachial coronary arteriography in Sones' own center was less than 0.1% as far back as 1963–1964 [22].

Judkins and Gander [27] maintained that an incomplete or nondiagnostic study adversely affected patient management and should be regarded as a complication of coronary arteriography. Complete diagnostic studies require multiple projections to demonstrate each section of each epicardial artery at right angles to the X-ray beam and free of overlapping branches. The importance of caudal and cranial angulations in these respects becomes increasingly obvious [35] and they are most easily obtained with the leg approach, which leaves the patient's arms to be freely moved out of the X-ray beam (and removes the operator from the immediate vicinity of the radiation).

These various factors seemed responsible for the trend towards the Judkins technique during the 1970s, but they also suggest that coronary arteriography is equally safe by either approach in skilled and practised hands. A center must contain expertise in femoral and brachial routes if a comprehensive coronary arteriography service is to be provided, and even then the ravages of peripheral vascular disease and sometimes of previous catheterizations will, in very rare circumstances, demand axillary artery [36] or even translumbar aortic [37] access for coronary catheterization.

Summary

The latest available published information from continuing USA and UK audits indicates a mortality of 0.11% for diagnostic cardiac catheterization and angiocardiography. In most instances, death is due to MI which, like a stroke, is usually embolic in this setting. The rates of nonfatal MI and CVA are approximately 50% of that for mortality. Mortality for PTCA is at least double that of diagnostic studies and it is yet higher for more complex interventions.

Complications of vascular access

The complications of cardiac catheterization include those of arterial and venous entry, and of catheter passage to the target. A falling rate of access complications for diagnostic angiography has been accompanied by an increase from the growing numbers of interventions with relatively massive catheters and intensive, often prolonged, heparinization.

Recognition or occurrence of vascular complications can be delayed and their incidence is probably underestimated in laboratory based surveys such as the SCAI Registry, which gave a rate of 0.43% in its 1990 report [24]. Two large retrospective analyses confined to complications needing surgery gave overall figures of 0.9% [38] and 0.45% [39]. A smaller but prospective study [40] found a 1.6% total incidence of vascular complications requiring blood transfusion ($\geqslant 2$ U), surgery, or antibiotics; the rate was 0.6% for diagnostic procedures, 2.6% for PTCA, and 6.6% for more complex interventions. Only 50% of the diagnostic and about 25% of the PTCA complications required surgery, which suggests possible underestimation in retrospective surgical studies.

Generally, cut-downs have a higher occlusion rate and Seldinger catheterizations have a higher incidence of bleeding complications [23,29]. Risk factors for both bleeding and occlusion include extremes of age, female gender, peripheral vascular disease, catheter/sheath size of 8-F or more, the length and the complexity of procedures. Small body surface area [38] and also obesity [41] have both been implicated. There is no doubt that intense anticoagulation during interventional procedures increases the bleeding risk and this is especially so with prolonged postprocedural heparinization [42]. Coronary stent insertion carries a particularly high rate of femoral bleeding complications [43]: percutaneous aortic valvotomy [44] and any procedures requiring intraaortic balloon counterpulsation have high rates of femoral arterial occlusion [45].

Hemorrhage/hematoma

Nine catheter entry site hemorrhages, four of which were in infants, appear in the 1968 Cooperative Study of 12 367 cardiac catheterizations, i.e., 0.07%; troublesome bleeding during actual catheterization occurred in only one of the adults — during a 6-hour procedure [22]. Procedural bleeding is thus rare in diagnostic studies; hemostasis on completion being secured by suture after cut-down and manual pressure after percutaneous catheterization. Pressure hemostasis is usually achieved within 5–10 minutes, but there is no prescribed time. Pressure must be renewed if there is any sign of continuing bleed (the site should not be covered by "pressure" dressings, which seldom press and always obscure). Surgical intervention is rarely required at this stage and the advice in troublesome cases must be "keep pressing" — provided that the presser is experienced enough to maintain both control and distal flow. In 1974, Semler [46] published experience with an external clamp that can give consistent and appropriate prolonged pressure. This had limited popularity then, but hemostasis problems associated with cardiac interventions have spawned a rash of similar devices in recent years and even a technique for collagen embolization of the catheter track [47].

Some degree of bruising is common after any vessel entry and hematoma is not usually recorded as a complication unless it necessitates transfusion or surgery, or prolongs hospital stay. Retrospective surgical studies therefore underestimate the occurrence. Wyman *et al.* [30] found hematomas described as "significant" but not requiring transfusion or surgical repair in 1.8% of a prospective series of diagnostic and interventional cases. This was skewed by relatively high vascular complications recorded in the diagnostic group, but I think most practitioners would agree that hematomas are more often underreported and accept the figure as representative. Resolution of hematoma may leave a small hard lump in the groin for many weeks and subcutaneous scarring often persists, to be encountered as an almost wooden hardness at any subsequent percutaneous catheterization.

Concealed hemorrhage can be of more concern than frank bleeding or hematoma. Major "silent" blood loss can occur into a grossly obese thigh or into the normal retroperitoneal space, and these possibilities should be considered if shock occurs during or after femoral catheterization. Displacement of the contrast-filled bladder can be an invaluable sign of a retroperitoneal collection both at catheterization and in the ensuing few hours; computed tomography (CT) confirmation [48] will usually be required at later stages. A particular risk factor for retroperitoneal hemorrhage is high puncture of the common femoral artery (or low puncture of the external iliac!). The inguinal ligament arches down from its bony attachments and is above, rarely at, the inguinal crease [49]; it should be identified before femoral puncture. Those who still use transfixion (with the inevitable double arterial puncture where only one is required) should avoid undue obliquity which can carry an anterior wall common femoral puncture out through the posterior wall of the external iliac artery [50].

Hemorrhage can complicate any cardiac catheterization and the patient's blood group should be known and serum retained against the possibility. Oral anticoagulation increases the risk of bleeding in proportion to the international normalized ratio (INR) for prothrombin time [51]. Elective procedures in patients on necessary long-term anticoagulation should therefore be deferred unless the INR is at the lower end of the therapeutic range, i.e., below 2.5. This is best achieved by temporary cessation of warfarin; reversal with parenteral vitamin K and perhaps fresh frozen plasma should be reserved for emergencies, during which essential anticoagulation can be "fine tuned" with parenteral heparin, by virtue of its short half-life of only 30–120 minutes [52] and, if absolutely necessary, its antidote protamine sulfate. Heparinization during such emergencies and interventions should be at the lowest therapeutic level necessary for the procedure and this is readily monitored by the activated coagulation time (ACT), which can be measured in the catheterization laboratory [53]. Heparin resistance induced by parenteral glyceryl trinitrate and increased sensitivity after its cessation [54] makes monitoring particularly important during and after PTCA.

False aneurysm (FA)

This is an extravascular collection of liquid blood communicating with the arterial lumen and limited exteriorly by thrombus and surrounding tissues. It results from failed closure, or reopening, of a vessel puncture site after catheterization. The rind of thrombus is of variable thickness and its content shows turbulent systolic/diastolic flow, often with a jet effect at the communication which is either flush with the artery or a defined neck within thrombus. On examination it is a pulsatile (expansile) tender hematoma which may have a systolic bruit; the fluid content differentiates it from massive simple hematoma and is most easily shown by duplex Doppler ultrasound [55], preferably with color-flow facility [56]; CT is an alternate if there is exquisite tenderness (Fig. 17.1) [57]. Arteriographic demonstration should be strictly limited to the occasional surgical need to see proximal and distal vessels before repair, and in such cases should be by intravenous digital subtraction (IVDSA) where possible. Patients are understandably disturbed by any mention of a repeat arterial catheterization!

FA complicating cardiac catheterization is predominantly related to the percutaneous femoral approach and variously reported to occur in 0.07% [39] to 0.38% [58] of such diagnostic procedures. An incidence of 0.04% has been seen with brachial cut-down [39]. Interventions are associated with much higher figures — an annual rate of 1.6% for femoral FA in a retrospective study [58], 6.3% in a prospective analysis of 144 PTCAs [59].

Low femoral puncture with catheterization of common femoral branches rather than the larger parent artery was implicated as the major factor in FA formation by Rapoport *et al.* [60] on the basis of superficial femoral puncture in five of six cases, and profunda femoris puncture in the sixth. Altin *et al.* [61] supported this, reporting seven branch against four common femoral punctures in 11 cases. No control groups were given for these or for the larger study of 73 FAs [58], in which 60% were associated with superficial femoral artery puncture. Kresowik *et al.* [59] found no relation to branch puncture in nine cases, and seven out of 10 aneurysms in another series were from the common femoral artery [57]. The role of low puncture is, thus, far from clear but it would seem prudent to aim for the common femoral (which can be subsequently compressed against its posterior bony relations) rather than its lower and smaller branches, particularly when large catheters/sheaths are to be used. The point of best pulsation below the inguinal

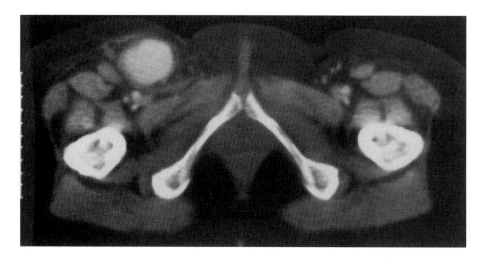

Fig. 17.1 CT, groin region, showing a large FA of the right superficial femoral artery following cardiac catheterization.

ligament has been suggested as a reliable guide for common femoral artery (CFA) puncture [62]; the inguinal crease is usually below both the ligament and the common femoral bifurcation [49], and is an unreliable guide to either. The bony landmarks should therefore be defined and, if this is not possible, skin entry at the fluoroscopically determined level of the lower margin of the femoral head, with needle angulation to puncture the artery about 2 cm above, will find the common femoral artery in 95% of punctures according to Kim *et al.* [58]. Unduly high puncture, i.e. above the ligament, carries its own danger of retroperitoneal hemorrhage and must be avoided.

Surgical closure was formerly advocated for all FAs but many thrombose spontaneously [63], and ultrasound-guided external compression is an effective treatment early in their course [64]: this has also been reported for brachial FA [65]. Surgery is still necessary for those FAs that expand or fail to resolve under observation, and the risk of rupture must not be underestimated — McCann *et al.* [38] refer to three ruptures of which two were fatal, and there were 12 ruptures in a series of 50 FAs reported by Graham *et al.* [66]. Kresowick *et al.* [59] suggest physical examination of all patients after catheter removal and again before discharge, with color-flow duplex scan of any suspected femoral complication. The need for such a formal policy is illustrated by Graham *et al.*'s series — 10 of the 12 ruptures were of undiagnosed FAs, two of the patients had been discharged from hospital [66].

The emphasis here is on cardiac catheterization, but radiologists note: three of Graham *et al.*'s 50 FAs followed radiologic procedures with 5-F catheters — and they all ruptured [66]!

Femoral arteriovenous fistula (AVF)

AVF is relatively uncommon, with less than 50% of the recorded incidence of FA. They occasionally coexist (Fig. 17.2), and their etiology is similar but simultaneous arterial and venous catheterization or inadvertent puncture of both artery and vein are considered additional causative factors for AVF.

The anterior relationship of the superficial femoral artery to its vein is well known and provides a valid reason for avoidance of low puncture (particularly for transfixers), but the common femoral artery does not always have the side to side relation to the femoral vein quoted by Kim *et al.* [58] and more often overlaps the vein [67].

AVF is usually associated with hematoma and may have a continuous murmur on auscultation. Diagnosis is confirmed by duplex ultrasound [68]. An AVF is of no initial hemodynamic significance, and although it may progress to this, spontaneous closure within the first 2 months seems more likely [63]. Immediate surgical repair is therefore unnecessary and the need for later elective surgery must be lessened by the reported success of ultrasound-guided compression in early closure [64].

Occlusion

Occlusion of a catheterized vessel will be due to thrombosis, spasm, or dissection. These may occur alone or in any combination, but thrombosis is the predominant cause. Incidence varies with entry site and operator experience, patient age, coexistent peripheral vascular disease, and both the nature and length of the procedure.

In the early days of left heart catheterization, brachial cutdown was the favored approach and its occlusion rate was lower than that for percutaneous femoral puncture — 0.3% versus 1.1% in the 1968 Cooperative Study [22]. The trend towards the femoral approach has been accompanied by a rise in brachial and a fall in femoral occlusion rates in large surveys — 1.9% versus 0.2% in the 1979 CASS [29], and 2.9% versus 0.4% in the 1989 VA study [23]. It seems that practice makes perfect and that learning curves can be reversed; it must be emphasized that these figures are not

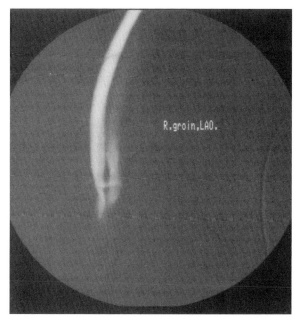

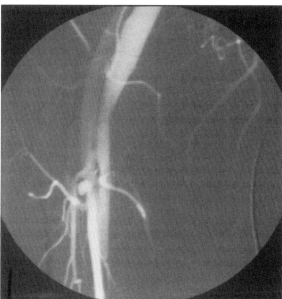

Fig. 17.2 IVDSA showing an AVF of the femoral vessels with a clearly defined neck in the early phase and an associated small FA filling later. These followed arterial and venous catheterizations for balloon mitral valvotomy.

representive of the few centers that continue to use a majority brachial approach.

The incidence of femoral occlusion increases with increasing numbers of interventional procedures (but not as dramatically as do the bleeding complications — heparinization has its upside and downside). Messina *et al.* [69] reported an incidence of 0.97% arterial thrombosis for all interventions against 0.2% for diagnostic catheterizations, but it is notable that the occlusion rate was only 0.06% in 4988 PTCAs at

Emory University Hospital [42]. Aortic balloon valvotomy and intraaortic balloon pump (IABP) insertion are associated with particularly high rates of leg ischemia in adults [44,45], as is any balloon dilatation procedure in children [70].

Systemic heparinization for diagnostic catheterization was advocated by Judkins and Gander [27], but the CASS report [29] did not show that it reduced the incidence of thrombosis and there is no clear consensus for femoral procedures. Heparin is, however, almost universally added (e.g., 1000 U/ 500 ml) to the saline or dextrose solutions used for flushing cardiac catheters.

Surgical embolectomy is the standard treatment for arterial thrombosis complicating cardiac catheterization, although thrombolysis has advantages in neonates and infants [71]. Arterial spasm at the entry site is not a problem in adult femoral catheterization but can be so in children [72], and may require oral, intravenous, or local intraarterial nitrates. Catheter or guidewire-induced nonocclusive dissections can resolve spontaneously and the need for emergency or delayed surgery or endovascular treatment (angioplasty, stent insertion) will depend on the degree of distal ischemia.

Infection

Cardiac catheterization is carried out with sterile precautions and most of the instruments used are disposables. Local infection is rarely noted as a complication, although all practitioners will be familiar with an occasional pustular memorial to their efforts. Serious local infection was cited in 10 of the 12 367 patients (0.08%) of the 1968 Cooperative Study [22], and antibiotic therapy for access site sepsis was required in 0.29% of Muller *et al.*'s [40] prospective study of 2400 cases. Studies of catheter complications have become almost a regular feature of the *Journal of Vascular Surgery* in the 1990s and the many published papers include only one on septic complications [73], which describes nine cases, all of whom had had repeat puncture of their same femoral artery or prolonged femoral artery sheath placements. The organism of infection was *Staphylococcus aureus* in all but one. The authors advise avoidance of the obvious risk factors where possible, and antibiotic therapy against *S. aureus* pending culture results when infection occurs. One of their cases developed a psoas abscess and this complication of femoral catheterization was also reported from the UK in the same year [74]. The proximity of the hip joint to the femoral artery (and the unnecessary 7 cm length of many proprietary "femoral" needles) makes occasional hip-joint puncture almost inevitable in femoral catheterizations, and it is no surprise that septic arthritis has been recorded [75].

Infective endocarditis was a rare complication (0.02%) in the 1968 Cooperative Study [22], despite the invasion of patients with congenital or valvular heart disease in many cases. Bacteremia during catheterization is, however, so unusual that it has been categorically stated that: "... prophylactic antibiotics are not required in diagnostic cardiac catheterisation or angiocardiography" [76].

Nerve damage

The femoral nerve is not contained in the femoral sheath but is otherwise an immediate lateral relation of the common femoral artery in the femoral triangle. It is occasionally touched with the local anesthetic needle or even the puncture needle during femoral catheterization, but the effect is transitory (prior warning of a possible momentary thigh shock earns patient trust in the event).

Bilateral femoral nerve palsy has complicated bilateral retroperitoneal bleeds after bilateral femoral catheterizations (for coronary arteriography/PTCA) in a luckless heparinized patient [77]; these were attributed to nerve compression by hematoma beneath the inguinal ligaments. Motor function recovered within 4 weeks but neuralgia persisted. Femoral neuralgia may be an indication for FA repair [63] and has also been reported as the most frequent persisting complaint following surgery of catheter-related vascular trauma, particularly FA [78].

Embolization

Needles, wires and catheters, and blood vessels traumatized by them, are fertile areas for thrombus formation and potential seed beds for distal embolization. Fragments can also be released from atherosclerotic arteries, diseased heart valves, vegetations, or mural thrombus during catheter manipulations; catheters, wires, interventional devices, or fragments thereof have themselves also been recorded as emboli. Systemic embolization is a particular complication of both mitral and aortic balloon valvuloplasties, occurring in over 2% in each case [44,79].

Avoidance of embolic complications rests more on meticulous technique than anticoagulation, and particular attention must be paid to frequent catheter flushing and minimizing guidewire time in catheters. Continuous drip flush is the norm for cardiac catheters, but this is only completely effective for those with single end holes; the more side holes (particularly with pigtail catheters), the less the distal orifices will be flushed clear of blood, and the greater the chance of thrombus formation in the terminal segment — waiting to be blasted off with the next angiographic pressure injection. A catheter must be handflushed every few minutes — after ensuring patency by aspiration. A catheter that cannot be aspirated must not be injected and has to be changed — but not over a wire! If a sheath is in place, the catheter should be simply withdrawn, if not the catheter should be cut and a matching sheath advanced over it to allow catheter removal without sacrificing access.

Embolic events are rare, but distal pulses should be routinely checked before starting and before completing arterial catheterization, and operators should be constantly alert to the possibilities of coronary and cerebral embolization when manipulating cardiac catheters. Such practice has become all the more relevant with the emergence of catheter-based treatments (suction, lysis, retrieval) for some of these.

Peripheral arterial embolism

This is the least common vascular complication in reports that separately identify it (most do not). Messina *et al.* [69] give an incidence of 0.04% in diagnostic procedures and 0.11% in interventions. Oweida *et al.* [42] found 0.08% in their large PTCA series. The CASS report [29] showed no significant difference between brachial (0.08%) and femoral (0.06%) catheterizations for such emboli.

Massive cholesterol embolization is a disastrous complication of femoral catheterization [80], but is rare and not listed in the large cardiac catheter surveys quoted here. There is some evidence that it is becoming more frequent with increasing numbers of procedures in the elderly [81]. In this context, it is due to the release of aortoiliac atheromatous material during catheterization, but it is a well-known complication of aortic surgery and may occur spontaneously. It is characterized clinically by severe lower limb pain during or shortly after the procedure. This is associated initially with a white leg, or legs, shortly followed by a reddish blue mottling — livedo reticularis — which may extend to involve the trunk, typically with an upper demarcation at about umbilical level. Despite these gross signs of ischemia it is striking that pulses are preserved, distinguishing the condition from aortoiliac dissection or thromboembolism. There is no specific therapy and mortality is high. Pathologically there is evidence of widespread cholesterol crystal microembolization.

Cerebral embolism

This is the usual culprit for stroke or transient ischemic attack complicating invasive cardiac studies. Its occurrence in 0.43% of femoral procedures versus 0.23% for the brachial route in the patients surveyed by Adams *et al.* [26], raised considerable concern as has been detailed above. The CASS report 6-years later [29] showed no difference between the two techniques, with a total incidence down to 0.03% (two patients, one from each group, both heparinized at catheterization). These figures refer to nonfatal events; cerebrovascular accidents also contribute to the mortality of these procedures.

Coronary embolism

Emboli actually observed during coronary arteriography are usually air bubbles introduced into what should be a closed injection system by faulty technique. The filling defects

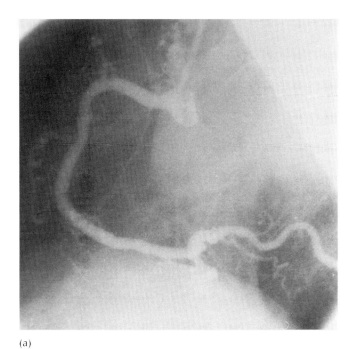

(a)

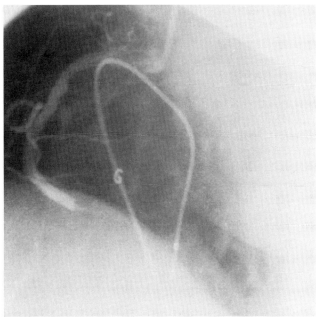

(b)

Fig. 17.3 Coronary thromboembolism. (a) Initial right coronary artery arteriogram. (b) The diagnostic procedure was then complicated by occlusive thromboembolism which is clearly shown here and which led to asystole (note pacing catheter now in right ventricular cavity).

travel distally with the contrast column, usually to break up and become lost to view in small vessels. Adverse effects are rare but occasionally an air lock is created in a large epicardial artery with resulting myocardial ischemia. Spontaneous resolution within 5–10 minutes can be expected (the resorption of the bubble may be accelerated by 100% oxygen via a face mask), but in that time the patient is at risk and the team must be alert to the possibility of arrhythmia or collapse. The more complex catheter systems used in PTCA appear to increase the possibility of air embolism [82].

Coronary thromboembolism is more likely to result in myocardial ischemia (Fig. 17.3); its incidence is usually hidden in the overall figures for mortality and nonfatal myocardial infarction, but Bourassa and Noble [28] recognized three coronary embolisms in 5250 coronary arteriographies (0.07%).

Pulmonary embolism

Pulmonary thromboembolism was only recorded in 11 (0.09%) of the patients in the 1968 Cooperative study [22], conducted when right heart catheterization was relatively common; in four, it complicated transseptal left heart catheterization from difficult femoral vein punctures, with clinical femoral venous thrombosis in three of these. One ad-

ditional pulmonary infarct was due to prolonged wedging of a pulmonary artery catheter.

New pulmonary perfusion defects on radionuclide scans have been detected in about 8% of patients undergoing right and left heart studies from the groin [83], but modern practice is dominated by coronary studies with no right heart catheterization, and clinical pulmonary embolism seems so rare that it is not even listed in the recent surveys.

Transseptal catheterization has been resurrected for balloon mitral valvuloplasty and a registry report of complications for adult cases contains one procedural death from pulmonary embolus (0.1%) and two cases of pulmonary emboli (0.3%) in the recovery period [79].

Catheter trauma to the heart, great vessels, and coronary arteries

Heart and great vessels

Perforation of the heart or great vessels was reported in 100 patients (0.8%) of the 1968 Cooperative study [22]. Thirty perforations were related to transseptal catheterization.

A transseptal needle aimed at the interatrial septum (preferably after exclusion of a probe patent foramen ovale — 29% of us have them [84]!) can inadvertently stab the ascending aorta or pericardium, but tamponade is unlikely unless the catheter is also advanced. This is usually avoided by monitoring needle-tip pressure and only sleeving the catheter on when a left atrial trace is seen (see also pp. 286, 326).

The validity of indirect left atrial pressures (pulmonary artery "wedge"), ability to cross nearly all stenotic aortic valves retrogradely, and the increasing use of echocardiography for native and prosthetic valve assessment, led to diminishing use of transseptal catheterization through the 1970s to the mid-1980s — and fewer cardiac perforations. The technique had to be learned again when mitral balloon valvuloplasty became feasible and the 1990 SCAI Registry [24] records a 0.3% perforation rate; none was seen in the previous two reports [24]. Cardiac tamponade and/or perforation was recorded in 8% of mitral valvuloplasties in the National Heart, Lung and Blood Institute (NHLBI) Registry [79], although death from this cause usually followed a left ventricular perforation rather than one directly due to the transseptal puncture. Such perforations are also seen with aortic balloon valvuloplasty [46].

Transseptals and valvuloplasties are not the only villains: 23 of the 100 perforations described above were complications of angiocardiography (and 14 additional patients showed "significant" myocardial stain after contrast injection). Eleven of the 23 required pericardiocentesis. Such figures for angiocardiography are unheard of today due to better catheter materials and shapes (notably side-holed pigtails for flush studies), reliable pressure injectors, and better fluoroscopy. Small myocardial stains, together with resultant early coronary venous filling (Fig. 17.4), are occasional sequelae of left ventricular injection, even with pigtails, and a preliminary test injection to ensure a free position is mandatory. Flow rates should be low (10–12 ml/s) to minimize catheter whip, and central catheter placement is

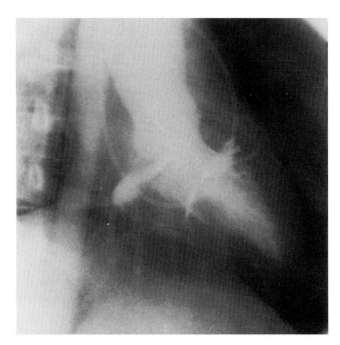

Fig. 17.4 Left ventricular angiogram showing myocardial extravasation of contrast medium. Note coronary sinus opacification due to the typical early venous filling from the myocardium in such accidents.

more reliably obtained with an angled rather than a straight-shaft pigtail [85].

Excluding transseptal injuries, the right ventricle was the most frequent site of perforation in the Cooperative report [22], and this can be attributed to its relatively thin wall and the stiff right heart catheters then in use. Right heart catheterization is now the exception rather than the rule in adult cardiology practice and is more frequently performed for right atrial contrast injections in digital subtraction peripheral arteriography (where extravasation is extremely rare, although tamponade has been reported [86]). It is still commonly employed in pediatric studies, but the only right heart perforation recorded in 1037 catheterizations by Cassidy *et al.* [87] was due to damage by a transseptal sheath.

Pulmonary arteriography is best performed by pulmonary artery catheterization and its complications are discussed fully in Chapter 16. It is interesting to note in relation to perforation that, despite the safety of the technique in a large study of acute pulmonary embolism [88], an important trial of thrombolytic therapy in this condition was halted because of an unacceptable number of perforations (five in 63 cases) attributed, even in the 1980s, to the use of stiff angiographic catheters [89].

Coronary arteries

Catheter trauma to a coronary artery can produce spasm, dissection, thrombosis, and even rupture of the vessel (Fig. 17.5). The first two can occur with diagnostic or interventional procedures; thrombosis or rupture are virtually confined to PTCA and related procedures (stenting, atherectomy). Acute occlusion from one or a combination of these occurs during or shortly after PTCA in up to 11% of cases, and is the major cause of its morbidity and mortality [90].

Spasm of a coronary artery in response to intubation at diagnostic coronary arteriography typically involves the right coronary artery (RCA) at or near the offending catheter tip. It resolves with catheter removal in most instances but may need an oral or parenteral vasodilator to prevent its recurrence during continued examination. It is usually asymptomatic and not recorded as a complication. Gensini [91] noted RCA spasm in 3%, and main left coronary spasm in only one of over 3000 arteriograms in his laboratory. Its importance lies in its recognition and avoidance of a misdiagnosis of coronary disease.

Some degree of coronary spasm in response to angioplasty is an expected event [92], and a parenteral nitrate infusion is routinely commenced before, and continued during and after PTCA, supplemented as necessary by intracoronary nitrates or calcium antagonists. This is the first line of therapy for acute occlusion complicating PTCA.

Dissection at diagnostic coronary arteriography was recorded in 0.07% of cases by Bourassa and Noble [28] and

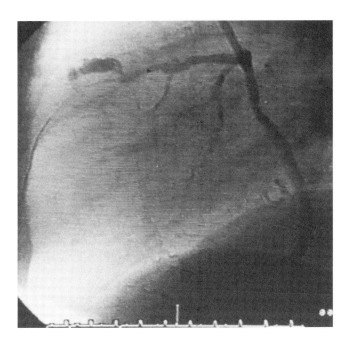

Fig. 17.5 Left coronary artery arteriogram following PTCA balloon inflation in the anterior descending branch — which ruptured!

primarily involved the RCA; the only death occurred in a patient with atresia of the left coronary artery (LCA) ostium. Dissection is recognizable angiographically at PTCA in about 5% of cases [93] and is probably the major cause of acute occlusion. The dissection may itself occlude the artery or may trigger occlusive spasm and/or thrombosis. These events carry a high risk of infarction and a high mortality. Facilities for emergency bypass surgery and interim support by intra-aortic ballon pump must therefore be available to any laboratory undertaking PTCA. The NHLBI Registry has shown a reducing need for emergency surgery [93], but it is still required in 3.5% of cases. Treatment of dissection by "tacking-up" with repeat long, low-pressure balloon inflations, maintenance of distal flow with "perfusion" balloon catheters (side holes proximal and distal to the balloon), and stenting are some of the catheter remedies that may avert the need for surgery [94].

Thrombus formation is closely related to dissection during PTCA but can occur in isolation. The clinical relevance of the differing anticoagulant properties of ionic and nonionic low-osmolar contrast media (LOCM) is widely debated and one paper suggests that thrombotic events during PTCA are significantly less when an ionic rather than a nonionic LOCM is used [95]. There is, however, experimental evidence that endothelial damage as judged by platelet deposition is significantly greater with the ionic LOCM [96], and no consensus exists as to the best LOCM for PTCA or diagnostic coronary arteriography (see also pp. 260, 342).

Arrhythmias (see also Chapter 4)

Bradyarrhythmia

Vasovagal reaction — pallor, sweating, nausea with bradycardia, and hypotension — occurs more commonly in our laboratory than is generally reported, and we find the figures given by the prospective study of Wyman *et al.* [30] representative. They report a 2.1% incidence in diagnostic studies, 0.7% in PTCA, and 2.0% in balloon valvotomy [30]. A vasovagal "faint" is within everyone's personal experience, but it may have severe consequences at cardiac catheterization, particularly in patients with coronary artery disease or aortic stenosis. The patient is already supine and thus beyond one of the usual remedies. Attempts at vessel entry (it typically occurs early in the procedure) or catheter manipulation must stop immediately and parenteral atropine sulfate must be given urgently in aliquots of 0.6 mg until the situation is controlled. One dose usually suffices, but up to four are occasionally required. If hypotension is marked, the patient's legs should be elevated. The importance of early recognition is vital as heart block, asystole, or circulatory collapse can supervene. It is salutary to read that four of six deaths in an early experience of coronary arteriography were due to vasovagal collapse [97]. This should not occur in modern practice.

Sinus bradycardia of some degree is expected with selective coronary injection of high-osmolar contrast media (HOCM) and may proceed to heart block or asystole. Contrast-induced bradyarrhythmia was found in only 2% of patients given nonionic LOCM but occurred in 21% with ionic media [98]. Wisneski *et al.* [99] found no significant change in the RR interval with ionic or nonionic LOCM.

Right-bundle branch block may occur with right ventricular catheterization, and complete heart block is therefore a risk in patients with preexisting left-bundle branch block [100].

Complete heart block or severe bradycardia can therefore complicate cardiac catheterization, and facility for immediate placement of an endocardial pacing system must be available in the laboratory. In high-risk patients this may be required prophylactically.

Tachyarrhythmia

Ventricular premature beats (VPB), even short runs of ventricular tachycardia (VT), occur with nearly all ventricular catheterizations and a "quiet" catheter placement is sought for pressure measurement and angiocardiography. Even so, VPBs mar about 50% of left ventriculograms [85].

Atrial fibrillation or flutter complicating right atrial catheter manipulation are recognized. They usually revert spontaneously within a few hours, but antiarrhythmic drug therapy or cardioversion may occasionally be necessary.

VT or ventricular fibrillation can occur with any intra-cardiac catheter placement or contrast injection, but are reported in 0.5% or less of recent studies [23,24,28]. The electrophysiologic changes associated with coronary injection of contrast media are complex; nonionic media cause significantly less prolongation of the QT interval than ionics, but it is debatable whether there is any difference between them in the frequency of ventricular fibrillation [101].

It is obvious that any catheter or vascular radiology laboratory must be equipped to deal immediately with VT or ventricular fibrillation; facilities for cardioversion are mandatory.

Contrast-medium toxicity

The adverse effects of intravascular contrast media are considered in detail in Chapter 13, and their relationship to thrombosis and to arrhythmia during diagnostic and interventional cardiac catheterization has also been referred to above.

It is worth noting here that the effects of HOCM on left ventricular end-diastolic pressure and on mitral valve gradient are such that they have been utilized as alternates to pacing and exercise stress tests in ischemic and valvular heart disease respectively [102,103]. The minimal response to LOCM gives these no such "value". Their lesser adverse electrophysiologic and hemodynamic effects are generally acknowledged, although the clinical significance is debated [8]. The symptomatic effects of HOCM in angicardiography are far greater than for LOCM and, of the LOCM, nausea, vomiting, and allergic reactions occur more frequently with ionic (ioxaglate) than nonionic preparations [104].

These factors leave me in no doubt as to which family of contrast media I would choose to receive for angiocardiography, and indeed I would regard any physician electing to have HOCM as mildly eccentric. Where LOCM are available, such personal views forbid me to administer HOCM despite their significantly lower cost. Economics cannot be ignored, but rather than attempting to justify continued, albeit limited, use of HOCM, attention should perhaps be directed at:

1 the savings to be made in angiocardiography by using lower concentrations of LOCM (i.e. 300 mg.I/ml, radiographically effective and theoretically safer) rather than arbitrarily selected and more costly high concentrations;

2 the variations in cost between a given LOCM in different countries and, in a given country, the apparent uniformity of cost per milligram of iodine among comparable nonionic LOCM.

Conclusion

The possible complications of angiocardiography and cardiac interventions are endless; only the surface has been scratched in this chapter. "What can go wrong will go wrong" is quoted with feeling by many writers on the subject. Despite the possibilities, complication rates of under 1% and a mortality rate of about 0.1% are currently achieved in patient populations known to have similar morbidity and mortality in the 24 hours preceding catheterization [105]!

References

1 Forssmann W. Die Sondierung des rechten Herzens. *Klin Wschr* 1929;8:2085–2087.

2 Moniz E, de Carvalho L, Lima A. Angiopneumographie. *Presse Med* 1931;53:996.

3 Castellanos A, Pereiras R, Garcia A. L'angio-cardiographie chez l'enfant. *Presse Med* 1938;46:1474–1477.

4 Robb GP, Steinberg I. Visualisation of chambers of heart, pulmonary circulation, and great blood vessels in heart disease; preliminary observations. *Am J Roentgenol* 1939;42:14–37.

5 Chavez I, Dorbecker N, Celis A. Direct intracardiac angiocardiography: its diagnostic value. *Am Heart J* 1947;33:560–593.

6 Seldinger SI. Catheter replacement of the needle in percutaneous arteriography. A new technique. *Acta Radiol* 1953;39:368–376 (reproduced with permission in *Am J Roentgenol* 1984;142:368–376).

7 Bunnell IL, Greene DG, Tandon RN, Arani DT. The half axial projection. A new look at the proximal left coronary artery. *Circulation* 1973;48:1151–1156.

8 Nissen SE, Douglas JS, Dreifus LS *et al.* ACC position statement. Use of nonionic or low osmolar contrast agents in cardiovascular procedures. *J Am Coll Cardiol* 1993;21:269–273.

9 Rashkind WJ. Atrioseptostomy by balloon catheter in congenital heart disease. *Radiol Clin N Am* 1971;9(2):193–202.

10 Porstmann W, Wierny L, Warnke H, Gerstberger G, Romaniuk PA. Catheter closure of patent ductus arteriosus. 62 cases treated without thoracotomy. *Radiol Clin N Am* 1971;9(2):203–218.

11 Dotter CT, Judkins MP. Transluminal treatment of arteriosclerotic obstruction. *Circulation* 1964;30:654–670.

12 Gruntzig A, Hopff H. Perkutane Rekanalisation chronischer arterieller Verschlusse mit eineum neuen dilatations Katheter. Modifikation der Dotter-technik. *Dtsch Med Wschr* 1974;99:2502–2510.

13 Gruntzig AR. Transluminal dilatation of coronary artery stenosis. *Lancet* 1978;i:263.

14 van den Brand M (for the European Angioplasty Survey Group). Utilisation of coronary angioplasty and cost of angioplasty disposables in 14 western European countries. *Eur Heart J* 1993;14:391–397.

15 Freisinger GC, Adams DF, Bourassa MG *et al.* Optimal resources for examination of the heart and lungs: cardiac catheterisation and radiographic facilities. *Circulation* 1983;68:891A–930A.

16 Murphy KP, Wilde P. The current position of cardiac radiology in the United Kingdom. *Clin Radiol* 1989;40:455–456.

17 Cameron A, Sheldon WC, Balter S. Cardiac catheterisation laboratory survey: 1990. Society for Cardiac Angiography and Interventions. Laboratory Performance Standards Committee. *Cathet Cardiovasc Diagn* 1992;27:267–273.

18 Ryan TJ, Faxon DP, Gunnar RN *et al.* ACC/AHA Task Force Report. Guidelines for percutaneous transluminal coronary angioplasty. *J Am Coll Cardiol* 1988;12:529–545.

19 Bourassa MG, Alderman EL, Bertrand M, *et al*. Report of the Joint ISFC/WHO Task Force on Coronary Angioplasty. *Circulation* 1988;78:780–789.

20 Gray HH, Balcon R, Dyet J, *et al*. Guidelines for training in percutaneous transluminal coronary angioplasty. *Br Heart J* 1992;68:437–439.

21 Chamberlain DA, Pentecost BL, Brooks NH *et al*. Provision of service for the diagnosis and treatment of heart disease. Fourth Report of a Joint Cardiology Committee of the Royal College of Physicians of London and the Royal College of Surgeons of London. *Br Heart J* 1992;67:106–116.

22 Braunwald E, Swan HJC (eds). Cooperative study on cardiac catheterisation. *Circulation* 1968;37(Suppl. 3):1 113.

23 Folland ED, Oprian C, Giacomini J *et al*. (VA Cooperative Study on Valvular Heart Disease). Complications of cardiac catheterisation and angiography in patients with valvular heart disease. *Cathet Cardiovasc Diagn* 1989;17:15–21.

24 Noto TJ, Johnson LW, Krone R *et al*. Cardiac catheterisation 1990: a report of the Registry of the Society for Cardiac Angiography and Interventions (SCA&I). *Cathet Cardiovasc Diagn* 1991;24:75–83.

25 de Bono D (for organising committee). Confidential enquiry into cardiac catheter complications. *Br Heart J* 1992;68:68.

26 Adams DF, Fraser DB, Abrams HL. The complications of coronary arteriography. *Circulation* 1973;48:609–618.

27 Judkins MP, Gander MP. Editorial — prevention of complications of coronary arteriography. *Circulation* 1974;49:599–602.

28 Bourassa MG, Noble J. Complication rate of coronary arteriography. *Circulation* 1976;53:106–114.

29 Davis K, Kennedy JW, Kemp HG, Judkins MP, Gosselin AJ, Killip T. Complications of coronary arteriography from the Collaborative Study of Coronary Artery Surgery (CASS). *Circulation* 1979;59:1105–1112.

30 Wyman RM, Safian RD, Portway V *et al*. Current complications of diagnostic and therapeutic cardiac catheterisation. *J Am Coll Cardiol* 1988;12:1400–1406.

31 Sones FM Jr, Shirey EK. Cine coronary arteriography. *Mod Concepts Cardiovasc Dis* 1962;31:735–738.

32 Ricketts HJ, Abrams HL. Percutaneous selective coronary cine arteriography. *J Am Med Assoc* 1962;181:620–624.

33 Judkins MP. Selective coronary arteriography. Part 1: a percutaneous transfemoral technique. *Radiology* 1967;89:815–824.

34 Amplatz K, Formanek G, Stanger P, Wilson W. Mechanics of selective coronary catheterisation via femoral approach. *Radiology* 1967;89:1040–1047.

35 Guthaner DF, Wexler L. New aspects of coronary angiography. *Radiol Clin N Am* 1980;18:501–514.

36 Weidner W, MacAlpin R, Hanafee W, Kattus A. Percutaneous transaxillary selective coronary arteriography. *Radiology* 1965;85:652–657.

37 Argenal AJ, Baker MS. Selective coronary arteriography via translumbar catheterisation. *Am Heart J* 1991;121:198–199.

38 McCann RL, Shwartz LB, Piper KS. Vascular complications of cardiac catheterization. *J Vasc Surg* 1991;14:375–381.

39 Babu SC, Piccorelli GO, Shah PM, Stein JH, Clauss RH. Incidence and results of arterial complications among 16 350 patients undergoing cardiac catheterization. *J Vasc Surg* 1989;10:113–116.

40 Muller DWM, Shamir KJ, Ellis SG, Topol EJ. Peripheral vascular complications after conventional and complex percutaneous coronary interventional procedures. *Am J Cardiol* 1992;69:63–68.

41 Skillman JJ, Kim D, Baim DS. Vascular complications of percutaneous femoral cardiac interventions. *Arch Surg* 1988;123:1207–1212.

42 Oweida SW, Roubin GS, Smith RB, Salam AA. Postcatheterisation vascular complications associated with percutaneous coronary angioplasty. *J Vasc Surg* 1990;12:310–315.

43 Carrozza JP, Kuntz RE, Levine MJ *et al*. Angiographic and clinical outcome of intracoronary stenting: immediate and long-term results from a large single-center experience. *J Am Coll Cardiol* 1992;20:328–337.

44 McKay R, MSAVR Investigators. The Mansfield Scientific Aortic Valvuloplasty Registry: overview of haemodynamic results and procedural complications. *J Am Coll Cardiol* 1991;17:1188–1191.

45 Eltchaninoff H, Dimas AP, Whitlow PL. Complications associated with percutaneous placement and use of intraaortic balloon counterpulsation. *Am J Cardiol* 1993;71:328–332.

46 Semler HJ. Experience with an external clamp to control bleeding following transfemoral catheterisation. *Radiology* 1974;110:225–226.

47 Ernst SMPG, Tjonjoegin RM, Schrader R *et al*. Immediate sealing of arterial puncture sites after cardiac catheterisation and coronary angioplasty using a biodegradable collagen plug: results of an international registry. *J Am Coll Cardiol* 1993;21:851–853.

48 Trerotola SO, Kuhlman JE, Fishman EK. Bleeding complications of femoral catheterisation: CT evaluation. *Radiology* 1990;174:37–40.

49 Lechner G, Jantsch H, Wancck R, Kretchmer G. The relationship between the common femoral artery, the inguinal crease, and the inguinal ligament: a guide to accurate angiographic puncture. *Cardiovasc Intervent Radiol* 1988;11:165–169.

50 Kaufman JL. Pelvic hemorrhage after percutaneous femoral angiography. *Am J Roentgenol* 1984;143:335–336.

51 Fennerty A, Campbell IA, Routledge PA. Anticoagulants in venous thromboembolism. *Br Med J* 1988;297:1285–1288.

52 Hirsh J. Heparin. *New Engl J Med* 1991;324:1565–1574.

53 Scott JA, Berenstein A, Blumenthal D. Use of the activated coagulation time as a measure of anticoagulation during interventional procedures. *Radiology* 1986;158:849–850.

54 Habbab MA, Haft JA. Heparin resistance induced by intravenous nitroglycerin. *Arch Int Med* 1987;147:857–860.

55 Helvie MA, Rubin JM, Silver TM, Kresowik TF. The distinction between femoral artery pseudoaneurysms and other causes of groin masses: value of duplex doppler ultrasonography. *Am J Roentgenol* 1988;150:1177–1180.

56 Mitchell DG, Needleman L, Goldberg BB *et al*. Femoral artery pseudoaneurysm: diagnosis with conventional duplex and color doppler US. *Radiology* 1987;165:687–690.

57 Fitzgerald EJ, Bowsher WG, Ruttley MST. False aneurysm of the femoral artery: computed tomographic and ultrasound appearances. *Clin Radiol* 1986;37:585–588.

58 Kim D, Orron DE, Skillman JJ *et al*. Role of superficial femoral artery puncture in the development of pseudoaneurysm and arteriovenous fistula complicating percutaneous transfemoral cardiac catheterisation. *Cathet Cardiovasc Diagn* 1992;25:91–97.

59 Kresowik TF, Khoury MD, Miller BV *et al*. A prospective study of the incidence and natural history of femoral vascular complications after percutaneous transluminal coronary angioplasty. *J Vasc Surg* 1991;13:328–336.

60 Rapoport S, Sniderman KW, Morse SS, Proto MH, Ross GR. Pseudoaneurysm: a complication of faulty technique in femoral arterial puncture. *Radiology* 1985;154:529–530.

61 Altin RS, Flicker S, Naidech HJ. Pseudoaneurysm and arteriovenous fistula after femoral artery catheterization. *Am J Roentgenol* 1989;152:629–631.

62 Grier D, Hartnell G. Percutaneous femoral puncture: practice and anatomy. *Br J Radiol* 1990;63:602–604.

63 Kent KC, McArdle CR, Kennedy B, Baim DS, Anninnos E, Skillman JJ. A prospective study of the clinical outcome of femoral pseudoaneurysms and arteriovenous fistulas induced by arterial puncture. *J Vasc Surg* 1993;17:125–133.

64 Fellmeth BD, Buckner NK, Ferreira JA, Rooker KT, Parsons PM, Brown PR. Postcatheterisation femoral artery injuries: repair with color flow US guidance and C-clamp assistance. *Radiology* 1992;182:570–572.

65 Skibo L, Polak J. Compression repair of a post catheterization pseudoaneurysm of the brachial artery under sonographic guidance. *Am J Roentgenol* 1993;160:383–384.

66 Graham ANJ, Wilson CM, Hood JM, Barros D'Sa AAB. Risk of rupture of postangiographic femoral false aneurysm. *Br J Surg* 1992;79:1022–1025.

67 Baum PA, Matsumoto AH, Teitelbaum GP, Zuurbier RA, Barth KH. Anatomic relationship between the common femoral artery and vein: CT evaluation and clinical significance. *Radiology* 1989;173:775–777.

68 Igidbashian VN, Mitchell DG, Middleton WD, Schwartz RA, Goldberg BB. Iatrogenic femoral arteriovenous fistula: diagnosis with color doppler imaging. *Radiology* 1989;170:747–752.

69 Messina LM, Brothers TE, Wakefield TW *et al.* Clinical characteristics and surgical management of vascular complications in patients undergoing cardiac catheterisation: interventional versus diagnostic procedures. *J Vasc Surg* 1991;13:593–600.

70 Burrows PE, Benson LN, Williams WW *et al.* Iliofemoral arterial complications of balloon angioplasty for systemic obstructions in infants and children. *Circulation* 1990;82:1697–1704.

71 Brus F, Witsenburg M, Hofhuis WJD, Hazelzet JA, Hess J. Streptokinase treatment for femoral artery thrombosis after arterial cardiac catheterisation in infants and children. *Br Heart J* 1990;63:291–294.

72 Franken EA Jr, Girod D, Sequeira FW, Smith WL, Hurwitz R, Smith JA. Femoral artery spasm in children: catheter size is the principal cause. *Am J Roentgenol* 1982;138:295–298.

73 McCready RA, Siderys H, Pittman JN *et al.* Septic complications after cardiac catheterisation and percutaneous transluminal coronary angioplasty. *J Vasc Surg* 1991;14:170–174.

74 Loveday EJ, Tonge KA, du Peloux Menage HG. Iliopsoas abscess: an unusual complication of femoral artery catheterisation. *Br J Radiol* 1990;63:224–226.

75 Resnik CS, Sawyer RW, Tisnado J. Septic arthritis of the hip: a rare complication of angiography. *J Can Assoc Radiol* 1987;38:299–301.

76 Shulman ST, Amren DP, Bisno AL *et al.* Prevention of bacterial endocarditis; a statement for health care professionals by the Committee on Rheumatic Fever and Infective Endocarditis of the Council on Cardiovascular Disease in the Young. *Circulation* 1984;70:1123A–1127A.

77 Puechal X, Liote F, Kuntz D. Bilateral femoral neuropathy caused by iliacus haematomas during anticoagulation after cardiac catheterisation. *Am Heart J* 1992;123:262–263.

78 Hallett JW, Wolk SW, Cherry KJ, Gloviczki P, Pairolero PC. The femoral neuralgia syndrome after arterial catheter trauma. *J Vasc Surg* 1990;11:702–706.

79 Complications and mortality of percutaneous balloon mitral commissurotomy. A Report from the National Heart, Lung and Blood Institute Balloon Valvuloplasty Registry. *Circulation* 1992;85:2014–2024.

80 Gaines PA, Cumberland DC, Kennedy A, Welsh CL, Moorhead P, Ruttley MS. Cholesterol embolisation: a lethal complication of vascular catheterisation. *Lancet* 1988;i:168–170.

81 Ong HT, Elmsly WG, Friedlander DH. Cholesterol atheroembolism: an increasingly frequent complication of cardiac catheterisation. *Med J Aust* 1991;154:412–414.

82 Kahn JK, Hartzler GO. The spectrum of symptomatic coronary air embolism during balloon angioplasty: causes, consequences, and management. *Am Heart J* 1990;119:1374–1377.

83 Gowda S, Bollis AM, Haikal AM, Salem BI. Incidence of new focal pulmonary emboli after routine cardiac catheterization comparing the brachial to the femoral approach. *Cathet Cardiovasc Diagn* 1984;10:157.

84 Thompson T, Evans W. Paradoxical embolism. *Q J Med* 1930;23:135–150.

85 Lehmann KG, Yang JC, Doria RJ *et al.* Catheter optimization during contrast ventriculography: a prospective randomized trial. *Am Heart J* 1992;123:1273–1278.

86 Gallant MJ, Studley JGN. Delayed cardiac tamponade following accidental injection of non-ionic contrast medium into the pericardium. *Clin Radiol* 1990;41:139–140.

87 Cassidy SC, Schmidt KG, Van Hare GF, Stanger P, Teitel DF. Complications of pediatric cardiac catheterization: a 3-year study. *J Am Coll Cardiol* 1992;19:1285–1293.

88 Stein PD, Athanasoulis C, Alavi A *et al.* Complications and validity of pulmonary angiography in acute pulmonary embolism. *Circulation* 1992;85:462–468.

89 Meyer G, Sors H, Charbonnier B *et al.* Effects of intravenous urokinase versus alteplase on total pulmonary resistance in acute massive pulmonary embolism: a European multicenter double-blind trial. *J Am Coll Cardiol* 1992;19:239–245.

90 de Feyter PJ, van den Brand M, Jaarman G, van Domburg R, Serruys P, Suryapranata H. Acute coronary artery occlusion during and after percutaneous transluminal coronary angioplasty. Frequency, prediction, clinical course, management, and follow-up. *Circulation* 1991;83:927–936.

91 Gensini GG. Coronary arteriography. In: Braunwald E, ed. *Heart Disease. A Textbook of Cardiovascular Medicine*. Philadelphia: WB Saunders, 1980:308–362.

92 Fischell TA, Derby G, Tse TM, Stadius ML. Coronary artery vasoconstriction routinely occurs after percutaneous transluminal coronary angioplasty: a quantitative arteriographic analysis. *Circulation* 1988;78:1323–1334.

93 Holmes DR, Holubkov R, Vlietstra RE *et al.* Comparison of complications during percutaneous transluminal coronary angioplasty from 1977 to 1981 and from 1985 to 1986. The National Heart, Lung and Blood Institute Percutaneous Transluminal Coronary Angioplasty Registry. *J Am Coll Cardiol* 1988;12:1149–1155.

94 Cripps TR, Morgan JM, Rickards AF. Outcome of extensive coronary artery dissection during coronary angioplasty. *Br Heart J* 1991;66:3–6.

95 Piessens JH, Stammen F, Vrolix MC *et al.* Effects of an ionic versus a nonionic low osmolar contrast agent on the thrombotic complications of coronary angioplasty. *Cathet Cardiovasc Diagn* 1993;28:99–105.

96 Riemann CD, Massey CV, McCarron DL, Borkowski P, Johnson

PC, Ziskind AA. Ionic contrast agent-mediated endothelial injury causes platelet deposition to vascular surfaces. *Am Heart J* 1993;125:71−78.

97 Petch MC, Sutton R, Jefferson KE. Safety of coronary arteriography. *Br Heart J* 1973;35:377−380.

98 Murdock CJ, Davis MJE, Ireland MA, Gibbons FA, Cope GD. Comparison of meglumine diatrizoate, iopamidol, and iohexol for coronary angiography and ventriculography. *Cathet Cardiovasc Diagn* 1990;19:179−183.

99 Wisneski JA, Gertz EW, Dahlgren M, Muslin A. Comparison of low osmolality ionic (ioxaglate) versus nonionic (iopamidol) contrast media in cardiac angiography. *Am J Cardiol* 1989;63:489−495.

100 Gupta PK, Haft JI. Complete heart block complicating cardiac catheterization. *Chest* 1972;61:185−187.

101 Brogan WC, Hillis LD, Lange RA. Contrast agents for cardiac catheterisation: conceptions and misconceptions. *Am Heart J* 1991;122:1129−1135.

102 Cohn PF, Horn HH, Teicholz LE, Kreulen TH, Herman MV. Effects of angiographic contrast medium on left ventricular function in coronary artery disease. Comparison with static and dynamic exercise. *Am J Cardiol* 1973;32:21−26.

103 Brown AK, Epstein EJ, Coulshed N, Clarke JM, Doukas NG. Haemodynamic changes after angiocardiography. *Br Heart J* 1969;31:233−245.

104 Gertz EW, Wisneski JA, Miller R *et al.* Adverse reactions of low osmolality contrast media during angiography: a prospective randomized multicenter study. *J Am Coll Cardiol* 1992;19:899−906.

105 Hildner FJ, Javier RP, Tolentino A, Samet P. Pseudo complications of cardiac catheterization. *Cathet Cardiovasc Diagn* 1982;8:43−47.

Complications of percutaneous angioplasty

Louise S. Wilkinson and Robert A. Wilkins

Introduction

Even for the most experienced operator, exercising the highest level of care, complications are ultimately inevitable during angioplasty. Prior knowledge of the potential pitfalls and how to avoid them, together with attention to detail, will go some way to reducing the rate of adverse effects. Detailed history taking, familiarity with the results of previous studies and careful planning allow the most appropriate procedure to be performed. Complications are increasingly likely during difficult procedures with prolonged manipulation times, so it is vital that operators are aware of their limitations, know when to terminate the procedure, and know how to extricate themselves from difficulties encountered.

As catheter, balloon, and guidewire technology improves and more interventionists acquire skills, angioplasty success rates are rising. In addition, there are probably fewer complications, although this has not been fully documented. Indeed, it is difficult to make satisfactory comparisons of reported complications for several reasons: (i) there is a wide variation in definition of what are major and minor complications [1]; (ii) some complications may be successfully treated at the time of angioplasty, and it is unclear whether such complications are reported in all publications; and (iii) the lack of definition in many publications of the site of angioplasty, and of the site at which a complication occurred makes interpretation of some reported complications difficult [2].

Peripheral angioplasty

Complications are most usefully defined as those which:

1 need surgical intervention as a result of the complication (major complication);

2 prolong hospital stay without requiring further intervention (minor complication);

3 make no difference to the clinical management (reporting varies).

For example, hematoma formation at the puncture site is relatively common. It very rarely requires surgical intervention; but, these cases could fall into group (1). It may cause the patient's hospital stay to be extended (group 2), or may not affect the clinical management (group 3). Reporting, particularly in the latter case, is variable. Similarly, dissection at the site of angioplasty is considered by some to be a necessary consequence of angioplasty ("controlled injury"), but may be reported by others as a complication [3].

Complications should be minimized by selecting patients carefully and choosing the most appropriate interventional technique. There is a growing trend for angioplasty to be seen as an opportunity for limb salvage when patients are deemed unfit for surgery; not surprisingly, the complication rate is increased in such patients [4]. As with all interventional procedures, there is a learning curve for the operator in which the complication rate falls as experience is acquired. In order to minimize complications that are unforeseen due to lack of experience, there should be a high level of supervision of trainees during all procedures. Above all, a good angioplasty service relies on close cooperation between the radiologist and the vascular surgeon; not only to select patients, but also to facilitate the rapid surgical treatment of major complications should the need arise [5].

The aftercare of the patient is also critical and delayed complications must be recognized at the earliest opportunity. Good communication with experienced ward staff is essential to allow early detection of complications after the patient has left the radiology department. With increasing pressure on resources, more patients are being treated as outpatients, but provided that these patients are carefully selected there does not seem to be an increased risk of major complications in this group [6]. Hirschl *et al.* [7] have recommended the following indications for outpatient angioplasty:

1 lesions above the knee only;
2 exclusive catheter recanalization;
3 absence of complications during the procedure;
4 radiologic and vascular surgical standby;
5 patient compliance;
6 adequate social environment;
7 suitable transport arrangements.

Table 18.1 lists figures for outcome and complication rates from several of the larger studies.

Complications can be grouped as follows:
1 complications at the catheter entry site;
2 complications at the angioplasty site;
3 late complications at the angioplasty site;
4 problems distal to the angioplasty site;
5 equipment failure;
6 systemic and remote complications;
7 complications related to contrast medium.

Table 18.1 Success rates and complication rates

Number of patients	Procedures	Sites	Initial success rate (%)	Complication rate (%)	Surgery rate (%)*	Remote complications[†]	Deaths[‡]	Reference
352	453	All	89.0	13.0	3.0	1	1	[1]
	318	All	83.0	9.0	3.1		1	[8]
	202	All		32.7	10.9		12	[4]
902	985	All	88.6	9.5	1.1		4	[5]
3650	4750	All	91.0	2.9	2.6	4	3	[9]
107	142	Periph	91.4	20.0	2.8		1	[10]
370	500	Periph	85.0	8.8	1.8		4	[11]
	147	Periph	88.0	10.2	4.0		1	[12]
135	148	Periph	95.2	14.2	1.5	3	1	[13]
1141	1642	Periph	91.0	2.6	1.3	4	2	[14]
	100	Periph	91.0	8.0	2.0			[15]
	49	Periph	61.2	26.7		4		[16]
152	217	Periph	80.0	10.0	4.1		3	[17]
127	134	Periph		21.0	1.4			[18]
	376	Periph	95.7		2.1			[19]
129	129	Periph	84.5	17.1				[20]
175	206	Periph	88.3	25.2	5.8	5		[21]
32	58	Aorta	94.8	6.9	1.7			[22]
27	27	Aorta	100.0	7.4	7.4			[23]
28	32	Aorta	100.0		0.0			[24]
200	340	Aortoiliac	94.7	10.5	1.5	4		[25]
154	194	Iliac	96.0	2.0	0.0			[26]
50	56	Iliac	71.4	12.0				[27]
150	174	Iliac	93.0	18.0	2.0			[28]
106	126	Fem/pop	95.0	2.0			1	[29]
129	164	Fem/pop	84.0	6.0	1.2			[30]
98	145	Fem/pop	97.0	2.1	0.0			[31]
25	29	Prof-fem	89.7		6.9			[32]
40	55	Infrapop	95.0		0.0			[33]
111	168	Infrapop	90.0	14.0	3.0	4		[34]
168		Infrapop		18.4		1	5	[35]
53	57	Infrapop	97.0	40.4	3.5	2	1	[36]

* Rate of complications requiring surgery.
† Angina, bowel ischemia, myocardial infarction, cerebrovascular accident, sepsis, pulmonary embolus, deep vein thrombosis, renal failure.
‡ Cholesterol embolus, aortoiliac thrombosis, cardiorespiratory arrest, sepsis, disseminated intravascular coagulopathy.
Fem/pop, superficial femoral and popliteal arteries; infrapop, below-knee; periph, iliac/femoral/below-knee; prof-fem, profunda femoris.

Although complication rates may seem high in some series, most complications are minor, and percutaneous angioplasty remains the treatment of choice for many patients.

Complications at the catheter entry site

Entry site complications are similar to those described for angiography (see Chapter 14). The particular problems related to angioplasty mainly concern the larger catheter systems and arterial sheaths required to permit passage of the angioplasty balloon. However, as technology improves, the size of the catheter diminishes, and the majority of angioplasties can be performed with a 5-F system. Puncture site complications, principally hematoma formation and local dissection or thrombosis, can therefore be expected to have reduced in recent years, although for reasons described above, this is not well documented.

The percutaneous arterial puncture should be in the common femoral artery, and the angle at the skin should be such that there are no unnecessary curves to the catheter path. The use of single-wall and double-wall punctures is discussed in Chapter 14. An introducer sheath should be used if a lengthy procedure, or more than one or two catheter exchanges are anticipated.

The significance of hematoma formation at the puncture site is variable. A simple femoral hematoma is often of little clinical significance, although extension above the inguinal ligament with retroperitoneal hemorrhage may be fatal. Conversely, a small hematoma following an axillary or high brachial puncture may cause vascular and nerve compression; early surgical intervention may be necessary.

The largest recorded series (1141 patients) to address complication rates during angioplasty [14] describes two wound hematomas requiring surgical evacuation and two retroperitoneal hematomas; one false aneurysm is also listed. Ultrasonography is useful to assess and monitor the progress of false aneurysms; on occasion these may be managed conservatively if asymptomatic [21]. Alternately, a method of treating false aneurysms by graded compression at ultrasound has been described [37−39]. Other entry site complications reported include arteriovenous fistulae and femoral nerve damage [14,18,40] (see Table 18.2).

Table 18.2 Entry site complications

Patients	Procedures	Sites	Hematoma or hemorrhage*	False aneurysm	Arteriovenous fistula	Thrombosis	Femoral nerve damage	Reference
902	985	All	57	1	1			[5]
	318	All	9					[8]
3650	4750	All	26					[9]
	202	All	16					[4]
352	453	All	16	1			3	[1]
175	206	Periph†	7	3	2			[21]
127	134	Periph	4			1		[18]
135	148	Periph	8					[13]
	376	Periph	4					[19]
370	500	Periph	3	1				[11]
129	129	Periph	12					[20]
152	217	Periph			1			[17]
	100	Periph						[15]
1141	1642	Periph	2	1		3	1	[14]
	147	Periph	3					[12]
	49	Periph	2					[16]
200	340	Aortoiliac	4	1			3	[25]
32	58	Aorta	1	1				[22]
50	56	Iliac					1	[27]
150	174	Iliac	25					[28]
154	194	Iliac	2				1	[26]
129	164	Fem/pop	3					[30]
98	145	Fem/pop	1					[31]
25	29	Prof-fem†	1				1	[32]
53	57	Infrapop†	11					[36]
111	168	Infrapop	2				2	[34]
168		Infrapop	2					[35]

* Reporting varies as some reports only include major hematomas.
† Periph includes iliac and femoropopliteal vessels.
Fem/pop, superficial femoral and popliteal arteries; infrapop, infrapopliteal artery; prof-fem, profunda femoris artery.

A review of the incidence of hematomas in the Cardio-vascular and Interventional Radiology Research and Education Foundation (CIRREF) Contrast Registry (74 496 diagnostic and interventional procedures) showed that hematomas are more common following interventional procedures than diagnostic studies [41] (see Table 18.3).

Puncture site hematomas are seen more commonly with femoropopliteal angioplasty than with iliac angioplasty because of the need for a high antegrade puncture [5]. As with conventional angiography, hemostasis following withdrawal of the catheter should be controlled manually, preferably by the radiologist. The pressure applied should be over the arterial, rather than the skin, puncture site. It should be constant and sufficient to stop the bleeding without occluding the artery. The length of time required to prevent hematoma formation may be prolonged by the use of anticoagulants or thrombolytic therapy. Significant retroperitoneal bleeding may occur in the absence of a visible hematoma, and should be actively excluded by careful monitoring of the patient in the postangioplasty period [14,42]. Severe hemorrhage may require transfusion or surgery [21].

Complications at the angioplasty site

influenced by the complications of the procedure. In particular, complications are more commonly seen with occlusions than stenoses [17] and in heavily calcified lesions [3]. Complications are seen more often during angioplasty distal to the inguinal ligament than with iliac angioplasty [8]. The incidence of complications occurring at the angioplasty site is shown in Table 18.4.

The most commonly reported and most important complication arising at the angioplasty site is early *reocclusion of the lesion*. This may be due to thrombosis, dissection, spasm, or elastic recoil. The latter does not usually cause total obstruction.

There are many causes of *thrombus formation*. It may be accelerated by the necessary endothelial damage that occurs at angioplasty. It is more likely when there is low flow at low pressure; a normal blood pressure should therefore be

Table 18.3 Incidence of hematomas

Intervention	Incidence of hematomas (%)
Angiography of extremities	2.50
Angioplasty of extremities	6.90
Renal–visceral angioplasty	4.90
Atherectomy	8.19
Stent insertion	4.58
Thrombolysis	6.94

maintained during the procedure. Thrombus may form around the catheter itself. Very rarely, the patient may have an underlying thrombogenic disorder such as systemic lupus erythematosus which predisposes to thrombus formation [40]. Pretreatment with aspirin, an antiplatelet agent, is recommended prior to angioplasty. A bolus dose of intra-arterial heparin 1000–5000 U immediately prior to dilatation has been shown to reduce the incidence of thrombus formation [3]. If thrombus formation occurs despite these measures, it may be successfully treated with local thrombolysis [1].

Dissection of the arterial wall, particularly when treating an occluded vessel, may not be reported as a complication. However, when dissection results in occlusion of the vessel — especially if it converts a previously stenosing lesion to an occlusion — it represents a significant complication. In the femoropopliteal vessel the dissection may be exacerbated by the flow of blood holding open and widening the intimal flap. The blood flow has the opposite effect in the iliac segments, when the arterial puncture is retrograde. Iliac dissections are often less significant as the flow of blood closes the dissection flap.

Dissection may be caused by subintimal passage of the guidewire (more commonly seen with straight wires [43]), or by trauma from the catheter (Fig. 18.1). Dissection may also occur when contrast is injected immediately following angioplasty if there is intimal damage at the site of the lesion [44]. If dissection at the lesion occurs prior to angioplasty, e.g., during manipulation of the guidewire, it may be advisable to delay intervention for 4–6 weeks to allow healing of the dissection flap [1,44]. Significant dissection is often preceded by severe pain: if the patient complains of undue pain, the possibility of dissection should be considered.

In patients with severe atheromatous disease, special care should be taken throughout the procedure as intimal flaps are readily formed. When this occurs in the iliac region, it may lead to iliac, or even aortic occlusion with fatal outcome as a consequence [18].

Dissection may be treated during angioplasty by recanalizing the true lumen, and inflating the angioplasty balloon, effectively "welding" the dissection flap together [44,45]. This may require prolonged inflation times. The arterial lumen may also be restored by atherectomy of the lesion, effectively removing the dissection flap [46]. Alternately, the lumen may be kept open by a prosthetic stent [47]. If treatment of the acute occlusion is not successful, then urgent surgical intervention may be needed, particularly if the limb is critically ischemic.

Perforation of the vessel at the angioplasty site may occur either by the guidewire or due to vessel rupture during balloon inflation. Perforation by the guidewire is not usually serious in the superficial femoral artery, and does not normally require surgical management. However, perforation or rupture of the iliac vessels may be life-threatening because the surrounding retroperitoneal tissues are only loosely

Table 18.4 Angioplasty site complications

Patients	Procedures	Sites	Occlusion*	Thrombosis	Dissection	Spasm	Guidewire perforation†	Vessel rupture	Embolization	Collateral occlusion†	Equipment failure	Renal insufficiency	Reference
352	453	All		9	17			2	7				[1]
202	202	All		12				2	3				[4]
902	985	All	15	6				1					[5]
3650	4750	All		33	42			14					[9]
	318	All		4	1			4	10				[8]
370	500	Periph			30				7				[11]
1141	1642	Periph	28				2	1					[14]
135	148	Periph			7				3				[13]
	376	Periph					2						[19]
129	164	Periph		2		1			4				[30]
175	206	Periph		14	11		2		7		1		[21]
	49	Periph		1	1				1				[16]
	147	Periph		2					7				[12]
98	145	Periph											[31]
152	217	Periph	1	4	4				2	3			[17]
	100	Periph		3					1	2			[15]
200	340	Periph						1	3			4	[25]
50	56	Periph					1	4					[27]
154	194	Periph			1						1		[26]
150	174	Periph					1		5				[28]

* This includes thrombosis and dissection, when the cause of occlusion is not specified.
† Perforation and collateral occlusion are not necessarily considered complications and therefore are not universally reported.
All, all sites; periph, iliac, femoral, or popliteal.

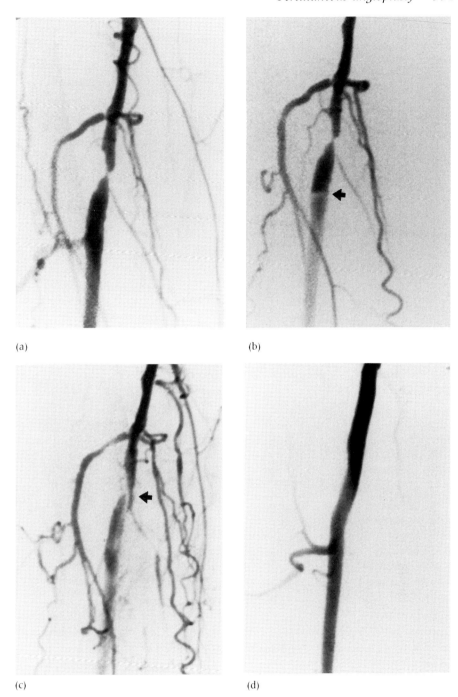

Fig. 18.1 (a) Superficial femoral artery prior to angioplasty. (b) Angioplasty projection showing dissection flap (arrow). (c) Oblique projection showing dissection flap (arrow). (d) Superficial femoral artery following angioplasty.

(a)

(b)

(c)

(d)

adherent and there may be considerable hematoma formation. Rupture of the vessel is usually related to the use of an oversized balloon and is heralded by severe pain at the angioplasty site, due to damage of the adventitia. It is diagnosed by demonstrating contrast medium outside the vessel wall (Fig. 18.2). If the hemorrhage is severe, it should be interrupted either by inflating a balloon across the lesion [1], followed by surgical repair or bypass of the vessel. Alternately, the artery may be occluded by embolization coils prior to a bypass procedure [48].

Occlusion of branch vessels may also occur. This may be insignificant if the branch vessel is a collateral that is no longer required following a successful angioplasty. However, if the angioplasty is not successful and the origin of the collateral vessel is occluded, clinical deterioration may be observed; this may precipitate the need for surgery. Careful technique and advance planning are required in locations such as the aortic bifurcation and tibial origins to ensure that branches are not occluded. This is frequently accomplished by introducing two catheters or wires, one into the branch

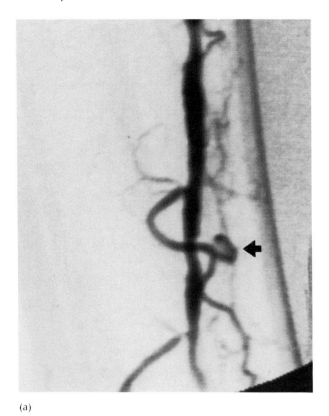

(a)

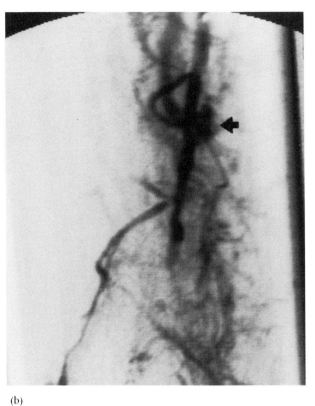

(b)

Fig. 18.2 (a) Superficial femoral artery prior to angioplasty (arrow marks site of later perforation). (b) Arterial perforation following attempted angioplasty (arrow).

that is vulnerable and one into the vessel that is to be angioplastied. This is the so-called "kissing balloon technique". It is seldom necessary in the aortoiliac region. Angioplasty is not recommended above the level of the renal arteries, as occlusion of renal and mesenteric vessels is critical. Several studies show favorable results of infrarenal aortic angioplasty [24].

Arterial spasm may cause subsequent thrombosis. It may be precipitated by manipulation of the guidewire or catheter, or by injection of a high concentration of contrast medium. It is more frequent in the renal arteries and infrapopliteal vessels. It may be prevented to some extent by a sublingual dose of nifedipine (10 mg) immediately prior to the procedure, and may be treated with an intraarterial bolus of glyceryltrinitrate (0.1 mg) or papaverine (25 mg) delivered proximal to the site of spasm [3]. The use of local anesthetic has largely been abandoned.

Late complications at the angioplasty site

The main late complication is *restenosis* at the angioplasty site. This presents with recurrent symptoms and may be diagnosed at diagnostic angiography. Recurrent symptoms

may equally well be due to progression of the disease away from the angioplasty site. There is no contraindication to repeat angioplasty. Stent placement may reduce the rate of restenosis in large vessels, but results in the superficial femoral artery are poor. *Aneurysm formation* is also recognized at the site of previous angioplasty [49,50]. Such aneurysms may be managed surgically or conservatively, depending on the clinical setting.

Problems distal to the angioplasty site

The major problem occurring distal to the angioplasty site is *occlusion*; this may be due to embolization or damage to the vessel extending from the angioplasty site. The latter includes continuation of a *false passage* created at the angioplasty site by poor control of the guidewire or by creation of a dissection flap by contrast injection at the site of angioplasty.

Embolic phenomena include microembolization, which may be visible radiologically, but do not usually compromise the vascular supply as they occlude small distal vessels. Larger emboli may occlude larger, more proximal vessels causing significant ischemia. If this is recognized at the time of the procedure, it may be treated by aspiration and/or thrombolysis of the embolus (Fig. 18.3). This risk is increased in patients who present with the "blue digit syndrome", indicating thromboembolic episodes [44]. Embolization occurs more commonly during treatment of recently formed long occlusions.

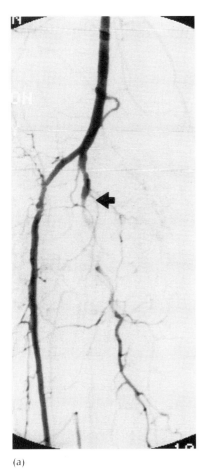

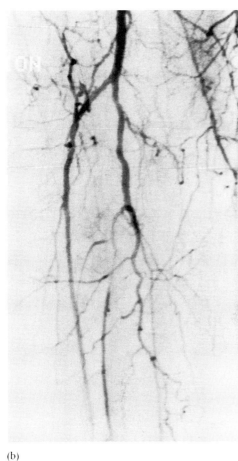

Fig. 18.3 (a) Embolization of common peroneal artery following angioplasty of superficial femoral artery. (b) Patent common peroneal artery following percutaneous aspiration of thrombus.

(a)

(b)

Cholesterol emboli caused by rupture of an atheromatous plaque carry a poor prognosis and may result in loss of an affected limb and fatality.

Equipment failure

Occasionally an angioplasty balloon may fail to deflate; transcutaneous puncture is possible in the femoropopliteal arteries, but is inappropriate in more proximal vessels which do not afford direct access [51]. It may be possible to puncture the balloon with a Chiba needle passed carefully through the introducer sheath [19], but surgical intervention is often required.

Balloon rupture may cause local spasm, and trauma may be caused at the puncture site as the ruptured balloon is removed, although as a rule a longitudinal split does not cause significant problems. However, a transverse rupture may cause considerable trauma, necessitating the use of a sheath which must be passed over the original catheter to facilitate withdrawal [44]. A recent report describes circumferential rupture and separation of the angioplasty balloon. This was successfully retrieved using grasping forceps and a basket [52]. The incidence of equipment failure — mainly rupture of balloons — is diminishing as technology improves.

Guidewire and catheter problems are dealt with in Chapter 14.

Systemic and remote complications

The incidence of systemic complications following angioplasty is influenced by the general health of patients undergoing the procedure. By the nature of their disease, such patients tend to be elderly, with widespread arteriovascular disease, and multiple pathologies. This is reflected in the 30-day mortality rate which is reported as around 1% in most series, and which is usually the consequence of *myocardial infarction* rather than as a direct result of the procedure. These patients are also prone to cerebrovascular disease.

During the angioplasty procedure, monitoring with pulse oximetry, particularly in sedated patients, is recommended. *Vasovagal episodes* are not uncommon, and should be treated with atropine (0.6 mg intravenously). A normal blood pressure should be maintained to maximize perfusion of the angioplasty site. Blood pressure and fluid balance should be monitored rigorously following renal artery angioplasty, as this may result in severe hypotensive episodes.

Sepsis, either local or systemic is uncommon following angioplasty, but has been reported in several publications

[9,35]. Prophylactic antibiotics may be used to prevent local sepsis after graft puncture [48].

Problems related to contrast medium

Most angioplasties are performed using digital subtraction angiography. The improved resolution allows use of dilute contrast medium and, hence, reduces the dose of contrast medium required. However, many patients selected for angioplasty are elderly with widespread atheromatous disease which often involves the renal arteries. *Renal failure* may be induced or exacerbated by high doses of contrast medium. A careful check on cumulative contrast dose must be kept, particularly when the angioplasty involves extensive lesions or multiple sites, and when the patient has had a recent angiogram, or other procedure requiring contrast. Angioplasty of the renal arteries delivers high doses of contrast directly to the kidney, and carries a high risk of consequent transient or irreversible renal damage. Carbon dioxide has been used as a contrast medium during renal angioplasty to prevent this complication [53].

For further consideration of contrast-related complications refer to Chapter 13.

Drug-related problems

Anticoagulants

The endothelial damage caused during angioplasty is thrombogenic. This can be counteracted to some extent by pretreatment with aspirin, which reduces platelet aggregation. Hence, *aspirin* is recommended prior to angioplasty in all patients. As it prolongs bleeding time, it is contraindicated in patients with active peptic ulcer disease, and those with a previous history of adverse reactions to aspirin or other nonsteroidal antiinflammatory drugs. The optimal dose of aspirin needed has not been identified [3]; the dose most commonly recommended ranges from 75 to 300 mg daily.

Heparin is an anticoagulant which is used both in the saline flush solution and as an intraarterial bolus (1000–5000 U) immediately prior to angioplasty [3]. The magnitude of the effect of a single bolus is somewhat unpredictable; the half-life is approximately 6 hours, but is increased in patients with renal or hepatic dysfunction. Heparin has the effect of prolonging clotting time, hence hemostasis at the entry site may take longer to achieve. This does not usually present a problem, but if a hematoma continues to accumulate, despite adequate compression, the effect of heparin may be reversed with protamine sulfate [45], although this in itself is potentially hazardous (see p. 247). The time of administration of the heparin bolus should be recorded, as a repeat dose may be needed in prolonged procedures. Various commercially available clotting time monitors may be used to assess the degree of anticoagulation.

Antispasmodics

Nifedipine is a calcium channel blocking agent used to relieve arterial spasm. It is no longer available for intravascular use, but a sublingual dose of 10 mg is advocated to prevent arterial spasm, particularly when the infrapopliteal or renal arteries are involved. Nifedipine may cause *hypotension* and *reflex tachycardia*, thus precipitating *angina* in patients with ischemic heart disease (see p. 32).

Glyceryl trinitrate (GTN) is also used as an antispasmodic, given as an intraarterial bolus of 100 µg [3]. It is inactivated on first pass through the liver, and repeated doses may be given. Like nifedipine, GTN can cause hypotension and a reflex tachycardia (see p. 41).

Fibrinolytics

Fibrinolytic agents are used in patients with critical lower limb ischemia, particularly those in whom surgery is likely to have a poor outcome, in those with acute emboli or thrombus formation, or in thrombus formation at the site of a recent angioplasty [48]. The most commonly used agents are *urokinase*, *streptokinase*, and *tissue plasminogen activator*. Fibrinolytic agents are contraindicated in patients with:

1 active bleeding from any source;
2 a stroke in the previous 2–3 months;
3 major surgery within 10–14 days;
4 major trauma within 10–14 days;
5 a known bleeding diathesis;
6 a potential bleeding site such as a peptic ulcer;
7 severe hypertension;
8 pregnancy and recent delivery;
9 long-term anticoagulant treatment;
10 hepatorenal failure [48].

Systemic complications associated with use of fibrinolytic agents include hemorrhage, particularly cerebrovascular [54]. Hypersensitivity reactions are associated with the use of streptokinase, especially if the patient has previously received it. The incidence of such complications increases with prolonged perfusion times and higher doses, hence perfusion times should be kept to a minimum [45].

Local complications of thrombolysis include hemorrhage at the puncture site or at the angioplasty site. False aneurysm formation at the arterial puncture site may occur following local hemorrhage [55]. In addition, leakage through the interstices of Dacron grafts has been described [48]. Embolization may occur; this is usually transient but occasionally requires surgery. Paradoxical thrombus may form around the catheter or at the lesion, but the incidence of this is reduced by the use of heparin. It is important to maintain an adequate blood pressure to establish good flow through the angioplasty site in order to minimize the risk of rethrombosis.

Reperfusion of critically ischemic tissue may cause *compartment syndrome* and the limb should be carefully observed following the procedure. Finally, revascularization of necrotic tissue may cause release of myoglobin, resulting in renal impairment [45].

Special sites (see Table 18.5)

Infrapopliteal vessels

The *tibial arteries* are essentially end arteries, hence occlusion as a complication has serious consequences. To minimize complications in crural artery percutaneous transluminal angioplasty (PTA), small balloons on small shafts, e.g., 3 or 4 mm balloons on 3.5-F shafts are needed with fine, e.g., 0.457-mm wires. Infrapopliteal vessels are particularly susceptible to spasm and thrombosis, therefore manipulation of the guidewire and catheter should be kept to a minimum. Pretreatment with antispasmodics is important to reduce the risk of spasm and subsequent thrombosis. Thrombolytic therapy may reverse an acute occlusion with satisfactory outcome.

Renal angioplasty

Renal angioplasty has been used to treat both fibromuscular dysplasia and atherosclerotic lesions. The success rate is low and the complication rate high in atherosclerotic lesions, particularly when plaque causes ostial stenosis [63]. The etiology should be considered when patients are selected for angioplasty.

The majority of renal artery angioplasties are performed to treat renovascular hypertension, although PTA is increasingly used to try and prevent deterioration of renal function in renal artery stenosis. Prior to the procedure, the patient's therapy should be changed from long-acting to short-acting antihypertensives, but the drugs should be determined together with the referring physician. The patient should be well hydrated during and after the procedure, and rigorous monitoring of the blood pressure following angioplasty is mandatory. To this end it is recommended that an intravenous infusion is maintained during renal artery angioplasty.

The main problems to consider are *arterial spasm, arterial rupture, embolization,* and *renal failure* secondary to contrast-medium toxicity. The incidence of complications related to renal angioplasty is shown in Table 18.5.

The renal arteries are particularly susceptible to *spasm,* and care must be taken during manipulation of both the guidewire and the catheter. Subintimal damage distal to the angioplasty site can result in occlusion of both the main renal artery and also the segmental branches, causing *renal infarction* and subsequent hypertension. *Rupture* of the renal artery, which is more likely with an oversized balloon, may lead to severe or fatal *retroperitoneal hemorrhage* [64]. The length of the balloon used for renal PTA is critical. A balloon that is too long may extend beyond the site to

be angioplastied, into a branch artery, hence producing a rupture. As with the peripheral arteries, imminent rupture is heralded by severe *pain* due to adventitial damage.

As contrast is delivered directly to the renal parenchyma, the risk of inducing or causing exacerbation of *renal failure* is higher than in other angioplasty sites. Therefore, the concentration and dose of contrast must be carefully monitored.

Renal transplant vessels are prone to *stenosis* as a result of hyperplasia at the anastamosis site. The significance of an observed stenosis should be confirmed by the presence of a pressure gradient across the lesion. Renal artery spasm may lead to thrombosis, and should be treated promptly with antispasmodics. Close cooperation with a surgeon is mandatory, to prevent loss of a transplant kidney should complications arise [45].

Supraaortic angioplasty

Supraaortic angioplasty is being used more frequently as an alternate to surgery, in both the cerebral and subclavian arteries. It is chosen for patients in whom the operative risk is high, such as those with coronary heart disease. The patients should receive aspirin prior to the procedure, unless there is an absolute contraindication, and peroperative anti-coagulation is recommended with heparin. This should be continued for 48 hours after the procedure has been carried out [65]. Sedative drugs are not recommended as this may obscure neurologic symptoms. A small caliber catheter with hydrophilic coating should be used. The balloon should be able to withstand pressures of 6–8 atm, and should not deform on inflation. Any air bubbles in the balloon should be fully aspirated to prevent air embolus should the balloon rupture. An additional balloon to prevent embolization is not recommended as this is likely to prolong the procedure and cause additional intimal damage. If the stenosis cannot be adequately treated by angioplasty alone, stenting may be necessary [65].

Carotid body stimulation may occur during dilatation of the carotid arteries, resulting in bradycardia and hypotension. This may be treated prophylactically by the intravenous injection of 0.6 mg of atropine. Nifedipine may be given if vasospasm occurs.

It is important to keep the duration of the procedure to a minimum so that the cerebral blood flow is not interrupted for any longer than necessary. The patient's neurologic status should be observed throughout the procedure; *transient neurologic disturbance* is not uncommon during angioplasty. This should be monitored by continuous electroencephalo-gram, and by talking to the patient throughout the procedure. The cerebral blood flow may be observed using transcranial Doppler. Rarely, patients may suffer a *hyperperfusion syndrome,* as the unaccustomed increase in flow and blood pressure in cerebral arteries may not respond to autoregulation

Table 18.5 Special sites

Patients	Procedures	Sites	Initial success rate (%)	Complication rate (%)	Surgery rate (%)	Remote complications*	Deaths	Entry site complications			Angioplasty site complications										Reference
								Hematoma or hemorrhage	False aneurysm	Thrombosis	Occlusion	Thrombosis	Dissection	Spasm	Guidewire perforation	Vessel rupture	Embolization	Equipment failure	Renal insufficiency	
288	388	Renal	78.6	4.6	3.6	1		5					7			5	2		2	[56]
78	101	Renal	89.0	64.0	5.1	9	1	2			4	2	12		2	7	6	6	14	[42]
202	250	Renal	83.0	11.0	3.0	1		4	1		3		2	6	2		6		6	[57]
17	19	Renal	89.5	52.6	0.0		5	4				1	1				3			[58]
18	24	T-renal†	58.0	25.0	11.1				1								1		2	[59]
28	32	Aorta	100.0	0.0	0.0															[24]
32	58	Aorta	94.8	6.9	1.7			1						1			1			[22]
27	27	Aorta	100.0	7.4	7.4				1								2			[23]
25	29	Prof-fem†	89.7		6.9			1		1										[32]
53	57	Infra-pop†	97.0	40.4	3.5	2	1	11			6				2		6		3	[36]
168		Infra-pop†	77.0	18.4	2.4	4	5	2				2			1		3	1	1	[35]
111	168	Infra-pop†	90.0	14.0	3.0	4		2		2	1		1				4		4	[34]
40	55	Infra-pop†	95.0	0.0	0.0															[33]
7	9	SCA†	44.4	33.0	0.0	1														[60]
50	50	SCA†	90.0	10.0	4.0					3		1					1			[61]
10	19	Visceral	89.5	5.3	0.0								1							[62]

* Surgery rate, rate of complications requiring surgery.

† T-renal, renal transplant artery.

Infra-pop, infrapopliteal arteries; prof-fem, profunda femoris artery; SCA, subclavian arteries.

processes. This is also seen after surgery, and is manifest as a stroke secondary to a cerebral hematoma [65].

A recent large series reported by Mathias *et al.* [66] included 192 PTA attempts. Twelve neurologic complications were described, including transient ischemic attacks, prolonged reversible ischemic neurologic deficit, partial middle cerebral artery infarction, anterior–medial cerebral artery infarction, and a cerebral hemorrhage.

Atherosclerotic vertebral artery stenoses are generally ostial and inaccessible to surgery; the associated morbidity and mortality is high. Complications are infrequent at angioplasty.

Dilatation of the intracranial arteries has been described, although the procedure may produce spasm, rupture, occlusion, and fatality [65].

Subclavian and *brachiocephalic angioplasty* are performed for atherosclerotic disease, fibromuscular hyperplasia, and arteritis; these usually present as a subclavian steal. Complications include hemiparesis, transient arm paresis, and transient ischemic attack in addition to the complications encountered with angioplasty at other sites [65].

Angioplasty of the subclavian arteries is usually successful, with a low complication rate, even when the lesion is proximal to the origin of the vertebral artery [3]. Patients with antegrade vertebral flow are at high risk of cerebral embolization during angioplasty [60]. The presence of residual plaque at the lesion may be resolved by use of a stent [9].

Mesenteric angioplasty

Angioplasty of the *mesenteric vessels* is occasionally performed for mesenteric ischemia. The diagnosis may be difficult to establish, and there should be good clinical indications for intervention. Surgical management usually yields good results, but balloon dilatation may be satisfactory [45]. Celiac artery stenosis that is secondary to median arcuate ligament compression is unlikely to respond to angioplasty [62]. As with renal arteries, ostial stenoses are difficult to dilate successfully.

Special techniques (see Table 18.6)

Atherectomy devices

Atherectomy devices may be used to recanalize a vessel prior to angioplasty; the major complications are those of perforation and dissection [90]. Other reports describe complications as minor and involving the entry site [67]. Reid *et al.* [71], found that use of the transluminal extraction catheter was associated with a higher incidence of occlusion and restenosis compared to the Kensey and Simpson catheters. The low-speed rotational (Rotablator) catheter caused gross hemoglobinuria in 63% of patients in a recent study

[70]. Compared to angioplasty, there seems to be little or no reduction of restenosis rates following atherectomy [91] (see also Chapter 19).

Laser angioplasty

Lasers have been used for recanalization of occluded vessels. The most common complication is perforation, which may not be a major complication in a totally occluded vessel. The risk is diminished by the use of lasers with a hemispherical metal tip, which converts the laser energy to heat, and causes less local tissue damage [90,92]. Care should be taken to maintain the laser in coaxial alignment with the vessel to minimize the risk of perforation (see also Chapter 12).

Ultrasound recanalization

Recanalization of occlusions with an *ultrasound angioplasty ablation system* has been described [88,89]. Perforation is the major complication, but the risk of this is reduced by using an over-the-wire, monorail-type probe. Arterial spasm distal to the recanalization site may be treated by application of the energized ultrasound ablation catheter [88].

Intravascular stents

Intravascular stents are used to maintain a patent vessel either as a primary treatment or following a failed percutaneous angioplasty [93]. They are particularly useful in the iliac region and have also been successfully placed in the aorta [83]. Associated complications are at the entry site, related to the size of the system required to deliver the stent [18], and at the site of the lesion, related to stent positioning and early thrombosis. Suspected perforation of the vessel is an absolute contraindication to stenting, since the defect will be enlarged as the stent is expanded [80]. Positioning the stent may prove difficult, particularly with the Wallstent which has low radiographic contrast and asymmetric shortening. The Strecker and Palmaz stents have better radiographic contrast and are easier to see fluoroscopically [82]. Protrusion of iliac stents into the aorta should be avoided as this results in thrombosis around the proximal end of the stent [85]. The Palmaz stent is rigid, and therefore unsuitable for tortuous vessels [78].

Stent insertion carries a risk of distal embolization which is more common with extensive, calcified, and eccentric plaque [85]. Predilatation to the full diameter of the vessel prior to stent insertion may predispose to embolization [84].

Thrombosis of the stent is the most common complication, but long-term anticoagulant treatment is recommended unless patients have a hypercoaguability state [80]. Thrombus formation is related to low flow, and therefore adjacent stenoses should be dilated at the time of stent insertion [80]. Further advantages of stenting include management of

Table 18.6 Complications associated with atherectomy, laser, stents, thrombolysis, and ultrasound recanalization

| | | | | | | | | | Entry site complications | | | Intervention site complications | | | | | | | | | |
Patients	Procedures	Sites	Techniques	Initial success rate (%)	Complication rate (%)	Surgery rate (%)*	Remote complications	Deaths	Hematoma or hemorrhage	False aneurysm	Arteriovenous fistula	Occlusion	Thrombosis	Dissection	Spasm	Guidewire perforation	Vessel rupture	Embolization	Collateral occlusion	Protrusion of stent into aorta	Reference
77	85	Periph	Ather	92.0	21.0	3.9			11	3		1						3			[67]
30		Fem/pop	Ather	93.3	10.0	0.0			60					3				1			[68]
1252		All	Ather	80.0	13.6	–								100							[69]
43	82	All	Ather	88.0	–	5.0	27†		10			2			10						[70]
52	52	Periph	Ather	60.0	9.6	1.9			1				1					2			[71]
112	140	SFA	Ather	95.0	7.1	2.7		1	6	1				4		3		2			[72]
129		Periph	Laser	68.0	32.0	–			6				5			25		5			[73]
28		Fem/pop	Laser	67.0	25.0	–										7					[74]
69	77	Fem/pop	Laser	81.0	–	11.6			6												[75]
40	40	Fem/pop	Laser	77.5	17.5	–										4		3			[76]
17		Fem/pop	Laser	59.0	17.6	0.0										3					[77]
10		Iliac	Stent	100.0	0.0	0.0															[78]
19	27	Iliac	Stent	74.0	11.1	5.3						1	2								[79]
154	171	Iliac	Stent	97.1	11.7	6.5			6	1			2	1		2	1	4	1		[80]
49	53	Iliac	Stent	–	10.0	–	1						1				1	3	1		[81]
79	82	Iliac	Stent	98.0	12.0	6.0			3		1		1					3	1		[82]
7		Aorta	Stent	100.0	0.0	0.0															[83]
68	68	Iliac	Stent	71.0	8.8	0.0	2		1					2				1			[84]
43	50	Iliac	Stent	100.0	10.0	2.0			3				1					1		2	[85]
91	100	Iliac	Stent	97.0	2.0	–							2								[86]
	82	All	Thrombo	82.0	36.5	2.4	2	2	21												[54]
	15	Fem/pop	Thrombo	100.0	33.3	26.7		1	4												[87]
32	32	Periph	U/S	81.0	18.0	–			4						2						[88]
45	50	Periph	U/S	86.0	20.0	0.0			4					4	2	4					[89]

* Surgery rate, rate of complications requiring surgery.

† Gross hemoglobinuria with no long-term effects.

Ather, atherectomy; fem/pop, superficial femoral and popliteal arteries; periph, iliac/femoral/below-knee; SFA, superficial femoral artery; thrombo, thrombolysis; U/S, ultrasound recanalization.

arterial dissection occurring as a complication of angioplasty [93]. Careful technique is required during stent insertion, in accordance with the manufacturers instructions for each prosthesis. The use of heparin is vital to minimize stent thrombosis (see also Chapter 19).

References

1 Gardiner GA, Meyerovitz MF, Stokes KR, Clouse ME, Harrington DP, Bettmann MA. Complications of transluminal angioplasty. *Radiology* 1986;159:201—208.

2 Adar R, Critchfield GC, Eddy DM. A confidence profile analysis of the results of femoropopliteal percutaneous transluminal angioplasty in the treatment of lower extremity ischaemia. *J Vasc Surg* 1989;10(1):57—67.

3 Becker GJ, Catson BT, Dake MD. Non coronary angioplasty. *Radiology* 1989;170:921—940.

4 Hasson JE, Acher CW, Wojtowycz M, McDermott J, Crummy A, Turnipseed WD. Lower extremity percutaneous transluminal angioplasty: multifactorial analysis of morbidity and mortality. *Surgery* 1990;108(4):748—752.

5 Johnstone KW, Rae M, Hogg-Johnstone SA *et al.* 5-year results of a prospective study of percutaneous transluminal angioplasty. *Ann Surg* 1987;206(4):403—412.

6 Struk DW, Rankin RN, Eliasziw M, Vellet AD. Safety of outpatient peripheral angioplasty. *Radiology* 1993;189(1):193—196.

7 Hirschl M, Urbanek A, Tischler R. Outpatient percutaneous transluminal angioplasty: preconditions and results. *Wien Klin Wochenschr* 1991;103(22):673—677.

8 Armstrong MW, Torrie EP, Galland RB. Consequences of immediate failure of percutaneous transluminal angioplasty. *Ann Roy Coll Surg Engl* 1992;74(4):265—268.

9 Beck AH, Muhe A, Ostheim W, Heiss W, Hasler K. Long term results of percutaneous transluminal angioplasty: a study of 4750 dilatations and local lyses. *Eur J Vasc Surg* 1989;3:245—252.

10 Cambria RP, Faust G, Gusberg R, Tilson MD, Zucker KA, Modlin IM. Percutaneous angioplasty for peripheral arterial occlusive disease. *Arch Surg* 1987;122:283—287.

11 Morse MH, Jeanes WD, Cole SEA, Grier D, Ndlovu D. Complications in percutaneous transluminal angioplasty relationships with patients age. *Br J Radiol* 1991;64(757):5—9.

12 Lancashire MJ, Torrie EP, Galland RB. Percutaneous angioplasty in a district general hospital: impact and implications. *J Roy Coll Surg Edinb* 1992;37(3):183—186.

13 Rooke TW, Stanson AW, Johnson CM *et al.* Percutaneous transluminal angioplasty in the lower extremities: a 5-year experience. *Mayo Clin Proc* 1987;62:85—91.

14 Belli A-M, Cumberland DC, Knox AM, Procter ER, Welsh CL. The complication rate of percutaneous peripheral balloon angioplasty. *Clin Radiol* 1990;41:380—383.

15 Kashdan BJ, Trost DW, Jagust MB, Rackson ME, Sos TA. Retrograde approach for contralateral iliac and infrainguinal percutaneous transluminal angioplasty: experience in 100 patients. *J Vasc Intervent Radiol* 1992;3(3):515—521.

16 Mosley JG, Gulati SM, Raphael M, Marston A. The role of percutaneous transluminal angioplasty for atherosclerotic disease of the lower extremities. *Ann Roy Coll Surg Engl* 1985;67:83—86.

17 Capek P, Mcklean GK, Berkowitz HD. Femoropopliteal angioplasty. Factors influencing long term success. *Circulation* 1991;83(2) (Suppl. 1):70—80.

18 Weibull H, Bergqvist D, Jonsson K, Karlsson S, Takolander R. Complications after percutaneous transluminal angioplasty in the iliac, femoral and popliteal arteries. *J Vasc Surg* 1987;5(5):681—686.

19 Harris RW, Dulawa LB, Andros G, Oblath RW, Salles-Cunha SX, Apyan RL. Percutaneous angioplasty of the lower extremities by the vascular surgeon. *Ann Vasc Surg* 1991;5(4):345—353.

20 Wilson SE, Wolff GL, Cross AP. Percutaneous transluminal angioplasty versus operation for peripheral arteriosclerosis. *J Vasc Surg* 1989;9(1):1—8.

21 Samson RH, Sprayregen S, Veith FJ *et al.* Management of angioplasty complications, unsuccessful procedures and early and late failures. *Ann Surg* 1984;199:234—240.

22 Tegtmeyer CJ, Kellum CD, Kron IL, Mentzer RM. Percutaneous transluminal angioplasty in the region of the aortic bifurcation. *J Radiol* 1985;157:661—665.

23 Ravimandalam K, Rao VR, Kumar S *et al.* Obstruction of the infrarenal portion of the abdominal aorta: results of treatment with balloon angioplasty. *Am J Roentgenol* 1991;156(6):1257—1260.

24 Morag B, Garniek A, Bass A, Schneiderman J, Walden R, Rubinstein ZJ. Percutaneous transluminal aortic angioplasty: early and late results. *Cardiovasc Intervent Radiol* 1993;16(1):37—42.

25 Tegtmeyer CJ, Hartwell GD, Selby JB, Robertson R Jr, Kron IL, Tribble CG. Results and complications of angioplasty in aortoiliac disease. *Circulation* 1991;83(Suppl. 2):153—160.

26 van Andel GJ, van Erp WFM, Krepel VM, Breslau PJ. Percutaneous transluminal dilatation of the iliac artery: long term results. *Radiology* 1985;156(2):321—323.

27 Gupta AK, Ravimandalam K, Rao VR *et al.* Total occlusion of iliac arteries: results of balloon angioplasty. *Cardiovasc Intervent Radiol* 1993;16(3):165—177.

28 Jorgensen B, Skovgaard N, Morgard J, Karle A, Holstein P. Percutaneous transluminal angioplasty in 226 iliac artery stenoses: role of the superficial femoral artery for clinical success. *Vasa* 1992;21(4):382—386.

29 Hunink MG, Donaldson MC, Meyerovitz MF *et al.* Risks and benefits of femoropopliteal percutaneous balloon angioplasty. *J Vasc Surg* 1993;17(1):183—192.

30 Krepel VM, van Andel GJ, van Erp WFM, Breslau PJ. Percutaneous transluminal angioplasty of the femoropopliteal artery: initial and long term results. *Radiology* 1985;156(2):325—328.

31 Schwarten DE, Cutcliff WB. Arterial occlusive disease below the knee: treatment with percutaneous transluminal angioplasty performed with low-profile catheters and steerable guidewires. *Radiology* 1988;169:71—74.

32 Dacey JE, Daniell SJ. The value of percutaneous transluminal angioplasty of the profunda femoris artery in threatened limb loss and intermittent claudication. *Clin Radiol* 1991;44(5):311—316.

33 Brown KT, Moore ED, Getrajdman GI, Saddekni S. Infrapopliteal angioplasty: long-term follow-up. *J Vasc Intervent Radiol* 1993;4(1):139—144.

34 Dorros G, Lewin RF, Jamnadas P, Mathiak LM. Below-the-knee angioplasty: tibioperoneal vessels, the acute outcome. *Cathet Cardiovasc Diagn* 1990;19(3):170—178.

35 Bull PG, Mendel H, Hold M, Schlegl A, Denck H. Distal popliteal and tibioperoneal transluminal angioplasty: long-term follow-up. *J Vasc Intervent Radiol* 1992;3(1):45—53.

36 Bakal CW, Sprayregen S, Scheinbaum K, Cynamon J, Veith FJ.

Percutaneous transluminal angioplasty of the infrapopliteal arteries: results in 53 patients. *Am J Roentgenol* 1990;154(1): 171−174.

37 Fellmeth BD, Roberts AC, Bookstein JJ *et al.* Post angiographic femoral artery injuries: non surgical repair with US-guided compression. *Radiology* 1991;178:671−675.

38 Fellmeth BD, Baron SB, Brown PR *et al.* Repair of post catheterisation femoral pseudoaneurysms by color flow ultrasound guided compression. *Am Heart J* 1992;123:547−551.

39 Shibo L, Polak LF. Compression repair of a postcatheterisation pseudoaneurysm of the brachial artery under sonographic guidance. *Am J Roentgenol* 1992;160:383−384.

40 Becker G. Intravascular stents. General principles and status of lower extremity arterial applications. *Circulation* 1991;83(2) (Suppl. 1):122−136.

41 Lossef SV, Barth KH. *Incidence of haematomas in contemporary practice of vascular and interventional radiology: results of the SCVIR contrast registry.* Abstract. Presented at the Society of Cardiovascular and Interventional Radiology, San Diego, California, March 1994.

42 Weibull H, Bergqvist D, Jonsson K, Carlsson S, Takolander R. Analysis of complications after transluminal angioplasty of renal artery stenoses. *Eur J Vasc Surg* 1987;1:77−84.

43 Dyer R (ed.). *Handbook of Basic Vascular and Interventional Radiology.* New York: Churchill Livingstone, 1992.

44 Tegtmeyer CJ. Percutaneous transluminal angioplasty. *Curr Probl Diagn Radiol* 1987;16(2):75−139.

45 Kadir SB (ed.). *Current Practice of Interventional Radiology.* Philadelphia: BC Decker Inc, 1992.

46 Webb JG, Dodek AA, Allard M, Carere R, Marsh I. "Salvage atherectomy" for discrete arterial dissections resulting from balloon angioplasty. *Can J Cardiol* 1982;8(5):481−486.

47 Becker GJ, Palmaz JC, Rees CR *et al.* Angioplasty induced dissections in human iliac arteries: management with Palmaz balloon expandable intraluminal stents. *Radiology* 1990;176:31.

48 Belli AM (ed.). *Practical Interventional Radiology of the Peripheral Vascular System.* London: Edward Arnold, 1994.

49 Vive J, Bolia A. Aneurysm formation at the site of percutaneous transluminal angioplasty: a report of two cases and a review of the literature. *Clin Radiol* 1992;45(2):125−127.

50 Gehani AA, Ashley S, Kester RC, Brooks SG, Davies GA, Rees MR. Aneurysm formation after dynamic catheter assisted balloon angioplasty. *Clin Radiol* 1990;41(4):283−285.

51 Johnsrude IS. Percutaneous transluminal angioplasty. In: Johnsrude IS, Jackson DC, Reed Dunnick N, eds. *A Practical Approach to Angiography.* Little, Brown and Company, 1987.

52 Selby JB Jr, Oliva VL, Tegtmeyer CJ. Circumferential rupture of an angioplasty balloon with detachment from the shaft: case report. *Cardiovasc Intervent Radiol* 1992;15(2):113−116.

53 Thompson K. *Use of CO$_2$ as a contrast medium during renal angioplasty.* Presented at the Andreas Gruntzig Society, Sydney, 1994.

54 Browse DJ, Barr H, Torrie EP, Galland RB. Limitations to the widespread usage of low-dose intraarterial thrombolysis. *Eur J Vasc Surg* 1991;5(4):445−449.

55 Brown KT, Schoenberg NY, Moore ED, Saddekni S. Percutaneous transluminal angioplasty of infrapopliteal vessels: preliminary results and technical considerations. *Radiology* 1988;169:75−78.

56 Lohr E, Bock KD, Eigler F *et al.* Angioplasty of renal arteries: a report of ten years experience. *Angiology* 1991;42(1):44−47.

57 Baert AL, Wilms G, Amery A, Vermylen J, Suy R. Percutaneous transluminal renal angioplasty: initial results and long-term follow-up in 202 patients. *Cardiovasc Intervent Radiol* 1990; 13(1):22−28.

58 O'Donovan RM, Gutierrez OH, Izzo JL Jr. Preservation of renal function by percutaneous renal angioplasty in high risk elderly patients: short-term outcome. *Nephron* 1992;60(2):187−192.

59 Matalon TA, Thompson MJ, Patel SK, Brunner MC, Merkel FK, Jensik SC. Percutaneous transluminal angioplasty for transplant renal artery stenosis. *J Vasc Intervent Radiol* 1992;3(1):55−58.

60 Sharma S, Kaul U, Rajani M. Identifying high risk patients for percutaneous transluminal angioplasty of subclavian and innominate arteries. *Cardiol Clin* 1991;9(3):515−522.

61 Millaire A, Trinca M, Marache P, de Groote P, Jabinet JL, Ducloux G. Subclavian angioplasty: immediate and late results in 50 patients. *Cathet Cardiovasc Diagn* 1993;29(1):8−17.

62 Odurney A, Sniderman KW, Colapinto RF. Intestinal angina: percutaneous transluminal angioplasty of the celiac and superior mesenteric arteries. *Radiology* 1988;167:59−62.

63 Sos TA. Angioplasty for the treatment of azotemia and renovascular hypertension in atherosclerotic renal artery disease. *Circulation* 1991;83(2)(Suppl. 1):162−166.

64 Sharma S, Arya S, Mehta SN, Talwar KK, Rajani M. Renal vein injury during percutaneous transluminal renal angioplasty in non specific aorto arteritis. *Cardiovasc Intervent Radiol* 1993; 16(2):114−116.

65 Mathias KD. Percutaneous transluminal angioplasty in supraaortic artery disease. *Intervent Cardiovasc Med* 1994;00:745−776.

66 Mathias KD, Luth I, Haarmann P. Percutaneous transluminal angioplasty of proximal subclavian artery occlusions. *Cardiovasc Intervent Radiol* 1993;16:214−218.

67 Kim D, Gianturco LE, Porter DH, Orron DE. Peripheral directional atherectomy. 4 year experience. *Radiology* 1992;183(3):773−778.

68 Vroegindeweij D, Kemper FJ, Tielbeek AV, Buth J, Landman G. Recurrence of stenoses following balloon angioplasty and Simpson atherectomy of the femoro-popliteal segment. A randomised comparative 1 year follow-up study using colour flow duplex. *Eur J Vasc Surg* 1992;6(2):164−171.

69 Vallbracht C, Liermann DD, Landgraf H *et al.* Recanalization of chronic arterial occlusions: low-speed rotational angioplasty. 5 years experience in peripheral and coronary vessels. *Eur J Med* 1993;2(4):232−238.

70 Dorros G, Iyer S, Zaitoun R, Lewin R, Cooley R, Olson K. *Cathet Cardiovasc Diagn* 1991;22(3):157−166.

71 Reid JD, Hsiang YN, Doyle DL *et al.* Atherectomy. Early use of three different methods. *Can J Surg* 1992;35(3):242−245.

72 Graor RA, Whitlow PL. Transluminal atherectomy for occlusive peripheral vascular disease. *J Am Coll Cardiol* 1990;15(7):1551−1558.

73 Douek PC, Leon MB, Geschwind H *et al.* Occlusive peripheral vascular disease: a multicenter trial of fluorescence guided, pulsed dye laser assisted balloon angioplasty. *Radiology* 1991; 180(1):127−133.

74 White RA, White GH, Mehringer MC, Chain FL, Wilson SE. A clinical trial of laser thermal angioplasty in patients with advanced peripheral vascular disease. *Ann Surg* 1990;212(3): 257−265.

75 Harrington ME, Schwartz ME, Sanborn TA *et al.* Expanded indications for laser-assisted balloon angioplasty in peripheral arterial disease. *J Vasc Surg* 1990;11(1):146−154.

76 Arlart IP, Gerlach A, Grass HG. Laser-assisted balloon angioplasty in complete femoropopliteal occlusions: preliminary results. *Cardiovasc Intervent Radiol* 1991;14(4):233−237.

77 Veith FJ, Bakal CW, Cynamon J *et al*. Early experience with the smart laser in the treatment of atherosclerotic occlusions. *Am Heart J* 1991;121(5):1531−1538.

78 Kidney D, Murphy J, Malloy M. Balloon expandable intravascular stents in atherosclerotic iliac artery stenosis. Preliminary experience. *Clin Radiol* 1993;47:189−192.

79 Bonn J, Gardiner GA Jr, Shapiro MJ, Sullivan KL, Levin DC. Palmaz vascular stent: initial clinical experience. *Radiology* 1990;174:741−745.

80 Palmaz JC, Garcia OJ, Schatz RA *et al*. Placement of balloon-expandable intraluminal stents in iliac arteries: first 171 procedures. *Radiology* 1990;74:969−975.

81 Long AL, Page PE, Raynaud AC *et al*. Percutaneous iliac artery stent: angiographic long-term follow-up. *Radiology* 1991;180(3):771−778.

82 Hausseger KA, Lammer J, Hagen, Fluckiger F, Lafer M, Klein GE, Pilger E. Iliac artery stenting-clinical experience with the Palmaz stent, Wallstent and Strecker stent. *Acta Radiol* 1992;33:292−296.

83 Long AL, Gaux JC, Raynaud AC *et al*. Infrarenal aortic stents: initial clinical experience and angiographic follow-up. *Cardiovasc Intervent Radiol* 1993;16(4):203−208.

84 Vorwoerk D, Guenther RW. Mechanical revascularisation of occluded iliac arteries with use of self-expandable endoprostheses. *Radiology* 1990;175:411−415.

85 Dyet JF, Shaw JW, Cook AM, Nicholson AA. The use of the wallstent in aorto-iliac vascular disease. *Clin Radiol* 1993;48:227−231.

86 Gunther RW, Vorwerk D, Antonucci F *et al*. Iliac artery stenosis or obstruction after unsuccessful balloon angioplasty: treatment with a self-expandable stent. *Am J Roentgenol* 1991;156(2):389−393.

87 Seabrook GR, Mewissen MW, Schmitt DD *et al*. Percutaneous intraarterial thrombolysis in the treatment of thrombosis of lower extremity arterial reconstructions. *J Vasc Surg* 1991;13(5):646−651.

88 Monteverde-Grether C, Valez y Tello de Meneses M, Nava-Lopez G *et al*. Percutaneous transluminal ultrasonic angioplasty: preliminary clinical report of ultrasound plaque ablation in totally occluded peripheral arteries. *Arch Invest Med* 1991;22(2):171−179.

89 Siegel RJ, Gaines P, Cre JR, Cumberland DC. Clinical trial of peripheral ultrasound angioplasty. *J Am Coll Cardiol* 1993;22(2):480−488.

90 Michaels JA. Percutaneous arterial recanalization. *Br J Surg* 1990;77:373−379.

91 Fischell TA, Stadius ML. New technologies for the treatment of obstructive arterial disease (Review). *Cathet Cardiovasc Diagn* 1991;22(3):205−233.

92 Widlus DM, Osterman FA. Evaluation and percutaneous management of atherosclerotic peripheral vascular disease. *J Am Med Assoc* 1989;261(21):3148−3154.

93 Yang XM, Manninen H, Matsi P, Soimakallio S. Percutaneous endovascular stenting: development, investigation and application (Review). *Eur J Radiol* 1991;13(3):161−173.

Complications of the newer intravascular interventions

Robert P. Liddell, Randall J. Enstrom
and Michael D. Dake

Advances in biomedical engineering have contributed to an expanding list of promising new vascular interventional devices and procedures. The development of these new technologies represent a continued effort by peripheral interventionalists to provide less-invasive, more cost-effective therapies capable of achieving durable long-term results. The literature describing many of the new devices and techniques focuses on the authors' clinical and technical successes. Often, however, the risks and complications associated with these newer interventional procedures are overshadowed by the initial enthusiasm of the investigators and are not given the proper consideration [1].

Recently developed endovascular interventional procedures include atherectomy, laser angioplasty, arterial stenting, and transjugular intrahepatic portosystemic shunting (TIPS). Complications associated with these new procedures can occur at a variety of anatomic locations: the puncture site, the site of intervention, and distal to that site. Specific complications can also be categorized as attributable to the general procedure (groin hematoma, bleeding, azotemia related to the use of contrast media, etc.), or directly related to the device itself (vessel perforation, distal embolization, local thrombosis, migration, etc.). A clear distinction between these is often very difficult to delineate.

The more common risks and complications reported in newer interventional procedures are not unlike those previously described in the percutaneous transluminal angioplasty (PTA) literature [2–4]. Complications at the puncture site are described in most PTA series as the most common untoward effects. The incidence of hematomas, pseudoaneurysms, dissections, arteriovenous fistulas, as well as other access related complications has not been reduced by the use of the newer recanalization devices (Fig. 19.1). In fact, the larger profiles of many of the newer devices may be responsible for an increased frequency of complications associated with vascular access compared to PTA. Other complications remote from the puncture site, and possibly more closely related to the actual devices include embolization, thrombosis, dissection, perforation, and migration of the device.

Atherectomy

The specific complications associated with atherectomy catheters frequently depend on the device being discussed. Currently, there are at least 12 atherectomy catheters being modified or investigated, while only four are currently approved for clinical use by the USA Food and Drug Administration (FDA). All four of these devices were designed to remove atheroma from atherosclerotic arteries by one of two methods. The Simpson Atherocath (Devices for Vascular Intervention Inc., Redwood City, CA) and the Transluminal Extraction Catheter (TEC) (Interventional Technologies, Inc., San Diego, CA) use an extirpative technique, which involves cutting of atheromatous material with retrieval. The second technique employed by the Trac–Wright atherectomy catheter (formerly known as the Kensey catheter, Dow Corning Wright, Arlington, TX) and the Auth Rotoblator (Heart Technology, Bellvue, WA) involves the fragmentation or ablation of atheromatous material without its retrieval.

The Simpson Atherocath was the first atherectomy device to gain widespread use by interventionalists and is currently the most popular of the four approved devices. Simpson et al. [5] initially described their atherectomy experience on 61 patients with 136 lower extremity lesions. Dissection occurred in three of the 61 patients (6%), while distal embolization was noted in only one (3%), and was treated nonsurgically. No perforations were reported and no surgical salvages were necessary. The complications encountered in the larger clinical trials that followed were relatively few in number. In the series described by Dorros et al. [6], an 11% complication rate was reported in 131 patients who presented

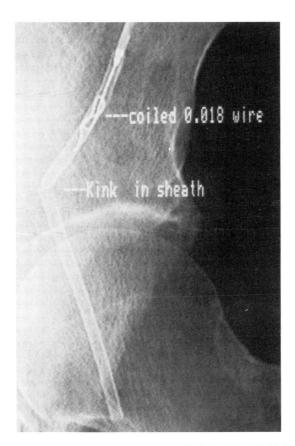

Fig. 19.1 Vascular access complication at the left groin with kinking of the angiographic sheath within the soft tissues of an obese individual. This kink was associated with coiling of the fixed wire tip of a Simpson directional atherectomy catheter. Resultant damage to the leading wire required refitting of the atherectomy catheter with a new nose cone. Antegrade vascular access for treatment of lower extremity occlusive disease may result in significant complications, especially in obese individuals.

with 139 stenoses and 56 occlusions. Specifically, eight cases (6%) of arterial tears, five cases (4%) of distal embolization without clinical significance, and two cases (2%) of groin hematomas were described (Fig. 19.2). Another trial done by Hinohara *et al.* [7], reported fewer complications associated with the procedure. In a series of 100 patients, they reported two cases of distal embolization and one case each of delayed occlusion, transient thrombosis, and groin hematoma. In contrast, a series of 77 patients described by Kim *et al.* [8] summarized a 21% complication rate primarily due to groin hematomas, but notably three (4%) puncture site pseudo-aneurysms required surgical repair and one (1%) case of retroperitoneal bleeding required transfusion.

The TEC catheter is the second extirpative atherectomy device that has found relatively widespread acceptance while having very few reported complications. The catheter employs rotational cutters at its distal tip to shave atheromatous plaque. The cuttings are suctioned through the catheter into an external vacuum bottle. A series by Wholey *et al.* [9] demonstrated the success of the catheter in preventing distal emboli (0%) in 95 patients treated with 126 lesions. Two of the 95 patients (2%) experienced temporary thrombotic occlusions at the site of intervention which were successfully treated with thrombolytic therapy. There were no cases of vascular perforation or significant distal microembolization reported in this series. Although there are currently no reported cases of excessive blood loss, investigators do point out that the suction required by the device to remove atheromatous material may eventually necessitate blood transfusions in patients who have longer stenoses.

The first ablative atherectomy device, the Trac–Wright atherectomy catheter, was developed and described by Kensey *et al.* [10] in 1987. Although the device was described initially by its developers with positive technical results, many studies have since described total complication rates of between 15 and 35% [11–15]. Perforation and subintimal dissection caused by the device's rotating cam accounted for many of the complications in these studies. The incidence of distal embolization has also been relatively high in these series. This may be due, in part, to the fact that ablative atherectomy catheters do not have provisions for collecting the particulate debris they produce. In theory, the ablative atherectomy devices pulverize the atheromatous material into microparticles that should not cause clinically significant embolization.

Coleman *et al.* [16], however, used cadaver atherosclerotic peripheral arteries to show that the Trac–Wright catheter does not sufficiently pulverize microemboli, to avoid causing clinically significant particle embolization. Cull *et al.* [11] treated 46 patients with the Trac–Wright catheter and experienced an overall complication rate of 35%. Perforations were seen in 11 patients (24%), while no clinically significant distal embolizations were noted. Snyder *et al.* [14] described perforated vessels in six of 113 cases attempted (5%), with subintimal dissections reported in 14 cases (12%), while Desbrosses *et al.* [15] had the lowest complication rate (15%). Specifically, four of the 46 lesions (9%) developed dissections and three cases (7%) had clinically significant microembolization. Most of the complications described as perforations occurred in lesions that were heavily calcified.

The last of the approved atherectomy devices is the Auth Rotoblator. Like the Trac–Wright catheter, the Rotoblator is an ablative atherectomy device that attempts to fragment atheromatous material by advancing a rotating, diamond-encrusted burr through the occluded arterial segment. Studies using this device had complication rates of 0–50% [17–19]. One unique complication documented with the use of this device was hemoglobinuria. The high-speed rotation (up to 180 000 rpm) of a large burr ($\geq$4 mm) has been directly correlated to a significant incidence of hemoglobinuria. Dorros *et al.* [17] reported 27 cases (63%) of hemoglobinuria in a series of 43 patients who had 82 lesions. Ahn

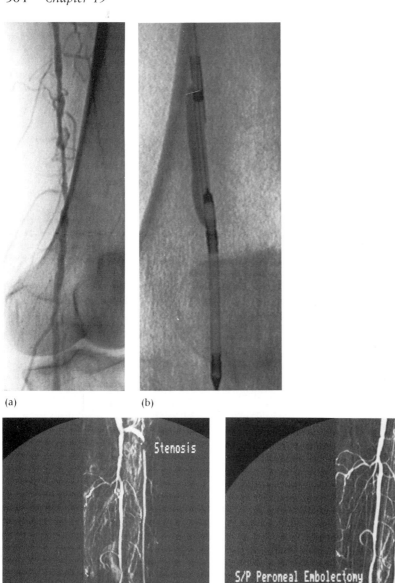

(a)   (b)

(c)   (d)

Fig. 19.2 (a) Diffusely diseased left superficial femoral artery at the adductor canal. (b) Simpson directional atherectomy catheter centered within the lesion. Note slight extrinsic impression upon the balloon at inflation pressure of 2 atm. The effectiveness of atherectomy can be monitored by observing a loss in this defect with subsequent passes of the cutter. In addition, the collection chamber is filled with compacted atheromatous shavings to the level of the cutting window. (c) Following atherectomy, filming over tibial vessels demonstrates an embolic occlusion of the left peroneal artery. (d) Improved patency is noted within the peroneal artery following transcatheter aspiration embolectomy. No untoward clinical sequelae were noted following the procedure.

et al. [18] described four cases (16%) of transient hemoglobinuria in the 25 atherectomies performed, while Zacca *et al.* [19] had two cases (33%) in the six patients treated in their series. In contrast to the results reported for the Trac−Wright catheter, the number of perforated and dissected vessels reported in these series was significantly less. In the three series reviewed, only two cases (5%) of perforation were reported by Dorros *et al.* [17] while only one case of intimal dissection was directly attributed to the Rotoblator [18]. As with the Trac−Wright catheter, distal embolization

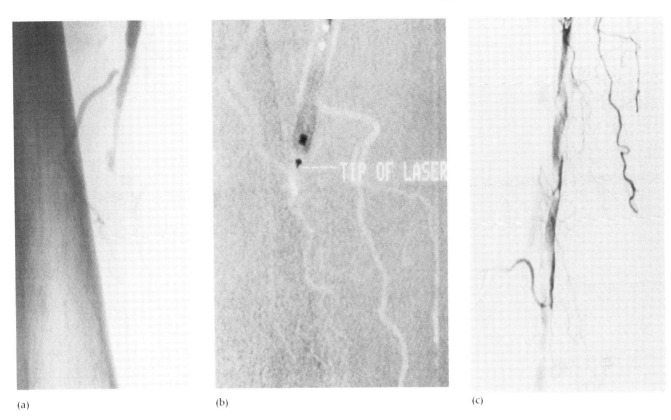

(a)   (b)   (c)

Fig. 19.3 (a) Occluded right distal superficial femoral artery at the adductor canal. (b) Excimer laser catheter engaging proximal margin of the occlusion. (c) Arteriographic appearance following application of laser energy demonstrates marked spiral dissection through the distal superficial femoral artery.

is inevitable. Three cases of clinically insignificant microemboli and one case of diffuse thromboembolism necessitating amputation occurred in one series, while no embolic events were reported in another [18,19].

Laser angioplasty

Laser recanalization of totally occluded peripheral arteries was initially met with much enthusiasm. Its documented ability to ablate atheromatous material and debulk a diseased vessel was seen as a step toward improved long-term patency over balloon angioplasty [20,21]. Metal and sapphire contact probes were developed in an attempt better to control the amount of thermal energy delivered and decrease the incidence of vessel injury. The initial enthusiasm subsided, however, in the wake of well-documented poor long-term patency figures (11–57% after 1 year) [22–28]. Complications associated with laser recanalization in these series carried an overall rate of 10–58%. A review of the literature reveals that perforation is clearly the most common consequence of attempted arterial recanalization with lasers. White *et al.* [22] reported the highest incidence of vessel perforation with seven instances directly attributed to the device in 28

vessels treated (25%). Not unlike atherectomy devices previously described, perforation with lasers during recanalization may be a consequence of their tendency to follow a path of least resistance. Unfortunately, in a hard, calcified atherosclerotic lesion, that path may lead to healthy tissue and cause a dissection or perforation. Indeed, subintimal dissections constitute the next most frequent group of complications experienced (< 1–4%) (Fig. 19.3). Embolic events occurred rarely (0–4%) (Fig. 19.4). In addition, Sanborn *et al.* [28] have reported four cases of mechanical probe tip detachment, with all but one successfully removed percutaneously.

Intravascular stents

Like other new interventional devices, the initial development of intravascular stents was in response to the limitations of balloon angioplasty, especially the incidence of abrupt closure and intimal dissection observed after PTA [29,30]. Stents provide a mechanical means of compressing dissected intima and atheromatous plaque against the vessel wall in an attempt to restore luminal diameter. Most of the large reported series of patients treated with stents have described results in the peripheral vasculature. Recently, however, there are reports of increasing success in treating renal [31,32], coronary, femoral, and brachiocephalic arterial lesions. European investigators have also documented success using stents in venous stenoses and occlusions [33].

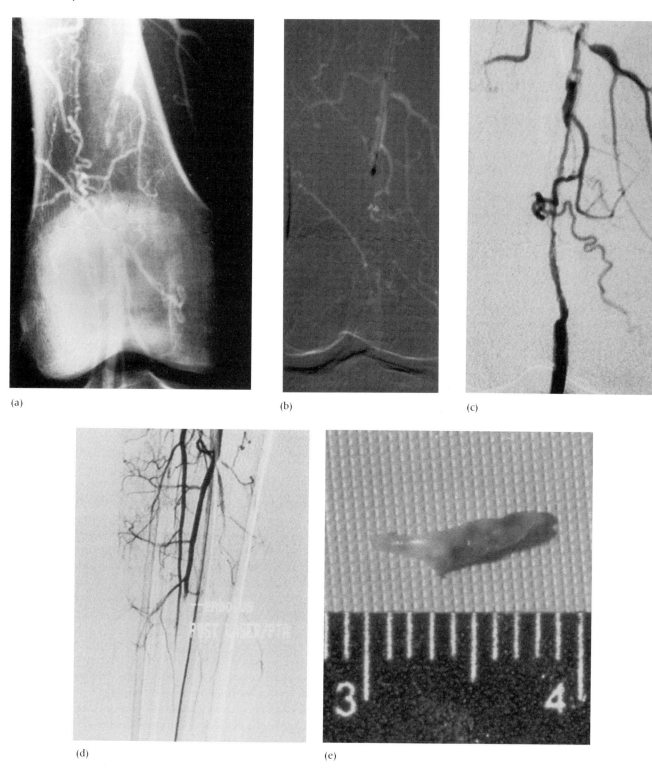

(a)

(b)

(c)

(d)

(e)

Fig. 19.4 (a) Irregular occlusion of proximal right popliteal artery. (b) Thermal laser probe advanced into occluded segment. (c) Arteriogram following recanalization of occluded popliteal artery with laser probe. (d) Distal extremity arteriogram demonstrates embolic occlusion of peroneal artery following laser PTA. (e) Embolectomy specimen recovered from peroneal artery at surgery.

There are a number of different designs to consider when describing the evolution of stents, but for simplicity, the three most widely used and investigated will be discussed. Intravascular stents and their associated complications can be classified into two general categories based on the means of their mechanical deployment. Balloon expandable stents include the Palmaz stent (Johnson & Johnson Interventional Systems, Warren, NJ) and the Strecker stent (Boston Scientific Corporation, Watertown, MA). In contrast, the Wallstent (Schneider AG, Zurich, Switzerland) is a self-expanding stent that uses a constraining catheter that, when retracted, allows the stent to expand radially.

In addition to outlining technical advances, initial articles describing stents have focused on improved clinical results in the setting of failed PTA. Progress made in improving recanalization results as well as long-term patency have not, however, been accompanied by improvements in overall complication rates. These rates should gradually decrease as interventionalists gain experience with this new technology. Vascular injuries occurring at the puncture site represent many of the reported complications. However, investigators are quick to attribute these consequences to the procedure and not the stent itself [29,33]. In an attempt to address the frequency of complications related to general vascular access, manufacturers have modified designs to allow a reduction in the diameter of some stent/delivery systems. Specific stent-related complications described in the literature include acute thrombosis of the stented segment, dissection, rupture, infection, pseudoaneurysm formation, migration, and delivery system failure.

In 1987, a multicenter study approved by the FDA was initiated by Palmaz et al. [34] to evaluate the efficacy and safety of the Palmaz balloon expandable stent. During the 4-year study, 587 procedures were performed on 486 patients with localized iliac artery disease. Patency and complication rates were both favorable. The overall complication rate was 10%. The most common complication encountered by the investigators was related to vascular access (8%), while only a small number of problems were directly attributed to the stent itself (2%). Acute thrombosis of the stented region was noted in five (1%) of the lesions treated, with four of the five thromboses successfully recanalized using local thrombolytic therapy. The remaining one underwent bypass surgery. Also reported were two (<1%) pseudoaneurysms that developed in the stented region. In both cases, the vessels were chronically occluded iliac arteries that had been recanalized using lasers before angioplasty and subsequent stenting. Dislodgment and migration of deployed stents was noted in four cases (1%) (Fig. 19.5). The circumstances of the migrations were not described in this series.

At the time of Palmaz stent delivery, the stent can migrate partially, or completely off the angioplasty balloon before it can be centered across the targeted lesion. Retrieval of the stent is then necessary. Migration of the stent during di-

latation can occur if the balloon inflates asymmetrically or ruptures. In addition, the rigid Palmaz stents are susceptible to mechanical forces which may lead to crushing or deformation of the prosthesis after deployment. Stents that are deployed near joints in peripheral vessels can be plastically deformed by contact with joints or bones in the region of treatment (Fig. 19.6). Other extrinsic mechanical forces, such as recurrent tumor or fibrosis, may also damage a deployed stent, while neointimal hyperplasia has recently been reported by investigators to be responsible for stenoses found within stents on follow-up [35].

In 1988 Strecker et al. [36] initially described the more flexible Strecker stent and its preliminary clinical results. Lierman et al. [37] implanted 100 Strecker stents in the iliac and femoral arteries. Stents placed in the iliac arteries had a patency rate of 97% after 8 months. In contrast, stented femoral arteries had only a 60% patency rate at follow-up. The most prevalent complication reported was thrombosis of the stented area due to the stent's inability to limit neointimal hyperplasia in the peripheral vasculature. This consequence has prompted further investigation into its underlying mechanism and has subsequently resulted in limited use of the stent in treating femoral occlusive disease. Acute complications, such as dissection, pseudoaneurysm formation, and dislodgment, are similar to those outlined for the Palmaz stent. Long-term complications, besides neointimal hyperplasia, have not been reported.

In contrast to both the Palmaz and the Strecker stents, the Wallstent is a flexible stent that uses an overlining catheter membrane that, when retracted, allows the stent to self-expand. Vorwerk et al. [38] treated 125 patients with 63 iliac occlusions and 62 iliac stenoses with the Wallstent. Patency was reported in 100% of the lesions after 6 months and 89% after 24 months. Complication rates were also rather low (<2%). Complications after stenting were observed in five patients (4%), with only two requiring surgical or percutaneous intervention. Three iliac reocclusions were described after stenting. There was also one stent that did not cover the entire diseased segment and subsequently was associated with distal embolization. Self-expanding stents, such as the Wallstent, are often difficult to deploy precisely in the intended area. When the stent is deployed, a considerable amount of foreshortening of the stent may occur, resulting in incomplete lesion coverage and placement of multiple stents. Wallstents have also been utilized in the venous system with considerable success, while experiencing similar complications to those reported for arterial lesions [33].

TIPS

The formation of a TIPS is a modification of a technique originally described in 1969 by Rosch et al. [39] and involves the deployment of a stent across a percutaneously created tract connecting the portal and hepatic veins to relieve portal

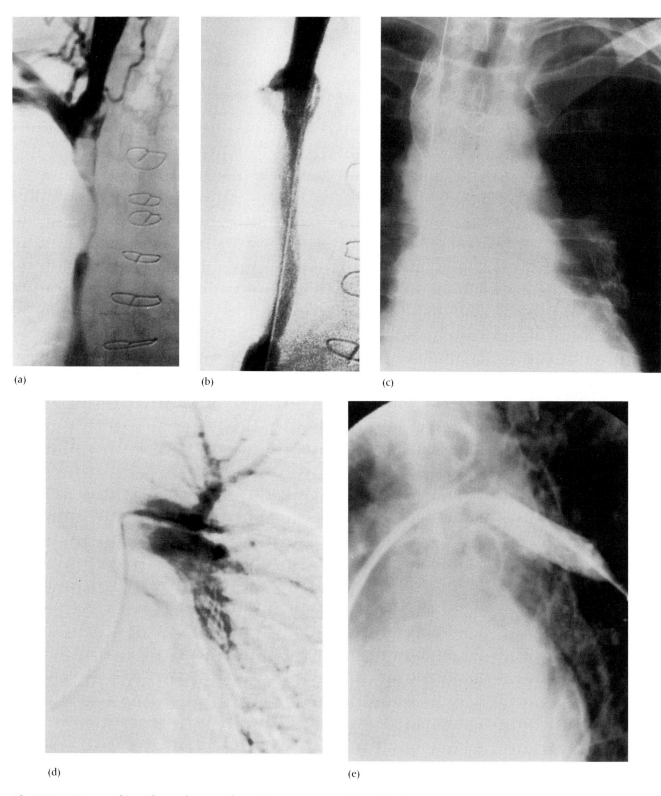

(a)

(b)

(c)

(d)

(e)

Fig. 19.5 (a) Venographic evidence of narrowed superior vena cava in patient with facial, neck, and upper extremity swelling. (b) Incremental improvement in venographic appearance following stenting of the superior vena cava with a series of Palmaz balloon expandable stents. (c) Migration of the most caudal stent to the descending left pulmonary artery was noted on a follow-up chest radiograph. (d) Pulmonary arteriography demonstrates the exact position of the stent within the arterial tree. (e) The prosthesis was cannulated with a balloon catheter and relocated into the right iliac vein.

Newer intravascular interventions

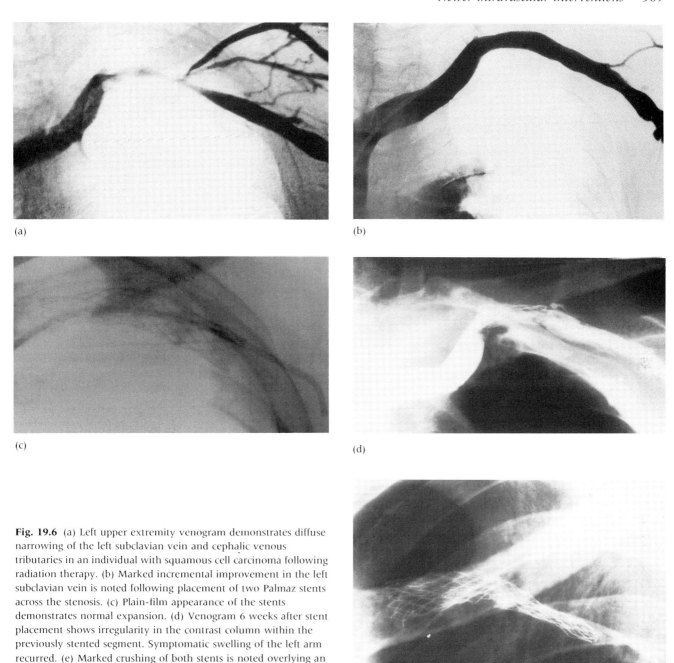

(a)

(b)

(c)

(d)

(e)

Fig. 19.6 (a) Left upper extremity venogram demonstrates diffuse narrowing of the left subclavian vein and cephalic venous tributaries in an individual with squamous cell carcinoma following radiation therapy. (b) Marked incremental improvement in the left subclavian vein is noted following placement of two Palmaz stents across the stenosis. (c) Plain-film appearance of the stents demonstrates normal expansion. (d) Venogram 6 weeks after stent placement shows irregularity in the contrast column within the previously stented segment. Symptomatic swelling of the left arm recurred. (e) Marked crushing of both stents is noted overlying an area of fluffy parenchymal lung infiltrates most compatible with radiation injury. The exact etiology of the extrinsic forces responsible for the plastic deformation of the stents is unclear; however, it is most likely associated with some effect from radiation tissue damage.

hypertension. The development of vascular stents has improved initially poor patency results reported by Colapinto *et al.* [40]. The past 10 years have seen a number of studies attempt to determine the efficacy and safety of stenting portohepatic venous shunts [41–43]. All have reported favorable results.

The incidence of complications in the reported series has

been relatively infrequent. The complications identified include intraperitoneal hemorrhage, hepatic artery injury, myocardial infarction, transient hemobilia, transient renal failure, fever, and stent migration. LaBerge *et al.* [41] described very good clinical and technical results in their first 100 TIPS procedures, with a 9% incidence of clinically significant complications. Stenosis or occlusion of the shunt were the most common complications described. In these situations, shunt patency has been successfully reestablished and stenoses treated by shunt dilatation and/or repeat stent placement.

In the process of creating a tract between the portal and hepatic veins, inadvertent needle punctures of the liver capsule may occur. LaBerge *et al.* [41] reported many extra-capsular punctures; however, only one intraperitoneal hemorrhage of clinical significance developed. Intrahepatic biliary duct transection and inadvertent gall-bladder puncture have also been described in a number of cases. Resultant consequences include transient hemobilia. Hepatic artery injuries have been noted and their consequences not fully understood. Haskal *et al.* [44] reported five cases of known hepatic artery punctures. Two of the five cases developed clinical symptoms. One puncture was deemed directly responsible for a subsequent hepatic artery occlusion and permanent liver damage. The second resulted in severe intraperitoneal bleeding that necessitated emergency surgery to identify and oversew its source. Migration of stents deployed in TIPS procedures has also been noted. Sanchez *et al.* [45] reported a case in which a stent was dislodged while an adjacent area was being dilated by a second stent. The dislodged stent was successfully retrieved from the right atrium percutaneously.

New endovascular interventional devices and procedures are continually being developed and investigated. The literature describing these advances has focused primarily on their ability to improve technical and clinical results established for PTA. In contrast, complications attributed to these newer devices and procedures have not been described in notable detail. Although the incidence of these complications is generally low, their consequences can be complex. As a result, they are not clearly reported, and are therefore difficult to understand. For investigators, this stresses the increasing importance of not only defining the more commonly reported complications associated with vascular access, but also complications specifically related to the device or procedure.

References

1 Ahn SS, Eaton D, Moore WS *et al.* Endovascular surgery for peripheral arterial occlusive disease. *Ann Surg* 1992;July,216(1): 3–16.

2 Weibull H, Berquist D, Jonsson K *et al.* Complications after percutaneous transluminal angioplasty in the iliac, femoral, and popliteal arteries. *J Vasc Surg* 1987;5:681–686.

3 Gardiner GA, Meyerovitz MF, Stokes KR *et al.* Complications of transluminal angioplasty. *Radiology* 1986;159:201–208.

4 Berquist D, Jonsson K, Webull H. Complications after percutaneous transluminal angioplasty of the peripheral, and renal arteries. *Acta Radiol* 1987;28:3–12.

5 Simpson JB, Selman MR, Roberson *et al.* Transluminal atherectomy for occlusive peripheral vascular disease. *J Am Cardiol*

6 Dorros G, Lewin RF, Sachdev N *et al.* Percutaneous atherectomy of occlusive peripheral vascular disease: stenoses and/or occlusion. *Cathet Cardiovasc Diagn* 1989;18:1–6.

7 Hinohara T, Selman MR, Robertson GC *et al.* Directional atherectomy. New approaches for the treatment of obstructive coronary and peripheral vascular disease. *Circulation* 1990;81(Suppl. IV): 79–90.

8 Kim D, Gianturco LE, Porter DH *et al.* Peripheral directional atherectomy: 4-year experience. *Radiology* 1992;183:773–778.

9 Wholey MH, Jarmolowski CR. New perfusion devices: the Kensey catheter, the atherolytic reperfusion wire device, and the transluminal extraction catheter. *Radiology* 1989;172: 947–952.

10 Kensey KR, Nash JE, Abrahams C *et al.* Recanalization of obstructed arteries with a flexible, rotating tip catheter. *Radiology* 1987;165:387–389.

11 Cull DL, Feinberg RL, Wheeler JR *et al.* Experience with laser-assisted balloon angioplasty and a rotary angioplasty instrument: lesson learned. *J Vasc Surg* 1991;14:332–339.

12 Triller J, Do DD, Madden G *et al.* Femoropopliteal artery occlusion: clinical experience with the Kensey catheter. *Radiology* 1992;182:257.

13 Wholey MH, Smith JAM, Godlewski BS *et al.* Recanalization of total arterial occlusions with the Kensey dynamic angioplasty catheter. *Radiology* 1989;172:95–98.

14 Snyder SO, Wheeler JR, Overlie PA *et al.* Kensey catheter a mechanical recanalization device: use in 113 patients with 157 lesions in peripheral circulation (abstract). *Radiology* 1990; 177(p):203.

15 Desbrosses D, Petit H, Torres E *et al.* Percutaneous atherectomy with the Kensey catheter: early and midterm results in femoro-popliteal occlusions unsuitable for conventional angioplasty. *Ann Vasc Surg* 1990;4:550–552.

16 Coleman CC, Posalaky IP, Robinson JD *et al.* Atheroablation with the Kensey catheter: a pathologic study. *Radiology* 1989; 170:391–394.

17 Dorros G, Lyer S, Zaitoun R *et al.* Acute angiographic and clinical outcome of high speed percutaneous rotational atherectomy (Rotoblator). *Cathet Cardiovasc Diagn* 1991;22:157–166.

18 Ahn SS, Eton D, Yeatman LR *et al.* Intraoperative peripheral rotary atherectomy: early and late clinical results. *Ann Vasc Surg* 1992;6:272–280.

19 Zacca NM, Raizner AE, Noon GP *et al.* Treatment of symptomatic peripheral atherosclerotic disease with a rotational atherectomy device. *Am J Cardiol* 1989;63:77–80.

20 Choy DSJ, Sterzer SH, Rotterdam HZ *et al.* Transluminal angioplasty. *Am J Cardiol* 1982;50:1206–1208.

21 Lee G, Ikeda RM, Kozina J *et al.* Laser dissolution of coronary atherosclerotic obstruction. *Am Heart J* 1981;102:1074–1075.

22 White RA, White GH, Mehringer MC *et al.* Clinical trial of laser thermal angioplasty in patients with advanced peripheral vascular disease. *Ann Surg* 1990;212:257–264.

23 Blebea J, Ouriel K, Green RM *et al.* Laser angioplasty in peripheral vascular disease: syptomatic versus hemodynamic results. *J Vasc Surg* 1991;13:222–230.

24 Segger JM, Abela GS, Silverman SH *et al.* Initial results of laser recanalization in lower extremity arterial reconstruction. *J Vasc Surg* 1989;9:10–17.

25 Wright JG, Belkin M, Greenfield AJ *et al.* Laser angioplasty for limb salvage: observations and results. *J Vasc Surg* 1989;10: 29–37.

1988;61:96–101.

26 Owen ERTC, Moussa SA, Lewis JD *et al*. Peripheral laser angio-plasty: results, complications and follow-up. *J Roy Coll Surg Edinb* 1990;35:75−79.

27 Lammer J, Pilger E, Karnel F *et al*. Laser angioplasty: results of a prospective, multicenter study at three year follow-up. *Radiology* 1991;178:335−337.

28 Sanborn TA, Cumberland DC, Greenfield AJ *et al*. Peripheral laser-assisted balloon angioplasty: initial multicenter experience in 219 peripheral arteries. *Arch Surg* 1989;124:1099−1103.

29 Sigwart U, Puel J, Mirkovitch V *et al*. Intravascular stents to prevent occlusion and restenosis after transluminal angioplasty. *New Engl J Med* 1987;316:701−708.

30 Becker GJ, Katzen BT, Dake MD. Non-coronary angioplasty. *Radiology* 1989;170:921−940.

31 Wilms GE, Peene PT, Baert AL *et al*. Renal artery stent placement with the use of the Wallstent endoprothesis. *Radiology* 1991;179: 457−462.

32 Richter GM, Roeren T, Noeldge G *et al*. Renal aorta stenting: European experience with the new type of Palmaz−Shatz two segmented articulated stent (abstract). *Radiology* 1990;177(p): 299.

33 Antonucci F, Salomanowitz E, Struckman G *et al*. Placement of venous stents: clinical experience with a self-expanding pros-thesis. *Radiology* 1992;183:493−497.

34 Palmaz JC, Caborde JC, Rivera FJ *et al*. Stenting of the iliac arteries with the Palmaz stent: experience from a multicenter trial. *Cardiovasc Intervent Radiol* 1992;15:291−297.

35 Do DD, Triller J, Walpoth BH *et al*. A comparison study of self-expandable stents versus balloon angioplasty alone in femoro-popliteal artery occlusions. *Cardiovasc Intervent Radiol* 1992;15: 306−312.

36 Strecker EP, Ber G, Schneider B *et al*. A new vascular balloon expandable prosthesis: experimental studies and first clinical results. *J Intervent Radiol* 1988;3:59−62.

37 Lierman D, Strecker EP, Peters J. The Strecker stent: indications and results in iliac and femoropopliteal arteries. *Cardiovasc Intervent Radiol* 1992;15:298−305.

38 Vorwerk D, Gunther RW. Stent placement in iliac arterial lesions: three years experience with the Wallstent. *Cardiovasc Intervent Radiol* 1992;15:285−290.

39 Rosch J, Hanafee WN, Snow H. Transjugular portal venography and radiological portocaval shunt: an experimental study. *Radiology* 1969;92:1112.

40 Colapinto RF, Stronell RD, Gildiner M *et al*. Formation of intra-hepatic portosystemic shunts using a balloon dilatation catheter: preliminary clinical experience. *Am J Roentgenol* 1983;140: 709−714.

41 LaBerge JM, Ring EJ, Gordon RL *et al*. Creation of transjugular intrahepatic portosystemic shunts with the Wallstent endo-prosthesis: results in 100 patients. *Radiology* 1993;187:413−420.

42 Noeldge G, Richter GM, Roessle M *et al*. Morphologic and clinical results of the transjugular intrahepatic portosystemic stent-shunt (TIPSS). *Cardiovasc Intervent Radiol* 1992;15: 342−348.

43 Mayner M, Cabera J, Palido-Duque JM *et al*. Transjugular intra-hepatic portosystemic shunt: early experience with a flexible Trocar/Catheter system. *Am J Roentgenol* 1993;161:301−306.

44 Haskal ZJ, Pentecost MJ, Rubin RA. Hepatic arterial injury after transjugular intrahepatic portosystemic shunt placement: report of two cases. *Radiology* 1993;188:85−88.

45 Sanchez RB, Roberts AC, Valji K *et al*. Wallstent misplaced during transjugular placement of an intrahepatic portosystemic shunt: retrieval with a loop snare. *Am J Roentgenol* 1992;159: 129−130.

CHAPTER 20

Complications of regional fibrinolytic therapy

David A. Kumpe and Janette D. Durham

Introduction

Transcatheter regional thrombolysis has become a standard technique for interventional radiologists. Local administration of a plasminogen activator greatly extends the range of endovascular techniques that can be offered to patients with acute and chronic peripheral arterial and venous occlusions, and enables the interventionalist to manage thrombotic complications of angioplasty, endovascular stent placement, atherectomy, and surgery. Familiarity with the various techniques of local thrombolysis is mandatory for any interventionalist.

Nonetheless, thrombolysis has received grudging acceptance by many clinicians because of the perception of a high complication rate. Apprehension about complications is not unjustified. Interventionalists in their enthusiasm to promote a valuable technique have often ignored or minimized the complications associated with this form of therapy. Only a few reviews on the complications of thrombolytic therapy have appeared in print [1–6].

This chapter will review the complications of regional thrombolytic therapy. The complications of systemic thrombolysis used to treat acute myocardial infarction, deep venous thrombosis, and pulmonary embolism will be covered only insofar as they are relevant to regional lysis.

Choice of fibrinolytic agent

Three plasminogen activators are commonly available in the USA for intraarterial thrombolysis: streptokinase (SK), urokinase (UK), and recombinant tissue plasminogen activator (r-tPA). Another plasminogen activator, anisoylated plasminogen streptokinase activator complex (APSAC) has recently become available.

Clinical differences in fibrinolytic agents

While logic would suggest that there should likely be differences in complication rates for comparable intraarterial doses of these three agents based on the differences in mechanism of action [7–10], very little comparative data for regional infusions are available. The investigators who have described their experience with fibrinolysis have fallen into two main camps, utilizing different plasminogen activators administered by different routes. The cardiology community has used either SK or tPA almost exclusively for systemic fibrinolytic therapy for acute myocardial infarction. On the other hand, in the USA, essentially all experience over the last decade with fibrinolytic agents among interventional radiologists is with UK. At the University of Colorado we have used UK exclusively since 1984. The motives for adopting UK include unsatisfactory results obtained in many early series utilizing SK [11–15], and the powerful influence of the original report in 1985 by McNamara and Fischer [16] of better results with lower complications using UK. The following is a brief review of complications in studies comparing the fibrinolytic agents.

UK versus SK

Many interventional radiologists believe that SK and tissue plasminogen activator have higher rates of hemorrhage than UK. The meager comparative documentation that exists supports this belief. McNamara and Fischer [16], in the first report of intraarterial thrombolytic infusions using UK in a high-dose protocol, compared their results using UK with five previously reported series of intraarterial SK infusions. They reported major bleeding in 4% of UK infusions, compared to a mean major bleeding rate of 13% for intraarterial SK. On the other hand, bleeding complications with intraarterial SK in the series they cited occurred using a SK dose of 5000 U/h, roughly the equivalent lytic power of 10 000−15 000 U/h of UK (A. Sasahara, personal communication), and far less than the lytic power of the infusion dose used by McNamara and Fischer [16] (240 000 U/h for ≤ 4 hours, followed by an infusion of 60 000−120 000 U/h until completion of lysis). In the series cited for SK, infusion times averaged 41 hours, versus 18 hours for UK [16]. It is therefore possible that at least part of the excess bleeding complications seen with SK reflect the dosage protocol and prolonged infusion times used, rather than the agent infused.

Intrainstitutional retrospective comparisons of the results of SK and UK infusions suggest that UK infusions produce results with fewer complications than SK [17−21].

In one of the largest reported single institution experiences with different plasminogen activators administered by catheter-directed intraarterial infusions, Graor et al. [17] retrospectively compared their experience with catheter-directed regional infusions of SK (n = 200), UK (n = 200), and tPA (n = 65). The dose rates for the three agents were: SK 5000 U/h; UK 240 000 U/h; and tPA either 0.05 mg/kg per h, or 0.1 mg/kg per h. Clinical success rates were 60% for SK, 95% for UK, and 91% for tPA. Major bleeding complications (defined as bleeds that produced hemodynamic instability, or which required transfusion or surgery, or which caused death) occurred in 28% of SK-treated patients, 6% of UK-treated patients, and 12% of tPA-treated patients. Intracranial bleeding occurred in 2% of patients treated with SK and with tPA, and did not occur in any of the UK-treated patients. Death rates were 4% in the SK group, 2% in the tPA group, and 0% in the UK group. Decreases in clottable fibrinogen at the end of the infusions was greater for SK than for either UK or tPA. This was a retrospective study, however, so statistical comparison is of limited value. Nonetheless, the differences in bleeding complications between SK and either tPA or UK were statistically significant, while those between UK and tPA did not reach statistical significance. These comparative results have the same problem mentioned above − that differing doses of lytic agent and different infusion times are uncontrolled factors.

There are few data on the use of SK in doses equivalent to current UK protocols for regional thrombolysis. Nonetheless, there was a difference in bleeding complications in the only prospective comparative study of which we are aware in which comparable intraarterial doses of UK and SK were administered. Tennant et al. [22] gave intraarterial (intracoronary) infusions of equivalent doses of SK (2000 U/min) and UK (6000 U/min) prospectively, in this instance for 2 hours or less, into 80 patients suffering from acute myocardial infarction. There was equal fibrinolytic success with the two agents (60% for UK versus 57% for SK). Bleeding complications occurred in 29% of the SK-treated patients and 11% of the UK-treated patients; major bleeding after early coronary artery bypass surgery was more frequent after SK (four out of five patients) than UK (zero out of five patients).

UK versus tPA

Meyerovitz et al. [23] compared regional infusions of UK and tPA in 32 acutely thrombosed native arteries and grafts. Early lysis (at 4 and 8 hours) of thrombus was greater with tPA, while at 24 hours, lysis was equal, as were clinical success rates at 30 days. Major bleeding complications (bleeding requiring surgery, two or more units of transfusion, or interruption of the fibrinolytic infusion) occurred in 12.5% of the UK patients and 31% of the r-tPA group, a difference which was not statistically significant (P = 0.39). In addition, minor bleeding occurred in 12.5% of tPA patients and in no patient treated with UK. Fibrinogen levels were significantly lower at 24 hours among the tPA patients than the UK patients.

Comparative studies of fibrinolytic agents in systemic treatment

Acute myocardial infarction

Subtle differences in complication rates among fibrinolytic agents have emerged from the much larger experience with systemic infusions to treat acute myocardial infarction, although overall bleeding complications among the agents

Table 20.1 Bleeding complications from systemic administration of thrombolytic agents to treat acute myocardial infarction. Combined data from Third International Study of Infarct Survival (ISIS-3) and Gruppo Italiano per lo Studio della Streptochinasi nell' Infarcto Miocardico (GISSI-2) on noncerebral bleeds associated with use of thrombolytic agents and heparin. (From de Bono & More [24])

	SK	r-tPA	APSAC	Heparin	No heparin
n	19 979	19 928	13 773	26 831	26 849
Total bleeds (%)	5.6	6.2	5.4	7.3	4.3
Major bleed (%)	0.9	0.7	1.0	1.0	0.8

tested are remarkably similar (Table 20.1). The treatment for acute myocardial infarction involves the administration in a short period of time of a much larger total dose of thrombolytic agent than is generally used in regional thrombolysis, producing an immediate systemic thrombolytic state. The overall incidence of nonintracranial bleeds was 5–7%, with major bleeding episodes (defined as a bleed that causes death or permanent disability, or which prolongs the patient's hospital stay) occurring in 1% of cases. The relative fibrin specificity of r-tPA does not protect against bleeding; on the contrary, there is a suggestion in separate studies that agents of greater thrombolytic potential, such as r-tPA, may be associated with a higher risk of intracranial hemorrhage (see Intracranial hemorrhage, below).

Deep vein thrombophlebitis (DVT)

A different dosage regimen of the fibrinolytic agent is used in the treatment of DVT. Infusion times used for DVT (12–48 hours) are comparable to those used for regional infusions [25], as opposed to the short-term (≤3 hours) infusions used to treat acute myocardial infarction. The dosage rate and total dose of intravenous (systemic) SK, UK, or r-tPA used for treating DVT usually exceed those administered for regional intraarterial treatment. With protracted infusions of plasminogen activators used for DVT, the relative uniformity of bleeding complication rates seen in short infusions of distinct fibrinolytic agents (Table 20.1) does not hold. Instead, the incidence of major bleeding (defined as resulting in discontinuance of therapy, blood transfusion, or death) varies by a factor of 15 — from 14% for SK infusions to 0.8% for UK infusions (Table 20.2). Thus, in systemic infusions of longer duration, the potential for development of a bleeding complication may be related to the fibrinolytic agent chosen.

Reported complications of intraarterial fibrinolytic therapy

Various investigators use different criteria to define a complication. Specific conclusions drawn from any data compilation are therefore dubious. Nonetheless, a number of important general points and principles emerge from such analyses.

Gardiner and Sullivan [5] summarized the incidence of

Table 20.2 Bleeding complication rate from systemic thrombolysis used to treat DVT. From Pilla & Comerota [25]; Goldhaber *et al.* [26,27]

	SK	UK	tPA	Heparin
Major bleeding	87/624 (14%)	1/171 (0.6%)	2/53 (4%)	21/217 (9.7%)

complications from 1787 published cases of regional thrombolysis used to treat arterial occlusions. These are shown in Table 20.3.

The papers used to compile these data were not listed; equally unclear were the fibrinolytic agent used, and the types of infusion techniques employed [5]. To assess the complication rate for regional infusion of a plasminogen activator using current techniques and the currently favored agent in the USA, we reviewed all reports of the use of regional UK infusions for treating arterial and arterial graft occlusions since 1985. Fifteen reports [28–42] detailed complications of 892 infusions in 789 patients. These are shown in Table 20.4. Major complications occurred in 5–37% of infusions in these series, and minor complications in 6–35%.

Hemorrhage

The most common and most appropriately feared complication of thrombolytic therapy is hemorrhage. In Gardiner and Sullivan's [5] survey of complications of intraarterial local lysis, either major hemorrhage (defined as bleeding requiring transfusions, surgical intervention, or discontinuation of the thrombolytic infusion) or minor hemorrhage occurred in 13% of cases (see Table 20.3). In our survey the combined incidence of major and minor hemorrhage was 19%. The total incidence of hemorrhage is undoubtedly higher since minor bleeding is not consistently reported. While most bleeding occurred at the catheter insertion site, in one-fourth to one-third of cases, major bleeding occurred at a remote site; intracranial bleeds occurred in 0.2–0.5% of cases.

The "baseline" bleeding complication rates which are to be expected from the systemic thrombolytic state produced by administration of a fibrinolytic agent are presented in Tables 20.1 and 20.2. Comparison with the complications of regional thrombolysis is instructive. Contrary to the generally held

Table 20.3 Complications of regional thrombolysis. (From Gardiner & Sullivan [5])

Complication	Incidence (%)
Major bleeding	6.6 (CNS 0.5)
Minor bleeding	6.3
Embolization	5.2
Thrombosis	3.1
Death	0.8
Reperfusion syndrome	0.7
Vessel wall dissection	0.6
Acute renal failure	0.3
Sepsis	0.2
Myocardial infarction	0.2

CNS, central nervous system.

Table 20.4 Complications for intraarterial/intragraft infusions of UK. (From [28–42])

	Overall percentage	Range (%)
Bleeding complications		
Major hemorrhage	5.9	3–17
Local	3.9	2–9
Remote	0.8	1–2
Intracranial hemorrhage	0.2	0–2
Minor hemorrhage	12.8	4–24
Local	12.1	4–23
Remote	0.7	1–4
Nonbleeding complications		
Embolization	7.2	2–40
Requiring therapy	1.8	1–12
Pericatheter thrombosis	1.9	2–10
Requiring therapy	0.8	0–6
Reperfusion syndrome	0.1	0–1
Compartment syndrome	0.9	1–8
Renal failure	1.7	1–5
Acute myocardial infarction	0.8	0–5
Miscellaneous major complications*	2.5	0–16
Mortality and amputation		
Death from procedure	0.9	0–2
All Deaths at 30 days	5.2	1–18
Amputations from procedure	0.8	0–4
All Amputations 30 days	11	2–18

* Total 22 miscellaneous major complications: stroke ($n = 2$) [35]; graft infection ($n = 1$) [35]; pseudoaneurysm ($n = 6$) [30,33,38]; sepsis ($n = 1$) [38]; arrhythmia ($n = 1$) [39]; pulmonary edema ($n = 1$) [39]; arteriovenous fistula ($n = 2$) [36,42]; groin infection ($n = 1$) [36]; arterial perforation ($n = 1$) [32]; cardiopulmonary complication ($n = 6$) [30].

belief [5], it is clear that the bleeding rate from regional thrombolysis is significantly *greater* than that seen with systemic thrombolysis, either from a large systemic dose of thrombolytic agent over a short period (treatment of acute myocardial infarction), or with systemic infusions of thrombolytic agents for DVT (at least using UK) using larger doses than those used for regional thrombolysis over comparable infusion times.

The difference is due to a high rate of local bleeding — in our survey, two out of three major bleeds and 12 out of 13 minor bleeds during regional thrombolysis occurred at the catheter insertion site. A similar finding has been reported in the experience with myocardial infarction. There is a marked difference in total bleeding complications between the cardiac trials in which there is early arterial intervention (total bleeding complications 20–47%) versus those in which there is no early arterial intervention (total bleeding complications 1–8%) [24].

Pericatheter hemorrhage

Pericatheter bleeding during an intraarterial fibrinolytic infusion is unusual during the first 4–12 hours of infusion, when using dosage rates of 4000 U/min for the intravascular infusion. The reason why pericatheter bleeding may begin after this time is not known. McNamara *et al.* [6] point out the lack of pericatheter bleeding around arterial catheters of similar size, which are used for infusion of cancer chemotherapy, vasodilators for mesenteric ischemia, or vasopressin for gastrointestinal hemorrhage, and have speculated pericatheter bleeding may begin when there is loss of a fibrin-platelet seal at the catheter entry site due to the thrombolytic state produced by the plasminogen activator after 4–12 hours.

Preventive measures for pericatheter bleeding

For intraarterial infusions, the first bleeding manifestation (and the best clinical warning sign that a more significant hemorrhage, either local or remote, may be pending) usually occurs at the catheter insertion site. Meticulous attention must be paid to initial catheter insertion, with all effort directed toward gaining access to the vessel on the first needle stick. A micropuncture set (Cook, Inc., Bloomington, IN) can be used for the initial arterial puncture when thrombolytic therapy is anticipated, as this produces a smaller needle hole and allows test insertion of the smaller inner catheter, supplied with the coaxial dilator, to check the status of the insertion site if necessary. In some circumstances, the small catheter may be used for the infusion. If the wrong vessel is punctured during initial catheter insertion (femoral vein instead of artery, or vice versa), a small catheter is left in for the duration of the infusion to avoid leakage from the fresh puncture site.

Bleeding around the catheter is common enough that it must be anticipated as part of regional fibrinolytic treatment. When pericatheter bleeding begins, simple local compression will usually control or halt the bleeding. Occasionally, a pledget of Gelfoam soaked with thrombin or with ε-aminocaproic acid pressed externally at the bleeding site will help. If pericatheter bleeding persists after these measures, the infusion rate of the thrombolytic agent can be halved, and heparin stopped. If bleeding still persists, infusion of the thrombolytic agent is halted. The size of catheter used for the infusion can often be important. Starting the infusion with the smallest possible catheter, and exchange to a larger catheter or sheath if local bleeding develops, may also control the bleeding. When pericatheter bleeding develops, McNamara *et al.* [6] recommend checking the activated partial thromboplastin time (aPTT) and fibrinogen levels. If coagulation parameters are not seriously disturbed (fibrinogen ≥ 100 mg/dl and aPTT ≤ 60 seconds), they ascribe the pericatheter bleeding to enlargement of the arteriotomy site and exchange to a larger catheter or sheath. For a fibrinogen level less than 100 mg/dl or an aPTT of greater than 150 seconds, they recommend decreasing heparin and/or UK dose without changing to a larger catheter.

If bleeding is severe and persistent despite the above measures, consultation with a hematologist expert in coagulation may be helpful. Reversal of the systemic lytic state can be accomplished by administration of cryoprecipitate (three to 10 bags), fresh frozen plasma, ε-aminocaproic acid (5 g intravenously (IV) followed by 1–1.25 g IV/h if necessary, maintaining the plasma level at 0.13 mg/ml), transexamic acid, or aprotinin [43,44]. The risks of administering these agents must be balanced against the risk posed by the continued bleeding.

Bleeding from a catheter insertion site in the femoral artery, in an extraanatomic PTFE graft, or in a hemodialysis access site, is usually of no consequence. In contrast, pericatheter bleeding from an axillary catheter insertion site is potentially much more severe, because an expanding hematoma in the axillary sheath may produce a permanent nerve paresis. In De Maioribus *et al.*'s [32] series, a major bleeding complication occurred in three of four cases in which the catheter had been inserted in an axillary site, leading them to abandon the axillary artery as a catheter insertion site for regional fibrinolytic therapy.

Intracranial hemorrhage

One of the most feared complications of the use of thrombolytic therapy is the occurrence of intracranial bleeding. The incidence of intracranial bleeding associated with intraarterial fibrinolysis is low: 0.2% in our survey, 0.5% in the Gardiner and Sullivan compilation [5], 0.1%, 0.2%, and 0.4–0.5% in three other large experiences [6]. In the combined experience of the University of Colorado Health Sciences Center and the Denver Veterans Administration (VA) Medical Center, two instances of intracranial hemorrhage have occurred in approximately 600 infusions (0.3%). The risk of intracranial hemorrhage may be less with intraarterial infusions of UK than with systemic infusions of large doses of thrombolytic agent for the treatment of acute myocardial infarction; during and immediately after which intracranial hemorrhage occurs in about 0.8% of cases [24], range 0.3–5.0% [45–52].

Such episodes, however rare, are deadly. Of eight patients at Mayo Clinic who had intracranial hemorrhage after systemic fibrinolytic treatment of acute myocardial infarction, seven died [53]. One of the two patients who had intracranial hemorrhage in our experience died.

There is no apparent relation during regional thrombolysis between the occurrence of intracranial hemorrhage and either the infusion rate of plasminogen activator or the duration of the infusion. Intracranial hemorrhages have occurred at doses of 1000–4000 U/min of UK [6]. Most

cases of intracranial hemorrhage associated with regional thrombolysis have occurred during the infusion — sometimes within hours of initiation of the infusion — while the intracranial hemorrhages associated with systemic infusions for acute myocardial infarction have occurred after the infusion; the latter phenomenon is no doubt related to the short infusion times (≤ 3 hours) for treating acute myocardial infarctions. Of the two intracranial hemorrhages in our experience, one occurred after an overnight (15-hour) infusion of UK at 120 000 U/h for a thrombosed hemodialysis access site (Fig. 20.1). A second occurred at the VA Hospital after approximately 3 hours of a second infusion (Fig. 20.2). One patient (see Fig. 20.1) underwent immediate operative evacuation of the hematoma and has made a satisfactory recovery 3 months after the event with essentially no neurologic deficit. The hemorrhage was fatal in the other patient (Fig. 20.2). Both episodes of intracerebral hemorrhage have occurred in the last year.

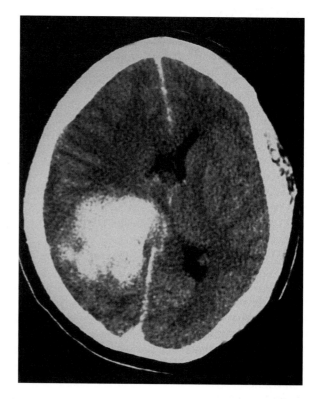

Fig. 20.1 A 38-year-old woman with diabetes and end-stage renal disease, on chronic hemodialysis. Her PTFE hemodialysis access graft had clotted and was not cleared sufficiently of thrombus with pulsed spray UK, clot maceration, and angioplasty. Overnight (15-hour) infusion of UK was performed at 120 000 U/h. Neurologic changes were noted approximately 2 hours after UK was discontinued, while the patient was on dialysis. Intracerebral hemorrhage in the right posterior parietal region was documented by computed tomography. Note the lobar distribution of the clot. Emergency clot evacuation was performed. Three months later the patient has recovered with no functional neurologic deficit.

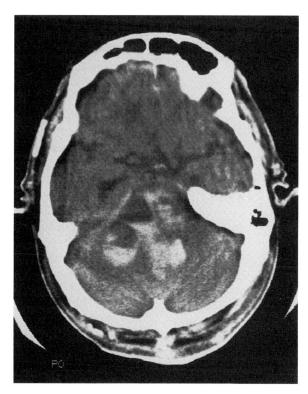

Fig. 20.2 A 73-year-old male with diabetes, hypertension, and longstanding end-stage renal disease, admitted with a thrombosed hemodialysis access site. He had had a fall 5-days previously without loss of consciousness. A head computed tomography (CT) the day after the fall showed no abnormality. He had received 1.25×10^6 U of UK 3 days previously without incident for the clotted access, with incomplete resolution of the thrombus. UK treatment was initiated with a 250 000 U bolus into the clot, followed by an infusion at 100 000 U/h. The patient developed a respiratory arrest after 3 hours of infusion. CT showed a multiloculated posterior fossa hemorrhage with fluid levels within the hematoma. Patient died the day after the hemorrhage.

For regional fibrinolysis, neither a risk factor profile for intracranial hemorrhage nor an assessment of the relative risk of intracranial hemorrhage with the use of different fibrinolytic agents is available. For systemic administration of thrombolytics, some risk factors have been established, particularly age greater than 70 years and hypertension. In the GISSI-2 trial the incidence of intracranial hemorrhage was four times as great in patients whose diastolic blood pressure exceeded 110 mmHg as opposed to those whose diastolic blood pressure was less than 100 mmHg [52]. In addition, a large dose of thrombolytic agent, prior neurologic disease, concomitant drugs including the use of calcium antagonists, female sex, prior cardiopulmonary resuscitation, low body weight, coincident head injury, previous stroke, and, curiously, previous coumarin anticoagulation are considered to be risk factors [50,52,54]. The type of thrombolytic agent employed may be of some importance. Surveys of large numbers of patients treated systemically with different agents in the coronary trials have revealed statistically significant but still minor differences in the incidence of intracranial hemorrhage and total stroke. In the Third International Study of Infarct Survival (ISIS-3) and GISSI-2 studies more than 39 000 patients who had acute myocardial infarction received SK (1.5×10^6 U) or r-tPA (100 mg), and another 13 773 received APSAC (30 U). The total rate for cerebral hemorrhage was higher for r-tPA than for SK (0.6% versus 0.3%; $P < 0.00001$) [46]. In ISIS-3 the frequency of intracerebral hemorrhage was also significantly higher with APSAC than with SK. Reports from separate trials [55] suggest a higher incidence of intracranial hemorrhage with r-tPA plus aspirin [56] than with either SK plus aspirin [57] or APSAC [58]. From these experiences, Topol and Califf [59], in an editorial, suggested that use of r-tPA had a higher bleeding complication rate, and that greater fibrin specificity in a fibrinolytic agent carried a higher risk of intracranial hemorrhage, particularly among elderly patients. They suggested that the dose of fibrinolytic agent be reduced in proportion to patient weight. Nonetheless, the relatively small differences in incidence of intracranial hemorrhage suggest to us that the risk of intracranial hemorrhage is more dependent on the presence of the (as yet not established) predisposing cause of intracranial hemorrhage rather than the specific drug chosen for infusion.

Gore *et al.* [50] point out that as many as 70% of cerebral hemorrhages associated with fibrinolysis occur in the cerebral lobes, frequently in multiple locations. This distribution is atypical of hypertensive hemorrhages, which are more common in the distribution of perforating vessels, such as basal ganglia, posterior lateral thalamus, pons, and cerebellar hemispheres [53]. Even in the treatment of acute stroke with systemic fibrinolysis, in one multicenter study, there is a preponderance of lobar hemorrhage in the 11% of patients who had intracerebral hemorrhage producing a parenchymal hematoma [60]. In comparison with intracranial hemorrhages of other etiologies (tumor, arteriovenous malformation, amyloid angiopathy), intracranial hemorrhages associated with systemic fibrinolytic therapy are more often multiple, in multiple intracranial compartments (intraventricular, subarachnoid, subdural, and parenchymal), and contain fluid levels inside the hematomas suggesting continuing or repeated bouts of hemorrhage (Fig. 20.2) [53].

There is evidence that cerebral amyloid angiopathy is at least partly responsible for intracerebral hemorrhage during fibrinolytic therapy [2,53,61−64]. However, it is recognized that lobar intracerebral hemorrhage associated with amyloid angiopathy has a good outcome in most patients [65], so that the grim outcome in thrombolytic patients [53] cannot be explained by the presence of amyloid angiopathy alone.

Because the risk profile for cerebral hemorrhage during regional fibrinolysis is so poorly defined, there are few recommendations for preventive measures. McNamara *et al.*

[6] recommend that hypertension be controlled aggressively during fibrinolytic infusion, keeping blood pressure less than 150/95 with nifedipine 10 mg sublingually every 15 minutes, as needed, for a maximum of four doses. If systolic pressure exceeds 200 mmHg or diastolic pressure exceeds 110 mmHg, the infusion is halted until blood pressure is under control. Elderly patients may be at greater risk for intracranial hemorrhage; age greater than 75 years should be considered a relative but not absolute contraindication for regional fibrinolytic therapy.

Remote nonintracranial hemorrhage

Other unusual sites and consequences of remote bleeding have been reported. These include:
1 femoral nerve palsy from an iliacus hematoma [66,67] (Fig. 20.3);
2 hemorrhage into a renal tumor [68];
3 the parapharyngeal space [69];
4 lung [70];
5 pituitary tumor [71];
6 the spinal epidural space [72,73];
7 the triceps compartment [74].
Intrathoracic hemorrhage after cardiopulmonary resuscitation and treatment with SK can be fatal [75]. Hematoma formation around a vein graft can simulate an intrinsic venous stricture [76]. Retroperitoneal hematoma may be the consequence of a dissection of blood upwards from a femoral puncture site, even in the absence of swelling in the groin [6].

Treatment of thrombosed hemodialysis access sites has become a frequent application of regional fibrinolysis in many centers. At the University of Colorado this problem accounted for 50% of all regional fibrinolytic treatments over the last 2 years. Interventionalists who treat thrombosed hemodialysis access sites will encounter extravasation of blood from recent puncture sites. There is most commonly swelling over the extravasation site without external bleeding. Seldom will there be more than a solitary bleeding point. The exact point of bleeding can be defined by the injection of a small amount of contrast near the external swelling under fluoroscopic observation — a puff of contrast through the wall of the graft will localize the point of extravasation (Fig. 20.4). Bleeding from a puncture site can be minimized, if not avoided entirely, if manual compression is applied at the bleeding site and flow is reestablished early using pulsed-spray crossed-catheter technique [77–80], with early angioplasty as appropriate. Local extravasation has become quite unusual in our experience since we introduced cross-catheter technique, falling from 12.9% with single-catheter technique to 1.4% with crossed-catheter technique [80].

Laboratory monitoring for hemorrhage

Disappointingly, laboratory studies have been of no value in predicting which patients will have successful thrombolysis or which will have a bleeding complication. Nonetheless, baseline laboratory measurements can become important during the course of intraarterial fibrinolysis if clinical difficulties arise. Before starting fibrinolysis, a complete blood count including platelet count, prothrombin time (PT), aPTT, and serum creatinine should be obtained, and possibly serum fibrinogen. Thrombin time is not obtained because it is prolonged by the presence of concomitant heparin administration. Since heparin is administered with most regional fibrinolysis, thrombin time has not provided any useful information during infusion of the fibrinolytic agent. The laboratory studies listed may become important as a baseline if clinical difficulties arise later in the treatment. However, they will seldom if ever need to be repeated (other than aPTT) during the course of an intraarterial fibrinolysis which proceeds to a successful result, within 24 hours. On the other hand, if the pretreatment prothrombin time is significantly prolonged (INR > 2), or the creatinine is elevated (putting the patient at risk for contrast-induced renal failure), or any of the other parameters listed are grossly abnormal, the use of fibrinolysis is reconsidered with the referring clinical service. If feasible, elevated creatinine, coagulopathy, and other metabolic disturbances are corrected prior to the fibrinolytic treatment. The aPTT is followed closely during the infusion of fibrinolytic agent and heparin; any hemorrhage that develops is likely to be more severe if the aPTT is more than 100 seconds. It is easier to correct an elevated aPTT by changing the rate of heparin infusion, than it is to correct a low fibrinogen.

Serum fibrinogen determinations during fibrinolysis were monitored by most investigators in the past to determine if the infusion dose should be changed. A serum fibrinogen of more than 100 mg/dl is still used by many as an indicator to halt fibrinolytic therapy. It is our experience, and that of others [6], that bleeding, once started, is more difficult to control if fibrinogen is less than 100 mg/dl or aPTT is greater than 100 seconds, but that such levels are not predictive of an impending hemorrhage. Furthermore, serum fibrinogen determinations during fibrinolysis are not as accurate as in other circumstances, since fibrinogen determinations are altered in the presence of fibrin split products [9] and heparin [81]. For fibrinogen determinations, the sulfite precipitation test provides higher and more accurate levels than the Clauss chronometric method, although the Clauss method is believed to provide the best indication of functional fibrinogen levels [81]. Despite the intrinsic problems of determining serum fibrinogen levels in the presence of systemic heparin, if a protracted or difficult thrombolysis is anticipated, pretreatment serum fibrinogen can be obtained. In our practice, serum fibrinogen is not routinely determined before

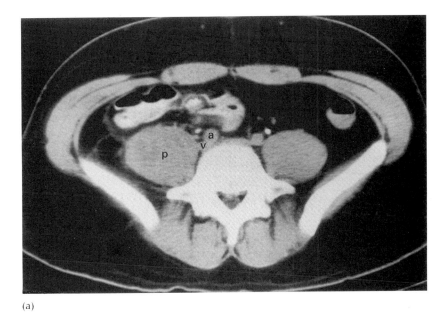

(a)

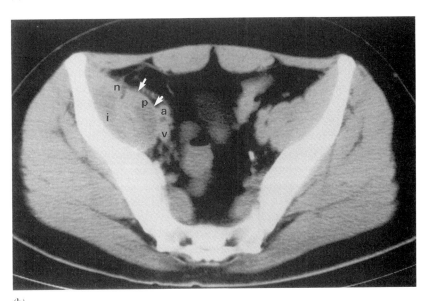

(b)

Fig. 20.3 Spontaneous right psoas and iliacus muscle hemorrhage resulting in right femoral neuropathy in a 35-year-old man 2 days following UK infusion and institution of heparin therapy for arterial occlusive disease in the left leg. Three computed tomographic images of the (a) upper, (b) middle, and (c) low pelvis. a, artery; v, vein; i, enlarged iliacus muscle; ip, enlarged iliopsoas muscle; n, location of femoral nerve; p, enlarged right psoas muscle; arrows, iliacus fascia. (From Durham & Rutherford [67].)

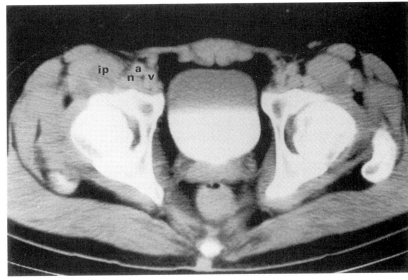

(c)

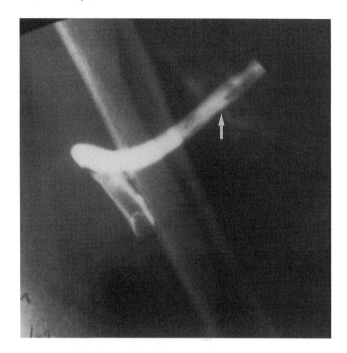

Fig. 20.4. Extravasation from a recent puncture site in a clotted PTFE hemodialysis access graft undergoing lysis. Extravasation site (arrow) can easily be localized under fluoroscopy after a small volume contrast injection to guide local compression.

fibrinolysis because pretreatment fibrinogen levels below 150 mg/dl are extremely rare. Likewise, fibrinogen levels are not determined during infusions when standard infusion dosage protocols are used and the infusion duration is less than 24 hours, since we have found that fibrinogen levels very seldom fall below 100 mg/dl. If an infusion is prolonged beyond 24 hours, we determine fibrinogen levels. If the fibrinogen is less than 100 mg/dl, we are more inclined to halt the infusion unless it appears that a final satisfactory result will be obtained with a further limited infusion (≤ 8 hours). As noted above, bleeding around the catheter at its insertion site usually precedes major remote hemorrhage when using UK, and can be used as an indicator to check aPTT and fibrinogen levels so that appropriate adjustments can be made (see Preventive measures for pericatheter bleeding, above).

Platelet counts should be obtained before initiating a thrombolytic infusion, particularly in patients who have been treated with heparin for periods of more than 1 week, to look for evidence of heparin-associated thrombocytopenia (HAT) due to the development of heparin-dependent anti-platelet antibodies [82–84]. A devastating "white clot syndrome" results when the presence of these antibodies is associated with arterial thrombosis [85]. Continued monitoring of platelet counts during and after completion of thrombolytic therapy, at least as long as the patient is being treated with heparin, is important for the same reason.

Measures for preventing and minimizing remote bleeding

Most remote bleeds occur at the site of previous vascular punctures. Invasive procedures (venipuncture, arterial puncture, intramuscular injections) should be scrupulously avoided. Blood for laboratory determinations must be obtained from indwelling lines. If no intravenous line is available for this purpose, one should be inserted before the infusion is initiated.

Vital signs, hematocrit, and aPTT should be monitored carefully. An increasing pulse rate frequently precedes a fall in blood pressure in the case of a continuing hemorrhage. A falling hematocrit may indicate an occult hemorrhage, although it is common to see a decrease of 2–4% without any apparent hemorrhage. The aPTT is used to monitor heparin infusion rates and is maintained at 60–100 seconds (see Preventive measures for pericatheter bleeding, p. 375).

Infusion time should be kept to a minimum. Measures that decrease infusion time include lacing a bolus of UK through the clot before starting the infusion, and use of a coaxial system to deliver UK simultaneously to more distal portions of the thrombus as well as the proximal end. As the infusion time exceeds 24 hours, and certainly 36 hours, the relative likelihood of improving the result with continuing the infusion must be balanced against the increasing probability of a complication. Generally, the dose of UK is decreased to 1000 U/min as infusion time increases. Alternate therapies, e.g., stopping the fibrinolytic infusion while continuing systemic anticoagulation, the use of aspiration thrombectomy, or surgical intervention, should be considered.

Surgery and fibrinolytic therapy

There are limited numbers of studies [86–90] on surgical intervention after systemic thrombolytic therapy, that generally indicate that surgery can be performed immediately after systemic thrombolytic therapy but at a cost of increased bleeding and more transfusions compared with patients who have not had thrombolytic therapy [91]. Control trials are not available. Current techniques of regional thrombolysis disturb the coagulation system less than systemic thrombolysis [22]. Most investigators have found that surgery can be performed immediately after cessation of regional thrombolysis without significant bleeding complications [23–92]. This is related to the short half-lives of the fibrinolytic agents. Clearance half-lives are listed as follows [24]: r-tPA 2–7 minutes, UK 10 minutes, SK 25 minutes, APSAC 80–90 minutes. With r-tPA, prolonged thrombolytic activity may occur within the thrombus. With SK, effective fibrinolysis may persist for 4–6 hours and may vary with the level of the antistreptococcal antibodies. It may be prudent to assume that some fibrinolytic activity will persist up to 24 hours after discontinuation of SK therapy.

It is also possible to treat patients in the recent postoperative period with short-term regional fibrinolysis at an acceptable risk. Molina *et al.* [93] successfully used thrombolytic therapy to lyse pulmonary emboli in 13 patients who had had surgery within the previous 14 days, without a clinically significant complication. The location of the recent surgery is obviously important. Lysis can be considered more seriously in the first 2 weeks after surgery if the surgical site is in the extremities or in a compressible location, as opposed to an intrathoracic or intraabdominal site.

Thrombosis

Pericatheter thrombus formation and measures to prevent it

Thrombosis during regional thrombolysis usually represents pericatheter thrombus formation, i.e., thrombus formation along the catheter shaft. It occurs when there is no flow around the shaft of the infusion catheter for prolonged periods. Causes include poor cardiac function, obturation of flow due to passage of the infusion catheter through a proximal critical stenosis, distal outflow occlusion due to persistent occlusive thrombus after start of the infusion, and the absence of a large collateral artery immediately proximal to the occlusion to allow continued arterial flow down to the point of occlusion.

A stenosis proximal to the thrombus should be detected on the preinfusion arteriogram. If no preinfusion arteriogram is performed (see Acute renal failure, p. 383), the presence of a proximal critical stenosis should be detected by indirect signs. A small amount of contrast injected just above the proximal meniscus of the offending clot should wash out rapidly. Similarly, if the tip of the infusion catheter has already been buried a few centimeters into the thrombus, contrast injected that refluxes back into the patent lumen should be rapidly washed out by flow through a collateral artery immediately adjacent to the proximal meniscus of the clot. Stasis of contrast in the lumen immediately proximal to the occlusion indicates either obturation of flow by the passage of the catheter shaft through a critical stenosis, or lack of a collateral outflow vessel at the proximal end of the occlusion. In either case, slow flow is a warning that the patient is at risk for pericatheter thrombus formation. Preinfusion measures should be taken to increase flow around the infusion catheter. The catheter is first withdrawn to look for a proximal critical stenosis, and preinfusion balloon angioplasty performed if one is present. Lacking a proximal stenosis, contrast stasis is almost assuredly due to poor collateralization at the proximal end of the occlusion. In the latter instance, pericatheter thrombosis formation during the infusion may be avoided by rapid reestablishment of flow through the occluded lumen, either by pulse spraying the length of clot, or at least lacing the fibrinolytic agent through the entire length of the clot.

Although very little supporting data are available, systemic heparinization is used by most interventional radiologists to help prevent pericatheter thrombus formation, keeping the aPTT in the range of 60–100 seconds. Lower aPTT values (60–80 seconds) are used when the infusion catheter has rapid flow around it; when the arterial segment proximal to the occlusion has slow flow or no flow, higher values are used (80–100 seconds).

Rethrombosis after successful recanalization

The rapidity of flow after recanalization can indicate whether the result is likely to remain successful. Slow flow through the recanalized segment after thrombolysis is usually the harbinger of rethrombosis. Systemic heparinization is of limited value to prevent rethrombosis in this circumstance. The cause of slow flow must be sought out and corrected if possible, with medical, catheter mediated, or surgical therapy as appropriate; causes most commonly include poor cardiac output, an uncorrected proximal flow-limiting lesion, residual thrombus, or a flow-limiting lesion (including a postangioplasty dissection) in the recanalized segment, or poor outflow due to underlying disease or multiple distal emboli.

Distal embolization

Embolization during fibrinolytic therapy occurs in two settings: (i) distal embolization from the thrombus/embolus being lysed; or (ii) among patients who are being treated for an acute embolus, recurrent embolization from the original embolic source.

Distal embolization during fibrinolytic infusion

During the early phases of thrombolytic infusion, a transient increase in clinical distal ischemia is common. In our survey (see Table 20.4) this occurred in 7% of cases overall, with a range of 2–40%. In recent series, it occurred in 5–15% of patients [5,30,94,95]. Increased ischemia is usually attributed to mobilization of clot and distal embolization, and should be anticipated when instructing the nursing personnel in the intensive care unit. The increase in distal ischemia (increased pain, colder temperature of the foot or hand) usually clears with continued administration of the fibrinolytic agent, generally in less than 1 hour. Increasing the rate of UK infusion for 1–2 hours may be of value. If clinical clearing of symptoms does not occur, angiography is performed. Demonstration that there is a new large distal embolus requires the rearrangement of the catheter infusion system. A coaxial system, if not employed previously, is established. The inner catheter is placed on the distal embolus, while the outer catheter is placed at the proximal end of the original occlusion. UK dosage is continued, either splitting the dose equally between the two catheters or, if anything, providing a higher infusion dose through the distal catheter. The distal embolus may also be laced with a bolus of fibrinolytic agent before beginning the infusion. If the ischemia persists or worsens, surgery may be necessary. In our survey, the need for surgical correction of an embolus occurred in a mean 1.8% of cases, with a range of 1−12%. In four recent series, the incidence of distal embolization requiring surgical intervention was 3.4% [96], 3.6% [32], 4.9% [94], and 7.5% [95].

Lacing of the thrombolytic agent through the thrombus before starting the infusion has been shown to decrease infusion times [96]. While it is the feeling of some investigators that the incidence of peripheral embolization is increased with preliminary lacing of fibrinolytic agent through the length of the thrombus before starting the infusion, the reported evidence to support this can be interpreted in several ways. The proponents of pulsed-spray technique have reported high embolization rates. Valji *et al.* [41] reported a 19% (four out of 21) incidence of distal embolization with pulsed-spray technique among patients who had clotted arteries and grafts. However, three of the four emboli could be attributed to aggressive percutaneous transluminal angioplasty performed in the presence of persistent thrombus, rather than the pulsed-spray technique itself. Kandarpa *et al.* [37] treated 25 patients who had acutely thrombosed native arteries and grafts with UK delivered by pulsed-spray technique initially, then with either continued pulsed-spray technique or infusion technique. There was a 40% incidence of angiographically detectable distal embolization (10 of 25), but only one (4%) required operative intervention. Nine of 10 emboli either resolved without special measures being taken ($n = 7$) or persisted but were asymptomatic ($n = 2$). These emboli were detected angiographically within 4 hours of initiation of fibrinolytic treatment and would likely have gone undetected if not for the early angiograms performed after fibrinolysis was initiated, as part of the study. Since angiograms at 4 hours are seldom performed during routine fibrinolysis, such (principally asymptomatic) emboli would likely have gone undetected in other investigators' hands.

Since there is evidence (see below) that use of techniques which produce more rapid lysis reduces the incidence of bleeding complications [28,96−99], it is an open question whether a possible increase in embolic complications, most of which will resolve with continued catheter treatment, is an acceptable price to pay for a lower incidence of bleeding.

Peripheral embolization from the embolic source

Peripheral emboli originate from the heart in 75−90% of

patients [100−103]. Even with current imaging techniques, however, the source of peripheral embolization is not detected in more than 10% of patients [90,100,104,105].

Approximately 70% of patients presenting with a peripheral embolus will have atrial fibrillation; atrial mural thrombus is presumed to be the source of the embolus in these patients [100,101,106]. Myocardial infarction is the second most common condition associated with peripheral embolization; it precedes 24% of peripheral embolic events [101]. Patients who have had a recent acute myocardial infarction, within 4 weeks, are at increased risk of peripheral embolization from a cardiac source [107−112]. In one series of 57 patients who had myocardial infarction [113], 13% had a late peripheral embolism (at a mean of 31 months) after the myocardial infarction. In that series there were no early embolizations. Stratton [113] also found that there was a higher likelihood of distal embolization if intraventricular thrombus were mobile, protruding, and large rather than flat and small.

In the patient who has acute peripheral embolism in whom there is a history of acute myocardial infarction or in whom a cardiac source is otherwise likely, there has been concern that repeat distal embolization from residual intracardiac thrombus might occur. Somewhat surprisingly, embolization from intracardiac thrombus seems to be quite rare during infusion of a thrombolytic agent either by local intraarterial infusion or by systemic administration. There are multiple reports that patients with intracardiac thrombus can be treated with regional and systemic fibrinolytic therapy without further embolization. Lonsdale *et al.* [114] treated 10 patients with peripheral intraarterial thrombolysis who had documented intracardiac thrombus. There were no embolic complications during the lysis or in the subsequent 30 days. They concluded that thrombolysis can be performed safely despite the presence of left heart thrombus. There are also reports of successful intentional thrombolysis of intracardiac thrombus, both left sided [115,116] and right sided [117−119]. Kremer *et al.* [116] reported that 14 of 16 intraventricular thrombi cleared either completely ($n = 10$) or partially ($n = 4$) after systemic UK (60 000 U/h for 2−8 days), with no occurrence of embolization during the fibrinolytic infusion, even though three of the 16 had had peripheral embolization prior to the fibrinolytic administration. In our experience, one 94-year-old patient with known intraventricular thrombus who had peripheral embolization and who was not a surgical candidate, underwent successful lysis of a common iliac embolus with a 14-hour infusion of UK at 100 000 U/h. At the same time, large intraventricular thrombi must not be taken lightly. One instance of fatal embolization during UK infusion was reported by Paulson and Miller [120] in a patient who had a large intraventricular thrombus associated with massive cardiomegaly due to cardiomyopathy.

Thus, in the patient presenting with an acute arterial

embolus, echocardiographic examination of the heart is advisable, if possible, before starting thrombolytic therapy. On the other hand, the experience reported in the literature suggests that the infusion should not be delayed if the echocardiogram is not immediately available. If intracardiac thrombus is encountered, lysis can still be performed unless the clot is large, mobile, free floating, or pedunculated. Simultaneous systemic heparin administration will help avoid further thrombus formation on the intracardiac thrombus during fibrinolytic treatment.

Amputation

Amputation is rarely precipitated by the use of fibrinolytic agents. In both Gardiner's and our surveys, unexpected amputation during the fibrinolytic infusion occurred in only 0.8% of cases. Amputation rate will depend on patient selection, since amputations occur almost exclusively among patients in whom the limb was at risk to begin with.

The overall incidence of amputation associated with the use of fibrinolytic therapy averages 11% [29,30,33−39,42] and varies from 3 [34] to 18% [33] (see Table 20.4). The incidence of amputation associated with the use of local fibrinolytic infusion to treat acute vascular occlusion is underestimated in many series because the data either exclude the 30-day amputation rate, or exclude the outcome of those patients in whom the fibrinolytic infusion failed (a "negative thrombolytic outcome") and who require surgery or primary amputation due to persistent ischemia. Patients who have a negative thrombolytic outcome usually constitute 20−25% of all patients infused; they have a much higher chance of undergoing amputation than those patients whose thrombolysis is successful. In three series in which the data were reported, the incidence of amputation specifically among patients who had a negative thrombolytic outcome was 50% [35,92,121]. As noted, when such patients are included in the overall data, the incidence of amputation associated with thrombolysis averages 11%, comparable with surgical thromboembolectomy.

Acute renal failure

By far the most common cause of acute renal failure during fibrinolytic infusions is contrast toxicity from repeated contrast studies. Transient renal failure is most common among patients who have preexisting renal failure, particularly those who have diabetes mellitus. Diabetic patients with acute arterial/graft occlusions who have elevated creatinines are at enough extra risk from contrast-induced renal failure that alternate means of treating their arterial occlusions, rather than using thrombolytic therapy, should be considered. If regional fibrinolysis is deemed to be the best option, patients should be as optimally hydrated before infusion as the clinical circumstances allow, and every effort

should be made to minimize contrast usage. Several changes in the routine work-up can be instituted in the patient with renal compromise to limit use of contrast. If the acutely ischemic lower extremity is viable (intact motor and sensory examination), we often eliminate the preinfusion angiogram. One can generally decide the anatomic approach for catheter placement by physical examination alone. During initial catheter placement, only enough contrast is used to determine that catheter placement for the infusion or bolus administration is satisfactory, and that there is adequate flow around the infusion catheter at the proximal end of the occlusion (see Pericatheter thrombus formation and measures to prevent it, p. 381). In marginal patients in whom limb viability is questionable, preinfusion diagnostic arteriography should be performed because it may have prognostic value (see Reperfusion syndrome, p. 384) [122]. If no preliminary arteriogram is obtained there is also the obvious risk that, should fibrinolysis fail, no preoperative arteriogram will be available. We thus eliminate the preliminary arteriogram only when contrast usage must be severely restricted. Likewise, during the fibrinolytic infusion in renal compromised patients, interim diagnostic arteriography to determine status of the graft should be employed only when there is a clinical problem, and otherwise avoided. Diagnostic arteriography should be performed only when it appears that a satisfactory clinical result has been obtained, prior to angioplasty or surgery.

As a general measure during all fibrinolytic infusions, patients should be adequately hydrated. A Foley catheter is helpful both to avoid bladder distension in supine patients while they are being infused and to monitor urinary output [5].

Other causes of renal failure after fibrinolytic therapy are much less common. Reperfusion syndrome (see below) is one [4]. This devastating syndrome is avoidable by proper patient selection. Acute renal failure due to cholesterol crystal embolization has occurred following intravenous tPA [123] and SK [124,125]. Cholesterol embolization, fortunately extremely rare, is probably unavoidable. Toupin and Blanchard [126] reported a novel case of genitourinary hemorrhage after combined thrombolytic and antithrombotic therapy, producing acute bilateral ureteral obstruction which led to acute anuric renal failure. A serum sickness-like syndrome of hematuria, proteinuria, and transient renal failure has been reported following SK administration [127].

Compartment syndrome

After revascularization, significant swelling of the treated extremity can occur resulting in compartment compression, particularly the anterior compartment of the lower extremity. Ischemic damage to the arterial wall allows fluid leakage into the interstitium. In a fascia-enclosed compartment such as the anterior compartment of the calf, increased intracompartmental pressure produces nerve compromise and compresses vessels, which results in decreased tissue perfusion, vascular thrombosis, and muscle necrosis. Venous thrombosis, if present, may exacerbate the situation [103]. An early clue to nerve dysfunction with anterior compartment syndrome is the presence of sensory loss between the web space of the great and second toes, due to compression of a branch of the peroneal nerve. As the syndrome progresses, peroneal nerve function is further compromised, leading to loss of motor function and inability to dorsiflex the foot. The increasing tissue pressure eventually compromises arterial flow, leading to muscle necrosis. The patient's ability to dorsiflex the foot should therefore be documented before starting the infusion, reconfirmed during the infusion, and monitored for several days after completion of fibrinolytic therapy. Compartment syndrome can occur up to 3 days following revascularization [5]. If evidence of compartment syndrome develops, the treatment is emergency fasciotomy of the appropriate compartment(s).

Reperfusion syndrome

Reperfusion syndrome (myonephropathic metabolic syndrome) is the occurrence of lactic acidosis, hyperkalemia, and myoglobinuria producing renal failure and cardiorespiratory decompensation, following revascularization of an ischemic extremity in which there has been a substantial volume of muscle necrosis. It is due to the washout into the systemic circulation of platelet aggregates, thrombotic debris, and the metabolic products of muscle infarction, including high concentrations of potassium, lactic acid, myoglobin, and cellular enzymes such as creatinine phosphokinase, lactate dehydrogenase, and serum glutamate oxalacetic transaminase (SGOT). This produces a significant fall in blood pH resulting from anaerobic metabolism, paralysis of the sodium—potassium cellular pump, and rhabdomyolysis [103,128]. The pathophysiology is complex and incompletely understood [129]. It is often a fatal complication in the patient with acute lower limb ischemia.

It is imperative, therefore, in the clinical evaluation of the patient who presents with acute lower limb ischemia, to ascertain that a significant volume of infarcted muscle is not present. Clinically, muscle infarction is present when there is rigor (stiffness) of the affected extremity. This is associated with loss of sensation and a cold, white appearance of the affected area. There is a problem in patients who have sensorimotor dysfunction without stiffness — this situation can sometimes be salvaged if revascularization is accomplished promptly [130], although compartment syndrome may result. The mass of muscle affected is important for obvious reasons: a larger volume of reperfused infarcted muscle will provide a large quantity of noxious metabolites to the systemic circulation. If only small volumes of infarcted

muscle are present, it is possible to revascularize the affected extremity without producing the myonephropathic syndrome. The syndrome is uncommon if revascularization is performed in patients whose acute ischemia is confined to the calf and to the arm [6,131].

Not only physical examination, but the angiographic findings may be important in the evaluation of the patient who has a borderline ischemic situation (sensorimotor dysfunction without rigor). McNamara *et al.* [6,122] have emphasized that the lack of visualization of collateral pathways around the occlusion on a properly performed arteriogram, in a patient who has sensorimotor dysfunction, may portend rapid progression to muscle infarction despite the lack of rigor upon presentation, and that consideration should be given to excluding the patient from treatment. If the decision is made to treat these patients, efforts should be directed to reestablishing perfusion as quickly as possible (pulse spray or bolus lacing of the clot, followed by high dose (250 000 U/h) infusion of UK in an attempt to restore antegrade arterial flow through the occluded region within 1—2 hours) [130]. Concomitant heparin infusion, maintaining PTT at 80—100 seconds, is recommended to prevent further clot propagation in the ischemic bed [6,122].

Acute myocardial infarction

The occurrence of an acute myocardial infarction during and/or after a regional fibrinolytic infusion for an acutely occluded artery or graft is extremely rare, as opposed to the treatment of similar lesions with surgery [132,133]. This fact was recently documented in a randomized prospective study. Ouriel *et al.* [30] prospectively compared operative revascularization and thrombolytic therapy for acute lower limb ischemia; 57 patients each were randomized to surgical and fibrinolytic limbs. The 30-day "event-free survival" (alive, no amputation) favored the fibrinolytic group compared with the surgical patients (eight of 57 = 14% versus 17 of 57 = 30%; $P = 0.04$), although neither the individual differences between amputation at 30 days nor mortality at 30 days reached statistical significance. Cumulative limb salvage at 12 months was similar in both groups (82%), while cumulative survival was significantly higher in the patients treated with thrombolysis (84% versus 58%; $P = 0.01$). The differences in mortality were primarily attributable to an increased inhospital frequency of cardiopulmonary complications in the operative group; 49% of the operative group versus 16% of the fibrinolytic group had a cardiopulmonary complication. They also found that plasma fibrinogen concentration decreased during fibrinolytic infusion, reaching a nadir of 288 ± 22 mg/dl ($24\% \pm 7\%$ below initial concentration) at 24 hours, whereas fibrinogen increased in the operative group to 473 ± 69 mg/dl ($32\% \pm 5\%$ above baseline) at 24 hours after entrance into the study. McNamara *et al.* [6] theorize that the difference in fibrinogen response to the two methods of treatment may partly or completely account for the lesser incidence of posttreatment myocardial infarction, since fibrinogen concentration is an independent risk factor for acute myocardial infarction and stroke [134].

Myocardial infarction occurring during management of this high-risk population has a high mortality [132,133]. Acute myocardial infarction during fibrinolysis, although rare, is as deadly when it occurs as it is among the patients treated surgically, and is an important contributor to the procedure-related mortalities that do occur [21,35,121,135]. It is therefore obvious that basic monitoring measures should be followed to minimize further risk of myocardial infarction in a population that has an intrinsically high risk. These include prevention of hypotension, careful monitoring of hematocrit, with transfusions as appropriate (usually for hematocrit < 30%), and maintenance of adequate hydration with intravenous fluids so that there is a positive fluid balance of about 500 ml/day.

Shaking chills with UK

Since 1990, physicians using UK systemically or intraarterially in bolus doses of 250 000 IU or more [26,136–138], have encountered an increasing frequency of shaking chills in patients receiving intraarterial bolus doses of UK. For example, Matsumoto *et al.* [138] reviewed 86 UK infusions between January, 1988 and July, 1992. Bolus doses were given in 83 of the 86 treatments. In patients treated between January, 1988 and July, 1990, no episode of rigor occurred. Between July, 1990 and July, 1992, 28% of patients developed rigors. The development of rigors was not clearly associated with the method of bolus administration, the amount of bolus given, or prior exposure to UK. These investigators demonstrated that there was no evidence for the presence of an endotoxin in UK. In two recent editorial letters, the suggestion has been made that the rigors may develop during regional thrombolysis at the time when antegrade flow is reestablished [139,140]. The cause of the shaking chills remains elusive. The chills are generally of little permanent consequence, are usually self-limited, lasting 3–40 minutes.

Suggested preventive treatments [139] have included premedication with acetaminophen (1000–1500 mg), diphenhydramine hydrochloride (50 mg intravenously or by mouth), or an H_2-receptor blocker such as cimetidine (300 mg intravenously), famotidine (20 mg intravenously), or ranitidine (50 mg intravenously). However, these measures are not always effective. In a recent study using large systemic boluses of UK to treat patients with DVT [26], three separate systemic boluses of UK were given in 10 minutes each. Patients received 1 000 000 U of UK in each

bolus. There were 27 treatment courses in 25 patients. Despite premedication before each bolus with 100 mg hydrocortisone, 50 mg diphenhydramine intravenously, and 650 mg of acetaminophen orally, rigors developed in at least one of the three boluses in 16 of 27 treatment courses (59%). After shaking chills develop, they can generally be mitigated or eliminated by the administration of intravenous meperidine (Demerol) (25–50 mg), famotidine (20 mg), or diazepam (5–10 mg).

Fever without shaking chills during systemic administration of UK, although rare, has also been reported [141–145]. Fever occurs more commonly during administration of SK because of its antigenicity [143,146].

Duration of infusion as a risk factor

All complications increase with increasing time of infusion, either with systemic or regional administration. In the treatment of pulmonary embolism with systemic fibrinolysis Goldhaber *et al.* [97,98] found a significant correlation between the adoption of a "short-term high-dose" approach to systemic thrombolysis and a reduction in bleeding complications. In our early experience with intraarterial SK infusion, we found that all major complications occurred after 48 hours of infusion [147]. In another series of 58 consecutive regional infusions in 49 patients treated for arterial and bypass graft thrombosis, the cumulative probability of *all* major complications rose from 4% at 8 hours to 34% at 40 hours of infusion time [96]. The investigators compared results with two different bolus-lacing doses of UK delivered through the clot — "low dose" (mean 52 000 U of bolus) and "high dose" (mean 230 000 U of bolus) — before regional infusion of UK. However, in that series three of 10 total complications were acute renal failure, which occurred after infusions of 17–40 hours: the renal failure was likely related to higher doses of contrast material due to a higher number of interim angiograms associated with protracted infusion times. It is less clear from their data whether there was a lower rate of *bleeding* complications with shorter infusion times, although two findings from that study — that both infusion time and total UK dose were lower in the high-dose group — would logically support the presence of lower bleeding complications with a high-dose bolus-lacing technique. Average time to complete thrombolysis (10.4 hours for high dose, 33.6 hours for low dose) and total dose of UK (1.26×10^6 U for high dose, 2.75×10^6 U for low dose) favored the high-dose group. Additional evidence that lessening the time of infusion lessens the incidence of bleeding is the low bleeding complication rate — two of 69 cases treated (2.9%) — reported by the group of investigators who developed pulsed-spray fibrinolysis, the fastest known technique of fibrinolysis [28,99].

Unusual complications of thrombolytic therapy

Other less common complications of thrombolytic therapy have included extension of aortic dissection misdiagnosed as an acute myocardial infarction [148], cardiac rupture [149], cholesterol embolization producing renal failure [123–125, 150] and extrarenal manifestations [151], renal failure secondary to renal hemorrhage producing acute bilateral ureteral obstruction [126]. Complications related to use of SK have included median and ulnar nerve palsy produced by a toxic effect of local extravasation of SK [152], jaundice [153], development of Guillain–Barré syndrome [154], fatal bronchospasm [155]. Development of shaking chills (discussed above) following bolus administration is a problem peculiar to the use of UK.

Patient selection

Patient selection is one of the most important factors in avoiding complications, and requires considerable judgment, clinical experience, and common sense. The lists of absolute and relative contraindications for fibrinolytic therapy vary little between authors. One such example is shown in Table 20.5.

As with any list, these are inclusive, judicious guidelines that tabulate circumstances when the risk of a complication (often more severe than the patient's original condition) makes the use of regional fibrinolytic therapy unacceptable or at least inadvisable. Individual case judgments must be made considering the known risks of proceeding in the face of the listed conditions. Is another treatment available? The patient can suffer from overaggressive use of catheter-directed fibrinolysis when there are less risky options. On the other

Table 20.5 Contraindications to regional fibrinolysis. (From Gardiner & Sullivan [5])

Absolute
Active internal bleeding
Recent (< 3 months) intracranial, intraocular, or intraspinal surgery
Intracranial pathology (neoplasm, aneurysm, cerebrovascular event (< 3 months))
Devitalized limb manifested by sensory deficit and motor paresis
Pedunculated left ventricular thrombus

Relative
Recent abdominal or thoracic surgery (< 14 days)
Recent organ biopsy (14 days)
Recent gastrointestinal bleeding
Uncontrolled hypertension
Recent trauma
Left heart thrombus
Diabetic retinopathy
Postpartum (< 10 days)

hand, when the clinical condition is severe, potentially reversible, and otherwise untreatable, the risks of using regional fibrinolysis may be warranted. For example, trans-catheter regional intracranial therapy of acute stroke is a developing treatment option [156–160]. In our mind, the potential to resolve an ongoing acute major embolic stroke in the entire middle cerebral artery distribution using a short-term local infusion of a fibrinolytic agent justifies its use even in the presence of the relevant "absolute contraindications" listed in Table 20.5. This is a controversial proposal, however, which must be evaluated. Similarly, patients in the recent postoperative period who have pulmonary emboli can be treated with short-term regional fibrinolysis at an acceptable risk [93], although there is obviously a greater and perhaps unacceptable risk when the operative site is intrathoracic or intraabdominal. The greater the risk of a complication, particularly bleeding, the more imperative it is that the duration of fibrinolysis be kept short.

In addition, clinical judgment is vital in deciding when an ischemic condition can be reversed. If a leg is cadaveric, no application of fibrinolysis, no matter how rapidly applied or how successful, will be effective. The patient will only be exposed to the risks of reperfusion syndrome.

Another factor in patient selection that has been under-emphasized is the ability of the patient to tolerate regional fibrinolysis. This generally implies spending a minimum of 8 hours (rarely less), and usually overnight, in an intensive care unit. Patients who cannot tolerate this requirement should not be started on a fibrinolytic infusion unless there are literally no therapeutic alternates. Patients who are psychotic, mentally retarded, uncooperative, or are likely candidates for delerium tremens, are more likely to fail because the infusion must be aborted, or to cause a complication, e.g., by pulling out the catheter.

Summary

Pathologic thrombus, arterial or venous, is always an expression of an underlying disease. The severe consequences of pathologic clot — critical extremity ischemia, amputation, stroke, myocardial and other organ infarction, cardiovascular collapse from massive pulmonary embolism, death — may be more devastating than the underlying disease, but are, nonetheless, a secondary consequence of the underlying disease.

The learning curve in the use of regional fibrinolytic therapy during which the treating physician must develop both clinical judgment and specific technical skills, is long. The complication rates, as well as the success rates, of treating pathologic clot depend not only on the treating physician's technical skill and judgment, but on the natural history of the consequences of the pathologic thrombus as well as on the natural history of the underlying condition that produced it. Regional fibrinolytic therapy has significant intrinsic risks in a high-risk patient population. Current data suggest that the risks are less than those offered by surgical alternates. Clearly, patients who are candidates for this form of treatment require careful monitoring, usually in an intensive care unit. The risk of many complications can be minimized by careful patient selection and meticulous attention to detail and to technique. These complications include local bleeding at the catheter insertion site, acute renal failure due to excessive contrast dosage, reperfusion syndrome, compartment syndrome, white clot syndrome, remote hemorrhage from puncture sites, hemorrhage from recent puncture sites in PTFE dialysis accesses, distal embolization from intracardiac thrombus, and pericatheter thrombus formation. For some potential complications, however, there are currently no means of detecting which patients are at excess risk. These complications include intracranial bleeding, distal embolization from the thrombus, shaking chills with bolus use of UK, and cholesterol embolization. Complication rates in the treatment of some conditions (acute stroke, acute myocardial infarction, acute thrombosis of an infrainguinal graft, acute popliteal embolism) will be intrinsically higher than in others (clotted hemodialysis access sites, effort thrombosis of the subclavian vein). Despite the considerable experience with systemic and regional fibrinolytic therapy, much needs to be learned about the influence of the underlying disease on complication rates of fibrinolytic treatment, and the specific use of fibrinolytic agents in many of the wide variety of pathologic conditions which produce the offending thrombus.

References

1 Graor R, Risius B, Young J. Low dose streptokinase for selective thrombolysis: systemic effects and complications. *Radiology* 1984;152:35–39.

2 Palaskas C, Totty W, Gilula L. Complications of local intra-arterial fibrinolytic therapy. *Semin Intervent Radiol* 1984;2: 396–404.

3 Hirshberg A, Schneiderman J, Garnick A *et al.* Errors and pitfalls in intraarterial thrombolytic therapy. *J Vasc Surg* 1989;10: 612–616.

4 Lang E. Streptokinase therapy: complications of intraarterial use. *Radiology* 1985;154:75–77.

5 Gardiner GJ, Sullivan K. Complications of regional thrombolytic therapy. In: Kadir S, ed. *Current Practice of Interventional Radiology*. Philadelphia: BC Decker, 1991:87–91.

6 McNamara T, Goodwin S, Kandarpa K. Complications of thrombolysis. *Semin Intervent Radiol* 1994;11(2):134–144.

7 Bell W, Meek A. Guidelines for the use of thrombolytic agents. *New Engl J Med* 1979;301:1266–1270.

8 Loscalzo J. An overview of thrombolytic agents. *Chest* 1990;97: 117S–123S.

9 Lucas F, Miller M. The fibrinolytic system-recent advances. *Cleve Cl J Med* 1988;55:531–541.

10 Holden R. Plasminogen activators: pharmacology and therapy. *Radiology* 1990;174:993–1001.

11 Dotter CT, Rösch J, Seaman AJ. Selective clot lysis with low-dose streptokinase. *Diagn Radiol* 1974;111:31–37.

12 Totty WG, Gilula LA, McClennan BL *et al.* Low-dose intra-vascular fibrinolytic therapy. *Diagn Radiol* 1982;143(1):59–69.

13 van Breda A. Regional thrombolysis in the treatment of peripheral arterial occlusions. *Appl Radiol* 1982;5:63–72.

14 Becker GJ, Rabe HE, Richmond BD *et al.* Low-dose fibrinolytic therapy: results and new concepts. *Radiology* 1983;148(3): 663–670.

15 Mori KW, Bookstein JJ, Heeney DJ *et al.* Selective streptokinase infusion: clinical and laboratory correlates. *Radiology* 1983; 148(3):677–682.

16 McNamara TO, Fischer JR. Thrombolysis of peripheral arterial and graft occlusions: improved results using high dose urokinase. *Am J Roentgenol* 1985;144(April):769–775.

17 Graor RA, Olin JW, Bartholomew JR *et al.* Efficacy and safety of intraarterial local infusion of streptokinase, urokinase, or tissue plasminogen activator for peripheral arterial occlusion: a retrospective review. *J Vasc Med Biol* 1990;2(6):310–315.

18 Traughber P, Cook P, Micklos T, Miller F. Intraarterial fibrinolytic therapy for popliteal and tibial artery obstruction: comparison of streptokinase and urokinase. *Am J Roentgenol* 1987; 149:453–456.

19 Belkin M, Belkin B, Bucknam C *et al.* Intraarterial fibrinolytic therapy. Efficacy of streptokinase vs. urokinase. *Arch Surg* 1986;121:769–773.

20 van Breda A, Katzen B, Deutsch A. Urokinase vs streptokinase in local thrombolysis. *Radiology* 1987;165:109–111.

21 Sicard G, Schier JJ, Totty W *et al.* Thrombolytic therapy for acute arterial occlusion. *J Vasc Surg* 1985;2:65–76.

22 Tennant S, Dixon J, Venable T *et al.* Intracoronary thrombolysis in patients with acute myocardial infarction: comparison of the efficacy of urokinase with streptokinase. *Circulation* 1984; 69:756–760.

23 Meyerovitz M, Goldhaver S, Reagan K *et al.* Recombinant tissue-type plasminogen activator versus urokinase in peripheral arterial and graft occlusions: a randomized trial. *Radiology* 1990;175:75–78.

24 de Bono DP, More RS. Prevention and management of bleeding complications after thrombolysis. *Int J Cardiol* 1993;38:1–6.

25 Pilla T, Comerota A. Basic data related to thrombolytic therapy for venous thrombosis. *Ann Vasc Surg* 1989;3(1):81–85.

26 Goldhaber S, Polak J, Feldstein M *et al.* Efficacy and safety of repeated boluses of urokinase in the treatment of deep venous thrombosis. *Am J Cardiol* 1994;73(Jan 1(1)):75–79.

27 Goldhaber SZ, Meyerovitz MF, Green D *et al.* Randomized controlled trial of tissue plasminogen activator in proximal deep venous thrombosis. *Am J Med* 1990;88:235–240.

28 Valji K, Roberts AC, Davis GB, Bookstein JJ. Pulsed-spray thrombolysis of arterial and bypass graft occlusions. *Am J Roentgenol* 1991;156(3):617–621.

29 Parent FIII, Piotrowski JJ, Bernhard VM *et al.* Outcome of intraarterial urokinase for acute vascular occlusion. *J Cardiovasc Surg (Torino)* 1991;32(5):680–689.

30 Ouriel K, Shortell C, DeWeese J *et al.* A comparison of thrombolytic therapy with operative revascularization in the initial treatment of acute peripheral arterial ischemia. *J Vasc Surg* 1994;19:1021–1030.

31 Miller BV, Sharp WJ, Hoballah JJ *et al.* Management of infrainguinal occluded vein bypasses with a combined approach of thrombolysis and surveillance. A prospective study. *Arch Surg* 1992;127(8):986–989.

32 DeMaioribus CA, Mills JL, Fujitani RM *et al.* A reevaluation of intraarterial thrombolytic therapy for acute lower extremity ischemia. *J Vasc Surg* 1993;17(5):888–895.

33 Clouse M, Stokes K, Perry L, Wheeler H. Percutaneous intraarterial thrombolysis: analysis of factors affecting outcome. *J Vasc Intervent Radiol* 1994;5:93–100.

34 Eisenbud DE, Brener BJ, Shoenfeld R *et al.* Treatment of acute vascular occlusions with intra-arterial urokinase. *Am J Surg* 1990;160(2):160–164.

35 Durham JD, Geller SC, Abbott WM *et al.* Acceleration of thrombolysis with a high-dose transthrombus bolus technique. *Radiology* 1989;173(3):805–808.

36 LeBlang S, Becker G, Benenat J. Low-dose urokinase regimen for the treatment of lower extremity arterial and graft occlusions: Experience in 132 cases. *J Vasc Intervent Radiol* 1992;3:475–483.

37 Kandarpa K, Chopra P, Aruny J *et al.* Intraarterial thrombolysis of lower extremity occlusions: prospective, randomized comparison of forced periodic infusion and conventional slow continuous infusion. *Radiology* 1993;188:861–867.

38 McNamara TO, Bomberger RA, Merchant RF. Intra-arterial urokinase as the initial therapy for acutely ischemic lower limbs (see comments). *Circulation* 1991;83(Suppl.):1106–1119.

39 Sullivan KL, Gardiner G Jr, Kandarpa K *et al.* Efficacy of thrombolysis in infrainguinal bypass grafts. *Circulation* 1991; 83(Suppl. I):99–105.

40 Smith D, McCormick M, Jensen D, Westengard J. Guide wire traversal test: retrospective study of results with fibrinolytic therapy. *J Vasc Intervent Radiol* 1991;2:339–342.

41 Valji K, Bookstein J, Roberts A, Sanchez R. Occluded peripheral arteries and bypass grafts: lytic stagnation as an end point for pulse-spray pharmacomechanical thrombolysis. *Radiology* 1993;188:389–394.

42 Cragg A, Smith T, Corson J *et al.* Two urokinase dose regimens in native arterial and graft occlusions: initial results of a prospective, randomized clinical trial. *Radiology* 1991;178: 681–686.

43 Kumpe D, Rutherford R. *Thrombolysis: Clinical Applications.* Chicago: Discovery International, 1994.

44 Becker G, Holden R. Fibrinolytic therapy. In: Castañeda-Zúñiga W, Tadavarthy S, eds. *Interventional Radiology*, Vol. 1. Baltimore: Williams and Wilkins, 1992:599–634.

45 The International Study Group. In-hospital mortality and clinical course of 20 891 patients with suspected acute myocardial infarction randomised between alteplase and streptokinase with or without heparin. The International Study Group (see comments). *Lancet* 1990;336:71–75.

46 ISIS-3 (Third International Study of Infarct Survival) Collaborative Group. ISIS-3 a randomized comparison of streptokinase vs tissue plasminogen activator vs anistreplase and of aspirin plus heparin vs aspirin alone among 41 299 cases of suspected acute myocardial infarction. *Lancet* 1992;339:753–770.

47 Bovill EG, Terrin ML, Stump DC *et al.* Hemorrhagic events during therapy with recombinant tissue-type plasminogen activator, heparin and aspirin for acute myocardial infarction. Results of the thrombolysis in myocardial infarction (TIMI), phase II trial. *Ann Int Med* 1991;115:256–265.

48 Kase CS, Pessin MS, Zivin JA *et al.* Intracranial hemorrhage after coronary thrombolysis with tissue plasminogen activator. *Am J Med* 1992;92:384–390.

49 Althouse R, Maynard M, Cerqueira M *et al.* The Western Washington myocardial infarction registry and emergency department tissue plasminogen activator treatment trial. *Am J Cardiol* 1990;66:1298–1303.

50 Gore JM, Sloan M, Price TR *et al.* Intracerebral hemorrhage, cerebral infarction, and subdural hematoma after acute myocardial infarction and thrombolytic therapy in the thrombolysis in myocardial infarction study. Thrombolysis in myocardial infarction, phase II, pilot and clinical trial. *Circulation* 1991;83: 448–459.

51 Anderson J, Karagounis L, Allen A *et al.* Older age and elevated blood pressure are risk factors for intracerebral hemorrhage after thrombolysis. *Am J Cardiol* 1991;68:166–170.

52 Maggioni A, Franzosii M, Santoro E *et al.* The risk of stroke in patients with acute myocardial infarction after thrombolytic and antithrombotic treatment. *New Engl J Med* 1992;327:1–6.

53 Wijdicks E, Jack C. Intracerebral hemorrhage after fibrinolytic therapy for acute myocardial infarction. *Stroke* 1993;24: 554–557.

54 De Jaegere PP, Arnold AA, Balk AH, Simoons ML. Intracranial hemorrhage in association with thrombolytic therapy: incidence and clinical predictive factors. *J Am Coll Cardiol* 1992;19:289–294.

55 Marder VJ. Comparison of thrombolytic agents: selected hematologic, vascular and clinical events. *Am J Cardiol* 1989; 64:2A–7A.

56 Van de Werf F, Arnold AER. Intravenous tissue plasminogen activator and size of infarct, left ventricular function, and survival in acute myocardial infarction. *Br Med J* 1988;297: 1374–1379.

57 ISIS-2 (Second International Study of Infarct Survival) Collaborative Group. Randomised trial of intravenous streptokinase, oral aspirin, both, or neither among 17 187 cases of suspected acute myocardial infarction: ISIS-2. *Lancet* 1988;ii: 349–360.

58 AIMS. Trial Study Group. Effect of intravenous APSAC on mortality after acute myocardial infarction: preliminary report of a placebo-controlled clinical trial. *Lancet* 1988;i:545–549.

59 Topol E, Califf R. Thrombolytic therapy for elderly patients (editorial). *New Engl J Med* 1992;327:45–47.

60 Wolpert S, Bruckmann H, Greenlee R *et al.* Neuroradiologic evaluation of patients with acute stroke treated with recombinant tissue plasminogen activator. *AJNR* 1993; 14(Jan/Feb):3–13.

61 Molinari G. Lobar hemorrhages. Where do they come from? How do they get there? *Stroke* 1993;24:523–526.

62 Ramsay D, Penswick J, Robertson D. Fatal streptokinase-induced intracerebral haemorrhage in cerebral amyloid angiopathy. *Can J Neurol Sci* 1990;17:336–341.

63 Wakai S, Kumakura N, Nagai M. Lobar intracerebral hemorrhage. *J Neurosurg* 1992;76:231–238.

64 LeBlanc R, Haddad G, Robitaille Y. Cerebral hemorrhage from a myeloid angiopathy and coronary thrombolysis. *Neurosurgery* 1992;31(3):586–590.

65 Kase C, Robinson R, Stein R *et al.* Anticoagulant-related intracerebral hemorrhage. *Neurology* 1985;35:943–948.

66 Piazza I, Girardi A, Giunta G, Pappagallo G. Femoral nerve palsy secondary to anticoagulant induced iliacus hematoma. A case report. *Int Angiol* 1990;9:125–126.

67 Durham J, Rutherford R. Hemorrhagic compressive neuropathies: nerve injury without direct trauma or regional ischemia. *Semin Vasc Surg* 1991;4:26–30.

68 Kaplan S, Kohn I, Amis EJ *et al.* Renal angiomyolipoma presenting as a retroperitoneal mass following thrombolytic

therapy for acute myocardial infarction. *N Y State J Med* 1992; 92:217−219.

69 Scuba J, Parrado C. Parapharyngeal hemorrhage secondary to thrombolytic therapy for acute myocardial infarction. *J Oral Maxillofac Surg* 1992;50:413−415.

70 Nathan P, Torres A, Smith A *et al.* Spontaneous pulmonary hemorrhage following coronary thrombolysis. *Chest* 1992;101: 1150−1152.

71 Hyer S, Soo S, Taylor W, Nussey S. Spontaneous haemorrhage into a pituitary tumor after streptokinase therapy (letter). *Postgrad Med J* 1993;69:244.

72 Onishchuk J, Carlsson C. Epidural hematoma associated with epidural anesthesia: complications of anticoagulant therapy. *Anesthesiology* 1992;77(Dec):1221−1223.

73 Dickman C, Shedd S, Spetzler R *et al.* Spinal epidural hematoma associated with epidural anesthesia: complications of systemic heparinization in patients receiving peripheral vascular thrombolytic therapy. *Anesthesiology* 1990;72(May):947−950.

74 Segal L, Adair D. Compartment syndrome of the triceps as a complication of thrombolytic therapy. *Orthopedics* 1990;13: 90−92.

75 Oakley C. Fatal intrathoracic haemorrhage after cardio-pulmonary resuscitation and treatment with streptokinase and heparin (letter; comment). *Br Heart J* 1990;63(Jan):69.

76 Sprayregen S, Bakal C, Cynamon J. Compression of vein graft by hematoma during fibrinolytic therapy simulating intrinsic venous stricture − a case report. *Angiology* 1993;44:81−84.

77 Davis GB, Dowd CF, Bookstein JJ *et al.* Thrombosed dialysis grafts: efficacy of intrathrombic deposition of concentrated urokinase, clot, maceration and angioplasty. *Am J Roentgenol* 1987;149:177−181.

78 Valji K, Bookstein J. Fibrinolysis with intrathrombic injection of urokinase and tissue-type plasminogen activator: results in a new model of subacute venous thrombosis. *Invest Radiol* 1987;22:23−27.

79 Valji K, Bookstein JJ, Roberts AC, Davis GB. Pharmaco-mechanical thrombolysis and angioplasty in the management of clotted hemodialysis grafts: early and late clinical results. *Radiology* 1991;178:243−247.

80 Cohen M, Kumpe D, Durham J, Zwerdlinger S. Crossed catheter technique increases the salvage rate of thrombosed hemodialysis access sites with urokinase infusions and angio-plasty. *Kidney Int* 1994;46:1375−1380.

81 Sloan M, Price T. Intracranial hemorrhage following thrombolytic therapy for acute myocardial infarction. *Semin Neurol* 1991;11:385−399.

82 Ey F. Hematologic conditions predisposing to deep venous thrombosis. In: Strandness D Jr, van Breda A, eds. *Vascular Diseases: Surgical and Interventional Therapy*, Vol. 2. New York: Churchill Livingstone, 1994:853−865.

83 Warkentin T, Kelton J. Heparin-induced thrombocytopenia. *Ann Rev Med* 1992;40:31.

84 Chong B, Fawaz I, Chesterman C, Berndt M. Heparin-induced thrombocytopenia: mechanism of interaction of the heparin-dependent antibody with platelets. *Br J Haematol* 1989;73:235.

85 Stanton P, Evans J, Lefemine A *et al.* White clot syndrome. *S Med J* 1988;81:616.

86 Skinner JR, Phillips SJ, Zeff RH, Kongtahworn C. Immediate coronary bypass following failed streptokinase infusion in evolving myocardial infarction. *J Thorac Cardiovasc Surg* 1984; 87:567−570.

87 Kay P, Ahmad A, Floten S, Starr A. Emergency coronary

artery bypass surgery after intracoronary thrombolysis for evolving myocardial infarction. *Br Heart J* 1985;53:260−264.

88 Anderson JL, Battistessa SA, Clayton PD *et al.* Coronary bypass surgery early after thrombolytic therapy for acute myocardial infarction. *Ann Thorac Surg* 1986;41:176−183.

89 Mantia AM, Lolley DM, Stullken EH Jr *et al.* Coronary artery bypass grafting within 24 hours after intracoronary strepto-kinase thrombolysis. *J Cardiol Anesth* 1987;1:392−400.

90 Lee KF, Mandell J, Rankin JS *et al.* Immediate versus delayed coronary grafting after streptokinase treatment. Postoperative blood loss and clinical results. *J Thorac Cardiovasc Surg* 1988;95: 216−222.

91 TIMI Research Group. Immediate vs delayed catheterization and angioplasty following thrombolytic therapy for acute myocardial infarction: TIMI IIA results. *J Am Med Assoc* 1988; 260:2849−2858.

92 McNamara TO, Bomberger RA, Merchant RF. Intra-arterial urokinase as the initial therapy for acutely ischemic loser limbs. *Circulation* 1991;83(Suppl. I):1106−1119.

93 Molina J, Hunter D, Yedlicka J, Cerra F. Thrombolytic therapy for postoperative pulmonary embolism. *Am J Surg* 1992;163: 375−381.

94 Morag B, Garniek A, Setton A *et al.* Intra-arterial thrombolytic therapy; a combined approach with angioplasty and/or minor surgery. *Isr J Med Sci* 1993;29(Nov(11)):707−713.

95 Smith C, Yellin A, Weaver F *et al.* Thrombolytic therapy for arterial occlusion: a mixed blessing. *Am Surg* 1994;60: 371−375.

96 Sullivan K, Gardiner G, Shapiro M *et al.* Acceleration of thrombolysis with a high-dose transthrombus bolus technique. *Radiology* 1989;173:805−808.

97 Goldhaber SZ, Heit J, Sharma GVRK *et al.* Randomised trial of recombinant tissue plasminogen activator versus urokinase in the treatment of acute pulmonary embolism. *Lancet* 1988;2: 293−298.

98 Goldhaber SZ, Kessler CM, Elliott CG *et al.* Recombinant tissue-type plasminogen activator versus a novel dosing regimen of urokinase in acute pulmonary embolism: a randomised controlled multicenter trial. *J Am Coll Cardiol* 1992;20:24−30.

99 Valji K, Bookstein JJ, Roberts AC, Sanchez RB. Intraarterial thrombolysis of lower extremity occlusions: prospective, randomized comparison of forced periodic infusion and con-ventional slow continuous infusion. *Radiology* 1993;188(3): 861−867.

100 Mackey W. Peripheral embolization and thrombosis. In: Strandness D Jr, vanBreda A, eds. *Vascular Diseases: Surgical and Interventional Therapy*, Vol. 1. New York: Churchill Livingstone, 1994:341−354.

101 Mills J, Porter J. Basic data related to clinical decision making in acute limb ischemia. *Ann Vasc Surg* 1991;5:96.

102 Abbott W, Maloney R, McCabe C *et al.* Arterial embolism: a 44 year perspective. *Am J Surg* 1982;143:460.

103 Brewster D, Chin A, Fogarty T. Arterial thromboembolism. In: Rutherford R, ed. *Vascular Surgery*, Vol. 1, 3rd edn. Philadelphia: WB Saunders, 1989:548−564.

104 Cujec B, Polasec P, Boll C, Schuaib A. Transesophageal echo-cardiography in the detection of potential cardiac sources of embolism in stroke patients. *Stroke* 1991;122:727−733.

105 Wakefield T. Noninvasive methods of diagnosing cardiac sources for macroemboli. In: Ernst C, Stanley J, eds. *Current Therapy in Vascular Surgery*, 2nd edn. Philadelphia: BC Decker,

1991:264−267.

106 Cambria R, Abbott W. Acute arterial thrombosis of the lower extremity: its natural history contrasted with arterial embolism. *Arch Surg* 1984;119:784.

107 Weinreich D, Burke J, Pauletto F. Left ventricular mitral thrombi complicating acute myocardial infarction: long-term follow-up with serial echocardiography. *Ann Intern Med* 1984; 100:789−794.

108 Freidman M, Carlson K, Marcus F. Clinical correlations in patients with acute myocardial infarction and left ventricular thrombus detected by two-dimensional echocardiography. *Am J Med* 1982;72:894−898.

109 Spirito P, Bellotti P, Chiarella F. Prognostic significance and natural history of left ventricular thrombi in patients with acute anterior myocardial infarction: a two-dimensional echocardiography. *Circulation* 1985;72:774−780.

110 Tramarin R, Pozzoli M, Gebo O. Two-dimensional echocardiographic assessment of anticoagulant therapy in left ventricular thrombosis early after acute myocardial infarction. *Eur Ht J* 1986;7:482−492.

111 Gottdiener J, Gay J, van Voorhes L. Frequency and embolic potential of left ventricular thrombus in dilated cardiomyopathy infarction. *Am J Cardiol* 1983;52:1281−1285.

112 Johannessen K, Nordrehaug J, von der Lippe G. Left ventricular thrombosis and cerebral accident in acute myocardial infarction. *Br Heart J* 1984;51:553−556.

113 Stratton J. Embolic risk due to left ventricular thrombi. *Cardiol Board Rev* 1988;5:81−91.

114 Lonsdale R, Berridge D, Makin G *et al*. Detection of left heart thrombus by echocardiography is not essential before peripheral arterial thrombolysis. *J Roy Coll Surg Edinb* 1992;37:19−22.

115 Krogmann O, Von Kries R, Rammos S *et al*. Left ventricular thrombus in a 2-year-old boy with cardiomyopathy: lysis with recombinant tissue-type plasminogen activator. *Eur J Pediat* 1991;150:829−831.

116 Kremer P, Fiebig R, Tilsner V *et al*. Lysis of left ventricular thrombi with urokinase. *Circulation* 1985;72:112−118.

117 Kemennu L, Riggs T. Tissue plasminogen activator lysis of right ventricular thrombus. *Am Heart J* 1992;123:1057−1058.

118 Kasama M, Nakayama M, Shimizu K *et al*. A case of right atrial mobile thrombus complicating multiple pulmonary emboli. *Jpn Heart J* 1992;33:395−401.

119 Matana A, Mavri Z, Fischer F. Right-sided cardiac thromboembolism and its successful treatment with streptokinase: case report. *Angiology* 1992;43:697−700.

120 Paulson E, Miller F. Embolization of cardiac mural thrombus: complication of intaarterial thrombolysis. *Radiology* 1988;168:95−96.

121 Gardiner GJ, Harrington DP, Koltun W *et al*. Salvage of occluded arterial bypass grafts by means of thrombolysis. *J Vasc Surg* 1989;9(3):426−431.

122 McNamara T. Thrombolysis treatment for acute lower limb ischemia. In: Strandness D Jr, van Breda A, eds. *Vascular Diseases: Surgical and Interventional Therapy*, Vol. 1. New York: Churchill Livingstone, 1994:355−377.

123 Gupta B, Spinowitz B, Charytan C, Wahl S. Cholesterol crystal embolization − associated renal failure after therapy with recombinant tissue-type plasminogen activator. *Am J Kidney Dis* 1993;21:659−662.

124 Schwartz M, McDonald G. Cholesterol embolization syndrome: occurrence after intravenous streptokinase therapy for myocardial infarction. *J Am Med Assoc* 1987;258:1934−1935.

125 Glassock R, Bommer, J, Andrassy K, Waldherr R. Acute renal failure, hypertension, and skin necrosis in patient with streptokinase therapy. *Am J Nephrol* 1984;4:193−200.

126 Toupin L, Blanchard D. Acute anuric renal failure: a complication of combined thrombolytic and antithrombotic therapy. *Int J Cardiol* 1993;40:283−285.

127 Alexopoulos D, Raini A, Cobbi S. Serum sickness complicating intravenous streptokinase therapy in acute myocardial infarction. *Eur Heart J* 1984;5:1010−1012.

128 Fischer R, Fogarty T, Morrow A. Clinical and biochemical observations of the effect of transient femoral artery occlusion in man. *Surgery* 1970;68:323.

129 Belkin M. Pathophysiology of acute extremity ischemia. In: Strandness D Jr, van Breda A, eds. *Vascular Diseases: Surgical and Interventional Therapy*, Vol. 1. New York: Churchill Livingstone, 1994:305−310.

130 Lang E, Stevick C. Transcatheter therapy of severe acute lower extremity ischemia. *J Vasc Intervent Radiol* 1993;4:481.

131 Stallone R, Blaisdell F, Cafferata H, Levin S. Analysis of morbidity and mortality from arterial embolectomy. *Surgery* 1969; 65:207−213.

132 Blaisdell F, Steele M, Allen R. Management of acute lower extremity ischemia due to embolism and thrombosis. *Surgery* 1978;84:822−834.

133 Jivegård L, Holm J, Scherstén T. Acute limb ischemia due to arterial embolism or thrombosis: influence of limb ischemia vs. pre-existing cardiac disease on postoperative mortality rate. *Cardiovasc Surg* 1988;29:32−36.

134 Wilhelmsen L, Svardsbudd K, Dorsan-Bengtsen K *et al*. Fibrinogen as a risk factor for stroke and myocardial infarction. *N Engl J Med* 1984;311:501−505.

135 Koltun W, Gardiner G Jr, Harrington D *et al*. Thrombolysis in the treatment of peripheral arterial vascular occlusions. *Arch Surg* 1987;122:901−905.

136 Matsis P, Mann S. Rigors and bronchospasm with urokinase after streptokinase. *Lancet* 1992;340(December):1552.

137 Matsumoto A, Selby J Jr, Farr B *et al*. Shaking rigors during regional infusion of urokinase: a recent development (abstract). *J Vasc Intervent Radiol* 1993;4:24.

138 Matsumoto A, Selby J Jr, Tegtmeyer C *et al*. Recent development of rigors during infusion of urokinase: is it related to an endotoxin? *J Vasc Intervent Radiol* 1994;5:433−438.

139 Sasahara AA. Prophylaxis with urokinase thrombolysis. *J Vasc Intervent Radiol* 1994;5(5):787−788.

140 Kerns SR. Rigors with thrombolysis. *J Vasc Intervent Radiol* 1994;5(5):787.

141 Shibley M, Clifton G. Febrile reaction associated with urokinase. *Pharmacotherapy* 1994;14:123−125.

142 Sasahara A, Hyers T, Cole C *et al*. The urokinase pulmonary embolism trial. *Circulation* 1973;47:1−108.

143 Urokinase Pulmonary Embolism Trial Study Group. Urokinase−streptokinase embolism trial: phase 2 results: a cooperative study. *J Am Med Assoc* 1974;229:1606−1613.

144 Van de Loo J, Kriessmann A, Trubestein G *et al*. Controlled multicenter pilot study or urokinase-heparin and streptokinase in deep vein thrombosis. *Thromb Haemost* 1983;50:660−663.

145 Terada M, Satoh M, Mitsuzane K *et al*. Short-term intra-thrombotic injection of ultrahigh-dose urokinase for treatment of iliac and femoropopliteal artery occlusions. *Radiat Med* 1990;8:79−87.

146 Sasahara A, Sharma G, Parisi A *et al*. Fibrinolytic therapy: a

multicenter comparison of streptokinase and urokinase in acute pulmonary embolism. *Prog Resp Res* 1980;13:141−150.

147 Wolfson R, Kumpe D, Rutherford R. Role of intra-arterial streptokinase in treatment of arterial thromboembolism. *Arch Surg* 1984;119:697−702.

148 Mertens D, Herregods M, Van de Werf F. Thrombolytic therapy and acute aortic dissection. *Acta Cardiol* 1992;47:501−505.

149 Ishibashi-Ueda H, Imakita M, Fujita H *et al.* Cardiac rupture complicating hemorrhagic infarction after intracoronary thrombolysis. *Acta Pathol Jap* 1992;42((7)):504−507.

150 Pochmalicki G, Feldman L, Meunier P *et al.* Cholesterol embolisation syndrome after thrombolytic therapy for myocardjal infarction. *Lancet* 1992;339(Jan 4):58−59.

151 Shapiro L. Cholesterol embolization after treatment with tissue plasminogen activator. *New Engl J Med* 1989;321:1270.

152 Blankenship J. Median and ulnar neuropathy after streptokinase infusion. *Heart Lung* 1991;20:221−223.

153 Mager A, Birnbaum Y, Zlotikamien B *et al.* Streptokinase-induced jaundice in patients with acute myocardial infarction. *Am Heart J* 1991;121:1543−1545.

154 Barnes D, Hughes R. Guillain−Barre syndrome after treatment with streptokinase. *Br Med J* 1992;304:1225.

155 Shaw C, Easthope R. Fatal bronchospasm following streptokinase. *New Z Med J* 1993;106:207.

156 Barr J, Nathis J, Wildenhain S *et al.* Acute stroke intervention with intraarterial urokinase infusion *J Vasc Intervent Radiol* 1994;5:705−713.

157 Hacke W, del Zoppo G, Hirschberg M (eds). *Thrombolytic Therapy in Acute Ischemic Stroke.* Heidelberg: Springer Verlag, 1991.

158 del Zoppo G, Mori E, Hacke W (eds). *Thrombolytic Therapy in Acute Ischemic Stroke II.* Heidelberg: Springer Verlag. 1993.

159 Yamaguchi T, Mori E, Minematsu K *et al. Thrombolytic Therapy in Acute Ischemic Stroke III.* Heidelberg: Springer Verlag (in press).

160 Zeumer H, Freitag H-J, Zanella F *et al.* Local intra-arterial fibrinolytic therapy in patients with stroke: urokinase versus recombinant tissue plasminogen activator (r-tPA). *Neuroradiology* 1993;35:159−162.

CHAPTER 21

Complications of embolization

John F. Cockburn, James E. Jackson and David J. Allison

Introduction

When discussing the potential complications of vascular embolization, it is important to remember that any procedure during which vessel occlusion is being performed should include a comprehensive initial diagnostic study. While this may seem an obvious point, many of the complications and failures that occur are related to inadequate initial angiography, and it is worth emphasizing that vascular embolization should be performed only by angiographers who are experienced in superselective catheterization techniques. Simple diagnostic angiography is a very safe technique, even in relatively inexperienced hands and there is, therefore, a tendency among many radiologists in training to assume that there should be a natural and early progression into embolization. This is anything but the case; the angiographer performing embolization should not only be experienced in catheter manipulation, but should have extensive knowledge of the normal arterial anatomy, the variations which occur within the different organs with various disease processes, and the effect that embolization has on normal and abnormal tissues as well as the possible complications that may occur and how to avoid them. Fortunately, the likelihood of such complications is extremely small provided the operator is aware of all these caveats and follows the basic principles of embolization listed below.

General principles

The operator should:

1 have a thorough knowledge of the normal and variant anatomy;

2 always perform good quality angiograms of the vascular territory to be embolized so that the anatomy is fully appreciated;

3 always ensure a secure catheter position prior to the injection of embolic material;

4 choose the right embolic agent for the lesion being embolized;

5 always mix nonradiopaque embolic material with contrast medium prior to injection;

6 inject embolic material in small aliquots and under continuous fluoroscopy to ensure that it is passing only into those vessels that need to be embolized;

7 perform diagnostic angiograms at various times during embolization to assess the progress of the vascular occlusion, being careful not to overinject contrast material as this may cause the reflux of embolic material around the catheter into normal vessels;

8 always stop in case of uncertainty and perform a check arteriogram.

It is clear from points (7) and (8) that digital subtraction angiography (DSA) is almost mandatory during embolization procedures as it allows rapid angiography to be performed with immediate review. There is no doubt that DSA has made embolization considerably safer, both for this reason and because it allows the use of smaller quantities of contrast agent in patients who are often very unwell.

While it has been stressed above that a procedure involving vascular occlusion includes diagnostic arteriography, the complications discussed in this chapter relate specifically to embolization itself. The possible complications of angiography and selective catheterization such as puncture site hematoma, contrast-medium reaction, arterial dissection, etc. [1], will not be discussed, although it should be borne in mind that there is a higher incidence of such problems in patients undergoing complex interventional procedures than in those undergoing simple diagnostic studies.

Complications related to the type of lesion being embolized

The complications likely to occur in any particular procedure will be related in part to the nature of the lesion being embolized, regardless of its vascular territory; although anatomic location is of course critically important in determining the morbidity of complications related to the unintentional occlusion of vascular regions contiguous to the target lesion. Most vessels requiring occlusion can be broadly classified into one of the three following groups, although a combination of two or more of these abnormal vessels may coexist in any particular lesion.

1 Neoplastic vessels.
2 Arteriovenous communications.
3 Disrupted vessels with acute hemorrhage.
These will be discussed in turn.

Neoplastic vessels

The complications that occur during embolization of neoplastic vessels relate mainly to the nature of embolic agent required for their satisfactory occlusion. Few complications will result from the proximal occlusion of, e.g., a large hepatic arterial branch supplying a vascular tumor with a coil or pledget of absorbable gelatin sponge. There is also unlikely to be any benefit from such a maneuver, however, as the development of a collateral circulation in such circumstances is very rapid. In order to achieve infarction of neoplastic tissue, the smallest vessels supplying the lesion need to be occluded. Tumors may derive their vascular supply from a wide area, however, and in this situation it may not be feasible to identify and selectively occlude the multiple individual feeding vessels. The solution to this lies in blocking the tumor circulation at capillary level by introducing materials that will reach the capillary bed and stay there. Such agents include liquids such as absolute alcohol, cyanoacrylate, sodium tetradecyl sulfate, and small particulate materials such as polyvinyl alcohol and gelfoam powder. Such agents are, however, associated with a considerably greater incidence of severe complications than larger particulate emboli which cause a more proximal occlusion.

Complications may also occur in this group of patients because the general health of individuals requiring tumor devascularization is often poor and they are more likely to suffer one of the more serious adverse effects of embolization, such as organ failure.

Arteriovenous communications

The major complication specific to the embolization of an abnormal arteriovenous communication is the passage of the embolic agent through the shunt. When this shunt is on the systemic side of the circulation, as is the case, e.g., in a postbiopsy renal arteriovenous fistula, then emboli that pass through the communication will most probably lodge in the pulmonary circulation (Fig. 21.1). This is unlikely to be of any clinical significance when the embolic device is a metallic coil or small balloon but can be more serious in the case of, say, a large balloon causing proximal pulmonary artery occlusion, or a large amount of small particulate material causing peripheral pulmonary vascular bed occlusion.

If the shunt is in the pulmonary circulation, however (e.g. a pulmonary arteriovenous malformation), emboli of the incorrect size will pass directly into the left side of the heart and thence into the systemic arteries with potentially disastrous consequences.

Coils and balloons, particularly the newer designs, are very safe in practice, and nontarget embolization by migration of these devices during or after the procedure is unusual. Complications may occur, however, when an occlusion device of inappropriate size or type is employed, or when it is inserted into an incorrect position. For example, in a high-flow systemic arteriovenous fistula, too small an embolic agent will be swept through into the venous circulation. The same complication will result if an agent of the correct size is used but which has insufficient radial force to hold it within the fistula.

In certain vascular territories, such as the renal circulation, embolization of the renal artery branch just proximal to the fistula is usually successful in occluding the arteriovenous communication, as renal arteries are truly end vessels. This can only be done if the site of the fistula is sufficiently peripheral for the occlusion of its feeding vessel to have only a negligible effect on total renal perfusion. In most other territories, however, if proximal occlusion is performed the fistula will continue to fill via collateral vessels and occlusion of the fistula itself (or all potential vessels of supply) is therefore imperative in these circumstances. This example underlines the need to know the arterial anatomy of the area being embolized, and its response to embolization.

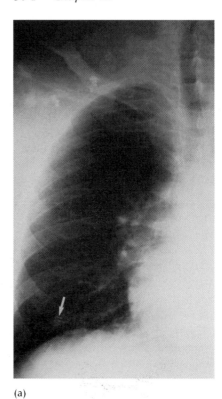

(a)

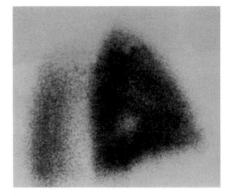

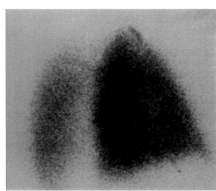

(b)

Fig. 21.1 Inadvertent pulmonary embolization through a high-flow shoulder arteriovenous malformation. (a) Postprocedure chest radiograph showing numerous metallic coils around the right shoulder and a single misplaced coil at the right lung base (arrow). (b) Perfusion (left) and ventilation (right) images showing mismatched perfusion defect due to iatrogenic pulmonary embolism.

Disrupted vessels and acute hemorrhage

There are many ways to achieve hemostasis using currently available materials. The exact method employed will depend on the site and severity of hemorrhage. In certain instances, the clinical state of the patient may be so poor that a relatively unselective embolization has to be performed in an attempt to prevent further blood loss but at the risk of causing ischemic complications in adjacent tissues. This is less important in some vascular territories than in others. For example, in pelvic trauma the occlusion of both internal iliac arteries with particulate material, which may occasionally be necessary, will only rarely cause pelvic organ infarction. In an organ such as the kidney, however, the nonselective embolization of a sizable vessel will cause infarction of a large proportion of the renal parenchyma. Fortunately, in most instances there is usually enough time to allow selective catheterization of the bleeding vessel, and the relatively recent improvements in coaxial catheter technology allow embolization to be performed very close to the bleeding point in the majority of cases. The type of agent used for occlusion will depend on the vascular territory being embolized and the risk of complications (e.g., bowel infarction when embolizing a bleeding small bowel artery) must be weighed against the potential benefits. This will be discussed in more detail under the separate organ headings below.

Complications according to vascular territory

A list of possible complications is given for each of the different vascular territories discussed below. The most common complications will be discussed in detail in the text.

Hepatic embolization (Table 21.1)

The widespread acceptance of embolization therapy in the liver is due not only to its success when employed for appropriate indications, but also to the relative safety of performing therapeutic devascularization in this territory. The liver is protected by its unique dual blood supply and by the rapidity with which a collateral circulation develops to devascularized hepatic parenchyma both from within the liver itself and from surrounding arteries.

The most common indication for hepatic embolization is the palliative treatment of vascular liver tumors. Neuroendocrine metastases and hepatocellular carcinoma account for the majority of these lesions worldwide. The majority of hepatic tumors derive their blood supply almost exclusively from the hepatic artery, while normal liver parenchyma derives 75% of its blood supply from the portal vein and is thus protected in the event of occlusion of hepatic arterial branches, provided that the portal vein is patent. Markowitz [37] is credited with first suggesting that liver tumors could be treated by depriving them of their arterial supply.

Table 21.1 Complications of hepatic embolization

Postembolization syndrome [2,3]
Septicemia [2,4]
Abscess [2,5,6]
Gangrenous cholecystitis [7–11]
Gall-bladder perforation [12]
Emphysematous cholecystitis [13]
Duodenal and gastric ulceration [14]
Pancreatitis [2,15–18]
Massive hepatic necrosis [19]
Biloma after chemoembolization [20,21]
Splenic infarction [22]
Acute liver atrophy [23]
Renal infarction [24]
Bile duct necrosis [25]
Portal venous gas [26]
Gallstones [27]
Disseminated intravascular coagulation [28]
Granulomatous arteritis [29]
Intraperitoneal bleed due to tumor rupture [30,31]
Neutropenia after chemoembolization [32]
Arterioportal fistula [33]
Neonatal death [34]
Death [4,35,36]

Because collateral vessels will rapidly develop if a distal arteriolar/capillary block is not achieved, embolization with particulate matter is mandatory in order to produce a satisfactory result. Before embarking on hepatic arterial embolization, the patency of the portal veins needs to be demonstrated. In the absence of a patent portal vein, or when the intrahepatic portal venous branches are severely compromised by tumor compression or invasion, arterial embolization will result in complete devascularization of the target parenchyma and extensive liver infarction will ensue.

The most common "complication" of hepatic embolization is the *postembolization syndrome*. This is best viewed as an expected sequel rather than a complication as, in some respects, it reflects the efficacy of the treatment. Pain over the liver and fever are the two most prominent symptoms. The pain often starts during the embolization procedure itself and is usually localized to the right upper quadrant and epigastrium but may also be felt in the back and shoulder tip. Some patients experience severe protracted vomiting which may begin in the angiography suite. Clinical signs are a low-grade fever with tenderness and guarding over the liver. A paralytic ileus may also develop. These symptoms are usually self-limiting but require symptomatic treatment with analgesics, antipyretics, and antiemetics. The maintenance of good hydration is essential in the management of this syndrome, particularly if the patient is vomiting.

A major worry is the similarity between this constellation of symptoms and signs and that of a developing *liver* abscess, although this relatively rare complication is made even less

likely by pretreatment with antibiotics. Ultrasound and plain abdominal films will show nonspecific collections of intrahepatic gas in both conditions (Fig. 21.2). The presence of high fevers, a marked leukocytosis or a second rise in C-reactive protein after an initial fall [38] should prompt blood cultures and early ultrasound or computed tomography of the liver with a view to guided percutaneous drainage. *Septicemia* due to multiple abscesses has been reported in a patient who was treated successfully with antibiotics and percutaneous drainage procedures [2].

Much less common, and perhaps avoidable in most cases, is *gall-bladder infarction* [7–10]. The clinical signs in this condition can also mimic those of an hepatic abscess and may masquerade as a postembolization syndrome. The ultrasound signs of mural thickening, gas within the gall-bladder wall, and localized fluid in the gall-bladder fossa aid in differentiating cholecystitis from the other conditions. Infarction of the gall-bladder can generally be avoided if the cystic artery is first identified on preliminary angiography. This vessel has a variable origin, most commonly arising from the right hepatic artery, and may be difficult to identify. If it is not visualized, it is the authors' opinion that embolization should proceed in any case, as gall-bladder infarction is rare. If it is identified, however, efforts should be made to preserve it by catheterizing the hepatic artery to a point beyond the cystic artery origin. Once satisfactory distal hepatic arterial occlusion has been performed, larger particles, such as pledgets of absorbable gelatin sponge may be introduced across the cystic artery origin to protect its distal branches from occlusion. Embolization of more proximal hepatic arterial branches will then be possible with smaller particulate emboli.

Reflux into the gastroduodenal artery is the likeliest mechanism for the *hyperamylasemia* (and acute pancreatitis), which have been reported following hepatic embolization [2,15–18].

Gastroduodenal erosions and frank ulceration have also been documented [14], albeit after chemoembolization. These complications should not occur if the introduction of small amounts of embolic material is interrupted by frequent angiographic assessment of the magnitude and direction of arterial flow beyond the catheter tip. If catheterization of the hepatic artery beyond the gastroduodenal artery (GDA) cannot be achieved, some authors advocate preliminary occlusion of the origin of the GDA with coils to protect its territory from embolization by small particles.

Infarction of other organs is a theoretical possibility if emboli escape from the hepatic artery into their vascular territories. For example, *splenic infarction* has been reported. This should be extremely rare provided that the actual process of injecting the emboli is closely monitored fluoroscopically and good technique is used.

Hepatic necrosis may occasionally occur in the presence of a normal portal venous supply. This is particularly likely if

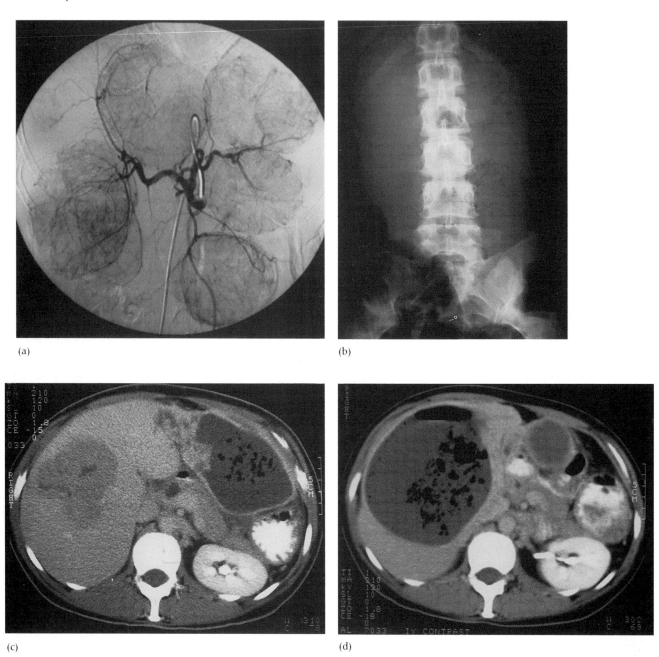

(a)

(b)

(c)

(d)

Fig. 21.2 Hepatic embolization for metastatic glucagonoma.
(a) Preembolization arteriogram showing numerous massive vascular metastases within both lobes of the liver.
(b) Postembolization plain abdominal radiograph (1 week following left hepatic arterial embolization). A large amount of speckled gas lucency is seen throughout the left side of the abdomen.
(c) Computed tomography scan at the same time as (b) demonstrates necrosis of the left lobe of liver metastasis and intratumoral gas. This settled without treatment. Note the right lobe of liver metastasis. (d) Two weeks post right hepatic arterial embolization (6 months after c). Note the left lobe of liver metastasis has almost completely resolved as evidenced by decreased size and density. The right lobe of liver lesion, previously seen in (c) is now necrotic and contains a large amount of gas. The patient was systemically unwell and this required percutaneous drainage.

liquid embolic agents such as absolute alcohol, or very small particles, such as *Gelfoam* powder, are used. These agents presumably pass through normal intrahepatic arterioportal communications, and thus interfere with sinusoidal perfusion. Hepatic necrosis has also been described in a patient with upper gastrointestinal bleeding following the embolization of a left gastric artery which also supplied the left lobe of liver [39]. It was suggested by the authors of this paper that this might have been attributable to a decreased resistance of the left lobe of liver to ischemic injury in the presence of an anomalous arterial supply.

Hepatic embolization is occasionally combined with the intraarterial injection of chemotherapeutic agents which, like particulate embolic materials, can cause *cholecystitis, pancreatitis, liver abscess, hepatic failure, gastrointestinal bleeding,* and *renal failure.*

Humoral effects may be observed in the case of neoplasms producing vasoactive amines such as carcinoid tumors, and it is therefore important to block the actions of these agents with appropriate drugs.

Hepatic arterial hemorrhage is most frequently due to accidental or iatrogenic trauma, and pseudoaneurysms and/or hepatic artery to portal vein fistulae are the lesions most commonly responsible for this. As mentioned earlier, it is vital when treating pseudoaneurysms and arterioportal fistulae to occlude the target vessel both distal and proximal to the lesion. An embolization procedure, in which only the vessel upstream of the lesion is occluded, may not only result in persistent hemorrhage owing to a downstream supply from intrahepatic collateral vessels, but may also prevent any subsequent successful embolization attempt as the proximal occlusion will prevent access to the bleeding point.

Table 21.1 lists the reported complications of hepatic embolization and it should be apparent from the above discussion that many of these are relatively easily avoided.

Renal embolization (Table 21.2)

Preoperative renal embolization for hypernephroma is a technique that has lost much of its initial popularity. This is mainly due to the increasing opinion of renal surgeons that little or no benefit is gained by the procedure. Palliative embolization, in patients who are inoperable, may be very beneficial but is associated with a relatively high morbidity and mortality owing to the large tumor bulk likely to be present in such individuals and their poor general health. Unlike liver, normal kidney is easy to infarct because the peripheral renal cortex is supplied by end arteries and undergoes rapid necrosis if devascularized. The consequences of inadvertent necrosis include renal failure [51] and *renin-dependent hypertension* [46–48]. Nakada *et al.* [47] demonstrated that embolization results in hyperplasia of the ipsilateral juxtaglomerular apparatus with a consequent increase

Table 21.2 Complications of renal embolization

Postembolization syndrome
Renal abscess [40]
Peripheral embolization [41,42]
Colonic infarction [41,43–45]
Renin-dependent hypertension [46–48]
Coil in right ventricular outflow tract [49]
Renal artery aneurysm [50]
Renal failure [51]
Celiac and superior mesenteric artery occlusion [52]
Intrarenal gas [53]
Skin necrosis [54]
Spinal cord damage [55,56]
Testicular infarction [57]
Death [41,38]

in plasma renin activity and hypertension. Embolization followed by early nephrectomy does not result in hypertension.

There is a greater risk of nontarget embolization occurring during renal interventional procedures than during hepatic procedures, partly because the main renal artery is shorter than the hepatic artery and partly because of the parasitic arterial supply that renal tumors frequently acquire from adjacent viscera. Organs particularly at risk of necrosis from refluxed embolic material include the colon (owing to inferior mesenteric artery (IMA) reflux) [41,43–45], the testis [57], and the spinal cord [55]. Much of the blame for the high complication rate associated with renal embolization can be attributed to the use of ethanol for tumor ablation and this point will be returned to later under complications related to type embolization material. A postembolization syndrome is common owing to the large bulk of tumor tissue which is usually present.

Bleeding after renal biopsy remains one of the most important indications for angiographic intervention in the kidney. Embolization of a bleeding point or pseudoaneurysm can be readily achieved using coils or balloons. In this situation the inadvertent embolization of normal renal arterial branches is a major potential complication. Coil migration to the pulmonary circulation may occur when embolizing a high-flow fistula, but this occurrence is usually of little clinical significance because of the size of the pulmonary vascular bed. Peripheral systemic arterial embolization with a coil as a result of its refluxing from the main renal artery has also been described [59,60]. In this situation, retrieval of the aberrant coil using percutaneous or cutdown techniques is usually straightforward.

Splenic embolization (Table 21.3)

It has long been hoped that the technique of "medical splenectomy" would supplant its surgical counterpart, at least in those patients deemed unfit for operation. Unfortunately, splenic abscess formation is common following embolization, particularly if total splenic infarction is attempted in one procedure, and if small particulate agents are used. Symptoms and signs suggestive of abscess formation include left flank pain, pleuritic chest pain, and a spiking pyrexia. There is often an associated left-sided pneumonia and pleural effusion. Disseminated intravascular coagulation and death have also been reported as complications of this procedure.

Some recent publications have drawn attention to disappointing long-term therapeutic results of splenic embolization: hypersplenism often responds initially with improvements in platelet count and hemoglobin values, but such benefit is usually short lived. Casteneda-Zuniga *et al.* [69] concluded that embolization for hypersplenism was indicated only in those patients for whom surgical splenectomy represented a very high risk, and that splenectomy should be carried out after embolization, as soon as the patient's condition allowed, to prevent infection of the infarcted tissue.

Patients at high risk from surgery include those with thalassemia (who may have a severe degree of hypersplenism and resultant thrombocytopenia), those with traumatic splenic injury, and those with coexisting bleeding abnormalities and/or portal hypertension. Splenectomy, either surgical or medical, deprives the patient of the opsonizing function of the spleen. This renders the patient liable to overwhelming sepsis due to infection, particularly with *Streptococcus pneumoniae*.

An increased awareness by radiologists of potential side-effects has led to changes in technique, such as the use of more distal catheterization of the splenic artery which spares the caudal pancreatic and short gastric branches, and the staging of an embolization over two or more procedures. This approach is successful provided that proximal (usually upper pole) branches of the splenic artery are not overlooked.

Table 21.3 Complications of splenic embolization

Postembolization syndrome
Splenic abscess [61,62]
Splenic pseudocyst [63]
Wedge-shaped infarction [22,64]
Splenic rupture [65]
Pneumonia, sepsis [66]
Renal failure [67]
Hyperamylasemia [68]
Pancreatitis [69,70]
Subcapsular hematoma [71]
Acute pseudo-obstruction of the colon [72]
Gastric wall necrosis [73]
Disseminated intravascular coagulation [69]
Progressive liver failure [66]
Splenic vein thrombosis [65,68]
Death due to overwhelming sepsis [69]

Some workers advocate the use of a balloon catheter to occlude the proximal splenic artery while distal embolization is performed. Others have proposed distal coil embolization of the superior or inferior polar branches and report a reduced incidence of side-effects using this technique, while still achieving splenic infarction. Antibiotics should be administered before and after embolization to obviate early infection of the infarcted tissue. The risk of pneumococcal infection is minimized by the administration of polyvalent pneumococcal vaccine a few days before embolization [74]. Despite these precautions, and despite the adoption of subtotal splenic embolization techniques, the mortality rate from this procedure approaches 10% and the morbidity 20%.

Bronchial arterial embolization (Table 21.4)

The most common indication for bronchial arterial embolization is life-threatening hemoptysis caused by conditions such as pulmonary tuberculosis, bronchiectasis, and aspergilloma. Hemorrhage is almost always from fragile vessels within peribronchial inflammatory tissue which have a systemic arterial supply from bronchial or "nonbronchial" vessels such as the internal mammary, lateral thoracic, and inferior phrenic arteries. Embolization is aimed at reducing the high perfusion pressure in these vessels and is therefore performed with small particulate embolic materials (e.g., polyvinyl alcohol) so as to achieve a distal occlusion and prevent early recurrence of hemoptysis through collateral vessels. All abnormal systemic feeding vessels should, if possible, be catheterized and occluded.

As in any other vascular territory, a thorough knowledge of normal anatomy is essential. Branches of the normal bronchial arteries supply the pulmonary arteries and aorta, the middle third of the esophagus, and the visceral pleura around the mediastinum as well as the major bronchi. They may also, rarely, communicate with the coronary circulation. Embolization of the bronchial arteries with liquid embolic

Table 21.4 Complications of bronchial arterial embolization

Dysphagia [75]
Chest pain and coughing [75]
Esophageal necrosis/ulceration [76]
Pulmonary infarction [77]
Bronchoesophageal fistula [78]
Bronchial stenosis [79]
Bronchial infarction [80]
Aortic dissection [75]
Aortic rupture [81]
Leg ischemia [75]
Hemiplegia [82,83]
Bronchoarterial fistula [76]
Myocardial infarction [76,84]

agents such as absolute alcohol therefore runs the risk of *pulmonary arterial* or *aortic wall ulceration/infarction, dysphagia* or *esophageal infarction, chest pain, myocardial infarction,* and *bronchial wall infarction.*

The anterior spinal artery may be supplied by a branch arising from the intercostal limb of a right intercosto-bronchial trunk, and inadvertent embolization of this artery may result in the catastrophic complication of *transverse myelitis.* The use of ionic contrast medium and a wedged catheter, positioned during angiography, make this complication more likely. Extreme care must, therefore, be taken to ensure that an anterior spinal artery does not arise from a prospective target vessel, and the use of DSA equipment greatly facilitates the detection of such important branches. It should be remembered, however, that bronchial artery hypervascularity might be such that there is a vascular "steal" from an anterior spinal artery which is therefore not visualized on the initial arteriogram, and Vujic *et al.* [82] reported a case where hemiplegia occurred even though a spinal vessel was not visible on preliminary angiography. As the embolization proceeds in such a case, the bronchial artery flow will obviously diminish and repeat arteriography, before total occlusion has been performed, may then demonstrate the spinal vessel, illustrating the importance of review studies to assess the progress of the procedure. The use of DSA equipment makes the detection of such important vessels easier.

Because hemiplegia is a catastrophic complication, some authors advise that, in a case in which a spinal artery has been demonstrated, the choice of embolization agents be restricted to those that are, by virtue of their size, incapable of entering small-caliber vessels. Other authors have suggested that embolization should not proceed at all. It is usually possible, however, to introduce a coaxial catheter or open-ended guidewire well beyond the spinal artery origin and perform bronchial artery embolization using small particulate emboli with little risk.

It is obvious from the foregoing comments that in the bronchial circulation it is particularly important for the fundamental rules of particulate embolization to be observed, i.e., multiple small aliquots of embolic material should be administered under screening control, monitored by frequent angiographic studies to detect any change in the pattern of arterial flow.

Pulmonary arterial embolization (Table 21.5)

Pulmonary artery embolization is most commonly undertaken for the treatment of congenital arteriovenous malformations. These lesions are usually found in association with hereditary hemorrhagic telangiectasia but may occur sporadically. Embolization of pulmonary arteriovenous malformations is usually performed in a specialist referral center and complications are fortunately unusual. The most serious

Table 21.5 Complications of pulmonary arterial embolization

Chest pain [85]
Pulmonary infarction [86]
Coil lodged in right ventricle [49]
Stroke [87]
Infection [86]
Endobronchial migration of coil [88,89]
Postembolization syndrome [89]
Systemic embolization
Cardiac arrhythmia
Air embolism

potential complication is the passage of an embolic device (coil or balloon) through a large shunt into a pulmonary vein and, thence, into the systemic circulation, with the resultant risk of occlusion of an important vessel such as the internal carotid artery. This complication is best avoided by using a detachable device (coil or balloon) that may be easily removed if too small or malpositioned.

Other possible complications include *lung infarction, chest pain, stroke,* and *deep venous thrombosis* — the latter problem being due to prolonged venous catheterization, bed rest, and the gross polycythemia (secondary to chronic hypoxemia) which is present in these patients.

Embolization of pelvic lesions (Table 21.6)

Embolization is most commonly performed in the pelvis for the treatment of arteriovenous malformations, or the control of hemorrhage associated with trauma, obstetric and gynecologic complications, or neoplastic disease. In the case of posttraumatic catastrophic hemorrhage, there may be insufficient time for superselective catheter placement, and bilateral internal iliac artery embolization may be necessary. In this situation, there is obviously a greater risk of nontarget devascularization than if a more selective catheter position can be achieved. Despite this, it is well established that

Table 21.6 Complications of embolization of pelvic lesions

Pulmonary migration and retrieval [90]
Abscess [91]
Leg ischemia [92]
Renal failure [92]
Bladder gangrene [93–95]
Vesicovaginal fistula [96,97]
Ureterovaginal fistula [97]
Urinary incontinence [98]
Impotence [92,99]
Cutaneous paresthesiae [99,100]
Lower limb hemiparesis [101]
Brown–Séquard syndrome [102]
Other neurologic complications [99,103,104]
Skin necrosis [99]
Death [99]

bilateral nonselective internal iliac artery embolization with polyvinyl alcohol or absorbable gelatin sponge may halt bleeding without necessarily resulting in significant injury to a pelvic viscus.

In the case of tumor palliation (e.g., bleeding due to inoperable gynecologic or bladder malignancy), embolization with particulate material after selective catheterization of the abnormal vessels is the technique of choice and has been shown to be more effective than embolization procedures using coils in these situations. Coil embolization in the pelvis, although safer (and less likely to produce a satisfactory clinical response), can produce critical ischemia of a vascular territory, particularly if bilateral occlusion of feeding arteries is undertaken [95].

It should be remembered that the internal iliac artery is an important source of collateral supply to the legs when there is severe femoral atheromatous disease. In such a situation, embolization of this vessel may produce acute lower limb ischemia.

Sciatic neuralgia may occur owing to the inadvertent reflux of embolic material into the sciatic artery — normally a small branch arising early from the anterior division of the internal iliac artery. The subsequent neural damage may lead to foot-drop and/or long-term severe pain in a sciatic distribution. The risk of these sciatic complications is highest with liquid embolic media which should be avoided in this situation.

Gastrointestinal embolization (Table 21.7)

Hemorrhage is the major indication for embolization therapy in the gastrointestinal tract. In the small bowel beyond the ligament of Treitz and the large bowel, there is a very poor potential collateral arterial supply and bowel necrosis is therefore a well-recognized complication of embolization. Modern coaxial catheters and superselective catheterization techniques, however, have enabled much more peripheral mesenteric vascular occlusions to be achieved than was formerly the case, with a resultant reduction in reports of ischemic complications. Because the selective catheterization

Table 21.7 Complications of gastrointestinal embolization

Gastric infarction [39,92,105]
Hepatic infarction [9,39]
Duodenal infarction [106,107]
Gall bladder necrosis [9]
Pancreatic necrosis [92,106]
Colonic infarction [92,108—110]
Colonic stricture [111]
Lumbar muscle infarction [92]
(Hemoperitoneum, hemothorax, pneumothorax, pulmonary embolism and portal vein thrombosis have all been reported after percutaneous portal sclerotherapy which has been largely abandoned.)

of a bleeding area of bowel involves positioning the catheter tip in distal mesenteric branches, the misplacement of embolic material jeopardizes the bowel rather than any other tissue. The list of potential complications of this procedure is therefore rather limited. The type of embolic agent that should be used in small and large bowel bleeding depends very much on the clinical situation and a detailed discussion of this lies outside the scope of this chapter. In view of the significant risk of *bowel ischemia/infarction*, mesenteric embolization should probably only be performed in patients who are unsuitable candidates for surgery and general anesthesia, and who have failed to respond to more conventional treatments such as intraarterial vasopressin. Arterial embolization above the ligament of Treitz (stomach and duodenum) is associated with considerably less risk of ischemic complications because of the extensive collateral vascular supply to this area. Occlusion of the left gastric arterial branches can be performed with fairly small caliber particulate materials in the treatment of localized or diffuse gastric hemorrhage, with little fear of causing necrosis of the stomach unless there has been previous surgery in the upper abdomen which might interfere with the potential collateral vascular supply (e.g., gastric surgery or splenectomy), or when there is severe atheromatous disease. Similarly, small branches of the pancreaticoduodenal arcades may be safely occluded when treating duodenal hemorrhage.

While the extensive vascular supply to this portion of the bowel makes embolization safer, it also means that successful control of hemorrhage is more difficult as an occlusion created in one vessel supplying a bleeding point is rapidly bypassed through collateral channels. The treatment of gastric or duodenal bleeding, therefore, often requires the use of small particulate embolic material to achieve a relatively distal block.

Peripancreatic arterial pseudoaneurysms are most commonly a sequel of acute or chronic pancreatitis and may be the cause of life-threatening bleeding. Treatment of these lesions by embolization requires their complete isolation from the arterial system, and this is usually best achieved by placing coils or balloons on either side of them. One of the most frequent complications of an inadequately conducted embolization is *recurrent bleeding* because of proximal arterial occlusion without distal occlusion. This lapse in technique usually results in continued retrograde perfusion of the pseudoaneurysm via collaterals.

Embolization of peripheral lesions (Table 21.8)

In clinical practice, embolization in the peripheral circulation (upper and lower limbs) is most commonly performed for the treatment of congenital arteriovenous malformations. The vascular route chosen to embolize these lesions will vary according to the nature of their abnormal vasculature; it may involve an arterial or venous approach, or the direct

Table 21.8 Complications of embolization of peripheral lesions

Severe local swelling [112]
Severe pain [113]
Pulmonary embolism [4,114–116]
Critical devascularization of an extremity [4]
Skin necrosis
Paresthesia [4]
Ischemic neuropathy — foot-drop [117]
Foot numbness [117]
Rectal ischemia [118]

percutaneous injection of sclerosants. Whichever approach is used, the most common serious complications are those of *digital ischemia* (which may result in amputation), *skin necrosis* (which may require grafting or amputation), and *neural damage. Pulmonary embolization* may also occur if there is a large arteriovenous fistula.

It should be clear from the foregoing comments that the decision whether or not to embolize a lesion in the periphery requires very careful consideration, and needs to be fully discussed with the patient beforehand as it is a sobering fact that many of the serious complications reported in the literature have occurred in patients whose relatively trivial symptoms probably did not merit embolization in the first place. A functional (albeit occasionally uncomfortable) limb is almost always preferable to a useless one due to neural damage, or an amputation stump.

Head and neck embolization (Table 21.9)

The interventional management of intracranial vascular malformations, tumors, and aneurysms is usually undertaken by neuroradiologists and lies outside the scope of this chapter. The embolization of lesions involving the external carotid artery territory is, however, performed by some nonneuroradiologists. It must be stressed once again that a thorough knowledge of normal anatomy is mandatory before embolization is even considered in this region. There are numerous potential communications between the internal

Table 21.9 Complications of external carotid artery territory embolization

Stroke [119]
Facial nerve palsy [120–122]
Ulceration of the tongue [123]
Retinal artery occlusion [124,125]
Skin necrosis [126]
Fatal intracerebral hemorrhage [127]
Nonfacial nerve palsies [119]
Dysphagia due to ascending pharyngeal artery embolization

and external carotid arterial systems which can (and often do) become much more apparent in vascular disease processes involving the head and neck. There are few things more disastrous than rendering a patient blind or hemiplegic during the treatment of a lesion causing a solely cosmetic deformity, because the angiographer is ignorant of normal vascular anatomy. The arterial supply to all external carotid vascular lesions should be fully documented prior to embolization by bilateral external carotid and (at the very least) ipsilateral internal carotid angiograms. In some instances, contralateral internal carotid and vertebral angiograms are also necessary. When embolization is being performed, it is important to ensure that the catheter is not wedged, as this allows embolic material to be forced retrogradely through other vessels supplying the lesion which may be arising from the internal carotid artery (e.g., the ophthalmic artery).

The majority of lesions treated in the external carotid territory are vascular malformations. As in other vascular territories the effective embolization of these lesions requires an agent that will penetrate into the substance or "nidus" of the malformation. Polyvinyl alcohol particles, bucrylate, and absolute alcohol (the latter usually reserved for direct puncture sclerotherapy of venous lesions) are the agents most commonly utilized. It should be emphasized that the use of liquid agents in the external carotid territory is extremely hazardous and should only be undertaken in selected cases by experts.

Complications related to type of embolization material

Coils

The coil has undergone relatively few changes since its introduction in 1975 by Gianturco *et al.* [128]. Its clot-promoting activity has been enhanced by the addition of silk, wool, and Dacron strands, but the fundamental principle of its design has not changed. Complications associated with the use of modern coils relate either to local misplacement or distal migration. They may also get stuck in the delivery catheter. Complications such as these arise when the size of coil chosen has been incorrect or when displacement of the catheter tip occurs during coil placement. Because a conventional coil is pushed out of the end of the catheter, and is not joined to the pushing wire, it cannot be retrieved once deployment has begun. Several new "detachable" coils have been designed in an attempt to overcome this problem.

A further line of interest has been the enhancement of coil thrombogenicity by soaking the devices in thrombin. Massive bleeding and disseminated intravascular coagulation has followed the use of systemic thrombin for embolization purposes, whereas soaking coils in a weak thrombin solution, while still promoting clotting, probably eliminates the risk of these side-effects [129].

Detachable balloons

The technology of the detachable balloon has reached a high level of sophistication. Its development and popularity have paralleled that of the coil. Serbinenko [130] first used a detachable balloon in 1974. Debrun [131] developed a coaxial detachable balloon system for neurosurgical work while White *et al.* [132] have directed their attention towards miniballoons for cardiovascular work. Some balloons can be propelled along a vessel by the injection of saline through the side arm of a coaxial catheter valve, allowing very distal positioning. There is no complication specific to the use of balloons other than premature deflation, although this occurs very infrequently particularly with the newer models. In certain circumstances, accurate positioning may be difficult to maintain with balloons because of their rounded shape. Their principal disadvantages are the need for multiple catheter exchanges and their expense.

Small particulate materials

Polyvinyl alcohol

Polyvinyl alcohol is supplied in a dried state which expands when it comes into contact with liquids. Particulate polyvinyl alcohol is marketed in exact size ranges and this allows the operator to choose a size of embolus appropriate to a particular level of vascular occlusion. It is nonresorbable and is therefore marketed as a permanent occlusive agent, although some recanalization does occur in clinical practice. The complications associated with particulate material parallel the degree of devascularization that can be achieved. Complete infarction of tissue is possible using particles, and infarction of nontarget tissue can therefore also be expected if regular "check" angiograms are not performed to confirm that appropriate flow patterns are being maintained as the embolization proceeds (Fig. 21.3). Nonradiopaque agents must be mixed with contrast medium in order to document flow patterns during embolization. As discussed earlier, embolic material should always be injected under continuous fluoroscopy.

Gelatin sponge and other resorbable materials

Gelatin acts as a matrix upon which thrombus can begin to form and propagate. Partial recanalization followed by complete recanalization takes place over a period of 30–35 days, but vascular occlusion can be expected to last for approximately 3 weeks. The degree of devascularization achievable with gelatin is less than that observed with other small particles, and complications associated with its use are therefore relatively uncommon. Other materials with broadly similar properties are oxidized cellulose Oxycel,

microfibrillar bovine collagen Avitene, and equine collagen flocculi Tachotop. The choice of an individual agent relates more to the operator's experience and training rather than any inherent advantage or disadvantage in the embolic material.

Liquids

Glue

Isobutyl-2-cyanoacrylate is a fascinating weapon in the interventional radiologist's armamentarium. The principle of its use is that it does not polymerize (set) unless it comes into contact with blood or another ionized medium, and the timing of its polymerization can be delayed by the addition of varying amounts of lipiodol. Because isobutyl-2-cyanoacrylate polymerizes so rapidly, catheter occlusion is common during its use and it is therefore best administered through a coaxial catheter. The complication unique to this material is gluing of the catheter to a vessel wall. This is avoided by a rapid injection of the material followed by the immediate withdrawal of the coaxial catheter through which it has been administered. Rapid injection has hazards of its own, the worst being migration of the catheter tip out of the target vessel as the injection is in progress, with potentially catastrophic consequences.

Alcohol and other sclerosants

Absolute alcohol produces permanent vessel occlusion and tissue infarction. In addition to its distal effects in a vascular territory, it causes spasm along the length of the feeding vessel. This has the potential effect of causing reflux into nontarget areas very soon after an injection has begun. Ethanol is ablative and recanalization of vessels through which it has passed does not occur. Because of its extreme toxicity and numerous reports of serious complications, it is rarely used in most centers.

Recently, however, there has been a resurgence of interest in this agent for the treatment of arteriovenous malformations, partly because of the increased use of coaxial catheters which allow very distal catheterization. While there is no doubt that the results of embolization with this agent can be dramatic, complications remain likely. It is to be hoped that the current increase in its popularity will not be paralleled by an increase in serious complications and associated cases of litigation.

Sodium tetradecyl sulfate is used by many radiologists in the treatment of varicoceles, either on its own or after the preliminary placement of coils or a balloon. It is marketed mixed with the anesthetic agent benzyl alcohol. It has no complications other than those associated with any sclerosing agent.

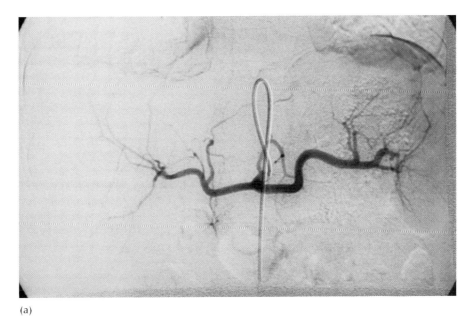

(a)

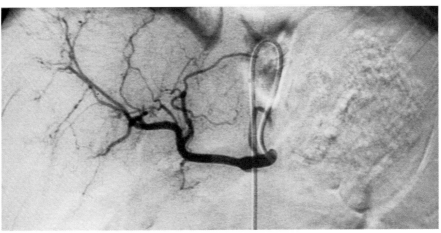

(b)

Fig. 21.3 Inadvertent splenic infarction and peripheral hepatic embolization during treatment of hemorrhage from the left gastric artery. (a) Celiac axis arteriogram demonstrates conventional arterial anatomy. (b) Postembolization celiac arteriogram demonstrates complete occlusion of the splenic artery and an intrahepatic arterial branch occlusion. (c) Contrast-enhanced computed tomography scan shows no splenic enhancement. The patient underwent subsequent splenectomy. Note the peripheral rounded areas of low attenuation in the right lobe of the liver consistent with embolic infarction.

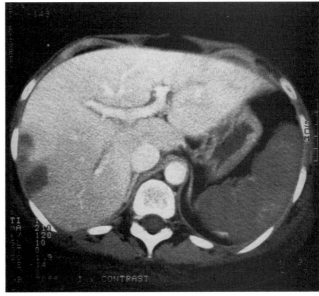

(c)

Conclusion

Therapeutic embolization is one of the most difficult and hazardous techniques in interventional radiology. The keys to success in this field are the skill, knowledge, and experience of the radiologist, access to an appropriate range of quality devices and materials, and the availability of modern imaging equipment. The risk of complications can be greatly reduced by a number of factors including good patient selection, good communication between the radiologist and patient, the provision of rapid surgical back-up where appropriate, and above all, adherence to the guiding maxim of good physicians through the ages: *"primum non nocere"*.

References

1 Allison DJ, Machan LS. Arteriography. In: Grainger RG, Allison DJ, eds *Diagnostic Radiology*. London: Churchill Livingstone, 1992:2205–2275.

2 Kolmannskog F, Kolbenstvedt AN, Schrumpf E, Hanssen LE. Side effects and complications after hepatic artery embolization in the carcinoid syndrome. *Scand J Gastroenterol* 1991;26(5): 557–562.

3 Clouse ME, Lee RG. Management of the posthepatic artery embolization syndrome (letter). *Radiology* 1984;152(1):238.

4 Hemingway AP, Allison DJ. Complications of embolization: analysis of 410 procedures. *Radiology* 1988;166(3):669–672.

5 Pueyo I, Guzman A, Fernandez F *et al*. Liver abscess complicating embolization of focal nodular hyperplasia. *Am J Roentgenol* 1979;133(4):740–742.

6 Okajima K, Kohno S, Tamaki M *et al*. Bilio-enteric anastomosis as a risk factor for postembolic hepatic abscesses. *Cardiovasc Intervent Radiol* 1989;12(3):128–130.

7 Kuroda C, Iwasaki M, Tanaka T *et al*. Gallbladder infarction following hepatic transcatheter arterial embolization. Angiographic study. *Radiology* 1983;149(1):85–89.

8 Onodera H, Oikawa M, Abe M, Goto Y. Gallbladder necrosis after transcatheter hepatic arterial embolization: a technique to avoid this complication. *Radiology* 1984;152(1):209–210.

9 Jacob ET, Shapira Z, Morag B, Rubinstein Z. Hepatic infarction and gallbladder necrosis complicating arterial embolization for bleeding duodenal ulcer. *Dig Dis Sci* 1979;24(6):482–484.

10 Takayasu K, Moriyama N, Muramatsu Y *et al*. Gallbladder infarction after hepatic artery embolization. *Am J Roentgenol* 1985;144(1):135–138.

11 Simons RK, Sinanan MN, Coldwell DM. Gangrenous cholecystitis as a complication of hepatic artery embolization: case report. *Surgery* 1992;112(1):106–110.

12 Sata T, Higashi Y, Ono Y. Sonography of gallbladder perforation: a complication of transcatheter hepatic arterial embolization. *J Ultrasound Med* 1986;5(12):715–718.

13 Nakamura H, Kondoh H. Emphysematous cholecystitis: complication of hepatic artery embolization. *Cardiovasc Intervent Radiol* 1986;9(3):152–153.

14 Hirakawa M, Iida M, Aoyagi K, Matsui T, Akagi K, Fujishima M. Gastroduodenal lesions after transcatheter arterial chemoembolization in patients with hepatocellular carcinoma. *Am J Gastroenterol* 1988;83(8):837–840.

15 Khan KN, Nakata K, Shima M *et al*. Pancreatic tissue damage by transcatheter arterial embolization for hepatoma. *Dig Dis Sci* 1993;38(1):65–70.

16 Beppu T, Ohara C, Yamaguchi Y *et al*. A new approach to chemoembolization for unresectable hepatocellular carcinoma using aclarubicin microspheres in combination with cisplatin suspended in iodized oil. *Cancer* 1991;68(12):2555–2560.

17 Kishimoto W, Nakao A, Takagi H, Hayakawa T. Acute pancreatitis after transcatheter arterial embolization (TAE) for hepatocellular carcinoma. *Am J Gastroenterol* 1989;84(11): 1396–1399.

18 Mendelson DS, Rubinoff SW, Dan SJ, Jones RB. Inadvertent pancreatic embolization as a complication of hepatic carcinoid treatment-computed tomography appearance. *Clin Imag* 1989; 13(3):212–214.

19 Stothert JC, Dubuque TJ, Srivisal S. Massive hepatic necrosis following selective arterial embolization, case report. *Mo Med* 1979;76(9):489–491.

20 Inoue Y, Nakamura H, Takashima S, Yamazaki K, Toyoshima H, Iwasaki M. Biloma following transcatheter oily chemoembolization. *Radiat Med* 1991;9(2):57–60.

21 Kobayashi S, Nakanuma Y, Terada T, Matsui O. Postmortem survey of bile duct necrosis and biloma in hepatocellular carcinoma after transcatheter arterial chemoembolization therapy: relevance to microvascular damage to peribiliary capillary plexus. *Am J Gastroenterol* 1993;88(9):1410–1415.

22 Takayasu K, Moriyama N, Muramatsu Y *et al*. Splenic infarction, a complication of transcatheter hepatic arterial embolization for liver malignancies. *Radiology* 1984;151(2):371–375.

23 Motoo Y, Okai T, Matsui O, Ohta H, Sawabu N. Liver atrophy after transcatheter arterial embolization and percutaneous ethanol injection therapy for a minute hepatocellular carcinoma. *Gastrointest Radiol* 1991;16(2):164–166.

24 Tegtmeyer CJ, Smith TH, Shaw A, Barwick KW, Kattwinkel J. Renal infarction: a complication of gelfoam embolization of a hemangioendothelioma of the liver. *Am J Roentgenol* 1977; 128(2):305–307.

25 Gotoh M, Monden M, Sakon M *et al*. Bile duct necrosis after partial hepatectomy and transcatheter hepatic arterial embolization (letter). *Am J Roentgenol* 1990;154(5):1124.

26 McCarthy P, Adam A, Jackson J, Benjamin IS, Allison D. Computed tomography demonstration of portal venous gas after hepatic artery embolization. *Br J Radiol* 1990;63(752): 647–648.

27 Jeng KS, Chiang HJ. Delayed formation of gallstone after transcatheter arterial embolization for hepatocellular carcinoma. Is elective cholecystectomy advisable during hepatectomy? *Arch Surg* 1989;124(11):1319–1322.

28 Katsushima S, Oi H, Nakagawa K *et al*. Hepatic neoplasms: effects of transcatheter arterial embolization on coagulation and fibrinolysis. *Radiology* 1990;174:747–750.

29 Ishikura H, Sotozaki Y, Adachi H, Sato M, Yoshiki T. Granulomatous arteritis with massive eosinophilic leukocyte infiltration and transient peripheral eosinophilia subsequent to transarterial embolization therapy with a gelatin sponge. *Acta Pathol Jap* 1991;41(8):618–622.

30 Bilbao JI, Ruza M, Longo JM, Lecumberri FJ. Intraperitoneal hemorrhage due to rupture of hepatocellular carcinoma after transcatheter arterial embolization with Lipiodol. A case report. *Eur J Radiol* 1992;15(1).68–70.

31 Nakao N, Kotake M, Miura K, Ohnishi M, Miura T. Rupture of hepatocellular carcinoma following transcatheter arterial embolization. *Radiat Med* 1988;6(4):147–149.

32 Furukawa H, Hara T, Hoshino K, Taniguchi T. An application of

recombinant human granulocyte colony-stimulating factor (rhG-CSF) in a case of hepatocellular carcinoma combined with liver cirrhosis in which leukopenia developed after chemoembolization. *Gastroenterol Jap* 1991;26(6):779—782.

33 Bedell JE, Keller FS, Rosch J. Iatrogenic intrahepatic arterial-portal fistula. *Radiology* 1984;151(1):79—80.

34 Repa I, Moradian GP, Dehner LP *et al.* Mortalities associated with use of a commercial suspension of polyvinyl alcohol. *Radiology* 1989;170(2):395—399.

35 Sjovall S, Hoevels J, Sundqvist K. Fatal outcome from emergency embolization of an intrahepatic aneurysm: a case report. *Surgery* 1980;87(3):347—350.

36 Trojanowski JQ, Harrist TJ, Athanasoulis CA, Greenfield AJ. Hepatic and splenic infarctions: complications of therapeutic transcatheter embolization. *Am J Surg* 1980;139(2):272—277.

37 Markowitz J. The hepatic artery. *Surg Gynaecol Obstet* 1952;95:642—646.

38 Hind CRK, Pepys MB. The role of serum C-reactive protein measurement in clinical practice. *Int Med Spec* 1984;5:112.

39 Brown KT, Friedman WN, Marks RA, Saddekni S. Gastric and hepatic infarction following embolization of the left gastric artery: case report. *Radiology* 1989;172(3):731—732.

40 Wallace S, Charnsangavej C, Carrasco CH, Richli WR, Swanson D. Renal tumours: clinical results. In: Dondelinger RF, Rossi P, Kurdziel JC, Wallace S, eds. *Interventional Radiology*. Suttgart: Thieme, 1990:468—477.

41 Hoogewoud HM, Petropoulos P. Renal embolization: a study of the interaction of contrast media and ethanol [published erratum appears in *Cardiovasc Intervent Radiol* 1987;10(5):313]. *Cardiovasc Intervent Radiol* 1987;10(4):219—222.

42 Woodside J, Schwarz H, Bergreen P. Peripheral embolization complicating bilateral renal infarction with gelfoam. *Am J Roentgenol* 1976;126(5):1033—1034.

43 Cox GG, Lee KR, Price HI, Gunter K, Noble MJ, Mebust WK. Colonic infarction following ethanol embolization of renal-cell carcinoma. *Radiology* 1982;145(2):343—345.

44 Mulligan BD, Espinosa GA. Bowel infarction: complication of ethanol ablation of a renal tumor. *Cardiovasc Intervent Radiol* 1983;6(1):55—57.

45 Sutherland PD, Howard PR, Marshall VR. Colonic infarction following ethanol embolisation of the kidney. *Br J Urol* 1986;58(3):337.

46 Alavi JB, McLean GK. Hypertension with renal carcinoma. An effect of arterial embolization. *Cancer* 1983;52(1):169—172.

47 Nakada T, Furuta H, Koike H, Akiya T, Katayama T, Wakaki K. Hyperplasia of juxtaglomerular cells and renomedullary interstitial cells after renal arterial embolization in patients with renal cell carcinoma. *Hinyo Kiyo* 1988;34(9):1561—1568.

48 Probert CS, Osborn DE, Watkin EM. Malignant hypertension due to embolisation of a clear cell renal carcinoma. *Br J Urol* 1992;70(1):95—96.

49 Radojkovic S, Kamenica S, Jasovic M, Draganic M. Catheter-aided extraction of a steel coil accidentally lodged in the right ventricle. *Cardiovasc Intervent Radiol* 1980;3(3):153—155.

50 Struthers NW, Samu P, Chalvardjian A. Renal artery aneurysm: a complication of Gianturco coil embolization of renal adenocarcinoma. *J Urol* 1980;123(1):105—106.

51 Lammer J, Justich E, Schreyer H, Pettek R. Complications of renal tumor embolization. *Cardiovasc Intervent Radiol* 1985;8(1):31—35.

52 Mukamel E, Hadar H, Nissenkorn I, Servadio C. Widespread dissemination of gelfoam particles complicating occlusion of renal circulation. *Urology* 1979;14(2):194—197.

53 Navio NS, Jimenez CJ, Zubicoa S, Garcia AJ, Boronat TF, Aguirre R. Appearance of gas in renal tissue after therapeutic embolization. *Urology* 1986;28(4):316—317.

54 Twomey BP, Wilkins RA, Mee AD. Skin necrosis: a complication of alcohol infarction of a hypernephroma. *Cardiovasc Intervent Radiol* 1985;8(4):202—203.

55 Milewski JB, Malewski AW, Malanowska S *et al.* Spinal cord damage as a complication of renal artery embolization in patients with renal carcinoma. *Int Urol Nephrol* 1981;13(3):221—229.

56 Gang DL, Dole KB, Adelman LS. Spinal cord infarction following therapeutic renal artery embolization. *J Am Med Assoc* 1977;237(26):2841—2842.

57 Siniluoto TM, Hellstrom PA, Paivansalo MJ, Leinonen AS. Testicular infarction following ethanol embolization of a renal neoplasm. *Cardiovasc Intervent Radiol* 1988;11(3):162—164.

58 Garel L, Mareschal JL, Gagnadoux MF, Pariente D, Guilbert M, Sauvegrain J. Fatal outcome after ethanol renal ablation in child with end-stage kidneys. *Am J Roentgenol* 1986;146(3):593—594.

59 Ekelund L, Karp W, Mansson W, Olsson AM. Palliative embolization of renal tumors: follow-up of 19 cases. *Urol Radiol* 1981;3(1):13—18.

60 Tisnado J, Beachley MC, Cho SR, Amendola M. Peripheral embolization of a stainless steel coil. *Am J Roentgenol* 1979;133(2):324—326.

61 Eron LJ, Clark L. Gelfoam embolization complicated by splenic abscess. *Va Med* 1980;107(9):624—626.

62 Jones KB, de Koos PT. Postembolization splenic abscess in a patient with pancreatitis and splenic vein thrombosis. *S Med J* 1984;77(3):390—393.

63 Reynolds M, Donaldson JS, Vogelzar RL. Giant iatrogenic splenic pseudocyst. *J Pediat Surg* 1989;24(7):700—701.

64 Weingarten MJ, Fakhry J, McCarthy J, Freeman SJ, Bisker JS. Sonography after splenic embolization: the wedge-shaped acute infarct. *Am J Roentgenol* 1984;142(5):957—959.

65 Wholey MH, Chamorro HA, Rao G, Chapman W. Splenic infarction and spontaneous rupture of the spleen after therapeutic embolization. *Cardiovasc Radiol* 1978;1(4):249—253.

66 Vujic I, Lauver JW. Severe complications from partial splenic embolization in patients with liver failure. *Br J Radiol* 1981;54(642):492—495.

67 Owman T, Lunderquist A, Alwmark A, Borjesson B. Embolization of the spleen for treatment of splenomegaly and hypersplenism in patients with portal hypertension. *Invest Radiol* 1979;14(6):457—464.

68 Alwmark A, Bengmark S, Gullstrand P, Joelsson B, Lunderquist A, Owman T. Evaluation of splenic embolization in patients with portal hypertension and hypersplenism. *Ann Surg* 1982;196(5):518—524.

69 Castaneda-Zuniga W, Hammerschmidt DE, Sanchez R, Amplatz K. Nonsurgical splenectomy. *Am J Roentgenol* 1977;129(5):805—811.

70 Spigos DG, Jonasson O, Felix E, Capek V. Transcatheter therapeutic embolization in the treatment of hypersplenism. *Am J Roentgenol* 1979;132:777—782.

71 Back LM, Bagwell CE, Greenbaum BH, Marchildon MB. Hazards of splenic embolization. *Clin Pediat Phila* 1987;(26)6:292—295.

72 Lo TJ, Lin KC. Acute pseudo-obstruction of the colon following partial splenic artery embolization: report of a case. *Taiwan I*

Hsueh Hui Tsa Chih 1992;91(3):351–355.

73 Mineau DE, Miller FJ, Lee RG, Nakashima EN, Nelson JA. Experimental transcatheter splenectomy using absolute ethanol. *Radiology* 1982;142:355–359.

74 Kumpe DA, Rumack CM, Pretorius DH, Stoecker TJ, Stellin GP. Partial splenic embolization in children with hypersplenism. *Radiology* 1985;155(2):357–362.

75 Uflacker R, Kaemmerer A, Picon PD *et al*. Bronchial artery embolization in the management of haemoptysis: technical aspects and long-term results. *Radiology* 1985;157:637–644.

76 Remy J, Jardin M. Bronchial bleeding. In: Dondelinger RF, Rossi P, Kurdziel JC, Wallace S, eds *Interventional Radiology*. Stuttgart: Thieme, 1990:325–341.

77 Remy J, Jardin M, Wattinne L. Transcatheter occlusion of pulmonary arterial circulation and collateral supply: failures, incidents, and complications. *Radiology* 1991;180:699–705.

78 Munk PL, Morris DC, Nelems B. Left main bronchial–esophageal fistula: a complication of bronchial artery embolization (see comments). *Cardiovasc Intervent Radiol* 1990;13(2):95–97.

79 Girard P, Baldeyrou P, Lemoine G, Grunewald D. Left main-stem bronchial stenosis complicating bronchial artery embolization. *Chest* 1990;97(5):1246–1248.

80 Ivanick MJ, Thorwarth W, Donohue J, Mandell V, Delany D, Jaques PF. Infarction of the left main-stem bronchus: a complication of bronchial artery embolization. *Am J Roentgenol* 1983;141(3):535–537.

81 Steckel RJ, Doppmann JL, Roiley RT, Martos EJ. Rupture of the aorta after mechlorethamine HCl infusion into a bronchial artery. *J Am Med Assoc* 1967;199:936–939.

82 Vujic I, Pyle R, Parker E, Mithoefer J. Control of massive hemoptysis by embolization of intercostal arteries. *Radiology* 1980;137(3):617–620.

83 Kardjiev V, Symeononov A, Chankov I. Etiology, pathogenesis and presentation of spinal cord lesions in selective angiography of the bronchial and intercostal arteries. *Radiology* 1974;112:81–83.

84 Miyazono N, Hiroki I, Akira H, Ichiroh KSJ, Masayuki N. Visualization of left bronchial to coronary communication after distal bronchial artery embolization for bronchiectasis. *Cardiovasc Intervent Radiol* 1994;17:36–37.

85 Mitchell SE, Kan JS, White RI. Interventional techniques in congenital heart disease. *Semin Roentgenol* 1985;20:290–311.

86 Remy JM, Wattinne L, Remy J. Transcatheter occlusion of pulmonary arterial circulation and collateral supply: failures, incidents, and complications (see comments). *Radiology* 1991;180(3):699–705.

87 Morgan MK, Biggs MT. Direct embolectomy of the basilar artery bifurcation. Case report. *J Neurosurg* 1992;77(3):463–465.

88 Abad J, Villar R, Parga G *et al*. Bronchial migration of pulmonary arterial coil. *Cardiovasc Intervent Radiol* 1990;13(6):345–346.

89 Gomes AS, Mali WP, Oppenheim WL. Embolization therapy in the management of congenital arteriovenous malformations. *Radiology* 1982;144(1):41–49.

90 Chomyn JJ, Craven WM, Groves BM, Durham JD. Percutaneous removal of a Gianturco coil from the pulmonary artery with use of flexible intravascular forceps. *J Vasc Intervent Radiol* 1991;2(1):105–106.

91 Choo YC, Cho KJ. Pelvic abscess complicating embolic therapy for control of bleeding cervical carcinoma and simultaneous radiation therapy. *Obstet Gynecol* 1980;55:77S–78S.

92 Jander HP, Russinovich NA. Transcatheter gelfoam embolization in abdominal, retroperitoneal and pelvic hemorrhage. *Radiology* 1980;136(2):337–344.

93 Braf ZF, Koontz WJ. Gangrene of bladder. Complication of hypogastric artery embolization. *Urology* 1977;9(6):670–671.

94 Hietala SO. Urinary bladder necrosis following selective embolization of the internal iliac artery. *Acta Radiol Diagn Stockh* 1978;19(2):316–320.

95 Schuur KH, Bouma J. Palliative embolization in gynaecological patients. *Eur J Radiol* 1983;3:9.

96 Behnam K, Jarmolowski CR. Vesicovaginal fistula following hypogastric embolization for control of intractable pelvic hemorrhage. *J Repro Med* 1982;27(5):304–306.

97 Lang EK. Transcatheter embolization in management of hemorrhage from duodenal ulcer: long-term results and complications. *Radiology* 1992;182(3):703–770.

98 Mann D, Satin R, Gordon PH. Neurologic sequelae following transcatheter embolization to control massive perineal hemorrhage. *Dis Colon Rectum* 1984;27(3):190–192.

99 Sclafani SJ, Weiss K, Glanz S, Scalea TM, Duncan AO, Atweh N. Posttraumatic impotence: resulting from transcatheter embolization. *Urol Radiol* 1988;10(3):156–159.

100 Bree RL, Goldstein HM, Wallace S. Transcatheter embolization of the iliac artery in the management of neoplasms of the pelvis. *Surg Gynecol Obstet* 1976;143:597–601.

101 Hare WS, Holland CJ. Paresis following internal iliac artery embolization. *Radiology* 1983;146(1):47–51.

102 Giuliani L, Carmignani G, Belgrano E, Puppo P. Gelatin foam and isobutyl-2-cyanoacrylate in the treatment of life-threatening bladder haemorrhage by selective transcatheter embolisation of the internal iliac arteries. *Br J Urol* 1979;51(2):125–128.

103 Quinn SF, Frau DM, Saff GN *et al*. Neurologic complications of pelvic intraarterial chemoembolization performed with collagen material and cisplatin. *Radiology* 1988;167(1):55–57.

104 Diamond NG, Casarella WJ, Bachman DM, Wolff M. Microfibrillar collagen hemostat: a new transcatheter embolization agent. *Radiology* 1979;133:775.

105 Bradley E, Goldman ML. Gastric infarction after therapeutic embolization. *Surgery* 1976;79(4):421–424.

106 Shapiro N, Brandt L, Sprayregen S, Mitsudo S, Glotzer P. Duodenal infarction after therapeutic Gelfoam embolization of a bleeding duodenal ulcer. *Gastroenterology* 1981;80(1):176–180.

107 Okazaki M, Higashihara H, Ono H *et al*. Embolotherapy of massive duodenal haemorrhage. *Gastrointest Radiol* 1992;17(4):319–323.

108 Gerlock AJ, Muhletaler CA, Berger JL, Halter SA, O'Leary JP, Avant GR. Infarction after embolization of the ileocolic artery. *Cardiovasc Intervent Radiol* 1981;4(3):202–205.

109 Shenoy SS, Satchidanand S, Wesp EH. Colonic ischemic necrosis following therapeutic embolization. *Gastrointest Radiol* 1981;6(3):235–237.

110 Rosenkrantz H, Bookstein JJ, Rosen RJ, Goff WB, Healy JF. Postembolic colonic infarction. *Radiology* 1982;142(1):47–51.

111 Mitty HA, Efremidis S, Keller RJ. Colonic stricture after transcatheter embolization for diverticular bleeding. *Am J Roentgenol* 1979;133(3):519–521.

112 Stanley RJ, Cubillo E. Nonsurgical treatment of arteriovenous malformations of the trunk and limb by transcatheter arterial embolization. *Radiology* 1975;115:609–612.

113 Katzen BT, Said S. Arteriovenous malformations of bone: an

experience with therapeutic embolization. *Am J Roentgenol* 1981;136:427−429.

114 McCarthy P, Kennedy A, Dawson P, Allison D. Pulmonary embolus as a complication for therapeutic peripheral arterio-venous malformation embolization. *Br J Radiol* 1991;64(758):177−178.

115 Verhagen P, Blom JM, van RP, Lock MT. Pulmonary embolism after percutaneous embolization of left spermatic vein. *Eur J Radiol* 1992;15(3)190−192.

116 Moriel E, Mehringer C, Schwartz M, Rajfer J. Pulmonary migration of coils inserted for treatment of erectile dysfunction caused by venous leakage. *J Urol* 1993;149(5):1316−1318.

117 Chuang VP, Soo CS, Wallace S, Benjamin RS. Arterial occlusion: management of giant cell tumour and aneurysmal bone cyst. *Am J Roentgenol* 1981;136:1127−1130.

118 Carrasco CH, Charnsangavej C, Richli WR, Wallace S. Bone tumours. In: Dondelinger RF, Rossi P, Kurdziel JC, Wallace S, eds. *Interventional Radiology*. Stuttgart: Thieme, 1990:489−497.

119 Frame JW, Putnam G, Wake MJ, Rolfe EB. Therapeutic arterial embolisation of vascular lesions in the maxillofacial region. *Br J Oral Maxillofac Surg* 1987;25(3):181−194.

120 deVries N, Versluis RJ, Valk J, Snow GB. Facial nerve paralysis following embolization for severe epistaxis (case report and review of the literature). *J Laryngol Otol* 1986;100(2):207−210.

121 Wehrli M, Lieberherr U, Valavanis A. Superselective embolization for intractable epistaxis: experiences with 19 patients. *Clin Otolaryngol* 1988;13(6):415−420.

122 Metson R, Hanson DG. Bilateral facial nerve paralysis following arterial embolization for epistaxis. *Otolaryngol Head Neck Surg* 1983;91(3):299−303.

123 Saydjari R, Saydjari R, Guinto FJ, Wolma FJ. Arteriovenous malformation of the tongue. *S Med J* 1990;83(11):1335−1337.

124 Soong HK, Newman SA, Kumar AA. Branch artery occlusion. An unusual complication of external carotid embolization. *Arch Ophthalmol* 1982;100(12):1909−1911.

125 Mames RN, Snady ML, Guy J. Central retinal and posterior ciliary artery occlusion after particle embolization of the external carotid artery system. *Ophthalmology* 1991;98(4):527−531.

126 Leikensohn JR, Epstein LI, Vasconez LO. Superselective embolization and surgery of noninvoluting hemangiomas and A-V malformations. *Plast Reconstr Surg* 1981;68(2):143−152.

127 Kondoh T, Tamaki N, Takeda N, Suyama T, Oi SZ, Matsumoto S. Fatal intracranial hemorrhage after balloon occlusion of an extracranial vertebral arteriovenous fistula. Case report. *J Neurosurg* 1988;69(6):945−948.

128 Gianturco C, Anderson JH, Wallace S. Mechanical devices for arterial occlusion. *Am J Roentgenol* 1975;124(3):428−435.

129 Nicholson DA, Cockburn JF, Bradshaw AE, Dawson P. Thrombin soaked embolization coils: the effect on whole blood clotting time. *Clin Radiol* 1992;46(2):108−110.

130 Serbinenko FA. Balloon catheterization and occlusion of major cerebral vessels. *J Neurosurg* 1974;41:125.

131 Debrum GM, Vinuela FV, Fox AJ, Kan S. Two different calibrated-leak balloons: experimental work and application in humans. *Am J Neuroradiol* 1982;3(4):407−414.

132 White RJ, Lynch NA, Terry P et al. Pulmonary arteriovenous malformations: techniques and long-term outcome of embolotherapy. *Radiology* 1988;169(3):663−669.

Complications of inferior vena cava filters

John A. Kaufman

Introduction

Partial interruption of the inferior vena cava (IVC) is an effective means of preventing pulmonary emboli from the lower extremities. The original techniques for IVC interruption required a major surgical procedure for ligation, plication, stapling, or clipping of the cava. The high morbidity and mortality of these interventions stimulated the development of endoluminal filtering devices that could be placed through smaller incisions. The first commercially available IVC filters (the Mobin–Uddin (MU) and stainless steel Greenfield (SSG)) were originally designed for insertion through surgically created jugular or femoral venotomies. Techniques for percutaneous placement of these filters were described in the 1970s [1]. The large (29-F) outer diameter of the sheath required for insertion of these filters prompted the development of percutaneous devices with smaller, less traumatic introducer sheaths in the mid-1980s [2]. Insertion of IVC filters is now a common procedure in many radiology departments.

There are currently six filters commercially available in the USA (Fig. 22.1): the SSG, the 12 French stainless steel Greenfield, the modified-hook Titanium Greenfield (MHTG), the modified Bird's Nest filter (MBN), the Simon Nitinol (SN), and the Vena-Tech (VT) [3]. The latter five filters were designed from inception for percutaneous insertion through sheaths with external diameters ranging from 9–15-F. These filters are routinely inserted through a variety of peripheral access routes, including the femoral, internal jugular, external jugular, subclavian, and brachial veins. The basic principles of percutaneous filter placement are similar for all devices, although the details of the delivery mechanisms vary. A mandatory prerequisite is fluoroscopic image quality adequate to visualize the cava and the filter during the procedure. Venous access is established with the Seldinger technique,

and a cavagram is performed. The cava is evaluated for patency, the presence of anatomic variants, and the location of the renal veins. The latter can be confirmed by selective catheterization if necessary. An appropriate site for placement of the filter is selected, usually just below the renal veins, and landmarks are noted. Serial dilatation of the percutaneous tract and the venotomy over a wire allows insertion of an introducer sheath and dilator assembly into the cava. The sheath is positioned so that the filter will be deployed at the desired level, and then the dilator, and frequently the wire, are removed. The filter is loaded into the sheath, advanced to the tip, and deployed. A postplacement cavagram, or as a minimum a plain film of the abdomen should be obtained to document the position of the filter. The venous access site is compressed in the standard fashion.

IVC filters are widely viewed as safe, effective devices that can be placed quickly, with minimal risk, and for an increasing range of indications [4]. The number of implantations has increased steadily, although precise figures are unavailable [5]. The basic indications for IVC filter placement are either contraindication to, or failure of, anticoagulant therapy in a patient with documented venous thromboembolic disease [3]. Because of the perceived safety of these devices, some authors have urged "extending" the role of filters to include prophylaxis in patients at risk for developing thromboembolic disease [4]. Yet, our understanding of many aspects of IVC filters, particularly complications, remains incomplete. Filters are permanent devices; temporary filters remain developmental. An appreciation of the complications of IVC filters is important for both the physicians who place filters and for those who care for the patients afterwards.

The published data on complications is inhomogeneous in type, quality, and completeness. There are many uncontrolled variables in these reports, such as operator experience, patient populations, and methods of follow-up. Interpret-

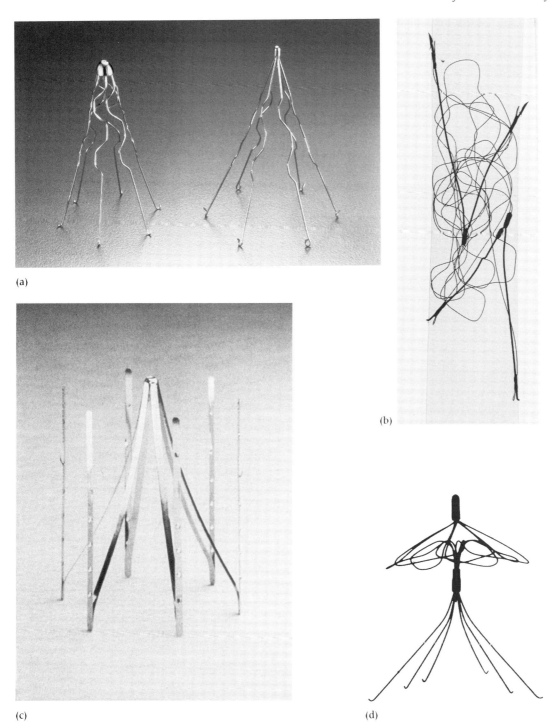

Fig. 22.1 (a) The SSG filter (left), and the modified-hook Titanium Greenfield filter (right). (Photograph courtesy of Medi-tech/Boston Scientific Corporation, Watertown, MA.) (b) The modified Bird's Nest filter. (Photograph courtesy of Cook Incorporated, Bloomington, IN.) (c) The Vena-Tech filter. (Photograph courtesy of B Braun/Vena Tech, Evanston, IL.) (d) The Simon Nitinol filter. (Photograph courtesy of Bard Incorporated, Billerica MA.)

ation of this data is confounded by the relatively short experience that exists with the newer, widely available filter designs. The filter with the longest and most complete follow-up, the 24-F SSG filter, is used infrequently in most radiology departments because of the ease of insertion of devices with 9–15-F sheaths [6]. Furthermore, experience with the SSG spans only slightly more than 20 years [7], a length of time that does not yet provide adequate data on late complications in patients who live 30 or 40 years after filter placement. Only scanty information has been accumulated about filters in unusual positions, such as above the renal veins or in the superior vena cava (SVC).

The complications associated with IVC filters can occur immediately during insertion, or years later. Many of the procedural complications are related to the venipuncture and contrast injections, and are not unique to IVC filters. These standard angiographic complications are not addressed in this chapter but should be kept in mind when placing filters. Air embolism, a rare but sometimes fatal complication during surgical cut-down upon the jugular vein for insertion of the SSG filter, is not a threat when this filter is placed from the femoral route [8], and is unlikely with percutaneous jugular insertion of filters with small diameter introducers. Table 22.1 is a summary of the major complications reported with the filters currently available in the USA.

Insertion site thrombosis

Thrombosis of the vein through which the filter is placed is the most common complication in the immediate periprocedural period. The etiology of this complication is multifactorial, and includes such variables as method of dilatation of the access site, size of the filter sheath, and the presence of a hypercoagulable state. Frequently, insertion site thrombosis is asymptomatic, or indistinguishable from symptoms of preexisting deep vein thrombosis. All of these factors make interpretation of rates of occurrence listed in Table 22.1 difficult.

The size of the introducer sheath is clearly linked to the incidence of insertion site thrombosis. The early enthusiasm for percutaneous insertion of the SSG filter was dampened by the high rate of thrombosis of the vein through which it was placed. This problem was attributed to both trauma to the vein during insertion of the large sheath and device, and the prolonged compression required to achieve hemostasis at the end of the procedure (9,10). Substituting balloon dilatation for serial dilators, and limiting the extent to which the introducer sheath was inserted into the vein, resulted in fewer episodes of access site thrombosis [9,10]. Although this complication occurs in as many as 40% of patients, the rate of symptomatic postinsertion thrombosis is much lower, ranging from 4 to 16% [9,11].

The incidence of insertion site thrombosis is lower with filters with smaller profile introducer sheaths [6]. In a prospective study by Molgaard *et al.* [12] asymptomatic occlusive thrombosis occurred in 10%, while asymptomatic nonocclusive thrombosis developed in 25% of patients in whom filters were placed through sheaths varying from 12 to 14-F in outer diameter. Only 3% of patients were symptomatic, of which one represented progression of nonocclusive thrombosis 2 weeks after filter placement.

In the study by Molgaard *et al.* [12], the prevalence of occlusive insertion site thrombosis was increased among patients with preexisting partially occlusive iliofemoral thrombus or extrinsic compression of the veins above the access site. This finding has been corroborated by other authors [13]. Presumably, the combination of slow venous flow and fresh intimal injury results in thrombus formation at the site of insertion. When possible, filters should be placed through access routes that are known or expected to be free of proximal thrombus or obstruction in order to minimize this complication.

Patients with malignancy are in a hypercoagulable state, and are therefore more prone to thrombotic complications from IVC filters [12,13]. These patients should be considered at high risk for insertion site thrombosis. Close clinical follow-up is recommended.

Anticoagulation has been suggested as a means of preventing insertion site thrombosis [14], particularly with the SSG filter. Unfortunately, this is not an option in those patients who receive filters for the classic indication of a contraindication to anticoagulation. Many times this is a temporary condition, however, and anticoagulation can be resumed later in patients at risk.

Patients who become symptomatic with pain at the insertion site or swelling of the ipsilateral extremity should be evaluated with either duplex ultrasonography or venography. If insertion site thrombosis is identified, anticoagulation should be initiated whenever this is feasible. Regardless, patients with documented insertion site thrombosis should be followed carefully. Although the reported case of fatal phlegmasia cerulea dolens (PCD) after femoral placement of

Table 22.1 Major complications. (References in brackets)

Filter	Insertion site thrombosis (%)		IVC thrombosis (%)		Recurrent pulmonary embolism (%)		Migration (%)	
SSG	14–41	[10,67]	2–15	[13,23]	4–7	[17,31]	0–26	[26]
MHTG	2–15	[12,45,68]	1–3	[68]	3–3.5	[45,68]	6–11	[6,45]
MBN	3–20	[6,69]	1.5–3	[18,30]	0.5–3	[18,30]	0	[6]
VT	6–32	[6,20]	0–30	[21,60]	3–4	[21,70]	3–36	[6,70]
SN	6–27	[6,19]	7–21	[19,22]	2	[19]	0–12	[6,19]

a MBN filter described thrombosis of the IVC extending to both popliteal veins [15], we have had one case of unilateral PCD on the side of insertion of a filter through a 14-F sheath.

IVC thrombosis

Asymptomatic occlusive IVC thrombosis probably occurs with a higher frequency than is reported in the literature. There are few large, prospective, comprehensive, imaging based studies that have addressed this question. The issue is further obfuscated by studies that report the incidence of caval thrombus without distinguishing between partial or complete thrombotic occlusion of the IVC [6,15]. Partial occlusion of the filter by thrombus may well represent trapped emboli, which is the intended function of the filter. In most cases, asymptomatic IVC occlusion is not a concern clinically.

IVC thrombosis may occur because of outright thrombosis of the filter, extrinsic compression of the cava, or occlusion of the filter by trapped thrombus. The latter case may alternately be considered a filter success; a volume of emboli large enough to occlude the IVC filter might have had severe consequences in the pulmonary circulation.

IVC thrombosis may present as new onset or progression of bilateral lower extremity swelling and venous insufficiency, or recurrent pulmonary embolus (PE) after IVC filter placement. Patients with these symptoms present a diagnostic challenge, as many causes other than IVC thrombosis can explain these symptoms and clinical findings. When IVC thrombosis is suspected, confirmatory studies should be obtained such as ultrasonography (US), computed tomography (CT), magnetic resonance imaging (MRI), or venography of the cava (Fig. 22.2).

The SSG is the standard to which other filters are compared when evaluating caval patency rates. Its predecessor, the MU umbrella filter, had an unacceptable caval occlusion rate that exceeded 60% [16]. This was attributed to a filter design that greatly impeded IVC flow. The rate of symptomatic IVC occlusion with the SSG from the series with the longest follow-up is approximately 4% in 127 patients over a 12-year period [17]. The 44% incidence of persistent lower extremity edema was attributed to underlying venoocclusive disease. In a small series, Kolachalam et al. [13] noted a 14% symptomatic IVC occlusion rate. The rate of asymptomatic IVC occlusion with the SSG is not known.

Reported IVC thrombosis rates for filters with small diameter introducer sheaths vary widely depending upon the type and size of the study. From Table 22.1, it is apparent that the incidence of all IVC thromboses (symptomatic and asymptomatic) ranges from 0 to more than 30%. In general, symptomatic IVC thrombosis rates range from 2.9 to 9% [18−21], with the exception of one small series reporting a rate of 21% with the SN [22]. Asymptomatic IVC thrombosis

may be more prevalent than suspected, as Crochet et al. [21] found a rate of 30% at 5 years with the VT filter. In this study, there was no statistically significant relationship between IVC occlusion and lower extremity venous insufficiency or trophic skin changes [21]. Given the relatively small published experience with these newer filters in comparison with the SSG, these rates are acceptable for current practice. It is expected that trends will become more apparent as the literature grows.

As with insertion site thrombosis, IVC thrombosis seems to occur more often in patients with hypercoagulable conditions. This has been noted with both the SSG and the SN filters in patients with malignancy [13,22].

The route of insertion does not appear to play a role in IVC thrombosis, as Pais et al. [23] noted a 2% symptomatic IVC thrombosis rate with percutaneous femoral insertion of the SSG. This compares well with the 4% incidence reported by Greenfield and Michna [17] with jugular insertions. Similarly, Hye et al. [24] found no difference in IVC thrombosis rates between surgical jugular and percutaneous femoral insertion routes for the SSG. The presence of nonocclusive thrombus in the IVC prior to placement of a filter has been related to progression to complete occlusion [25].

To minimize the incidence of IVC thrombosis, filters should be placed just below the level of the renal veins. Several filter designs, such as the MBN, VT and SN are designed to rest entirely below the renal vein orifices. The MHTG can be placed so that the apex of the filter is above the inferior edge of the renal veins, and therefore in an area of increased venous flow. Should thrombosis of these filters occur, the lack of a "dead space" between the top of the filter and the renal veins may reduce the chance of propagation of the thrombus above the filter.

Although IVC thrombosis has not been statistically linked to access site thrombosis, the same measures can be used to prevent both complications. If there is extensive preexisting thrombosis or compression of the infrarenal IVC, the filter can be placed in a suprarenal position where flow is more normal. Anticoagulation should be resumed in high-risk patients when possible, but is of uncertain benefit [26]. Placement of a filter into IVC thrombus should be avoided, as the risk of occlusion of the filter is probably high, and the filter may not open properly or engage the walls of the IVC.

The treatment of symptomatic IVC thrombosis is anticoagulation when possible, although thrombolytic therapy has been reported [17]. Many patients will not be a candidate for either of these options due to an underlying condition that had necessitated placement of the IVC filter rather than anticoagulation for the original thromboembolic event. Supportive therapy for lower extremity symptoms, such as elevation and elastic stockings may provide symptomatic relief. The incidence of venous stasis ulcers in these patients is not well established [3,17,21]. If recurrent pulmonary

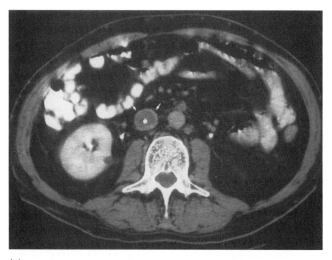

(a)

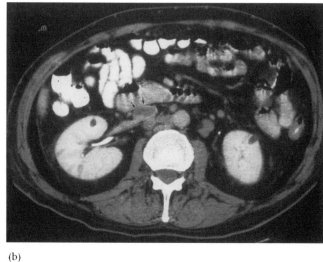

(b)

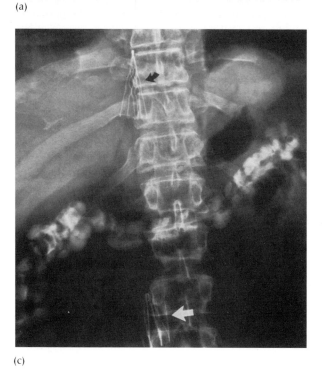

(c)

Fig. 22.2 (a) Contrast-enhanced abdominal CT scan with low attenuation within the IVC consistent with thrombus (arrows). The tip of a VT filter is present in the centre of the thrombus. (b) A higher slice at the level of the right renal vein in the same patient demonstrating propagation of thrombus above the filter (arrows). (c) Plain film of the abdomen after placement of a second filter in the suprarenal IVC. (Straight arrow, original VT filter; curved arrow, second filter (MHTG).)

embolization is an issue, placement of another filter above the first is required if the patient cannot be anticoagulated [27].

Recurrent PE

One of the qualities of the ideal IVC filter would be a 0% rate of recurrent PE, as this is the very condition for which the filter is inserted [28]. However, this would require a filter that would trap with such efficiency that patency rates would be adversely affected. Most manufacturers acknowledge that small thrombi (a few millimeters in radius) may not be trapped well, although there is no accepted definition

of a "clinically insignificant" embolus. Even if 100% of the emboli from the lower extremities were trapped, thrombus formation on the filter can result in PE [29]. Recurrent PE, albeit infrequent, appears to be an unavoidable outcome of IVC filtration.

The incidence of documented recurrent PE after IVC filter placement is uniformly low for all of the devices listed in Table 22.1, ranging from 0.5 to 7% [30,31]. No single design is clearly better or worse than the others. The 4% rate of recurrent PE with suprarenal SSG filters (based on limited experience) compares favorably with infrarenal filters [27]. The rate of asymptomatic PE cannot be estimated, as comprehensive angiographic or pathologic studies have not been performed. The clinical importance of asymptomatic emboli is unknown, but probably minor.

PE can occur at any time after IVC filter placement. Patients who present with symptoms suggestive of recurrent PE require the same diagnostic evaluation as patients without filters. A common misconception is that the presence of an IVC filter excludes PE from the differential diagnosis. Conversely, diagnosis of recurrent PE based on symptoms, lower extremity venous studies, or arterial blood gases is not adequate. An abdominal plain film will allow assessment of the position and integrity of the device. Ventilation/perfusion scans or pulmonary angiograms should be obtained on these patients. Pulmonary angiography can be safely performed through the filter [32], or from an upper extremity or jugular approach. The filter itself should be studied by US, CT, or cavography as a potential source of the emboli (Fig. 22.3).

When symptomatic recurrent PE has been confirmed, the first step in management is to determine the patient's risks for anticoagulation. If the condition of the patient has changed since the filter was placed, such that heparin and coumarin are no longer contraindicated, then anticoagulation is the treatment of choice.

In every case, the position of the filter in the IVC should be confirmed. Filter migration into a location in which it no longer provides protection from PE is a rare but well-documented occurrence. Ferris *et al.* [6] described a SN that embolized to the left pulmonary artery, Sidawy *et al.* [33] reported a case of distal migration of a SSG filter such that its base became oriented towards the orifice of the left iliac vein, allowing recurrent PE from thrombus in the right iliac vein. Chest and pelvic radiographs should be obtained when the filter cannot be found in the abdomen. If filter migration has allowed recurrent PE, then placement of a second filter should be considered.

The physical integrity of the filter can be easily assessed from a plain film, but in most cases is of uncertain importance. Multiple views (anterior–posterior and lateral, centered on the filter), or fluoroscopy may be necessary to evaluate asymmetric distribution or crossing of struts, incomplete opening, or fracture of the device. Filter tilt cannot be accurately assessed without knowledge of the course of the IVC. *In vitro* studies utilizing a variety of simulated IVCs and thrombi, and *in vivo* animal studies, indicate that trapping of small thrombi is affected by tilting, distribution of struts, and wire prolapse for the SSG, VT, SN, and BN [34–39]. The ability to trap large emboli by the filters was generally preserved in the *in vivo* animal studies [35,37,39]. Although the appearance of the filter may be esthetically unpleasant, there is little clinical evidence linking the factors described above to symptomatic recurrent PE. Nevertheless, a second filter can be placed if the filtering ability of the existing device is suspected to be inadequate.

Missed anatomic variants of the IVC can be responsible for recurrent PE [40]. A filter placed in only one limb of a double cava, or between communicating circumaortic left renal veins can allow emboli unrestricted access to the pulmonary circulation. Review of cavagrams obtained during insertion of the filter, cross-sectional imaging, or repeat cavography (preferably from the left femoral approach) may be required to clarify IVC anatomy. Placement of a second filter in a location that will trap emboli that bypass the first filter is the treatment of choice if anticoagulation is not feasible (Fig. 22.4).

Chronic IVC occlusion leads to the formation of large retroperitoneal collateral veins. Rarely, these veins can become alternate pathways for PE. Filter placement within an enlarged hemiazygous vein has been described [41].

Recurrent PE may be a presenting symptom of acute IVC thrombosis [13]. Thrombus can propagate through the filter, with subsequent embolization. Thrombus in a filter does not necessarily imply that the filter itself is a source of emboli, unless it extends above the filter.

Recurrent PE does not always represent failure of the existing filter. If the filter appears satisfactory in all respects, and no lower extremity or infrarenal venous source for emboli can be found, alternate sites of venous thrombosis should be considered. PE can result from upper extremity venous thrombosis [42,43], or from renal vein thrombosis due to malignancy or glomerulonephritis. In these cases, suprarenal or SVC filter placement may be considered.

Experience with filters in the SVC is extremely limited [44,45]. One should bear in mind that all of the currently available filters were designed for placement in the IVC. Because of the length of the BN filter and the tendency of the wires to prolapse (possibly into the atrium), this filter design is not optimal for this venous segment. The long-term outcome of SVC filters is unknown.

Filter migration

The tendency of a filter to move cephalad or caudad in the IVC is one of the characteristics often assessed when evaluating filters. This interest is in part a legacy of the experience with earlier filters, particularly the original 23-mm diameter MU filter. This filter proved too small for some IVCs, allowing migration into the chest [28]. The problem was corrected by increasing the diameter of the filter to 28 mm.

In practice, migration of a filter over a small distance is not only of little clinical importance, but it is also difficult to document [3]. Many factors can affect the appearance of a filter on an abdominal film, including respiration, positioning of the patient, and parallax (Fig. 22.5). When movement does occur, it is acceptable if it is only a few centimeters, and does not compromise the function of the filter. The percentages in Table 22.1 reflect primarily these minor changes in position.

Migrations into the iliac, renal, or hepatic veins, or the

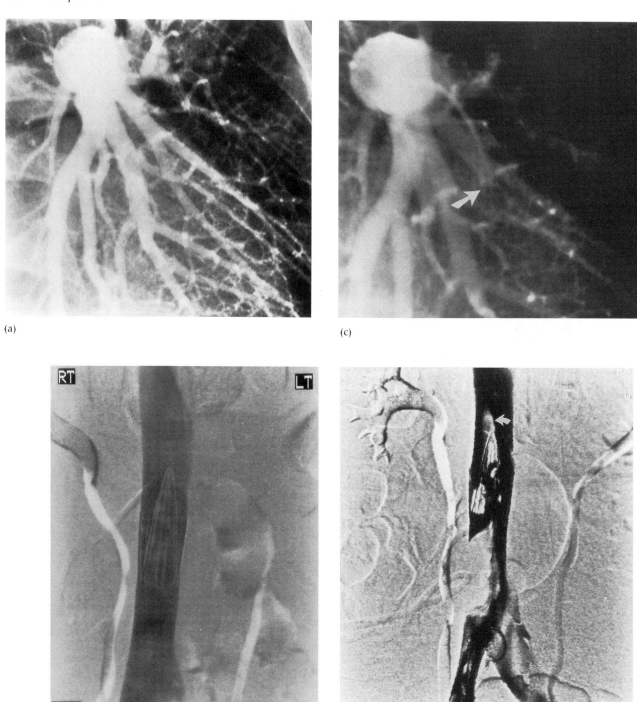

(a)

(c)

(b)

(d)

Fig. 22.3 Recurrent PE 2 days after placement of an IVC filter. (a) Selective left pulmonary angiogram from the time of placement of the original filter for right-sided PE. There is no evidence of PE on the left. (b) Control IVC cavagram after filter deployment. The filter is free of thrombus. (c) Two days later, a repeat pulmonary angiogram demonstrates a new segmental left lower lobe PE (arrow). (d) There is now thrombus trapped in the filter, with extension above the filter (arrow).

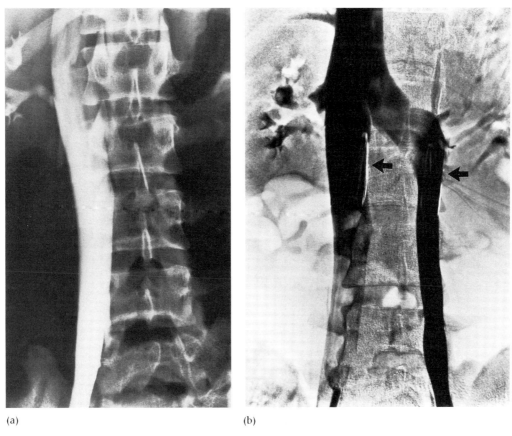

(a)   (b)

Fig. 22.4 (a) Cavagram performed with a pigtail catheter at the expected confluence of the iliac veins in a patient with a duplicated IVC. Inflow from the left iliac vein is absent. (b) Postfilter cavagram from the same patient after placement of a filter in each cava (arrows). Modified with permission from Kaufman *et al.* [40].

Fig. 22.5 Filter migration can be difficult to assess. Two abdominal films, one obtained at the time of filter insertion (a), and the other 14 days later (b) demonstrating apparent proximal migration of the filter. Note the difference in patient position on the two films (arrows on right iliac crests).

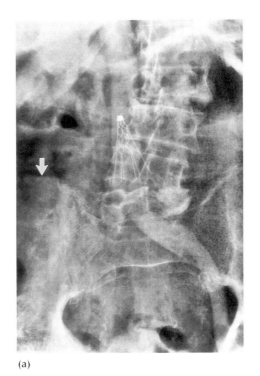

(a)

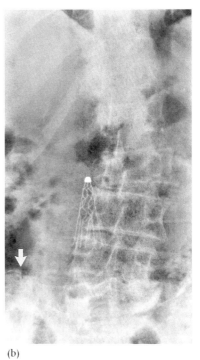

(b)

heart and pulmonary arteries are rare events. Many times, filters in these locations have been placed there by mistake [17] (Fig. 22.6). Filters in the iliac, renal, and hepatic veins are generally asymptomatic, and can be left alone. If the patient requires continued protection against PE, and anti-coagulation is not an option, the filter should be assessed for its ability to perform this function. If the migration has rendered the filter ineffective, a second filter is indicated.

The unusual patient with a filter in the heart or pulmonary artery represents a major management dilemma. With the newer filters, this usually represents embolization of the filter from the IVC, possibly due to failure to adequately engage the walls of the cava or in conjunction with a massive PE [46,47]. Inadvertent deployment directly into the heart is most commonly seen with the older SSG placed from the jugular vein [3]. This occurs due to difficulty negotiating the Eustachian valve with the large 24-F filter carrier, even over a wire [48]. Misplacement of the MHTG, VT, SN, and BN from the jugular approach is less likely as these filters are deployed through 15-F and smaller sheaths that are less difficult to advance through the right atrium into the IVC.

Patients with intracardiac and intrapulmonary filters are typically asymptomatic [49], but life-threatening arrhythmias, intimal dissection of the right coronary artery, and pericardial tamponade have been reported with the SSG

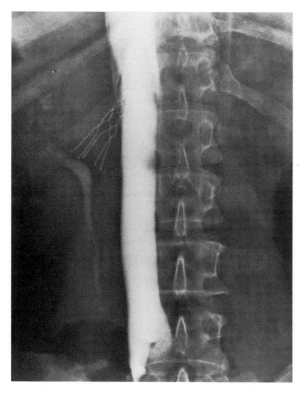

Fig. 22.6 SSG filter inadvertently deployed into the right renal vein via the right internal jugular approach.

[50–52]. Because of concern for these complications, some authors advocate either surgical removal or percutaneous repositioning of the filter in asymptomatic patients [47,48]. Most of the percutaneous techniques involve grasping the filter with a snare device or tip-deflecting wire and pulling it back into the IVC or into a large sheath [6,46–48]. In all cases, if the filter is not functional after repositioning, placement of another filter in the IVC may be necessary.

Other complications

The literature is replete with isolated case reports of unusual complications related to IVC filters (Table 22.2). The true incidence of these complications is difficult to gauge. It is important to recognize that a filter may cause seemingly unrelated symptoms at a time that is temporally remote from date of insertion. However, even after careful evaluation with cross-sectional imaging and angiography, it may not be possible to determine if the filter is the source of the symptoms.

Perforation of structures adjacent to the IVC by filter components has been widely reported, including the aorta, iliac artery, duodenum, bowel, lumbar artery, ureter, nerve ganglion, and vertebral body [6,53–58]. Intracardiac filters can penetrate the myocardium, as described in the preceding section [51,52]. When a perforation is symptomatic, surgical removal of the filter is necessary, but can be difficult in cases where the filter has become incorporated into the wall of the IVC [53]. If continued protection against embolization is required, the IVC can be clipped or plicated at the same time [57]. Asymptomatic perforations into non-critical structures should be managed expectantly [6].

Various technical problems may be encountered during filter placement, such as inability to advance the filter into the IVC, tilting of the filter, misplacement, thrombus formation in the filter, and incomplete opening [3,6,40,45,47, 59–62] (Figs 22.7 & 22.8). These can be due to inherent qualities of the device, patient specific anatomic variables, or operator inexperience. In some cases, perceived technical

Table 22.2 Unusual complications

Complication	Reference
Migration to heart and myocardial infarction	[51]
Migration to pulmonary artery	[71]
Lumbar artery laceration by strut	[57]
Small bowel obstruction by strut	[56]
Filter fracture	[55]
Aortic perforation	[54]
Vertebral perforation	[54]
Perforation of aortic aneurysm	[72]
Duodenal perforation	[53]
Entrapment of guide wire	[65]

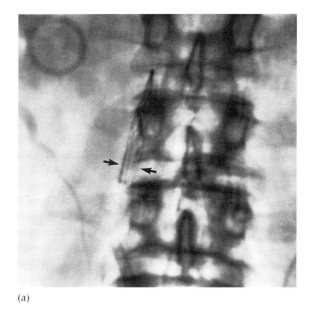

(a)

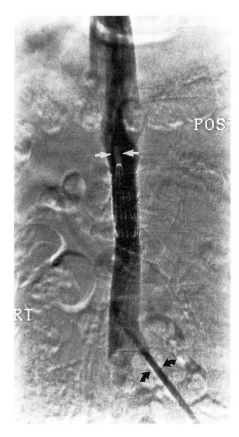

Fig. 22.7 Postplacement cavagram demonstrating a small cylindrical thrombus attached to the apex of the filter (straight arrows) that matches the diameter of the introducer sheath (curved arrows). Deployment of the filter was delayed after introduction of the filter into the sheath due to uncertainty about the level of the renal veins.

problems may not actually affect filter performance, such as prolapse of wires with the BN filter [38,39,59]. The true significance of other problems, such as tilting of the filter, also remain unresolved. Many technical issues can be avoided by a thorough familiarity with the device before attempting insertion. Adequate fluoroscopy is essential, and careful inspection of the cavagram will minimize the incidence of misplacements. In general, the right femoral approach is the easiest for all filter designs.

Fracture of filter elements is occasionally seen on abdominal films obtained for other indications [6,16,17,21,63,64] (Figs 22.9 & 22.10). No cases of recurrent PE have been attributed to fractured filters, suggesting that conservative management is indicated [6]. However, broken filter elements may impinge on adjacent structures and require removal [55]. Periodic evaluation with abdominal plain

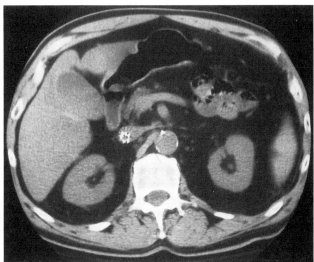

(b)

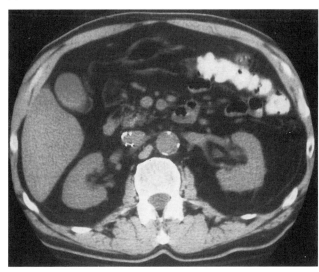

(c)

Fig. 22.8 (a) Intraprocedural appearance of an incompletely opened MHTG filter (arrows). (b,c) Two slices from an abdominal CT scan without contrast enhancement in the same patient confirming incomplete opening of the filter.

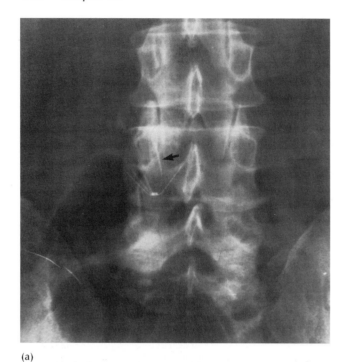

(a)

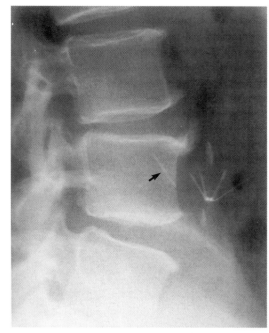

(b)

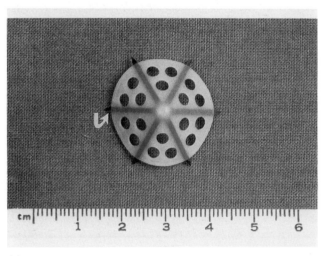

(c)

Fig. 22.9 (a,b) Asymptomatic fracture of a 15-year-old MU filter noted on lumbar spine films. One filter strut has detached and is in the paravertebral soft tissues (straight arrows). Four struts can be counted within the IVC. The sixth strut has disappeared, and could not be seen on either abdominal or chest films. The ability of this filter to trap emboli is now questionable. (c) A photograph of an intact MU filter, illustrating the arrangement of the six struts (curved arrow).

films, perhaps yearly, is recommended to confirm the stability of the fragments.

Primary septic complications of IVC filters, with the exception of the rare infected insertion site hematoma, are virtually unknown [3]. This may be due to either underreporting, or some feature of the filters or IVC that prevents bacterial contamination of the devices. In patients with sepsis and a patent IVC filter, the filter should not be considered infected until an exhaustive search for another source is negative. If thrombus is present within the filter, and a trapped septic embolus is suspected, intravascular biopsy of the thrombus may permit a microbiologic diagnosis.

Dislodgement of IVC filters by guidewires during blind placement of central venous catheters has been described

recently [65,66]. One filter in particular, the Vena Tech, has dominated these case reports. The filter appears to entrap the curved ends of J-tipped guidewires; continued traction on the guidewire can lead to avulsion of the device and fracture of the legs [65,66].

Deaths directly attributable to IVC filters are rare [3,15,18,23]. Periprocedural deaths may represent a concurrent process such as anaphylaxis, decompensation of preexisting disease, or a technical error. Death attributed to acute occlusion of the IVC has been described [15]. The estimated overall mortality rate of IVC filters of 0.12% may be lower than the actual rate, but corresponds closely to the anecdotal experience of most operators [3].

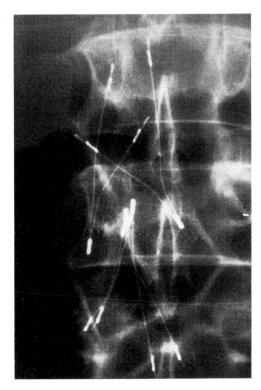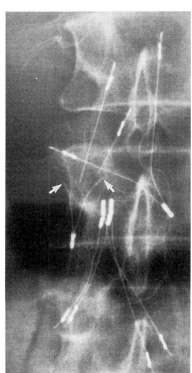

Fig. 22.10 (a) Abdominal film of a patient with two BN filters; the second filter was placed for suspected failure of the first filter. (b) Abdominal film 2-years later revealing asymptomatic fracture of the cephalad legs of the original filter (arrows).

Conclusion

Despite inconsistent documentation in the literature, complications of IVC filters appear to be generally infrequent and minor in severity. When a complication is suspected, the first step is documentation. Next, an assessment should be made regarding the ability of the filter to provide continued protection against PE. If the filter no longer appears effective as an antiembolic device, either anticoagulation or placement of another filter should be considered. Removal of the filter should be the final resort, and only in cases where the filter is the cause of a life-threatening complication that cannot be treated in any other way.

As our understanding of IVC filters grows, and more data is accumulated about the newer filters, one filter may prove safer than another. Currently, all filters appear approximately equal in the incidence and severity of complications. The indications for the filter placement should be clear, and the risks of alternate therapy should be carefully weighed whenever implantation is contemplated. IVC filters should not be considered innocent devices, nor should clinicians diagnose a complication of a filter without firm documentation. A complication from an IVC filter inserted for appropriate indications may be an acceptable alternate to the morbidity associated with either operative caval interruption or no protection from PE.

References

1 Rizk GK, Amplatz K. A percutaneous method of introducing the caval umbrella. *Am J Roentgenol* 1973;117:903.

2 Roehm JOF Jr, Gianturco C, Barth MN, Wright KC. Percutaneous transcatheter filter for the inferior vena cava: a new device for treatment of patients with pulmonary embolism. *Radiology* 1984;150:255–257.

3 Becker DM, Philbrick JT, Selby JB. Inferior vena cava filters: indications, safety, effectiveness. *Arch Int Med* 1992;152: 1985–1994.

4 Rohrer MJ, Scheidler MG, Wheeler HB, Cutler BS. Extended indications for placement of an inferior vena cava filter. *J Vasc Surg* 1989;10:44–50.

5 Athanasoulis CA. Complications of vena cava filters. *Radiology* 1993;188:614–615.

6 Ferris EJ, McCowan TC, Carver DK, McFarland DR. Percutaneous inferior vena cava filters: follow-up of seven designs in 320 patients. *Radiology* 1993;188:851–856.

7 Greenfield LJ, McCurdy JR, Brown PP, Elkins RC. A new intracaval filter permitting continued flow and resolution of thrombi. *Surgery* 1973;73:599–606.

8 Pais SO, Mirvis SE, De Orchis DF. Percutaneous insertion of the Kimray–Greenfield filter: technical considerations and problems. *Radiology* 1987;165:377–381.

9 Mewissen MW, Erickson SJ, Foley WD *et al.* Thrombosis at venous insertion sites after inferior vena caval filter placement. *Radiology* 1989;173:155–157.

10 Dorfman GS, Cronan JJ, Paolella LP *et al.* Iatrogenic changes at

the venotomy site after percutaneous placement of the Greenfield filter. *Radiology* 1989;173:159–162.

11 Rose BS, Simon DC, Hess ML, Van Aman ME. Percutaneous transfemoral placement of the Kimray–Greenfield vena cava filter. *Radiology* 1987;165:373–376.

12 Molgaard CP, Yucel EK, Geller SC, Knox TA, Waltman AC. Access-site thrombosis after placement of inferior vena cava filters with 12-14 F delivery sheaths. *Radiology* 1992;185:257–261.

13 Kolachalam RB, Julian TB. Clinical presentation of thrombosed Greenfield filters. *Vasc Surg* 1990;9:666–670.

14 Dorfman GS. Evaluating the roles and function of vena caval filters: will data be available before or after these devices are removed from the market? *Radiology* 1992;185:15–17.

15 Aruny JE, Kandarpa K. Phlegmasia cerulea dolens, a complication after placement of a Bird's Nest vena cava filter. *Am J Roentgenol* 1990;154:1105–1106.

16 McCowan TC, Ferris EJ, Carver DK, Molpus WM. Complications of the Nitinol vena cava filter. *J Vasc Intervent Radiol* 1992;3:401–408.

17 Greenfield LJ, Michna BA. Twelve-year clinical experience with the Greenfield vena caval filter. *Surgery* 1988;104:706–712.

18 Roehm JO Jr, Johnsrude IS, Barth MH, Gianturco Cesare. The Bird's Nest inferior vena cava filter: progress report. *Radiology* 1988;168:745–749.

19 Simon M, Athanasoulis CA, Kim D *et al*. Simon Nitinol inferior vena cava filter: initial clinical experience. *Radiology* 1989;172:99–103.

20 Murphy TP, Dorfman GS, Yedlicka JW *et al*. LGM vena cava filter: objective evaluation of early results. *J Vasc Intervent Radiol* 1991;2:107–115.

21 Crochet DP, Stora O, Ferry D *et al*. Vena Tech – LGM filter: long term results of a prospective study. *Radiology* 1993;188:857–860.

22 Grassi CJ, Matsumoto AH, Teitelbaum GP. Vena caval occlusion after Simon Nitinol filter placement: identification with MR imaging in patients with malignancy. *J Vasc Intervent Radiol* 1992;3:535–539.

23 Pais SO, Tobin KD, Austin CB, Queral L. Percutaneous insertion of the Greenfield inferior vena cava filter: experience with ninety-six patients. *J Vasc Surg* 1988;8:460–464.

24 Hye RJ, Mitchell AT, Dory CE, Freischlag JA, Roberts AC. Analysis of the transition to percutaneous placement of Greenfield filters. *Arch Surg* 1990;125:1550–1553.

25 Ricco JB, Crochet D, Sebilotte P *et al*. Percutaneous transvenous caval interruption with the "LGM" filter: early results of a multicenter trial. *Ann Vasc Surg* 1988;3:242–247.

26 Lang W, Schweiger H, Hofmann-Preiss K. Results of long-term venacavography study after placement of a Greenfield vena caval filter. *J Cardiovasc Surg* 1992;33:573–578.

27 Greenfield LJ, Cho KJ, Proctor MC, Sobel M, Shah S, Wingo J. Late results of suprarenal Greenfield vena cava filter placement. *Arch Surg* 1992;127:969–973.

28 Grassi CJ. Inferior vena caval filters: analysis of five currently available devices. *Am J Roentgenol* 1991;156:813–821.

29 Geisinger MA, Zelch MG, Risius B. Recurrent pulmonary embolism after greenfield filter placement. *Radiology* 1987;165:383–384.

30 Dorfman GS. Percutaneous inferior vena caval filters. *Radiology* 1990;174:987–992.

31 Golueke PJ, Garrett WV, Thompson JE, Smith BL, Talkington CM. Interruption of the vena cava by means of the Greenfield filter: expanding the indications. *Surgery* 1988;103:111–117.

32 Hansen ME, Geller SC, Yucel EK, Egglin TK, Waltman AC. Transfemoral venous catheterization through inferior vena caval filters: results in seven cases. *Am J Roentgenol* 1991;157:967–970.

33 Sidawy AN, Menzoian JO. Distal migration and deformation of the Greenfield vena cava filter. *Surgery* 1986;99:369–372.

34 Katsamouris AA, Waltman AC, Delichatsios MA, Athanasoulis CA. Inferior vena cava filters: *in vivo* comparison of clot trapping and flow dynamics. *Radiology* 1988;166:361–366.

35 Thompson BH, Cragg AH, Smith TP, Bareniewski H, Barnhart WH, Dejong SC. Thrombus-trapping efficiency of the Greenfield filter *in vivo*. *Radiology* 1989;172:979–981.

36 Greenfield LJ, Proctor MC. Experimental embolic capture by asymmetric Greenfield filters. *J Vasc Surg* 1992;16:436–444.

37 Millward SF, Marsh JI, Pon C, Moher D. Thrombus-trapping efficiency of the LGM (Vena Tech) and titanium Greenfield filters *in vivo*. *J Vasc Intervent Radiol* 1992;3:103–106.

38 Shlansky-Goldberg R, Wing CM, Leveen RF, Cope C. Effectiveness of a prolapsed bird's nest filter. *J Vasc Intervent Radiol* 1993;4:505–511.

39 Carlson JE, Yedlicka JW Jr, Castaneda-Zuniga WR, Hunter DW, Amplatz K. Acute clot-trapping efficiency in dogs with compacted versus elongated wires in Bird's Nest filters. *J Vasc Intervent Radiol* 1993;4:513–516.

40 Kaufman JA, Geller SC, Rivitz SM, Wattman AC. Operator errors during percutaneous placement of vena cava filters. *Am J Roentgenol* 1995;165:1281–1287.

41 Teitelbaum GP, McKay RH, Katz MD. Bird's nest filter placement within an enlarged hemiazygos vein for prevention of pulmonary embolism. *Cardiovasc Intervent Radiol* 1993;16:119–121.

42 Monreal M, Lafoz E, Ruiz J, Valls R, Alastrue A. Upper-extremity deep venous thrombosis and pulmonary embolism: a prospective study. *Chest* 1991;99:280–283.

43 Black MD, French GJ, Rasuli P, Boushard AC. Upper extremity deep venous thrombosis: underdiagnosed and potentially lethal. *Chest* 1993;103:1887–1890.

44 Pais SO, De Orchis DF, Mirvis SE. Superior vena caval placement of a Kimray–Greenfield filter. *Radiology* 1987;165:385–386.

45 Greenfield LJ, Cho KJ, Proctor M *et al*. Results of a multicenter study of the modified hook-titanium Greenfield filter. *J Vasc Surg* 1991;14:253–257.

46 Rogoff PA, Hilgenberg AD, Miller SL, Stepham SM. Cephalic migration of the Bird's Nest inferior vena caval filter: report of 2 cases. *Radiology* 1992;184:819–823.

47 Cynamon J, Bakal CW, Gabelman G. Percutaneous removal of a titanium Greenfield filter. *Am J Roentgenol* 1992;159:777–778.

48 Malden ES, Darcy MD, Hicks ME *et al*. Transvenous retrieval of misplaced stainless steel Greenfield filters. *J Vasc Intervent Radiol* 1992;3:703–708.

49 Gelbfish GA, Ascer E. Intracardiac and intrapulmonary Greenfield filters: a long term follow-up. *J Vasc Surg* 1991;14:614–617.

50 Bach JR, Zaneuski R, Lee H. Cardiac arrythmias from a malpositioned Greenfield filter in a traumatic quadraplegic. *Am J Phys Med Rehab* 1990;69:251–253.

51 Puram B, Maley TJ, White NM, Rotman HH, Miller G. Acute myocardial infarction resulting from migration of a Greenfield filter. *Chest* 1990;98:1510–1511.

52 Lahey SJ, Meyer LP, Karchmer AW *et al*. Misplaced caval filter and subsequent pericardial tamponade. *Ann Thorac Surg* 1991;51:299–301.

53 Appleberg M, Crozier JA, Doudenal perforation by a Greenfield caval filter. *Aust N Z J Surg* 1991;61:960−962.

54 Kim D, Porter DH, Siegal JB, Simon M. Perforation of the inferior vena cava with aortic and vertebral penetration by a suprarenal Greenfield filter. *Radiology* 1989;172:721−723.

55 Taheri SA, Kulaylat MN, Johnson E, Hoover E. A complication of the Greenfield filter: fracture and distal migration of two struts — a case report. *J Vasc Surg* 1992;16:96−99.

56 Kupferschmid JP, Dickson CS, Townsend RN, Diamond DL. Small-bowel obstruction from an extruded Greenfield filter strut: an unusual late complication. *J Vasc Surg* 1992;16:113−115.

57 Howerton RM, Watkins M, Feldman L. Late arterial hemorrhage secondary to a Greenfield filter requiring operative intervention. *Surgery* 1991;109:265−268.

58 Carabasi RA III, Moritz MJ, Jarrell BF. Complications encountered with the use of the Greenfield filter. *Am J Surg* 1987;154:163−168.

59 Vesely T, Darcy M, Picus D, Hicks M. Technical problems associated with placement of the Bird's Nest inferior vena cava filter. *Am J Roentgenol* 1992;158:875−880.

60 Cull DL, Wheeler JR, Gregory RT, Snyder SO, Gayle RG, Parent FN III. The Vena Tech filter: evaluation of a new inferior vena cava interruption device. *J Cardiovasc Surg* 1991;32:691−696.

61 Reed RA, Teitlebaum GP, Taylor FC *et al.* Incomplete opening of LGM (Vena Tech) filters inserted via the transjugular approach. *J Vasc Intervent Radiol* 1991;2:441−445.

62 Millward SF, Marsh JI, Peterson R *et al.* LGM (Vena Tech) filter: clinical experience in 64 patients. *J Vasc Intervent Radiol* 1991;2:429−433.

63 Bury TF, Barman AA. Strut fracture after Greenfield filter place-ment. *J Cardiovasc Surg* 1991;32:384−386.

64 Awh MH, Taylor FC, Lu C-T. Spontaneous fracture of a Vena-Tech caval filter. *Am J Roentgenol* 1991;157:177−178.

65 Loesberg A, Taylor FC, Awh MH. Dislodgement of inferior vena caval filters during blind insertion of central venous catheters. *Am J Roentgenol* 1993;161:637−638.

66 Urbaneja A, Fontaine AB, Brucker M, Spigos DG. Evulsion of a Vena Tech filter during insertion of a central venous catheter. *J Vasc Intervent Radiol* 1994;5:783−785.

67 Kantor A, Glanz S, Gordon DH, Sclafani SJ. Percutaneous insertion of the Kimray−Greenfield filter: incidence of femoral vein thrombosis. *Am J Roentgenol* 1987;149:1065−1066.

68 Greenfield LJ, Proctor MC, Cho KJ, Cutler BS, Ferris EJ, McFarland D, Sobel M, Tisnado J. Extended evaluation of the titanium Greenfield vena caval filter. *J Vasc Surg* 1994;20:458−465.

69 Hicks ME, Middleton WD, Picus D, Darcy MD, Kleinhoffer MA. Prevalence of local venous thrombosis after transfemoral placement of a Bird's Nest vena caval filter. *J Vasc Intervent Radiol* 1990;1:63−68.

70 Taylor FC, Awh MH, Kahn CE, Lu C-T. Vena Tech vena cava filters: experience and early follow-up. *J Vasc Intervent Radiol* 1991;2:435−440.

71 LaPlante JS, Contractor FM, Kiproff PM, Khoury MB. Migration of the Simon Nitinol vena cava filter to the chest. *Am J Roentgenol* 1993;160:385−386.

72 Kurgan A, Nunnelee J, Auer AI. Penetration of the wall of an abdominal aortic aneurysm by a Greenfield filter prong: a late complication. *J Vasc Surg* 1993;18:303−306.

CHAPTER 23

Complications of venous vascular stents

Mark D. Jacobson, Neil J. Solomon, Mark H. Wholey and Chester R. Jarmolowski

Introduction

The use of intravascular stents for venous applications, although considered investigational, is gaining widespread clinical acceptance. The overwhelming number of indications are related to malignancies, hemodialysis access, and central line complications. The anatomic sites are most frequently the superior vena cava, inferior vena cava, the brachiocephalic veins, and to a lesser extent subclavian and iliac veins.

Complications can be classified as acute or chronic. Acute complications are ordinarily related to those problems occurring during the stent deployment or within the first 3 weeks [1]. Long-term complications are those related primarily to stent patency. Our stent experience includes the balloon expandable Palmaz Stent (J&J Interventional Systems, Warren, NJ), the self-expanding Wallstent (Schneider, Minneapolis, MN), and the self-expanding Cook Gianturco (Cook, Bloomington, IN) stent. Complications occurring in the veins are quite different from those encountered in arteries considering the dissimilar hemodynamics, underlying pathologic processes, and compliance of the intima, media, and adventitia of these two types of vessels. Although venous stenting is usually initially successful (Figs 23.1–23.3), Table 23.1 [2–17] (N.J. Solomon, M.H. Wholey, & M.D. Jacobson, unpublished observations) summarizes the outcomes of some 301 cases of venous stenting documented in the radiology literature, and includes 20 cases from our personal experience.

Methods

The approach to venous stenting is quite variable depending on the stenotic or occluded site. Those patients with thrombotic occlusive disease involving the brachiocephalic veins or superior vena cava ordinarily receive a 24-hour period of intensive urokinase. Following some degree of recanalization, the vessel is then dilated with a conventional balloon. The dimensions of the balloon are ordinarily 10 mm with length variations from 2 to 4 cm. Rarely, this results in an adequate lumen and the residual stenotic segment is stented. Because of the increased radial force of the Palmaz stent, and its ability to be precisely positioned, it has been

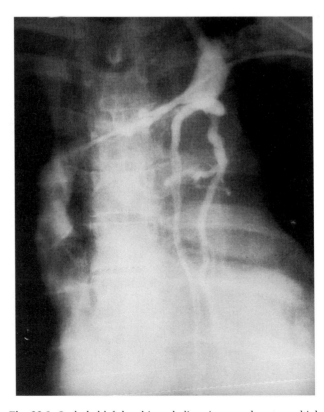

Fig. 23.1 Occluded left brachiocephalic vein secondary to multiple hemodialysis catheter placements.

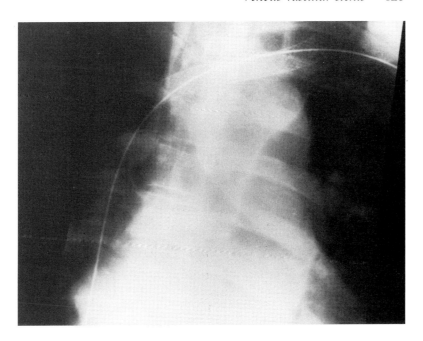

Fig. 23.2 Successful placement of Wallstent in left brachiocephalic vein.

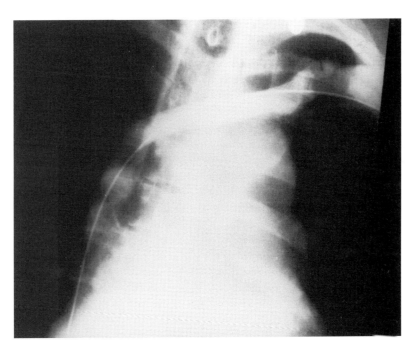

Fig. 23.3 Venogram demonstrating restored patency of the stented left brachiocephalic vein.

our stent of choice for superior vena cava syndromes. On certain occasions, the stent has been expanded to 18 mm utilizing the larger valvuloplasty balloons. In those stents where some motion still exists following deployment, the 0.035 Wholey steerable wire (Mallinckrodt, St Louis, MO) should be maintained through the lumen and the balloon replaced with one of larger dimensions. Most of the migration complications occur at the junction of the superior vena cava with the right atrium, where an increase in junctional diameter occurs. For these reasons, when the occlusive process extends to the level of the right atrium, a lengthy stent should be chosen so that there is adequate fixation proximally at a higher superior vena cava level to avoid the possibility of migration. Migration is rarely a problem at higher levels where the venous dimensions are frequently only 10–12 mm. In these situations, the self-expanding Wallstent is an option. These patients are anticoagulated during the procedure with approximately 10 000 U of heparin, maintaining an activated clotting time (ACT) at the 300 s level. Patients are then heparinized for a 24–48-hour period followed by long-term coumarin.

The Wallstent, considering its versatile 7-F delivery

Table 23.1 Summary of the outcome of 301 cases of venous stenting

Stent	Number of sites	Acute	Recurrence	Follow-up	Reference
Wallstent	20	2	6	14.9	Antonucci *et al.* [2]
Gianturco	28	12	N/A	N/A	Carrasco *et al.* [3]
Gianturco	2	1	0	5	Charnsangavej *et al.* [4]
Variety	98	3	11	9.1	Dake *et al.* [5]
Palmaz	6	4	0	4	Elson *et al.* [6]
Gianturco	9	2	0	3.5	Furui *et al.* [7]
Wallstent	22	1	3	2	Gray *et al.* [8]
Wallstent	6	2	3	4	Gunther *et al.* [9]
Gianturco	17	0	3	N/A	Lakin *et al.* [10]
Palmaz	6	0	3	6	Landwehr *et al.* [11]
Gianturco	16	0	4	11	Petersen *et al.* [12]
Gianturco	25	3	14	10	Quinn *et al.* [13]
Gianturco	28	0	4	8.5	Roesch *et al.* [14]
Palmaz/Gianturco	6	1	2	2	Solomon *et al.* [15]
Wallstent	9	0	5	15	Turmel-Rodrigues *et al.* [16]
Wallstent	3	1	1	7	Zollikofer *et al.* [17]
Total	301	32	59		
					N.J Solomon, M.H. Wholey, & M.D. Jacobson,
P2 W3	5	1	1	5	unpublished observations
P11 W4	15	5	N/A	N/A	SSH, Shadyside Hospital.
Overall total	321	38	60		

N/A, not applicable; P, Palmaz stent; W, Wallstent.

catheter dimensions, may be positioned from either a brachial or femoral approach. One should be aware, however, of the geometry of the self-expanding stent and problems that might occur with overlap at ostial junctions.

The Palmaz stent, however, because of its limited flexibility, has been difficult to position via brachial or axillary approaches, but is ideally suited for delivery from the femoral approach. Larger stents are incorporated into a 10-F delivery system. The sheath is positioned in the midright atrium, and with the steerable wire passed through the lesion this stent is accurately positioned and subsequently expanded. Following the reestablishment of flow, and a return of the ACT to the 150–200s range, the sheaths are removed and hemostasis is established.

Acute complications

The acute complications most frequently described include: thrombotic occlusion, failure of the stent to expand adequately, stent collapse, migration of the stent, perforation with associated hemorrhage at the stent site, stent misplacement and/or displacement, and finally vessel perforation. These complications are summarized in Table 23.2.

The most frequently documented early complication of intravenous stenting is occlusion by thrombus. As summarized by Palmaz [1], this is multifactorial and includes the

Table 23.2 Complications

Type	Number
Thrombotic occlusion	10
Failure of initial expansion	8
Migration	5
Systemic bleeding	4
Stent collapse	2
Stent fracture	3
Access site bleeding	2
Misplacement (premature delivery)	2
Perforation	1
Displacement (iatrogenic)	1
Total	38*

* See Table 23.1.

structural material of the stent, inflow/outflow relationships, failure to endothelialize, and flow dynamics that exist in the venous system.

Although biocompatible, intravascular stents, regardless of design or composition, are inherently thrombogenic. Several measures, however, can be initiated to minimize risk. Beginning with the diagnostic angiographic evaluation, the potentially stentable vessel should be traversed and manipulated with the utmost of care so as to minimize the degree of iatrogenic endothelial trauma. Next, one must ensure that the stent is properly expanded at the time of its deployment. This often requries the adjunctive use of an angioplasty balloon of slightly larger diameter than the native vessel. Once the stent has been deployed, the balloon is inflated so as to produce slight overdistension of the stent, imbedding its metal struts into the vessel wall such that the endothelial surface fills the stent interstices. This, in turn, directly reduces the amount of exposed metal surface of the stent and ultimately facilitates its incorporation by the vascular endothelium. Furthermore, because thrombus deposition is inversely related to flow velocity, patency rates are generally higher in larger diameter veins in which blood flow through the stent is fairly rapid [1]. Finally, anti-coagulants (heparin, coumarin) and platelet inhibitors (aspirin, dipyridamole) may also help prevent acute thrombotic occlusion, especially in vessels in which flow is suboptimal. Nonetheless, at least 50% of the reported in-stances of acute thrombosis occurred while patients were receiving such drugs. Ineffective stent placement can also lead to rethrombosis upstream of the stent, with relapse and/or progression of the presenting symptoms of venous occlusive disease [3]. The ideal antithrombotic regimen remains to be determined and must often be tailored to individual clinical circumstances and patient requirements (Figs 23.4–23.8).

Another problem that is immediately apparent is in-complete expansion of the stent once it is deployed. Complete expansion depends on the relative degree of vessel rigidity, elastic recoil, and extrinsic compression, versus the expansile force generated by the stent. The latter is directly related to stent diameter and inversely related to its length [3].

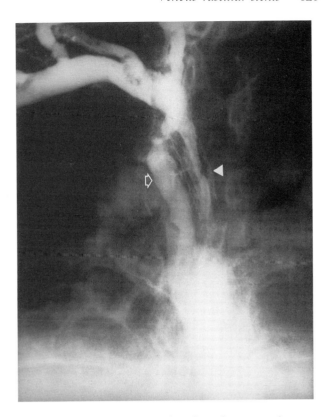

Fig. 23.5 Right arm venogram 1 day after Palmaz stent placement in the superior vena cava (arrowhead) showing acute thrombosis despite systemic heparinization. There is also retrograde filling of the azygos vein (open arrow).

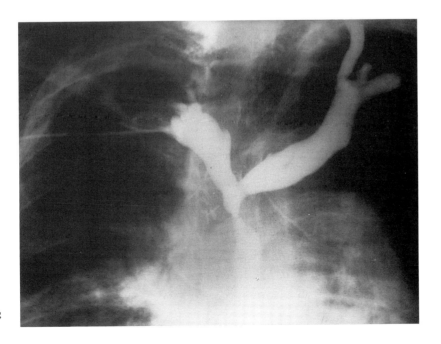

Fig. 23.4 Bilateral arm venograms demonstrating superior vena cava stenosis.

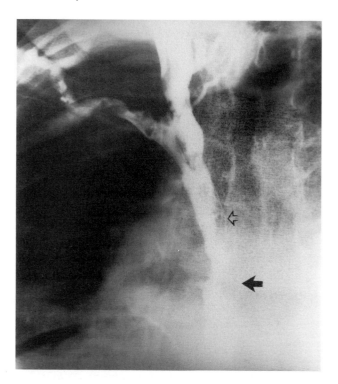

Fig. 23.6 Right arm venogram following 15.5 hours of urokinase infusion (1.5×10^6 U) through a coaxial system showing the stent (open arrow) and residual superior vena cava stenosis (solid arrow).

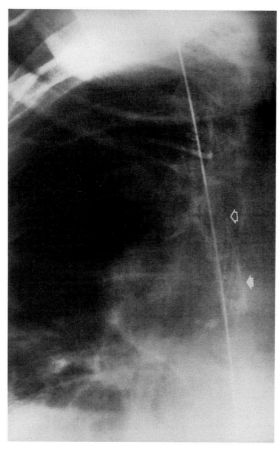

Fig. 23.7 A second stent (solid arrow) was placed by a right common femoral venous approach through an area of residual stenosis in the superior vena cava, below the initial stent (open arrow). There is minimal overlapping of the two stents.

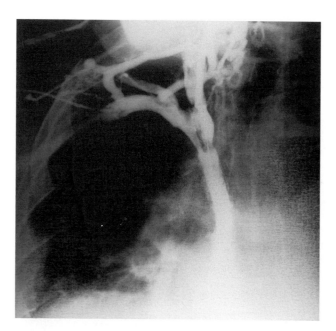

Fig. 23.8 Follow-up venogram shows restored patency of the superior vena cava.

Stent geometry and material composition also determine expansibility, with thicker struts having greater radial force but also being more susceptible to fracture. Several of the cited cases of incomplete expansion involve the junction site or joining struts bridging tandem stents [3]. The additional reported cases of incomplete stent expansion were attributed to extrinsic compression either by neoplasm [3] or by adjacent osseous structures [6]. In these situations, even overdilatation or dual balloon application may be unsuccessful, increasing the likelihood of acute thrombosis or stent migration.

Stent migration can result from incomplete expansion of a stent, incorrect stent selection (Figs 23.9–23.15), and improper positioning of a stent (Figs 23.16–23.22). Mechanical failure, such as fracture of struts adjoining tandem stents, may also lead to migration. By way of observation, the collected data as well as our own experience indicates that most often, stent migration was of little apparent consequence even in those patients where stent embolization to the right ventricle and pulmonary artery had occurred (see

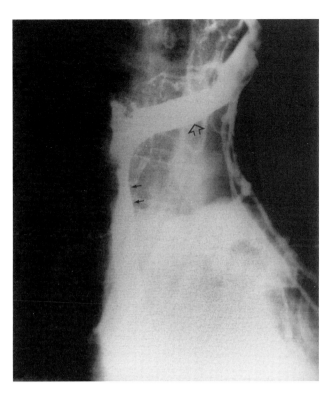

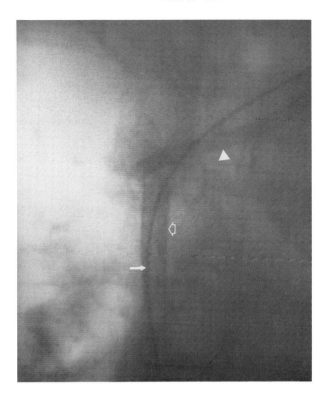

Fig. 23.9 Venogram following urokinase and percutaneous angioplasty of superior vena cava (small arrows) and left brachiocephalic vein occlusion (open arrow) secondary to indwelling central venous catheter.

Fig. 23.10 Initially deployed Palmaz stent (open arrow), insufficiently expanded secondary to balloon rupture. An indwelling left subclavian Hickman catheter (arrowhead) and common femoral vein guidewire (small arrow) are also noted.

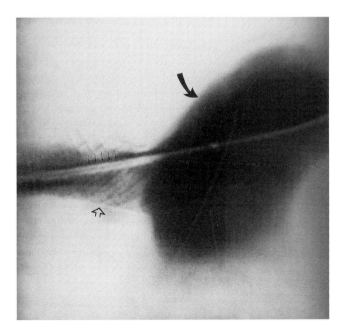

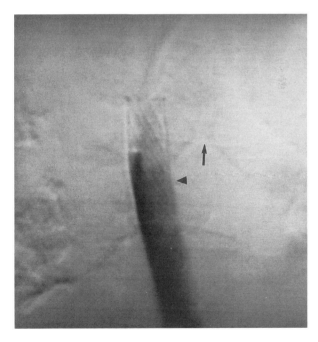

Fig. 23.11 The initial stent (open arrow) was recaptured using an angioplasty balloon (small arrows), but migrated from the superior vena cava to the inferior vena cava following attempts at repositioning. Curved arrow indicates right atrium.

Fig. 23.12 Second Palmaz stent (arrowhead) successfully positioned across the superior vena cava stenosis. (Arrow indicates tracheal bifurcation.)

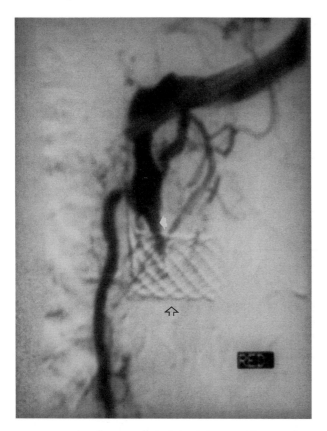

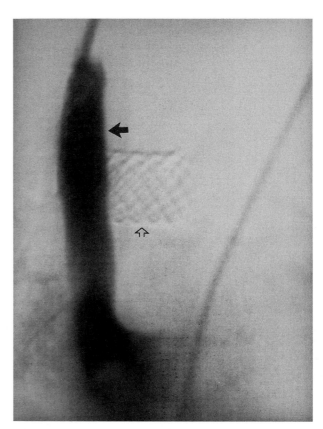

Fig. 23.13 Venogram through the left subclavian Hickman catheter 1 week poststenting showing acute thrombosis of the superior vena cava stent (solid arrow) and right pulmonary artery embolization of the initial stent (open arrow), which had been redeployed in the inferior vena cava.

Fig. 23.14 Superior venacavogram following 1.5×10^6 U of urokinase infusion demonstrating patency of the superior vena cava and stent (solid arrow). Open arrow indicates initial stent, which embolized to right main pulmonary artery.

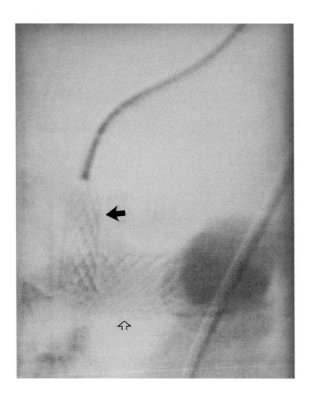

Figs 23.13–23.15) (N.J. Solomon, M.H. Wholey, & M.D. Jacobson, unpublished observations). Nevertheless, if stent embolization is imminent, one should undertake every reasonable effort to contain the stent either by retrieving it and expanding it within the desired site or a related "safe" area (see Fig. 23.11), retrieving it and removing it via venotomy, or permanently containing the potential intravascular projectile beneath a vena cava filter (see Figs 23.20–23.22) [3,6,8]. In addition, recent case reports involving migrated Wallstents following transjugular intrahepatic portosystemic shunt procedures have shown that these may be successfully retrieved with the use of loop snares [10,18]. Perhaps subsequently developed stents designed specifically for intravenous application will in-

Fig. 23.15 Pulmonary arterial phase of the superior venacavogram demonstrating patency of the right pulmonary artery with the embolized stent positioned parallel to the pulmonary artery lumen (open arrow). Solid arrow indicates second stent successfully deployed in the superior vena cava.

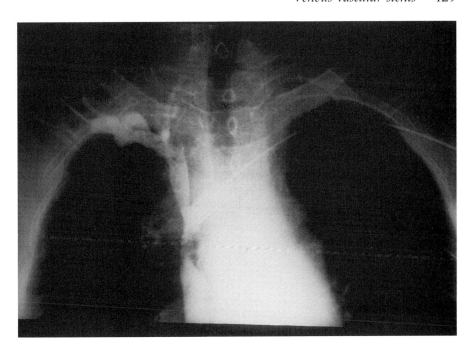

Fig. 23.16 Bilateral arm venograms showing superior vena cava compression by a right paratrachial mass.

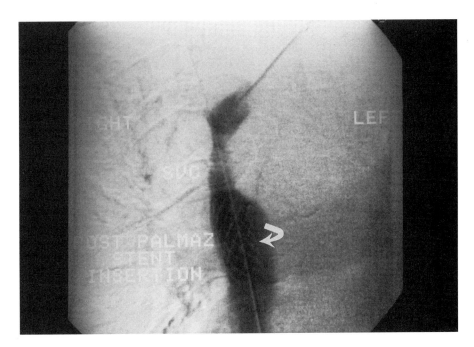

Fig. 23.17 Superior venacavogram with Palmaz stent (curved arrow) having migrated inferior to the area of stenosis following balloon withdrawal.

corporate microbarbs or fasteners designed to anchor them effectively in the desired position. Furthermore, considering the dimensions of the superior and inferior vena cava, greater expansile capabilities to 2–3 cm may ultimately be necessary.

Hemorrhagic complications may arise as a consequence of venous stenting and can be categorized as systemic or local. The former usually result from preliminary fibrinolytic therapy or concurrent anticoagulation (heparin/coumarin) and can range in severity from hematuria [5] or gastro-

intestinal bleeding [15] to hemothorax and intracranial hemorrhage [3].

Localized bleeding usually consists of a hematoma at the puncture site and could conceivably be the result of vessel manipulation and/or concurrent anticoagulation or fibrinolytic therapy [3] (N.J. Solomon, M.H. Wholey, & M.D. Jacobson, unpublished observations).

Stent collapse and fracture are intimately related to one another and to the tensile strength of the material comprising the stent. Larger diameter elements, although providing

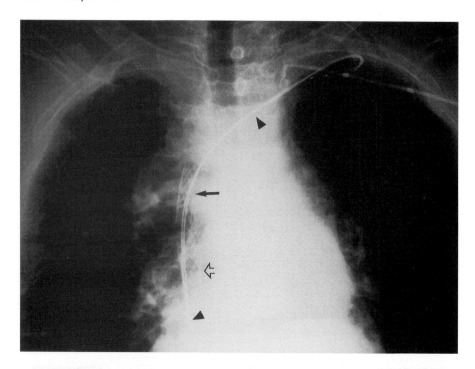

Fig. 23.18 Second Palmaz stent successfully deployed at site of superior vena cava stenosis by a left brachial venous approach (solid arrow). A right femoral guidewire (arrowheads) retains the initially deployed stent (open arrow).

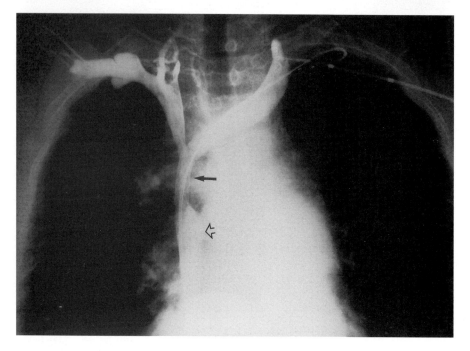

Fig. 23.19 Venogram demonstrating superior vena cava patency. Open arrow indicates initially deployed, migrated stent. Solid arrow is subsequently placed stent across prior area of superior vena cava stenosis.

greater radial stiffness, are also more susceptible to fracture on overexpansion. Fractures most commonly involve the struts adjoining tandem stents, especially at stress angles [3]. Stent fracture by decreasing radial expansile force, ultimately predisposes the stent to collapse as does overwhelming extrinsic compressive force.

Unusual acute complications of venous stenting include stent misplacement and vessel perforation [6,13] (N.J. Solomon, M.H. Wholey, & M.D. Jacobson, unpublished observations). The former may be related to difficulty accessing the diseased vessel, usually because of anatomic considerations (tight stenosis, tortuous vessels, stent delivery system too large or short to reach the intended placement site) (Figs 23.23–23.26).

It is conceivable that overdistension with an angioplasty balloon to seat a stent firmly within a thin-walled vein could result in vessel perforation even in the absence of underlying disease. This risk is potentially greater in the pathologic vein.

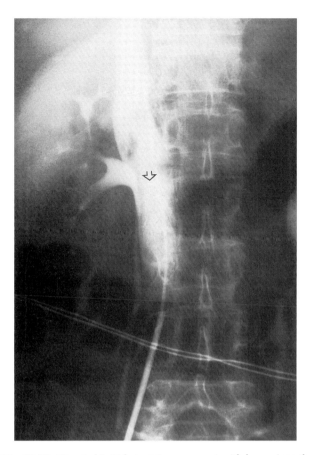

Fig. 23.20 Migrated initial stent (open arrow) withdrawn into the inferior vena cava with angioplasty balloon. A wire remains across the stent to prevent stent embolization.

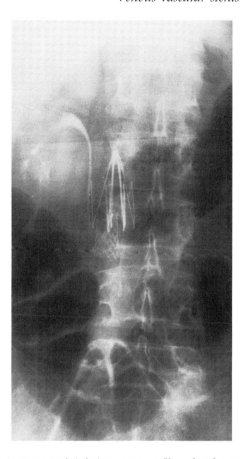

Fig. 23.21 Vena-Tech inferior vena cava filter placed superior to stent and below renal vein ostia via right common femoral venous approach.

Nevertheless, the only reported case of such transmural vascular injury was not immediately evident either radiographically or clinically, but was noted at autopsy in which the cause of death was not attributable to the stenting [13].

Newly deployed stents should be traversed with steerable wires and selective catheters only when necessary. One must be certain that the wire is within the stent lumen and not between the interstices of the stent and vessel wall. In such events, the wire and/or the catheter may be entrapped within the interstices, resulting in stent displacement or shearing forces resulting in catheter fragmentation and embolization (Figs 23.27–23.31).

Long-term patency

Occlusion or stenosis of the stented lumen occurring more than 3 weeks following placement of the stent is ordinarily an issue of patency. The patency in the venous system is

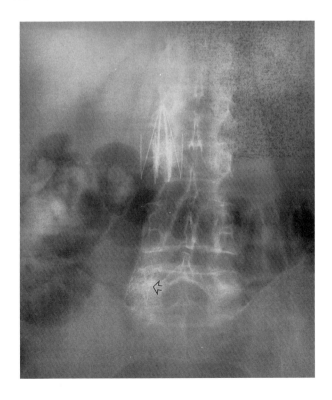

Fig. 23.22 Stent (open arrow) withdrawn and wedged in right common iliac vein using angioplasty balloon.

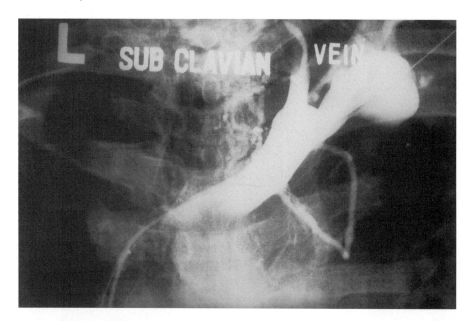

Fig. 23.23 Left subclavian venogram showing occlusion of the left proximal brachiocephalic vein.

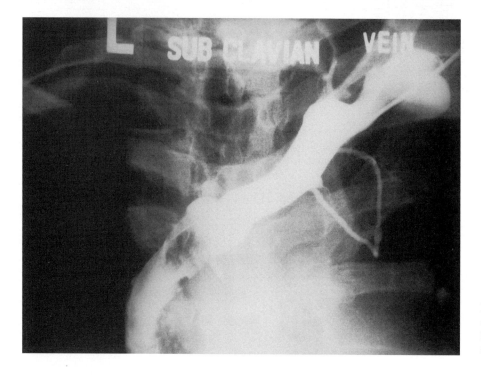

Fig. 23.24 Left brachial venogram showing persistent narrowing of the left brachiocephalic vein following fibrinolytic therapy with urokinase.

quite complex, but ordinarily relates to disorderly thrombus deposition, intimal hyperplasia, flow dynamics, and the underlying pathologic process. Intimal hyperplasia has primarily been studied in arteries; therefore, accurate conclusions from these studies and applying them to the venous system is an assumption. As indicated in Table 23.1, according to the reviews of the literature and personal experience, the overall span of follow-up ranges between 2 and 14.9 months. The primary patency rate as indicated by a diameter of at least 50% of the original stented lumen was 60%. Lesser degrees of intimal hyperplasia not requiring secondary procedures could not be assessed.

The neointimal lining is formed by the endothelialization process which occurs in the stented lumen. Complete endothelialization of the stent is necessary to reduce its thrombogenicity, and has been shown to take 3 weeks in canine arteries [19]. The more rapid the endothelialization process, the thinner the new intimal lining and, therefore, the larger the stented lumen. As previously stated, mechanical considerations, blood-flow characteristics, including turbulence,

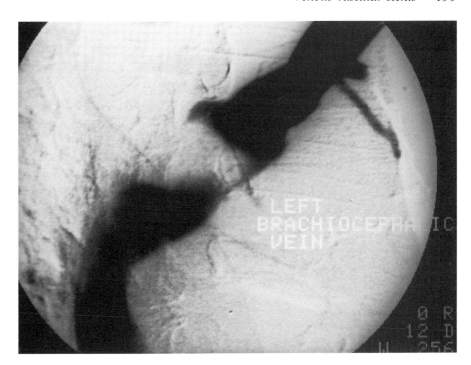

Fig. 23.25 Postangioplasty venogram with persistent stenosis of the left brachiocephalic veins secondary to extrinsic compression. Angioscopy and intravascular ultrasound showed no intraluminal thrombus.

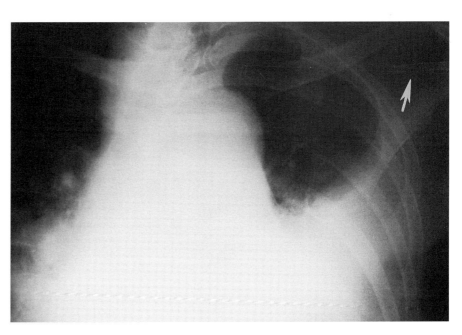

Fig. 23.26 Following unsuccessful attempts at stent placement, the balloon-mounted stent was withdrawn, the stent slipped off the balloon and became misplaced in the left axillary vein (solid arrow).

and use of anticoagulation and antiplatelet drugs are important factors in determining the rate of endothelialization.

Inherent in the long-term patency of the stented vein is the underlying pathologic process. In arteries, atherosclerosis is the primary lesion; however, in veins this is not the case. Fibrous scanning or neoplasia, either by direct invasion or external compression, are most often the underlying disease processes.

In patients with benign disease such as fibrous strictures in any central veins, or at venous graft anastomoses and hemo-dialysis shunts, long-term patency is a critical issue. Especially in hemodialysis patients, careful follow-up with regard to recirculation measurements, hemodynamic changes in the graft, and physical examination needs to be done to assess for recurrent stenosis [20–23]. Secondary treatments with thrombolytics, angioplasty, atherectomy, and further stenting may be utilized to preserve the hemodialysis access site and patency of the outflow vein.

Patients with a malignancy are often inoperable or have received maximum radiation therapy. Stent placement in

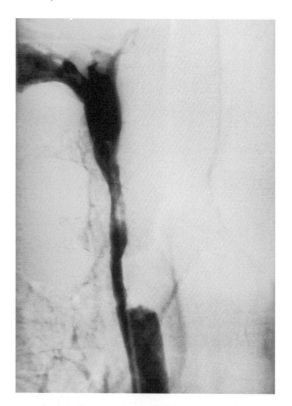

Fig. 23.27 Superior venacavogram following urokinase administration and percutaneous angioplasty with residual superior vena cava stenosis secondary to compression by mediastinal mass.

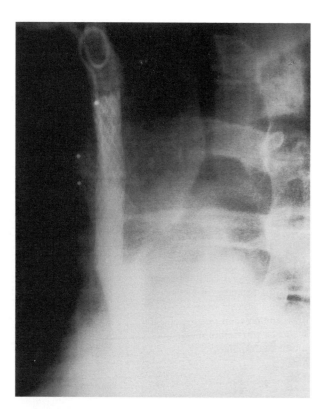

Fig. 23.28 Superior venacavogram showing initial placement of Palmaz stents (× 2) with restored superior vena cava patency.

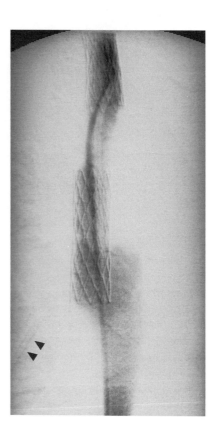

these instances is strictly for palliation. Long-term patency, although still important on an individual basis, is not as crucial an issue as achieving immediate success in relieving symptoms, since many of these patients have a limited life expectancy. Disease progression with tumor growth may compress the stent extrinsically. Alternately, tumor proliferation at the stent margin also may result in recurrent stenosis and possible occlusion. These recurrences can be effectively treated with thrombolytics, angioplasty, atherectomy, and/or further stenting.

Conclusions

Potential complications notwithstanding, intravenous placement of vascular stents is often the only effective means of alleviating debilitating symptoms in patients suffering from central venoocclusive disease.

Fig. 23.29 Freshly placed stent traversed with wire and catheter combination in an effort better to visualize right subclavian vein, resulting in entanglement of the wire and catheter in the interstices of the most inferior stent. During removal of the catheter, its tip was sheared and embolized to the right lower lobe pulmonary artery (arrowheads). Guidewire removal resulted in displacement of the lower stent inferiorly.

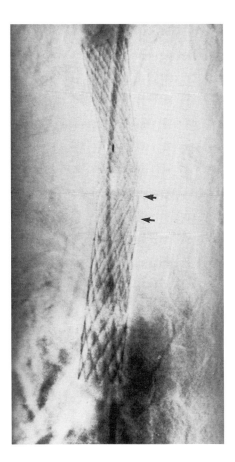

Fig. 23.30 Third stent (solid arrows) positioned bridging first two stents.

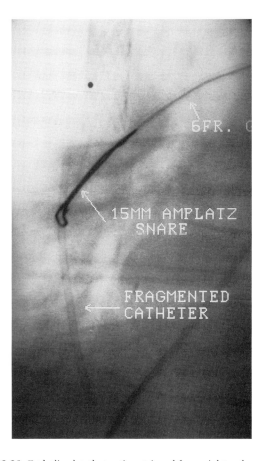

Fig. 23.31 Embolized catheter tip retrieved from right pulmonary artery using loop snare.

The most significant problem related to intravascular venous stents remains recurrent thrombosis. This is true for all prosthetic devices on the venous side. Hopefully, future stents will incorporate timed-release drug-delivery systems that would minimize the progressive intimal hyperplasia and/or the superimposed thrombotic change.

References

1 Palmaz J. Intravascular Stents. In: Muller P, van Sonnenberg E, Becker G, eds. *A Categorial Course in Diagnostic Radiology: Interventional Radiology*. Oak Brook: Il: RSNA Publications, 1991; 185–192.

2 Antonucci F, Salomonowitz E, Stuckman G, Stiefel M, Largiader J, Zollikofer C. Placement of venous stents: clinical experience with a self-expanding prosthesis. *Radiology* 1992;183:493–497.

3 Carrasco C, Charnsangavej C, Wright K, Wallace S, Gianturco C. Use of the Gianturco self expanding stent in the stenosis of the superior and inferior vena cava. *J Vasc Intervent Radiol* 1992;3: 409–419.

4 Charnsangavej C, Carrasco C, Wallace S *et al*. Stenosis of the vena cava: preliminary assessment of treatment with expandable metallic stents. *Radiology* 1986;161:295–298.

5 Dake M, Semba C, Enstrom R, Skeens J, Venugopal C, Wittich G. *Percutaneous treatment of venous occlusive disease with stents.*

Presented at the Annual Meeting of the SCVIR, New Orleans, February 22–March 4, 1993.

6 Elson J, Becker G, Wholey M, Ehrman K. Vena caval and central venous stenoses: management with Palmaz balloon – expandable intraluminal stents. *J Vasc Intervent Radiol* 1991;2: 215–223.

7 Furui S, Sawada S, Irie T *et al*. Hepatic inferior vena cava obstruction: treatment of two types with Gianturco expandable metallic stents. *Radiology* 1990;176:665–670.

8 Gray R, Horton K, Dolmatch B. *Wallstents for hemodialysis access.* Presented at the Annual Meeting of the SCVIR, New Orleans, February 27–March 4, 1993.

9 Gunther R, Vorwerk D, Bohndorf K *et al*. Venous stenoses in dialysis shunts; treatment with self-expanding metallic stents. *Radiology* 1989;170:401–405.

10 Lakin P, Petersen B, Barton R, Keller F, Rosch J. *Combined local urokinase thrombolysis with expandable Z stents in the treatment of major venous obstruction.* Presented at the Annual Meeting of the SCVIR, New Orleans, March, 1993.

11 Landwehr P, Lackner K, Ruediger G. *Middle term results of Palmaz stent versus conventional percutaneous transluminal angioplasty for treatment of central vein obstructions in hemodialysis patients.* Presented at the Annual Meeting of The Radiologic Society of North America, Chicago, November 26, 1990.

12 Petersen B, Rosch J, Uchida B, Antonovic R, Barton R, Keller F. *Expandable Z stents in treatment of large vein obstruction of benign*

origin: long term follow-up. Presented at the Annual Meeting of the SCVIR, New Orleans, February 27–March 4, 1993.

13 Quinn S, Schuman E, Hall L *et al.* Venous stenoses in patients who undergo hemodialysis: treatment with self expandable endovascular stents. *Radiology* 1992;183:409–504.

14 Roesch J, Uchida B, Hall L *et al. Gianturco expandable wire stents in treatment of venous obstructions.* Presented at the Annual Meeting of the Radiological Society of North America, Chicago, November 26, 1990.

15 Solomon N, Wholey M, Jarmolowski C. Intravascular stents in the management of superior vena cava syndrome. *Cathet Cardiovasc Diagn* 1991;23:245–252.

16 Turmel-Rodrigues L, Pengloan J, Blanchier D *et al.* Insufficient dialysis shunts: improved long-term patency rates with close hemodynamic monitoring, repeated percutaneous balloon angioplasty and stent placement. *Radiology* 1993;187:273–278.

17 Zollikofer C, Largiader I, Bruhlmann W, Uhlschmid G, Marty A. Endovascular stenting of veins and grafts: preliminary clinical experience. *Radiology* 1988;167:707–712.

18 Cekirge S, Foster R, Weiss J, McLean G. Percutaneous removal of an embolized Wallstent during a transjugular intrahepatic portosystemic shunt procedure. *J Vasc Intervent Radiol* 1993;4: 559–560.

19 Schatz R, Palmaz J, Tio F, Garcia F, Cascia O, Reuter S. Balloon-expandable intracoronary stents in the adult dog. *Circulation* 1987;76:450–457.

20 Gaylord G, Taber T. Long term hemodialysis access salvage problems and challenges for nephrologists and interventional radiologists. *J Vasc Intervent Radiol* 1993;4:103–107.

21 Sullivan K, Besasab A, Bonn J, Shapiro M, Gardinor G, Moritz M. Hemodynamics of failing dialysis grafts. *Radiology* 1993;196: 867–872.

22 Cohen G, Ball D. Delayed Wallstent migration after a trans-jugular intrahepatic portosystemic shunt procedure: relocation with a loop snare. *J Vasc Intervent Radiol* 1993;4:561–563.

23 Sullivan K, Besasab A, Bonn J, Shapiro M, Gardiner G, Moritz M. Hemodynamics of failing dialysis grafts. *Radiology* 1993;96: 867–872.

Complications of diagnostic neuroangiography

Brian Kendall

Introduction

The diagnostic role of neuroangiography has decreased progressively over the past two decades with the increasing sophistication and availability of computed X-ray tomography (CT) and magnetic resonance imaging (MRI). Even current application in the detailed study of cerebrovascular disease, arteriovenous malformations, fistulas, and aneurysms, apart from in the control of interventional procedures, is being limited by the advances in magnetic resonance angiography [1,2] and spiral CT [3].

In all modern radiologic departments, digital subtraction angiography has replaced conventional studies and the increased contrast discrimination permits adequate visualization with low intravascular iodine concentrations. In general, the major arteries and the venous sinuses are adequately visualized using central intravenous injection of contrast medium. More selective injection into cervical arteries is often necessary to avoid confusing overlap in detailed visualization of the smaller intracranial vessels. Low contrast-medium concentrations (about 150 mg iodine/ml) are very adequate for such studies, and are easily delivered through fine (4-F) soft catheters.

Nonionic nondissociable contrast media, with which general toxicity and neurotoxicity have been markedly reduced, should now be used routinely for neuroangiography by the intraarterial routes and, economic considerations apart, are preferable for the intravenous route also.

Contrast-media toxicity

The toxic effects of contrast media on the central nervous system are dependent on two factors:

1 passage through a permeable region of the blood−neural tissue barrier (blood−brain barrier, BBB);
2 toxic effects from direct contact with neural tissue.

Contrast medium within the brain parenchyma may produce inhibitory effects related to hypertonicity or excitatory effects related to the chemical structure.

Certain regions of the brain, such as the area postrema in the floor of the fourth ventricle and the tuber cinereum, normally lack a BBB. Neuronal toxicity is responsible for vomiting, hyperthermia, bradycardia due to direct contrast-media stimulation of chemoreceptive zones in these regions of the brain stem, or hypothalamus [4].

It is possible for a defect in the normal BBB to be induced by certain contrast media, especially in high dosage [5]: cellular toxicity of such contrast media may explain cases of encephalopathy reported after selective cerebral angiography [6].

A defective BBB may also be due to pathologic processes, including brain tumors, infarcts, or inflammatory lesions.

Abnormal permeability of the BBB varies in degree; in some cases, small molecules may pass through and cause edema and even neurologic complications, while large molecules, such as contrast media and macromolecular dyes may be retained by the barrier [7].

BBB toxicity

Two factors are involved in blood neural barrier toxicity of contrast media.

1 Hypertonic contrast media may produce shrinkage of endothelial cells with opening of tight junctions. Since it is no longer necessary to use significantly hypertonic contrast media, this factor is no longer of clinical significance.

2 Chemotoxicity may cause increased pinocytosis or interference with enzymatic processes in vascular endothelium.

Macromolecules pass through the capillary wall of a pathologically opened BBB: they are transported by astrocytes to the neurons or extravasated into the extracellular spaces. Histologically, there is an increase in endothelial pinocytic vesicles, which may proceed on to swelling, or even rupture of pericapillary astrocytes. These cellular reactions have not been observed with the use of contrast media of low hypertonicity. These include nonionic monomers, such as iopamidol (osmolality 0.61 m.osmol/kg) and iohexol (osmolality 0.64 m.osmol/kg), with concentrations up to 300 mg iodine/ml. Since it is no longer necessary to achieve concentrations above 150 mg iodine/ml, BBB toxicity due to the injection of the contrast medium should not occur [8–13].

The clearance of contrast media from the parenchyma is by flow through the interstitial spaces towards the ventricular system, by absorption into the parenchymal capillaries, or by pinocytosis.

Cellular toxicity

Modern contrast media do not injure the BBB when injected in the highest concentrations used in clinical practice, but they do pass through when it is disrupted by pathologic conditions; neurotoxic reactions may then be induced, depending upon the cellular toxicity of the contrast medium.

Margolis *et al.* [14], using retrograde aortography on the dog, have provided much of the basic knowledge to explain the harmful effects of angiography on neural tissues. The toxic effects observed in the animals can be divided into the following.

1 Immediate convulsive muscular spasms. These could be due, in part, to contrast perfusion of muscle [15], but are mainly neurogenic. Although potentially reversible, they are sometimes accompanied by petechial hemorrhages and edema in the spinal cord substance.

2 Persistent neurologic defects that are associated with histopathologic evidence of cord necrosis.

The pathology of the injury to the spinal cord has been documented throughout its development in material obtained from such experiments designed specifically to study the effects of contrast toxicity on the central nervous system [16]. The contrast media caused cord necrosis of varied severity (Fig. 24.1); in the early phases there was, in ad-

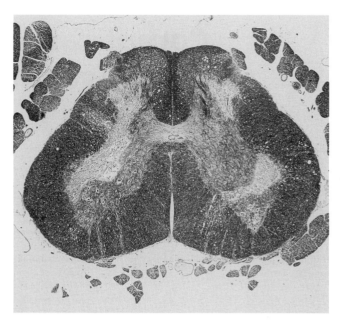

Fig. 24.1 Sharply marginated foci of necrosis in gray matter are demarcated by their pallor in this example of moderate focal injury. Mild involvement of white matter is indicated by the vacuolar areas. (Photograph courtesy of G. Margolis.)

dition, extensive edema and/or hemorrhage progressing to myelomalacia (Fig. 24.2). The central gray matter was particularly affected, but the lesion extended through the white matter (Fig. 24.3) and into the nerve roots in the more severe cases; several segments of the spinal cord were commonly involved. This type of cord damage has been shown to follow disruption of the blood–neural barrier, which occurs so rapidly after injection that it must be due to direct contrast-medium toxicity (Fig. 24.4) and is concentration dependent [17–19]. The critical concentration varies with the toxicity of individual contrast media [20]. Neurotoxicity is least with the nonionic media, which are sufficiently benign to be placed in direct contact with neural tissues, as in myelography. If used exclusively for aortography, toxic contrast-media complications on the cord will cease to occur.

Cellular toxicity is now estimated by reaction to pericerebral or cisternal injections of contrast media [21,22]. Ionic compounds precipitate convulsions and induce inflammatory reactions and cellular necrosis. Nonionic compounds, such as iohexol and iopamidol, which are used for myelography and cisternography, do not induce convulsions or tissue reaction, but there are changes on electron micrographs which indicate that the compounds are not totally inert. In the concentrations used for intraarterial digital subtraction angiography, these compounds neither damage the BBB nor show clinical evidence of cellular toxicity.

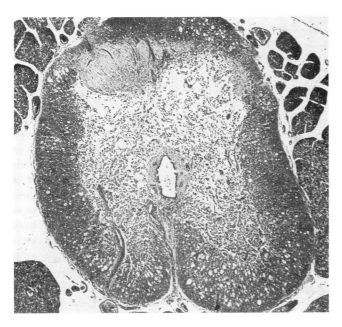

Fig. 24.2 Myelomalacia involving virtually all gray matter bilaterally and scattered injury of surrounding white matter. The necrotic zone is disintegrated and occupied by macrophages. (Photograph courtesy of G. Margolis.)

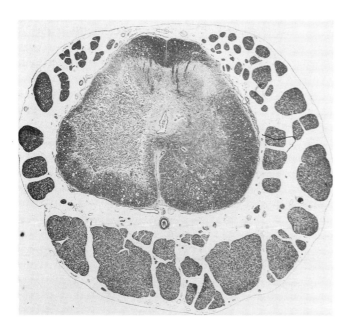

Fig. 24.3 Severe but essentially unilateral injury is illustrated in this section which has the distribution of an anterior sulcal artery. Almost all gray matter is destroyed. Surrounding white matter is severely involved. Scattered vacuoles appear in other areas of white matter. The necrotic zone is heavily infiltrated with phagocytic cells. (Photograph courtesy of G. Margolis.)

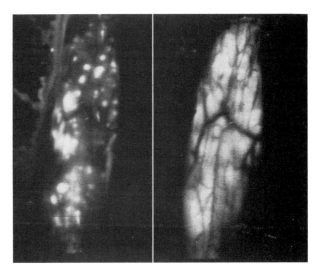

Fig. 24.4 (a) Frame from a fluorescein angiography record enlarged from a 16-mm film of the flow of a toxic dose of contrast agent (70% Hypaque) through the vascular bed of the cord. The mass had been injected via retrograde aortography and rendered neurotoxic by the neuripetal shunt induced by levarterenol. This photograph, made 15 seconds after the arrival of the fluorescent injection mass in the cord, illustrates the instantaneous onset of fluorescence due to the disruptive action upon the BBB. (b) Frame from the same film sequence 90 seconds after entry of the fluorescein-labeled contrast agent into the vascular bed of the cord. The parenchyma is now diffusely fluorescent, and the surface vessels appear in dark contrast against the light background. The rapidity and severity of breakdown of the BBB clearly demonstrated that the contrast-medium injury was a direct histotoxic effect, rather than a consequence of ischemia. It was this observation that pointed to the need for a search for prophylactic rather than remedial approaches. (Photograph courtesy of G. Margolis.)

Other factors related to toxicity

Viscosity

With contrast medium previously in use that could injure the BBB, the length of contact time between the contrast medium and the barrier was potentially significant. Viscous solutions reduce blood flow and increase contact time. In dogs, the intracarotid blood flow was reduced and the number of BBB lesions increased when contrast medium was injected at 23°C in comparison to 37°C [23].

Red blood cell rigidity

Increased erythrocyte rigidity, deformity, and tendency to aggregation may impair the microcirculation. The effects of contrast medium on red cell rigidity are a direct function of osmolality and can be reproduced with hyperosmolar saline solutions [24]. The modern nonionic contrast media in the concentrations used for cerebral angiography do not cause changes in red cell rigidity.

Embolization

Concentrated solutions of some contrast media may become supersaturated. Crystalline material may precipitate and cause both mechanical and chemical effects on vessels [25]. Glass particles produced during opening of ampoules may also become emboli [26,27].

Particular risk factors during neuroangiography

Technical factors

The significant neurologic complications of angiography are mainly due to ischemia, generally on an embolic basis. Embolism may result in temporary or permanent neurologic signs including global amnesia [28–30].

The significance of meticulous attention to details of technique is evident from the fact that complications are more frequent in teaching hospitals in which less experienced radiologists are performing many angiograms, than in non-teaching hospitals [31–33].

Neurologic complications are more frequent with the transaxillary than the transfemoral approach [34]. The number of adverse reactions increases with procedure time, use of more than one catheter, number of injections made, and volume of contrast medium injected.

The use of small soft catheters is associated with reduction of clinically evident embolic phenomena. These are usually due to thrombus forming near the catheter tip. Routine precautions to avoid this include:

1 perfusion continuously or intermittently with heparinized saline;

2 if intermittent perfusion is used, withdrawal of blood from the catheter before reperfusion with heparinized saline or contrast medium;

3 the use of syringes composed of the least thrombogenic type of plastic rather than glass, which is more likely to induce clotting;

4 the use of polythene catheters, preferably heparin treated, although these are relatively expensive.

Ionic contrast media have more anticoagulant effect than nonionic contrast media, but this factor is far outweighed by the advantages of the nonionic contrast media; attention to good angiographic technique is the cardinal factor in avoiding the majority of embolic complications. Cholesterol crystals, platelet aggregates, foreign particles including glass from ampoules and talc from glove powder contaminating contrast media, or crystals precipitating from supersaturated contrast medium have caused emboli in a few instances [24–26].

Very rapid injection of fluid into cerebral vessels may increase the pressure in cerebral capillaries: this may cause opening of the BBB. This is more likely in premature newborns and in the presence of preexisting hypertension [35].

Clinical factors

The incidence of neurologic complications is higher in the following.

1 In the presence of cerebrovascular disease, in elderly patients suffering from severe systolic hypertension, and in younger patients with fibromuscular hyperplasia [36]. Permanent complications in patients with symptomatic cerebrovascular disease are usually recorded in between 0.5 [36] and 0.63% of examinations [37]. However, in a recent prospective study confined to patients with cerebrovascular disease, ischemic events occurred in the unusually high proportion of 11% and persistent neurologic deficit was present after 1 month in 5% [38].

There is no additional increase in risk in cases with a history of recent stroke or transient ischemic attacks [39], but in such cases clinical deterioration is frequent whether or not angiography is performed [40].

2 In the presence of severe extracranial vessel stenosis [41] if the catheter is passed through the stenotic region [42].

3 In patients with gross vertebrobasilar ectasia undergoing vertebral angiography [43].

It is important in all patients, but particularly in the presence of cerebrovascular disease, that adequate hydration is maintained in order to avoid the potentially adverse effects of systemic hypotension.

Very rarely, rupture of an aneurysm occurs during selective angiography, but otherwise there is no increased risk of permanent neurologic complication due to the angiographic procedure itself in patients with aneurysm or subarachnoid hemorrhage [37]. However, transient deficits may occur if severe spasm is noted, and in such cases the procedure should be limited to study of the site of hemorrhage.

In our experience, there is no increase in angiographic complications in migraineurs, although angiography is not performed during a migraine attack because of the theoretical risk of increasing the severity of any neurologic sequelae [44].

Commoner complications of neuroangiography

Complications of neuroangiography fall into three categories:
1 local;
2 general;
3 neurologic.

Local complications

1 Hematoma at the puncture site is not infrequent, particularly in hypertensive patients or if large catheters or extensive manipulation are used. It usually absorbs spontaneously, but it may require evacuation. This is particularly so in the axilla because prolonged pressure on the axillary plexus may result in permanent neurologic deficit.

Direct cervical puncture is rarely necessary, but cervical hematoma may cause tracheal compression and respiratory obstruction necessitating tracheotomy.

If communication of the hematoma with the artery persists (pulsating hematoma or false aneurysm), the puncture may require suturing to avoid continued growth and possible rupture of the false aneurysm.

2 Arteriovenous fistula may require closure by surgery or interventional radiology. In the neck, between the carotid artery and jugular vein, or the vertebral artery and vertebral vein, closure by embolization is usually preferred.

3 Subintimal or intramural injection of contrast medium may result in arterial narrowing or occlusion, which may or not be symptomatic, depending on the adequacy of collateral flow. It may resolve spontaneously or precipitate thrombosis of the injured vessel.

4 Embolism may result from dislodgment of thrombus from the catheter, which is more likely on withdrawal of a large catheter. Less often, cholesterol or platelet aggregates on atheromatous plaques on the wall of the vessel may be the source.

5 Obstruction of blood flow due to catheter occlusion of the lumen is more likely in a small artery, such as the vertebral. More frequently, a catheter induces spasm, which causes cessation of flow and retention of contrast medium. This may be asymptomatic, and with the important proviso that perfusion is maintained with heparinized saline so as to avoid any thrombus formation, the angiogram may be completed quickly before withdrawing the catheter.

General complications

Nausea, vomiting, hypotension, laryngospasm, and renal failure occur less frequently with intraarterial than with intravenous injection, and with nonionic than with ionic contrast media. The distressing discomfort and heat experienced with the ionic contrast media is also much reduced when using the nonionic contrast media [6,45−47].

Neurologic complications of intracranial angiography

For documentation purposes, any neurologic deterioration occurring within 24 hours of an angiogram is considered to be a complication of the procedure.

1 The fatality rate is in the region of 0.03%. It is usually related to technical complications, mainly embolization or obstruction of a cerebral vessel, either by the catheter or by dissection.

2 Permanent or severe neurologic complications occur in 0.25% overall, but are recorded to be around 0.7% in a careful prospective teaching hospital study [48], and as low as 0.04% in a retrospective nonteaching center study [49]. The cause of stroke is embolism in the great majority of cases. Emboli have been visualized during angiography [50], new peripheral middle cerebral infarcts have been shown on CT in patients developing neurologic deficits during angiography [48], and silent infarcts have been shown on MRI after selective carotid and vertebral angiography [51]. The risk of embolic stroke is equally great with aortic arch injection (0.7%) as with selective catheterization (0.8%) [48], again suggesting that thrombus in or around the catheter tip is the usual source of emboli. Severe and distressing deficit may be motor with or without aphasia, sensory, or visual, or there may be amnesia or seizures.

Because of the unstable neurologic condition of many patients, the incidence of transient neurologic defects is difficult to assess, especially in retrospective surveys, but it is probably about 1% and possibly less with the newer nonionic contrast media.

Spinal cord complications of angiography

Detailed descriptions of the cord vasculature are given by Lazorthes *et al.* [52] and reviewed by Djindjian *et al.* [53].

The anterior spinal artery consists of anastomosing ascending and descending branches of radiculomedullary arteries. Typically, two or three of these arise in the cervical region from the vertebral arteries and/or the deep cervical branches of the costocervical trunks; one arises from an upper intercostal artery and a large one, the artery of Adamkiewicz, from a lower intercostal or upper lumbar artery. However, the origins of the radiculomedullary arteries are inconstant and a major one can arise at any level between the upper cervical and lumbosacral regions. The posterolateral spinal arteries supply only part of the dorsal columns and posterior horns of gray matter. The arteries feeding them are the posterior radiculomedullary branches of the segmental arteries which are small and numerous. Occlusion of these vessels rarely causes symptoms, but injection of toxic or polymerizing substances that may reach and/or occlude the capillary bed supplied by one of these vessels can produce a significant and permanent neurologic deficit.

In nonneurologic angiography, the spinal cord is particularly at risk during injection into the deep cervical artery or costocervical trunk when seeking the inferior thyroid artery for thyroid and parathyroid angiography, and into the intercostals supplying bronchial arteries [54]. The inconstancy of the origin of the artery of Adamkiewicz [55] renders it vulnerable in lower thoracic and lumbar aortography, especially in cases of aortic occlusive disease [56]; in some, the risk may be compounded if the vesssel giving rise to the artery of Adamkiewicz is also acting as a collateral channel bypassing an aortic obstruction.

In a survey of complications of abdominal aortography [57,58], damage to the spinal cord was recorded in 0.2% of the procedures, with subsequent fatality in 0.03%. These results included many studies performed with relatively toxic contrast media [59] which are no longer used, and the figures are undoubtedly too high for modern practice. However, complications continue to be recorded [60,61]. The most frequently observed is transient spasticity of the lower extremities with hyperreflexia, which in series subjected to detailed observation may reach an incidence as high as 0.5% [62]. The most severe complication, permanent paraplegia, is now very rare, but is reported sporadically [63].

Severe cord damage has been described as a complication of vertebral angiography [64,65], bronchial angiography [66], renal angiography [67], and parathyroid angiography. In all these nonneurologic studies, induction of cord damage was generally related to unintentional injection of excessive or highly concentrated contrast medium into important vessels supplying the spinal cord [68].

Avoidance of cord damage is a particular consideration in selective spinal angiography, especially in cases where spinal cord function may already be compromised, and in the treatment of angiomatous malformations and arteriovenous fistulae by embolization. The experience of Djindjian *et al.* [69] and Doppman *et al.* [70] attests to the reasonable safety of these procedures when carefully performed; with the introduction of modern nonionic contrast media, the transient deterioration that previously was a not infrequent accompaniment of the investigation of spinal angiomatous malformations, is no longer a significant problem [71,72]. Nevertheless, disabling complications do occasionally occur and angiography is only indicated when the result may influence patient management.

For spinal angiography, injections of up to 4 ml contrast medium containing up to 300 mg iodine/ml are made into the segmental arteries. No toxic effects were noted using this concentration of modern ionic contrast media, apart from the not infrequent transient deterioration in patients with spinal angiomatous malformations; this does not occur when nonionic contrast media are used. Increased susceptibility of the traumatized spinal cord to aortography with ionic media has been shown experimentally [73]. The much diminished direct neurotoxicity of the nonionic media, as well as the lesser effects on the circulatory dynamics [74], makes their use mandatory for any angiogram in which a diseased spinal cord may be perfused either deliberately or incidentally.

In aortography, the volume and concentration of the contrast medium entering the vessels supplying the spinal cord is dependent on several factors, including the following.
1 The relation of the catheter tip to the origins of the vessels supplying the anterior spinal artery.
2 The position of the patient. Hyperbaric contrast medium tends to gravitate towards the dependent wall of the aorta. The orifices of the intercostal and lumbar arteries arise from the posterolateral aspect of the aorta and, therefore, flow into them is increased in the supine position and relatively diminished in the prone position. Postural changes markedly influence the induction and severity of experimentally produced lesions [16].
3 Contrast perfusion of the spinal cord can also be influenced pharmacologically by injection of vasoconstrictor and vasodilator drugs [75], which produce more marked effects on visceral than systemic vessels [76]. The former agents cause deviation of contrast medium towards the spinal cord and the latter away from it.
4 The performance of a Valsalva maneuver causes reduction in aortic outflow: intraaortic injections are therefore diluted to a lesser degree than usual and the concentration of contrast medium entering the cord vessels is increased.

Spinal cord ischemia may be precipitated during angiography by the following.
1 Dissection of the orifices of segmental arteries during catheter manipulation, or by intramural hematoma or extravasation of perfusion fluid or contrast medium during injection.
2 The catheter occluding the orifice of the segmental artery supplying the arteria radicularis magna. This is normal procedure in spinal angiography, and in all but the most exceptional circumstances there is ample collateral circulation from adjacent vessels to fill the artery and all its branches beyond the catheter occlusion. Only in rare cases of extensive vascular occlusive disease is there likelihood of occlusion by the catheter tip causing ischemia.
3 Embolization: by indigenous thrombus, atheroma, or the other agents mentioned previously as well as during therapeutic occlusion of spinal arteriovenous fistulae or angiomatous malformations.

Arteriovenous fistulae or malformations connecting with the venous plexuses draining the spinal cord cause increased pressure within the plexuses. This may lead to edema of the cord and to reduction of the normal arteriovenous pressure gradient in the vessels supplying the cord substance. Consequently, there is diminution in flow through these vessels, causing ischemia of the cord [77]. Changes in pressure within the plexus are thought to be the basis of the typical transient variations in the severity of symptoms of angiomatous malformation, that may occur spontaneously, or following exercise, or prolonged maintenance of certain postures. The alternate possibility of stealing of blood by the fistula or malformation from the arteries supplying the spinal cord, thus precipitating ischemia, may be a factor in cases in which the anterior spinal artery itself feeds the fistula. However, in the great majority of patients, the fistula is related to the dura and is supplied by arteries that are isolated from those supplying the spinal cord. Also, although there is a much higher incidence of subarachnoid hemorrhage and hematomyelia when the fistula is within or on the surface of the spinal cord, the slowly progressive symptoms and variation of intensity of disabilities is similar whether the fistula is dural or within the cord substance, which gives support to the concept of venous hypertension being an important common etiologic factor.

In our experience, transient deterioration in neurologic symptoms occurred in 7.7% of patients with spinal angiomatous malformations examined using an ionic contrast medium; these were considered to be due to the vasodilator effects of the contrast medium, causing an increase in blood flow through the angiomatous malformation. No such deterioration has occurred following injection of iohexol; this is presumably because the systemic vasodilator effects of this contrast medium are less than those of the ionic media [72]. Iohexol has been shown experimentally to constrict the large cerebral vessels [74]; since it presumably affects those of the spinal cord in a similar fashion, its use could theoretically augment the effects of steal in malformations supplied by vessels also contributing to neural substance.

Very uncommonly, extravasation of contrast medium may occur into a spinal tumor due to rupture of a pathologic vessel during spinal angiography. Moseley and Tress [78] recorded such a case being examined under general anesthesia, in which extravasation of an ionic medium into a cystic hemangioblastoma of the cervical spinal cord was noted immediately following injection of the artery supplying it. Immediate lumbar puncture yielded heavily blood-stained cerebrospinal fluid and this was replaced with normal saline until the blood cleared, which required about 40 ml of fluid exchange. Marked deterioration of cord function was evident and this persisted. Surgical exploration 4 days after the angiogram revealed hemorrhage into small glial-lined cavities above and below a tumor nodule.

Clinical indicators of spinal cord damage

A warning sign that the cord may be at risk during angiography is the occurrence of back pain and/or of involuntary twitching, tonic, or clonic movements of the lower limbs during or immediately after an injection of contrast medium. Such an event usually lasts only a few seconds and is unlikely to be followed by delayed neurologic sequelae; nevertheless, the patient should be treated with systemic steroids as though cord damage has occurred. The angiographic series should be carefully inspected to see if the catheter has been placed unintentionally close to the origin of the artery of Adamkiewicz [55], and, if so, the tip should be moved to a satisfactory location. Further injections at the same site carry an increased risk of cord damage [79].

More prolonged hyperexcitability of the lower limbs, myoclonic movement, or tonic and clonic contraction of the lower limbs, often associated with considerable pain and with hyperextension of the back, are indicative of cord damage from which there may or may not be clinical recovery. The procedure should be terminated and the patient placed on steroid and nimodipine drugs. The contractions are treated with systemic diazepam in dosage adequate to relieve them.

Further evidence of damage to the spinal cord includes paraparesis or paraplegia, loss of sensation, and incontinence. Neurologic defect without preliminary hyperirritability may be the first sign of cord damage, especially in patients who have been examined under general anesthetic.

Prognosis should be guarded; in about one-third of cases there will be progression of the immediate symptoms, but improvement can be expected in about 50% [80]. In addition to treatment with systemic steroids and intravenous diazepam, if ionic contrast medium has been injected, the patient should be placed in the head-up position to assist gravitation towards the lumbar sac of any contrast medium that has penetrated the BBB; cerebrospinal fluid should be withdrawn in 10-ml increments and replaced with isotonic saline in order to reduce the concentration of contrast medium within the extracellular spaces of the spinal cord which are in continuity with the cerebrospinal fluid [81]. This treatment is unnecessary if modern nonionic contrast media, suitable for injection into the subarachnoid space, have been used.

Neurologic complications of intravenous contrast medium for cerebral CT scanning and digital subtraction angiography

The degree of enhancement achieved on CT depends on the concentration of contrast medium in the blood: larger doses are frequently administered than are used for urography. Claims that large intravenous doses of hyperosmolar contrast medium break down the BBB and produce brain edema [82] have been disproved [83,84]. Neurologic complications of CT scanning are mainly epileptic seizures [85]. These mostly occur when there is BBB damage, and have been recorded using ionic contrast media in up to 15% of patients with brain metastasis [86] and glioblastomas [87]. Status epilepticus and prolonged retention of contrast medium within the brain have also been recorded in neonatal anoxic encephalopathy [88], in herpes simplex encephalitis [89], and postmeningitic ependymitis [90]. BBB disruption associated with acute vascular lesions may be associated with contrast-medium-induced seizures [91].

In scanning the spine with modern machines, intravenous contrast medium may be of value in the diagnosis of enhancing inflammatory and tumor masses, and for showing their relationship to the spinal theca and cord. Large blood vessels associated with angiomatous malformations and aneurysms may be diagnosed. Intravenous contrast medium is also of value in the differentiation of postoperative fibrosis from recurrent disk protrusion.

Complications involving the spinal cord have not been recorded with intravenous injections of contrast media in general, with the exception of two cases in which extensor spasms of the trunk and limbs developed towards the end of an intravenous infusion of 30% meglumine iothalamate [92] and angiographin [93]. In the first case they lasted for 1 hour. Spasms were precipitated by minor stimuli such as movement of CT scanner table. The other patient developed a severe paraplegia with sensation absent below the 10th dorsal level. Subsequent myelography revealed angiomatous malformations of the spinal cord in both cases. The occurrence of any symptoms related to the spinal cord during or soon after the administration of intravenous contrast medium should therefore be taken as a possible indication of spinal cord pathology, and the patient should be submitted to detailed neurologic examination.

Stable xenon is a chemically inert gas that does not undergo biotransformation. It has been used intrathecally for spinal cord enhancement which occurs by absorption of the heavy gas into the cord substance [94]. It is more usually administered by inhalation. It is freely diffusible and highly soluble in lipids, which renders it suitable for enhancement of the central nervous sytem and also for determination of regional cerebral blood flow. There are two major drawbacks to the use of xenon:

1 it is expensive;
2 it is an anesthetic — a 50% concentration induces sleep and a 70% concentration produces general anesthesia.
However, no spinal symptoms or signs have ensued from its use.

Neurologic episodes are extremely rare with intravenous digital subtraction angiography if modest volumes up to 56 g of iodine per examination of nonionic contrast media are used [45,95–97]. The angiographic detail necessary for clinical management of cerebrovascular disease remains controversial [45,98–100], but in combination with magnetic resonance angiography and/or doppler ultrasound, adequate information can be achieved in over 90% of cases. In a situation in which about 3% of patients overall may benefit from surgery [101], a diagnostic procedure like transarterial angiography which carries a not insignificant incidence of neurologic complications, is an inappropriate screening test for large populations of arteriopaths.

Conclusions

The modern contrast media used in neuroangiography do not injure the BBB in doses and concentrations much greater than those necessary for clinical investigation. The cellular toxicity of nonionic contrast media is very low, and penetration into neural substance through a damaged BBB does not precipitate permanent neurologic complications. In addition, the low osmolality and diminished cardiovascular effect cause less subjective effects and less discomfort and therefore facilitate and reduce the examination time for patients undergoing angiographic procedures.

References

1 Wesby GE, Bergan JJ, Moreland SI. Cerebrovascular magnetic resonance angiography: a critical verification. *J Vasc Surg* 1992; 16:619–632.
2 Pan XM, Anderson CM, Reilly LM. Magnetic resonance angiography of the carotid artery combining two- and three-dimensional acquisitions. *J Vasc Surg* 1992;16:609–618.
3 Schwartz RB, Jones KM, Chernoff DM. Common carotid artery bifurcation: evaluation with spiral CT. *Radiology* 1992;185: 513–519.
4 Lalli AF. Contrast media reactions: data analysis and hypothesis. *Radiology* 1980;134:1–12.
5 Junck L, Marshall WH. Fatal brain oedema after contrast medium overdose. *Am J Neuroradiol* 1986;7:522–525.
6 Haley EC Jr. Encephalopathy following arteriography: a possible toxic effect of contrast agents. *Ann Neurol* 1984;15: 100–102.
7 Sage JI, Van Uitert RL, Duffy TE. Early changes in blood–brain barrier permeability to small molecules after transient cerebral ischaemia. *Stroke* 1984;15:46–50.
8 Gonsette RE, Liesenborgh I. New contrast media in cerebral angiography: animal experiments and preliminary clinical studies. *Invest Radiol* 1980;15:270–274.
9 Gospos C, Koch HK, Mathias K, Seemann W, Tan KG, Papacharalampous X Scanning electron microscopic studies on the effect of X-ray contrast media on aortic endothelium in the rat. *Invest Radiol* 1983;18:382–386.
10 Rainiko R. Role of hypertonicity in the endothelial injury caused by angiographic contrast media. *Acta Radiol (Diagn)* 1979;20:410–416.
11 Rainiko R. Endothelial permeability increase produced by angiographic contrast media. *Fortschr Roentgenstr* 1979; 131: 433–438.
12 Nyman U, Almen T. Effects of contrast media on aortic endothelium. Experiments in the rat with non-ionic monomeric and monacidic dimeric contrast media. *Acta Radiol* 1980; 362(Suppl.):65–71.
13 Laerum F, Borsum T, Reisvaag A. Human endothelial cell culture as an evaluation system for the toxicity of intravascular contrast media. *Invest Radiol* 1983;18:199–206.
14 Margolis G, Bourne HM, Bogdanowicz W, Ellington EE. Pathogenesis of contrast medium injury: *in vivo* studies with intra-arterial injection of contrast media. *J Neuropathol Exp Neurol* 1969;28:155.
15 Hilal SK. Haemodynamic changes associated with the intra-arterial injection of contrast media. *Radiology* 1966;86: 615–633.
16 Margolis G, Tarazi AK, Grimson KS. Contrast medium injury to the spinal cord produced by aortography: pathologic anatomy of the experimental lesion. *J Neurosurg* 1956;13:349–365.
17 Margolis G, Griffin AT, Kenan PH, Tindall GT, Riggins R, Fort L. Contrast-medium injury to the spinal cord: the role of altered circulatory dynamics. *J Neurosurg* 1959;16:390–406.
18 Margolis G, Griffin AT, Kenan PD, Tindall GT, Riggins R, Fort L. Contrast-medium injury to the spinal cord: the role of altered circulatory dynamics. *J Neurosurg* 1959;16:390–406.
19 Margolis G. Pathogenesis of contrast media injury: insights provided by neurotoxicity studies. *Invest Radiol* 1970;5: 392–406.
20 Albertson KW, Doppman JL, Ramsey R. Spinal seizures induced

by contrast media. *Radiology* 1973;107:349–351.

21 Gonsette RE. Biological tolerance of the central nervous system to Metrizamide. *Acta Radiol* 1973;335(Suppl.):25–44.

22 Gonsette RE, Brucher JM. Neurotoxicity of novel water-soluble contrast media for intrathecal application. *Invest Radiol* 1980; 15:254–259.

23 Morris TW, Kern MA, Katzbert RW. The effects of media viscosity on hemodynamics in selective arteriography. *Invest Radiol* 1982;17:70–76.

24 Dawson P, Harrison MJG, Weisblatt E. Effect of contrast media on red cell filtrability and morphology. *Br J Radiol* 1983;56: 707–710.

25 Dawson P, Pitfield J, Skinnemoen K. Isomeric purity and supersaturation of Iopamidol. *Br J Radiol* 1983;56:711–713.

26 Winding O. Foreign bodies in contrast media for angiography. *Am J Hosp Pharm* 1977;34:705–708.

27 Winding O. Intrinsic particles in angiographic contrast media. *Radiology* 1980;134:317–320.

28 Wales LR, Nov AA. Transient global amnesia: complication of cerebral angiography. *Am J Neurol* 1981;2:275–277.

29 Cochran JW, Morrell F, Huckman MS, Cochran EJ. Transient global amnesia after cerebral angiography. Report of seven cases. *Arch Neurol* 1982;39:593–594.

30 Pexman JHW, Coates RK. Amnesia after femorocerebral angiography. *Am J Neurol* 1983;4:979–983.

31 Mani RL, Eisenberg RL, McDonald EJ Jr, Pollack JA, Mani JR. Complications of catheter cerebral arteriography: analysis of 5000 procedures. I Criteria and incidence. *Am J Roentgenol* 1978;131:861–865.

32 Mani RL, Eisenberg RL. Complications of catheter cerebral procedures. II. Relation of complication rates to clinical and arteriographic diagnoses. *Am J Roentgenol* 1978;131:871–874.

33 Mani RL, Eisenberg RL. Complications of catheter cerebral arteriography: analysis of 5000 procedures. III. Assessment of arteries injected, contrast medium used, duration of procedure, and age of patient. *Am J Roentgenol* 1978;131:871–874.

34 Hessel SJ, Adams DR, Abrams HL. Complications of angiography. *Radiology* 1981;138:273–281.

35 Rapoport SI. Blood–brain barrier opening by isotonic saline infusion in normotensive and hypertensive animals. *Acta Radiol (Diagn)* 1978;19:921–932.

36 Huckman MS, Shenk GL, Neems RL, Tinor T. Transfemoral cerebral arteriography versus direct percutaneous carotid and brachial arteriography. A comparison of complication rates. *Radiology* 1979;132:93–97.

37 Earnest F, Forbes G, Sandok BA *et al.* Complications of cerebral angiography: prospective assessment of risk. *Am J Neuroradiol* 1983;4:1191–1197.

38 McIvor J, Steiner TJ, Perkin GD, Greenhalgh RM, Clifford Rose F. Neurological morbidity of arch and carotid arteriography in cerebrovascular disease. *Br J Radiol* 1987;60:117–122.

39 Caplan LR, Wolpert SM. Angiography in patients with occlusive cerebrovascular disease. *Am J Neuroradiol* 1991;12:593–601.

40 Baum S, Stern GN, Kuroda KK. Complications of "no arteriography." *Radiology* 1966;86:835–838.

41 Faught E, Trader SD, Hanna GR. Cerebral complications of angiography for transient ischaemia and stroke. Predication of risk. *Neurology* 1979;29:4–15.

42 Eisenberg RL, Bank WO, Hedgcock MW. Neurologic complications of angiography in patients with critical stenosis of the carotid artery. *Neurology* 1980;30:892–895.

43 Smoker WRK, Corbett JJ, Gentry LR, Keyes WD, Price MJ,

McKusker S. High resolution computed tomography of the basilar artery: 2. Vertebrobasilar dolichoectasia: clinical-pathologic correlation and review. *Am J Neuroradiol* 1986;7: 61–72.

44 Ekbom K, Grietz T. Carotid angiography in cluster headaches. *Acta Radiol Diagn (Stockh)* 1970;10:177–186.

45 Grainger RG. Osmolality of intravascular radiological contrast media. *Br J Radiol* 1980;53:739–746.

46 Robetson WD, Nugent RA, Russel DB *et al.* Clinical experience with Hexabrix in cerebral angiography. *Invest Radiol* 1984; 19(Suppl.):308–311.

47 Valk J, Crezee F, Olislagers-De Slegte RGM. Comparison of Iohexol 300 mgI/ml and Hexabrix 320 mgI/ml in central angiography. A double-blind trial. *Neuroradiology* 1984;26:217–221.

48 Stevens JM, Barter S, Kerslake R, Schneidau A, Barber C, Thomas DJ. Relative safety of intravenous digital subtraction angiography over other methods of carotid angiography and impact on clinical management of cerebrovascular disease. *Br J Radiol* 1989;62:813–816.

49 Mani RL, Eisenberg RL, McDonald JR, Pollack JA, Mani JR. Complications of catheter cerebral arteriography I–III. *Am J Roentgenol* 1978;131:861–874.

50 Olivecrona H. Complications of cerebral angiography. *Neuroradiology* 1977;14:175–181.

51 Mamourian A, Drayer BP. Clinically silent infarcts shown by MR after cerebral angiography. *Am J Neuroradiol* 1990;11:1084.

52 Lazorthes G, Ooulhes J, Bastide G, Chancholle AR, Zadeh O. *La vascularisation de la moelle eipniere. Pathologie vasculaire de la moelle.* XXVe Reunion Neurologique International Paris, Masson et Cie, Paris, 1962:5–27.

53 Djindjian R, Merland JJ, Djindjian M, Stroeter P. Revision of the blood supply of the spine. In: *Angiography of the spinal column and Spinal Cord Tumours.* Stuttgart: Georg Thieme Verlag. 1981:1–3.

54 Kardijiev V, Symeonov A, Chandkov I. Etiology, pathogenesis and prevention of spinal cord lesions in selective angiography of the bronchial and intercostal arteries. *Radiology* 1974;112: 81–83.

55 Adamkiewicz A. Blood vessels of the human spinal cord. Sitzungsverichte der Heidelberger Akademie der Wissenschaften. *Mathematische-naturwissenschaftliche Klasse* 1982;85:101–130.

56 Tornell G. Spinal cord tolerance to roentgen contrast media, particularly during aortography, with temporary occlusion of the aorta. An experimental investigation in dogs. *Acta Radiol (Diagn)* 1969;8:257–283.

57 McAfee JG, Wilson JKV. A review of the complications of translumbar aortography. *Am J Roentgenol* 1956;75:956–970.

58 McAfee JG. A survey of complications of abdominal aortography. *Radiology* 1957;68:825–835.

59 Lance EM, Killen DA. Experimental appraisal of the agents employed as angiocardiographic and aortographic contrast media. I Neurotoxicity. *Surgery* 1959;46:1107–1117.

60 Ansell G. A national survey of radiological complications: interim report. *Clin Radiol* 1968;19:175–191.

61 Editorial. Spinal cord damage after angiography. *Lancet* 1973;8: 1067–1068.

62 Cornell SH. Spasticity of the lower extremities following abdominal aortography. *Radiology* 1969;93:377–379.

63 Brodey PA, Doppman JL, Bisaccia LJ. An unusual complication of aortography with the pigtail catheter. *Radiology* 1974;110: 711–715.

64 Ederli A, Sassaroli S, Spaccarelli G. Vertebral angiography as a

cause of necrosis of the cervical spinal cord. *Br J Radiol* 1962; 35:261–264.

65 Killen DA, Foster JH. Spinal cord injury as a complication of contrast angiography. *Surgery* 1966;59:969–981.

66 Feigelson HH, Ravin HA. Transverse myelitis following selective bronchial arteriography. *Radiology* 1965;85:663–665.

67 Evans AT. Renal arteriography. *Am J Roentgenol* 1954;72: 574–585.

68 Di Chiro G. Unintentional spinal cord arteriography: a warning. *Radiology* 1974;112:231–233.

69 Djindjian R, Hurth M, Houdart R, Labovit G, Julian H, Mamo H. L'angiographie de la Moelle Epiniere. Paris: Masson et Cie, 1970.

70 Doppman JL, Di Chiro G, Ommoya AK. *Selective arteriography of the Spinal Cord*. St Louis MO: Green, 1969.

71 Kendall BE. Radiological investigation. In: Aminoff MJ, ed. *Spinal Angiomas*. Oxford: Blackwell Scientific Publications, 1976:109.

72 Kendall B. Spinal angiography with Iohexol. *Neuroradiology* 1986;28:72–73.

73 Fox AJ, Kricheff II, Goodgold J, Spielholz N, Tegerman L. The effect of angiography on the electrophysiological state of the spinal cord. A study in control and traumatized cats. *Radiology* 1976;118:343–350.

74 du Boulay GH, Wallis A. Cerebral artery constriction due to contrast media. *Acta Radiol (Diagn)* 1987;369:518–520.

75 Yerasimeds TG, Margolis G, Ponton HJ. Prophylaxis of experimental contrast medium injury to the spinal cord by vasopressor drugs. *Angiology* 1963;14: 394–403.

76 Margolis G, Yerazimides TG. Vasopressor potentiation of neurotoxicity in experimental aortography: implications regarding pathogenesis of contrast medium injury. *Acta Radiol (Diagn)* 1966;5:388–412.

77 Aminoff MJ, Bernard RO, Logue V. The pathophysiology of spinal vascular malformations. *J Neurol Sci* 1974;23:255–263.

78 Moseley IF, Tress BM. Extravasation of contrast medium during spinal angiography: a cause of paraplegia. *Neuroradiology* 1977; 13:55–57.

79 Rhea WG Jr, O'Neill JA, Killen DA, Foster JH. Toxic reactions incident to aortography. The hazard of repeat injection. *Circulation* 1964;29(Suppl.):161–164.

80 Killen DA, Foster JH. Spinal cord injury as a complication of aortography. *Ann Surg* 1960;152:211–230.

81 Mischkin MM, Baum S, Di Chiro G. Emergency treatment of angiography-induced paraplegia and tetraplegia. *New Engl J Med* 1973;288:1184–1185.

82 Fischer HW. Occurrence of seizure during cranial computed tomography. *Radiology* 1980;137:563–564.

83 Hayman LA, Panani JJ, Serur JR, Hinck VC. Impermeability of the blood–brain barrier to intravenous high-iodine-dose Meglumine Diatrizoate in normal dog. *Am J Neuroradiol* 1984; 5:409–411.

84 Wilcox J, Sage MR, Evill CA. Effect of intravenous contrast material on the integrity of the blood–brain barrier: experimental study. *Am J Neuroradiol* 1984;5:41–43.

85 Lozito JC. Convulsions: a complication of contrast enhancement in computerised tomography. *Arch Neurol* 1977;34: 649–650.

86 Pagani JJ, Hayman LA, Bigelow RH, Libshitz HI, Lepke RA, Wallace S. Diazepam prophylaxis of contrast-media induced seizures during computed tomography of patients with brain metastases. *Am J Neuroradiol* 1983;4:67–72.

87 Pagani JJ, Hayman LA, Bigelow RH, Libshitz HI, Lepke RA. Prophylactic diazepam in prevention of contrast media-associated seizures in glioma patients undergoing cerebral computed tomography. *Cancer* 1984;54:2200–2204.

88 Naheedy MH, Naidu S, Griffin AJ. Prolonged rentention of contrast medium in an hypoxic neonatal brain. *Surg Neurol* 1983;20:369–372.

89 Junck L, Enzmann DR, DeArmond SJ, Okerlund M. Prolonged brain retention of contrast agent in neonatal herpes simplex encephalitis. *Radiology* 1981;140:123–126.

90 Sullivan WT, Dorwart RH. Leakage of iodinated contrast material into the cerebral ventricles in an adult with ependymitis. *Am J Neuroradiol* 1983;4:1251–1253.

91 Benear JB, Vannatta JB, Jpstu TA, Hughes WL. Contrast-induced seizure associated with thrombotic thrombocytopenic purpura. Case report. *Arch Int Med* 1985;145:363–364.

92 Uhl GR, Martinez CR, Brooks BR. Spinal seizures following intravenous contrast in a patient with a cord AVM. *Ann Neurol* 1981;10:580–581.

93 Casazza M, Bracchi M, Girotti F. Spinal myoclonus and clinical worsening after IV contrast medium in a patient with spinal AVM. *Am J Neuroradiol* 1984;6:965–966.

94 Coin CG, Coin JT. Contrast enhancement by xenon gas in computed tomography of the spinal cord and brain. *J Comput Assist Tomogr* 1980;4:217–221.

95 Seyferth W, Dilbat G, Seitter E. Efficacy and safety of digital subtraction angiography with special reference to contrast agents. *Cardiovasc Intervent Radiol* 1983;6:265–270.

96 Sackett JF, Bergsjordet B, Seeger JF, Keiffer SA. Digital subtraction angiography: comparison of meglumine-Na diatrizoate with iohexol. *Acta Radiol* 1985;366(Suppl.):81–84.

97 Pinto RS, Manuel M, Kricheff II. Complications of digital intravenous angiography in replacing carotid arteriography. *Ann Int Med* 1986;104:572–574.

98 Warlow C. Carotid endarterectomy: does it work. *Stroke* 1984; 15:1068–1076.

99 Moseley I. *Diagnostic Imaging in Neurological Disease*. London: Churchill Livingstone, 1986:125.

100 Kricheff II. Arteriosclerotic ischaemic cerebrovascular disease. *Radiology* 1987;162:101–109.

101 European Carotid Surgery Trialists' Group. MRC European Carotid Surgery Trial: interim results for symptomatic patients with severe (70–99%) or with mild (0–29%) carotid stenosis. *Lancet* 1991;337:1235–1243.

Complications of neuroradiology: intrathecal studies

Robert D. Boutin, Frederick W. Rupp and William W. Orrison, Jr

Introduction

Intrathecal examinations — lumbar puncture and myelography — are the most commonly performed invasive neurodiagnostic procedures today. Over one million such examinations are performed each year by physicians with diverse goals and training: radiologists, pediatricians, family practitioners, internists, oncologists, psychiatrists, neurologists, neurosurgeons, and emergency medicine physicians. Each of these physicians should be cognizant of the potential complications associated with intrathecal procedures and how to minimize the frequency of such complications.

History

Puncture of the subarachnoid space dates back to 1764 when Cotugno conducted studies of cerebrospinal fluid (CSF) on cadavers [1]. In 1891, Quincke demonstrated the technique of inserting a styletted needle into the subarachnoid space for the purpose of removing CSF [2,3]. A contrast material was first injected into the subarachnoid space to outline the spinal cord in 1918 by Dandy [4]. In 1924, Ayer [5] identified several factors that could influence CSF dynamics, including the elasticity of the dura, intracranial arterial pressure, intracranial venous pressure, CSF secretion pressure, and CSF absorption rate. Cephalgia was the first reported adverse effect associated with myelography [6]. Indeed, Dandy stated: "So constant and characteristic is this pain that it seems to be positive evidence that there is no complete block of the spinal canal." The lateral C1−2 puncture for the purposes of myelography was described by Amundsen and Skalpe in 1975 [7,8].

Indications

Lumbar puncture (LP)

Indications for LP most commonly revolve around the removal of CSF for laboratory analysis. CSF analysis is most frequently done as part of the work-up when meningitis or subarachnoid hemorrhage is suspected. CSF samples are also useful for evaluating patients for central nervous system (CNS) malignancy (e.g., metastases), demyelinating disease (e.g., multiple sclerosis), and treatable causes of dementia (e.g., neurosyphilis). Therapeutically, LP is indicated for removal of CSF to reduce intracranial pressure in pseudotumor cerebri, chronic meningitis, normal pressure hydrocephalus, and posthemorrhagic hydrocephalus. Other interventions requiring LP include intrathecal chemotherapy and antibiotic therapy. LP, of course, is also performed as a prerequisite to myelography from the lumbar approach.

Myelography

Myelography — the injection of contrast material into the subarachnoid space — is designed to outline the spinal cord and nerve roots for diagnostic purposes. Presently, there is a strong trend away from using plain myelography without subsequently performing computed tomography (CT). Although myelography was the gold standard for years, several studies conclude that magnetic resonance imaging (MRI) is now the examination of choice for spinal pathology [9–12], largely because of its increased diagnostic sensitivity and noninvasive nature. Other specific factors that favor the trend toward MRI (and away from myelography) include: no ionizing radiation, no intrathecal contrast material, and often no needle or contrast at all.

MRI, however, will not completely replace diagnostic intrathecal procedures in the near future. MRI is a costly examination and is not universally available to patients in rural USA communities, developing countries, and even several developed countries. Furthermore, contraindications to MRI will continue to preclude its use in patients who have cardiac pacemakers, intraocular metallic foreign bodies, and ferromagnetic implants such as aneurysm clips. A small but significant number of patients will also be unable to undergo MRI due to claustrophobia, obesity, or bulky traction devices. Magnetic field inhomogeneity artifact from spinal instrumentation can also severely limit the utility of MRI in some cases. CT myelography is often of diagnostic benefit in these patient populations, as well as in those patients who are suspected of having lateral cervical disk herniations [13], arachnoiditis [9], or leptomeningeal metastases that do not enhance with gadolinium [14].

The C1–2 puncture for myelography has been advocated as a valuable adjunct to the lumbar approach for a variety of reasons: (i) the contrast is diluted less; (ii) the contrast is less likely to enter the cranium; (iii) a C1–2 puncture is helpful in defining the superior margin of a complete spinal canal block; and (iv) an LP is impractical or impossible in some patients (e.g., those with severe degenerative spondylosis, operative bony fusion, complete block between the LP level and the cervical region of interest) [15–19].

Cisternography

Metrizamide cisternography via suboccipital puncture was described by Grepe in 1975 [20]. This technique, however, requires inserting a needle in close proximity to the brainstem. Also, conventional cisternography reportedly caused headaches in 76% of patients [21]. The advent of CT cisternography markedly reduced the amount of intrathecal contrast needed and permitted contrast administration via a lumbar approach, both of which decreased the incidence of headache and other hazards [22]. Gas (2–5 ml) can also be injected into the lumbar subarachnoid space in order to examine the cerebellopontine angle by CT [23]. Although both types of CT cisternography may be performed as outpatient procedures and typically cause only brief headaches, they have been almost totally supplanted by MRI. As with cisternography, ventriculography and pneumoencephalography have essentially been eliminated with the advent

of CT and MRI, which are superior in the evaluation of ventricular configuration and skull base tumors. Readers interested in these earlier techniques are referred to previous editions of this book.

Thus, intrathecal examinations have a long history and continue to have numerous indications. These procedures are invasive, however, and adverse side-effects are not uncommon. The vast majority of the side-effects are *minor* in that they are transient and self-limited; examples include headache, nausea, vomiting, and dizziness. *Major* adverse effects are much less common but can cause extended hospital stays (e.g., meningitis), permanent neurologic deficits (e.g., hearing loss, paraplegia), or be life threatening (e.g., intracranial hemorrhage).

Precautions and contraindications

Dural puncture

The risks involved with performing dural puncture may outweigh the potential benefits of the procedure in certain clinical situations. When intracranial mass effect is suspected, dural puncture is contraindicated unless the amount of mass effect is judged to be safe by ophthalmologic examination, CT [24], and/or MRI. If an intraspinal mass is suspected, LP should not be performed. (If a myelogram must be performed, contrast should be administered via a C1–2 puncture rather than the lumbar route.) Dural puncture is also contraindicated if suppurated soft tissues must be transgressed; puncture in this setting could result in direct contamination of the subarachnoid space. The manufacturers of iohexol recommend that myelography not be performed in the presence of systemic infection when bacteremia is likely. Caution is also advised for patients with a known coagulopathy [25]. Dural puncture in uncooperative, combative patients is contraindicated for obvious reasons.

Myelography

Myelography should not be performed in patients with hepatorenal insufficiency unless the potential benefits clearly outweigh the added risks in these patients (see Adverse effects, p. 456).

Although anaphylactoid reactions from intrathecal contrast are rare, the need for myelography in patients with a known sensitivity to iodinated contrast should be evaluated carefully. If myelography is performed in these patients, the risk of repeated reaction is thought to be very low with premedication [26]. A premedication regimen used for intravascular studies may also be employed prior to myelography: prednisone (50 mg orally every 6 hours times three beginning 13 hours before myelography), diphenhydramine (50 mg orally or intramuscularly 1 hour before myelography), and ephedrine (50 mg orally 1 hour before myelography) [27].

Precautions must also be taken for patients with a history of seizures. Patients who are receiving anticonvulsants should continue on their therapy. Drugs that are known to lower the seizure threshold should be discontinued for at least 48 hours before and 24 hours after the procedure. These drugs include phenothiazine derivatives, monoamine oxidase inhibitors, tricyclic antidepressants, CNS stimulants, antipsychotic and psychoactive drugs. Anticonvulsants can be prescribed prophylactically for nonelective procedures in patients who must remain on these drugs, or in patients who receive a large or concentrated intracranial bolus of contrast.

Another relative contraindication to myelography is pregnancy. Although no harm to animal fetuses has been demonstrated with up to 100 times the recommended human dose of intravascular iohexol, no controlled studies have been performed in pregnant women. Furthermore, the radiation exposure during a fluoroscopically guided procedure is 30–100 mSv/min, suggesting that fluoroscopy should only be performed in this setting when absolutely necessary. Lumbar myelography with one lateral, two anterior–posterior, and four oblique radiographs yields a total radiation dose of 1.8 mSv to the gonads, 0.13 mSv to the thyroid, and 5.66 mSv to active bone marrow [28].

Technique

Since Quincke's description of the LP one century ago, the basic methods involved with dural puncture have not changed significantly, including patient positioning, use of a styletted needle, manometry, CSF removal, and postprocedure care. The technical details, however, are almost as variable as the number of physicians performing the procedure. Certain refinements in preprocedure, procedural, and postprocedural patient management are helpful in improving the intrathecal examinations and minimizing complications (Table 25.1).

Table 25.1 Standardized technique for LP and myelography

1 Patient education (written informed consent, if required)
2 Patient positioning (spine alignment)
3 Sterile technique
4 Identification of level of initial puncture (L2–3, L3–4, or L4–5)
5 Local anesthesia (slow injection rate)
6 Needle advancement (cephalad angulation, bevel oriented parallel to dural fibers, slow advancement, awareness of tenting)
7 Remove stylet (if "dry tap", slowly withdraw needle 3–4 mm)
8 Manometric and Queckenstedt tests (optional)
9 CSF collection (optional)
10 Injection of nonionic contrast medium
11 Reinsertion of stylet
12 Moderately slow, smooth needle withdrawal
13 Postprocedure care (hydration, positioning)

LP

Preprocedure

Proper preparation of the patient includes explaining why and how the procedure is performed, as well as reassuring the patient that the incidence of serious complications from LP is extremely low. Only scattered case reports of severe untoward effects exist in the literature after several million procedures (see Adverse effects, p. 456). The incidence of persistent morbidity or mortality from LP is estimated to be less than 0.5%. The issue of whether or not patients should be advised of very rare, but potentially lethal, complications from LP (and myelography) must be addressed by each of us. Written informed consent may be part of the procedure in some institutions, and all physicians should be aware of their institution's policy.

The procedure

Puncture site

L3–4 and L4–5 are the interspaces of choice for LP, with repeat attempts at more cephalad levels following dry taps. LP above the L2–3 interspace increases the risk of spinal cord damage. However, needle puncture of the cord alone, without injection of contrast or other material, does not necessarily cause neurologic damage, even in the cervical cord [29].

Whenever possible, the level where pathology is suspected should be avoided, since a hematoma or focal CSF collection could potentially cause a filling defect in the contrast column and be misinterpreted as a tumor or herniated disk.

Needle size

The use of a small-gage needle minimizes the potential for significant trauma to the dura. Minimizing such trauma reduces the likelihood of post-LP CSF leakage and postural headache. A small-gage needle may also help avoid such rare complications as a cerebrospinal fistula between the spinal canal and the skin [30]. Twenty-two-gage or smaller needles are recommended; the actual needle selection is dependent on such factors as physician preference and the volume of CSF needed.

Needle bevel

The size of the dural defect also varies according to the orientation of the bevel of the needle. Because the dural fibers are primarily aligned parallel to the long axis of the spine, the needle bevel should be oriented (longitudinally) to spread the fibers rather than cut across them (transversely). Consequently, the dural defect from a puncture performed

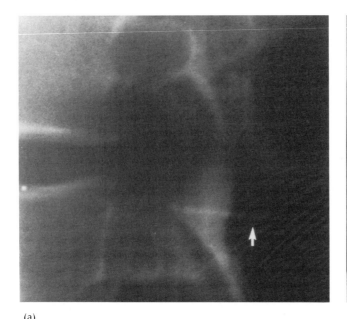

(a)

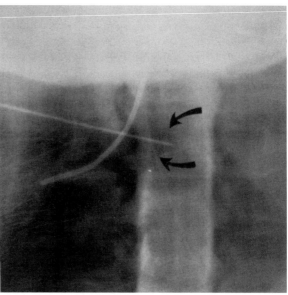

(b)

Fig. 25.1 Dural tenting. (a) Posterolateral lumbar approach (arrow indicates spinal needle). (b) Posterior cervical approach (arrows indicate tenting to midline prior to dural puncture). (From Orrison *et al.* [31].)

with the bevel face parallel to the direction of the dural fibers will be smaller and oblong, while a puncture with the bevel perpendicular to the fibers will cut across them and so be larger and rounded.

Tenting

An awareness of dural puncture dynamics is helpful in understanding how best to avoid procedural complications. Prior to the spinal needle puncturing the dura and entering the subarachnoid space, the needle momentarily indents or tents the dura inward [31] (Fig. 25.1). After the dura is punctured by the needle, the dura and CSF return to their prepuncture positions.

This tenting phenomenon is a factor in both traumatic and dry taps. Because of the transient inward tenting of the dura, the needle tip is actually deeper within the canal at the time of puncture than the physician might think. As the needle tip approaches the expected region of the spinal canal, the needle should be advanced slowly and cautiously. A "dural pop" — decreased resistance to needle advancement — characteristically signals penetration of the dura; this sensation may not be obvious with fine-gage needles or on neonates. The stylet should remain in place while advancing (or retracting) the needle, but removed frequently in order to assess for initial return of CSF, which indicates successful entry into the subarachnoid space. This technique may prevent penetration of the ventral dura and Batsons' plexus of veins,

thus significantly reducing the possibility of a traumatic tap and subsequent arachnoiditis. Slight advancement of the needle (1–2 mm) following initial CSF flow usually helps to assure proper positioning within the subarachnoid space. Rotation of the needle can also aid in optimizing CSF flow. If the physician is uncertain as to the depth of the needle tip, a crosstable lateral radiograph with the patient in the prone position may be obtained. If the needle has entirely traversed the spinal canal, slowly withdrawing the needle 3–4 mm often results in a free flow of CSF.

After access to the subarachnoid space is secured, the physician may then perform manometry, Queckenstedt testing [32], and/or CSF removal, if deemed clinically appropriate. If CSF analysis is indicated, approximately 9 ml are typically collected. If an unusual neurologic disorder is suspected, an extra 3 ml of CSF may be collected and refrigerated for additional studies that may not have been anticipated. After these steps are completed, myelography may be performed as well (see Myelography, p. 451).

Reverse tenting

When the spinal needle is removed from the subarachnoid space, the dura temporarily adheres to the needle causing retraction or reverse tenting. The pressure change created by the reverse tenting phenomenon causes a vortex and movement of CSF toward the needle. Rapid withdrawal of an unstyletted needle can initiate enough suction to herniate a nerve root or arachnoid into the needle. Even if the spinal needle is styletted, rapid removal may result in frictional damage to adjacent nerve roots from the cutting edge of the needle. Therefore, moderately slow and smooth withdrawal of the spinal needle — after the stylet has been reinserted — is important following dural puncture.

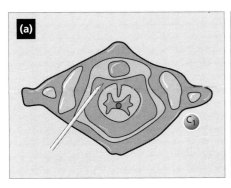
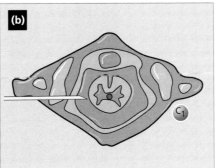
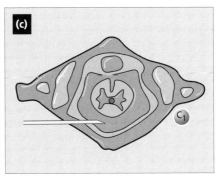

Fig. 25.2 C1−2 puncture needle positions (see text). (a) Anterior approach; (b) midplane approach; (c) posterior approach. (From Orrison *et al.* [31].)

Postprocedure

Following completion of the LP, semierect or supine patient positioning may help decrease the incidence of post-LP headache.

Myelography

Preprocedure

Patient preparation for myelography must incorporate the steps described above for LP, in addition to considering the potential risks and benefits of iodinated contrast media. Water-soluble contrast in the subarachnoid space, like CSF, is cleared by absorption through the arachnoid proliferations and lymphatics in the cranium and spine. Given that this absorption is a passive, pressure-dependent phenomenon, it is not surprising that removal of excessive CSF (for laboratory analysis or due to a dural leak) will reduce the subarachnoid space pressure driving clearance of contrast. Similarly, dehydration causes reduced CSF pressure in the subarachnoid space and therefore slower clearance of contrast [33]. Well-hydrated patients are therefore less likely to develop adverse effects following myelography than dehydrated patients. To ensure adequate hydration, fluids should be allowed until the time of the procedure. A normal diet may be maintained up to 2 hours prior to myelography.

Premedication with intravenous diazepam immediately before cervical myelography by the C1−2 approach may be used; however, consideration must also be given to the importance of an alert and cooperative patient when performing this procedure.

The procedure

Myelography via LP

After performing the LP as described above, contrast should be injected slowly over 1−2 minutes so as to avoid turbulent flow and premature dilution. Plain radiographs and CT scanning are subsequently performed, as desired. Routine radiography generally includes posterior−anterior, lateral, and bilateral oblique views with sufficient reverse Trendelenburg positioning to opacify the distal spinal canal. In addition, a prone or supine film of the conus medullaris is recommended to rule out an intrinsic lesion or extrinsic mass effect upon the distal spinal cord.

Myelography via cervical puncture

Lateral C1−2 puncture techniques are generally safe, but do have potentially serious complications and thus should only be performed by well-trained physicians. As seen with dural puncture in the lumbar spine, the spinal needle will often enter the subarachnoid space only after the tip has passed beyond the midpoint of the spinal canal due to dural flexibility and strength.

The cervical subarachnoid space can be accessed by three different types of lateral C1−2 puncture for the purposes of myelography: the midplane, the oblique anterior, and the posterior approaches (Fig. 25.2). The least favored technique is the *midplane approach* which aims the spinal needle directly at the cervical spinal cord [34], and results in an unnecessarily high risk of cervical spinal cord puncture. The *oblique anterior approach* directs the needle toward the anterior one-third of the spinal canal. This technique also results in an unacceptably high risk of injury to the cervical spinal cord because the subarachnoid space is smaller anteriorly (average 2.6 mm) than posteriorly (average 4.3 mm). In addition, the oblique anterior approach puts the vertebral artery at risk, because in 96% of patients it either projects anterior to the spinal canal or over the anterior one-third of the spinal canal when using lateral fluoroscopic guidance [35]. Puncture of the vertebral artery has resulted in death due to acute subdural hematoma in the craniocervical and posterior fossa regions [36].

The *posterior approach* to lateral C1−2 puncture is the safest and easiest of the three techniques. This approach minimizes the risk of vascular injury to a caudal loop of the posterior inferior cerebellar artery (PICA), which lies inferior to the foramen magnum in approximately 20% of patients [17]. Although significant tenting of the dura will occur regardless of the needle size used in the procedure, the extent of the needle "snowplow" effect while advancing into the spinal canal is directly proportional to the needle size. Regardless of needle size or angle of needle entry, however, the dura will be stretched over the needle tip for 5–10 mm before the dura will be penetrated. The tip of the dural tent will always project beyond the midpoint of the spinal canal prior to needle penetration of the dura [31] (Figs 25.3 & 25.4).

A scout radiograph should be obtained and the patient should be placed prone. Although the neck is classically positioned in extension, the procedure should be performed in a more neutral position if there is severe cervical spondylosis or a narrowed spinal canal. The central ray of the lateral fluoroscopic beam should be focused on the posterior one-third of the spinal canal, approximately 4–6 mm anterior to the spinolaminar line and 4–6 mm inferior to the arch of C1. The position of the spinal cord at the C1–2 level changes very little during flexion and extension of the neck or with prone or supine positioning of the patient [17].

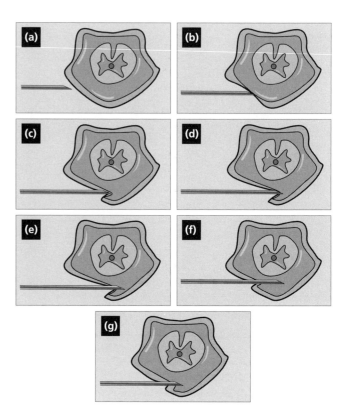

Fig. 25.4 "Snowplow" effect of cervical dural tenting. (a) Posterior C1–2 approach. (b) The needle makes contact with the dura. (c) The dural tent is formed. (d) The snowplow effect rolls the cord away from the needle tip. (e) The needle pierces the dura and enters the subarachnoid space. (f) The dural tent partially collapses. (g) As the needle is withdrawn, the dural tent collapses entirely. Further withdrawal leads to reverse tenting, not shown (see text). (From Orrison *et al.* [31].)

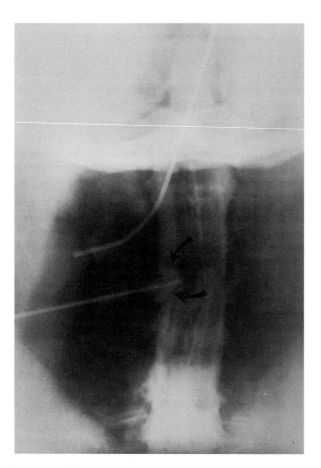

Fig. 25.3 Midplane C1–2 puncture approach with resultant spinal cord displacement to the right. (From Orrison *et al.* [31].)

The patient should be cautioned not to cough or swallow, if possible, until the needle is removed. The puncture is usually performed with a 22-gage needle, and close attention should be paid to needle position. Any anterior deviation of the needle during penetration should be corrected immediately to avoid contact with the cervical spinal cord. Initial contact with the subarachnoid space is confirmed by removing the stylet of the needle every 1–2 mm after reaching the level of the spinal canal, as evidenced on anteroposterior fluoroscopy. Typically, there will be blood return as the epidural space is traversed; CSF flow is then usually obtained by advancing the needle slightly. Once free flow of CSF is established, the needle may be advanced another 1–2 mm to ensure complete penetration of the dura and arachnoid. The needle may then be withdrawn 2–3 mm to ensure that the needle tip is not against the opposite side of the spinal canal or the cervical spinal cord.

Free flow of CSF should be reconfirmed before introducing contrast. Then, while monitoring fluoroscopically, the contrast is injected slowly. Following initial injection of a small amount of contrast, if a markedly enlarged ventral subarachnoid space is encountered, this should suggest posterior deviation of the cervical spinal cord due to a mass at or near the foramen magnum. As the incidence of a "dry tap" is increased in this scenario, the C1−2 puncture technique should be abandoned.

After injection of approximately 0.5 ml, attention should be addressed to the needle tip and any focal collection of contrast should be analyzed. Although injections of myelographic contrast outside the cervical subarachnoid space are unusual, failure to recognize such an injection could result in patient injury or misinterpretation of the myelographic findings [37] (Table 25.2). Epidural injections are characterized by a starburst configuration of contrast radiating outward from the injection site (Fig. 25.5). Subdural injections should produce a small, rounded pool of contrast collecting at the needle tip which very quickly dissects along the dura with increased injection volume (Fig. 25.6). Dentate ligament injections create fine lace-like configurations of contrast that remain within the midportion of the spinal cord and persist longer than would be expected. Subpial injections should be suspected when a fine, tapering line of contrast outlines the anterior or posterior margins of the cord and persists beyond the normal injection time (Fig. 25.7). Intramedullary injections into the spinal cord result in a distinct midline longitudinal stripe following the spinal tracts that extends both superiorly and inferiorly (Fig. 25.8). Increase in the volume of the contrast injected can also increase the cross-sectional diameter of the cord and compress the spinal tracts. If an intramedullary injection is inadvertently performed, the injection should be discontinued and a short course of steroid therapy initiated [38].

Once free flow of contrast is established, the cervical subarachnoid space should be opacified, but intracranial flow of contrast should be avoided. Following this, the stylet is replaced into the needle which is then withdrawn slowly and carefully. The patient should again be warned against any movement or swallowing during needle withdrawal.

Postprocedure

Position

The patient's head should be kept in a nondependent position.

Table 25.2 Myelographic artifacts of C1−2 misinjection

Site of misinjection	Myelographic appearance
Epidural	Starburst radiation
Subdural	Focal pooling
Dentate ligament	Lace-like collection
Subpial	Fine, tapering line
Intramedullary	Midline longitudinal stripe

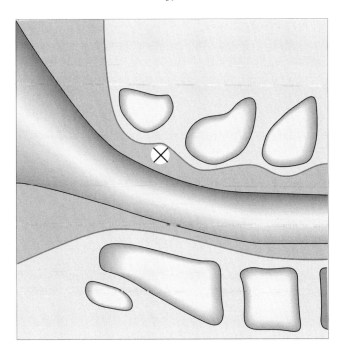

Fig. 25.5 The "X" marks the entry point for a posterior approach lateral C1−2 puncture for myelography in the prone position. (From Orrison *et al.* [31].)

Most practitioners advise the patient to remain in bed in a semisitting position (30−45°), especially in the first few hours following the procedure. Other authors, however, suggest that ambulation after the procedure should be allowed as it is not associated with increased headaches [39,40]. Both semirecumbent and upright positions delay intracranial dispersion of contrast and maximize absorption of the contrast in the spinal arachnoid; the upright position, however, is theoretically associated with dural leak and consequent headache. Regardless, contrast likely moves intracranially when the patient lies supine for CT myelography 2−6 hours following the instillation of contrast [41]. Although it is safe to perform myelography on an outpatient basis, the patient should not drive or be alone during the first 24 hours after myelography (see Adverse effects, p. 456).

Contrast media

Before 1970, oil-soluble iophendylate (Pantopaque) was the most commonly used intrathecal contrast medium. Unfortunately, iophendylate was associated with a relatively high potential for causing arachnoiditis and had to be reaspirated after myelography. Since the mid-1970s, only nonionic water-soluble contrast media have been utilized for myelographic examinations in the USA, Canada, and Europe [42]. Metrizamide (Amipaque) was the first nonionic contrast medium used for intrathecal injection. Although it represented a significant improvement over iophendylate, its intrathecal

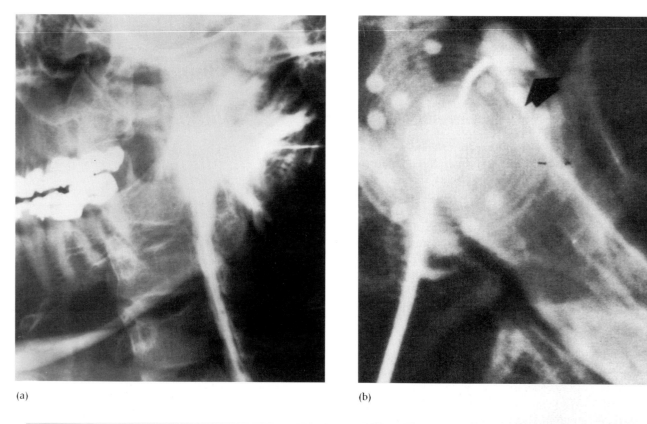

(a)

(b)

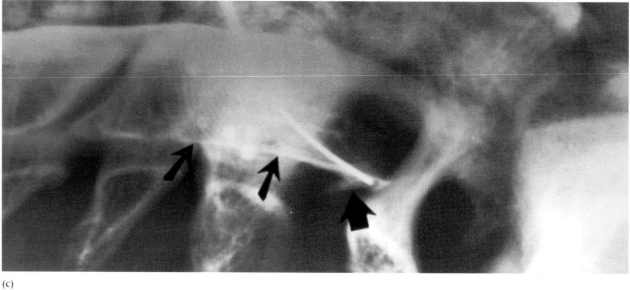

(c)

Fig. 25.6 (a) Epidural injection at C1−2 level with characteristic starburst pattern of contrast material. (b) Subdural injection at C1−2 level with localized pooling of contrast material posteriorly (arrow). (c) Partial subpial injection at C1−2 level with an irregular contrast collection at the needle tip (large arrow), and a thin tapering line of contrast material along the posterior aspect of the cervical spinal cord (small arrows). (From Orrison *et al.* [37].)

use was discontinued because of its relatively high incidences of headache, nausea, vomiting, dizziness, behavioral changes, and seizures. By comparison, the second-generation nonionic contrast agents (e.g., iohexol, iopamidol, iotrol) have a much lower incidence of general neurotoxicity and local chemotoxicity than older agents. The safety records of iohexol and iopamidol are roughly similar. Clinical comparisons between iohexol and iopamidol for myelography have shown iohexol to be safer in several studies [43−45], but

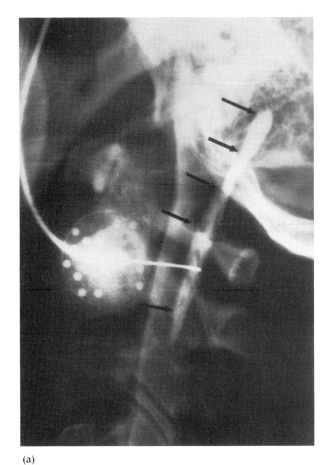

(a)

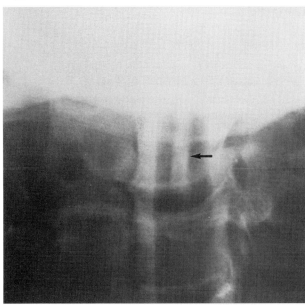

(b)

Fig. 25.7 Intramedullary injection at C1−2 level with a longitudinal collection of contrast material within the cervical spinal cord (arrows) in the lateral (a), and frontal (b) projections. (From Johansen *et al.* [38].)

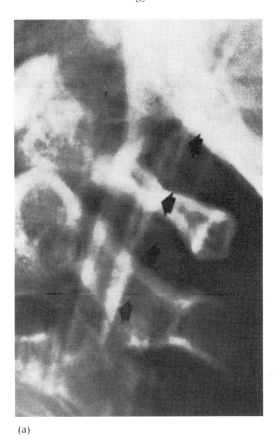

(a)

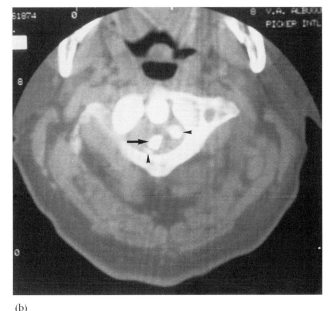

(b)

Fig. 25.8 (a) Lateral view of an intramedullary injection of 3 ml of metrizamide (300 mg iodine/ml) into the cervical spinal cord of a patient which resulted in a permanent monoparesis. (b) Transaxial CT scan of an intramedullary injection (arrow) of iohexol (180 mg iodine/ml) into the cervical spinal cord of a patient in which no deficit occurred. Also note smaller surrounding focal subdural injections (arrowheads).

other studies have shown it to be equivalent [41,46−48] or inferior [49].

Iohexol (Omnipaque) is transported to the bloodstream and typically reaches a peak serum concentration after 2 hours. Once in the serum, the half-life of iohexol is approximately 3.5 hours [50]. Over 80% of the contrast medium injected into the subarachnoid space is normally excreted in the urine within the first 24 hours. All myelographic examinations should now be performed with second-generation nonionic contrast media; intrathecal injection of ionic agents is strictly contraindicated. Misadministrations of ionic contrast into the subarachnoid space, however, do occur and can be fatal (see below).

The neurotoxicity of a contrast is not only determined by its intrinsic chemotoxicity, but also by its concentration and rate of clearance. In most cases, the lower concentration of iohexol (240 mg iodine (I)/ml) should be chosen over the higher concentration (300 mgI/ml); both concentrations produce myelograms of similar quality but the higher concentration causes more frequent side-effects [51]. In a study of 32 pediatric patients undergoing myelography with iohexol 210 mgI/ml and iohexol 180 mgI/ml [52], no side-effects were observed in either group. Although iohexol 210 mgI/ml may give superior visualization with no apparent added risk, these authors concluded that iohexol 180 mgI/ml is preferred for routine use [52].

Adverse effects

The complications related to dural puncture − with or without intrathecal contrast administration − are generally considered mild and self-limited. The most common side-effect is headache; other transient adverse effects include nausea, vomiting, dizziness, and focal neurologic symptoms (Table 25.3). Unfortunately, severe or permanent morbidity may also occur with complications such as meningitis, hemorrhage, and neurologic deficits. Rare cases of anaphylactoid reactions, encephalopathy, and death have also been reported. A summary of major complications related to cervical myelography is presented in Table 25.4.

Note must be made that clinical investigations in this area have generally used widely varying study designs and evaluated different aspects of the procedure (e.g., puncture

Table 25.4 Major complications of cervical myelography. (From Robertson & Smith [54])

Complication	Number of patients*
Related to C1−2 puncture	
Vertebral or PICA injury (occasional death)	3
Hematoma (epidural, subdural)	1
Cord puncture	5
Cord injection	16
Related to patient positioning (cervical hyperextension)	
Death	1
Paresis (quadriparesis, paraparesis, monoparesis)	15
Exacerbation of existing neurologic deficit	27
Total	68

* The total estimated number of procedures reported in this study was 187 300. The authors presumed the complications occurred over an average of 5 years with a range of 15 years.

technique, needle size, postprocedural instructions). Furthermore, many of the complications in the literature are in the form of case reports. Such variations not only make it difficult directly to compare study results, but also make it difficult to arrive at definitive conclusions regarding complication rates.

Headache

Significance

The most common adverse effect of dural puncture − other than the discomfort associated with needle insertion − is headache. Headaches occur after approximately 20% of LPs and myelograms [43,53,55], although the incidence is reported to vary from less than 10% to greater than 70% [56]. Cephalgia is usually mild to moderate in intensity, but can be severe. Headaches usually develop within the first 24 hours after the dural puncture [44,57] and remit by 24−48 hours, but have been reported to last for several weeks or months [58,59]. Intracranial hematoma should be considered in the differential diagnosis of protracted headaches following

Table 25.3 Adverse reaction profile in iohexol myelography. (From Shaw *et al.* [53])

	No reaction (%)	Headache (%)	Nausea (%)	Vomiting (%)	Pain (%)	Dizziness (%)	Mental status change (%)	Other (%)
Lumbar myelography (n = 677)	70	19	7	3	9	2	0	5
Cervical myelography (n = 368)	74	17	3	1	9	1	0	3

dural puncture, particularly if the patient is known to have a coagulation defect or cortical atrophy.

Etiology

The etiology of these headaches is multifactorial, and is influenced by several variables. Hypotension in the sub-arachnoid space caused by CSF leakage appears to be the major cause of most postural headaches. Variation among individuals in the production, circulation, and resorption of CSF probably influences the likelihood of any given patient experiencing a headache.

Strategies to minimize the incidence, severity, or duration of headache following dural puncture include: (i) using a small gage needle; (ii) proper needle orientation; (iii) limiting the volume of CSF removed and contrast injected (for myelography); and (iv) proper postprocedural positioning. The use of small-gage spinal needles results in a smaller defect in the dura, thus minimizing CSF leakage. For example, a coaxial system utilizing a 26-gage needle instead of a 22-gage needle results in a reduction of significant headaches from 23 to 13% [60]. Orienting the spinal needle bevel parallel to the long axis of the spine, as alluded to above, also tends to minimize the size of the dural rent. There is also evidence that excessive removal of CSF is correlated with an increased incidence of headaches, presumably secondary to CSF hypotension. Intrathecal contrast, when used in conventional doses, is not thought to be a significant factor causing headaches, because the frequency of headaches is roughly the same for both LP and lumbar myelography. However, at doses that exceed the recommended dose limit of 3.06 g of I (e.g., 17 ml of iohexol containing 180 mgI/ml) for adults, the frequency of headache, nausea, and vomiting increases [61].

Position. The postdural puncture headache is characteristically aggravated by erect posture and eased partially or completely by supine positioning. Postmyelogram headache, with its typical postural relationship, is thought to be related to the defect made in the dura during LP and not due to the subarachnoid contrast. The importance of postprocedural positioning is not universally accepted, however. In one study of 80 patients undergoing metrizamide myelography, the incidence of headaches was significantly higher in *non-ambulatory* patients (63%) who were restricted to complete bedrest for 24 hours as compared to *ambulatory* patients (43%) who were prescribed ambulation every 4 hours [39]. Another study prospectively investigated the influence of positioning on 110 patients after iohexol lumbar myelography and concluded that patients should be allowed to choose either ambulation or bedrest with their heads elevated because there was no significant difference in the frequency of postprocedural side-effects [40].

In addition to such technical and physical factors, psycho-logic factors may also influence the expression of side-effects such as headache [62]. Interestingly, some studies have found that postmyelogram headaches were significantly more common in patients with normal myelograms than in patients who were found to have an organic cause for their symptoms [60,62,63]. Perhaps patients with normal myelograms and subjectively severe headaches tend to have a lower threshold to pain [62]; alternately, patients with definite organic pathology may be relatively accustomed to pain and therefore have a higher pain threshold [60]. Post-myelogram headaches have also been correlated with other variables by some — but certainly not all — authors. Such controversial variables include hydration [62,64], gender [44,62,65], and age [62,65].

Treatment

The most commonly employed treatments for cephalgia are postprocedural positioning, hydration, and analgesics. When headaches are recalcitrant to such measures, an epidural blood patch is effective in relieving over 90% of headaches [59,66]. This treatment is performed by injecting approximately 10 ml of autologous blood into the region of the dural leak. The injection creates a gelatinous plug over the dural leak and promotes fibroblast activity and collagen deposition permanently to seal the dural tear. Less commonly used treatments include the subdural blood patch [67], epidural saline infusion [68], and surgical repair of the dural tear [69].

Pain, nausea, vomiting, dizziness

In the North American and European clinical trials of iohexol [53], 70% of 677 patients receiving iohexol for lumbar myelography reported no adverse reaction in the ensuing 24 hours after the procedure. Similarly, no adverse reactions were reported by 74% of the 272 patients undergoing cervical myelography with iohexol. Pain was reported by 9% of patients undergoing lumbar or cervical myelography. Nausea and vomiting were associated with lumbar myelography by approximately 7% and 3% of patients, respectively. By comparison, patients who had cervical myelography experienced nausea and vomiting with only 3% and 1% of the procedures, respectively. Dizziness was reported to occur with 1–2% of lumbar and cervical myelograms.

Inflammation and infection

Meningitis — both bacterial and chemical — may occur following dural puncture. Bacterial meningitis is rarely seen when aseptic technique is used, but can occur even when meticulous care is taken. Some investigators even recommend that all personnel involved in the procedure wear masks and hats, and draw contrast out of the bottle after disinfecting the cap's surface instead of just lifting the stopper out [70].

Chemical meningitis after myelography is far less common than it once was. Oil-based contrast agents (e.g., iophendylate), which are still used in some developing countries due to their relatively low cost [71], have a relatively high potential for causing meningeal inflammation and arachnoiditis (Fig. 25.9). Although chemical meningitis has been reported after intrathecal administration of the second-generation nonionic, water-soluble agents (e.g., iohexol [72], iopamidol [73], iotrol [74]), such cases are considered uncommon and are usually transient. The risk of permanent inflammatory alterations like arachnoiditis is likewise far lower with iohexol than with iophendylate or even metrizamide [75]. The risk of inducing arachnoiditis probably increases with contrast media when there is a hemorrhagic puncture [76] or concurrent administration of intrathecal steroids [77,78].

Treatment

Differentiating a true septic meningitis from a chemical inflammatory meningeal reaction to contrast is pivotal for choosing an appropriate treatment for the patient. Although the clinical signs of both types of meningitis are similar,

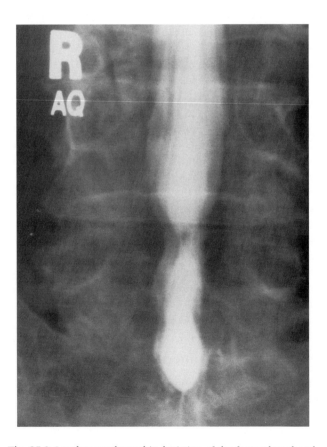

Fig. 25.9 Lumbar myelographic depiction of the featureless thecal sac of arachnoiditis.

bacterial meningitis typically results in CSF that has a protein level higher than 200 mg/100 ml and pleocytosis greater than 5000 white blood cells (WBC)/ml. Furthermore, the Gram's stain of the CSF is positive in 79% of cases and CSF culture is nearly always positive in cases of untreated bacterial meningitis [79]. Therefore, when signs of meningitis arise following myelography and the Gram's stain is positive, antibiotics are started immediately. If the Gram's stain is negative, corticosteroids and wide-spectrum antibiotics may be administered pending the results of the CSF and blood cultures. If the cultures are positive, the corticosteroids are discontinued and specific antibiotic therapy is given. Conversely, if cultures are negative, the corticosteroids are continued and the antibiotics are halted.

Anaphylactoid reaction

Anaphylactoid reactions — characterized by urticaria, bronchospasm, laryngeal edema, and/or vasomotor instability — are rarely caused by intrathecal administration of contrast. For example, no such reactions occurred in 2050 patients undergoing myelography with iohexol [53] or iopamidol [26]. Fifty of the patients receiving intrathecal iopamidol had previous histories suggestive of iodine intolerance, but none experienced any complication after premedication. Anaphylactoid reaction, however, has been reported [80]. This patient responded promptly and completely to 150 mg of prednisone intravenously. The mechanism of such anaphylactoid reactions probably involves the activation of complement sequences and the release of mediators such as histamine and bradykinin (see also Chapter 13, pp. 245, 285).

Hemorrhage

Hemorrhage is another recognized complication of dural puncture and myelography. Intraspinal hemorrhage following dural puncture most commonly occurs in the subarachnoid [81–88] or subdural spaces [88–92]; epidural hemorrhage is more rare [93,94]. Subarachnoid hemorrhage results from the spinal needle tearing a radicular vessel which enters the subarachnoid space together with a segmental nerve root. Subdural and epidural hemorrhage, conversely, are thought to occur when the ventral vertebral venous plexus is injured [81]. Iatrogenic intraspinal hemorrhage can cause pain, weakness, urinary retention, and even paraplegia [81,90,95].

A hematoma from LP can cause an extrinsic filling defect at myelography which can mimic pathology such as a disk protrusion. Therefore, LP for the purposes of myelography should not be performed at a level under clinical suspicion.

Hemorrhage can also occur with cervical punctures. In one case, intraspinal (epidural, subdural, and intramedullary) hematomas in a leukemic child resulted in temporary quadriplegia; complete recovery followed prompt surgical decompression and continued platelet support [25]. In another case, a patient with no known coagulation disorder developed a spinal subarachnoid hematoma that required surgical decompression [95]. Accidental puncture of an anomalous intraspinal vertebral artery has also been reported, resulting in death [36].

A survey of techniques and complications of cervical myelography estimated the risk of major complication during C1–2 puncture to be 0.045% (one of 2217) [54]. In this series, 25 cases of arterial hemorrhage or intramedullary spinal needle placement were reported; of these patients, two died, 10 had a persistent neurologic deficit, and 13 recovered completely. In addition, 43 major complications occurred due to cervical spine hyperextension in patients with preexisting severe cervical spondylosis and narrow spinal canals. In order to reduce these complications, these authors recommended premyelographic "scout" radiography, neutral positioning of the neck, and fluoroscopically guided needle placement.

Intracranial hemorrhage following dural puncture is a rare, but potentially catastrophic, complication. In most cases, the hematoma is subdural but intraparenchymal hemorrhage can also occur. In a literature review of 37 cases, intracranial hemorrhage was associated with the injection of spinal analgesia (29) or contrast (7) [96]. Less than 12 cases of intracranial hemorrhage have been reported involving myelography with iohexol [96–98]. Intracranial hemorrhage is thought to occur 12 hours to 7 days after myelography [97,98]. Late onset of headache after myelography is not always benign; patients with intracerebral hemorrhage after lumbar myelography have presented 1 week [96] to 2 months [99] after the procedure.

The pathogenesis of intracranial hemorrhage in these rare cases is debated. Decreased CSF pressure from LP may result in downward movement of the brain. Since the meningeal veins bridging the space between the leptomeninges and the dura lack a supportive stroma, the bridging veins can rupture and bleed [89,98,100]. Alternately, intracranial hemorrhage may reflect the neurotoxicity of the agents administered intrathecally [96].

Although no relevant preexisting disease can be found in many cases of intraspinal and intracranial hemorrhage, certain patient populations are probably at risk. In particular, patients who are elderly or have acquired immune deficiency syndrome (AIDS) commonly have cerebral atrophy; this may increase the possibility that bridging veins in the subdural space will shear when CSF pressure decreases as a result of dural puncture [99,100]. Patients with clotting abnormalities – including those with cirrhosis, thrombocytopenia, or on anticoagulant or myelosuppressive drugs – are obviously at increased risk for iatrogenic hemorrhage of all types. Rupture of a previously unsuspected aneurysm has also been reported as a cause of intracranial hemorrhage [101].

Prophylactic measures thought to minimize the possibility of hemorrhage include: (i) using needles as small as practically possible; (ii) only removing CSF that is needed; (iii) avoiding dehydration by encouraging adequate intake of oral fluids (or administering intravenous fluids, if necessary); and (iv) advising the patient to remain in the semirecumbent position for several hours after the procedure [96].

Progressive neurologic deficit or persistent pain should alert the physician to the possibility of hemorrhage, and a CT should be obtained promptly. If a hematoma is present, the patient's coagulation status should be optimized and surgical evacuation of the hematoma considered.

Neurologic symptoms

Dural puncture can cause a wide variety of neurologic symptoms, including: (i) dizziness; (ii) confusion; (iii) cranial nerve palsies; (iv) muscle weakness and spasm; (v) numbness and paresthesias involving the back, lower extremity, and coccygeal region; (vi) bladder and bowel symptoms; and (vii) paraplegia. Such morbidity is hypothesized to occur by several mechanisms, including: (i) direct injury to the spinal cord or a nerve root by the spinal needle; (ii) mass effect from hemorrhage or neck hyperextension in spondylotic patients; and (iii) contrast media causing an osmotic disturbance, direct neurotoxicity, or some unknown idiosyncratic reaction.

Cognitive and affective changes

Cognitive and affective changes after myelography have been studied by numerous investigators. Although some psychic side-effects have been described after iohexol myelography [102], they are significantly less frequent and less pronounced than after metrizamide [102,103]. Most clinical studies do not report any adverse mood changes (e.g., anxiety, anger, fatigue) or other mental disturbances with intrathecal iohexol [43,104].

Several electrophysiologic tests have been used to assess the neurotoxicity of contrast media, including electroencephalography (EEG), visual evoked potentials, and brainstem auditory evoked potentials. The epileptogenic effect of iohexol is low, especially when compared with other contrast media. Although sharp-wave activity on EEG has been reported after myelography by some [46], others have not found any epileptogenic activity after iohexol [41,53,65]. Iohexol does not cause any major or significant adverse effect on the neural pathways detected by visual evoked potentials [45] or brainstem auditory evoked potentials [45,105].

Cranial neuropathies

Impairment of cranial nerves III, IV, VI, VII, and VIII have been documented after LP and myelography [106–112]. Onset of symptoms *reportedly* can be immediate [110] or delayed for weeks [109] to years [112]. These uncommon complications are postulated to occur secondary to pressure changes in the subarachnoid space and/or the neurotoxicity of contrast media. When symptoms such as headache, nausea, and dizziness cause discomfort, such cranial nerve deficits may go unnoticed unless specific testing (e.g., audiography) is performed.

Hearing loss, in particular, is thought to occur in patients with a patent cochlear aqueduct which connects the subarachnoid and the perilymphatic spaces. When CSF pressure decreases (due to LP) or CSF osmolality increases (due to contrast injection), perilymph fluid can be released into the subarachnoid space if the cochlear aqueduct is patent. Such a shift in perilymph could drive down perilymph pressure and cause displacement of the basement membrane of the cochlea. In a series of nine cases of hearing impairment following myelography, LP, and spinal anesthesia [110], the hearing loss measured 30–70 dB and was found at lower frequencies. The impairment tended to be bilateral (six of nine) and self-limited (six of nine). Although there was a high rate of full recovery to normal hearing, a minority of patients (three of nine) complained of persistently impaired auditory acuity.

In most cases, resolution is spontaneous and complete. If such symptoms occur, however, treatment with intravenous fluids and an epidural blood patch should be considered promptly.

Severe neurologic deterioration

With current contrast media such as iohexol, seizures after myelography are rare in patients without certain predisposing factors. Risk factors for seizures include concurrent administration of drugs that lower the seizure threshold, a patient history of epilepsy, administration of an excessive contrast dose, and intracranial entry of a concentrated bolus of contrast. In the absence of these predisposing factors, few cases of seizures after iohexol [113,114] or iopamidol [115] myelography have been reported.

Encephalopathy is rarely reported in association with myelography [116–120]. When a patient does become unresponsive, it typically occurs within 1–2 days and can be heralded by disorientation and somnolence [118] or paresthesias and seizures [116]. The pathogenesis in many cases is unclear, but may be related to contrast neurotoxicity [116], plasma hypoosmolality [118], excessive fluid intake probably causing "water intoxication" [121], or renal failure [119]. Prognosis varies from complete resolution within days [118] to death [116,119]

One of these deaths was reported in a diabetic patient who experienced acute renal failure and encephalopathy after cervical myelography with 10 ml of iohexol [119]. Risk

factors for contrast-induced encephalopathy may include advanced age, diabetes, renal failure, dehydration, and myelography of the cervical spine [122,123]. The concomitant presence of diabetes and renal failure puts a patient at high risk for neurologic complications and further impairment of renal function if intrathecal contrast is administered.

Severe neurologic deterioration can also occur after dural puncture in patients with spinal subarachnoid block or increased intracranial pressure. Hollis *et al.* [124] reviewed 100 patients with complete spinal subarachnoid block at myelography, of whom 50 had an LP and 50 had a C1–2 puncture. They found that 14% of the patients who had *LP* had significant neurologic deterioration (e.g., paraplegia), whereas no deterioration occurred after *cervical* puncture. Other cases of paraplegia have been reported with LP alone or after myelography with iohexol and iopamidol [98,125–127].

LP in the setting of increased intracranial pressure is fraught with potential complications. In one series of 30 complications from LP performed in the setting of increased intracranial pressure, 13 patients (43%) lost consciousness immediately and 15 other patients (50%) experienced a progressively decreased level of consciousness within 12 hours [128]. Death occurred in 12 patients (40%) within 10 days of LP.

In patients with increased intracranial pressure or spinal tumors, removing CSF by LP is dangerous because it exacerbates already abnormal CSF pressure differentials in the cranium and the spine. In the case of increased intracranial pressure, this can result in tonsillar herniation. In the case of a spinal tumor, this can cause impaction of the mass against the spinal cord. Even if only a small amount of fluid is removed, or if volume is replaced, CSF can continue to leak out through the dural defect and perpetuate the pressure differential. In the event that a patient has a markedly elevated CSF pressure (normal range: 8–22 cmH$_2$O), therapeutic options include hyperventilation, steroids, hyperosmotic agents, and neurosurgical consultation.

Death is an extremely rare iatrogenic complication of LP and myelography when properly performed in appropriate patient populations. As alluded to above, fatalities can result secondary to hemorrhage, renal failure, or tonsillar herniation. In addition, inadvertent intrathecal injection of *ionic* contrast (e.g., meglumine diatrizoate) instead of *nonionic* compounds (e.g., iopamidol) [116,129] can be fatal, as well. The USA Food and Drug Administration received 19 reports over a 3-year period of contrast-media misadministrations, seven of which resulted in death [130]. In a series of seven misadministrations outside the USA, Rosati *et al.* [129] reported that ionic contrast media injected intrathecally was fatal for three out of seven patients.

The severity of a patient's reaction after contrast misadministration depends primarily on the osmolality and dosage of contrast [131]. Hyperosmolality tends to open the tight junctions between cells of the blood–brain barrier, thus promoting cerebral edema and limiting cerebral perfusion [132]. The contrast-media's ionicity or intrinsic neurotoxicity may change neurotransmitter metabolism, thus resulting in spasm or seizure.

To prevent misadministration, the radiologist performing the procedure should either draw up the contents of the syringe personally or witness that this is done from a bottle of nonionic contrast media. In addition, ionic and nonionic contrast media should be stored separately.

Therapeutic possibilities after such misadministrations are limited. Sedation and reverse Trendelenburg positioning may be helpful if only a few milliliters of ionic contrast have been injected. For larger volumes of ionic contrast, intrathecal lavage may be an effective intervention to dilute subarachnoid contrast [133] (see also Chapter 13, pp. 248, 285).

Pediatric patients

When performing an LP on infants and young children, some modifications in technique are necessary. Because the spinal cord may extend to the level of the L3–4 interspace, lower levels should be used. Furthermore, although unstyletted (e.g., butterfly) needles are still commonly used [134], they should be avoided because of the possibility of implanting epidermal tissue into the arachnoid and causing an iatrogenic epidermoid tumor [135]. Using a needle with a plastic hub (instead of a metal hub) allows earlier visualization of initial CSF flow and results in less weight pulling on the dura, thus helping to minimize the size of the dural defect. It is also prudent to support the spinal needle with the index finger of one hand during the procedure, since the dura in pediatric patients is not as strong as in adults.

Most of the adverse effects associated with dural puncture and myelography in children are similar to those in adults, including headache, nausea, and vomiting. In addition, adverse effects related to psychic agitation [136], anesthesia or narcotics [137], and epidermoid tumors [138] have been cited as major adverse effects. Epidermoid tumors are thought to occur when unstyletted needles (e.g., butterfly infusion needles) cut a core of epithelial tissue as they pass through the skin; the epithelial cells are then implanted in the spinal canal and grow into an intradural mass. Diagnosis is often delayed because epidermoid tumors are rare and several years usually pass between the patient's dural puncture and the onset of symptoms from the tumor [139,140]. Styletted spinal needles should always be used in order to prevent this complication [135].

When performing myelography, sedation is often given, usually with pentobarbital (Nembutal, 6 mg/kg intramuscularly or intravenously for patients <4 years old) or meperidine (Demerol, 1.5 mg/kg intramuscularly for children >4 years old) [52].

Conclusion

Hundreds of thousands of intrathecal procedures continue to be performed each year. With the advent of improved cross-sectional imaging methods and improved contrast media, both the number of intrathecal procedures and the incidence of subsequent adverse effects will probably continue to decrease. We have attempted to present the indications, contraindications, and technical considerations that physicians performing these procedures should be fully cognizant of. The above discussion also documents that the vast majority of adverse effects that occur with intrathecal procedures are minor, but severe complications are possible. Although there is clearly a need for physicians to be aware of the potential for significant — even catastrophic — complications associated with intrathecal procedures, it is equally important to place these potential hazards in proper perspective. The potential benefits of intrathecal procedures far outweigh the risks for a large number of patients. Indeed, if an overemphasis on the potential deleterious effects of these procedures led to inappropriate underutilization, many more patients would likely be harmed by a failure accurately to diagnose significant pathology than if responsible use of intrathecal procedures continues.

References

1 Sigerist HE (ed.) Domenico Cotugno: his description of the cerebrospinal fluid. *Bull Hist Med Johns Hopkins Univer* 1935;2: 701–738.

2 Quincke H. Über Hydrocephalus. Verhand Cong Med (Weisb) 1891;10:321–339. Translated in: Wilkins RH. Neurosurgical classics — XXXI. *J Neurosurg* 1965;22:294–308.

3 Quincke H. Die Lumbalpunction des Hydrocephalus. *Berl Klin Wochen Organ Pract Arzte* 1891;38:929–933.

4 Dandy WE. Ventriculography following the injection of air into the cerebral ventricles. *Ann Surg* 1918;70:397–403.

5 Ayer JB. Cerebrospinal fluid pressure from the clinical point of view. *Res Publ Assoc Res Nerv Ment Dis* 1924;41:159–171.

6 Dandy WE. Diagnosis and localization of spinal cord tumors. *Ann Surg* 1925;81:223–254.

7 Amundsen P, Skalpe IO. Cervical myelography with water soluble contrast medium (Metrizamide). *Neuroradiology* 1975; 8:209–212.

8 Skalpe IO, Amundsen P. Thoracic and cervical myelography with metrizamide. *Radiology* 1975;116:101–106.

9 Hesselink JR. Spine imaging: history, achievements, remaining frontiers. *Am J Roentgenol* 1988;150:1223–1229.

10 Thornbury JR, Fryback DG, Turski PA *et al.* Disk-caused nerve compression in patients with acute low-back pain: diagnosis with MR, CT myelography, and plain CT. *Radiology* 1993;186: 731–738.

11 Davis PC, Hoffman JC, Ball TI *et al.* Spinal abnormalities in pediatric patients: MR image findings compared with clinical, myelographic and surgical findings. *Radiology* 1988;166:679–685.

12 Kramer ED, Rafto S, Packer RJ *et al.* Comparison of myelography with CT follow-up versus gadolinium MRI for subarachnoid

metastatic disease in children. *Neurology* 1991;41:46—50.

13 Russel EJ. Cervical disk disease. *Radiology* 1990;177:313—325.

14 Rollins N, Mendelsohn D, Mulne A *et al.* Recurrent medulloblastoma: frequency of tumor enhancement on Gd-DTPA MR imaging. *Am J Neuroradiol* 1990;11:583—587.

15 Grepe A. Cisternography with metrizamide of the posterior fossa following lateral C1—2 puncture. *Acta Radiol (Stockh)* 1977;355(Suppl.):257—268.

16 Sackett JF, Strother CM, Quaglier CE, Javid MJ, Levin AB, Duff TA. Metrizamide — CSF contrast medium. *Radiology* 1977;123: 779—782.

17 Rice JF, Bathia AL. Lateral C1—2 puncture for myelography: posterior approach. *Radiology* 1979;132:760—762.

18 Leo JS, Bergeron RT, Kricheff II, Benjamin MV. Metrizamide myelography for cervical spinal cord injuries. *Radiology* 1978; 129:707—711.

19 Sortland O, Skalpe IO. Cervical myelography by lateral cervical and lumbar injection of metrizamide. *Acta Radiol (Stockh)* 1977; 355(Suppl.):154—163.

20 Grepe A. Cisternography with the non-ionic water-soluble contrast material metrizamide: a preliminary report. *Acta Radiol (Diagn) (Stockh)* 1975;16:146—160.

21 Sortland O, Nornes H, Djupesland G. Cisternography with metrizamide in cerebellopontine angle tumors. *Acta Radiol* 1977;355(Suppl.):345—356.

22 Greitz T, Hindmarsh T. Computer assisted tomography of intracranial CSF circulation using a water soluble contrast medium. *Acta Radiol* 1974;15:497—507.

23 Sortland O. CT combined with gas cisternography for the diagnosis of expanding lesions in the cerebellopontine angle. *Neuroradiology* 1979;18:19—22.

24 Gower DJ, Baker AL, Bell WO, Ball MR. Contraindications to lumbar puncture as defined by computed cranial tomography. *J Neurol Neurosurg Psychiat* 1987;50:1071—1074.

25 Mapstone TB, Rekate HL, Shurin SB. Quadriplegia secondary to haematoma after lateral C—1, C—2 puncture in leukaemic child. *Neurosurgery* 1983;12:230—231.

26 Ebersold MJ, Houser OW, Quast LM. Iopamidol myelography: morbidity in patients with previous intolerance to iodine derivatives. *J Neurosurg* 1991;74:60—63.

27 Bush WH, Swanson DP. Acute reactions to intravascular contrast media: types, risk factors, recognition, and specific treatment. *Am J Roentgenol* 1991;157:1153—1161.

28 Shapiro R. *Myelography*, 4th edn. Chicago: Yearbook Medical Publishers, 1984:71—72.

29 Farese MG, Martinez CR, Fisher CH. Inadvertent cervical cord puncture during myelography via C1—2 approach. *J Fla Med Assoc* 1990;77:91—93.

30 Morparia HK, Vontivillu J. Case report: cerebrospinal fluid fistula — a rare complication of myelography. *Clin Radiol* 1991; 44:205.

31 Orrison WW, Eldevik OP, Sackett JF. Lateral C1—2 puncture for cervical myelography. Part III: historical, anatomic, and technical considerations. *Radiology* 1983;146:401—408.

32 Gilland O. Cerebrospinal fluid dynamic diagnosis of spinal block: uniform lumbar electromanometrics. *Neurology* 1966; 16:1110—1117.

33 Potts DG, Gomez DG, Abbot GF. Possible causes of complications of myelography with water-soluble contrast media. *Acta Radiol* 1977;355(Suppl.):390—402.

34 Heinz ER, Goldman RL. The role of gas myelography in neuroradiologic diagnosis. *Radiology* 1972;102:624—629.

35 Katoh Y, Itoh T, Tsuji H *et al.* Complications of lateral C1—2 puncture myelography. *Spine* 1990;15:1085—1087.

36 Rogers LA. Acute subdural hematoma and death following lateral cervical spinal puncture: case report. *J Neurosurg* 1983; 58:284—286.

37 Orrison WW, Sackett JF, Amundsen P. Lateral C1—2 puncture for cervical myelography. Part II: recognition of improper injection of contrast material. *Radiology* 1983;146:395—400.

38 Johansen JG, Orrison WW, Amundsen P. Lateral C1—2 puncture for cervical myelography. Part I: report of a complication. *Radiology* 1983;146:391—393.

39 Smith CA, Chance KS. The effect of ambulation on post-myelography headache in patients injected with metrizamide. *J Neurosci Nurs* 1990;22:32—35.

40 Kuuliala IK, Goransson HJ. Adverse reactions after iohexol lumbar myelography: influence of postprocedural positioning. *Am J Neuroradiol* 1987;8:547—548.

41 Floras P, Deliac P, Gross C, Jouet P, Paty J, Caille JM. Neurotoxicity of iohexol vs iopamidol in lumbar myelography: clinical, electrophysiological and brain CT scan correlations. *J Neuroradiol* 1990;17:190—200.

42 Caille JM, Allard M. Contrast Media. In: Manelfe C, ed. *Imaging of the Spine and Spinal Cord.* New York: Raven Press Ltd, 1992: 195—219.

43 Lamb J. Iohexol vs. iopamidol for myelography. *Invest Radiol* 1985;20:S37—S43.

44 Davies AM, Evans N, Chandy J. Outpatient lumbar radiculography: comparison of iopamidol and iohexol and a literature review. *Br J Radiol* 1989;62:716—723.

45 Broadbridge AT, Bayliss SG, Brayshaw CI. The effect of intrathecal iohexol on visual evoked response: a comparison including incidence of headache with iopamidol and metrizamide in myeloradiculography. *Clin Radiol* 1987;38:71—74.

46 MacPherson P, Teasdale E, Coutinho C, MacGeorge A. Iohexol versus iopamidol for cervical myelography: a randomized double blind study. *Br J Radiol* 1985;58:849—851.

47 Molyneux AJ, Sheldon PW, Anslow P *et al.* A comparative trial of iohexol and iopamidol in cervical myelography. *Am J Neuroradiol* 1983;4:1145—1146.

48 Valk J, Crezee FC, de Slegte RGM *et al.* Iohexol 300 mgI/ml versus iopamidol 300 mgI/ml for cervical myelography double blind trial. *Neuroradiology* 1987;29:202—205.

49 Hoe JWN, Ng AMN, Tan LHA. A comparison of iohexol and iopamidol for lumbar myelography. *Clin Radiol* 1986;37:505—507.

50 Kido DK. *Adult lumbar myelography with iohexol (180 mgI/ml): pharmacokinetic and excretion study.* Report from the Department of Drug Metabolism and Disposition, Sterling-Winthrop Research Institute, February 3, 1984.

51 Belanger JC, Blair IG, Elder AM *et al.* Adult myelography with iohexol. *Can Assoc Radiol J* 1990;41:191—194.

52 Dube LJ, Blair IG, Geoffroy G. Paediatric myelography with iohexol. *Pediat Radiol* 1992;22:290—292.

53 Shaw DD, Bach-Gansmo T, Dahlstrom K. Iohexol: summary of North American and European clinical trials in adult lumbar, thoracic, and cervical myelography with a new nonionic contrast medium. *Invest Radiol* 1985;20:S44—S54.

54 Robertson HJ, Smith RD. Cervical myelography: survey of modes of practice and major complications. *Radiology* 1990; 174:79—83.

55 Kieffer SA, Binet EF, Davis DO *et al.* Lumbar myelography with iohexol and metrizamide: a comparative multicenter prospective

study. *Invest Radiol* 1985;20:S22—S30.

56 Bridenbaugh LD. Epidural blood patch for postmyelogram headache. *Reg Anaesth* 1977;2:4—5.

57 Sciarra D, Carter S. Lumbar puncture headache. *J Am Med Assoc* 1952;148:841—842.

58 Vandam LD, Dripps RD. Long-term follow-up of patients who received 10 098 spinal anesthetics. *J Am Med Assoc* 1956;161: 586—591.

59 Wilton NCT, Globerson JH, de Rosayro AM. Epidural blood patch for postdural puncture headache: it's never too late. *Anesth Analg* 1986;65:895—896.

60 Wilkinson AG, Sellar RJ. The influence of needle size and other factors on the incidence of adverse effects caused by myelography. *Clin Radiol* 1991;44:338—341.

61 Simon JH, Ekholm SE, Kido DK, Utz R, Erickson J. High-dose iohexol myelography. *Radiology* 1987;163:455—458.

62 Lee T, Maynard N, Anslow P, McPherson K, Briggs M, Northover J. Post-myelogram headache — physiological or psychological? *Neuroradiology* 1991;33:155—158.

63 Sand T, Stovner LJ, Myhr G, Sjaastad O. Lumbar iohexol myelography and diagnostic lumbar puncture. Headache and associated side effects in relation to neurological signs and diagnosis, previous mental symptoms and pain history. *Cephalalgia* 1990;10:9—16.

64 Eldevik OP, Nakken KO, Haughton VM. Effect of dehydration on the side effects of metrizamide myelography. *Radiology* 1978;129:715—716.

65 Maly P. Sex and age related differences in postmyelographic adverse reactions. A prospective study of 1765 myelographies. *Neuroradiology* 1989;31:331—335.

66 Cook MA, Watkins-Pitchford JM. Epidural blood patch: a rapid coagulation response. *Anesth Analg* 1990;70:567—568.

67 Shantha TR, Bisese J. Subdural blood patch for spinal headache (letter). *New Engl J Med* 1991;325:1252—1254.

68 Gibson BE, Wedel DJ, Faust RJ, Petersen RC. Continuous epidural saline infusion for the treatment of low CSF pressure headache. *Anesthesiology* 1988;68:789—791.

69 Gass H, Goldstein AS, Ruskin R, Leopold NA. Chronic post-myelogram headache. *Arch Neurol* 1971;25:168—170.

70 de Jong J, Barrs ACM. Lumbar myelography followed by meningitis (letter). *Infect Contr Hosp Epidemiol* 1992;13:74—75.

71 Mehta HJ, Ramakanta R, Piparia DH *et al*. Clinical implications of acute cerebrospinal fluid changes following iophendylate myelography. *J Postgrad Med* 1992;38:10—12.

72 Alexiou J, Deloffre D, Vandresse JH, Bouequey JP, Sintzoff S. Post-myelographic meningeal irritation with iohexol. *Neuroradiology* 1991;33:85—86.

73 Mallat Z, Vassal T, Naouri JF *et al*. Aseptic meningoencephalitis after iopamidol myelography. *Lancet* 1991;338:252.

74 Nakakoshi T, Moriwaka F, Tashiro K, Nakane K, Miyasaka K. Aseptic meningitis complicating iotrolan myelography. *Am J Neuroradiol* 1991;12:173.

75 Shaw DD, Potts DG. Toxicology of iohexol. *Invest Radiol* 1985; 20:S10—S13.

76 Haughton VM. The effect of myelography contrast media on the arachnoid. In: Amiel M, ed. *Contrast Media in Radiology*. Berlin: Springer-Verlag, 1982:149—153.

77 Roche J. Steroid-induced arachnoiditis. *Med J Aust* 1984;140: 281—284.

78 Johnson A, Ryan MD, Roche J. Depo-Medrol and myelographic arachnoiditis. *Med J Aust* 1991;155:18—20.

79 Schlesinger JJ, Salit IE, McCormack G. Streptococcal meningitis after myelography. *Arch Neurol* 1982;39:570—576.

80 Agildere AM, Haliloglu M, Cila A, Ozmen M. Laryngeal edema following the injection of iohexol into the subarachnoid space. *Neuroradiology* 1991;33:290.

81 Brem SS, Halfer DA, van Vitert RL, Ruff RL, Reichart WH. Spinal subarachnoid haematoma. A hazard of lumbar puncture resulting in reversible paraplegia. *New Engl J Med* 1981;304: 1020—1021.

82 Cooke JV. Hemorrhage into the cauda equina following lumbar puncture. *Proc Path Soc* 1911;14:104.

83 Diaz FG, Yock DH Jr, Rockswold GL. Spinal subarachnoid hematoma after lumbar puncture producing acute thoracic myelopathy: case report. *Neurosurgery* 1978;3:404—406.

84 Frager D, Zimmerman RD, Wisoff HS, Leeds NE. Spinal subarachnoid hematoma. *Am J Neuroradiol* 1982;3:77—79.

85 Hammes EM. Hemorrhage in the cauda equina secondary to lumbar puncture. *Arch Neurol Psychiat* 1920;3:595—596.

86 King OJ, Glas WW. Spinal subarachnoid hemorrhage following lumbar puncture. *Arch Surg* 1960;80:574—577.

87 Rengachary SS, Murphy D. Subarachnoid hematoma following lumbar puncture causing compression of the cauda equina: case report. *J Neurosurg* 1974;41:252—254.

88 Kirkpatrick D, Goodman SJ. Combined subarachnoid and subdural haematoma following spinal puncture. *Surg Neurol* 1975; 3:109—111.

89 Dunn D, Dhopesh V, Mobini J. Spinal subdural hematoma: a possible hazard of lumbar puncture in an alcoholic. *J Am Med Assoc* 1979;241:1712—1713.

90 Edelson RN, Chernik NL, Posner JB. Spinal subdural haematomas complicating lumbar puncture. Occurrence in thrombocytopenic patients. *Arch Neurol* 1974;31:134—137.

91 Gutterman P. Acute spinal subdural hematoma following lumbar puncture. *Surg Neurol* 1977;7:355—356.

92 Wolcott GJ, Grunnet ML, Lahey ME. Spinal subdural hematoma in a leukemic child. *J Pediat* 1970;77:1060—1062.

93 Laglis AG, Eisenberg RL, Weinstein PR, Mani RL. Spinal epidural hematoma after lumbar puncture in liver disease. *Ann Intern Med* 1978;88:515—516.

94 Stevens JM, Kendall BE, Gedroyc W. Acute epidural haematoma complicating myelography in a normotensive patient with normal blood coagulability. *Br J Radiol* 1991;64:860—864.

95 Abla AA, Rothfuss WE, Maroon JC, Deeb ZL. Delayed spinal subarachnoid haematoma: a rare complication of C1—2 cervical myelography. *Am J Neuroradiol* 1986;7:526—528.

96 Van de Kelft E, Bosmans J, Parizel PM, Van Vyve M, Selosse P. Intracerebral hemorrhage after lumbar myelography with iohexol: report of a case and review of the literature. *Neurosurgery* 1991;28:570—574.

97 Satoskar AR, Goel A, Desai AP, Usgaonkar TA. Intracranial haemorrhage and death after iohexol myelography (letter). *J Neurol Neurosurg Psychiat* 1991;54:1118—1119.

98 Bøhn HP. Intracranial haemorrhage and death after iohexol myelography (comment on letter). *J Neurol Neurosurg Psychiat* 1991;54:1119—1120.

99 Manji H, Birley H. Subdural haematoma — a complication of myelography in a patient with AIDS. *AIDS* 1990;4:698—700.

100 Dohrmann PJ, Elrick WL, Sin KH. Intracranial subdural hematoma after lumbar myelography. *Neurosurgery* 1983;12: 694—695.

101 Hart IK, Bone I, Hadley DM. Development of neurological problems after lumbar puncture. *Br Med J* 1988;296:51—52.

102 Cronqvist SE, Holtås SL, Laike T, Ozolins A. Psychic changes

following myelography with metrizamide and iohexol: a comparative investigation with psychologic tests. *Acta Radiol Diagn* 1984;25:369−373.

103 Radcliff G, Sandler S, Latchaw R. Cognitive and affective changes after myelography: a comparison of metrizamide and iohexol. *Am J Neuroradiol* 1986;7:683−687.

104 Maly P, Bach-Gansmo T, Elmqvist D. Risk of seizures after myelography: comparison of iohexol and metrizamide. *Am J Neuroradiol* 1988;9:879−883.

105 Yip PK, Chang YC, Liu HM. The effect of iohexol on brainstem auditory evoked potentials: a prospective study on 30 patients. *Neuroradiology* 1991;33:313−315.

106 Bell JA, Dowd TC, McIlwaine GG, Brittain GP. Postmyelographic abducent nerve palsy in association with contrast agent iopamidol. *J Clin Neuro-ophthalmol* 1990;10:115−117.

107 Ferrara VL. Letters to the editor (letter). *J Clin Neuro-ophthalmol* 1991;11:74.

108 Hardy PAJ. Influence of spinal puncture and injection on VIIIth nerve function. *J Laryngol Otol* 1988;102:452.

109 Kestenbaum A. *Clinical Methods of Neuro-ophthalmic Examination*, 2nd edn. New York: Grune and Stratton, 1961:287.

110 Michel O, Brusis T. Hearing loss as a sequel of lumbar puncture. *Ann Otol Rhinol Laryngol* 1992;101:390−394.

111 Miller EA, Savino PJ, Schatz NJ. Bilateral sixth-nerve palsy: a rare complication of water-soluble contrast myelography. *Arch Ophthalmol* 1982;100:603−604.

112 Mizuno M, Yamasoba T, Nomura Y. Vestibular disturbance after myelography. Contrast media in the internal auditory canal. *ORL J Otorhinolaryngol Relat Spec* 1992;54:113−115.

113 Altschuler EM, Segal R. Generalized seizures following myelography with iohexol (Omnipaque). *J Spinal Disord* 1990;3: 59−61.

114 Dalen K, Kerr HH, Wang AM, Olsen RE, Wesolowski DP, Farah J. Seizure activity after iohexol myelography (letter). *Spine* 1991;16:384.

115 Lipman JC, Wang AM, Brooks ML, Schick RM, Rumbaugh CL. Seizure after intrathecal administration of iopamidol. *Am J Neuroradiol* 1988;9:787−788.

116 Bøhn HP, Reich L, Suljaga-Petchel K. Inadvertent intrathecal use of ionic contrast media for myelography. *Am J Neuroradiol* 1992;13:1515−1519.

117 Ceylan S, Baykal S, Kuzeyli K, Akturk F, Komsuoglu S. A case of acute encephalopathy after iohexol lumbar myelography. *Clin Neurol Neurosurg* 1993;95:45−47.

118 Donaghy M, Fletcher NA, Schott GD. Encephalopathy after iohexol myelography. *Lancet* 1985;ii:887.

119 Ortiz A, Caramelo C, Fortes JR, Sarasa JL, Hernando J. Fatal coma and superimposed acute renal failure in a diabetic peritoneal dialysis patient following myelography [letter]. *Nephron* 1992;60:381−382.

120 Soriano-Soriano C, Jimenez-Jimenez FJ, Egido-Herrero JA *et al*. Acute encephalopathy following lumbar myelography with

iohexol. *Acta Neurol* 1992;14:127−129.

121 Ansell G. Radiological contrast media. In: Aronson JK, van Boxtel CJ, eds. *Side Effects of Drugs Annual 17*. Amsterdam: Elsevier Science, 1994:538.

122 Junck L, Marshall WH. Neurotoxicity of radiological contrast agents. *Ann Neurol* 1983;13:469−484.

123 Steiner E, Simon JH, Ekholm SE, Erickson H, Kido DK, Okarawa SW. Neurologic complications in diabetics after metrizamide lumbar myelography. *Am J Neuroradiol* 1986;7:323−326.

124 Hollis PH, Malis LI, Zappulla RA. Neurological deterioration after lumbar puncture below complete spinal subarachnoid block. *J Neurosurg* 1986;64:253−256.

125 Noda K, Miyamoto K, Beppu H, Hirose K, Tanabe H. Prolonged paraplegia after iohexol myelography. *Lancet* 1991;337:681.

126 Bain PG, Colchester ACF, Nadarajah D. Paraplegia after iopamidol myelography. *Lancet* 1991;338:252−253.

127 Rabinowitz JG (ed.) Woman paralyzed during myelogram. *Radiol Today* 1993;10:8.

128 Duffy GP. Lumbar puncture in the presence of raised intracranial pressure. *Br Med J* 1969;1:407−409.

129 Rosati G, Leto di Priolo S, Tirone P. Serious or fatal complications after inadvertent administration of ionic water-soluble contrast media in myelography. *Eur J Radiol* 1992;15:95−101.

130 American College of Radiology Bulletin. *FDA Seeks Boxed Warning Label on Contrast Agent Products*. July, 1993;49:3.

131 Hilz MJ, Huk W, Schellmann B, Sorgel F, Druschky KF. Fatal complications after myelography with meglumine diatrizoate. *Neuroradiology* 1990;32:70−73.

132 Velaj R, Drayer B, Albright R, Fram E. Comparative neurotoxicity of angiographic contrast media. *Neurology* 1985;35: 1290−1298.

133 Nakazawa K, Yoshinari M, Kinefuchi S, Amaha K. Inadvertent intrathecal administration of amidetrizoate. *Intens Care Med* 1973;15:55−57.

134 Halcrow SJ, Crawford PJ, Craft AW. Epidermoid spinal tumours after lumbar puncture. *Arch Dis Child* 1985;60:978−979.

135 Rawlinson MA, Coblentz CL, Franic S. Case of the month. A pearl of wisdom. *Br J Radiol* 1991;64:473−474.

136 Ruggiero R, Piscitelli G, Ambrosio A. Iopamidol for intrathecal use in pediatric neuroradiology. *Acta Radiol* 1986;(Suppl.): 532−536.

137 Kendall B. Iohexol in paediatric myelography. *Neuroradiology* 1986;28:65−68.

138 Manno NJ, Uihlein A, Kernohan JW. Intraspinal epidermoids. *J Neurosurg* 1962;19:754−765.

139 Caro PA, Marks HG, Keret D, Kumar SJ, Guille JT. Intraspinal epidermoid tumors in children: problems in recognition and imaging techniques for diagnosis. *J Pediat Ortho* 1991;11:288−293.

140 Visciani A, Savoiardo M, Balestrini MR, Solero CL. Iatrogenic intraspinal epidermoid tumor: myelo-CT and MRI diagnosis. *Neuroradiology* 1989;31:273−275.

CHAPTER 26

Complications in interventional neuroradiology

Robert D.G. Ferguson

Introduction

This chapter describes complications associated with neuro-interventional procedures and their consequences to patients and medical staff. Complications are unfavorable clinical outcomes that may result in patient injury. Whether injury occurs depends on endogenous and exogenous counter responses. If the counter response is ineffective, injury results by one or more of at least four mechanisms. This chapter focuses on complications that result in patient injury. In addition to its impact on patients, injury may adversely affect care givers by virtue of medicolegal action motivated by perceived negligence. Given the potentially devastating impact of patient injury, it is essential systematically to implement prevention of, and rapid response to, neuro-interventional complications.

Classification of complications resulting in injury

The unfavorable clinical outcomes that complicate neuro-interventional procedures are either a consequence of human error or unpredictable chance events. The latter may be due to the natural history of either the target disease, a comorbid condition, or the procedure itself (Fig. 26.1).

Mechanism of complications and their avoidance

The mechanism of complications that are directly attributable to neurointerventional procedures may be classified into one of four groups:
1 vascular obstruction;
2 vascular disruption;
3 local toxic effect;
4 systemic toxic effect.

Vascular obstruction producing ischemia

Vascular obstruction is the most common cause of neuro-interventional morbidity. Acute vascular obstruction, occurring in association with endovascular therapy, is usually due to thrombotic or thromboembolic occlusion, i.e., endothelial damage, spasm, and dissection, associated with guidewire or catheter manipulation, angioplasty balloon-induced vessel wall damage, or endovascular stent placement, which tends to produce *in situ* thrombosis at the target site (Fig. 26.2). Embolic obstruction is a consequence of distal endoluminal migration of endogenous or foreign debris. This includes thromboembolism from the surface of the vessel wall, guidewire, catheter, endovascular prosthesis, or from the margins of a therapeutically occluded vascular segment. Occasionally, the embolic debris comprises material other than thrombus,

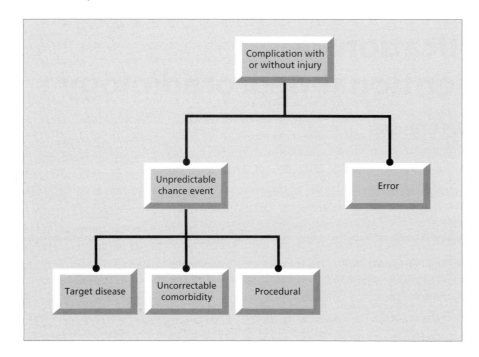

Fig. 26.1 Mechanisms of complications in neurointerventional procedures.

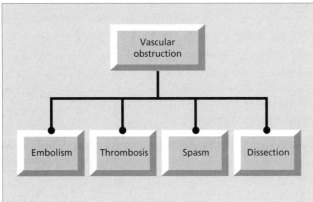

Fig. 26.2 Mechanisms of vessel obstruction.

i.e., air, catheter, or guidewire fragments, and fibers like cotton (Fig. 26.3).

Meticulous angiographic technique minimizes the potential for thrombotic and thromboembolic complications. Systemic heparinization has been advocated, but its routine use remains controversial except in revascularization therapy. Conversely, there is widespread use of continuous catheter perfusion with heparin during neurointerventional procedures. Pre- and postprocedure prescription of platelet antiaggregate drug is customary in most cerebral revascularization procedures. Postprocedure anticoagulation is less commonly advocated to prevent late thrombosis and thromboembolism.

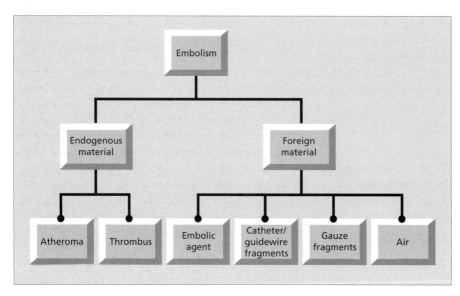

Fig. 26.3 Mechanisms of embolization.

Vascular disruption

Vascular disruption may be due to blood vessel perforation or rupture as a direct consequence of device manipulation, or as a result of induction of a coagulopathy, hemodynamic instability, or tissue necrosis. Perforation is most common with access devices (guidewires and catheters), as well as embolic agents like metallic coils. Rupture may follow balloon dilatation for atherocclusive disease and vasospasm or detachable balloon delivery.

Postlytic therapy

The exact pathophysiology of thrombolysis-associated hemorrhage in acute stroke patients is unclear. The time interval from ictus to reperfusion is thought to be a major determinant of the risk for cerebral bleeding. The increased bleeding rate with delayed reperfusion is believed to result from ischemic damage to the blood–brain barrier.

The incidence of intracranial bleeding, following local fibrinolysis for acute stroke, is uncertain. Hemorrhage may occur during or after drug infusion. The clinical manifestations can be subtle, and timely detection may be life saving. Therefore, it is essential to be familiar with the clinical manifestations of intracranial hemorrhage, which vary according to the nature and severity of the bleed. Marked contrast enhancement of brain parenchyma due to procedural contrast use may confound the computed tomographic diagnosis of parenchymal bleeding. Hyperdensity due to contrast enhancement should diminish, however, on serial scans at 4–8-hour intervals, while hyperdensity resulting from intracranial hemorrhage will remain stable over this period. Anticoagulation may increase the incidence of intracranial bleeding; however, this remains unproven.

Post-therapeutic embolization

Embolization procedures, that produce devascularization by design, may be complicated by ischemic and hemorrhagic complications. Cerebral ischemia may follow arterial or venous occlusion, culminating in infarction, depending on the extent and site of the involved territory. The infarct may then undergo hemorrhagic conversion as a result of tissue necrosis or reperfusion injury.

While excessive devascularization clearly causes unintentional ischemia, little is conclusively known about the pathogenesis of embolization-related hemorrhage. Rapid change in perfusion pressure (normal perfusion breakthrough), venous outlet occlusion, and specific agent characteristics have been implicated as causative factors.

Vascular perforation or rupture

Several endovascular therapeutic devices can produce perforation or rupture (Fig. 26.4). Thrombogenic intravascular coils, used for therapeutic vascular occlusion, may, on occasion, perforate vessels. Subarachnoid or intracerebral hemorrhage will result if the puncture is intracranial. This occurrence is more likely during coil placement in inherently weak vascular structures, particularly cerebral aneurysms and venous varices which are thin-walled compared to cerebral arteries. The other major cause of vascular perforation is intracranial guidewire manipulation. Although guidewire tips are designed to be atraumatic, they may, under certain conditions, exert sufficient force to breach the vessel wall. Maximum care must be exercised when pushing the tip of the guide out of the catheter, as the tip is supported while inside the distal most segment of the catheter, leading to reduced flexibility, i.e., the wire tip remains relatively rigid until it is advanced several millimeters beyond the tip of the catheter.

Local toxic effect

Toxic injury may be produced locally or systemically. Although the final common pathway for locally mediated toxicity is neuronal injury, a variety of stimuli initiate this process (Fig. 26.5). Direct toxic injury is most often seen following infusion of pharmacologic agents such as papavarine, various experimental chemotherapeutic agents, or contrast media. The

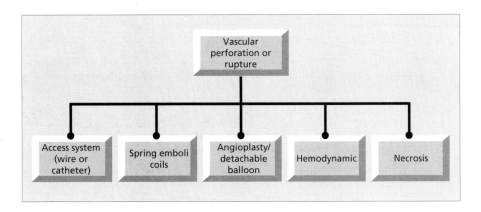

Fig. 26.4 Causes of vascular disruption.

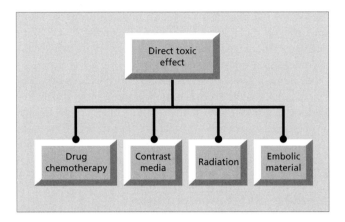

Fig. 26.5 Stimuli of local toxicity.

toxicity of these agents is related to their local tissue concentration. In addition to dosing error, hyperconcentration may also occur due to streaming or other hemodynamic peculiarities. Caution should be employed in catheter positioning to minimize the potential for such an occurrence.

Additionally, certain embolic materials, such as ethanol, produce direct cellular injury or death. The selection of an embolic agent requires careful consideration of the risks and benefits and demands judicious selection and cautious use.

Finally, radiation associated with prolonged fluoroscopy and radiography, may produce local injury, most commonly alopecia. Reduced dose fluoroangiography, now available on many machines, should be employed whenever possible. Maximum collimation should also be used, in association with optimized radiographic technique.

Systemic toxic effect

Systemic toxicity may occur during or following the procedure. Intraprocedural systemic toxicity may result from: (i) baroreceptor-induced, hemodynamically significant bradycardia associated with angioplasty or balloon occlusion of the internal carotid bulb; (ii) anaphylactoid contrast or anesthetic reactions, or malignant hyperthermia due to anesthesia; and (iii) respiratory depression associated with narcotic sedation (Fig. 26.6). Contrast-media-induced acute tubular necrosis (ATN), fluid overload, and infection are complications that, typically, are manifest after the procedure.

Incidence of complications for vascular interventions

The utilization of neuroendovascular therapy assumes that the risk of therapy is less than the risk of the target disease treated by alternate means, if alternates exist, or left untreated if they do not. However, the low incidence and prevalence of many serious conditions for which there is no effective therapeutic alternative, leads to reliance on imprecise studies that could not exclude potentially important biases. The relative immaturity of interventional neuroradiology as a clinical and scientific discipline further frustrates attempts to discern accurate rates of procedural complications. Hence, the incidence of complications in neuroradiology is difficult to estimate and the scientific basis for making risk–benefit assessments is often tenuous. There are no registries or systematic efforts to collect such data, yet.

Countermeasures for complications

Specific rescue technology and techniques

The choice of endovascular countermeasures depends on whether the adverse event is vasocclusive or hemorrhagic. Revascularization techniques are employed in cases of vasoocclusion, while devascularization technology and techniques are employed if bleeding occurs. These measures are used in conjunction with appropriate surgical or medical therapies, to assist in limiting the potential for patient injury.

Different technologies have evolved to address the two major categories of complication. For acute vascular occlusion with cerebral ischemia there are snares, retrievers, stents, stenting maneuvers, and lytic agents. For acute vascular injury with bleeding there is Amicar (ε-aminocaproic acid)

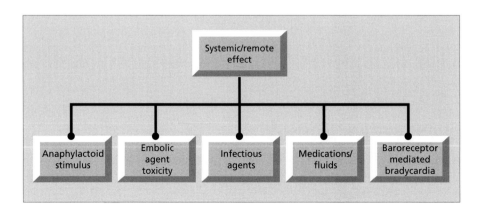

Fig. 26.6 Causes of systemic toxic effects.

and other procoagulants, and fresh frozen plasma (FFP), as well as vasocclusion devices and materials.

Hemorrhagic complications

Treatment is first directed at normalization of coagulation status. Protamine sulfate is employed to reverse the systemic effects of heparinization. An attempt should next be made to reestablish hemostasis at the site of vascular injury, be it within an aneurysm sac, varix, or other target vascular structure. In some cases, however, it may not be possible to restore vascular integrity locally, and treatment may then require control of inflow by occlusion of the parent vessel. Such a desperate measure should be employed if the effect of the resultant reduction in perfusion is likely to produce less harm than subarachnoid hemorrhage-related morbidity. In cases of vascular perforation, reversal of anticoagulation should be performed, followed by serial angiographic evaluation of the perforation site, using nonionic contrast media to avoid the cerebral irritation that is associated with extravasation of ionic media into the subarachnoid space. We have witnessed approximately 12 such incidents over the past 9 years, all of which were self-limited without additional instrumentation. This experience argues strongly against the remedial passage of the catheter across the site of vascular injury so as to permit placement of a thrombogenic coil through the breach in the vessel wall. Such therapy necessarily produces enlargement of the hole in the blood vessel, while also requiring the proximal end of the coil to be retained in the parent vessel lumen, thereby forming a potential embologenic stimulus. It is our belief that treatment by embolization should be reserved for incidents where bleeding is not self-controlled.

Ischemic complications

With exception of ischemia related to hypoperfusion due to cardiopulmonary arrest, acute ischemia occurring in association with, or as a consequence of, endovascular therapy is almost always thrombotic or thromboembolic in nature. Rarely, nonthrombotic atheroma may embolize. *In situ* thrombotic complications may result from angioplasty balloon- or catheter-induced vessel wall damage, or from implantation of an intravascular foreign body, such as a stent. The feared consequence of thrombotic or thromboembolic complications is tissue ischemia. In cases of acute vascular occlusion, endovascular and surgical countermeasures are directed at removing the offending stimulus, while medical measures are most commonly prescribed to mitigate the effects of tissue ischemia. In some cases, as in errant detachable balloon or coil delivery, it may be possible to extract the embolus. Similarly, other radiopaque foreign material may, occasionally, be retrieved using a variety of devices specifically designed for this purpose. This category of device includes snares and microforceps. Vasocclusion resulting from thrombus may be amenable to locally administered thrombolytic agents such as tissue plasminogen activator or urokinase. Preliminary experience suggests that this technique may be effective when little time has elapsed between the onset of occlusion and initiation of therapy, as is typically the case in treatment of iatrogenic vasocclusion.

Rarely, direct surgical exposure of the occluded vessel may also be used to restore flow in the cerebral circulation. Thrombectomy and embolectomy, however, are considered by most neuroscientists as heroic measures to be considered when endovascular measures fail or are impossible.

Certain medical therapies should be considered along with endovascular and surgical remedial measures. Additional medical therapy is directed at inhibiting further clot formation and propagation, increasing tissue perfusion via collateral inflow and the microvasculature, and maximizing oxygen saturation and delivery. Therefore, therapy with platelet antiaggregate drugs, anticoagulants, volume expanders, positive inotropic agents, vasopressors, and oxygen are warranted except in cases where an underlying condition precludes their use.

In cases of vascular obstruction, attributable to luminal compromise due to inward collapse of the vessel wall or its components, angioplasty, with or without intravascular stents or other implantable devices, may effect reperfusion with relief of ischemia. The simplest of these involves placing a stenting or perfusion catheter to allow perfusion through the catheter device as that catheter bridges the occluded segment. Alternately, balloon catheters have been employed to reappose intima in cases of occlusive dissection. Finally, implantable stents offer the potential to support collapsed vascular structures by means of placement of expandable cylindric metallic structures across a collapsed vascular segment.

The importance of familiarity with rescue maneuvers

Neurointerventionalists must be skilled in the use of remedial measures that can mitigate the adverse impact of complications. The choice of corrective measures depends on the ability to recognize significant clinical change, and correctly to identify its neurologic cause. The clinical presentation of certain complications makes this difficult in the arteriography suite, where the patient is relatively inaccessible and the clinical evaluation is constrained. Certain conditions, like dysphasia, may render the patient unable to communicate cogently. In addition, physical signs may escape detection because the patient is draped and kept immobile to maintain a sterile operative field. Furthermore, it may be impossible to interrupt the sequence of therapeutic maneuvers at sufficiently regular intervals to ensure immediate detection of all neurologic complications. A balance between detection of such complications and safe and timely performance of the therapeutic maneuvers is necessary. For example, a patient may not notice or report monocular blindness secondary to central retinal artery embolization during or immediately following therapy. Similarly, nondominant parietal brain injury may be asymptomatic and produce only subtle neurologic signs. It is therefore incumbent on the operator to maximize the potential for detecting subtle neurologic dysfunction. This can be approached by implementation of an effective clinical monitoring protocol that includes serial neurologic evaluation — except in cases performed under general anesthesia — in addition to routine monitoring of vital signs. If the monitoring is performed by allied health professionals, the interventionalist should ensure their competence.

If an adverse event occurs, timely response may prevent permanent tissue injury and a bad outcome. The operator's response should not be limited to remedial endovascular maneuvers. He/she must also optimize general patient care to achieve maximum risk reduction. Therefore, the neuro-interventionalist must initiate and maintain effective emergency supportive measures until the consultants arrive. These measures should be instituted in concert with specific remedial endovascular therapy and, if necessary, surgical correction. They include: volume expansion, therapeutic hyper- and hypotension, pharmacologic corrective measures, oxygen therapy, coagulation normalization, seizure management, pain control, and cardiac arrhythmia management.

Patient injury

Tissue injury occurring during neurotherapeutic vascular interventions may be a manifestation of unpredictable chance events, the result of deliberate action, or a consequence of human error (Fig. 26.7).

Unpredictable chance events

Target disease

Several anecdotes have confirmed the occurrence of target disease-related morbidity *prior* to the initiation of therapy. Many operators have witnessed preprocedural morbidity, including stroke and death, sometimes occurring only minutes prior to initiation of the procedure. It is a matter of probability that some patients who are about to undergo an intervention will suffer clinical deterioration prior to the procedure. Similarly, some patients will also deteriorate during the procedure, independent of the intervention and despite optimal technique. Since it is difficult to separate the effects of the target disease from those of the procedure under these circumstances, it is likely that some complications are erroneously attributed to the procedure when they are in fact a consequence of coincidental disease progression.

Procedure

Unknown factors that are beyond the control of the operator can affect the risk of procedural complication. For example, it appears that the risk of significant arterial dissection during angioplasty of atherosclerotic lesions depends on the volume of the plaque's necrotic core; however, there is currently no way of measuring or predicting this feature of the target lesion preoperatively. Device failure may also lead to unforeseeable negative patient consequences. For example, the loss of fluoroscopic guidance during a critical interventional maneuver, or the rupture of a catheter or balloon during embolization or angioplasty could produce significant patient injury through no fault of the operator.

Comorbidity

The occurrence of a comorbid event may either be independent of the neurointervention, or it may occur as a result of the procedure, as in contrast nephropathy in diabetics and multiple myeloma patients, or hemorrhage complicating neurointervention in patients with bleeding diatheses. Detailed preprocedure diagnosis and planning will alert the operator to the need for prophylactic therapy to reduce the risk of comorbid events.

Deliberate action

Planned or anticipated injury, undertaken with the patient's prior consent, while not a complication of the procedure, has the potential to produce harm. The sacrifice of tissue and function, as in the case of posterior cerebral artery embolization where a quadrantinopsia is predicted, and therefore anticipated, might reasonably be viewed as an acceptable concession to obtain a beneficial overall outcome. Deliberate tissue sacrifice should only be entertained after careful consideration and informed consent, and only if there is a reasonable prospect that such treatment will produce a net beneficial effect at the time, or confer sufficient reduction in the risk of future injury, to justify the anticipated loss (Fig. 26.7). Therefore, limited patient injury, even when deliberate, may sometimes be acceptable, if not desirable, if such action is taken with the intent to prevent even greater harm to the patient. This unusual situation, where sacrifice of tissue and/ or function is predicted, must always involve communication of the predicted adverse functional consequences and counseling as to the anticipated impact to the patient. The sole exception is in the case of a rapidly evolving emergency, where delay in obtaining such consent could reasonably be expected to result in harm to the patient.

Human error

All physicians are human. All humans commit errors. Some

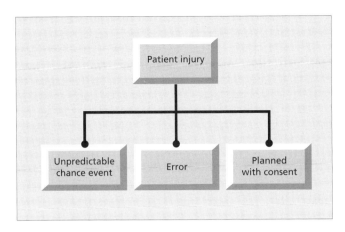

Fig. 26.7 Causes of injury during neurointerventional procedures.

errors cannot be reasonably anticipated and, hence, prevented, even by the most assiduous and careful of operators. Errors are of two types: (i) those that fall within the standard of care (nonnegligent); and (ii) those that occur in relation to treatment rendered outside of the legally accepted standard of care (negligence/malpractice) (Fig. 26.8). Whether error constitutes negligence in a particular case may be extremely difficult to establish scientifically and legally. Ultimately, this issue is arbitrated by the courts and decided by juries.

Although legal sophistry might occasionally confuse some jurors, only a dedicated misologist would equate error with negligence. Common sense tells us this is inappropriate, otherwise a physician would be held to an impossible standard of perfection. Yet, USA tort law provides little insight into specific measures that may be employed to determine responsibility in an individual case. Instead, the law has generally been interpreted as requiring the physician to perform to the standard of a similarly trained physician, according to either a local or national standard, depending on the jurisdiction. The lack of objective criteria implicit in such a system leaves considerable leeway to imply negligence in the case of physician error. Even the most zealous plaintiff attorneys would concede that not all suits that go to trial against physicians are meritorious, yet every suit that reaches such a point must necessarily be supported by a physician ready to provide presumably expert testimony that the defendant's alleged error was legally untenable. Verdicts therefore ultimately hinge on the jury's assessment of the credibility of the experts' opinions, which are necessarily contradictory on the issue of standard of care.

Relationship of error to patient injury

A complication may or may not result in an adverse event or bodily harm. The impact of a narrowly averted tragedy may, however, prompt considerable operator behavioral modification and ultimately have a substantial effect on the modification of therapy and technique. Such changes in practice are not necessarily progressive, however. The application of outcome analysis and failure avoidance strategies to interventional neuroradiologic procedures, even if methodical, rarely provides pristine enlightenment. The erroneous attribution of causality to a particular procedural factor may result in a less effective and no less dangerous therapy.

Medicolegal aspects of complications

Standard of care: error and negligence

Error is a *sine qua non* of negligence. Error, however, is not *de facto* proof of negligence (Fig. 26.9). Proof of malpractice requires that two conditions be met.

1 It must be established that an error occurred. This require-

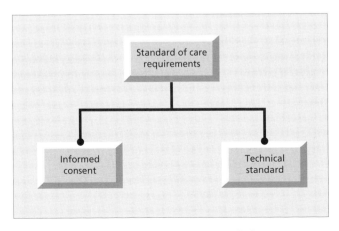

Fig. 26.8 Elements of the definition of standard of care.

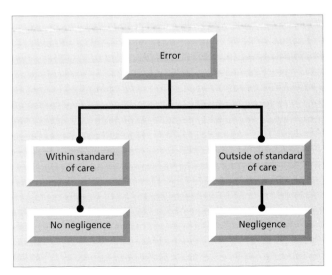

Fig. 26.9 The concept of error as a function of standard of care.

ment is satisfied by a determination of fact by the judge or jury.

2 The error leading to a complication must be of a nature that is sufficiently egregious to justify sanction by the court. In contrast, this determination is not one of fact but instead relies on the judgement of citizens to interpret the evidence and arrive at a conclusion regarding the magnitude and character of the error. This type of determination is by its very nature subjective, susceptible to bias, and inextricably linked to the notion of a standard. This standard presumes that such an individual will have the requisite training, affirmed through institutional credentialing, to be considered qualified to perform procedures specified by the credentialing process. Such a standard further requires that the practitioner be familiar with the standard of practice of peers. Information gathered through attendance at local, regional, and national meetings provides individual operators with the means to compare their performance with that of similarly qualified individuals in the local, regional, and national community. While this process ensures that the individual cannot be assailed by virtue of simple performance of specific procedures, it does not immunize him or her against claim of malpractice in specific instances.

The nature of the adversarial process is one that encourages and rewards those best able to convince the jury. The process of conquering a jury's collective heart, however, is divergent from the normal practice of scientific investigation and the search for truth. Sophistry and style may triumph over restrained objectivity and truth. The financial benefits for providing testimony in malpractice cases does not provide reassurance regarding the purity of motive. Documented hourly rates far in excess of what the expert would be expected to make in clinical practice raise concern regarding the potential for conflict of interest and bias.

Informed consent

It is the operator's legal and ethical responsibility to obtain informed consent. Specific requirements vary from state to state, according to applicable statutes. There is considerable uncertainty concerning the requirements for disclosing procedural success and complication rates that must be met to secure informed consent. In the absence of vast personal procedural experience, operators should offer the most conservative risk estimates available. This will obviate the need to justify the selection of more optimistic estimates that are based on the results obtained by more experienced operators.

In nonemergent cases, when the patient is unable to provide informed consent by virtue of neurologic dysfunction, as in severe head trauma or acute stroke, state law may permit surrogate consent, usually from the next of kin. Obtaining surrogate consent for investigational therapies is more complex. The procedure for doing so varies by state; however, not all jurisdictions permit surrogate consent by the next of kin in this situation. A policy regarding this matter should be formulated in concert with hospital administration. Finally, informed consent is not required in a neurologic emergency, when the anticipated delay in initiating therapy would harm the patient.

Special considerations in pediatric neurointervention

Although children may have a greater potential for recovery from neurologic injury than adults, they are more susceptible to the complications of some interventions. This is primarily because most devices and procedures were developed for adults and they are not easily downscaled for use in children, especially the very young. Contrast toxicity, thermal stress, intravenous fluid volume, ionizing radiation, and vessel trauma may have disproportionately harsh effects in this age group. Operators who treat young children should acquaint themselves with the idiosyncrasies of pediatric neuroendovascular therapy.

Nontreatment

The principle of *primum non nocere* — first do no harm — is one of the basic tenets that guide patient care. There may be occasions, however, when this philosophy may be misinterpreted. No treatment is without risks. The decision to treat must reflect the risk of the underlying condition versus, the net impact of the proposed therapy. In many circumstances, the risk of therapy will only be less than the risk of the underlying condition when considered in the context of an interval longer than that required to deliver therapy. Therefore, the decision to subject patients to such risk must be predicated on the belief that the patient's ultimate risk, measured over some time interval longer than that required to deliver treatment, will be lower than if therapy had been withheld. The interval used to compare the relative risk will vary as a function of the characteristics and severity of disease.

Complications of percutaneous intervention in the thorax

Simon P.G. Padley and Christopher D.R. Flower

Introduction

Percutaneous intervention in the thorax is an expanding area of interest to radiologists, with needle biopsy of focal lung disease still constituting the most commonly undertaken procedure. Initially, the practice of percutaneous needle biopsy was given great impetus by the classic work of Dahlgren and Nordenstrom over 25 years ago [1]. Since then, lung needle biopsy has been increasingly widely used and is now an accepted method of obtaining lung tissue with a high degree of accuracy and an acceptably low morbidity. More recently, percutaneous interventional techniques in the thorax have been extended to include biopsy of diffuse lung disease, pleural and mediastinal lesions, thoracentesis, and empyema drainage.

It is standard practice for percutaneous thoracic intervention to be performed using some form of imaging guidance. In the majority of cases, fluoroscopy is the most appropriate modality, but in certain circumstances computed tomography (CT) and ultrasonography are more suitable. Many of the complications that will be discussed are more likely to occur if biopsies are performed without imaging guidance.

Lung needle biopsy

Contraindications

Contraindications to lung needle biopsy include bleeding diathesis and anticoagulant therapy, patients with leukemia, underlying emphysema or bullae, contralateral pneumonectomy, pulmonary hypertension, and lack of patient cooperation. All are relative and depend upon the severity of the abnormality and the ability to correct it to reduce the likelihood of complications. More specific contraindications are a likely diagnosis of echinococcal cyst or pulmonary arteriovenous malformation.

Anticoagulant therapy must be adjusted to provide a satisfactory prothrombin index prior to intervention [2]. Some bleeding diatheses can be temporarily corrected. For example, localized pulmonary opacities in platelet-deficient patients can be biopsied with relative safety under cover of platelet transfusion. Although percutaneous biopsy of echinococcal cysts has been reported without serious consequences [3,4], it would seem prudent to avoid such a biopsy because of the risk of an anaphylactoid reaction following spillage of the cyst contents into the bronchial tree or pulmonary circulation. Similarly, although puncture of a vascular malformation is unlikely to produce severe bleeding because of the relatively low pressure within the pulmonary circuit, such lesions are best avoided by their prior recognition. It has been claimed that vascular malformations may be diagnosed by transcutaneous puncture and the injection of contrast medium [5]. However, this procedure is associated with a risk of air embolism and a preferable way of making the diagnosis is by CT or pulmonary angiography. Peripheral pulmonary masses can be biopsied relatively safely in the presence of pulmonary hypertension, but it is probably wise to avoid biopsy of juxtahilar masses where the hazard of inadvertent puncture of a major pulmonary artery with subsequent hemorrhage is greatest. The likelihood of producing a pneumothorax is obviously greater in patients with emphysematous lungs and/or bullae. Furthermore, the consequences of a pneumothorax in this group and in patients who have poor respiratory reserve, for whatever reason, are more severe. The prebiopsy use of CT to delineate bullous areas will enable the most suitable biopsy route to be chosen. By whichever technique biopsies are performed, it is essential for the patient to cooperate by lying still for 10–15 minutes and either suspending respiration at appropriate moments or breathing in a quiet controlled fashion. The risk of complications, particularly pneumothorax, is greatly increased if patients are not able to cooperate. Similarly, the hazard of pulmonary hemorrhage is increased in patients who have a depressed cough reflex, either because of debilitation or oversedation. For this reason we do not advise the use of premedication.

Complications of percutaneous lung biopsy

Reported complications of percutaneous lung biopsy are pneumothorax, pulmonary hemorrhage, hemothorax, tumor implantation, air embolism, tumor embolism, subcutaneous and mediastinal emphysema, empyema, and bronchopleural fistula (Table 27.1). The most important and potentially the most dangerous of these are pneumothorax and pulmonary hemorrhage. Overall mortality rate is extremely low (< 0.1% overall) [1,6–9], but deaths have been recorded due to massive pulmonary hemorrhage, tension pneumothorax, air embolism, and cardiac arrest [10–17]. The likelihood of such a catastrophe occurring is greatest in elderly or debilitated patients, with the use of cutting needles and biopsy of lesions adjacent to the central pulmonary vessels. The technique should not be performed in isolation from bronchoscopic facilities and the operator should be able to insert a chest tube drain.

Pneumothorax

In most large series, the likelihood of producing a pneumothorax is given as between 10 and 40% [6,7,9,14,17–22]. The increasingly common use of CT for lung needle biopsy has shown that the likelihood of a small pneumothorax is higher than previously appreciated on chest radiography (Fig. 27.1). Factors that increase the chances of producing a pneumothorax are:
1 the type of needle used — fine-gage (20–22-gage) needles

Table 27.1 Frequency of complications following lung needle biopsy

Complications	Incidence (%)
Pneumothorax	10–40
Pulmonary hemorrhage	5–15
Hemothorax, mediastinal emphysema	< 1
Others	≪ 0.1

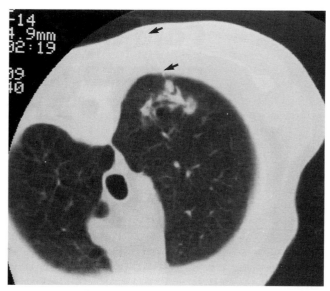

(a)

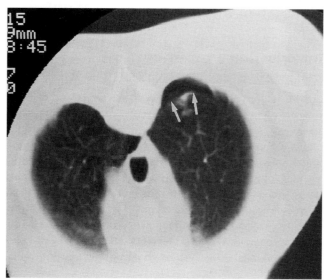

(b)

Fig. 27.1 (a) CT scan of a lesion in the left upper lobe of a 60-year-old male smoker, confirming correct placement of the needle (arrows). The patient is prone and a posterior approach has been used. (b) Immediate postbiopsy CT scan 2 cm cranial to the lung lesion. There is a small pneumothorax evident (arrows) that was not visible on the 4 hour postbiopsy chest radiograph. (Final diagnosis bronchioloalveolar cell carcinoma.)

are less likely to produce this complication than large-gage (16–18-gage) or cutting needles [4,6];
2 the number of times the pleura is transgressed (this includes not only the number of passes made by the biopsy needle but also inadvertent puncture of the pleura during infiltration with local anesthetic);
3 the size and depth of the lesion (as Sinner [6] has pointed

out, the biopsy of deep-seated lesions is more likely to result in a pneumothorax);

4 pre-existing lung disease, poor patient cooperation, and operator inexperience.

Experienced operators are more likely to obtain a satisfactory specimen at the first attempt and to spend less time with the needle in the lung, thereby diminishing the likelihood of pleural lacerations. It has been suggested that if a patient breathes oxygen during the procedure, both the likelihood and size of a pneumothorax are diminished [23].

The use of CT guidance rather than fluoroscopic guidance results in an increased period during which the needle transfixes the lung and an increased likelihood of a pneumothorax on the follow-up chest radiograph. As a result, CT guidance should be reserved for patients in whom the lesion is too small or too indistinct to be readily visible on fluoroscopy, and also where the lesion lies adjacent to vital structures such as the heart or great vessels.

The majority of pneumothoraces are small and do not require drainage. However, in approximately one of every five to eight patients who develop a pneumothorax, tube drainage will be required [1–7,14]. While a pneumothorax of greater than 30% of the volume of the affected lung is likely to require a chest drain, the size of the pneumothorax in itself is not an indication for drain insertion. The need for a chest drain is determined by the development of respiratory embarrassment, or progression in the size of the pneumothorax (Fig. 27.2).

It is usual for a very small amount of fluid to be associated with a pneumothorax and cause slight blunting of the costophrenic angle. However, the presence of any significant amount of pleural fluid should suggest an associated hemopneumothorax and prompt the immediate insertion of a chest drain.

Several techniques have been suggested to reduce the frequency and size of pneumothoraces. Injection of compressed collagen plugs into the needle tract as the needle is withdrawn has been shown to result in a reduced incidence of pneumothorax; however, there was no difference in the number of patients requiring chest drain insertion compared to a control group [24]. Other workers advocate the use of autologous blood clot injected into the needle tract as the needle is withdrawn, a practice known as the blood patch technique. Reports of the effectiveness of this technique are mixed [25] and overall it seems of doubtful clinical utility. Not surprisingly, a reduction in the rate of pneumothorax formation has been observed when the biopsy tract avoids aerated lung [26].

Attention to patient positioning following lung needle biopsy has been shown to reduce both the frequency of pneumothorax formation and the proportion of pneumothoraces subsequently requiring chest drain insertion [27–29]. In these series, the patients were placed with the biopsy site dependent and were restricted from coughing, moving,

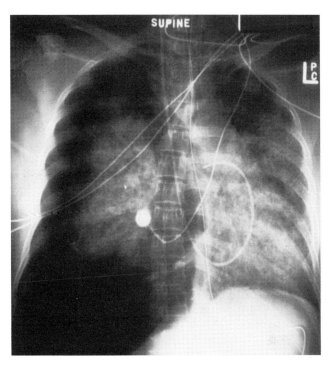

(a)

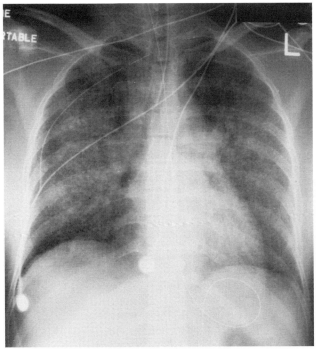

(b)

Fig. 27.2 (a) Supine chest radiograph of a 46-year-old male patient with acute diffuse lung disease, 20 minutes subsequent to a transbronchial biopsy. There is a large tension pneumothorax everting the right hemidiaphragm and shifting the mediastinum to the left. (b) Supine radiograph 15 minutes later following emergency insertion of an intercostal drain. (Final diagnosis pulmonary hemorrhage complicating Wegener's granulomatosis.)

or talking for at least 1 hour following the procedure.

When chest drain insertion is deemed necessary, it can be achieved by either the formal insertion of a standard chest drain, or by insertion of a radiographic catheter or narrow bore chest drain attached to a unidirectional air flow valve (Heimlich valve) [13,19,30–32]. This latter technique is preferred since it is relatively simple and safe, can be rapidly employed in the emergency situation, and causes the patient the minimum of discomfort and trauma compared to standard large-bore chest tube insertion. It is good practice to keep the patient in the radiology department for 10 minutes following biopsy, so that any rapidly progressive pneumothorax can be identified and managed. If there are no problems at this stage, check films are taken at 4 hours and first thing in the morning after an overnight stay. In some centers [8], the procedure is performed on an outpatient basis in suitably selected patients. Under these circumstances, the patient must be kept under observation for 4 hours following biopsy and only discharged if there is no radiographic evidence of a pneumothorax, and providing that he or she is conversant with the symptoms of a pneumothorax and has ready and rapid access to hospital care.

Pulmonary hemorrhage

A small blush at the site of the biopsied lesion is frequently seen at fluoroscopy following biopsy, due to a small focal pulmonary hemorrhage. Occasionally, this results in a small hemoptysis or in blood staining of sputum. With fine, 20–22-gage needles, this complication occurs in approximately 5–10% of patients [7,8,14,19]. The likelihood of significant pulmonary hemorrhage is increased by the use of 16–18-gage and cutting needles [4,13,33], although fatalities have also been described with: (i) the use of fine needles [12,16]; (ii) with biopsy in the presence of pulmonary hypertension; (iii) biopsy of juxtahilar masses [6]; and (iv) biopsy in diffuse lung disease. Any bleeding tendency greatly increases the risk of severe hemorrhage. Anticoagulant therapy is almost an absolute contraindication. The prothrombin time should not be extended by more than 3 seconds from the control. Leukemic patients who require a needle biopsy to establish the nature of a focal opacity are obviously at great risk if they are thrombocytopenic. In these circumstances, biopsy should be carried out during the transfusion of fresh plasma or platelets. Elderly and debilitated patients are particularly at risk from pulmonary hemorrhage because their relatively poor cough mechanism will prevent effective expectoration of blood, and increase the likelihood of respiratory embarrassment.

Massive pulmonary hemorrhage is the most feared complication of lung biopsy. Unlike the other major complication of the technique — tension pneumothorax — it is much less readily controlled and is the cause of most fatalities from biopsy. In most patients, pulmonary hemorrhage will cease soon after the biopsy and endobronchial blood will be coughed free. During this period, the patient should be retained on his or her side — the lung that has been biopsied being dependent. Continued hemorrhage will require bronchoscopic intubation and bronchial suction followed by occlusion of the appropriate bronchus with a balloon catheter. It is axiomatic that such facilities must be immediately available wherever biopsies are undertaken.

Proponents of the use of cutting needles claim that the risk of hemorrhage and pneumothorax is no greater than with fine needles if the technique is reserved for patients with masses that are reasonably superficial (3–8 cm from the skin surface) and are larger than 2–3 cm in diameter [34,35]. Cutting needles provide samples that are larger than those from fine-gage needles and they are more consistently suitable for histologic as opposed to cytologic interpretation.

Tumor implantation

Seeding of tumor along the needle track has been reported but is very rare [6,36–38]. The likelihood of this occurring is greatest following the use of cutting needles [35,39,40]. Mesotheliomas are particularly likely to seed to the skin. The incidence of tumor implantation following biopsy with fine-gage needles is very low, there being no recorded instances in most reported series. In a series of 4000 biopsies, Nordenstrom and Bjork [39] reported one definite case of seeding along a needle track and one possible case. Whether or not interference with the tumor by the needle tip is likely to increase the chances of hematogenous dissemination of the tumor is not known.

Air embolism

There are very few documented instances of this complication, which can be fatal [15,33,41,42]. In order to avoid the possibility of air embolus, patients should never be examined in the upright or semirecumbent position, but always when lying horizontally. This complication is also more likely when the lesion is adjacent to central pulmonary veins. The needle tip should never be allowed to remain in a pulmonary vein and care should always be taken to occlude the hub of the needle following removal of the stylet. Air embolism is possible if a communication is formed between a bronchus or lung cavity and an adjacent vein; this is more likely in patients with diffuse lung disease and a reduced lung compliance, particularly when cutting needles are used [33]. Air embolism should be suspected in patients who become acutely confused or obtunded during the biopsy procedure. The diagnosis of air embolus may be documented at the time of CT-guided biopsy by demonstration of intracardiac air or air within the cerebral circulation [42–44]; in the majority of cases, fluoroscopic guidance is likely to have been utilized, necessitating the diagnosis to be suspected clinically. Initial treatment should include placing the patient in a left-lateral decubitus position with the head dependent, administration of 100% oxygen and, if available, transfer to a hyperbaric oxygen unit, in addition to general supportive therapy [45,46].

Other complications

Subcutaneous and mediastinal emphysema are rare and almost invariably unimportant minor complications which are usually secondary to the production of a pneumothorax [6,18,21]. Mediastinal emphysema is more likely to occur following the biopsy of lesions in, or immediately adjacent to the mediastinum. Similarly, *mediastinal hematomas* may occur following the biopsy of mediastinal masses [47]. Only fine 21–22-gage aspirating needles should be used for the biopsy of mediastinal and hilar masses. Under these circumstances, the likelihood of serious mediastinal hemorrhage is remote [47].

Hemothorax occurs in under 1% of patients [6,8,14,18,21], and is most likely to occur with the use of cutting needles and following the inadvertent laceration of an intercostal or internal mammary vessel. Intercostal vessels can usually be avoided by not using an immediately subcostal approach. Although the production of an *empyema* is recorded [6], this is a very rare complication, even when biopsy is performed for the microbiology of localized pulmonary infections [2,48]. There have been two reported cases of *hemopericardium* leading to pericardial tamponade and cardiac arrest; both patients were resuscitated following pericardial aspiration [49].

Diffuse lung disease

Open lung biopsy is the best method for obtaining representative samples of tissue in diffuse lung disease. However, fiberoptic bronchoscopy with transbronchial biopsy gives a high yield in certain conditions, such as sarcoidosis and lymphangitis carcinomatosa. The likelihood of successful transbronchial biopsy can be predicted from the CT distribution of disease [50]. With appropriate patient selection, a diagnosis can be established by transbronchial biopsy or lavage in a high proportion of cases. For this reason, it is usually employed as the first technique in the investigation of diffuse lung disease. Fiberoptic bronchoscopy is also valuable in the assessment of immune suppressed patients with diffuse lung shadowing.

Fine needle aspiration is usually reserved for focal opacities in this group of patients, although it has been successfully employed in the diagnosis of *Pneumocystis carinii* pneumonia in patients with acquired immune deficiency syndrome (AIDS) when the diagnosis has not been reached by the usual means [33,51]. Increasing use of thoracoscopic lung biopsy will reduce the need for full open lung biopsy in selected patients.

Overall, there is little published data on the use of needle biopsy in noninfectious diffuse lung disease, and it is not at present a technique in wide use [52,53]. Contraindications are similar to contraindications for biopsy of focal lung disease, with these patients having a higher likelihood of pulmonary hypertension and severe respiratory impairment. In a series of 23 patients who underwent cutting needle biopsy for diffuse lung disease, infection was diagnosed in four patients, and diffuse noninfectious lung disease was diagnosed in the remainder. There was one tension pneumothorax and one hemoptysis [53]. Youmans *et al.* [33] reported a series of 151 patients with diffuse lung disease who underwent needle biopsy. After exclusion of 13% of these in whom the specimen was inadequate for analysis, a correct tissue diagnosis was made in 96%. Complications included a 36% pneumothorax rate, an 18% hemoptysis rate, one air embolism, and one fatal endobronchial hemorrhage [33].

Conclusion

Transthoracic needle biopsy is a safe procedure if correctly performed and if the contraindications are heeded. It should not be undertaken by anybody who is not able to deal with a pneumothorax by inserting a suitable chest drain, or performed in a department divorced from bronchoscopic facilities that enable bronchial hemorrhage to be controlled. Needle biopsy of discrete pulmonary masses is more likely to yield the diagnosis than transbronchial biopsy via the fiberoptic bronchoscope, which is also a more time-consuming and expensive procedure. However, transbronchial biopsy, accompanied where appropriate by bronchial lavage, is the preferred technique for the investigation of diffuse pulmonary shadowing.

Pleural intervention

Image-guided pleural intervention is an expanding area of radiology, and allows specific clinical problems to be accurately addressed. Pleural intervention may be therapeutic or diagnostic, and includes pleural thoracentesis, empyema drainage, pleural sclerosis, and pleural biopsy.

Diagnostic and therapeutic thoracentesis

Unguided pleural intervention as a bedside procedure — except in the case of large free pleural effusions — is now performed infrequently in hospitals with adequate radiologic facilities. Suspected pleural effusions down to a few milliliters in size can be accurately and sensitively diagnosed by ultrasound and CT. The authors feel that no patient should undergo thoracentesis without prior radiologic confirmation of the presence and site of pleural fluid. Unguided attempts at aspiration are more frequently unsuccessful than image-guided aspiration [54,55], and have a higher morbidity including chest wall pain, pulmonary hematoma formation, and laceration of the diaphragm, liver, or spleen [56].

As with lung needle biopsies, contraindications are relative and include poor patient cooperation and a bleeding diathesis. Unlike lung needle biopsy, pleural intervention under ultrasound guidance may be undertaken with the patient sitting since the probability of air embolus is negligible. Moreover, this position will encourage free pleural fluid to accumulate in a dependent position, allowing optimal access.

Complications of diagnostic and therapeutic pleural drainage include *hemothorax, pneumothorax, empyema,* and *re-expansion pulmonary edema.* Complication rates are lower than those associated with lung needle biopsy since usually only the parietal pleura is transgressed, rather than both pleural layers as well as aerated lung. A pneumothorax rate of less than 10% for therapeutic thoracentesis and 2% for diagnostic thoracentesis can be expected [57]. The monitoring of the development and the subsequent management of pneumothorax and other complications is similar to lung needle biopsy, although it is not our practice routinely to obtain additional radiographs after an uncomplicated diagnostic tap, and we only obtain a postdrainage film following therapeutic thoracentesis (Fig. 27.3). Care should be taken to minimize the introduction of air at the time of therapeutic drainage by occluding the cannula to the atmosphere at all times except when the patient is in the expiratory phase of respiration. To prevent the inadvertent introduction of air during subsequent catheter flushing, a stopcock is included in the drainage system. In patients who do develop a significant pneumothorax, the decision to treat by further tube drainage should be based on clinical grounds, particularly the development of respiratory symptoms, progression in the size of the pneumothorax, and the presence of preexisting lung disease. Hemothorax as a result of thoracentesis is very unlikely as long as a direct subcostal approach is avoided.

Re-expansion pulmonary edema is a rare but potentially fatal complication due to rapid drainage of a large pleural effusion or pneumothorax (Fig. 27.4). This complication seems more common when the underlying lung has been compressed or collapsed for some time (days or weeks) [58]. Re-expansion pulmonary edema can probably be avoided by limiting the rate of fluid removal to an empirical 1 l/h by use of a stopcock or gate clamp. The development of increasing breathlessness or distress during pleural drainage should prompt a further chest radiograph to exclude re-expansion edema or other potential complications.

Empyema drainage

Unguided empyema drainage, like diagnostic and therapeutic thoracentesis, is less likely to be successful and to have a higher complication rate than image-guided empyema drainage. Failure of surgical thoracentesis for empyema is most commonly due to tube malpositioning, or the presence of

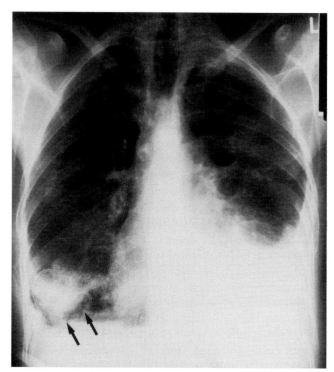

(a)

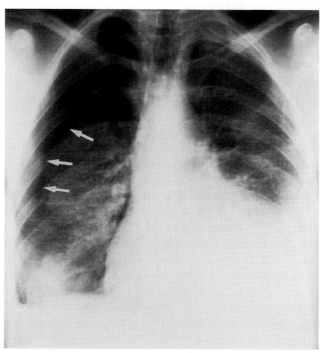

(b)

Fig. 27.3 (a) Postero−anterior chest radiograph of a 63-year-old female patient with bilateral effusions secondary to metastatic breast carcinoma. A narrow-bore chest drain has been inserted at the right base (arrows). (b) Chest radiograph following catheter removal after 24 hours of drainage demonstrates a moderate sized pneumothorax (arrows). This eventually resolved without further intervention.

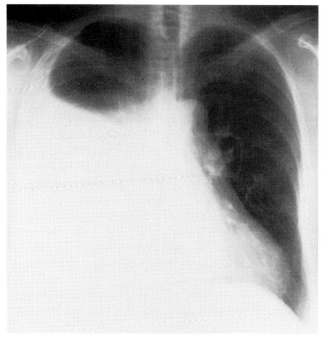

(a)

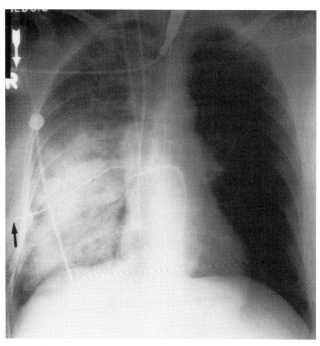

(b)

Fig. 27.4 (a) Postero−anterior chest radiograph of a 57-year-old female patient admitted for liver transplantation. There is a large right pleural effusion that had been present for some weeks. (b) Immediate postoperative film following transplantation. An intercostal drain has been inserted at the time of surgery. There is now extensive unilateral pulmonary edema following reexpansion. Note the malpositioned side hole of the drain lying in the soft tissues of the chest wall (arrow).

unrecognized pleural loculations [54,55,57]. Unguided tube thoracostomy success rates vary between 50 and 35%. Image-guided drainage, in a variety of series, and frequently following the failure of an unguided drainage procedure, has a success rate of between 92 and 75% [54,55,57,59−62].

Reported complications of image-guided empyema drainage are very rare, but include *hemothorax, pneumothorax, bacteremia*, and a single case of *cardiac arrest* [63]. Catheters with a diameter of 12−14-F are used and are more liable to block than larger surgical drains. They should be kept flushed with saline at 4−6-hour intervals.

Streptokinase or urokinase may be used to increase the successful drainage of empyemas, loculated pleural effusions, and selected cases of hemothorax. This technique has not been associated with an increase in general complications or in complications specific to the use of fibrinolytics [64,65].

Pleural biopsy

Fine-needle or cutting needle biopsy of the chest wall or of pleurally based masses may be undertaken safely under CT or ultrasound guidance [66−68]. Potential complications, which are uncommon in the reported series, include *hemothorax, hematoma* formation, and *pneumothorax*. Care should be taken to avoid the neurovascular bundle.

Lung abscess drainage

Most lung abcesses are adequately healed by antibiotic therapy. Failure to respond to antibiotics or persistence of an abscess due to lack of communication with the bronchial tree are indications for catheter drainage [69].

Possible complications include *pneumothorax, empyema, bronchopleural fistula, contamination of the remainder of the lung,* and *hemorrhage into the abscess cavity*. The catheter employed must be of relatively large caliber − usually 12−14-F − in order to drain successfully what may be tenacious abscess contents. Regular flushing of the catheter is usually required to prevent its occlusion.

Normal lung and pleura should not be transgressed by the catheter track since this increases the likelihood of complications, particularly hemorrhage [69]. Fortunately, most abscesses are in the lung periphery and abut the pleura. They can often be drained under fluoroscopic or ultrasound guidance, with CT reserved for potentially difficult or complicated cases.

Mediastinal biopsy

Fine needle aspiration of mediastinal disease has been used for diagnosis of primary and secondary carcinoma; neoplastic, reactive, and infectious nodal enlargement, and mediastinal abscess collections. However, the role of percutaneous biopsy in the diagnosis of mediastinal neoplastic disease is limited

[53,70]. For most primary mediastinal tumors, a mediastinoscopy or other open biopsy procedure is usually required. When percutaneous biopsy is used, e.g., to establish relapse in a patient with mediastinal lymphoma, a cutting needle should be used for reliable histology. This is a potentially hazardous undertaking and accurate radiologic guidance using dynamically enhanced CT is normally obtained to outline major vascular structures, including the internal mammary vessels.

A variety of approaches may be utilized depending on the nature of the lesion, with the safest and most suitable route being determined from the CT scan (Fig. 27.5). In addition to the usual paravertebral and parasternal routes, the use of a transsternal approach has been advocated in certain circumstances [71]. Subpleural injection of normal saline with a fine-gage needle, to displace aerated lung from the proposed needle tract, may also be employed [72]. Mediastinal biopsy under ultrasound guidance has been advocated [73], but requires special expertise in the use of mediastinal ultrasound.

The major complications of mediastinal biopsy are *pneumothorax, hemoptysis,* and *mediastinal hemorrhage* — including *hemopericardium, cardiac tamponade,* and *hemothorax*. With hemorrhagic complications constituting the major risk, bleeding diathesis should be an absolute contraindication, and extreme caution should still be employed when temporary correction of disordered clotting has been achieved by administration of blood products. It is clear that mediastinal biopsy should only be undertaken by persons capable of dealing with acute cardiac tamponade. Overall complication

rates are similar to other interventional procedures in the thorax. There is a reported pneumothorax rate of 8–23% and an incidence of hemoptysis of 2–10%, with other complications being rare [53].

Conclusions

The risk to the patient from percutaneous intervention in the thorax may be minimized or avoided by the use of appropriate imaging guidance, optimum technique, and the ability to deal rapidly and effectively with potential complications. This entails having all the necessary equipment to hand and being familiar with its use prior to commencement of the interventional procedure. If sensible precautions are undertaken and contraindications are observed, percutaneous intervention in the thorax has been shown to have an acceptably low morbidity and an extremely low mortality.

Complications of bronchography, including local anesthesia, are considered in the second edition of this book, pp. 273–287.

References

1 Dahlgren SE, Nordenstrom B. *Transthoracic Needle Biopsy.* Chicago: Year Book Publishers, 1966.
2 Bandt PD, Blank N, Castellino RA. Needle diagnosis of pneumonitis in high risk patients. *J Am Med Assoc* 1972,220:1578–1580.
3 Sanders DE, Thompson DW, Pudden BJE. Percutaneous aspiration lung biopsy. *Can Med Assoc J* 1971;104:139–142.
4 Berquist TH, Bailey PB, Cortese DA *et al.* Transthoracic needle biopsy. Accuracy and complications in relation to location and type of lesion. *Mayo Clin Proc* 1980;55:475–481.
5 Zelch JV, Lalli AF. Diagnostic percutaneous opacification of benign pulmonary lesions. *Radiology* 1973;108:559–561.
6 Sinner WN. Complications of percutaneous transthoracic needle aspiration biopsy. *Acta Radiol (Diagn)* 1976;17:813–828.
7 Dick J, Heard BE, Hinson KFW, Kerr IH, Pearson MC. Percutaneous needle biopsy of thoracic lesions; an assessment of 227 biopsies. *Br J Dis Chest* 1974;68:86–93.
8 Lalli S, McCormack LJ, Zelch M. Aspiration biopsy of chest lesions. *Radiology* 1978;127:35–39.
9 Herman PG, Hessel SJ. The diagnostic accuracy and complications of closed lung biopsies. *Radiology* 1977;125:11–13.
10 Meyer JE, Ferucci JT, Janower ML. Fatal complications of percutaneous biopsy. *Radiology* 1970;96:47–48.
11 Roncoroni AJ, Aquiles J. Fatal complications of percutaneous biopsy of the lung. *Chest* 1975;68:388.
12 Pearce JG, Patt NL. Fatal pulmonary hemorrhage after percutaneous aspiration lung biopsy. *Am Rev Respir Dis* 1974;110:346–349.
13 Norenberg R, Claxton CP, Takaio T. Percutaneous needle biopsy of the lung: report of two fatal complications. *Chest* 1974;66:216–218.
14 Sargent EN, Turner AF, Gordonson J, Schwinn CP, Pasky O. Percutaneous pulmonary needle biopsy: report of 350 patients. *Am J Roentgenol* 1974;122:758–768.
15 Westcott JL. Air embolism complicating percutaneous needle biopsy of the lung. *Chest* 1973;63:108–110.

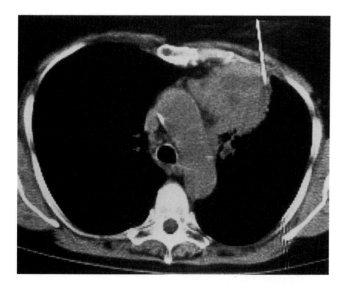

Fig. 27.5 CT-guided cutting needle biopsy of the periphery of a large partially necrotic mass abutting the mediastinum in a 60-year-old male smoker. Biopsy of the central part of a large tumor suspected of being partially necrotic is less likely to yield diagnostic material. (Eventual diagnosis, squamous cell carcinoma of the lung.)

16 Milner LB, Ryan K, Gullo J. Fatal intrathorax haemorrhage after percutaneous biopsy of the lung. *Am J Roentgenol* 1979;132: 280–281.

17 Weisbrod GL. Transthoracic percutaneous lung biopsy. *Radiol Clin N Am* 1990;23(3):647–655.

18 Flower CDR, Verney GI. Percutaneous needle biopsy of thoracic lesions: an evaluation of 300 biopsies. *Clin Radiol* 1979;30:215–218.

19 Westcott JL. Direct percutaneous aspiration of localised pulmonary lesions: results in 422 patients. *Radiology* 1980;137:31–36.

20 Jereb M. The usefulness of needle biopsy in chest lesions of different sizes and locations. *Radiology* 1980;134:13–15.

21 Stitik FP. *Percutaneous Lung Biopsy in the Pulmonary System: Practical Approaches to Pulmonary Diagnosis.* New York: Grune and Stratton, 1979:181–219.

22 Stevens GM, Jackman RJ. Outpatient needle biopsy of the lung: its safety and utility. *Radiology* 1984;22:329–330.

23 Cormier Y, Laviolette M, Tardif A. Prevention of pneumothorax in needle lung biopsy by breathing 100% oxygen. *Thorax* 1980; 35:37–41.

24 Engeler CE, Hunter DW, Castaneda-Zuniga W, Tashjian JH, Yedlicka JW, Amplatz K. Pneumothorax after lung biopsy: prevention with transpleural placement of compressed collagen foam plugs. *Radiology* 1992;184:787–789.

25 Herman SJ, Weisbrod GL. Usefulness of the blood patch technique after transthoracic needle aspiration biopsy. *Radiology* 1990;176:395–397.

26 Haramati LB, Austin HMA. Complications after CT guided needle biopsy through aerated versus non-aerated lung. *Radiology* 1991; 181:778.

27 Moore EH, Shepard JO, McLoud TC, Templeton PA, Kosiuk JP. Positional precautions in needle aspiration biopsy. *Radiology* 1990;175:733–735.

28 Moore EH, LeBlanc J, Montesi SA, Richardson ML, Shepard JO, McLoud TC. Effect of patient positioning after needle aspiration lung biopsy. *Radiology* 1991;181:385–387.

29 Cassel DM, Birnberg FA. Preventing pneumothorax after lung biopsy: the roll over technique (letter). *Radiology* 1990;174:282.

30 Sargent EM, Turner AF. Emergency treatment of pneumothorax. A simple catheter technique for use in the radiology department. *Am J Roentgenol* 1970;109:531.

31 Casola G, van-Sonnenberg E, Keightly A, Ho M, Withers C, Lee AS. Pneumothorax: radiologic treatment with small catheters. *Radiology* 1988;166:89–91.

32 Perlmutt LM, Braun SD, Newman GE *et al.* Transthoracic needle aspiration: use of a small chest tube to treat pneumothorax. *Am J Roentgenol* 1986;148:849–851.

33 Youmans CR, De Groot WJ, Marshall R *et al.* Needle biopsy of the lung in diffuse parenchymal disease: an analysis of 151 cases. *Am J Surg* 1970;120:637–643.

34 Zavala DC, Bedell GN. Percutaneous lung biopsy with a cutting needle. *Am Rev Respir Dis* 1972;106:186–193.

35 Harrison BDW, Thorpe RS, Kithchener PC *et al.* Percutaneous Trucut lung biopsy in the diagnosis of localised pulmonary lesions. *Thorax* 1984;39:493–499.

36 Berger RL, Dargan EL, Huang BL. Dissemination of cancer cells by needle biopsy of the lung. *J Thorac Cardiovasc Surg* 1972;63: 430–432.

37 Wolinsky H, Lischner MW. Needle track implantation of tumour after percutaneous lung biopsy. *Ann Int Med* 1969;71:359–362.

38 Sinner WM, Zajicek J. Implantation of metastases after percutaneous transthoracic needle aspiration biopsy. *Acta Radiol*

(Diagn) 1976;17:473–480.

39 Nordenstrom B, Bjork VO. Dissemination of cancer cells by needle biopsy of the lung. *J Thorac Cardiovasc Surg* 1973;65:671

40 Dutra FR, Geraci CI. Needle biopsy of the lung. *J Am Med Assoc* 1954;155:21–24.

41 Woolf CR. Applications of aspiration lung biopsy with review of the literature. *Dis Chest* 1954;25:286–289.

42 Aberle DR, Gamsu G, Golden JA. Fatal systemic arterial air embolism following lung needle aspiration. *Radiology* 1987;165: 351–353.

43 Tolly TL, Feldmeier JE, Czarnecki D. Air embolism complicating percutaneous lung biopsy. *Am J Roentgenol* 1988;150:555–556.

44 Cianci P, Posin JP, Shimshak RR *et al.* Air embolism complicating percutaneous thin needle biopsy of the lung. *Chest* 1987;92: 749–750.

45 Thomas AN, Roe BB. Air embolism following penetrating lung injuries. *J Thorac Cardiovasc Surg* 1973;66:533–539.

46 Murphy BP, Harford FJ, Cramer FS. Cerebral air embolism resulting from invasive medical procedures; treatment with hyperbaric oxygen. *Ann Surg* 1985;201:242–245.

47 Westcott JL. Percutaneous needle biopsy of hilar and mediastinal masses. *Radiology* 1981;141:323–328.

48 Castellino RA, Blank N. Etiologic diagnosis of focal pulmonary infection in immunocompromised patients by fluoroscopically guided percutaneous needle aspiration. *Radiology* 1979;132: 563–567.

49 Kucharczyk W, Weisbrod GL, Cooper JD *et al.* Cardiac tamponade as a complication of thin needle aspiration lung biopsy. *Chest* 1982;82:120–121.

50 Janzen DL, Adler BD, Padley SPG, Muller NL. Diagnostic success of bronchoscopic biopsy in immunocompromised patients with acute pulmonary disease: predictive value of disease distribution as shown on CT. *Am J Roentgenol* 1993;160:21–24.

51 Conces DJ, Clark SA, Tarver RD, Schwenk GR. Transthoracic aspiration needle biopsy: value in the diagnosis of pulmonary infections. *Am J Roentgenol* 1989;152:31–34.

52 McKenna RJ, Campbell A, McMurtrey M, Mountain CF. Diagnosis for interstitial lung disease in patients with acquired immunodeficiency syndrome (AIDS): a prospective comparison of bronchial washing, alveolar lavage, transbronchial lung biopsy, and open lung biopsy. *Ann Thorac Surg* 1986;41:318–321.

53 Gunther RW. Percutaneous interventions in the thorax. *J Vasc Intervent Radiol* 1992;3:379–390.

54 vanSonnenberg E, Nakamoto SK, Mueller PR *et al.* CT and ultrasound guided catheter drainage of empyemas after chest tube failure. *Radiology* 1984;151:349–353.

55 Westcott JL. Percutaneous catheter drainage of pleural effusion and empyema. *Am J Roentgenol* 1985;144:1189–1193.

56 Light RW. Parapneumonic effusions and empyema. *Clin Chest Med* 1985;6:55–61.

57 Silverman SG, Saini S, Mueller PR. Pleural interventions. Indications techniques and clinical applications. *Radiol Clin N Am* 1989;27:1257–1266.

58 Waqaruddin M, Bernstein A. Re-expansion pulmonary edema. *Thorax* 1975;30:54–60.

59 Stark DD, Federle MP, Goodman PC. CT and radiographic assessment of tube thoracostomy. *Am J Roentgenol* 1983;141:253–258.

60 Varkey B, Rose HD, Kutty Kesavan CP, Politis J. Empyema thoracis during a ten year period. *Arch Int Med* 1981;141:1771–1776.

61 Benfield GFA. Recent trends in empyema thoracis. *Br J Dis Chest* 1981;75:358–366.

62 Lemmer JH, Botham MJ, Orringer MB. Modern management of adult thoracic empyema. *J Thorac Cardiovasc Surg* 1985;90:849–855.

63 Merriam MA, Cronan JJ, Dorfman GS, Lambiase RE, Haas RA. Radiographically guided percutaneous catheter drainage of pleural fluid collections. *Am J Roentgenol* 1988;151:1113–1116.

64 Lee KS, Im J-G, Kim YH, Hwang SH, Won KB, Lee BH. Treatment of thoracic multiloculated empyemas with intracavitary urokinase: a prospective study. *Radiology* 1991;179:771–775.

65 Moulton JS, Moor PT, Mencini RA. Treatment of loculated pleural effusions with transcatheter intracavitary urokinase. *Am J Roentgenol* 1989;153:941–945.

66 Somers JM, Flower CDR. Percutaneous interventional techniques in the thorax. *J Intervent Radiol* 1990;5:49–55.

67 Mueller PR, Saini S, Simeone JF *et al.* Image-guided pleural biopsies: indications, technique, and results in 23 patients. *Radiology* 1988;169:1–4.

68 O'Moore PV, Mueller PR, Simeone JF *et al.* Sonographic guidance in diagnostic and therapeutic interventions in the pleural space. *Am J Roentgenol* 1987;149:1–5.

69 vanSonnenberg E, D'Agostino HB, Casola G, Halasz NA, Sanchez RB, Goodacre BW. Percutaneous abscess drainage: current concepts. *Radiology* 1991;181:617–626.

70 Herman JH, Holub RV, Weisbrod GL, Chamberlain DW. Anterior mediastinal masses: utility of transthoracic needle biopsy. *Radiology* 1991;180:167–170.

71 Swanson DC, Wittich GR. CT guided trans-sternal biopsy of a mediastinal mass. *J Intervent Radiol* 1990;5:163–164.

72 Klose KC, Gunther RW. CT-gesteuerte Biopsie. In: Gunther RW, Thelen M, eds. *Interventionelle Radiologie*. Stuttgart, Germany: Thieme, 1988:459–484.

73 Wernecke K, Vassallo P, Peters PE, von Basseswitz D-B. Mediastinal tumours: biopsy under ultrasound guidance. *Radiology* 1989;172:473–476.

CHAPTER 28

Complications of diagnostic studies of the gastrointestinal tract

Michael Y.M. Chen, George Ansell
and David J. Ott

Oral barium (Table 28.1)

Barium meal examinations, both single contrast and double contrast, are virtually the mainstay of radiology, and few

Table 28.1 Complications of oral barium

Types of complications [reference]	Prevalence (cases or %)	Death (cases or %)
Severe		
Barium aspiration [1,2]	6	6
Obstruction [1,3]	U	
Barium appendicitis [1,4]	U	
Perforation [5–11]	10	
Gastric dilatation [12]	3	
Poisoning [13,14]	1	1
Barium encephalopathy [15,16]	2	1
Other		
Constipation [17–20]	23%	
Nausea [17]	17%	
Rib fracture [21]	1	
Contamination [22]	U	

U, uncertain.

examinations have a higher margin of safety relative to their diagnostic yield. Nevertheless, for many patients they may still cause considerable anxiety. With the use of modern image intensification, fainting of the patient is perhaps less common than in the days of hot, dark, X-ray rooms, but it may still occur. The experienced radiologist anticipates the problem and often puts the examination table into the horizontal position to prevent injury to the patient. More important, the collapse may occasionally be caused by or may progress to cardiac arrest, particularly in elderly or debilitated patients, as well as those with heart ailments. In these cases, prompt resuscitation may avert a fatal outcome. Patients who have been confined to bed for even a few days may rapidly lose vasomotor tone and therefore be susceptible to sudden fainting. Loss of vasomotor tone may also occur in the pyrexial or toxic patient. Where there is any doubt, the patient should be examined in the recumbent or semierect position.

Barium aspiration

Six fatal cases of barium aspiration have been reported in elderly patients with poor respiratory function, bronchial neoplasm, or swallowing disorders caused by neurologic deficits (Fig. 28.1) [1,2]. In some cases, serious aspiration

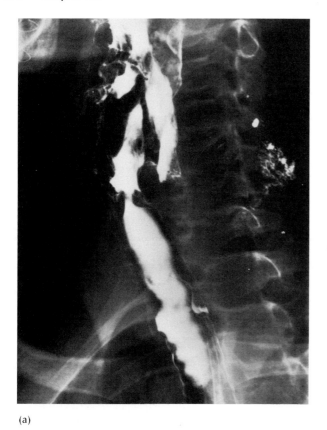

(a)

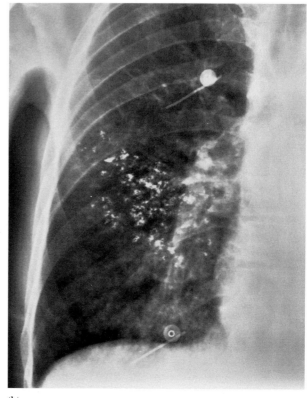

(b)

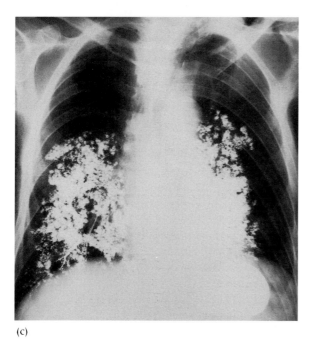

(c)

Fig. 28.1 (a) Severe aspiration after barium swallow in a patient with cerebrovascular disease. (b) Barium retained in the alveoli of the lung several weeks after aspiration via a tracheoesophageal fistula due to esophageal carcinoma. (From Gelfand [23].) (c) Male, age 80, in poor general condition with anemia and hypoproteinemic edema, felt faint during barium meal and barium was given with table horizontal. Inhaled a considerable amount of barium but not immediately distressed. Deteriorated and confused in the evening. Treated with physiotherapy; initial improvement but gradual deterioration, with death on the ninth day. Chest radiograph showing extensive bilateral "barium bronchogram". Barium is also present in the stomach. (From Ansell [1].)

prompted a tracheal obstruction that caused sudden death; in others, patients showed few symptoms initially and then developed fever, became comatose and hypotensive, and died 10 hours to 9 days later.

Small amounts of aspirated barium should be treated by physiotherapy with postural drainage. Retention of a small amount of barium in the lungs does not appear to cause fibrosis, but pulmonary infection may occur [24]. There is an impression that barium aspiration has become more common with the use of high-density barium preparations for double-contrast examinations and that swallowing difficulties may be exacerbated by effervescent mixtures or by anticholinergic drugs that may interfere with esophageal motility [1]. Accidental inhalation of sodium bicarbonate granules (Carbex) may precipitate an acute attack of asthma [25].

For patients with swallowing disorders caused by cerebrovascular diseases, neuromuscular diseases, or trauma, a special examination is conducted in many swallowing centers. The patient is first administered a small amount of low-viscosity barium suspension or low-osmolar water-soluble medium to reduce the chance of serious aspiration. If substantial aspiration of this material occurs, further administration is avoided. However, patients who aspirate the low-viscosity barium suspension may sometimes have improved swallowing function with a high-viscosity barium suspension, barium paste, or semisolid material.

Obstruction

With thicker barium or paste, there may be a risk of impaction and blockage at an esophageal stricture. Orally ingested barium may become impacted in the colon and precipitate an acute obstruction at the site of a carcinoma or diverticulitis [3]. In patients with severe dysphagia, a small amount of barium or low-osmolar water-soluble medium should be used initially to exclude obstruction and prevent substantial aspiration.

Constipation is the most common symptom (23%) after upper gastrointestinal and small-bowel studies [17]. Minor degrees of barium impaction are not uncommon in routine barium meal examinations, and patients may have considerable discomfort from the passage of hardened masses of barium. There may be prolonged retention of barium in the colon for 2−6 weeks without any obvious obstructing lesion [18]. There is probably little risk that a small bowel obstruction will be aggravated by barium, since the large accumulation of fluid in the obstructed bowel should prevent inspissation. However, impaction of barium in the small bowel has been reported in an infant with cystic fibrosis [19].

Barium suspension used in patients with Parkinson's disease should be evacuated from the intestine by means of a laxative to prevent the formation of a barium impaction [20]. If routine purgation and enemas fail to dislodge the barium, lactulose is generally effective.

Barium appendicitis

Barium retained in the appendix for a prolonged period may act as an obstructing fecalith and has caused acute appendicitis and perforation up to 6 months after a barium meal [4]. Therefore, appendectomy has been suggested in symptomatic patients with retained barium in the appendix [4].

Perforation

In general, perforation of the upper gastrointestinal tract after a barium meal is probably less hazardous than colonic perforation after a barium enema where there is associated peritoneal fecal contamination from the colon (Fig. 28.2).

Esophageal perforation was reported after a double-contrast examination in a patient with severe esophageal stenosis and ulceration [5]. The patient complained of diffuse chest pain, and air appeared in the mediastinal tissues on a chest film; the symptoms resolved rapidly, and there were no sequelae in this particular case.

Perforation of a pyloric ulcer was reported in a patient receiving steroids for primary amyloidosis, and symptoms developed shortly after the barium examination [6]. The perforation occurred when the gastric outlet was obstructed. Pressure from an effervescent agent may convert a walled off perforation into a free extravasation [7].

Three cases of perforation relating to duodenal ulcers were reported in a series of 10 250 barium meal examinations [8]. Manual palpation and air contrast techniques were employed during the examinations. Patients with giant duodenal ulcerations have a greater risk of perforation during barium studies.

A duodenal perforation caused by intubation during enteroclysis has been reported. Careful supervision of inexperienced persons and retraction of the guidewire 3−5 cm behind the tip of the catheter are advised [9]. Small bowel perforation with massive intraperitoneal leakage of barium during enteroclysis has also been reported [10]. The perforation occurred in an ischemic segment of partially obstructed ileum and was likely caused by rapid barium infusion and increased abdominal pressure when the patient rotated to prone position [10]. Limitation of fluoroscopic and radiographic evaluations to supine and oblique positions would prevent abdominal pressure associated with the prone position.

Colonic perforation after a barium meal has been reported in two cases [11]. One patient had an occult carcinoma of the colon, and although the other patient had no specific lesion in the colon, barium collection was the cause of perforation 10 days later.

Poisoning

The soluble salts of barium are highly poisonous, but the widespread use of commercial preparations of barium sulfate has largely eliminated this risk. However, a case of fatal barium poisoning occurred in India, where a pharmacist misread a prescription for barium sulfate and dispensed barium sulfide by mistake [13]. This accident caused corrosive changes, vomiting, and diarrhea followed by vascular paralysis and cardiac arrest.

In the emergency treatment of barium poisoning, sodium

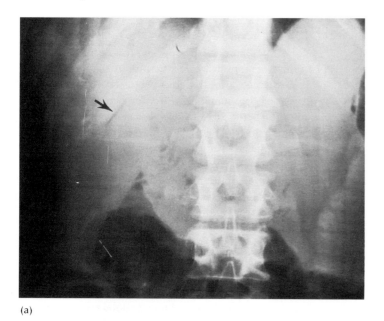

(a)

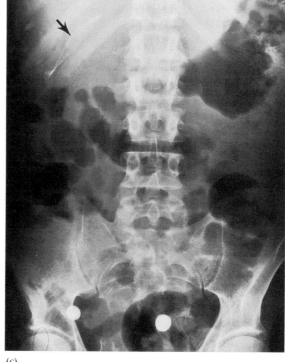

(c)

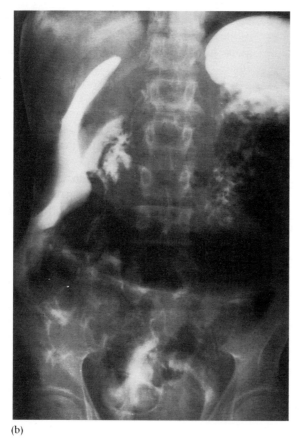

(b)

Fig. 28.2 (a) Small amount of free air in the peritoneal cavity (arrow) due to perforation of a gastric ulcer shown in the plain abdominal film but not recognized. (b) Barium extravasation into the peritoneal cavity after upper gastrointestinal examination. (c) Barium remains in the peritoneal cavity (arrow) 4 months after surgery (From Gelfand [23].)

sulfate or magnesium sulfate can be given orally in an attempt to form an insoluble precipitate of barium sulfate. An intravenous infusion of potassium to correct lowered serum potassium may be required, along with artificial respiration to counteract temporary paralysis of the skeletal muscles involved in respiration [14].

Barium encephalopathy

A patient who had undergone three barium examinations within 1 week, developed convulsions and encephalopathy with abnormal electroencephalogram (EEG) changes. The barium level in the blood was 260 µg/l [15]. In another case, myoclonic changes and mental deterioration occurred 16 days after intraperitoneal rupture during a barium enema, and barium assay of the cerebrospinal fluid showed a level of 180 µg/l [16].

Contamination

Growths of *Escherichia coli*, *Klebsiella*, *Streptococcus faecalis*, *Pseudomonas*, and *Clostridia* have been found in barium solutions that have been allowed to stand overnight in reservoirs after mixing [22]. However, newer prepackaged commercial barium preparations have eliminated contamination.

Mistakes may arise as a result of mislabeling. Plaster of Paris stored in a barium container was administered to four patients, and accidental administration of alkali-containing washing powders instead of barium caused acute corrosive poisoning [26].

Anticholinergic agent effects

Anticholinergic drugs may cause transient side-effects, such as tachycardia, dryness of the mucous membranes, difficulty in micturition, and mydriasis. Because of the latter effect, they are contraindicated in patients with glaucoma. Three cases of acute gastric dilatation have been reported after the administration of 30 mg of Pro-Banthine for hypotonic duodenography [12]. In two of these patients, partial obstruction of the third part of the duodenum by a pancreatic carcinoma was exacerbated by the anticholinergic agent, and a nasogastric suction was required. A partial duodenal obstruction should be regarded as a contraindication, and food should also be withheld for 8–12 hours after the examination. This complication would be unlikely with hypotonic agents of briefer duration, such as Buscopan or glucagon.

Minor reactions

Nausea occurred in 17% of patients receiving upper gastrointestinal series in one study [17]. Anterior rib fracture occurred in a patient receiving corticosteroid treatment. The fracture was caused by a compressing paddle with the patient in the prone oblique position [21].

Water-soluble media (Table 28.2)

Gastrografin (Schering AG, Berlin) is a 76% aqueous solution of sodium methylglucamine diatrizoate, 0.1% of the wetting agent Tween 80 and added flavoring. Water-soluble contrast material are useful to evaluate suspected gastrointestinal perforation or postoperative complications. Low-osmolar contrast media could with advantage replace the ionic, hyperosmolar agents but their current costs are prohibitive, particularly in the USA, (see also p. 285).

Hypovolemia

The major disadvantage of Gastrografin is its hypertonicity, since it has an osmolarity of 1900 mosmol/l, about six times that of normal serum [27]. This hypertonicity causes fluid to be drawn into the gastrointestinal tract causing a cathartic effect. Loss of fluid from the circulation causes hypovolemia, and increased serum osmolarity has been noted in adult patients following the oral administration of Gastrografin [28]. These changes can be particularly serious in dehydrated, malnourished children, or debilitated adults. Dehydration should be corrected prior to, and following, administration of Gastrografin.

Bowel damage

In an adult patient, inflammatory changes have been noted in the colonic mucosa after prolonged retention of a Hypaque

Table 28.2 Water-soluble media

Types of complications [reference]	Prevalence (cases or %)	Death (cases or %)
Severe		
Hypovolemia [27,28]	U	
Bowel damage: perforation, infarction [29–31]	3	
Aspiration, pulmonary edema [1,32]	2	2
Precipitation [33,34]	2	
Adverse reaction to iohexol [35]	1	
Allergic, anaphylactic (see Table 28.3)		
Other		
Ileus [36]	4%	
Diarrhea [37,39]	45%	

U, uncertain.

enema [29]. Histologic examination showed mucosal and submucosal edema, dilated blood vessels, and macrophages containing a brown-staining pigment. Cecal perforation occurred 24 hours after a Gastrografin enema administered to an adult patient with fecal impaction and a mass in the sigmoid colon [30]. A large volume of Gastrografin was retained in the proximal colon and progressive distension resulted from the hypertonic effect of the contrast medium. Acute abdominal distension and hypotension developed after administration of Gastrografin via a gastric tube in a patient with subacute bowel obstruction caused by secondary deposits [31]. Subsequently, a small bowel infarction developed.

Aspiration

Accidental aspiration of Gastrografin may cause a mild cough or immediate dyspnea. After a brief interval, there may be respiratory collapse and death from pulmonary edema [1,32]. The risks are higher in patients with preexisting pulmonary disease and cor pulmonale.

In a few cases, pulmonary edema and respiratory distress syndrome developed in patients with an esophageal fistula or perforation after a swallow with hyperosmolar medium. Prolonged positive pressure ventilation was required, and there was residual pulmonary impairment [38]. Where there is a risk of aspiration of contrast medium, small volumes of barium suspension or low-osmolar water-soluble media are preferable. Aspiration of iopromid or iotrolan may cause less respiratory distress [37].

Precipitation

Diatrizoate is precipitated in an acid environment at a strength of 0.1 normal hydrochloric acid to form water-insoluble carboxylic acid. In a patient with hyperchlorhydria, a solid putty-like precipitate occurred in the stomach after instillation of Gastrografin [33]. Gastrografin can apparently also be precipitated in the achlorhydric stomach after partial gastrectomy and vagotomy, if stomal obstruction is present. In a reported case, Gastrografin remaining in the gastric stump for 24 hours formed a solid precipitate, which caused multiple gastric erosions with a massive hematemesis. At surgery, the erosions were found to be restricted to the area of contact of the Gastrografin bolus [34].

Ileus and diarrhea

Postoperative administration of Gastrografin may have been a cause of *ileus* in 4% of patients in one study [36]. Gastrografin may induce serious diarrhea in 12% of patients [37].

Reactions to low-osmolar contrast

A severe reaction after oral administration of iohexol (Win-throp Pharmaceuticals, New York, NY) has been reported [35]. The reaction was characterized by cramping abdominal pain, nausea, vomiting, retching, hypotension, tightness of the throat, and difficulty in breathing. Symptoms responded to treatment with intravenous hydrocortisone, chlorphenira-mine, and plasma expanders [35]. Diarrhea was a complication in 18 of 40 patients receiving iohexol. The incidence of diarrhea was not related to the concentration of iohexol. Fever, nausea and vomiting, and urticarial reactions were also reported [39].

Barium enema (Table 28.3)

This section primarily describes complications related to single- and double-contrast barium enema. However, the cleansing enema if used may cause complications, such as tip trauma, perforation, and water intoxication, that are similar to complications caused by barium enema and are therefore included in this section.

Perforation

The most important and frequent complication of barium enema is that of perforation with extravasation of barium into the retroperitoneal tissues or the peritoneum, or intra-mural extravasation; the prevalence is 0.02−0.04% [23,40]. However, some minor cases of extraperitoneal leakage may remain undiagnosed. The overall mortality rate for barium enema perforation in adult patients has varied from 33 to 80% [1,41], but with prompt diagnosis and effective treatment, a high survival rate (>80%) can be achieved [6,78].

Pathogenesis

The causes of colonic perforation include high intraluminal pressure, or colon weakened by diseases or iatrogenic trauma, which impairs the tensile strength of the colonic wall. Older patients, those treated with long-term steroids or radiation, and those with diseases including neoplasms, diverticulitis, and inflammatory bowel diseases are more predisposed to perforation.

The bursting pressures of different areas of the colon removed at autopsy were measured in a series of patients [79]. The rectum has the highest bursting pressure whereas the cecum is the weakest area. The lowest bursting pressure in the series was found in a colon from a 30-year-old patient, in whom the cecum ruptured at a pressure of only 50 mmHg. The highest pressure was sustained in the rectum of a 5.5-year-old infant, in whom a pressure of 646 mmHg was required before rupture occurred. However, the condition of the bowel wall is important, and if it is thinned, ulcerated, or even unduly rigid, it will be more prone to perforation. When a section of colon is inflated by pneumatic pressure,

Table 28.3 Barium enema

Types of complications [reference]	Prevalence (cases or %)	Death (cases or %)
Severe		
Perforation [1,23,40,41] (Retroperitoneal emphysema, intramural extravasation, spontaneous dissection)	0.02−0.04%	33−80%
Barium granuloma [42−44]	U	
Peritonitis [40]	U	50%
Venous intravasation [1,45−53]	28	56%
Barium embolization [45−49]	20	74%
Portal vein embolization [45−49]	8	13%
Vaginal rupture [1,47−49]	11	70%
Portal vein gas [54,55]	U	
Water intoxication [56]	U	
Toxic dilatation [1]	U	
Septicemia [1,57]	4	2
Perforation related to colonic biopsy [58]	11	
Other		
Electrocardiogram changes [59]	U	
Bacteremia [60]	U	
Constipation [17,61]	20−36%	
Barium retention in the dysfunctional rectum [1]	5	
Abdominal pain [17]	U	
Diarrhea [17]	8%	
Allergic or anaphylactic reactions* [1,62−77] (Barium suspension, latex, water soluble contrast, glucagon, Buscopan)	1/1700−750 000	8

* Seen in upper or lower gastrointestinal studies.
U, uncertain.

perforation is preceded by a longitudinal split in the serosa and muscularis. Then, as the distension increases, the mucosa herniates through the split and eventually ruptures.

The presence of colonic haustra suggests that tone is still present in the colonic wall so that there is a capacity to respond to increased volume. In a relevant case, perforation of the ascending colon occurred when the enema reservoir was raised to 120 cm in an attempt to reflux barium into the terminal ileum when colonic haustra were absent [80].

The theoretical hydrostatic pressure resulting from a 20% w/v low-viscosity barium suspension is 71 mmHg when the reservoir is 90 cm above the rectum, and the pressure is 123 mmHg when the reservoir is at a height of 150 cm [1]. Transient colonic spasms or straining by the patient may increase the pressure by an additional 170 mmHg. When high-viscosity barium is used, the rate of flow is more sluggish and a height of 150 cm does not appear to cause colonic spasms. In general, when low-viscosity barium is used, a height of 60 cm is considered safe [80].

Diner *et al.* [81] measured the intraluminal pressures in patients receiving single- and double-contrast enemas and found little difference between the pressures generated by these two examinations. The maximum peak pressure with air insufflation was 66 mmHg, whereas that with the single-contrast barium was 60 mmHg.

The cleansing enema itself may result in perforation and, if the patient complains of undue symptoms, an abdominal plain film should be obtained before commencing the barium examination. The use of large doses of purgatives during the preparation for barium enema is not without hazard. Colonic perforation with fecal peritonitis and death occurred in two patients after the use of X-prep (Napp Laboratories Ltd, UK) [82]. Occasional skin reactions have been reported after use of Picolax (sodium picosulfate). In two cases, the patients were under treatment with sulfasalazine [83].

Iatrogenic causes: balloons and enema tips

In the majority of perforations reported during barium enema, a balloon catheter was used [42]. Overdistension of the balloon with air may damage the rectal wall, and in one case rupture of the balloon preceded colonic rupture (Fig. 28.3) [42]. After passing the enema tip through the anal canal, the tip should be directed posteriorly along the course of the rectum to prevent damage to the anterior rectal wall. Asymmetric inflation of a small rectal balloon may force the enema tip into the rectal wall [23]. If the enema tip is bent inadvertently during insertion, it may suddenly straighten during inflation causing rectal trauma. In one patient, involuntary expulsion of an inflated balloon catheter caused multiple mucosal tears in the anal canal, with perirectal and retroperitoneal emphysema [84]. If the balloon is placed at the rectosigmoid junction, where the wall is less distensible, it is more likely to cause damage.

The patient may develop high intracolonic pressure from spasm or stricture which limits the proximal flow of barium when a balloon is employed [85]. Although there are occasions when a balloon catheter is necessary, the routine use of such a catheter in every patient is *not* recommended.

The Weber catheter (Picker International Inc., Highland Heights, OH) is similar to the older Bardex catheter, which

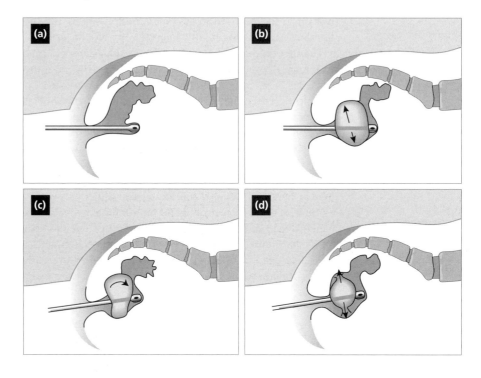

Fig. 28.3 Causes of rectal perforation related to enema tips and balloons. (a) Continuing the anterior direction of the tip after it has transversed the anus impales the anterior rectal wall. (b) Overdistension of the balloon tears the rectum. (c) Eccenteric inflation of the small rectal balloon on a disposal tip levels the tip into the rectal wall. (d) Balloon bursts in rectum causing tear. (From Gelfand [23].)

may cause perforation [86]. The Weber balloon should be inflated intermittently under fluoroscopic control, and there should be sufficient barium around the balloon to prevent contact with the rectal wall. When the balloon is adequately inflated, gentle traction on the catheter will bring the balloon backwards to occlude the anal canal [23]. This catheter is no longer being made and will not be available when the remaining stock of catheters runs out.

Endoscopic biopsy or polypectomy

Unrecognized trauma caused by endoscopy may predispose a patient to perforation during or following barium enema. Sigmoidoscopy may traumatize the rectal mucosa, particularly if a biopsy has been performed. In a survey, 50 radiologists reported 11 cases of perforation related to colonic biopsies in the rectum or sigmoid colon [58].

In a subsequent clinical investigation, transcolonoscopic forceps were found to produce only superficial biopsies, and there were no complications in the following barium enemas. However, the transproctoscopic forceps used for biopsies through a rigid proctoscope may produce a deep biopsy. Therefore, it was suggested that with the use of the rigid type instrument and biopsy forceps, barium enemas should be deferred for at least 6 days unless histologic analysis shows that the biopsy was superficial [58,87,88]. Barium enemas should also be deferred for at least 6 days after an electrosurgical polypectomy [88].

Colostomies

Barium enemas performed through a colostomy were a particular hazard and accounted for 12 of 53 perforations in one series [42]. Intraluminal balloon catheters are a particular danger in these cases. There may also be diminished distensibility of the nonfunctioning loop, and the attachment of the colostomy to the abdominal wall and peritoneum may be fragile. The colostomy can be occluded by pressing an inflated Foley catheter against its outside surface, or a special colostomy enema tip may be used and inserted gently for only a short distance into the colostomy.

Diagnosis of perforation

Intraperitoneal perforations usually cause sudden, severe abdominal pain and shock. When perforation occurs during a double-contrast enema, extravasation of air rather than barium is more likely (Fig. 28.4) [89]. The air may be visualized earlier on the decubitus views of the abdomen than on fluoroscopy (Fig. 28.5). It is also important to inspect the postevacuation film which may sometimes provide the first indication of perforation (Fig. 28.6).

Extraperitoneal extravasation is caused by transmural perforation occurring below the level of the peritoneal reflection into the sigmoid mesentery (Fig. 28.7), or transverse mesocolon, or posterior surfaces of the ascending or descending colon. Extensive extraperitoneal spread could occur without any appreciable discomfort in the early stages, since the rectal mucosa above the pectinate line is insensitive to pain.

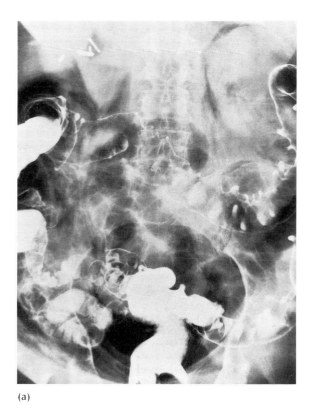

(a)

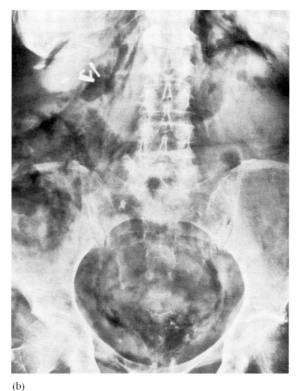

(b)

Fig. 28.4 Free air seen in the peritoneal cavity and retroperitoneal space during (a) and after (b) double-contrast barium enema. (Photograph courtesy of Dean D. T. Maglinte, Indianapolis, IN.)

Slight clinical symptoms such as rectal pain or spontaneous bleeding may be an indication of trauma, and may be followed by sudden cardiovascular collapse after several hours. Delayed retroperitoneal fibrosis and ureteral obstruction have been reported (Fig. 28.8) [90].

Retroperitoneal emphysema may be seen on delayed films, 12−24 hours after a double-contrast barium enema. The perforation may also be recognized as pneumomediastinum on a chest radiograph, and the patient's voice may change because of parapharyngeal emphysema [91,92]. In most cases, sigmoidoscopy is normal or reveals only mild superficial lesions. With retroperitoneal perforation, computed tomography (CT) delineates retroperitoneal perforation secondary to barium enema. Because of the high density of

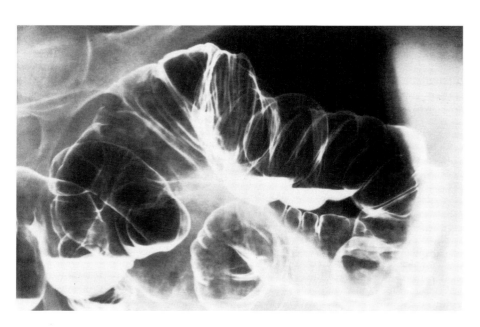

Fig. 28.5 A large amount of free air in the peritoneal cavity was detected by decubitus film during double-contrast barium enema. A 0.3-cm long perforation in the transverse colon was confirmed by surgery. (From Gelfand *et al.* [89].)

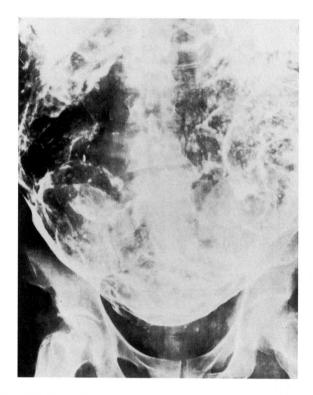

Fig. 28.6 Marked peritoneal barium contamination in a patient after barium enema.

barium it can be readily detected by CT in the rectal wall or perirectal tissue [93].

Intramural extravasation is caused by a partial tear of the colonic wall and is a relatively benign process. A thin longitudinal translucent line representing mucosa and muscularis displaced by intramural dissection, or a transverse striation pattern outlining the inner circular muscle fibers, may be present [94].

Spontaneous dissection of air into the transverse mesocolon may occur in an asymptomatic patient during double-contrast barium enema. Dissection of air and contrast material may occur in the rectum in association with anal fissure, mucosal inflammation, malignancy, mucosa abraded by catheter tip, inflated rectal balloon, or hardened feces. This is usually a self-limited complication, but barium dissection may interrupt the blood supply, causing secondary bowel necrosis or a fatal massive venous intravasation. Dissection in the sigmoid colon, transverse colon, or cecum has been reported with or without underlying colonic disease such as obstruction, carcinoma, or ulcerative colitis [95].

Consequences of perforation

Barium peritonitis

Peritonitis may immediately follow a severe intraperitoneal perforation; the mortality rate is 50% [40]. Bacteria are

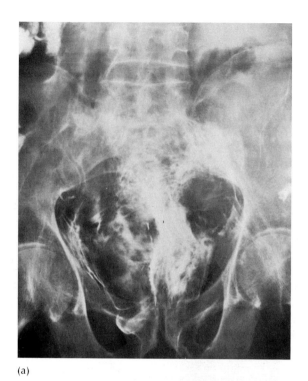

(a)

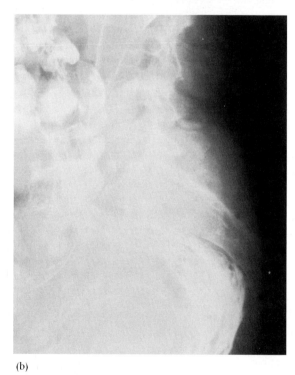

(b)

Fig. 28.7 Barium in the retroperitoneal tissues after rectal perforation during administration of a barium enema. Frontal (a) and lateral (b) views show streaky and granular appearance of extravasated barium. (From Gelfand [23].)

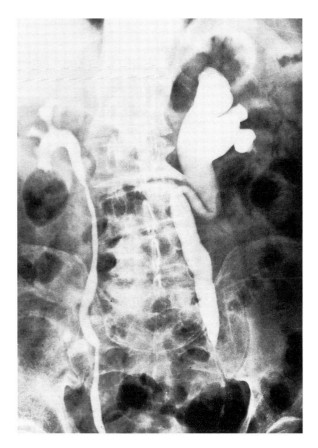

Fig. 28.8 Retrograde pyelograms showing left ureteral obstruction as a result of the rupture of a diverticulum of the sigmoid colon. (From Gelfand [23].)

absorbed rapidly from the peritoneal cavity. The intravascular release of intracellular endotoxins is a factor contributing to early shock and death. Chemical peritonitis causes a rapid accumulation of fluid in the peritoneal cavity that may induce hypovolemia; intravenous fluids have been shown to be of importance in eliminating endotoxin from the blood.

If possible, laparotomy should be undertaken as soon as the patient's condition permits. A diverting cecostomy or colostomy should be performed with peritoneal lavage, but major surgery should probably be avoided. In addition to wide-spectrum antibiotic therapy, there may be a case for injecting a nonabsorbable antibiotic such as kanamycin into the bowel to destroy the Gram-negative bacteria that are the source of the endotoxin. The value of steroids in the treatment of septic shock is controversial, and a higher incidence of superinfection has been reported in steroid-treated cases [96].

Even if laparotomy is performed promptly, it may be difficult to remove the barium completely by irrigation and it may adhere persistently to the peritoneal surface. Urokinase solution may aid in the removal of adherent barium from the peritoneum [97]. If the patient survives the initial shock

and sepsis, intraabdominal adhesions may develop and can cause bowel obstruction.

Mild extraperitoneal tears may heal spontaneously, but serious tears may develop into infections in the soft perirectal tissue a few hours or days later. Drainage of air, barium, and secretions locally are suggested in substantial lesions [98]. A serious extraperitoneal extravasation of barium should be treated similarly to an intraperitoneal perforation. In one review [40], the mortality from intra- and extraperitoneal perforations in adults was 27% in patients with surgical treatment and 60% for a conservatively treated group.

Barium granuloma (barytoma)

Small amounts of residual barium in the peritoneum may be asymptomatic, but in one study 30% of patients who survived an intraperitoneal extravasation of barium eventually developed peritoneal adhesions causing narrowing of the bowel, and sometimes required additional surgery [42].

Ureteral obstruction caused by periureteric barium granuloma may also occur as a late complication (see Fig. 28.8). A case of barium granuloma involving the left ureteral orifice of the bladder and mimicking a nonpapillary irregular tumor has been reported [43]. Ureteric endoprostheses have been used to treat a case of bilateral hydronephrosis resulting from barium-induced retroperitoneal fibrosis [99].

Small extravasations of barium may pass into the perirectal tissues and remain undiagnosed until symptoms develop from a few weeks to several years later [100]. A low-grade chronic infection and even abscess formation may occur, but symptoms usually subside with conservative treatment, even though barium persists in the soft tissues. The endoscopic findings of barium granuloma include ulcers, nodules, or plaques that mimic malignancy, but barium sulfate crystals causing a macrophage reaction can be detected in the interstitial tissues of the biopsy specimen using plain radiography [44].

Venous intravasation

Barium embolization is a rare complication of barium enema; a total of 28 cases have been reported with a mortality rate of 56% [45–49]. In the 28 reported cases, the average patient age was 63 years (range 25–86 years). Sites of mucosal injury were the rectum, sigmoid colon, transverse colon, colostomy, and vagina. Twelve patients had underlying diseases including diverticula (5), ulcerative colitis (3), carcinomas (2), Crohn's disease (1) and proctitis (1). Another 16 patients had no abnormalities of the colon, but venous intravasation occurred as a result of vaginal rupture in 11 cases. Elderly patients have more risk of embolization because of thinning and diminishing elasticity of the rectal wall with age [45].

Barium may enter the splenic and portal veins and lodge

in the intrahepatic branches of the right portal vein or in the systemic veins through the hemorrhoidal pelvic veins. Barium in the pelvic venous plexus causes a Medusa-head appearance [50], and barium may be seen in the inferior mesenteric vein, simulating a coloreteric fistula, or it may pass into the heart and pulmonary circulation [51,52]. Barium in the portal vein may be mistaken for a colobiliary fistula [46]. Increased density of the liver and spleen may be seen due to reticuloendothelial cell accumulation of barium [48]. In reviewing five previous reports [45–49], barium embolization in the systemic circulation occurred in 20 patients, 14 (74%) of whom died and one of whom was undocumented as to status. One in eight patients (13%) with portal vein embolization died 30 days after examination [45–49].

Transient bacteremia may occur after barium enema in patients with bowel inflammation resulting from small amounts of fecal-contaminated gas entering the venous system. A liver abscess following the intravasation of a small amount of barium into the portal circulation has been reported [53].

If venous intravasation is noted during barium enema, the examination should be terminated immediately. Lowering of the barium reservoir may siphon off barium and reduce the intraluminal pressure. If the patient is not hypotensive, it would be rational to reverse the procedure used for air embolism by tilting the table "feet down" and turning the patient onto the right side in an attempt to prevent the passage of barium into the pulmonary circulation. Oxygen may be required along with full supportive therapy and prophylactic antibiotics.

Vaginal rupture

Vaginal rupture with venous intravasation of barium has been reported in 11 cases, in which a barium enema had been inadvertently administered into the vagina by means of a balloon catheter [47,48]. With elderly patients in particular, a redundant vulva may lead to accidental insertion of the catheter into the vagina even by an experienced technologist. All patients in these reports were unaware of whether the catheter was in the vagina or rectum. If a self-retaining balloon catheter or tip is used, barium cannot escape and increasing pressure causes vaginal rupture. The barium may enter into paravaginal venous plexus and ultimately into the systemic circulation (Fig. 28.9). A massive pulmonary embolization is a major cause of sudden death in this situation. In 11 cases of vaginal rupture (mean age, 68 years), seven patients died from 30 minutes to 3 weeks later, three survived, and outcome for one was unstated [47–49].

In one case with vaginal rupture, the examination was discontinued when the patient complained of lower abdominal discomfort and blood was found on the X-ray couch. The radiograph was interpreted as showing an extraperitoneal leak of barium, which was assumed to be due to

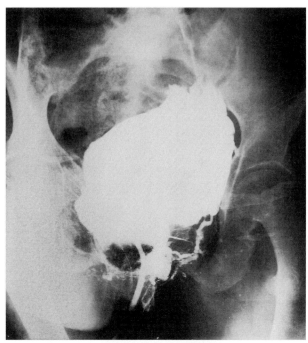

(a)

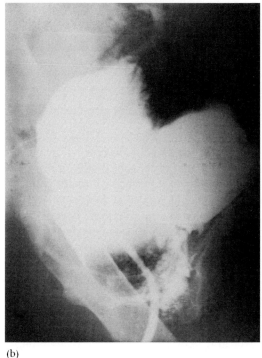

(b)

Fig. 28.9 Female, age 72 years. Misplacement of balloon catheter into vagina. The balloon is at the introitus. (a) Rupture of vagina with barium in pelvic soft tissues. There is venous intravasation of barium. (b) Lateral view shows barium in the iliac vein. The bladder is also shown filled with barium. Died 24 hours later. (From Ansell [1].)

bowel damage. Laparotomy and transverse colostomy were performed; but no lesion was detected in the sigmoid colon. The patient died 3-weeks later, and at autopsy a 5-cm tear was found on the posterior vaginal wall [1]. In another case, an obvious venous intravasation did not cause any symptoms and repeated chest radiographs did not reveal any barium in the lungs. The patient made an uncomplicated recovery [1].

Portal vein gas

The presence of gas in the portal venous system of the liver is usually an indication of invasion by gas-forming organisms, and the prognosis is grave. However, gas may occur in the portal venous system after air insufflation for double-contrast enemas in patients with chronic ulcerative or Crohn's colitis [54]. In one of these patients, there was also a coincidental bowel perforation with free intraperitoneal air. The patient responded to antibiotic therapy. The mechanism by which gas enters the portal vein is unclear, but gas entering a hypervascular ulcerated area in the colon or a tear of the mucosa is the most likely cause. In patients with portal vein gas resulting from air-contrast barium enema and no serious underlying condition, conservative treatment is suggested, but antibiotics may be necessary if symptoms of bacteremia are present [55].

Water intoxication

The hazard of water intoxication in megacolon is now well established. A large amount of water can be absorbed by the large surface area of the colonic mucosa with resulting hydremia, hyponatremia, pulmonary edema, and cerebral edema. Clinically, the patient becomes drowsy and apathetic with vomiting, abundant dilute urine, and flushed skin. Cardiac problems, convulsions, coma, and death may supervene. Water intoxication has also been reported in a child with impairment of renal function [56].

The most important preventive measure is to limit the volume of fluid administered by enema in patients with megacolon or chronic constipation. The addition of sodium chloride to the enema solution has been suggested, but the possibility exists that this may also be absorbed and cause pulmonary edema, particularly in patients with cardiac or renal insufficiency. In cases of acute water intoxication with cerebral edema, urgent intravenous infusion of hypertonic saline and intravenous furosemide are required. Worthley and Thomas [101] have administered 50 ml of 29.2% sodium chloride solution through a central venous catheter in adult patients with convulsions caused by water intoxication. Preparatory water enema should be avoided in children with suspected Hirschsprung's disease because of potential complications.

Tannic acid

For a number of years, tannic acid was widely used in barium enemas to improve the quality of the evacuation film. Subsequently, tannic acid was cited as a cause of hepatic damage [102]. Although low concentrations were claimed to be safe [103], use of tannic acid in enemas has virtually been abandoned. This subject is discussed in greater detail in the first edition of this book.

Electrocardiogram (EKG) changes

Studies of EKGs recorded by radiotelemetry in patients undergoing routine barium enema examinations showed that transient EKG changes commonly occurred, particularly in elderly patients or patients with heart disease [59]. These changes appeared to be common during the evacuation phase, the filling phase, and during gas insufflation. The abnormalities noted included arrhythmias, conduction defects, and depression of RS-T waves. Although there were frequently no accompanying symptoms, some of the EKG abnormalities were potentially hazardous. Acute myocardial infarction may result in arrhythmias and death. Delaying elective barium enema at least 4 weeks after a myocardial infarct is suggested [104].

Infection

During a routine barium enema, feces and mucus may be seen to float up the plastic tube and even to enter the enema reservoir. All of the enema equipment is, therefore, subject to contamination, and it may become a potential source for transmission of pathogenic organisms that are excreted in the bowel. Although contamination of the barium reservoir has been avoided by the use of disposable packaging, contamination may still be present in some areas where disposable bags and tubes are not available.

A transient and self-limited bacteremia may occur in patients during or after barium enema or colonoscopy. However, antibiotic prophylaxis is not necessary in most patients undergoing barium enema procedure [60]. Septicemia after barium enema in an immunocompromised patient and a case of bacterial endocarditis have been reported [1,57] (see also p. 111).

Barium retention and minor reactions

In a barium enema, unlike a barium meal, the amount of barium retained in the colon is less and the risk of barium impaction is reduced. Nevertheless, 20–36% of patients have complained of constipation after barium enemas [17,61]. In an atonic colon filled with feces, inspissated barium may persist for days or weeks after a barium enema, aggravating the problems of constipation and occasionally causing an acute obstruction [3]. A more intractable but less well-recognized problem arises when a barium enema is performed to examine the distal loop after a defunctioning colostomy. Inspissated barium may persist in the defunctioned rectum for weeks or months, giving rise to intermittent discomfort and excess mucus secretion (Fig. 28.10). Therefore, it is preferable to use a water-soluble medium when examining the distal colonic segment and to wash out any remaining contrast material at the completion of the examination to avoid irritation by the hypertonic medium [1].

Abdominal pain is common in elderly patients after barium enema [17], and diarrhea has been reported in 8% of patients after barium enema [17]. Protective shielding of the enema tip, if not removed before insertion, can remain in the colon. This shielding may be passed spontaneously or should be removed by proctoscopy [105].

Allergic and anaphylactic reactions

Pure barium sulfate is an inert substance. However, commercial preparations contain a variety of additives that may help coating and preservation, and are believed to be the cause of hypersensitivity. Allergic reactions to commercial barium products has been reported in one of every 1700–750 000 examinations [62–64]. Allergic and anaphylactic reactions from both barium products for either an upper or lower gastrointestinal tract, water-soluble contrast media, latex enema tips, and drugs are discussed in this section.

Allergic reactions to barium suspension

From a survey of gastrointestinal radiologists and from other sources, Janower [63] collected 106 cases of hypersensitivity reactions after barium examinations. Most of the reactions occurred with double-contrast techniques, and only 11 of these patients had received glucagon. Of all the reactions, 61% involved the skin, 8% of patients became unconscious, and one patient developed severe migraine.

Adverse reactions to barium preparations include erythema, periorbital edema, vertigo, loss of consciousness, severe anaphylactic collapse, and generalized urticaria. An unusual allergic reaction to a barium preparation was reported in a patient with a history of allergy to a variety of drugs [65]. Initially, esophageal and abdominal pain occurred 30 minutes after a barium meal. All symptoms, including shivering, headaches, joint pain, and pyrexia, improved over 3 days but recurred on rechallenge at 15 days.

In five other cases, allergic reactions occurred after barium meals or enemas, and it was suggested that methylparabens, used as a perservative, may have been responsible [66]. However, methylparabens has since been removed from some barium suspensions. Allergic angioedema of the stomach and small bowel showing thickening of the folds in the stomach and duodenum was attributed to red-dye additives in barium products [67]. These symptoms occurred in the same patient on two separate barium meals using E-Z-HD (E-Z-Em Co., Westbury, NY). As these ingredients are approved by the Food and Drug Administration (FDA), food allergies may be responsible.

Severe anaphylactic reactions are rare during barium enemas. One patient developed erythema, pruritus, respiratory and circulatory arrest after a barium enema [66]. A fatal reaction occurred in a 49-year-old woman with a history of asthma and allergy; during a single-contrast enema she complained of warmth and itching, then became dyspneic and collapsed. The autopsy showed severe mucous plugging in her bronchi [68]. Patients with asthma or with food allergies and eosinophilic gastroenteropathy may be at particular risk [106].

Latex balloon-equipped enema tips

Allergic and anaphylactic reactions to latex products is a growing problem that may occur with rectal manometry in which the finger of a latex glove is used to cover the transducer [69]. Similarly, with barium enemas reaction to the latex balloon-equipped enema tip has been reported to occur during the enema, or even after insertion of a balloon tip but before the administration of barium suspension [70].

Latex, a natural product derived from the sap of the rubber tree, consists of long-chain molecules. The liquid latex supplied to manufacturers contains small amounts of water-soluble proteins of low molecular weight. After the latex rubber product is formed by heating the liquid latex, water-soluble proteins remain in the product and may be absorbed by the rectal mucosa. This process can trigger allergic and anaphylactic reactions in sensitized patients. In 1990, seven fatal anaphylactic reactions related to the latex

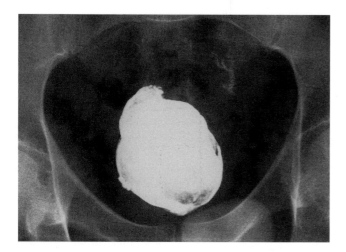

Fig. 28.10 Male, age 35 years. Transverse colostomy for perforated diverticulitis. Residual barium in the rectum 8 months after barium enema to demonstrate the distal loop. (From Ansell [1].)

balloon enema tip occurred; the E-Z-Em Company discontinued the use of latex to produce balloon tips in 1991. In 1991, there was only one fatal anaphylactic reaction reported ([70] E-Z-Em Co., personal communication).

The major manifestations of anaphylactic reactions are dyspnea, hypotension, edema, headache, and agitation. Other symptoms include urticaria to a varying extent, occurring on the head, trunk, or upper extremity. Some patients (40%) had a history of allergies or asthma, or use of bronchodilators [64]. *In vitro* studies show that the presence of immunoglobulin E antibodies specific for latex allergens can be detected by the radioallergosorbent (RAST) method showing more than 300% of negative control values (normal <300%), or by using enzyme-linked immunosorbent assay (ELISA) more than 140% (normal <140%) [71]. Skin tests may also be positive for the extracts of latex products [71].

The Weber catheter was made from latex but is no longer being manufactured. Anaphylactic reactions from Weber catheters have not been reported, possibly because the Weber balloon is used less often than the E-Z-Em catheter or was made from a latex with less water-soluble proteins on the surface of the catheter (Picker Company, personal communication). Currently, silicone balloon enema tips are now available but are of smaller size than the Weber or Bardex-like tips (see also p. 91).

Hypersensitivity to water-soluble media

Water-soluble iodinated contrast media were not believed to be absorbed from the gastrointestinal tract in the absence of a perforation, but this is no longer considered true. Measurable amounts of diatrizoate can be detected in the blood after intraduodenal administration [72]. An idiosyncratic reaction has been reported in a 66-year-old man who received 2 ml of Gastrografin during the course of a jejunal biopsy. He developed acute angioneurotic edema and this was followed by a cerebrovascular accident [1].

Glucagon

Glucagon (Eli Lilly Co., Indianapolis, IN) is extracted from porcine and bovine pancreas. Where glucagon has been used prior to double-contrast barium examinations, it was suggested that allergic reactions may be due to either glucagon or barium suspension [62]. Glucagon has been reported to cause allergic and anaphylactic reactions including skin rashes, periorbital edema, erythema multiforme, and anaphylaxis. The producer, Eli Lilly Company, estimates the likelihood of an adverse reaction to glucagon to be 1:1 × 10^6 million doses [73]. In February 1985, the manufacturer had received 11 reports of allergic and anaphylactic reactions. In 1986, Eli Lilly Company developed a more purified glucagon product by hydrophobic ion-exchange chromatography (over 90% purity). Since introduction of new purified

products, only one anaphylactic reaction was reported related to a radiologic procedure (Eli Lilly Research Laboratories, Eli Lilly Co., personal communication).

Erythema multiforme with arthralgia has been reported after intravenous glucagon in a double-contrast barium meal [74]. Cardiopulmonary arrest after a barium enema with glucagon has also been reported [75]. The patient who had a history of allergy to chocolate and atopic dermatitis, had itching, vomiting, diaphoresis, and cardiopulmonary arrest immediately after glucagon was administered. Cardiopulmonary resuscitation was started immediately, but the patient did not respond.

Buscopan

Buscopan has been claimed to cause angioneurotic edema [76] and a severe asthmatic attack [77].

It is important that resuscitation facilities should be immediately available.

Cholecystography and cholangiography

Oral cholecystography (OCG) (Table 28.4)

The gall bladder was first opacified by Graham and Cole in 1924 [117]. In the early 1950s, OCG became the standard procedure for examining the gall bladder with the introduction of iopanoic acid [118]. Iopanoic acid and other

Table 28.4 Cholecystography

Types of complications [reference]	Prevalence (cases or %)	Death (cases or %)
Severe		
Hypotensive collapse, myocardial infarction [1]	5	U
Anaphylactic reaction [107]	1/600 000	
Renal failure [108]	80	U
Overdose [107,110]	U	7
Thrombocytopenic purpura [1,121]	5	
Thyrotoxicosis [1]	2	
Other		
Minor reactions [111,112]	5–75%	
Nausea, vomiting [111,112]	10–33%	
Diarrhea [113]	14–30%	
Headache [111,112]	U	
Dysuria [114,115]	1–19%	
Skin rash [111,112,116]	0.5–2%	

U, uncertain.

cholecystographic media have been widely used since then, but in the early 1980s, the availability of ultrasonography, percutaneous cholangiography, CT, endoscopic retrograde cholangiopancreatography, and improved nuclear biliary imaging agents resulted in a marked reduction in the use of OCG. In the late 1980s, the use of OCG rebounded because of its more precise assessment of the size and number of gallstones in conjunction with biliary lithotripsy.

Major reactions

Serious or life-threatening reactions to OCG agents are rare. Major reactions include anaphylactic shock, cardiovascular complications, hepatorenal toxicity, and overdose, all of which may cause death.

Anaphylactic shock is rare and has been reported in one of 600 000 doses of ipodate [107]. Cardiovascular complications include hypotension, coronary insufficiency, or infarction. Hypovolemia induced by dehydration secondary to vomiting and diarrhea could also contribute to hypotension [119].

Renal toxicity has been the most frequent serious reaction to the OCG agents, and at least 80 cases of renal failure had been reported to 1972 [108]. All of the OCG media have been incriminated. In most of these patients, excess dosage or concomitant use of iodipamide meglumine (Cholografin) for intravenous cholangiography, or liver and gall-bladder diseases were associated. The etiology of renal damage caused by cholecystographic media is not clear [109,119,120]. High blood levels of contrast agent due to excessive dosage and decreased hepatic clearance caused by liver derangement may be important [109,119]. Other proposed mechanisms include a direct toxic effect on the renal tubules [120], intratubular block by crystalluria or urinary protein, and constriction of the preglomerular vessels with subsequent renal ischemia [109].

Massive overdoses have been reported, the largest being accidental ingestion of 75 g of iopanoic acid without permanent ill-effects [110]. On the other hand, seven deaths from overdoses have been reported in association with 22×10^6 doses of iopanoic acid [107]. Four deaths resulted from renal damage, and one each was related to myocardial insufficiency, hepatic disease, and overdose.

Severe thrombocytopenic purpura may occur as a rare complication of OCG with either iopanoic acid, ipodate, or iocetamic acid [121] (see also p. 261).

Minor reactions

Minor reactions have a reported incidence varying from less than 5% and up to 57% [111,112]. The most common complaints include nausea, vomiting, abdominal cramping, diarrhea, dysuria, headache, and skin rash. Nausea and vomiting occurred in 10−33% of cases [111,112]. Diarrhea has been noted in 14−30% of patients, particularly with iopanoic acid [113]. Iocetamic acid (3.0-g dose) has the lowest reported incidence of gastrointestinal side-effects but a higher incidence of skin rashes (see below) [116].

Dysuria has been noted in 1−19% of cases [114,115]. Approximately 35% of absorbed iopanoic acid is excreted in the urine, and the higher incidence of dysuria following iopanoic acid ingestion may relate to its greater urinary load. Pseudoalbuminuria may occur. Cholegraphic media are uricosuric agents and fluctuations in the serum urate may precipitate an attack of gout [1,110].

Skin reactions, itching, erythema, urticaria, and angioneurotic edema are less common in patients receiving iopanoic acid, tyropanoate, and ipodate [115,116]. The incidence of skin reactions associated with iocetamic acid, however, has been higher (0.5−2%) [116]. Alterations in thyroid function may occur, and at least two cases of thyrotoxicosis have been reported [1].

Intravenous cholangiography (IVC)

In 1954, iodipamide meglumine (Cholografin, E.R. Squibb Co., NY) was introduced as a radiographic contrast material for IVC. Other cholangiographic agents include meglumine ioglycamate (Biligram, Schering, UK), meglumine iodoxamate (Cholovue), and meglumine iotroxate (Biliscopin, Schering, UK), which are chemically similar to Cholografin except for a variation in the interconnecting polymethylene chain. However, the use of IVC has been dramatically curtailed in the last decade to a total of eight cases per year in 30 academic radiology departments according to a 1989 survey [122]. In one review of 3711 cases, the overall incidence of reactions to iotroxate ranged from 3.5 to 12%, ioglycamate ranged from 9 to 30%, and iodoxamate ranged from 5 to 15% [123].

Major reactions

Serious reactions to iodipamide include severe cutaneous reactions, cardiorespiratory manifestations, hypotension, hepatorenal toxicity, and anaphylaxis. Deaths have occurred in one of 3000−5000 cases, a significantly higher mortality rate than with the urographic contrast agents [124,125]. In an analysis of 28 deaths following IVC, 15 were attributed to cardiac arrest or myocardial infarction, and four to pulmonary edema. Pretesting and premedication with antihistamines or steroids have no proven effect on preventing major reactions or death. In seven patients, fatal reactions began with nausea and vomiting [126] (see also p. 261).

Potential *hepatic toxicity* relates to the type and amount of agent used; there was elevation of SGOT by 18.3% in patients receiving 40 ml of iodipamide, in comparison to elevation of 8.7% SGOT in patients receiving 20 ml of iodipamide [127]. Slow intravenous infusion of cholangiographic contrast material (>30 minutes) reduced reactions to one-third the frequency than when an equal amount of the same contrast material was injected (6—10 minutes) [123]. Infusion of iotroxate caused the lowest incidence of reactions: minor reactions 3%; moderate reactions 0.3%; severe reactions 0.2% [123].

The causes of iodipamide-associated *nephrotoxicity* include dose-related phenomena, simultaneous administration of other contrast agents, direct effect on the kidney resulting from either tubular toxicity or preglomerular vasoconstriction, contribution of enhanced uric acid excretion, and possibility of urate nephropathy. IVC is not indicated when serum bilirubin levels are above 3—4 mg%, or when significant hepatorenal disease, dehydration, or globulinopathies are present [128]. IVC should not follow examinations using other iodinated contrast media within 24—48 hours, because of a possible increase in the risk of serious morbidity and mortality. Considering all factors, 20 ml of iodipamide with slow administration appears to be the optimum dose to allow satisfactory biliary opacification and to minimize side-effects. If iotroxate is available, this is preferable.

Minor reactions

The overall reported incidence of minor reactions (to iodipamide) has varied from 4.1 to 23.9% [127,129]. Gastrointestinal side-effects include nausea, vomiting, diarrhea, and hepatic pain. Cutaneous reactions include flushing, itching, and urticaria. A slow infusion rate of 10 minutes or more, or use of an antihistamine may reduce minor side-effects. The complications from OCG and IVC are described in greater detail in the previous edition of this book [1].

For treatment of reactions, see p. 280.

Operative and T-tube cholangiography

Since the 1930s, wide experience with operative and T-tube cholangiography indicates that severe adverse effects associated with these procedures are relatively rare [128,130].

A fatal reaction to diatrizoate was reported during the performance of intraoperative cholangiography. Although the patient did not have biliary obstruction, contrast material entered the bloodstream [131]. Other potential problems include liver damage, abscess formation, sepsis in an obstructed biliary tract, pancreatitis, nausea and vomiting, fever, cholangitis, and contrast reactions.

Biliary peritonitis caused by leakage of contrast material during T-tube cholangiography may resolve spontaneously, but bacterial infection of the bile can cause septic peritonitis. The incidence of biliary peritonitis was reported in four (14%) of 28 patients with a radiologic leak during T-tube cholangiography [132]. The T-tube should be retained for another 7—10 days to prevent bile spillage into the peritoneal cavity if a contrast leak is found during the T-tube study [132]. There is no reported incidence of bile peritonitis in patients with no leak during T-tube cholangiography. Dellinger *et al.* [133] have followed up 170 T-tube cholangiograms in 139 patients. The incidence of febrile reactions in the 24 hours following cholangiography was 5.3%, with two cases of endotoxic shock [133]. Hand injection into the T-tube may produce transient bile-duct pressures up to 80 cm of water with reflux of biliary contents into the venous system.

Since 1987, *laparoscopic cholecystectomy* has become more popular due to an early lower complication rate, lower cost, and shorter recovery time when compared to conventional cholecystectomy. Intraoperative cholangiography is routinely performed during the laparoscopic procedure. The major complications associated with laparoscopic cholecystectomy are hepatic duct injuries or strictures and problems related to bile leak and bilomas [134].

References

1 Ansell G. Oral and intravenous cholegraphy: Alimentary tract. In: Ansell G, Wilkins RA, eds. *Complications in Diagnostic Imaging*, 2nd edn. Oxford: Blackwell Scientific Publications, 1987:205—246.

2 Gray C, Sivaloganathan S, Simpkins KC. Aspiration of high-density barium contrast medium causing acute pulmonary inflammation — report of two fatal cases in elderly women with disordered swallowing. *Clin Radiol* 1989;40:397—400.

3 Killingback M. Acute large-bowel obstruction precipitated by barium X-ray examination. *Med J Austr* 1964;2:503—508.

4 Palder SB, Dalessandri KM. Barium appendicitis. *W J Med* 1988;148:462—464.

5 Rohrmann CA Jr, Acheson MB. Esophageal perforation during double-contrast esophagram. *Am J Roentgenol* 1985;145:283—284.

6 Grobmyer AJ III, Kerlan RA, Peterson CM, Dragstedt LR II. Barium peritonitis. *Am Surg* 1984;50:116—120.

7 Shimi SM. Peptic ulcer perforation: a complication of double contrast barium meal examination. *Scott Med J* 1989;34:500.

8 Gillespie P, Riley J, Hunt J. Perforation of duodenal ulcer during barium meal. *Australas Radiol* 1977;21:241—242.

9 Diner WC. Duodenal perforation during intubation for small bowel enema study. *Radiology* 1988;168:39—41.

10 Ginaldi S. Small bowel perforation during enteroclysis. *Gastrointest Radiol* 1991;16:29—31.

11 Walker AJ. Case report: perforation of the colon after barium meal examination. *Clin Radiol* 1989;40:530.

12 Gelfand DW, Moskowitz M. Massive gastric dilatation complicating hypotonic duodenography. A report of three cases. *Radiology* 1970;97:637—639.

13 Govindiah D, Bhaskar GR. An unusual case of barium poisoning. *Antiseptic* 1972;69:675—677.

14 Berning J. Letter: hypokalaemia of barium poisoning. *Lancet* 1975;1:110.

15 Dupuy F, Bestagne MH, Rodor F, Poyen B, Jouglard J. Encéphalopathie convulsive et sulfate de barium. *Therapie* 1980;35:447—449.

16 Deixonne B, Baumel H, Mauras Y *et al.* Un cas de barytopéritoine avec atteinte neurologique intérêt du dosage du barium dans les liquides biologiques. *J Chir (Paris)* 1983;120:611—613.

17 Smith HJ, Jones K, Hunter TB. What happens to patients after upper and lower gastrointestinal tract barium studies? *Invest Radiol* 1988;23:822−826.

18 Prout BJ, Datta SB, Wilson TS. Colonic retention of barium in the elderly after barium-meal examination and its treatment with lactulose. *Br Med J* 1972;4:530−533.

19 Fischer WW, Nice CM Jr. Barium impaction as a cause of small bowel obstruction in an infant with cystic fibrosis. *Pediat Radiol* 1984;14:230−231.

20 Umeki S. Caution in upper gastrointestinal X-ray study in constipated parkinsonian patients. *S Med J* 1982;82:1589.

21 Jackson DM. A word of caution to radiologists (letter). *New Engl J Med* 1978;298:856.

22 Amberg JR, Unger JD. Contamination of barium sulfate suspension. *Radiology* 1970;97:182−183.

23 Gelfand DW. Complications of gastrointestinal radiologic procedures: I. Complications of routine fluoroscopic studies. *Gastrointest Radiol* 1980;5:293−315.

24 Erickson LM, Shaw D, MacDonald FR. Prolonged barium retention in the lung following bronchography. *Radiology* 1979;130:635−636.

25 Griffith J, White P. Acute asthma precipitated by accidental inhalation of sodium bicarbonate granules (Carbex). *Clin Radiol* 1994;49:435.

26 Felson B. Radiologist on the rocks (letter). *Semin Roentgenol* 1973;8:361−363.

27 Harris PD, Neuhauser EBD, Gerth R. The osmotic effect of water soluble contrast media on circulating plasma volume. *Am J Roentgenol* 1964;91:694−698.

28 Elman S, Palayew MJ. Assessment of biochemical and hematologic changes related to oral administration of an iodinated contrast medium. *Invest Radiol* 1973;8:322−325.

29 Creteur V, Douglas D, Galante M, Margulis AR. Inflammatory colonic changes produced by contrast material. *Radiology* 1983;147:77−78.

30 Seltzer SE, Jones B. Cecal perforation associated with Gastrografin enema. *Am J Roentgenol* 1978;130:997−998.

31 Hogan TF. Gastrografin and bowel necrosis. *Ann Int Med* 1977;87:382−383.

32 Chiu CL, Gambach RR. Hypaque pulmonary edema. A case report. *Radiology* 1974;111:91−92.

33 Ross LS. Precipitation of meglumine diatrizoate 76% (Gastrografin) in the stomach. Observations on the insolubility of diatrizoate in the normal range of gastric acidity. *Radiology* 1972;105:19−22.

34 Gallitano AL, Kondi ES, Phillips E, Ferris E. Near-fatal hemorrhage following Gastrografin studies. *Radiology* 1976;118:35−36.

35 Glover JR, Thomas BM. Case report: severe adverse reaction to oral iohexol. *Clin Radiol* 1991;44:137−138.

36 Davies NP, Williams JA. Tubeless vagotomy and pyloroplasty and the "Gastrografin test." *Am J Surg* 1971;122:368−370.

37 Gmeinwieser J, Erhardt W, Reimann HJ *et al.* Side effects of water-soluble contrast agents in upper gastrointestinal tract. *Invest Radiol* 1990;25:S27−S28.

38 Blanloeil Y, Colomb P, Vairon A, Paineau J, Dixneuf B. Syndrome des détresse respiratoire aiguë aprés inhalation accidentelle de produit de contrast hydrosoluble. *Semaine Hôpit Paris* 1983;59:762−764.

39 Cohen MD, Towbin R, Baker S *et al.* Comparison of iohexol with barium in gastrointestinal studies of infants and children. *Am J Roentgenol* 1991;156:345−350.

40 Williams SM, Harned RK. Recognition and prevention of barium enema complications. *Curr Probl Diagn Radiol* 1991;20:123−151.

41 Cordone RP, Brandeis SZ, Richman H. Rectal perforation during barium enema: report of a case. *Dis Colon Rectum* 1988;31:563−569.

42 Zheutlin N, Lasser EC, Rigler LG. Clinical studies on the effect of barium in the peritoneal cavity following rupture of the colon. *Surgery* 1952;32:967−979.

43 Yanagi S, Ishii T, Tsuji Y, Ariyoshi A. Barium granuloma involving urinary bladder. *Urol Int* 1989;44:249−251.

44 De Mascarel A, Merlio JP, Goussot JF, Coindre JM. Radiohistology as a new diagnostic method for barium granuloma. *Arch Pathol Lab Med* 1988;112:634−636.

45 Fowlie S, Barton JR, Fraser GM. Barium embolisation during barium enema examination: a report of a case and a review of the literature. *Br J Radiol* 1987;60:404−406.

46 Wheatley MJ, Eckhauser FE. Portal venous barium intravasation complicating barium enema examination. *Surgery* 1991;109:788−791.

47 Jaluvka V, Cammann U. Versehentliche vaginale Applikation des Kolonkontrastmittels. *Zentralbl Gynakol* 1991;113:115−118.

48 Chan F-L, Tso W-K, Wong L-C, Ngan H. Barium intravasation: radiographic and CT findings in a nonfatal case. *Radiology* 1987;163:311−312.

49 Taylor DB, Yoong P. Non fatal barium intravasation during barium enema. *Australas Radiol* 1990;34:165−167.

50 Zatzkin HR, Irwin GAL. Nonfatal intravasation of barium. *Am J Roentgenol* 1964;92:1169−1172.

51 Rosenberg LS, Fine A. Fatal venous intravasation of barium during a barium enema. *Radiology* 1959;73:771−773.

52 Kanehann LB, Caroline DF, Friedman AC, Lev-Toaff AS, Radecki PD. CT findings in venous intravasation complicating diverticulitis. *J Comput Assist Tomog* 1988;12:1047−1049.

53 Isaacs I, Nissen R, Epstein BS. Liver abscess resulting from barium enema in a case of chronic ulcerative colitis. *N Y St J Med* 1950;50:332−334.

54 Sadhu VK, Brennan RE, Madan V. Portal vein gas following air-contrast barium enema in granulomatous colitis: report of a case. *Gastrointest Radiol* 1979;4:163−164.

55 Moss ML, Mazzeo JT. Pneumoperitoneum and portal venous air after barium enema. *Va Med Q* 1991;118:233−235.

56 Peterson CA, Cayler GG. Water intoxication. Report of a fatality following a barium enema. *Am J Roentgenol* 1957;77:69−70.

57 Hammer JL. Septicemia following barium enema. *S Med J* 1977;70:1361−1363.

58 Harned RK, Consigny PM, Cooper NB, Williams SM, Woltjen AJ. Barium enema examination following biopsy of the rectum or colon. *Radiology* 1982;145:11−16.

59 Berman CZ, Jacobs MG, Bernstein A. Hazards of the barium enema examination as studied by electrocardiographic telemetry: preliminary report. *J Am Geriat Soc* 1965;13:672−686.

60 Butt J, Hentges D, Pelican G *et al.* Bacteremia during barium enema study. *Am J Roentgenol* 1978;130:715−718.

61 Russell JGB. Patients' complaints after barium enema. *Br J Radiol* 1986;59:294−295.

62 Gelfand DW, Sowers JC, DePonte KA, Sumner TE, Ott DJ. Anaphylactic and allergic reactions during double-contrast studies: is glucagon or barium suspension the allergen? *Am J Roentgenol* 1985;144:405−406.

63 Janower ML. Hypersensitivity reactions after barium studies of the upper and lower gastrointestinal tract. *Radiology* 1986;161:

139−140.

64 Feczko PJ. Increased frequency of reactions to contrast materials during gastrointestinal studies. *Radiology* 1990;174:367−368.

65 Aznauryase MS, Shryov MK. An incident of allergy to barium sulphate (in Russian). *Klin Med (Mosc)* 1978;56:122−123.

66 Wasser MNJM, Chandie Shaw MP, Holten-Verzantvoort A, de Pont ACJM, Toet AE. Anaphylaxis as a rare complication of a barium enema examination. *Neth J Med* 1989;35:147−150.

67 Shaffer HA Jr, Eckard DA, de Lange EE, Ramakrishnan MR. Allergy to barium sulfate suspension with angioedema of the stomach and small bowel. *Gastrointest Radiol* 1988;13:221−223.

68 Feczko PJ, Simms SM, Bakirci N. Fatal hypersensitivity reaction during a barium enema. *Am J Roentgenol* 1989;153:275−276.

69 Sondheimer JM, Pearlman DS, Bailey WC. Systemic anaphylaxis during rectal manometry with a latex balloon. *Am J Gastroenterol* 1989;84:975−977.

70 Gelfand DW. Barium enemas, latex balloons, and anaphylactic reactions. *Am J Roentgenol* 1991;156:1−2.

71 Ownby DR, Tomlanovich M, Sammons N, McCullough J. Anaphylaxis associated with latex allergy during barium enema examinations. *Am J Roentgenol* 1991;156:903−908.

72 Sable RA, Rosenthal WS, Siegle J, Ho R, Jankowski RH. Absorption of contrast medium during ERCP. *Digest Dis Sci* 1983;28:801−806.

73 Schuh M, Petrelli NJ, Herrera L. Systemic hypersensitivity reaction following a barium enema examination. *N Y State J Med* 1988;88:86−87.

74 Edell SL. Erythema multiforme secondary to intravenous glucagon. *Am J Roentgenol* 1980;134:385−386.

75 Harrington RA, Kaul AF. Cardiopulmonary arrest following barium enema examination with glucagon. *Drug Intell Clin Pharm* 1987;21:721−722.

76 Thomas AK, Kubie AM, Britt RP. Acute angioneurotic oedema following a barium meal (letter). *Br J Radiol* 1986;59:1055−1056.

77 Treweeke P, Barrett NK. Allergic reaction to Buscopan (letter). *Br J Radiol* 1987;60:417−418.

78 Masel H, Masel JP, Casey KV. A survey of colon examination techniques in Australia and New Zealand, with a review of complications. *Australas Radiol* 1971;15:140−147.

79 Burt CAV. Pneumatic rupture of intestinal canal with experimental data showing mechanism of perforation and pressure required. *Arch Surg* 1931;22:875−902.

80 Noveroske RJ. Perforation of a normal colon by too much pressure. *J Indiana State Med Assoc* 1972;65:23−25.

81 Diner WC, Patel G, Texter EC Jr *et al*. Intraluminal pressure measurements during barium enema: full column vs. air contrast. *Am J Roentgenol* 1981;137:217−221.

82 Galloway D, Burns HJG, Moffat LEF, MacPherson SG. Faecal peritonitis after laxative preparation for barium enema. *Br Med J* 1982;284:472.

83 McBride K. Sodium picosulphate: drug reaction or drug interaction? *Clin Radiol* 1992;45:290.

84 Peterson N, Rohrmann CA Jr, Lennard ES. Diagnosis and treatment of retroperitoneal perforation complicating the double-contrast barium-enema examination. *Radiology* 1982;144:249−252.

85 Kapote S, Nazareth HM, Bapat RD. Barium peritonitis (a case report). *J Postgrad Med* 1988;34:103−104.

86 Noveroske RJ. Perforation of the rectosigmoid by a Bardex balloon catheter. Report of 3 cases. *Am J Roentgenol* 1966;96:326−331.

87 Merrill CR, Steiner GM. Barium enema after biopsy: current practice and opinion. *Clin Radiol* 1986;37:89−92.

88 Harned RK, William SM, Maglinte DDT *et al*. Clinical application of *in vitro* studies for barium−enema examination following colorectal biopsy. *Radiology* 1985;154:319−321.

89 Gelfand DW, Ott DJ, Ramquist NA. Pneumoperitoneum occurring during double-contrast enema. *Gastrointest Radiol* 1979;4:307−308.

90 Vandendris M, Giannakopoulos X. Retroperitoneal barytoma. *Urology* 1981;17:358−359.

91 Beerman PJ, Gelfand DW, Ott DJ. Pneumomediastinum after double-contrast barium enema examination: a sign of colonic perforation. *Am J Roentgenol* 1981;136:197−198.

92 Rabin DN, Smith C, Witt TR, Holinger LD. Voice change after barium enema: a clinical sign of extraperitoneal colon perforation. *Am J Roentgenol* 1987;148:145−146.

93 Gardner DJ, Hanson RE. Computed tomography of retroperitoneal perforation after barium enema. *Clin Imag* 1990;14:208−210.

94 Seaman WB, Bragg DG. Colonic intramural barium: a complication of the barium−enema examination. *Radiology* 1967;89:250−255.

95 Cho KC, Simmons MZ, Baker SR, Cappell MS. Spontaneous dissection of air into the transverse mesocolon during double-contrast barium enema. *Gastrointest Radiol* 1990;15:76−77.

96 Sprung CL, Caralis PV, Marcial EH *et al*. The effects of high-dose corticosteroids in patients with septic shock. A prospective, controlled study. *New Engl J Med* 1984;311:1137−1143.

97 Yamamura M, Nishi M, Furubayashi H, Hioki K, Yamamoto M. Barium peritonitis. Report of a case and review of the literature. *Dis Colon Rectum* 1985;28:347−352.

98 Terranova O, Meneghello A, Battocchio F *et al*. Perforations of the extraperitoneal rectum during barium enema. *Int Surg* 1989;74:13−16.

99 Von Stosch M, Steinhohh H. Iatrogene sekundäre retroperitoneale Fibrosierung (sekundarer Morbus Ormond) durch Kontrastmitteleinlauf und bei Behandlung der enstandenem Harnstaungsmieren mit der endoureteralen Schienung ("endoprosthese"). *Z Urol Nephrol* 1981;74:571.

100 Subramanyam K, Rajan RT, Hearn CD. Barium granuloma of the sigmoid colon. *J Clin Gastroenterol* 1988;10:98−100.

101 Worthley LIG, Thomas PD. Treatment of hyponatraemic seizures with 29.2% saline. *Br Med J* 1986;292:168−170.

102 Zboralske FF, Harris PA, Riegelman S, Rambo ON, Margulis AR. Toxicity studies on tannic acid administered by enema. III. Studies on the retention of enemas in humans. IV. Review and conclusions. *Am J Roentgenol* 1966;96:505−509.

103 Harper RA, Pemberton J, Tobias JS. Serial liver function studies following barium enemas containing 1% tannic acid. *Clin Radiol* 1973;24:315−317.

104 Smith HJ. Performance of barium examinations after acute myocardial infarction: report a survey. *Am J Roentgenol* 1987;149:63−65.

105 Zeligman BE, Feinberg LE, Johnson ED. A complication of cleansing enema: retained protective shield of the enema tip. *Gastrointest Radiol* 1986;11:372−374.

106 Stringer DA, Hassall E, Ferguson AC, Cairns R, Nadel H, Sargent M. Hypersensitivity reaction to single contrast barium meal studies in children. *Pediat Radiol* 1993;23:587−588.

107 Shehadi WH. Clinical problems and toxicity of contrast agents. *Am J Roentgenol* 1966;97:762−771.

108 Gaudet M, Cortet P, Rifle G, Villand J. L'insuffisance rénale

aigue après cholécystographie orale. Revue générale à propos de deux observations. *Rev Fr Gastro-enterol* 1974;102:47−58.

109 Ansari Z, Baldwin DS. Acute renal failure due to radio-contrast agents. *Nephronology* 1976;17:28−40.

110 Gelfand DW, Ott DJ, Klein A. Massive iopanoic acid (Telepaque) overdose without ill effects. *Am J Roentgenol* 1978;130:1174−1175.

111 Stanley RJ, Melson GL, Cubillo E, Hesker AE. A comparison of three cholecystographic agents. A double-blind study with and without a prior fatty meal. *Radiology* 1974;112:513−517.

112 Juhl JH, Cooperman LR, Crummy AB. Oragrafin, a new cholecystographic medium. *Radiology* 1963;80:87−91.

113 Tishler JM, Gold R. A clinical trial of oral cholecystographic agents: telepaque, sodium oragrafin and calcium oragrafin. *Can Assoc Radiol J* 1969;20:102−105.

114 Krook PM, Bush WH Jr. Single dose oral cholecystography. *Radiology* 1978;127:643−644.

115 White WW, Fischer HW. A double blind study of oragrafin and telepaque. *Am J Roentgenol* 1962;87:745−748.

116 Parks RE. Double-blind study of four oral cholecystographic preparations. *Radiology* 1974;112:525−528.

117 Graham EA, Cole WH. Visualizing of gallbladder by the sodium salt of tetrabromphenolphthalein. *J Am Med Assoc* 1924;82:1777−1778.

118 Hoppe JO, Archer S. Observations on a series of aryl triiodo alkanoic acid derivatives with particular reference to a new cholecystographic medium, Telepaque. *Am J Roentgenol* 1953;69:630−637.

119 Teplick JG, Myerson RM, Sanen FJ. Acute renal failure following oral cholecystography. *Acta Radiol* 1965;3:353−369.

120 Harrow BR, Sloane JA. Acute renal failure following oral cholecystography. *Am J Med Sci* 1965;249:26−35.

121 Insauti CLG, Lechin F, van der Dijs B. Severe thrombocytopenia following oral cholecystography with iocetamic acid. *Am J Hematol* 1983;14:285−288.

122 Scott IR, Gibney RG, Becker CD, Fache JS, Burhenne HJ. The use of intravenous cholangiography in teaching hospitals: a survey. *Gastrointest Radiol* 1989;14:148−150.

123 Nilsson U. Adverse reactions to iotroxate at intravenous cholangiography. *Acta Radiol* 1987;28:571−575.

124 Shehadi WH. Adverse reactions to intravascularly administered contrast media. A comprehensive study based on a prospective survey. *Am J Roentgenol* 1975;124:145−152.

125 Ansell G. Adverse reactions to contrast agents. Scope of problem. *Invest Radiol* 1970;5:374−391.

126 Lalli AF. Contrast media deaths. *Australas Radiol* 1984;28:133−135.

127 Scholz FJ, Johnston DO, Wise RE. Intravenous cholangiography. Optimum dosage and methodology. *Radiology* 1975;114:513−518.

128 Ott DJ, Gelfand DW. Complications of gastrointestinal radiologic procedures. II. Complications related to biliary tract studies. *Gastrointest Radiol* 1981;6:47−56.

129 Johnson JH Jr, Wise RE. Intravenous cholangiography: a study of reactions to iodipamide methylglucamine. *Lahey Clin Bull* 1964;13:245−250.

130 Berci G, Hamlin JA. Operative and postoperative cholangiography. In: Berk RN, Ferrucci JT Jr, Leopold GR, eds. *Radiology of the Gallbladder and Bile Ducts.* Philadelphia: WB Saunders, 1983:401−431.

131 Sakahira K, Ebata T, Tsunoda Y, Amaha K, Meno K. Serum diatrizoate level during intraoperative cholangiography in patients without choledochal obstructions. *Digest Dis Sci* 1990;35:1085−1088.

132 Mosley JG, Barron JA, Holbrook MC, Desai A. An association between leakage of contrast seen on T-tube cholangiogram and subsequent biliary peritonitis. *Br J Radiol* 1992;65:185−186.

133 Dellinger EP, Kirshenbaum G, Weinstein M, Steer M. Determinants of adverse reaction following postoperative T-tube cholangiogram. *Ann Surg* 1980;191:397−403.

134 Trerotola SO, Savader SJ, Lund GB *et al.* Biliary tract complications following laparoscopic cholecystectomy: imaging and intervention. *Radiology* 1992;184:195−200.

CHAPTER 29

Complications of transhepatic biliary procedures

Philip C. Pieters and Michael A. Bettmann

Introduction

Technologic advances in instrumentation over the past two decades have led to significant advances in percutaneous transhepatic procedures. Major improvements in catheters, guidewires, and drainage catheters as well as the introduction of expandable metallic stents have allowed for improved management of biliary tract diseases. The advent of metallic stents has also had a major impact on the care of patients with portal hypertension, adding percutaneous creation of portosystemic shunts (transjugular intrahepatic porto-systemic shunt, TIPS) to the armamentarium of the interventional radiologist. The TIPS procedure has been shown to have lower morbidity and mortality rates than those of surgical shunting. Because of the invasive nature of the TIPS procedure and other transhepatic biliary procedures, how-ever, complications do occur and are relatively common in comparison to most radiologic procedures. It is essential for all radiologists involved in interventional transhepatic pro-cedures to have a thorough knowledge of the complications that may occur, the precautions that should be taken to minimize them, and their subsequent management should they occur.

Percutaneous liver biopsy

Percutaneous liver biopsy has come to play a central role in diagnosing various liver abnormalities. Refinements in tools and guidance by means of computed tomography (CT) and ultrasound have allowed precise placement of the biopsy needle, even in very small targets. Although percutaneous liver biopsies are considered safe, rare complications do occur, including severe and even fatal ones. Two large surveys, conducted by Smith in 1984 [1] and in 1991 [2], concerned complications following percutaneous fine needle biopsies of abdominal lesions. These surveys revealed four deaths after 63 108 biopsies (0.006%) and five deaths after 16 381 biopsies (0.031%), respectively. Two similar European questionnaires [3,4] revealed mortality rates of 0.008% ([3] $n = 66397$) and 0.018% ([4] $n = 10766$). Of the 33 total deaths documented in these four surveys, 21 involved biopsies of liver lesions.

Hemorrhage

Of the 21 deaths in the above mentioned surveys, 17 were secondary to hemorrhage, and these occurred principally in patients with a bleeding diathesis or a liver tumor. In several of these cases, a bleeding disorder was known to exist, and in others it may not have been looked for. The minimum work-up prior to a liver biopsy in a patient with no bleeding history should include a platelet count and prothrombin time. Thrombocytopenia and prolonged prothrombin time are clearly associated with a higher risk of bleeding [5,6]. Percutaneous liver biopsy is usually considered undesirable if the platelet count is less than 80 000/ml or if the pro-thrombin time is prolonged more than 3 seconds above the normal value [7]. Platelet concentrate and/or coagulation factors, in the form of fresh frozen plasma, may be transfused prior to the procedure, but the efficacy of such prophylactic treatment has not been evaluated. Patients who fall within these high-risk groups and are in need of a biopsy should have consideration given to transjugular liver biopsy, to percutaneous biopsy with embolization of the biopsy tract as described below, or even to an open biopsy [35,36].

Eleven of the 21 fatal liver biopsies in the above mentioned surveys occurred in patients with primary liver tumors, and nine occurred in patients with liver metastases from various sites [2]. Of the primary hepatic tumors that resulted in fatal liver biopsies, two were angiosarcomas which are relatively rare hepatic lesions. Only two deaths following biopsy of hepatic hemangiomas, a common hepatic lesion, were reported which is consistent with the experience related in the recent radiology literature [8–12]. Among the cases of fatal hemorrhage, in several patients the liver lesion was located superficially, making it possible that the biopsy needle did not traverse normal liver parenchyma prior to entering the lesion. This may explain why, in some instances, bleeding persisted despite surgical exploration [4,13]. It is clear that biopsy of vascular lesions such as hemangiomas is common and generally safe. Experience suggests, then, that it is prudent to direct the biopsy needle through normal liver tissue before entering the lesion, allowing normal liver tissue to tamponade the bleeding. As an additional control, Martino *et al.* [14] have suggested that CT-guided liver biopsies should be performed following bolus contrast injection and dynamic scanning, in order to evaluate the vascularity of the lesion. If the abnormality is considered vascular (e.g., if it enhances to the same degree as the aorta), it may be prudent to perform fine needle aspiration only, without using larger cutting needles. Consideration should also be given to embolization of the biopsy tract when biopsying a vascular lesion.

Intuitively, it would be expected that the risk of bleeding should increase in relation to the number of punctures performed. The fewest number of passes possible, therefore, should be performed to obtain an adequate specimen of tissue. As such, it is helpful to have a pathologist readily available to evaluate the specimen for diagnostic adequacy. If the initial pass results in an adequate specimen, then no further passes are necessary and the inherent increased risk with multiple passes is avoided.

Several studies have demonstrated that the complication rate (chiefly from bleeding) increases as needle size increases [14–19]. Authors have reported good results with CT-guided skinny needle aspiration, and some have stated that there is no need for the use of large cutting needles. Others [14,15] have reported the advantages of larger caliber needles. On the other hand, Martino *et al.* [14] concluded that the cutting needle biopsy provides a high yield of diagnostic tissue as compared to fine needle aspiration biopsy. Welch *et al.* [20] also reported greater diagnostic accuracy with specimens obtained with cutting needles (98.5% accuracy) when compared to fine needle biopsies, but also showed that the complication rate varied with needle size: 3.3% incidence of complications with a 15-gage needle, 2.1% with a 16-gage needle, 0.3% with an 18-gage needle, and 0.36% with a 21-gage needle. The choice of needle size involves a balance between the need to obtain a diagnostic specimen and the probable increased risk of larger needles. A choice of a needle should, therefore, be tailored to each individual case, with factors such as lesion vascularity, coagulation profile, and availability of a pathologist figuring prominently in the decision-making process.

In patients with suspected diffuse liver disease, transjugular liver biopsy is now the method of choice. This method is not practical, however, for biopsy of focal hepatic lesions. Zins *et al.* [7] reported a series of patients classified as high risk because of severe coagulation disorders, who underwent percutaneous biopsy with plugging of the biopsy tract. An 18-gage metal sheath was placed into the liver, through which the biopsy was performed with a 19-gage cutting needle. The sheath was left in place while the specimen was evaluated for adequacy. If the specimen was unsatisfactory, a cutting needle was reinserted for a second pass. After an adequate specimen was obtained, a mixture of surgical gelatin sponge particles and thrombus was injected during slow withdrawal of the needle. Major bleeding occurred in 2.8% of these high-risk patients, a higher incidence than with the transjugular method. These authors concluded that in patients with severe coagulation disorders, plugging liver biopsy should be performed only in focal lesions or after failure of transjugular liver biopsy.

Tract seeding

Needle-tract seeding following biopsy of a malignant hepatic lesion appears to be exceedingly rare. In Smith's accumulation of questionnaires and literature review [2] only three cases of tract seeding following biopsy of the liver were found. In multiple large series from individual institutions [3,21–23] no occurrence of needle-tract seeding was reported.

Ascites

Ascites has been considered a contraindication to percutaneous liver biopsy by some [24–26], but no large studies designed to compare the complication rates of biopsies in patients with and without ascites have been reported. A small study [27] designed to answer this question concluded that the complication rate in liver biopsies guided by CT or sonography in the presence of ascites is no higher than similar biopsies done in the absence of ascites. This question remains to be answered in a large series. At this time, most consider massive ascites to be an indication for a transjugular liver biopsy.

Transjugular liver biopsy

With this well-established technique, major complications have been reported with an incidence ranging from 1.3 to 6% [28–31]. The most common complication is intraperitoneal hemorrhage secondary to capsular perforation with the biopsy needle. Most often capsular perforation results in subclinical bleeding, but deaths from major intraperitoneal hemorrhage have been reported [28–30]. In patients at high risk for bleeding, several techniques to decrease the likelihood of capsular perforation and hemorrhage have been described. Because of its size, the right lobe is the most favorable site for biopsy. Biopsy should be performed with the catheter in the free position within the hepatic vein, not in the wedged position [32]. Although the needle is more likely to penetrate hepatic parenchyma with the catheter wedged, it is also more likely to lead to perforation because the needle tip lies more peripherally and therefore, closer to the capsule (Fig. 29.1). Injection of contrast medium through the guiding catheter can identify perforation following passage of the biopsy needle. If capsular perforation is identified, the tract can be embolized with gelfoam fragments or steel coils [30,33,34].

Other complications reported with the transjugular technique include cardiac arrhythmias, carotid artery puncture, and bleeding/hematoma at the vascular access site. Transient supraventricular tachycardia is easily recognized with electrocardiographic (EKG) monitoring (which should routinely be performed during the procedure) and will usually resolve with removal of the catheter/guidewire from the right atrium. Corr *et al.* [31] found ultrasound-guided puncture of the jugular vein helpful in patients in whom venous access is difficult and this helped reduce the incidence of carotid artery puncture. It is helpful to perform initial puncture with a small needle (e.g., using a micropuncture set) in those patients with bleeding tendencies, so that in the event of inadvertent puncture of the carotid artery, a major bleeding event can be avoided. The likelihood of hematoma formation at the puncture site can be reduced by adequate compression following catheter removal and by placing the patient in the

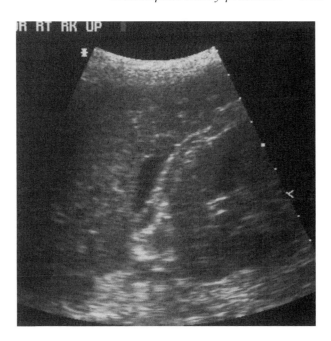

Fig. 29.1 Perinephric hematoma secondary to a transcapsular puncture during transjugular liver biopsy. A 28-year-old female with liver failure and severe coagulopathy; a transjugular liver biopsy was performed. The Colapinto needle was advanced from the *wedged* position. The pathology report noted "normal renal parenchyma." The patients hemoglobin dropped 3.0 g/dl over 24 hours and this ultrasound was obtained showing a heterogeneous region of increased echogenicity compressing the superior pole of the right kidney.

sitting position to reduce jugular venous pressure. The only other complication of concern following this procedure is transient pyrexia [29,30].

Percutaneous transhepatic cholangiography (PTC)

Fine needle PTC using a 22 or 23-gage needle is widely employed for direct opacification of the biliary tree. This method has supplanted the 18-gage sheathed needle technique of PTC because of the latter's higher complication rate: using the fine needle technique for PTC decreases the overall complication rate by a factor of 3.8 and the mortality rate by a factor of 2.6 [37]. There is no statistical difference between the PTC morbidity and mortality rates (3% and 0.1%, respectively) and the endoscopic retrograde cholangiopancreatography (ERCP) morbidity and mortality rates (3% and 0.3%, respectively) [37]. Although ERCP has the advantage of demonstrating the biliary and pancreatic ducts, PTC is less expensive and is more readily available in smaller hospitals. Additionally, the 90–99% success rate for demonstrating the bile ducts with PTC [37,38] compares favorably with ERCP's success rate of 70% [39–41]. The success rate using fine needle PTC increases with the number of passes, and increasing the number of passes does not increase the incidence of serious complications [37].

Sepsis

Sepsis is the most frequent significant complication of fine needle PTC, occurring in 1.5—3.5% of patients [42—44]. The incidence of sepsis is higher in patients with choledocholithiasis [43], reflecting the higher incidence of pre-existing infected bile in these patients (70—90%), compared to the incidence of infected bile in patients with malignant obstruction [45,46].

Sepsis occurring during the PTC procedure is due to microorganisms and related endotoxins entering the circulation, either through biliary—vascular communications along the needle tract, or due to overvigorous injection of contrast media during cholangiography. As discussed below (see p. 507), the most frequently encountered organisms in bile are *Escherichia coli*, *Pseudomonas aeruginosa*, *Klebsiella pneumoniae*, enterococci, *Enterobacter aerogenes*, and *Candida albicans* and wide-spectrum antibiotics should be given prophylactically to cover this broad range of flora in order to minimize the incidence of bacteremia and septicemia. During the procedure, the biliary system should not be overdistended with contrast medium so as not to force bacterial products into the circulation. If the PTC demonstrates significant biliary obstruction, the risk of cholangitis and sepsis is high. Immediate percutaneous biliary drainage is, therefore, generally indicated.

The most common manifestation of systemic sepsis is the development of rigors and fever. The patient may complain of light headedness, nausea, or malaise. This may progress to endotoxic shock with hypotension. Should these signs occur, blood cultures should be drawn and intravenous antibiotic therapy rapidly instituted.

Bile leakage

Bile leakage may occur in the peritoneal cavity or be localized to form a biloma. The incidence of bile peritonitis is reported as 0.2—0.6% [37,43]. The most common cause of this complication is inadvertent puncture of the extrahepatic bile ducts or the gall bladder. More than 50% of patients with intraperitoneal bile leakage, however, remain asymptomatic and do not develop biliary peritonitis [37]. To help minimize the possibility of this complication, the fine needle should be advanced superiorly and away from the porta hepatis, from the right lateral approach. The subxiphoid (left lobe) approach can be done using sonographic guidance to assure the puncture is performed within the liver. In patients with significant biliary obstruction and dilated bile ducts, the best protection against bile leakage, as in preventing sepsis, is the insertion of a biliary drainage catheter to decompress the system. If percutaneous biliary drainage is not performed in this group of patients, the complication rate may be as high as 38% [48].

Bleeding complications: intraperitoneal hemorrhage

The incidence of intraperitoneal hemorrhage following fine needle PTC is variously reported as ranging from 0 to 0.6% [43,44]. There are no reported deaths from this complication using the fine needle technique. The incidence of subcapsular and intraparenchymal hepatic hematomas is difficult to define, since these are usually asymptomatic and are only discovered incidentally during subsequent CT or ultrasound. Bleeding complications can be kept to a minimal incidence by attention to the preprocedural coagulation tests: the prothrombin time, partial thromboplastin time, and platelet count should be assessed in all patients, particularly since coagulation abnormalities are likely to exist in patients with biliary obstruction, due to decreased absorption of the fat-soluble vitamin K. If coagulation abnormalities are present, these can generally be corrected before the procedure.

Other complications

Intrahepatic arteriovenous fistulae discovered incidentally at hepatic arteriography following fine needle PTC have been reported in 3.8% of cases [49]. These are rarely of any clinical significance.

Allergy-like contrast reactions such as skin rash, bronchospasm, and hypotension occur with an incidence of 0.15% with PTC [37]. Other complications of fine needle PTC including pneumothorax, hemothorax, and needle breakage are extremely rare. Vasovagal reactions occur in 1.15% of patients [37], but are readily treated with atropine. However, this stresses the importance of constant hemodynamic monitoring of the patient during this invasive procedure.

Percutaneous transhepatic biliary drainage (PTBD) (Table 29.1)

Several authors initially described a technique of simple external drainage of the biliary system using a sheathed needle in the mid and late 1970s [49,55]. With the subsequent technologic advances in instrumentation, areas of stricture and obstruction of the bile ducts can now be negotiated, and combined internal—external drainage can be achieved. Palliative decompression of the bile ducts in both benign and malignant disease is possible with a technical success rate of 94—99%, and PTBD is now widely used, principally in patients with inoperable cancer causing symptomatic obstruction. This technique is an extension of PTC, and the acute complications that may occur are similar. The incidence of complications, however, is higher because larger needles and catheters are used and manipulation is necessary

Table 29.1 Complications of PTBD

	Mueller *et al.* [50]	Carrasco *et al.* [51]	Hamlin *et al.* [52]	Yee and Chia-Sing [53]	Gunther *et al.* [54]	Total
Number of patients in series	200	161	118	206	311	996
Technical success	188 (94%)	a	114 (97%)	a	(99%)	94–99%
Acute deaths	3 (1.5%)	9 (5.6%)	3 (2.5%)	4 (1.9%)	2 (0.7%)	21 (2.1%)
Major complications: acute						
Bleeding	6 (3%)	1 (0.6%)	2 (1.7%)	1 (0.5%)	3 (1.0%)	13 (1.3%)
Septicemia/septic shock	7 (3.5%)	3 (2.0%)	1 (0.8%)	5 (2.4%)	8 (2.6%)	24 (2.4%)
Bile peritonitis	0	0	0	3 (1.5%)	5 (1.6%)	8 (0.8%)
Minor complications: acute						
Fever	21 (10.5%)	NR	16 (14%)	NR	23 (7.3%)	7.3–14%
Hemobilia	18 (9.0%)	12 (7.0%)	19 (16%)	NR	0	0–16%
Pleural complications	1 (0.5%)	5 (3.0%)	0	2 (1%)	0	8 (0.8%)
Delayed complications						
Catheter dislodgment or migration	11 (5.5%)	29 (18%)	(3.4%)	48 (23.3%)	26 (8.3%)	3.4–23.3%
Cholangitis*	48 (24%)	75 (47%)	b	50 (24.3%)	NR	24–47%
Tube obstruction	7 (3.5%)	22 (14%)	b	21 (10.2%)	35 (11.3%)	3.5–14%
Arteriovenous fistula or pseudoaneurysm[†]	0	0	1 (0.8%)	0	0	1 (0.1%)
Acute cholecystitis	0	0	0	0	0	0
Subphrenic or retroperitoneal abscess	0	0	1 (0.8%)	0	1 (0.3%)	2 (0.2%)
Metastatic spread of tumor along tract	0	0	1 (0.8%)	0	0	1 (0.1%)
Bile leakage around tube	8 (3.0%)	26 (16%)	b	7 (3.4%)	9 (2.9%)	2.9–16%

* Either after clamping a well-positioned internal catheter or in patients with segmental obstruction of a left hepatic duct which was underdrained.

[†] Symptomatic.

a, Retrospective study in successful procedures; b, poor follow-up long term; NR, not reported.

in the biliary tree. The complications from PTBD procedures can be divided into those that are acute and those that are delayed in onset. Major complications and procedure-related deaths of biliary drainage procedures are more common in patients with malignant versus benign obstruction. This was demonstrated in a large series reported by Yee *et al.* [53] who found a major complication rate of 2% in the benign group and 7% in the malignant group. Mortality did not occur in patients with benign lesions, but there was 3% incidence in the malignant group. The actual difference in the incidence of complications between the two groups is not surprising considering that patients with malignant obstruction are, in general, older, in poorer physical health, debilitated, and, in many cases, are immunocompromised because of the underlying disease and therapy.

Acute complications

Death

The death rate following PTBD ranges from 0.5 to 5.6%. Death immediately following the procedure is usually the result of septic shock or severe hemorrhage. Bile peritonitis following premature removal of the drainage tube has been reported as a cause of death in one patient in Yee *et al.*'s series [53] and in two patients reported by Gunther *et al.* [54]. Other less common causes of death resulting from complications of PTBD include hypersecretion of bile [51], peritonitis [51], and pleural complications (pneumothorax and biliary pleural fistulae) [50,51].

Bacteremia/sepsis

The most frequent acute complication of PTBD is bacteremia or sepsis. The high incidence of these complications is not surprising, since a large per cent of obstructed biliary systems are already infected. On routine cultures of bile obtained at the time of drainage. Yee *et al.* [53] found positive cultures in 43% of patients with malignant obstruction, and 68% of patients with benign obstruction. This is consistent with previous reports that showed a higher percentage of infected bile in patients with benign causes of biliary obstruction [45,46]. As noted in the previous section, the most frequently encountered organisms are *E. coli, P. aeruginosa, K. pneumoniae,* enterococci, *E. aerogenes,* and *C. albicans.* As many as 14% of patients will develop transient fever due to bacteremia which does not require therapy beyond the routinely administered prophylactic antibiotics. Hamlin *et al.* [52] found that 12% of their patients had an increase in the white blood cell count of greater than 5000/m^3 within 48 hours of PTBD, but very few required further therapy.

Sepsis with hypotension (defined as a fall of 50% in systolic blood pressure) within the first 24 hours has an incidence of 0.8−3.5%. Severe septicemia can be life threatening and prevention is important. Septic complications can be minimized as mentioned previously, by using combined prophylactic antibiotic therapy (e.g., ampicillin or a cephalosporin plus an aminoglycoside such as gentamicin) beginning 2−4 hours prior to the procedure and continuing for 24−48 hours afterwards. Usual dose is 1 g of ampicillin and 80 mg of gentamycin intravenously three times per day. Parenteral antibiotics do not enter the obstructed biliary system in concentrations significant enough to influence the bacterial content, but they do serve to combat bacteremia occurring during cholangiography and catheter manipulation [56]. After decompression, higher biliary antibiotic concentrations can be anticipated. During PTC, a minimal amount of contrast should be injected to opacify the ducts satisfactorily to permit catheterization. Injection of large volumes of contrast medium into a high-pressure system is unnecessary and may precipitate biliovenous and biliolymphatic backflow [47], leading to bacteremia and sepsis [57]. Mueller *et al.* [50] stressed the importance of minimizing catheter and guidewire manipulation in the biliary tree during PTBD, especially in patients with clinical evidence of ascending cholangitis. Although no study has been done to compare the incidence of sepsis in the two-stage (initial external drainage followed by conversion to internal−external drainage after clearance of cholangitis) versus the one-stage (placement of internal−external stent during the initial study) procedures, it was felt that prolonged catheter manipulations in an infected biliary system may cause mucosal damage which, together with transient pressure elevations due to contrast injection, may contribute to septicemia. Proponents of the one-stage approach reason that if the catheter initially used for gaining access to the biliary tree easily passes the obstructing lesion, placement of an internal−external drainage tube (or an expandable metallic stent) across the stricture is readily accomplished with little additional manipulation. Since colonization of any external drainage tube from skin contami-

nation occurs within days of placement, it can be further argued that establishing internal drainage quickly is likely to decrease later infectious complications.

Hemobilia

This is a relatively common complication, both early and delayed, and may present as intestinal bleeding, blood in a drainage bag, or a thrombus cast in the biliary tree on cholangiography. Hoevels and Nilsson [58] performed hepatic angiography after PTBD in a series of 83 patients and demonstrated intrahepatic vascular lesions in 33%, although clinical evidence of hemorrhage developed in only 6%. Likewise, Okudo *et al.* [49], reported intrahepatic vascular lesions in 26.2%, and Monden *et al.* [59] in 19.1% of patients undergoing PTBD. Transient hemobilia requiring no therapy was the most frequent complication in Hamlin *et al.*'s [52] series, occurring in 16% of patients undergoing PTBD. Patients with asymptomatic hemobilia (i.e., non-pulsatile bleeding through the drainage tube with stable blood pressure and hematocrit) should initially be evaluated with cholangiography to ensure that the catheter is properly positioned and that no side holes are adjacent to venous radicals within the hepatic parenchyma. If side holes are within the hepatic parenchyma, either secondary to improper initial placement or because of inadvertent partial withdrawal of the tube, the tube should be repositioned or replaced by one with fewer proximal side holes. If no side holes are seen within the parenchymal tract, but blood tracks along the tubing, the catheter size should be increased to tamponade the bleeding.

Patients with symptomatic bleeding demonstrated by tachycardia, hypotension, falling hematocrit, or pulsatile blood loss through the PTBD catheter, and with properly positioned catheters, most likely have an arterial source of hemorrhage and should undergo immediate arteriography (Fig. 29.2). This complication was seen in 0.5−3.0% of patients in the cited series (see chart). Hemobilia, even if severe, is rarely a cause of death in these patients. Prompt

Fig. 29.2 *(facing page)* Hematobilia status post biliary drainage. Elderly white male underwent PTBD due to pancreatic carcinoma obstructing distal common bile duct. Two weeks later during preoperative radiation, melanotic stools were noted, and subsequently rectal bleeding. (a) Tube cholangiogram demonstrates extensive clot formation in the biliary tract. (b) Hepatic arteriogram with biliary drainage tube in does not demonstrate a bleeding site. (c, d) Two views from selective hepatic arteriography performed after drainage catheter has been exchanged for a 5-F straight catheter. An active bleeding site is seen with bleeding along catheter drainage tract. (e) Release of coil in branch vessel after selective coil occlusion of two other branch vessels. (f) Selective arteriogram after embolization shows occlusion of three branches and no further bleeding.

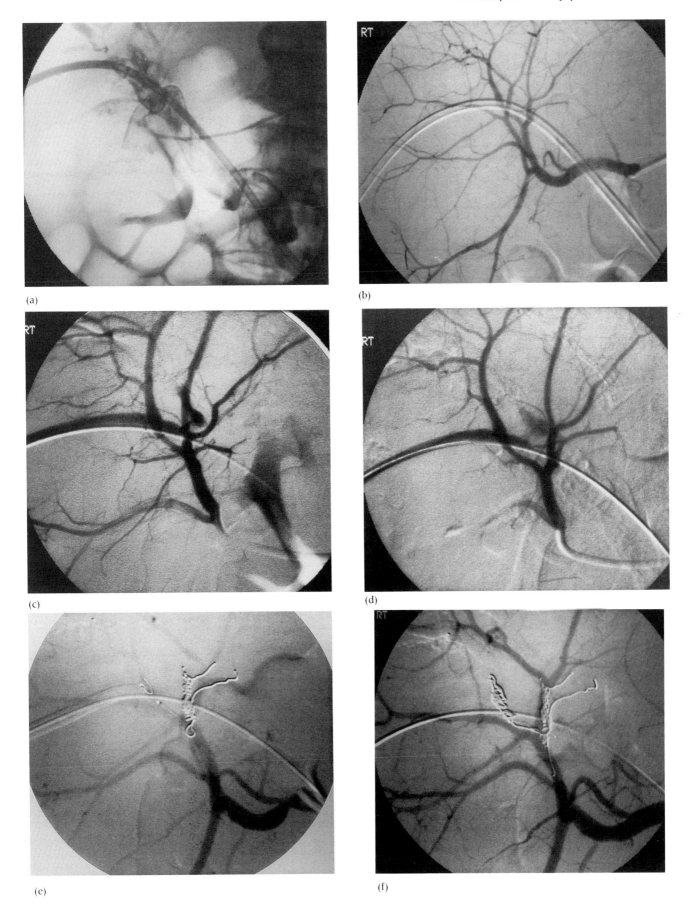

(a)

(b)

(c)

(d)

(e)

(f)

angiographic evaluation, however, including superior mesenteric artery (SMA), celiac axis, and selective hepatic artery injections, and transcatheter embolic therapy is warranted to avert a life-threatening situation, particularly in the debilitated individual. Lesions commonly responsible for symptomatic bleeding include hepatic artery pseudoaneurysm, hepatic artery–bile duct fistula, and, less commonly, hepatic artery–portal vein fistula. Angiography is very good at identifying the source of bleeding in patients with severe hemobilia [59], although in nearly 50% of the patients the arterial injury may not be identified unless the catheter is removed, leaving a guidewire in place to maintain access [60]. Patency of the portal vein should also be confirmed before performing hepatic artery embolization. Embolization of hepatic artery lesions has been performed with a variety of agents, but embolization coils and detachable balloons have been shown to be the safest [60,61]. These agents offer both a high level of control in terms of delivery and the greatest degree of preservation of the peripheral circulation. By placing the balloon or coils across the neck of the arterial injury ("straddling the lesion") the lesion can be isolated and excluded from the circulation while allowing collaterals to reconstitute the peripheral branches, thus decreasing the possibility of hepatic infarct.

The incidence of hepatic artery injury can be minimized by attention to technique during the initial placement of the drainage catheter. Puncture of the biliary ducts near the porta hepatis may increase the chance of damaging larger hepatic artery branches close to the liver hilus. This is a possible explanation for Savader *et al.*'s [61] finding that patients with nondilated ducts at the time of PTBD had 1.7 times the incidence of hepatic artery injury as patients with dilated ducts. As with other invasive procedures, including percutaneous liver biopsy, patients' coagulation parameters should be checked and corrected prior to the procedure. Increasing the number of liver punctures with an 18-gage needle increases the incidence of hemorrhagic complications. In the majority of cases in patients with dilated ducts, access is possible with no more than three punctures. If more than one puncture is required, it is important not to remove the needle entirely from the liver between successive attempts, but rather to redirect the needle each time without withdrawing it from the liver capsule. An alternate technique is to use a small-bore (22-gage) needle for puncture of an appropriate duct, and then convert to a larger catheter without further puncture, or with directed puncture with an 18-gage needle following contrast opacification, thus minimizing the number of punctures necessary with the larger needle.

Bile peritonitis

Bile leakage leading to peritonitis is an uncommon complication provided adequate drainage is established in an ob-

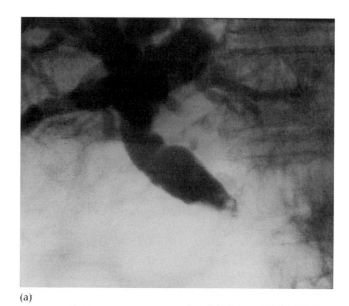

(a)

(b)

Fig. 29.3 Failed conversion to internal drainage. An 86-year-old female with metastatic colon carcinoma leading to biliary obstruction. Successful percutaneous cholangiography and establishment of external drainage (a), but obstruction could not be crossed. On reattempt 2 days later, a false passage was established, and contrast injection (b) demonstrated extravasation in the region of the duodenum. Patient remained asymptomatic from this but expired several days later from complications of widespread metastases.

structed biliary tree. If there is failure to establish biliary drainage in such patients, the incidence of bile peritonitis rises dramatically to 23% [48]. Gunther *et al.* [54] reported two deaths from bile peritonitis, both of which occurred after dislocation of the drainage catheter. This emphasizes the importance of maintaining drainage once established (Fig. 29.3). If the catheter is dislodged and the biliary system is no longer decompressed, the tube tract provides a readily accessible outlet for bile to drain into the peritoneum. Tube dislodgment occurs most frequently in patients in whom it was necessary to place the catheter tip above an obstructing lesion. Clearly, it is critical to maintain external drainage in these patients (see Tube dislodgment, p. 512). Inadvertent puncture of the extrahepatic biliary tree also predisposes to bile leakage and peritonitis. The hilum of the liver must, therefore, be avoided with the definitive puncture for drainage. A single puncture of the liver capsule with the 18-gage needle with redirection of the needle without complete withdrawal from the liver capsule helps to minimize the likelihood of a bile peak. Rarely, a bile leak may loculate to form a biloma [62]. These collections are best identified on CT or sonography, and percutaneous drainage of the collection is an effective therapeutic measure. Bilomas should be considered in patients with persistent leak and those with persistent or worsening right upper quadrant symptoms, such as pain.

Pancreatitis

Although Luska and Poser [63] reported acute pancreatitis complicating PTBD in 4.7% of a series of 85 patients, in the experience of most authors this is a rare complication. To evaluate the effects of PTBD on the pancreas, however, Savader *et al.* [64] measured amylase levels for 7 consecutive days following PTBD procedures and demonstrated a significant rise in 34%. Ten per cent of the patients in this series had hyperamylasemia with associated symptoms of abdominal pain, fever, and nausea/vomiting. Most of these patients had resolution of the symptoms within 4 days. The mechanism may be obstruction of the pancreatic duct by the drainage catheter lying adjacent to it, either directly or by inflammation resulting from the catheter. Trauma to the region of the ampulla of Vater during passage of the guidewire or catheter may also play a part. The acute pancreatitis may present either immediately after the procedure or several days later.

Pleural complications

The incidence of pleural complications occurring in PTBD is generally low, with no such complications reported in several large series. However, several biliopleural fistulae complicating PTBD [51,65,66], hemothoraxes [54,67–71], and pneumothoraxes have been reported with at least two deaths resulting [54,67]. Biliopleural fistulae complicated PTBD in three patients in a series reported by Strange *et al.* [65]. The biliopleural fistulae developed as a complication of inadvertent catheter removal in two patients and of catheter dysfunction in a third patient, all with malignant obstruction of

the biliary tree. Early reinstitution of biliary drainage and successful drainage of the pleural space led to complete recovery in all cases.

The common radiologic practice of trying to assess the inferior recess of the pleura by fluoroscopy does not delineate the extent of the pleural space, but rather the inferior excursion of the lung. In the midaxillary line, the parietal reflection occurs at the level of the tenth rib. Thus, punctures in the ninth intercostal space (a common site) will almost invariably traverse the pleural [72]. In most instances, this does not lead to any serious complications because the biliary drainage catheter obturates the tract. Performing the procedure through the tenth intercostal space or lower is safer, but is technically much more difficult because of the acute angle with the branch of the right hepatic duct. An anterior (subxiphoid) approach with puncture of a left hepatic duct, can be performed under ultrasound guidance and avoids the risk of a transpleural puncture. In addition, an anteriorly placed catheter appears to give less discomfort to the patient. Considering this, many preferentially use an anterior approach, performing right-sided drainage only in cases of poor visualization of the left hepatic ducts [73]. As noted, when the right approach is utilized, it must be recognized that the pleura is generally traversed, and the patient must be monitored for pleural complications.

Contrast reaction

Contrast-medium reactions are unusual during PTBD, but they can occur, presumably due to injection of contrast into the vascular system during the diagnostic transhepatic cholangiogram.

Delayed complications

Cholangitis

The most frequent complication of PTBD is cholangitis which may occur under several circumstances, most commonly with clamping of external drainage in patients with inadequate internal drainage. An important caveat in all patients in whom a drainage tube is successfully placed across the obstruction into the duodenum is that initial drainage should be external. With chronic obstruction of the biliary tree, the bile is of increased viscosity (as well as frequently infected), and the trauma of inserting the catheter may cause hemobilia with intraductal thrombi. These factors increase the risk of tube obstruction and cholangitis in the early days of drainage. External drainage allows for careful monitoring of the adequacy of drainage and provides the opportunity for early intervention — be it flushing the catheter or replacing it — if there is slow or inadequate drainage, thus lessening the risk of cholangitis. If a 10-F catheter is placed initially, this can be successfully converted to internal drainage after 2–5 days in most patients. If an 8-F catheter is initially used, this should not be placed for internal drainage, but rather should be exchanged for the larger 10-F or 12-F catheter. The incidence of cholangitis occurring after attempted conversion of an 8-F ring catheter to internal drainage was 63% in Mueller *et al.*'s series [50]. However, when the 8.3-F catheter was exchanged for a 10-F or 12-F catheter with larger side holes and larger internal diameter, conversion to internal drainage resulted in an incidence of cholangitis of 11%. Since a significant number of patients will develop cholangitis even with 10-F or larger tubes, all patients should be carefully monitored after conversion to internal drainage for signs of sepsis, such as fever and chills, and the tube should immediately be unclamped if such symptoms occur. A difficult clinical balance must be maintained in regard to internal versus external drainage. While the risk of cholangitis is clearly lower with the latter, prolonging external drainage leads to altered digestion due to loss of bile salts. Furthermore, drainage tubes are fairly rapidly colonized with skin bacteria; prolonged external drainage may actually raise the risk of cholangitis with manipulations such as tube cholangiography or tube change.

Recurrent episodes of delayed cholangitis are common, and are usually due to obstruction of the drainage catheter by debris, to obstruction of an intrahepatic duct by the catheter, or, more commonly, by progression of the primary disease process. Obstruction of the drainage catheter can be minimized by routine catheter exchanges every 2–3 months. If the catheter does become obstructed, it is best to replace it rather than merely clearing it with a guidewire or high-pressure flushing. With every routine tube exchange, a cholangiogram should be performed and carefully compared to previous cholangiograms in order to identify branches of the intrahepatic ducts that may no longer be drained. If there is an undrained duct in the presence of sepsis, it is essential that this duct be drained by placing a second catheter into the undrained duct. Cholangitis may be further complicated by multiple intrahepatic abscesses which can precipitate unexpected patient deterioration; if clinical suspicion exists (e.g., because of cholangitis with no evidence of new obstruction), CT should be obtained.

Acute cholecystitis

As noted in the previous section, sepsis, heralded by fever, is a common complication during long-term PTBD. Most often, this is due to cholangitis secondary to tube or duct obstruction, and can be managed with antibiotics and by changing the catheter or resuming external drainage. The possibility of a hepatic abscess should also be considered in these patients. Acute cholecystitis, however, should be considered as a source of sepsis in patients in whom antibiotics and catheter manipulation do not provide relief. Although the large series cited in Table 29.1 do not report a single case of post-PTBD cholecystitis, Lillemoe *et al.* [74] reported an incidence of 2.7% among patients on long-term biliary drainage. They postulated that the acute cholecystitis was caused by mechanical obstruction of the cystic duct, leading to stagnant bile which combined with the usual chronic colonization to lead to acute infection. Although cholecystitis is a rare cause of sepsis in patients with indwelling PTBD catheters, a high index of suspicion should be maintained, especially if antibiotics and catheter manipulation have failed to improve the clinical condition. Further diagnostic examinations including sonography and/or radionuclide scans should be performed in this setting. Successful management can be expected if early recognition and surgical or percutaneous management are provided.

Catheter obstruction

Catheter obstruction, in addition to leading to cholangitis, may also result in recurrent jaundice. In this case, replacement of the catheter is again necessary. Obstruction of either the left or right hepatic duct on its own will not cause jaundice, since adequate drainage through either one of these ductal systems will be sufficient to prevent the accumulation of bilirubin. Bile leak around the catheter entry site is probably a more common complication of catheter obstruction. This usually can be readily resolved simply by catheter exchange.

Tube dislodgment

This is a complication that depends on the type of catheter used. With an 8.3-ring biliary drainage catheter, Carrasco *et al.* [51] reported catheter dislodgment in 18% of patients. Using the Cope self-retaining catheters, with or without fixation to the skin, catheter dislodgment should be an uncommon occurrence. Hamlin *et al.* [52] found that tube dislodgment occurred almost exclusively in those patients in whom the catheter tip could not be placed beyond an obstructing lesion. With the tube anchored in the intercostal space, there is a tendency for the catheter to be withdrawn from the liver, and buckle between the liver and abdominal wall due to hepatic excursion during respiration. Use of a pigtail catheter rather than a straight catheter may help prevent withdrawal of the tube and dislodgment. If the indwelling catheter has been in place long enough for a good tract to form (i.e. ≥3 weeks), reinsertion of the catheter along the same tract is generally possible if attempted within 48–72 hours.

Delayed hemorrhage

Delayed hemorrhage is an unusual but potentially serious complication. A pseudoaneurysm caused by insertion of the biliary drainage catheter, possibly with superimposed infection, may later be eroded by the indwelling drainage catheter, resulting in rupture of the aneurysm into the bile duct. The resulting hemorrhage may prove to be fatal. Hepatic arteriography and embolization should be performed as discussed in the section on Acute bleeding (see p. 508 & Fig. 29.2).

Hypersecretion of bile

With patients on external drainage, high-volume bile output has been reported by Carrasco *et al*. [51] with an incidence up to 5%. The pathophysiology of this phenomenon is unknown [75]. Hypersecretion of bile may lead to significant fluid and electrolyte loss, sufficient to produce hypotension and symptomatic hyponatremia. Aggressive replacement therapy may be necessary. At least one death has resulted, at least in part, from this complication [51].

When catheters are placed to external drainage, there may be loss of considerable fluid volume due to reflux of intestinal secretions via catheter side holes within the duodenum [76]. This may be due to peristaltic duodenal pressure exceeding the secretory pressure of bile in the biliary tree. These complications do not occur with internal drainage, which is one of the major reasons why internal drainage is always preferable, albeit not always possible.

Extension of neoplasm along the tract

Several reports of malignant seeding along the catheter tract in patients who underwent PTBD for malignant obstruction have been published, but such events are rare. They include subcutaneous and peritoneal tumor implants of cholangiocarcinoma [77,78], as well as seeding by pancreatic carcinoma [79]. Anschuetz and Vogelzang [80] reported a patient with cholangiocarcinoma who developed a malignant pleural effusion after long-term biliary drainage. The duration of catheter placement, together with the propensity of cholangiocarcinoma to invade locally is undoubtedly the cause of this complication. It is also possible that multiple catheter exchanges may predispose to malignant seeding [81]. Placement of internal plastic or metallic expandable stents should lessen the likelihood of the occurrence of this complication.

Local complications

Local complications at the catheter entry site are not of any serious consequence, but they may cause considerable discomfort to the patient. The use of soft, relatively biocompatible catheter materials such as a siliconized compound (USCI, Billerica, MA) or a modified polyurethane compound (Cook Inc., Bloomington, IN) will decrease the incidence of these complications and allow greater comfort when compared to the use of rigid polyethylene catheters (e.g., a ring catheter). Catheter erosion of the adjacent ribs has been reported in association with the right intercostal approach

[82]. This complication is circumvented when a subxyphoid approach is used. Local entry site infections are common, and can be treated with topical antibiotics, although systemic antibiotics may occasionally be necessary. Any local collection of pus must be drained. A granuloma arising at the catheter entry site can be effectively treated with local application of silver nitrate [83].

Percutaneous transhepatic biliary endoprosthesis

Plastic prostheses

The initial treatment of choice for nonoperative biliary drainage — endoscopic placement of a stent — can be achieved in a single session in most patients with low morbidity and mortality. Such stents cannot always be placed endoscopically, however, and may need to be placed percutaneously. The complications of placement of a biliary endoprosthesis from a percutaneous transhepatic approach are similar to the complications of PTBD, since the former is merely an extension of the drainage procedure. In the past, it was customary first to place a biliary drainage tube with exchange for an endoprosthesis after a variable period of time, usually approximately 2 weeks, after an adequate tract had developed. More recently, stents have been placed in a single-stage procedure unless the patient has preexisting biliary sepsis [84]. After the stent is deployed, a self-retaining drainage catheter (8-F or 10-F) should be left in the biliary tree above the stent as an external drain. Cholangiography should be performed 2–3 days after placement of the endoprosthesis to check for adequate positioning of the stent and good antegrade flow into the duodenum. If these conditions are satisfied, the catheter can be removed over a guidewire, leaving the guidewire in place for several minutes to check for bleeding. If mild bleeding is noted following removal of the catheter, the catheter should be replaced into the biliary system to tamponade bleeding and left in place for 1–2 weeks, at which time the bleeding should no longer be seen. If brisk bleeding is demonstrated, hepatic arterial bleeding should be suspected and arteriography performed. In a series of 113 patients [85], there was a 7% incidence of early complications (within the first 30 days) directly attributable to stent placement. The most common early complication, with an incidence of 3.5%, was malpositioning of the stent leading to biliary cutaneous fistula after removal of the safety catheter. The biliary cutaneous fistula can be prevented by leaving the drainage (safety) catheter until the biliary tree is cleared of blood clots.

Although biliary endoprostheses avoid the delayed local complications at the catheter entry site associated with external/internal drainage, and the complications of electrolyte imbalance in patients on external drainage, the major problems with endoprostheses lie in the difficulty or even the impossibility of accomplishing exchange should occlusion or migration occur. There is a 6–31% incidence of delayed complications [84–86], the most common (23%) being obstruction by debris or food particles [85]. The other delayed complications are migration of the endoprostheses either proximally or distally (3–6%), and obstruction due to tumor progression (3%). The symptoms that indicate stent obstruction or migration are recurrent jaundice, cholangitis, or the formation of an external biliary fistula along the previous transhepatic tract. If there is evidence of delayed cholangitis, antibiotic therapy for 2–3 weeks relieves symptoms within a few days and in most cases prevents premature occlusion of the stent because of debris [86]. It is also imperative to reestablish drainage, usually requiring a repeat biliary drainage procedure. After any acute sepsis has subsided on external drainage, an attempt may be made to reestablish patency of the obstructed endoprosthesis by passing a guidewire or wire brush through it. If this fails, the endoprosthesis may be removed by pushing it into the duodenum with a large catheter, attempting to pull it back through the tract using a balloon catheter inflated inside the stent [85], or pulling it out through the mouth using a catheter and snare wire placed perorally into the duodenum. If these measures fail, the stent may be removed either endoscopically or surgically. The difficulty in managing postplacement migration of the stent and stent occlusion, combined with the high radiation dose to the operator, have led some authors to abandon the use of endoprosthesis, especially since the advent of self-expanding metallic biliary stents.

Self-expanding metallic biliary stents (Table 29.2)

The use of metallic self-expanding endoprostheses has changed percutaneous stent placement substantially. Self-expanding stents have several advantages over plastic stents. The Wallstent is introduced on a 7-F delivery catheter and the smaller transhepatic tract makes insertion easier, less painful, and probably safer than placement of plastic stents. When expanded, the metallic stents have a relatively large inner diameter which reduces the rate of occlusion by encrusted bile. The self-expanding stent, because of constant radial forces, is fixed in position after release, thus eliminating the problem of migration. Finally, reintervention is more easily accomplished with metallic stents than with plastic stents. Despite these many advantages, complications do occur with insertion of self-expanding metallic stents (Table 29.2). The early complications are predominantly those seen with any transhepatic technique such as septicemia, bleeding, and pleural complications. Very few procedure-related mortalities have been reported. As with plastic stents, the major late complication is obstruction.

Early complications

Septicemia

Yee *et al.* [53], on routine cultures of bile obtained at the time of drainage, found positive cultures in 43% of patients with malignant obstruction and 68% of patients with benign

Table 29.2 Complications of expandable metallic biliary stents

	Stoker *et al.* [87]	Gordon *et al.* [88]	Adam *et al.* [89]	Lammer *et al.* [90]	Gillams *et al.* [91]	Range (mean) (%)
Number of patients in series	176	50	41	61	45	Total 373
Procedure-related deaths	3 (2%)	0	0	0	2 (4%)	0–3 (1.3)
Early complications						
Septicemia	6 (3%)	2 (4%)	2 (5%)	0	4 (9%)	0–9 (3.8)
Hemobilia	1 (0.5%)	4 (8%)	0	0	0	0–8 (1.3)
Severe bleed	0	1 (2%)	0	1 (2%)	1 (2%)	0–2 (0.8)
Acute reobstruction	4 (2%)	0	0	0	0	0–2 (1.1)
CBD/duodenal perforation	1 (0.6%)	0	0	0	0	0–0.6 (0.3)
Hepatic abscess	1 (0.6%)	1 (2%)	0	0	0	0–2 (0.5)
Pleural complications	1 (0.6%)	0	0	1 (2%)	2 (4%)	0.4 (1.1)
Cholecystitis	1 (0.6%)	0	0	0	0	0–0.6 (0.3)
Biliary peritonitis	0	0	1 (2%)	0	0	0–2 (0.3)
Late complications						
Late obstruction	33 (19%)	12 (24%)	3 (7%)	8 (13%)	24 (53%)	7–53 (21.4)
Cholecystitis	4 (2%)	0	0	0	0	0–2 (1.1)
Duodenal pressure ulcer	2 (1%)	0	0	0	0	0–1 (0.5)
Bleeding	3 (2%)	0	0	0	0	0–2 (0.8)

CBD, common bile duct.

obstruction. As previously discussed, manipulations in an infected biliary tree carry significant risk and should be kept to a minimum. The incidence of septicemia appears significantly higher with placement of self-expanding metallic biliary stents as opposed to internal/external or simple external drainage, occurring in most series with an incidence of 3–9%. As such, a two-stage procedure with initial internal/ external drainage, followed by stent placement after resolution of cholangitis is preferred by many. Adams *et al.* [89] agreed that manipulations should be kept to a minimum in such patients, but felt that if the catheter initially used for drainage passes the obstructing lesion easily, it is justifiable to release a Wallstent across the stricture. They reason that the Wallstent can be introduced very easily with very few additional manipulations, and dilatation of the intrahepatic tract is unnecessary. The one-step procedure allows placement of the stent, and its inherent manipulations and trauma to be performed prior to colonization of the tract with bacteria. Broad-spectrum antibiotics should routinely be administered prophylactically (see Percutaneous transhepatic biliary drainage, pp. 507–508 for discussion).

Bleeding

As with other transhepatic biliary drainage procedures, bleeding is to be expected as a complication with placement of self-expandable stents. Self-limited bleeding into the drainage tube not requiring transfusion has been observed with an incidence as high as 8% [88]. Self-limited bleeding may be treated by placing a larger tube and leaving the tube in place for 2 weeks [92]. Severe bleeding requiring transfusion has been reported sporadically [88,90–92]. Because of the small numbers of patients in these series, it is difficult to estimate the true incidence of severe bleeding, although, as with PTBD, 1–2% can be expected. Gordon *et al.* [88] and Lammer *et al.* [90] each described patients with pseudoaneurysms which were treated with embolization with resolution of bleeding. Gillams *et al.* [91] reported a death from hemorrhage from the puncture site. As with PTBD, the incidence of hepatic artery injury can be minimized with attention to technique during the initial placement. This subject is covered in detail in the PTBD section but, in summary, the definitive puncture of the biliary ducts should be as peripheral in the liver as possible to avoid injury to large hepatic artery branches near the porta hepatis. The number of liver punctures with an 18-gage needle should be minimized with only one puncture of the liver capsule, redirecting the needle with successive attempts without withdrawing from the liver. Finally, coagulation parameters should be evaluated and, if necessary, corrected prior to the procedure.

Common bile duct perforation

Stoker *et al.* [87] and Lameris *et al.* [92] each reported a patient in whom biliary stents caused perforation of the common bile duct, which proved fatal in each case. The sharp wires on either end of the stent are felt to be responsible for this complication. In addition, Lameris *et al.* [92] speculate that the straightening force of a short stent may lead to acute angulation at the junction of the stent and the normal bile duct. This may cause not only stent occlusion, but also significant damage to the bile duct epithelium. In a distal stenosis, this can be prevented by using a stent of adequate length, which maintains a gradual curve in the common bile duct by extending beyond the lesion proximally or, if necessary, in both directions.

Pleural complications

Biliary pleuritis has been reported in a patient, most likely secondary to a high transpleural approach [90]. A fatality occurred from a pleural empyema following placement of a biliary Wallstent after a transpleural approach. As with PTBD, the anterior (subxyphoid) approach is often the preferable approach when placing an expandable metallic biliary stent in order to avoid pleural complications. Right intercostal approaches if above the tenth rib invariably traverse the pleural space, although pleural complications are rare. Nevertheless, if the intercostal approach is used, the patient should be carefully monitored for pleural complications.

Late complications

Late obstruction

Reobstruction is the major late complication following placement of an expandable metallic biliary stent, occurring with an incidence of 7–53% [87–91]. The most common cause of late obstruction is tumor overgrowth, especially proximal to the stent. Stoker *et al.* [87] reported 33 late obstructions in their series of 176 patients (19%) after a median period of 135 days (range, 6–395 days). Of the 33 patients in this series with reobstruction, 27 occurred in patients with hilar stenoses predominantly in patients with cholangiocarcinoma ($n = 12$) and gall-bladder carcinoma ($n = 7$). Tumor ingrowth directly into the stent has been reported as a rare cause of stent obstruction [90,91]. Unlike plastic prostheses, sludge rarely accumulates in metallic stents and is a rare cause of stent obstruction. Reintervention was performed in 25 of the patients in Stoker *et al.*'s series [87] with placement of another Wallstent or an internal/external drain. Nineteen of the 25 patients who underwent reintervention benefited from the procedure.

Proximal overstenting of hilar stenoses can prevent, or at least delay, proximal overgrowth of tumor. However, the number and size of segmental ducts limits the ability sufficiently to overextend the stent proximally. A potential drawback of proximal overstenting is the potential for obstructing side branches with the stent itself. The work of Lameris *et al.* [92], however, suggests that side branches continue to drain through the wire mesh. Another consideration of proximal overstenting is the possibility that, if reintervention is necessary, it may be more difficult if important side branches of the biliary tree are covered by the stent.

As previously discussed in response to common bile duct perforation, a short Wallstent has the tendency to straighten the normally smoothly curved common bile duct. Occlusion of the proximal end of the stent by the overlying bile duct wall can occur because of the acute angle that is created [87,93]. In a distal stenosis, this can be prevented by a stent of adequate length and "overstenting" the lesion at the proximal site. Reobstruction has also been reported because of the tendency of the stent to shorten secondary to its self-expanding qualities (i.e., as the stent expands over time to its maximum diameter, it simultaneously foreshortens). This foreshortening may lead to uncovering of a portion of the lesion and, hence, to reobstruction. This complication may also be avoided by overstenting. Regardless of the cause of reobstruction, most patients can benefit from reintervention, with introduction of a second prosthesis through the first.

Percutaneous transhepatic biliary dilatation

Since transhepatic biliary drainage is used to gain access for dilatation and is maintained for a variable period of time following the procedure, complications are much the same as described for transhepatic biliary drainage [95,96]. There is the potential for perforation of the duct being dilated due to a transmural tear, but this has not been reported. In a small series of 13 patients [97], there were no major complications directly related to the dilatation procedure; however, all patients did experience chest and abdominal pain during the balloon inflation and this pain was occasionally associated with a vasovagal reaction. This again emphasizes the importance of constant blood pressure monitoring and EKG monitoring during the procedure.

Percutaneous stone extraction

Extraction via T-tube tract

The incidence of retained calculi following cholecystectomy and common bile duct exploration is as high as 8% [98]. Reexploration for retained common bile duct stones is associated with increased morbidity and mortality relative to initial surgery [99]. A nonoperative means to remove stones is, therefore, desirable. Removing biliary stones through the

T-tube tract has proven effective and has markedly decreased the need for reoperation [98,100−103]. A second operation for choledocholithiasis should be undertaken only if percutaneous extraction fails. Percutaneous stone extraction through the T-tube tract has a 95% success rate, and a 4.1% complication rate [101].

Mortality

No deaths were reported in the two largest series [99,101], although a single death was reported in another large series [102].

Fever and sepsis

The most common complication is sepsis and fever, with a reported incidence of 2% in a large series of patients [101], and a 15% incidence in a smaller one [104]. Bile cultures in patients with T-tubes have been positive for at least one bacterium (62% Gram-negative aerobes, 27% Gram-positive aerobes, 9% anaerobes) in 90% of patients, and broad-spectrum antibiotics covering both Gram-positive and Gram-negative organisms should be administered. The most effective antibiotic combination is ampicillin plus an aminoglycoside, such as gentamycin or tobramycin [104]. The use of prophylactic antibiotics is controversial; some authors recommend their use routinely, whereas others reserve their use for procedures that are expected to be difficult and prolonged, e.g., in patients with a history of postoperative pancreatitis. Certainly, if evidence of sepsis occurs during or after the procedure, blood cultures should be drawn and urgent and vigorous treatment with intravenous antibiotics is necessary.

Tract perforation

Leakage of contrast medium from the sinus tract occurs in 1% of procedures [101], but this is usually of little clinical significance; leakage into the peritoneal cavity (0.3%) may be more serious, but treatment with antibiotics and drainage has proven to be adequate [101]. Even extensive tract perforation with communication with the abdomen usually has no sequelae (see Fig. 29.3). Since forceful extraction of large stones through the tract may cause damage and perforation, these stones should first be reduced in size either by physical fragmentation or by dissolution with a chemical agent such as monooctanoin [105]. In addition, dilatation of the tract to a large size (from 24-F to 30-F) with placement of a working sheath permits exchange of instruments and extraction of stones with minimal trauma to the tract.

Subhepatic bile collection

In Burhenne's series [101] of 661 patients, subhepatic bile

collections occurred in two patients (0.3%). A subhepatic bile collection may require drainage if sufficiently large and this can generally be accomplished percutaneously. Sub diaphragmatic abscesses have not been reported [101].

Pancreatitis

Postprocedural pancreatitis has an incidence of 0.3% [102], probably due to manipulation in the region of the ampulla with resultant edema and partial pancreatic duct obstruction. The single reported mortality from percutaneous stone extraction was due to concomitant pancreatitis, thought to have been caused by reflux of bile into the pancreatic duct [102].

Vasovagal reaction

These may also occur during manipulation in the biliary tree (0.2%), but are readily treated with atropine. Pushing stones through the ampulla and pulling stones through a small tract causes abdominal pain, and a vasovagal reaction may result. The patient must be closely monitored throughout the procedure and appropriate therapy (intravenous fluids, sedation, and atropine) quickly administered.

Extraction without surgical tract

Patients with common bile duct stones with a prior history of cholecystectomy but without a T-tube tract, or patients who are poor surgical risks for cholecystectomy, may have their bile duct calculi removed percutaneously through a transhepatic tract. The risks of this procedure are largely related to the biliary drainage procedure. If the intention is to withdraw the stone through the transhepatic tract, then it is essential to allow this tract to mature around the biliary drainage catheter for several weeks to avoid or limit direct hepatic damage. Even with such precautions, large stones should not be withdrawn in this way because of the possibility of liver laceration. An alternate is to engage the stone in a modified Dormia basket, to the end of which has been attached a flexible guidewire, and to push the stone through into the duodenum [103]. This technique may be employed at the time of the primary biliary drainage procedure. The reported complications have been sepsis, hemorrhage, and pancreatitis [103]. As with any major intrahepatic manipulations, patients should be on prophylactic broad-spectrum antibiotics. It is essential subsequently to leave a biliary drainage tube in place for 24−48 hours because of ampullary edema resulting from the manipulation.

Dissolution of bile duct stones

Attempted dissolution of retained bile duct stones using infusions of various chemical agents has, until recently,

required prolonged hospitalization and has had unpredictable results. Bile acid infusions have enjoyed some popularity, but have only a slightly higher success rate than the 50% success achieved by flushing with saline. In addition, bile acid infusions often cause diarrhea, which may require cholestyramine for control [106]. More recently, these agents have been superseded by monoctanoin, a mixture of medium-chain triglycerides, which is an effective cholesterol solvent. Still, the dissolution of cholesterol stones with this agent may take 1−2 weeks and is associated with side-effects such as nausea, vomiting, anorexia, and diarrhea. These reported side-effects of monoctanoin infusion are most likely related to increased intraductal pressure caused by the infusion in a system with partial obstruction. An infusion rate that is too high may also lead to abdominal cramps and diarrhea. When the rate of infusion was kept to 2−4 ml/h in a series of 24 patients [107], no significant complications were encountered. One patient developed diarrhea, but this resolved spontaneously; three patients developed transient biliary colic, probably because of partial biliary obstruction. Minor abdominal discomfort occurred in several patients, but this subsided on temporary cessation of the infusion. Increasing the rate of infusion above 4 ml/h increased the side-effects of nausea, vomiting, biliary colic, and diarrhea, without increasing the dissolution rate. If there is partial or complete biliary obstruction, it may be necessary to place a second biliary drainage catheter to allow a route of egress of the infused fluid. Other reported complications of monoctanoin infusion include duodenal ulceration leading to serious hemorrhage [108], and systemic side-effects of facial flushing, metallic taste, dyspnea, and hypoxemia [109]. These systemic symptoms were attributed to absorption of the monoctanoin from the biliary tree, due to denuded biliary epithelium resulting from previous cholangitis. There has been a single reported death following the infusion of monoctanoin into the gall bladder after cholecystostomy for perforated cholecystitis; acute pancreatitis and cholangitis occurred with the histologic finding of toxic epithelial necrosis in the bile ducts (necrotizing choledochomalacia) [110].

Methyl-tert-butyl ether (MTBE), an aliphatic ether that remains liquid at body temperature, appears to dissolve cholesterol stones rapidly. This agent has been shown to dissolve cholesterol stones 50 times faster (v/v) than monoctanoin. MTBE, however, is an explosive anesthetic agent similar to diethyl ether, and absorption of this agent leads to sedation. If not used carefully, it can induce anesthesia in the patient as well as nearby medical personnel. Although there is limited clinical experience with MTBE, complications have been shown to include hemorrhagic duodenitis if there is overflow into the duodenum. Such overflow may also result in systemic absorption which can lead to intravascular hemolysis [111].

Percutaneous gall-bladder interventions

Needle aspiration of bile

Various diagnostic and therapeutic gall-bladder procedures are now performed by percutaneously inserting needles and catheters into the gall bladder. Diagnostic procedures include needle aspiration of bile, needle aspiration biopsy of the gall bladder, and transcholecystic angiography. The most common therapeutic procedure is percutaneous cholecystostomy.

Nuclear medicine studies can usually confirm the gall bladder as the source of infection in patients with calculous cholecystitis. In some patients with calculous cholecystitis and in patients with suspected acalculous cholecystitis, however, percutaneous aspiration of bile may be indicated when sonography and scintigraphy are inconclusive. The procedure may be performed under ultrasound or CT guidance in the radiology department or with the use of mobile sonographic equipment at the bedside. A positive bile culture is consistent with the diagnosis of acute cholecystitis, but negative cultures do not exclude cholecystitis in patients already receiving antibiotic therapy. Two large series of 36 [112] and 60 patients [113] report no major complications of percutaneous needle aspiration. One patient did develop transient bacteremia (fever and chills) after a needle aspiration biopsy [113]. A small risk of bile peritonitis exists and care should be taken not to puncture the back wall of the gall bladder, which would increase the risk of bile spillage. To this end, a small-bore needle (20–22-gage) is inserted into the gall bladder by the most direct anterior or anterior lateral route [113], attempting in general to enter the gall bladder via the liver rather than through a free wall.

Transcholecystic cholangiography

Patients with suspected biliary disease in whom ultrasound or CT do not show dilated intrahepatic ducts, may be evaluated safely with transcholecystic cholangiography. Illescas *et al.* [114] reported a series of five patients, and van Sonnenberg [115] 10 patients, in whom transcholecystic cholangiography was performed without complications. Teplick *et al.* [113], in a series of 33 patients, reported on four patients (12%) with minor complications consisting of transient mild abdominal or right shoulder pain which subsided shortly after the procedure without need for treatment. Two of the patients in Teplick *et al.*'s series [113] (6%) had more serious complications (probably local peritonitis) consisting of abdominal pain, tenderness, and fever lasting 1–2 days. These patients were maintained on antibiotics and pain-relieving drugs and recovered completely. To date, there are no reports of hemorrhage or vasovagal reactions with transcholecystic cholangiography.

Percutaneous cholecystostomy

Percutaneous cholecystostomy has become an acceptable and even preferred alternate to surgical cholecystostomy for patients with acute cholecystitis who are poor surgical candidates. In addition, cholecystostomy can be performed in patients with common bile duct obstruction with minimal or absent intrahepatic bile duct dilatation, in whom a percutaneous transhepatic drainage procedure would be difficult or impossible. Teplick *et al.* [113] reviewed the English-language literature and found reports of 231 percutaneous cholecystostomies as of 1989. Pearse *et al.* [116] mentioned the only occasion on which an attempted percutaneous cholecystostomy failed. Of the 231 percutaneous cholecystostomies reported, only three cases of bile peritonitis (1%) and one death have been reported [116]. Other reported complications are four cases of severe vasovagal reactions [115]; one case of acute cholecystitis when a stone became lodged in the cystic duct [115]; five patients with hemobilia, none of whom required treatment [117,118], and one patient with transient decrease in blood pressure [118]. The overall reported complication rate in this review was 8% (18 out of 231).

Because of the high incidence of infected bile in patients with acute cholecystitis [112] and cholangitis, manipulation in the gall bladder may seed organisms into the bloodstream, leading to bacteremia or even septicemia. For this reason, broad-spectrum antibiotic coverage (e.g., ampicillin plus an aminoglycoside), should be administered for at least several hours prior to the procedure and continued for at least 48 hours afterwards. Manipulation in the gall bladder and contrast-medium injections should be kept to a minimum [116]. Vogelzang and Nemcek [119] found the use of the Hawkin's Needle Guide (Cook Inc., Bloomington, IN) very helpful because it permitted catheterization of the gall bladder without any catheter or guidewire exchanges, thus reducing the number of manipulations through the gall-bladder wall. It is best to defer diagnostic contrast studies until the cholecystitis or cholangitis have resolved due to the risk of inducing worsening sepsis. A small amount of contrast should be injected to confirm position of the needle and/or tube after complete aspiration of gall-bladder contents.

Life-threatening vagal reactions with severe hypotension and bradycardia have been reported in patients with underlying cardiac disease and markedly distended gall bladders who undergo percutaneous cholecystostomy [115]. These vagal reactions occur with guidewire manipulation within the gall bladder, or with bile aspiration. They can be minimized by prophylactic administration of atropine, although other authors report no significant vasovagal episodes without pretreatment with atropine [119]. Again, manipulations within the gall bladder should be kept to an absolute minimum. Finally, cardiac monitoring, appropriate supportive measures (e.g., administration of fluids, atropine, and dopamine), and availability of assistance from clinicians are essential [115].

Puncture of adjacent organs, such as the colon may occur, but this can be avoided by using ultrasound guidance.

Bile leakage may occur during or following cholecystostomy, but this is uncommon. There has been no controlled study to assess the relative safety of inserting the catheter into the gall bladder through the liver versus directly through the peritoneal cavity. Some authors have used both approaches [113,115] without an apparent difference in prevalence of bile peritonitis. However, the transhepatic approach is advocated by most authors, via an anterior approach so that the gall bladder is entered extraperitoneally. This extraperitoneal approach would seem to minimize the possibility of bile peritonitis should bile leak occur. In order to ensure placement of the drainage catheter in the gall bladder, the procedure should be performed using both ultrasound and fluoroscopic guidance. A major cause of bile leakage is inadvertent catheter removal; to prevent this, self-retaining accordion or pigtail catheters that retain their curves (Hawkin's Accordion or Cope Loop, Cook Inc., Bloomington, IN) should be used. When removing the drainage catheter, experience suggests that development of a well-formed tract along the path of the percutaneous cholecystostomy catheter may prevent bile leakage. A period of 20 days usually suffices for development of a well-formed tract, providing the patient has adequate nutrition, there is no infection or tumor along the tract, and there is no distal obstruction [120]. It has been suggested that it may be useful to visualize the tract at the time of removal of the drainage tube, leaving a safety wire in place. If the tract is poorly formed, and there is leakage into the peritoneum, the tube can be replaced until a tract is well developed.

TIPS

Variceal hemorrhage is a life-threatening complication of portal hypertension. Current therapeutic options include endoscopic sclerotherapy, surgical creation of a portosystemic shunt, liver transplantation, and a relatively new non-operative procedure, TIPS. The TIPS procedure has been shown to have lower morbidity and mortality rates than those of surgical shunting, but complications do occur. The following categorization of complications of TIPS was proposed by Freedman *et al.* [121], and the procedural morbidity and mortality rates as reported in some of the larger TIPS series are shown in Table 29.3, also adapted and updated from the comprehensive review of these authors.

Some consider hepatic encephalopathy and chronic narrowing of the shunt as inevitable long-term complications which must be closely monitored and quickly treated when they occur. New or worsening hepatic encephalopathy can be expected in 5–35% of patients who have undergone TIPS. Delayed stenosis or occlusion due to pseudointimal hyperplasia has been shown to occur in up to 75% of TIPS patients. Excluding these two complications, an overall complication rate of less than 10% can be expected for TIPS [121]. Direct procedural mortality rates of less than 2% have been reported, with most deaths resulting from intra-procedural myocardial infarction or intraperitoneal hemorrhage as described below.

Table 29.3 Complications associated with TIPS. (From Freedman *et al.* [121])

	UCSF [122]	MVI [123]	UH/UF [124,125]	MCV [126]
Number of patients	100	76	120	64
Technical success	96*	76	111	59
Direct procedural mortality (%)	0	0	<1	1.5
Procedural morbidity (%)	NR	15	NR	20
Transcapsular puncture (%)	Many†	NR	NR	30
Portal venous rupture (%)	0	1.3	0	0
Splenoportal venous thrombosis (%)	NR	5	NR	9
Acute stent thrombosis (%)	NR	NR	NR	3
Delayed shunt occlusion (%)	9	3 at 1 yr	5	5
Delayed shunt stenosis	6‡	36	30	60–75
Stent shortening/incomplete placement (%)	2	NR	NR	1.5
Puncture site hematoma/bleeding (%)	4.5	NR	4	1.5
New/worsening hepatic encephalopathy (%)	17	13	New 5	25
Fever/sepsis (%)	10	NR	<1	10

* TIPS was successfully performed in seven of 10 patients with portal venous occlusion.
† One patient with intraperitoneal hemorrhage required 2 U of packed red blood cells.
‡ Includes cases with 50% or greater stenosis.
MCV, Medical College of Virginia (Richmond); MVI, Miami Vascular Institute (Baptist Hospital, Miami, Florida); NR, not reported; UCSF, University of California in San Francisco; UH/UF, Ruprect-Karls-University (Heidelberg, Germany)/Albert Ludwig University (Freiburg, Germany).

Intraperitoneal hemorrhage

Transcapsular puncture is frequently noted, but only infrequently results in intraperitoneal hemorrhage. Traversal of the liver capsule is particularly likely in patients with small livers and has been noted in up to 30% of cases in some series [121]. Serious hemoperitoneum, however, is rare [121,122], which is perhaps surprising in light of the high incidence of coagulation abnormalities among these patients. Nonetheless, prophylactic correction of clotting abnormalities with infusion of fresh frozen plasma and platelets is advisable. Some prefer to use a small needle (an 18-gage needle instead of the 16-gage Colapinto needle) in an attempt further to decrease the likelihood of bleeding. The disadvantages of the 18-gage Brockenbrough USCI Division, Bard, Billerica, MA) are its decreased stiffness and the necessity of using a 0.018-in (0.45 mm) guidewire.

In order to confine the needle to the hepatic parenchyma (i.e., avoid transcapsular puncture), the needle puncture should be started close to the junction of the hepatic vein with the inferior vena cava, and the needle should be advanced only 3–4 cm into the hepatic parenchyma [122]. Nevertheless, transcapsular punctures are inevitable and, when possible, it is reasonable to embolize the transcapsular needle tract with a pledget of gelatin sponge [121]. In general, the fewer passes made with the needle while attempting to cannulate the portal vein, the safer the procedure. Interventional radiologists today are familiar enough with transhepatic cannulation of the portal vein so that, in most cases, few passes are required and procedure time is short. Wedged hepatic venography with retrograde opacification of the portal vein (using water-soluble contrast or carbon dioxide) is a low-risk maneuver initially to localize the portal vein, thus guiding the transhepatic puncture and helping to limit the number of passes. This technique with water-soluble contrast is successful in opacifying the portal vein 76% of the time [127], and using carbon dioxide may opacify the portal vein even more readily [128]. Some authors [129] prefer initial arterial mesenteric portography or ultrasound guidance. In cases in which cannulation of the portal vein is especially difficult, transhepatic insertion of a 0.018-in (0.45 mm) guidewire into the portal vein under ultrasound guidance has been found to be helpful [129].

Intraperitoneal hemorrhage may also result from rupture of the portal vein. This can occur if the extrahepatic portal vein is punctured and, subsequently, balloon dilated. Without surrounding hepatic parenchyma to tamponade bleeding, immediate massive hemoperitoneum can result. Therefore, only cannulation of the right or left portal vein branches (which are reliably intrahepatic) should be used to create the shunt. After the portal vein or one of its branches is cannulated, a portal venogram should be performed carefully to assess the entrance site into the portal vein.

Hepatic artery injury and fistula formation

The proximity of the hepatic artery, portal vein, and bile ducts accounts for the reports of hepatic arterial injuries and significant hemobilia that can occur after repeated transhepatic punctures. Patients with cirrhosis may be at increased risk of hepatic arterial injury because of enlargement and increased flow in the hepatic artery [130]. Hepatic arterial occlusion has been reported following inadvertent arterial puncture [130]. This proved to be devastating in a patient whose hepatic blood supply was already compromised by the portal venous shunt, and the patient developed accelerated liver failure, with death 3-days later. Angiography (with hepatic and superior mesenteric arterial injections) to evaluate for hepatic artery occlusion or bleeding, should be performed in patients whose condition deteriorates following a TIPS, with evidence of worsening liver function or blood loss not caused by variceal bleeding. In such circumstances, intervention may be possible with selective embolization of a bleeding site or recannulization of an occluded hepatic artery. It should be emphasized that if embolization of a hepatic arterial injury is performed in a cirrhotic patient following TIPS, the embolization must be superselective because ischemia to a large part of the liver could otherwise result, with the danger of worsening liver failure.

Fistulae may develop between hepatic arteries, hepatic veins, portal veins, and bile ducts. As previously discussed, intrahepatic vascular lesions have been shown to occur in 20–33% of patients following PTBD [49,58,59], although most are asymptomatic. It is likely that TIPS will result in an incidence of vascular lesions at least as great and possibly greater than PTBD, secondary to both anatomic proximity and increased hepatic artery and hepatic vein flow. Undoubtedly, most of these lesions will remain asymptomatic. However, if a fistula involving the hepatic artery becomes symptomatic, arteriography should be performed with the intention of performing percutaneous arterial embolization.

Complications related to the transvenous access to the portal vein

These complications have already been discussed under the topic of Transjugular liver biopsy, p. 505.

Complications related to cannulation of the portal vein

Splenoportal venous thrombosis

Splenoportal venous thrombosis is likely to result only with extended cannulation and manipulation. However, thrombus may already be present within the portal vein prior to the procedure, as portal hypertension alone is an independent risk factor [121,130]. This emphasizes the importance of obtaining pre-TIPS studies, such as arterial portography, enhanced abdominal CT, or ultrasound to assess portal vein patency. During the course of the TIPS procedure, with catheter manipulation in the portal vein, thrombus may propagate resulting in decreased flow in the shunt. It is therefore important to minimize catheter manipulation in the portal vein. Furthermore, when balloon dilatation of the parenchymal tract is performed, care should be taken to minimize the portion of the balloon that projects into the portal vein [121].

Complications related to the stent

Acute thrombosis

Early thrombosis of the stent usually is the result of technical error, such as incomplete coverage of the parenchymal tract with the stent or a stenosis of the hepatic vein. However, thrombosis can occur as a result of extended cannulation and manipulation as discussed in the previous section. Regardless of the cause, treatment options include suction embolectomy with a large end-hole catheter such as the 9-F Colapinto guiding catheter [121], or dislodgment of the thrombus with an occlusion balloon. Although technically more difficult to perform, it is preferable to "bulldoze" the thrombus into the coronary vein, thereby simultaneously occluding the varices. This is performed by cannulating the occluded portal vein and selectively placing the catheter and guidewire into the coronary vein or varix. The catheter is removed leaving the guidewire in place. The occlusion balloon is inflated proximal to the thrombus and the thrombus is pushed along the path of the guidewire into the coronary vein. Alternately, the balloon can be inflated beyond the thrombus and pulled back through the stent, pulling the thrombus into the inferior vena cava and right atrium. This maneuver is contraindicated in patients with severe lung disease and with right to left cardiac shunts.

Delayed occlusion

Delayed occlusion of the stent is thought to be the result of myointimal proliferation, although technical factors such as incomplete coverage of the parenchymal tract with the stent (possibly secondary to shortening of the stent) may play a role. Superimposed thrombosis is likely to be present as well. Delayed occlusion with resultant recurrent bleeding secondary to insufficient stent placement is avoidable. The stent, particularly if a Wallstent is used, should be placed with at least a 1-cm margin of stent above and below the parenchymal tract to ensure that the tract is adequately covered and that any stent shortening that may occur over time will not result in a lack of stent coverage of the tract [122]. Stenosis of the hepatic vein may be related to utilization of a small hepatic vein. Initial selection of the largest hepatic vein is the best guaranty against this problem [121], and the stent may even be placed all the way through the hepatic vein to the junction with the inferior vena cava. Delayed stenosis/occlusion due to development of intimal hyperplasia within the shunt cannot currently be effectively prevented. Close follow-up with serial duplex ultrasound and direct portal venography with pressure measurements when stenosis is suspected, should, therefore, be undertaken in all patients with the assumption that this complication is inevitable and should be diagnosed and treated before becoming clinically significant (i.e., resulting in rebleeding). Doppler ultrasonography has proven to be a good method of screening to depict the patency of a TIPS, and the maximum velocity is an accurate, noninvasive parameter for assessing shunt patency [126,127].

Gordon *et al.* [124], have reported on 11 of 135 patients who have returned with occluded stents, necessitating recannulization of the shunt. In some of these patients, the material occluding the stent offered considerable resistance to passage of guidewires. The authors suggested use of the Colapinto needle, which in their experience provided the necessary support to enable a wire to be forced through the occlusion. Following recannulization of the occluded shunt, urokinase infusion may be necessary to remove thrombus, followed by angioplasty or placement of another stent to keep the shunt patent. Assisted primary patency (i.e., correction of a stenosis) appears to be better than secondary patency, although results at 1 year and greater are good in both groups [132].

Hepatic encephalopathy

When creating a portosystemic shunt, the diameter of the shunt must be carefully considered. On the one hand, the shunt must be large enough adequately to decompress the portal venous system in order to prevent rebleeding from varices. On the other hand, if the diameter of the shunt is too large, an abundance of portal venous blood is shunted away from the liver, and hepatic encephalopathy results. The experience with surgically created shunts has shown that smaller selective shunts are less likely to cause hepatic encephalopathy than larger, nonselective shunts [132–139], although rebleeding is more likely with the former. Surgical shunting results in hepatic encephalopathy in 5–67% of patients, depending on the type of shunt created and the size of the shunt [132–139].

As with surgical shunts, the incidence of hepatic encephalopathy in TIPS increases with the diameter of the stent. Therefore, the stent should be dilated to the diameter that adequately decompresses the portal venous system (a portosystemic gradient of ≤ 13 mmHg) and no greater. Other factors that increase encephalopathy are patient age greater than 62 years and advanced liver disease. Following TIPS, hepatic encephalopathy has been seen in 5−35% of patients [121,122,125,133−135]. However, *de novo* hepatic encephalopathy (occurring in patients with no sign of hepatic encephalopathy prior to TIPS) develops in less than 10% of patients. Careful assessment of the presence of encephalopathy based on clinical grounds is essential because it is generally possible effectively to treat the condition with diet and lactulose.

References

1 Smith EH. The hazards of fine-needle aspiration biopsy. *Ultrasound Med Biol* 1984;10;629−634.

2 Smith EH. Complications of percutaneous abdominal fine-needle biopsy. *Radiology* 1991;178:253−258.

3 Weiss H, Weiss A, Scholl A. Todliche Komplication einer Fennodelbiopsie der Liber. *Deutsch Med Wochenschr* 1988;113:139−142.

4 Fornari F, Civardi G, Cavanna L *et al.* Complications of ultrasonically guided fine-needle abdominal biopsy: results of a multicenter Italian study and review of the literature. *Scand J Gastroenterol* 1989;24:949−955.

5 Mahal AS, Knaver CM, Gregory PB. Bleeding after liver biopsy: how often and why? (abstract). *Gastroenterology* 1979;76:1192.

6 Sharma P, MacDonald GB, Banaji M. The risks of bleeding after percutaneous liver biopsy: relation to platelet count. *J Clin Gastroenterol* 1982;4:451−453.

7 Zins M, Vilgrain V, Gayno S, Rolland Y *et al.* US guided percutaneous liver biopsy with plugging of the needle tract: a prospective study in 72 high-risk patients. *Radiology* 1992;184:841−843.

8 Taavitsainen M, Kivisaari L. Is fine-needle biopsy of liver hemangioma hazardous? *Am J Roentgenol* 1987;148:231−232.

9 Solbiati L, Livraghi T, De Pra L *et al.* Fine needle biopsy of hepatic hemangioma with sonographic guidance. *Am J Roentgenol* 1985;144:471−475.

10 Cronan JJ, Esparza AR, Dorfman GS, Ridlen MS, Paolella LP. Cavernous hemangioma of the liver: role of percutaneous biopsy. *Radiology* 1988;166:135−138.

11 Charboneau J, Reading C, Welch T. CT and sonographically guided needle biopsy: current techniques and new innovations. *Am J Roentgenol* 1990;154:1−10.

12 Tung GA, Cronan JJ. Percutaneous needle biopsy of hepatic cavernous hemangioma. *J Clin Gastroenterol* 1993;16(2):117−122.

13 Terriff B, Gibney R, Scudamore C. Fatality from fine-needle aspiration biopsy of a hepatic hemangioma. *Am J Roentgenol* 1990;154:203−204.

14 Martino C, Haaga J, Bryan P *et al.* CT guided liver biopsies: eight years experience. *Radiology* 1984;152:755−757.

15 Pagani JJ. Biopsy of focal hepatic lesions: comparison of 18 and 22 g. needles. *Radiology* 1983;147:673−675.

16 Bernardino ME. Percutaneous biopsy. *Am J Roentgenol* 1984;142:41−45.

17 Wittenberg J, Mueller PR, Ferrucci JT Jr *et al.* Percutaneous core biopsy of abdominal tumors using 22 g. needles: further observations. *Am J Roentgenol* 1982;139:75−80.

18 Palestrant AM. *CT Guided Large Needle Biopsy.* Presented at the 13th Annual Meeting of the Society of Cardiovascular and Interventional Radiology, Orlando, FL, March 21−24, 1988.

19 Andriole JG, Haaga JR, Adams RB, Nunez C. Biopsy needle characteristics assessed in the laboratory. *Radiology* 1983;148:659−662.

20 Welch TJ, Sheedy PF, Johnson CD, Johnson CM, Stephans DH. CT guided biopsy: prospective analysis of 1000 procedures. *Radiology* 1989;171:493−496.

21 Gebel M, Horstkotte H, Koster C, Brunkhorst R, Brandt M, Atay Z. Ultraschallgezielte Feinnadelpunktion abdomineller Organe: Indikationen, Ergebnisse, Risiken. *Ultraschall Med* 1986;7:198−202.

22 Nolsoe C, Nielsen L, Torp-Pedersen S, Holm HH. Major complications and deaths due to interventional ultrasonography: a review of 8000 cases. *JCV* 1990;18:179−184.

23 Bret P, Labadie M, Bretagnolle M, Paliard P, Fond A, Vallette PJ. Hepatocellular carcinoma: diagnosis by percutaneous fine needle biopsy. *Gastrointest Radiol* 1988;13:253−255.

24 Velt PM, Choy OG, Shimkin PM, Link RJ. Transjugular liver biopsy in high risk patients with hepatic disease. *Radiology* 1984;153(1):91−93.

25 Colapinto RF. Transjugular biopsy of the liver. *Clin Gastroenterol* 1985;14(2):451−467.

26 Perrault J, McGill DB, Ott BJ, Talor WF. Liver biopsy: complications in 1000 inpatients and outpatients. *Gastroenterology* 1978;74:103−106.

27 Murphy F, Barefield K, Steinberg H, Bernardino M. CT or sonography-guided biopsy of the liver in the presence of ascites: frequency of complications. *Am J Roentgenol* 1988;151:485−486.

28 Lebrec D, Goldfarb G, Degott C, Rueff B, Benhamou JP. Transvenous liver biopsy: an experience based on 1000 hepatic tissue samplings with this procedure. *Gastroenterology* 1982;83:338−340.

29 Bull HJM, Gilmore IT, Bradley RD, Mangold JH, Thompson RPH. Experience with transjugular liver biopsy. *Gut* 1983;24:1057−1060.

30 Gamble P, Colapinto RF, Stronel R, Colman J, Blendis L. Transjugular liver biopsy: a review of 461 biopsies. *Radiology* 1985;157:589−593.

31 Corr P, Beningfield SJ, Davey N. Transjugular liver biopsy: a review of 200 biopsies. *Clin Radiol* 1992;45:238−239.

32 Lebrec D, Degott C, Rueff B, Benhamou J-P. Transvenous (transjugular) liver biopsy: an experience based on 100 biopsies. *Am J Digest Dis* 1978;23:302−304.

33 Allison D, Adam A. Percutaneous liver biopsy and tract embolization with steel coils. *Radiology* 1988;169:261−263.

34 Braillon A, Revert R, Remond A, Auderbert M, Capron J. Transcatheter embolization of liver capsule perforation during transvenous liver biopsy. *Gastrointest Radiol* 1986;11:277−279.

35 Gazelle GS, Haaga JR, Neuhauser D. Hemostatic protein−polymer sheath: new method to enhance hemostasis of percutaneous biopsy. *Radiology* 1990;175:671−674.

36 Chezmar J, Keith L, Nelson R, Plair J, Hetzler G, Bernardino M. Liver transplant biopsies with a biopsy gun. *Radiology* 1991;179:447−448.

37 Hardin WP, Mueller PR, Ferrucci JT Jr. Transhepatic cholangiography: complications and use patterns of the fine needle technique. *Radiology* 1980;135:15−22.

38 Ferrucci JT, Wittenberg J. Refinements in chiba needle transhepatic cholangiography. *Am J Roentgenol* 1977;129:11.

39 Bilbao MK, Potter CI, Lee TG, Katon RM. Complications of endoscopic retrograde cholangiopancreatography (ERCP): a study of 10 000 cases. *Gastroenterology* 1976;70:314.

40 Nebel OT, Fornes MF. Endoscopic pancreaticocholangiography. *Digest Dis* 1973;18:1042.

41 Katon RM, Lee TG, Parent JA, Bibao MK, Smith FW. Endoscopic retrograde cholangiopancreatography (ERCP) experience with 100 cases. *Am J Digest Dis* 1974;19:295.

42 Ferrucci JT, Wittenberg J, Sarno RA *et al*. Fine needle THC, a new approach to obstructive jaundice. *Am J Roentgenol* 1976; 127:403.

43 Ariyama J, Shirakabe H, Ohasi K, Roberts GM. Experience with percutaneous transhepatic cholangiography using the Japanese needle. *Gastrointest Radiol* 1978;2:359−365.

44 Okuda K, Tanikawa K, Emura T *et al*. Nonsurgical percutaneous transhepatic cholangiography-diagnostic significance in medical problems of the liver. *Am J Digest Dis* 1974;19:21−36.

45 Keighley MRB, Lister DM, Jacobs SI, Giles GR. Hazards of surgical treatment due to micro-organisms in the bile. *Surgery* 1974;75:578−583.

46 Keighley MRB. Micro-organisms in the bile. A preventable cause of sepsis after biliary surgery. *Ann Roy Coll Surg Engl* 1977;59:328−344.

47 Hultborn A, Jacobson B, Rosengreen B. Cholangiovenous reflux during cholangiography. An experimental and clinical study. *Acta Chir Scand* 1962;123:111−124.

48 Nilsson V, Evander A, Ihse I, Lunderquist A, Mocibob A. Percutaneous transhepatic cholangiography and drainage: risks and complications. *Acta Radiol* 1983;24:433−439.

49 Okuda M, Musha H, Nakajima Y *et al*. Frequency of intrahepatic arteriovenous fistula as a sequella to percutaneous needle puncture of the liver. *Gastroenterology* 1978;74:1204−1207.

50 Mueller P, Van Sonnenberg E, Ferrucci JT. Percutaneous biliary drainage: technical and catheter related problems in 200 procedures. *Am J Roentgenol* 1982;138:17−23.

51 Carrasco CH, Zornoza J, Bechtel WJ. Malignant biliary obstruction: complications of percutaneous biliary drainage. *Radiology* 1984;152:343−346.

52 Hamlin J, Friedman M, Stein M, Bray J. Percutaneous biliary drainage: complications of 118 consecutive catheterizations. *Radiology* 1986;158:199−202.

53 Yee ACN, Chia-Sing Ho. Complications of percutaneous biliary drainage: benign vs malignant diseases. *Am J Roentgenol* 1987; 148:1207−1209.

54 Gunther RW, Schild H, Thelen M. Review article: percutaneous transhepatic biliary drainage: experience with 311 procedures. *Cardiovasc Intervent Radiol* 1988;11.65−71.

55 Hansson JA, Hoevels J, Simert G *et al*. Clinical aspects of nonsurgical percutaneous transhepatic bile drainage in obstructive lesions of the extrahepatic bile ducts. *Ann Surg* 1977;189: 58−61.

56 Lou Mas, Mandal AK, Alexander JL *et al*. Bacteriology of the human biliary tract and the duodenum. *Arch Surg* 1977;112: 965−967.

57 Kadir S, Baassiri A, Barth K, Kaufman S, Cameron J, White R. Percutaneous biliary drainage in the management of biliary sepsis. *Am J Roentgenol* 1982;138:25−29.

58 Hoevels J, Nilsson U. Intrahepatic vascular lesions following non-surgical percutaneous transhepatic bile duct intubation. *Gastrointest Radiol* 1980;5:127−135.

59 Monden M, Okamura J, Kobayashi N *et al*. Hemobilia after percutaneous transhepatic biliary drainage. *Arch Surg* 1980; 115:161−164.

60 Mitchell SE, Shuman LS, Kaufman SL *et al*. Biliary catheter drainage complicated by hemobilia: treatment by balloon

embolotherapy. *Radiology* 1985;157:645−652.

61 Savader SJ, Trerotola SO, Merine DS, Venbrux AC, Osterman FA. Hemobilia after percutaneous transhepatic biliary drainage: treatment with transcatheter embolotherapy. *J Vasc Intervent Radiol* 1992;3:345−352.

62 Vasquez JL, Thorsen MK, Dodds WJ *et al*. Evaluation and treatment of intra-abdominal bilomas. *Am J Roentgenol* 1985; 144:933−938.

63 Luska G, Poser H. Acute pancreatitis in obstructive jaundice following combined internal and external percutaneous transhepatic bile duct drainage (PTBD). *Eur J Radiol* 1983;3: 112−114.

64 Savader SJ, Venbrux AC, Robbins KV, Gittelsohn AM, Osterman FA. Pancreatic response to percutaneous biliary drainage: a prospective study. *Radiology* 1991;178:343−346.

65 Strange C, Allen ML, Freedland PN, Cunningman J, Sahn SA. Biliopleural fistula as a complication of percutaneous biliary drainage: experimental evidence for pleural inflammation. *Am Rev Respir Dis* 1988;137:959−961.

66 Dosik MH. Bile peritonitis − another complication of percutaneous liver biopsy. *Am J Digest Dis* 1975;20:91−93.

67 Dawson SL, Neff CC, Mueller PR, Ferrucci JT Jr. Fatal hemothorax after inadvertent transpleural biliary drainage. *Am J Roentgenol* 1983;141:33−34.

68 Nakayama T, Ikeda A, Okuda K. Percutaneous transhepatic drainage of the biliary tract: technique and results in 104 cases. *Gastroenterology* 1978;74:554−559.

69 Berquist TH, May GR, Johnson CM, Adson MA, Thistle JL. Percutaneous biliary decompression: internal and external drainage in 50 patients. *Am J Roentgenol* 1981;136:901−906.

70 Clark RA, Mitchell SE, Colley DP, Alexander E. Percutaneous catheter biliary decompression. *Am J Roentgenol* 1981;137: 503−509.

71 Oleaga JA, Ring EJ. Interventional biliary radiology. *Semin Roentgenol* 1981;16:116−134.

72 Neff CC, Muellar PR, Ferrucci JT *et al*. Serious complications following transgression of the pleural space in drainage procedures. *Radiology* 1984;152:335−341.

73 Lameris JS, Obertop H, Jeekel J. Biliary drainage by ultrasound-guided puncture of the left hepatic duct. *Clin Radiol* 1985;36: 269−274.

74 Lillemoe KD, Pitt HA, Kaufman SL, Cameron JL. Acute cholecystitis occurring as a complication of percutaneous transhepatic drainage. *Surg Gynecol Obstet* 1989;168:348−342.

75 Taber DS, Stroehlein JR, Zornoza J. Work in progress: hypotension and high volume biliary excretion following external percutaneous transhepatic biliary drainage. *Radiology* 1982; 145:639−640.

76 Ferrucci JT Jr, Mueller PR, Harbin WP. Percutaneous transhepatic biliary drainage: technique, results and applications. *Radiology* 1980;135:1−13.

77 Miller GA Jr, Heaston DK, Moore AV Jr, Mills SR, Dunnick NR. Peritoneal seeding of cholangiocarcinoma in patients with percutaneous biliary drainage. *Am J Roentgenol* 1983;141: 561−562.

78 Oleaga JA, Ring EJ, Freiman DB, McLean GK, Rosen RJ. Extension of neoplasm along the tract of a transhepatic tube. *Am J Roentgenol* 1980;135:841−842.

79 Kim WS, Barth KH, Zinner M. Seeding of pancreatic carcinoma along the transhepatic catheter tract. *Radiology* 1982;143: 427−428.

80 Anschuetz S, Vogelzang RL. Malignant pleural effusion: a

complication of transhepatic biliary drainage. *Am J Roentgenol* 1986;146:1165−1166.

81 Chapman WC, Sharp KW, Weaver F, Sawyers JL. Tumor seeding from percutaneous biliary catheters. *Ann Surg* 1989; 209(6):708−713.

82 Severini A, Bellomi M, Cozzi G, Bellegotti L, Lattuada A. Rib erosion: late complication of longstanding biliary drainage catheters. *Radiology* 1984;150:666.

83 Ring EJ, Kerlan RK. Interventional biliary radiology. *Am J Roentgenol* 1984;142:31−34.

84 Dick BW, Gordon RL, Laberge JM, Doherty MM, Ring EJ. Percutaneous transhepatic placement of biliary endoprosthesis: results in 100 consecutive patients. *J Vasc Intervent Radiol* 1990; 1:97−100.

85 Mueller P, Ferrucci J Jr, Teplick S *et al.* Biliary stent endoprosthesis: analysis of complications in 113 patients. *Radiology* 1985;156:637−639.

86 Lammer J, Neumayer K. Biliary drainage endoprosthesis: experience with 201 placements. *Radiology* 1986;159:625−629.

87 Stoker J, Lameris JS, Veeze-Kuijpers B, Bot F. Delayed biliary and duodenal perforation after wallstent insertion in irradiated biliary malignancy. *J Intervent Radiol* 1991;6:127−130.

88 Gordon RL, Ring EJ, LaBerge JM, Doherty MM. Malignant biliary obstruction: treatment with expandable metallic stents — follow-up of 50 consecutive patients. *Radiology* 1992;182: 697−701.

89 Adam A, Chetty N, Roddie M, Yeung E, Benjamin IS. Self-expandable stainless steel endoprostheses for treatment of malignant bile duct obstruction. *Am J Roentgenol* 1991;156: 321−325.

90 Lammer J, Klein GE, Kleinert R, Hausegger K, Einspieler R. Obstructive jaundice: use of expandable metal endoprosthesis for biliary drainage. *Radiology* 1990;177:789−792.

91 Gillams A, Dick R, Dooley JS, Wallsten H, El-Din A. Self-expandable stainless steel braided endoprosthesis for biliary structures. *Radiology* 1990;174:137−140.

92 Lameris JS, Stoker J, Nijs HGT *et al.* Malignant biliary obstruction: percutaneous use of self-expandable stents. *Radiology* 1991;179:703−707.

93 Davids PHP, Groen AK, Rauws EAJ, Tytgat GNJ, Huibregtse K. Randomized trial of self-expanding metal stents vs polyethylene stents for distal malignant biliary obstruction. *Lancet* 1992;340: 1488−1492.

95 Salomonowitz E, Castaneda WR, Lund G *et al.* Balloon dilatation of benign biliary strictures. *Am J Roentgenol* 1984;151:613.

96 Weyman PJ, Balfe DM. Percutaneous dilatation of biliary structures. *Semin Intervent Radiol* 1982;2:50−59.

97 Gallacher DJ, Kadir S, Kaufman SL *et al.* Non-operative management of benign post-operative biliary strictures. *Radiology* 1985;156:625−629.

98 Smith SW, Engel C, Averbrook B, Longmire WB Jr. Problems of retained and recurrent common bile duct stones. *Surgery* 1969;66:291−298.

99 Mazzariello R. Removal of residual biliary calculi without re-operation. *Surgery* 1970;67:556.

100 Herrara M, Colemann CC, Castaneda WR, Amplatz K. New techniques for replacing dislodged T-tubes. *Am J Roentgenol* 1984;142:102.

101 Burhenne HJ. Complications of non-operative extraction of retained common bile duct stones. *Am J Surg* 1976;131: 260−262.

102 Polack EP, Fainsinger MH, Bonnano SV. A death following

complications of roentgenologic non-operative manipulation of common bile duct calculi. *Radiology* 1977;123:585−586.

103 Clouse ME, Falchuck KR. Percutaneous transhepatic removal of common duct stones: report of ten patients. *Gastroenterology* 1983;85:815−819.

104 Wayne PH, Whelan JG Jr. Susceptibility testing of biliary bacteria obtained before bile duct manipulation. *Am J Roentgenol* 1983;140:1185−1188.

105 Haskin PH, Teplick JK. Percutaneous management of biliary stones. *Semin Intervent Radiol* 1985;2:81−96.

106 Motson RW. Dissolution of common bile duct stones. *Br J Surg* 1981;68:203−208.

107 Jarrett LN, Balfour TW, Bell GD, Knapp DR, Rose DH. Intra-ductal infusion of mono-octanoin: experience in 24 patients with retained common duct stones. *Lancet* 1981;1:68−70.

108 Train JS, Dan SJ, Cohen LB, Mitty HA. Duodenal ulceration associated with mono-octanoin infusion. *Am J Roentgenol* 1983; 141:557−558.

109 Minuk GJ, Hoofnagle JH, Jones EA. Systemic side effects from the intrabiliary infusion of mono-octanoin for the dissolution of gallstones. *J Clin Gastroenterol* 1982;4:133−135.

110 Crabtree TS, Dykstra R, Kelly J, Preshaw RM. Necrotizing choledochomalacia after use of mono-octanoin to dissolve bile duct stones. *Can J Surg* 1982;25:644−646.

111 Williams HJ Jr, Bender CE, LeRoy AJ. Dissolution of choles-terol gallstones using methyl tert-butyl ether. *Cardiovasc Inter-vent Radiol* 1990;13:272−277.

112 McGahan JP, Lindfors KK. Acute cholecystitis: diagnostic accuracy of percutaneous aspiration of the gallbladder. *Radiology* 1988;167:669−671.

113 Teplick SK. Diagnostic and therapeutic interventional gall-bladder procedures. *Am J Roentgenol* 1989;152:913−916.

114 Illescas FF, Braun SD, Cohan RH, Bowie JD, Dunnick NR. Ultrasonically guided percutaneous transhepatic transchole-cystocholangiography in the non-dilated biliary tree. *Gastrointest Radiol* 1986;11:77−80.

115 van Sonnenberg E, Wittich GR, Casola G *et al.* Diagnostic and therapeutic percutaneous gallbladder procedures. *Radiology* 1986;160:23−26.

116 Pearse DM, Hawkins IF, Shaver R, Vogel S. Percutaneous cholecystostomy in acute cholecystitis and common duct ob-struction. *Radiology* 1984;152:365−367.

117 Makucchi M, Yamazaki S, Hasegawa H. Ultrasonically guided cholangiography and bile drainage. *Ultrasound Med Biol* 1984; 10(5):617−623.

118 Lohela P, Soiva M, Suramo I, Taavitsainen M, Holopainen O. Ultrasound guidance for percutaneous puncture and drainage in acute cholecystitis. *Acta Radiol (Diagn)* 1986;27(5):543−546.

119 Vogelzang RL, Nemcek HA Jr. Percutaneous cholecystostomy: diagnostic and therapeutic efficacy. *Radiology* 1988;168:29−34.

120 D'Agostino HB, vanSonnenberg E, Sanchez RB, Goodacre BW, Casola G. Imaging of the percutaneous cholecystostomy tract: observations and utility. *Radiology* 1991;181:674−675.

121 Freedman A, Sanyal A, Tisnado J *et al.* Complications of trans-jugular intrahepatic portosystemic shunt: a comprehensive review. *Radiographics* 1993;13:1185−1210.

122 LaBerge JM, Ring EJ, Gordon RL *et al.* Creation of transjugular intrahepatic portosystemic shunts with the wallstent endo-prosthesis: results in 100 patients. *Radiology* 1993;187: 413−420.

123 Lafortune M, Martinez J-P, Denys A *et al.* Short and long-term hemodynamic effects of transjugular intrahepatic portosystemic

shunts: a Doppler/manometric correlative study. *Am J Roentgenol* 1995;164:997−1002.

124 Gordon RL, LaBerge JM, Ring EJ, Doherty MM. Recanalization of occluded intrahepatic portosystemic shunts. use of the colapinto needle. *J Vasc Intervent Radiol* 1993;4:441−443.

125 Freedman AM, Sanyal AJ, Tisnado J *et al*. Results with percutaneous transjugular intrahepatic portosystemic stent-shunts for control of variceal hemorrhage in patients awaiting liver transplantation. *Transplant Proc* 1993;25:1087−1089.

126 Chong WK, Malisch TA, Mazer MJ, Lind CD, Worrell JA, Richards WO. Transjugular intrahepatic portosystemic shunt: US assessment with maximum flow velocity. *Radiology* 1993;189:789−793.

127 Bonn J, Soulen MC, Eschelman DJ *et al*. Techniques for portal vein localization during transjugular portosystemic shunt (abstract). *Radiology* 1992;185:104.

128 Rees CR, Niblett RL, Lee SP, Diamond NG, Crippin JS. Use of carbon dioxide as a contrast medium for transjugular intrahepatic portosystemic shunt procedures. *J Vasc Intervent Radiol* 1994;5:383−386.

129 Harman JT, Reed JD, Kopecky KK, Harris VJ, Haggerty MF, Strzemosz AS. Localization of the portal vein for transjugular catheterization: percutaneous placement of a metallic marker with real-time ultrasound guidance. *J Vasc Intervent Radiol* 1992;3:545−547.

130 Haskal ZJ, Pentecost MJ, Rubin RA. Hepatic arterial injury after transjugular intrahepatic portosystemic shunt placement: report of two cases. *Radiology* 1993;188:85−88.

132 Rikkers LF, Jin G. Variceal hemorrhage: surgical therapy. *Gastroenterol Clin N Am* 1993;22:821−842.

133 Zemel G, Katzen BT, Becker GJ, Benenati JF, Salee S. Percutaneous transjugular portosystemic shunt. *J Am Med Assoc* 1991;266:390−393.

134 Noeldge G, Richter GM, Roessle M *et al*. Morphologic and clinical results of the transjugular intrahepatic portosystemic stent-shunts (TIPS). *Cardiovasc Intervent Radiol* 1992;342−348.

135 Richter GM, Noeldge G, Palmaz JC *et al*. Transjugular intrahepatic portocaval stent-shunt: preliminary clinical results. *Radiology* 1990;174:1027−1030.

136 Rikkers LF, Jin G. Variceal hemorrhage: surgical therapy. *Gastroenterol Clin N Am* 1993;22:821.

137 Rikkers LF, Jin G. Surgical management of acute variceal hemorrhage. *World J Surg* 1994;18:193−199.

138 Collins JC, Rypins EB, Sarfeh IJ. Narrow diameter portocaval shunts for management of variceal bleeding. *World J Surg* 1994;18:211−215.

139 Zakim D, Boyer TD, eds. *Hepatology: a Textbook of Liver Disease*. Philadelphia, PA: Saunders, 1990:599−601.

CHAPTER 30

Complications in the gastrointestinal tract: hollow organs and abscesses

C. Christopher Pittman, Steven B. Oglevie,
Risteard M. O'Laoide, Horacio B. D'Agostino,
and Eric vanSonnenberg

Abscess drainage

Introduction

Image-guided catheter drainage is the treatment of choice for intraabdominal fluid collections and abscesses, regardless of etiology [1–6]. Infected and noninfected pancreatic collections, multiloculated abscesses [7–10], multiple abscesses [8,10], abscesses with internal communications, hematomas [1,6,8], lymphoceles, enteric-related abscesses [1,5,7–9, 11–13], necrotic tumors [1,14], benign cysts, amebic and echinococcal abscesses, splenic and tuboovarian abscesses, and occasionally phlegmon [3,7,8,10] — cases for which percutaneous abscess drainage (PAD) was previously considered inappropriate — are currently treated with percutaneous methods. PAD is especially suitable in severely ill patients who are not surgical candidates [10]. PAD has proven to be as efficacious as surgical drainage [4]. In addition, PAD obviates general anesthesia and laparotomy and generally results in decreased postoperative hospitalization and in cost-savings [5,9,15].

Over the past decade, the newly expanded role of PAD has illuminated different aspects in which complications may occur. These complications will be individually addressed and discussed. Complications of PAD may be separated into two main categories. Those complications that occur during

the performance of PAD and others that occur during the management of the PAD catheter.

Complications during aspiration and/or drainage

Patient selection and contraindications

There are no specific ultrasonography (US) or computed tomography (CT) features of an intraabdominal collection that predict successful percutaneous drainage [6,16]. Thus, there are no specific imaging features that portend PAD failure. Both CT and US are sensitive for detecting intraabdominal fluid collections, but imaging does not reliably distinguish infected from noninfected collections. A variety of fluid collections appear similar on CT and US, e.g., loculated ascites, hematomas, urinomas, bilomas, lymphoceles, necrotic tumors, as well as abscesses. Only diagnostic aspiration can establish the need for PAD and the probability of successful drainage [6]. All patients with intraabdominal fluid collections should be considered candidates for percutaneous drainage [16].

A relative contraindication to PAD is uncorrectable coagulopathy. Patient candidates for PAD are often very ill [10,13, 17] and frequently have a rapidly changing hemostatic status because of sepsis, cancer, liver disease, renal disease, immunosuppression, and acquired immune deficiency syndrome (AIDS). An identified hemostatic abnormality may or may not be correctable. Most bleeding disorders can be improved with some kind of replacement therapy. Patients should be managed individually, however, and physicians have the right and the responsibility to deviate from guidelines if the clinical situation warrants it, particularly in the case of emergency or life-saving procedures. Hemorrhage is a well-recognized potential complication of PAD and of any interventional radiologic procedure [3,7,18]. Transgression of vessels may occur during performance of PAD [5,7,9]. Vascular anatomy is usually well defined by a CT scan. Review of a previously obtained CT scan during PAD, or performance of PAD under CT guidance assists in avoidance of vascular structures *en route* to a fluid collection. Color Doppler US prior to or during PAD shows the vascularity of the proposed access route and also aids in avoidance of the most vascular portion of a lesion [19].

The only absolute contraindication to PAD is lack of a safe access route [2,9,10]. Failure to identify or plan a safe access route is a recognized cause of PAD morbidity. Identification of a safe access route is seldom a problem, however, when utilizing some combination of CT, US, and fluoroscopy. In general, transgression of overlying organs during aspiration and drainage should be avoided. On occasion, organ transgression is unavoidable, especially with deep abdominal aspiration and drainage procedures. Adjacent solid organs such as the liver, kidney, or spleen may be traversed both to achieve and optimize drainage. Noninfected and infected pancreatic fluid collections have been successfully drained via transhepatic, -gastric, -splenic, -jejunal, and -duodenal routes [17,18,20]. Accurate localization of a collection is critical for both diagnosis and planning an access route for aspiration and possible drainage. The principal cause for failure of both PAD and surgical drainage is the misdiagnosis of the magnitude, extent, complexity, location, and response of the abscess [7]. It is important to scan the entire abdomen, especially for pancreatic and postoperative collections [18]. When only US guidance will be used for abdominal PAD, it is prudent to obtain a CT scan prior to the procedure for more definitive diagnosis and planning an access route.

Nontarget organ and sterile cavity transgression

Transgression of the colon during PAD may cause cystocolonic or cystocolocutaneous fistulae, peritonitis, or infection of a sterile fluid collection. The colon should never be punctured, even with a small-gauge needle. If the colon is punctured with a 20-gauge or smaller needle, the patient may be given an appropriate antibiotic and observed. If the colon is transgressed with larger than a 20-gauge needle, a percutaneous colostomy using the inadvertent tract may be performed. If a catheter is placed through the colon in error, its tip is withdrawn to lie within the colon producing a catheter colostomy [21]. The colostomy catheter is left in place for 3–4 weeks to allow establishment of a mature tract. The tract should heal after the catheter is pulled if there is no distal obstruction. This sequence hopefully prevents intraperitoneal spillage of colonic contents and peritonitis.

Conversely, the small bowel is sometimes punctured intentionally, preferably with a small-gauge needle, *en route* to a deep abdominal biopsy. Usually, this occurs without ill-effect. The small bowel should not be transgressed during fluid aspiration if catheter drainage is a possibility. If small bowel is punctured with a large-gauge needle or catheter (e.g., during PAD, intraperitoneal catheter placement, percutaneous gastrostomy (PG)), a percutaneous enterostomy may be performed or the offending catheter withdrawn into the small intestine, as described above [3]. With the transvaginal approach to pelvic abscesses, a potential increased risk of bowel perforation exists because of the presence of dependent bowel loops in the pouch of Douglas [22,23]. In general, inadvertent hollow organ puncture by a large instrument is converted to an enterostomy for treatment and prevention of complications such as peritonitis.

Bowel transgression during PAD has been considered a complication; however, a recent study has brought this belief into question. The small or large bowel of 12 pigs was transgressed during intraperitoneal percutaneous catheter placement. CT follow-up and autopsy 9 days after catheter placement showed no bowel leakage, peritonitis, or abscess [2]. However, neither infected nor noninfected fluid collections were drained during the experiment.

Transgression of previously sterile cavities (e.g., pleura, peritoneum) also should be avoided when possible [7,9]. The incidence of transgression of the parietal pleura during abdominal interventions is low, but the severity of this complication can be great [24]. Transient violation of the parietal pleura with a needle during biopsy or percutaneous transhepatic cholangiography (PTC) is usually without significant risk to the patient. Transgression of the pleura with a catheter (e.g., abscess, biliary) may lead to significant complications, even death [25]. Use of an improper route during subphrenic PAD can result in pneumothorax [5], bilothorax, hemothorax, pleural effusion [3,5], or empyema [4,7,18]. The interventional radiologist should take responsibility for these complications as they usually respond to percutaneous pleural drainage. If symptomatic pneumothorax occurs, a small-bore chest tube can be placed. If pleural effusion develops, it may be monitored by periodic thoracentesis to identify possible empyema formation [24]. Empyema may also be treated percutaneously.

Methods to avoid transgressing the pleura during a totally CT-guided procedure include the triangulation method [26], although it can be complex to perform [24]. Combined imaging using a prior CT and/or US as an aid to localization and fluoroscopy for needle guidance can be used to access lesions high in the dome of the liver or in the subphrenic space. The patient is asked to inspire deeply to demonstrate full diaphragmatic excursion. The aspiration of pus confirms the diagnosis and a catheter can be placed using fluoroscopic guidance. If one is facile with US guidance using "freehand" technique [27], a needle may be placed below the tenth rib while using US to direct it cephalad into the lesion.

Surgical principles dictate that retroperitoneal abscesses (e.g., perirenal, pancreatic) are drained via a retroperitoneal approach to prevent contamination of a sterile body cavity and this principle should be adhered to whenever possible during PAD. However, sectional imaging demonstrates highly accurate access routes through the anterior abdominal wall and flanks, and realtime monitoring of guidewire and catheter placement minimizes the risk of peritoneal contamination and injury to interposed vital structures [6].

Operator hazards

Performance of an interventional radiologic procedure is fraught with potential hazards to both interventional radiologists and radiology personnel. An inadvertent needlestick or puncture injury during an interventional radiologic procedure should be considered a serious complication. Accidental infection by blood-borne viruses (e.g., human immunodeficiency virus (HIV) and hepatitis B) is a potential reality for the interventional radiologist and ancillary personnel. Simple devices have been devised to ensheath all sharp objects used during an interventional procedure [28,29]. The routine use of a protective cannister on all instrument trays has contributed to a negligible incidence of needlestick injury after thousands of interventional procedures at University of California, San Diego (UCSD). Radiation exposure during a radiologic procedure is a liability to both physician and patient. The use of US guidance whenever feasible benefits operator and patient because of the absence of ionizing radiation [27].

Diagnostic aspiration

After diagnostic imaging, a site for needle puncture is selected. The skin is marked using indelible ink or pressure from a needle hub. The skin site is prepared and draped using sterile technique. Local anesthetic is infiltrated and diagnostic aspiration is performed generally with a 22-gauge spinal or Chiba needle.

During CT-guided procedures particularly, initial needle placement is often shown to be inaccurate. To confirm that site of puncture coordinates have been transcribed to the patient accurately, we usually begin with a 1.5 in 22-gauge venipuncture needle to determine the best route. If the follow-up CT scan shows that a needle has been suboptimally placed, we leave the needle in position as a marker and guide for subsequent needle placements [17]. The tenet is:

"Bad needles make good markers" (E. vanSonnenberg, personal communication). When appropriate marker needle position is confirmed, diagnostic needle insertion follows utilizing tandem technique. Alternately, a 1.5 in 18-gauge venipuncture needle can be used followed by coaxial placement of a 22-gauge Chiba needle.

The depth of puncture is determined from imaging studies and the appropriate distance marked on the shaft of the needle with sterile tape. To avoid puncturing the backwall of a collection and possibly underlying organs, it is safest to mark the depth of puncture, regardless of guidance modality or width of access route. If fluoroscopic guidance is used, prior imaging studies are almost always available from which depth can be calculated [9]. Although realtime capability is the major advantage of US guidance, it is sometimes difficult to appreciate the needle tip [19,27]. The preprocedure US scan allows depth measurement and this should be taken advantage of and obtained. Color Doppler imaging demonstrates vascular portions of a lesion, which should be avoided, and may aid in needle tip visualization [19]. With CT guidance, the needle is sequentially advanced with serial CT scanning to confirm a safe course.

A basic principle is always to aspirate fluid (or air) to confirm proper needle or tube placement. After diagnostic needle placement, extension tubing is attached between the needle hub and syringe for added safety during aspiration. This step allows minimal disturbance of needle position during aspiration and easy needle manipulation, if required. A 60-ml syringe is utilized for suction because the larger surface area of the plunger generates more powerful suction. If fluid (or air) cannot be initially aspirated from the 22-gauge needle, the needle tip position is reassessed. It is also determined whether the needle lumen is occluded by clot or tissue fragments. Patency is most easily assured by using a needle with a stylet (e.g., spinal or Chiba) during insertion. If the needle is well positioned, unoccluded, and no fluid returns, a larger gauge needle is inserted using tandem technique. Initially, a 20-gauge needle is placed and then an 18-gauge needle, if still unsuccessful. Needles larger than 18-gauge are not generally used for diagnostic aspiration; instead, biopsy specimens may be obtained via the needles already in position.

Although it is fundamental to aspirate fluid (or air) to confirm proper needle or tube placement, occasionally, a fluid collection may be initially unaspirable yet still deserve a trial of catheter drainage. If imaging studies are convincing that a fluid collection is present, catheter placement combined with aggressive irrigation and catheter care may soften thick or inspissated material with eventual egress of material and percutaneous cure. With a nonaspirable fluid collection, easy passage of a guidewire through a drainage catheter and into the collection (i.e., protective guidewire technique, see p. 530), prior to catheter advancement, ensures safe catheter introduction [30]. Partial success of PAD should not be regarded as a failure. Percutaneous radiologic drainage may serve as a beneficial temporizing manuever permitting elective low-morbidity surgery [10,13−15,17,18,31,32]. Surgery is never precluded by PAD and the patient usually benefits, even if drainage is partially successful.

Usually, fluid is recovered using the initial 22-gage needle. If the fluid is not grossly purulent, several milliliters are sent to the laboratory for immediate Gram stain. As small a volume as possible is aspirated for diagnosis to ensure that the collection remains as large as possible [9]. If drainage is subsequently required, it is easier and safer to insert a catheter into a large collection. If the fluid appears grossly purulent, catheter drainage is performed. Inspection of aspirated fluid is not invariably indicative of infection [17] or lack of infection, however.

Gram stain of an abscess specimen typically reveals leukocytes and bacteria. A specimen from a patient receiving antibiotics may have white blood cells but no bacteria, the so-called "sterile abscess" [1]. Transenteric diagnostic needle aspiration may lead to the false-positive diagnosis of abscess or infection; traversing bowel loops may yield a false-positive Gram stain and culture or contaminate uninfected fluid collections [9,17]. Inadvertently aspirated bowel contents may resemble pus, but can usually be distinguished on Gram stain by the presence of bacteria without white blood cells. An immunosuppressed patient, who may not mount a leukocytic response, may also show this Gram stain appearance, however. CT guidance is crucial to avoid traversing adjacent bowel during interloop or deep abdominal abscess drainage [17,27,31]. Occasionally, a false-negative diagnosis of abscess after needle aspiration can result from sampling of the supernatant portion of a layered fluid collection [6,9]. The needle or diagnostic catheter may need to be directed into the dependent sediment for an accurate diagnosis.

If grossly purulent material is not aspirated and the Gram stain is negative (no organisms and no or few white blood cells), the fluid collection is evacuated as completely as possible and the diagnostic needle or catheter withdrawn. Occasionally, the exact nature of a fluid collection cannot be determined on initial diagnostic aspiration. There is generally little risk to a trial of PAD. The catheter can be removed after the etiology of the fluid collection has been determined. All percutaneous catheters and the fluid collections they drain eventually become colonized, however. Thus, it is inadvisable to leave a catheter in a noninfected, asymptomatic fluid collection longer than 24−48 hours [9], except in those cavities in which sclerosis is planned (e.g., lymphocele, hepatic cyst, renal cysts).

Most patients are already receiving antibiotics when referred for PAD. If a patient is not on antibiotics and a fluid collection is suspected or confirmed to be infected after diagnostic aspiration, broad-spectrum intravenous antibiotics are instituted. Gram-stain results may help guide the choice of antibiotics. Prophylactic antibiotics are administered prior to wire and/or catheter manipulation to minimize the consequences of possible induction of bacteremia [9]. If clinical infection is discovered or suspected during an aspiration or drainage, or at any time after a drainage procedure, overdistension of the system or cavity and manipulation are kept to a minimum [6,9,13].

Catheter choice

Poor choice of catheter usually leads to the complication of unsuccessful PAD. The most important determinant for catheter selection is the character of the aspirated fluid. Additional factors are the size of the collection and the margin of safety of the access route [1,6,13,18]. In general, the more viscous the collection, the larger the catheter bore should be. Catheters of 7−9-F are adequate for less viscous fluid collections (e.g., cysts, lymphoceles, and noninfected pseudocysts). A 12−14-F catheter provides adequate drainage for most abscesses; a 16-F catheter or larger may be necessary for evacuation of thick hematomas, advanced empyemas, or necrotic tissue from pancreatic collections [1,33]. A large-caliber (24−28-F) catheter system using Seldinger technique has been advocated for drainage of processes such as complex abscesses with loculations or debris, pancreatic abscesses, and infected hematomas.

Sump catheters allow the ingress of air so that the cavity wall does not collapse around the catheter and prevent drainage when suction is applied [9,18,34]. Sump catheters also allow application of low, continuous suction; single-lumen catheters are placed to low, intermittent suction to prevent continuous occlusion of catheter side holes from tissue encroachment.

Catheter insertion

Following diagnostic aspiration and initiation of intravenous antibiotics, a deep skin incision is made with a (#11) blade adjacent to and including the diagnostic needle. The incision includes the needle such that the blade and needle come into contact while incising. The skin incision should be wide enough easily to accept the diameter of the catheter. It is important to penetrate deeply enough so that the catheter need not be advanced with excessive force [17]. This usually requires scalpel penetration of several centimeters so that the deep fascia and even pleura or peritoneum is incised. If a safe and accurate catheter route has been chosen, there is no risk to deep penetration with a blade tandem to the diagnostic needle. This principle greatly facilitates catheter placement. Next, blunt dissection of the soft tissues is performed with a hemostat, which may also need to be buried several centimeters to ease catheter passage. Failure to adhere to the principle of adequate incision and dissection of the soft tissues may result in inability to advance the catheter, catheter buckling, and often increased patient discomfort. This potential problem is particularly relevant to transvaginal aspiration and drainage when tenting of the pliable vaginal wall may occur during needle advancement. A blade affixed to a long clamp may be required for transvaginal needle or catheter passage [22,23]. Use of a Colapinto needle over a guidewire or coaxially through a fascial dilator has been advocated to facilitate passage of catheters during transvaginal drainage procedures [35].

The two primary methods of catheter insertion are via Seldinger or trocar technique. Seldinger technique is usually performed with fluoroscopic guidance. Following initial detection and needle or wire localization in the US or CT suite, the patient is generally moved to the fluoroscopy suite. Progressive tract dilatation is performed prior to final catheter placement over a guidewire. A soft or flexible-tipped guidewire (e.g., "floppy," J-tipped) is preferred for atraumatic introduction into a fluid collection. With the Seldinger technique, there may be leakage of contaminated fluid around the guidewire between dilatations and catheter placement, possibly leading to the spread of infection.

Most catheters are designed for either trocar or Seldinger placement. At our institution, the vast majority of fluid collections and abscesses are accessed using trocar puncture guided with tandem technique. Direct catheter insertion, without the need for sequential dilatation of the soft tissues, greatly simplifies PAD. The tandem trocar technique can be done using a single modality for guidance, obviating moving the patient to the fluoroscopy suite for completion of the procedure. Use of the trocar technique eliminates unnecessary and painful soft tissue dilatation [1], and decreases the potential for leakage of contaminated fluid and spread of infection.

The standard trocar puncture method, however, may lead to back-wall perforation [3] and possible transgression of underlying organs. Improper measurement of catheter-insertion depth is usually contributory to this complication [5]. Kinking of the catheter may also follow trocar insertion. The protective guidewire technique aids in prevention of these complications and facilitates catheter positioning within a cavity [17,30]. On an appropriate guidewire (e.g., "floppy", J-tipped), sterile tape is placed at the same total length as the drainage catheter. It will then be apparent when the tip of the guidewire exits the catheter within the collection. The guidewire is then advanced (the tape is removed) and permitted to coil within the cavity. If the guidewire does not exit the catheter tip easily, the catheter is *not* advanced. It is presumed that the catheter tip is against a wall (inside or outside wall) of the cavity or that the puncture did not correctly enter the cavity. It is also possible that the puncture did not enter the cavity at all or that the catheter is indenting the outside wall of the cavity. A CT scan is obtained to determine which situation exists. If catheter manipulations fail to correct the situation, a repuncture is usually necessary. If US guidance is utilized, a properly placed guidewire can be

seen to coil within the cavity. The protective guidewire technique also prevents kinking of a redundant catheter within a cavity. Moreover, if a catheter tip is placed within a fluid collection but the contents are too viscous to be aspirated, easy passage of a guidewire ensures safe catheter introduction.

Losing access to a collection during performance of PAD is usually an avoidable complication. Lost access is likely to occur during PAD of small collections and especially during transvaginal drainage. Lost access is prevented by use of a "safety" wire [36,37]. An access set (e.g., Cook, Meditech) is initially placed followed by insertion of both a "working" wire (e.g., 0.038 in) for catheter placement and a "safety" wire (e.g., 0.018 in), which is left in the cavity to preserve access. The safety wire is not removed until the conclusion of the procedure. A safety catheter (4–6-F) can also be placed. If access to a collection or cavity is lost, a soft-tip guidewire can be used to probe the tract in conjunction with a small dilator to opacify the tract [38]. A fresh tract is often impossible to renegotiate and a new puncture is usually required. Occasionally, a catheter may be defective such that the inner cannula may not be removable or the catheter may have a hole in it that is discovered after placement. This situation can be remedied using a guidewire for catheter exchange. If a safety wire is present in tandem, a new catheter can be placed following exchange for a stiffer working wire.

Immediate postdrainage management

Immediate, gentle irrigation of the abscess cavity with copious amounts of sterile saline is important and is performed after complete evacuation of all obtainable purulent material. This principle minimizes the chances of bacteremia and endotoxemia [6,9,13]. Irrigant volumes of 25–50% of the volume evacuated from the cavity are used. Irrigation with sterile saline is executed until the fluid is clear; this might require several hundred milliliters in small aliquots. Aspiration should be slow and deliberate. Overvigorous aspiration of a freshly drained abscess may result in bloody effluent, indicating irritation of the friable and vascular abscess wall. Although significant vessel damage and hemorrhage is rare, this minor complication is avoidable.

The volumes of both irrigant and aspirate are carefully noted to prevent overdistension of the cavity. Occasionally, a portion or all of the irrigation fluid cannot be aspirated. Volumes of both irrigant and aspirate can be easily monitored using extension tubing, a three-way stopcock, and two large (e.g., 60 ml) syringes; volumes of irrigant fluid and aspirate fluid should be nearly equal. If the volume aspirated becomes significantly less than the volume instilled, irrigation should be discontinued to prevent overdistension of the cavity. The catheter may need to be repositioned within the cavity, sometimes with the aid of fluoroscopic guidance.

After initial catheter aspiration or catheter irrigation, the area of the fluid collection is reimaged with either CT or US to ascertain collapse of the cavity and the absence of residual collections. Abscesses that are complicated, extensive, or contain thick fluid frequently require multiple and large (14–28-F) catheters for adequate drainage and cure [33]. Use of multiple and/or large catheters should be considered essential for success in these types of cases. Multiple and large drains are frequently placed during surgical treatment of abscesses; the same principles apply to percutaneous drain placement. After initial placement, indwelling PAD catheters can be exchanged and upsized at any time. Failure to recognize and respond to loculation or septations is one of the most common causes of abdominal PAD failure [7]. Contrast diffusion study at initial PAD has been advocated to identify compartmentalization [7]. However, the decision to place an additional catheter(s) into an undrained or loculated fluid collection should be tempered by the character of the fluid, the size of the collection, and the clinical status of the patient.

Immediate postprocedure imaging demonstrates the adequacy of PAD, including the presence of undrained locules, catheter position and the need for catheter manipulation, and the need for additional catheters [15]. Multiple catheters are indicated when post-PAD imaging demonstrates a persistent collection of undrained locules [3,7,10,17,18]. A catheter is required in each of multiple noncommunicating collections seen on diagnostic imaging, tempered by the clinical status of the patient. The surgical adage is, "drainage of the first abscess makes the patient feel better; drainage of the last abscess cures the patient." Inadequate drainage can also result from a malpositioned catheter [3,5,11,18].

A nondependent catheter position may contribute to poor drainage [7,9]. The surgical tenet of dependent drainage should be followed whenever possible [9]. However, PAD may be performed effectively from nondependent routes because imaging guidance allows manipulation of the catheter and optimal placement within the cavity. Placement of drainage catheters to suction also diminishes the importance of dependent drainage. Moreover, the patient can be turned, positioned, and maneuvered to maximize drainage.

Immediate postdrainage sinography has been advocated to optimize catheter positioning and to aid in identification of communications and fistulas [10,12]. For successful treatment, multiple fistulae require multiple catheters to drain all fistulous tracts [11]. Routine post-PAD imaging will help to avert the complications of poor or inadequate drainage.

There is a variety of methods for catheter fixation. The catheter should be well secured to the skin despite the use of locking catheters. Satisfactory catheter fixation can be accomplished without the need for suturing to the skin. Our preference is the Percufix kit from Meditech (Boston Scientific Corporation, 480 Pleasant Street, Watertown, MA 02172, USA). Decline in the use of suture fixation to the skin has paralleled a decrease in incidence of pericatheter infection. In addition, a generous adhesive tape "mesentery" is fashioned by first taping around the catheter and then onto the skin to absorb unwanted traction [1]. Our preference is to use silk tape which has superior adhesive properties. Whenever possible, catheters are secured *horizontally*, across the patient's body, to prevent kinking from the patient bending at the waist.

Complications during catheter management

Although catheter placement requires skill and experience, it is catheter management that frequently determines percutaneous drainage cure or failure. Patient visitation by the interventional radiologist, catheter irrigation and manipulation, and repeat radiologic evaluations are critical to achieve high rates of success from PAD. Poor catheter management unquestionably will contribute to the complication of failed PAD.

Infection

The possibility of infecting a noninfected fluid collection is a concern whenever the Gram stain is negative and the aspirated fluid is not grossly purulent. As noted above, a trial of drainage for 24–48 hours pending culture results is not contraindicated. The possibility of infecting a noninfected fluid collection is theoretically increased with transvaginal and -rectal drainage procedures because sterilization of the operative field is virtually impossible. Furthermore, the catheter maintains a communication with these nonsterile body lumena. The incidence of colonization increases with the time a catheter is indwelling. Despite the high likelihood of ultimate colonization of a catheter and the drained fluid collection, infection is unlikely if adequate drainage is established and maintained; an immunocompromised patient being a possible exception [5,6,39]. Meticulous catheter care to assure catheter patency is essential to prevention of secondary infection.

Irrigation of the catheter with sterile saline is performed every 4–12 hours depending on the viscosity of the fluid collection. Irrigant volumes are correlated with the decompressed cavity size; 10–20 ml sterile saline every 8 hours is typical. The irrigation interval is gradually lengthened and the irrigant volume is decreased as the cavity shrinks. A nurse or a family member (if managed as an outpatient) may perform irrigation following strict sterile technique. Irrigant fluid is deposited directly into the body and adherence to sterile procedures is mandatory to reduce the chance of secondary infection. A three-way stopcock placed between catheter hub and suction tubing (or drainage bag) helps to assure sterility because the catheter system is then accessed for irrigation only via the side port. The side port of the stopcock (or catheter hub) is cleansed with alcohol prior to syringe attachment. Adequacy of suction can easily be checked by closing the port to the patient and opening the side port; adequate suction produces an audible hissing sound. Performing this step prior to irrigation also clears the drainage tubing of debris or potentially coagulating fluid.

Catheter dislodgment, obstruction, and removal

Catheter dislodgment is a common complication during the course of percutaneous therapy [3,14]. Replacement of a dislodged or prematurely withdrawn tube is an emergency because the tract closes as a function of time. The tract must be probed and a tractogram performed quickly to increase the chances for successful reentry of the cavity [38]. If undue delay occurs, the entire catheter placement procedure may need to be repeated.

At least once daily irrigation and catheter check by the interventional radiologist is required to confirm catheter patency and to detect real or potential catheter problems. The catheter is evaluated for kinking and impending obstruction. Kinking is often associated with an improperly secured catheter and also occurs when the patient lays (often unavoidably) on the catheter. Tape adhesiveness decreases over time; the catheter(s) is resecured if necessary.

An obstructed tube is heralded by increased resistance during irrigation or sinography, decreased output, pericatheter leakage, or infection. Obstruction and pericatheter leakage may be caused by thick fluid and/or debris, or by the presence of side holes outside the cavity. A catheter may merely require repositioning within the cavity to reestablish patency; catheter side holes should be positioned within the cavity [9]. Pericatheter leakage of pus may also be a normal occurrence. Aggressive irrigation may unocclude a blocked catheter, but catheter exchange may be necessary.

Several transcatheter and pericatheter maneuvers have been described to achieve exchange of an occluded catheter [40]. Transcatheter methods are easiest to perform and should be attempted initially. They include probing with a small-dimension guidewire or the stiff end of a guidewire. If the catheter end hole is blocked, a curved-tip guidewire will frequently exit the side hole of a multiple-hole catheter. The stiff end of a very stiff guidewire may be used to perforate a curved-tip catheter. Extreme caution must be exercised to avoid perforating an underlying organ or viscus. Once a guidewire exits a side hole or a newly created side hole, the catheter is removed and replaced. Pericatheter methods include entering the tract of an occluded catheter in tandem with a guidewire or a guidewire inserted through a small dilator. Soft-tipped guidewires are preferred (e.g., 15-mm J, Bentson (Cook Inc., Bloomington IN), Glidewire (Teruno Corporation, Tokyo, Japan)). A tractogram performed through a dilator aids in depicting the appropriate route. Alternately, the hub of an occluded catheter is cut off, followed by outer coaxial placement of a sheath. The occluded catheter is removed and a new catheter replaced over a guidewire which has been introduced into the tract through the sheath. The tandem guidewire–dilator approach is preferred for more mature tracts; the sheath method is useful for occlusions of recently placed catheters. Occasionally, a catheter cannot easily be withdrawn. Not uncommonly, the suture within a Cope locking catheter will not release tension on the catheter pigtail because of hardened secretions within the catheter lumen. The catheter hub can be cut off, one end of the suture secured with a hemostat (to prevent loss of suture within the tract), and the catheter is usually easily removed. A guidewire may also be advanced to help break up concretions, while using a hemostat to secure one end of the suture to prevent suture occlusion of the catheter lumen. If further difficulty is encountered, the catheter can be removed coaxially through a sheath under fluoroscopic guidance.

Premature catheter withdrawal is a common and avoidable complication of PAD [6–7,18]. It was the most common technical error in a series of 136 abdominal PAD patients [7]. Criteria for removal of the PAD catheter include parameters that are clinical (defervescence, normal leukocyte count, decreased pain, resumption of appetite), catheter related (minimal — <10 ml/day — or no drainage, clearing of debris, resistance to injection, and/or pericatheter leakage of small amounts of saline), and radiologic (diminished cavity size, no evidence of loculation or multiple collections, closure of communication depicted on prior sinogram) [1]. Gradual or sequential catheter withdrawal, a surgical tenet, has been recommended but has no proved benefit at this time over abrupt catheter withdrawal [9,12,18,29].

The above criteria must be modified in certain circumstances by several caveats. In patients with known necrotic tumor, neither catheter output (usually low) nor catheter injection to visualize the size of the abscess (usually small) are necessarily good indicators of when to remove the catheter [14]. It is prudent to leave the catheter in place until surgery, or indefinitely for palliation. It is important to note that some PAD patients respond clinically, despite little or even no catheter output.

An abscess cavity may shrink and heal in several days, but an associated fistula often takes much longer to close. The cavity may decrease in size, but catheter output usually remains high with an associated fistula. It is critical to monitor catheter output in this scenario. Monitoring cavity size alone with CT or US in this situation could result in failure of PAD [11]. Obliteration of the abscess cavity should not be the sole criterion for catheter removal. Serial sinography may demonstrate resolution of the cavity and a persistent communication. Alternately, in place of sinography, the catheter(s) could be clamped for several days prior to removal and the patient studied with CT or US to detect any evidence of fluid reaccumulation [5,18]. The catheter should not be pulled until the communication of fistula closes.

Conversely, the misconception, usually by the clinical service, that cessation of drainage means complete obliteration of the abscess cavity may initiate the unwarranted removal of the PAD catheter. Routine use of follow-up CT has been advocated to identify loculation or residual abscess cavities which, unrecognized, might lead to failed PAD [7]. Any patient who is not responding to catheter drainage should be reimaged. If the post-PAD patient is improved and doing well clinically, however, routine follow-up imaging is probably unnecessary.

If at any time during percutaneous therapy uncertainty or confusion develops regarding catheter status or the patient's clinical condition is not improving, the patient and catheter are reimaged, usually by CT, sinography, or both [7,18,32]. The catheter(s) may need repositioning or undrained fluid collections may be discovered. Catheter irrigation and volume of drainage assessment by a single person (e.g., interventional radiologist) will almost always resolve confusing catheter output data.

Poor catheter output

Initially, the more common causes of poor catheter output should be excluded. The entire catheter drainage apparatus is meticulously examined to exclude possibilities such as kinking, blockage by debris, closed stopcock, or malfunctioning suction device. Patency is assessed by aspiration, forward flush of sterile saline, and reaspiration. The catheter dressing should be removed entirely and the catheter exit site examined.

A collection may be unaspirable or contain very thick, pasty, or tenacious fluid. In this situation, small volumes of irrigant (2–5 ml) may be instilled frequently (e.g., 3–4 hours), and the catheter(s) left to gravity drainage; suction or aspiration is usually futile. This regimen may succeed over several days in dissolving these initially undrainable collections. The catheter(s) may be placed to suction following liquefaction of the fluid collection.

Various proteolytic, mucolytic, and thrombolytic agents have been used to promote liquefaction and removal of viscous pus, debris, and hematoma [6–8,41–43]. Conscientious and meticulous irrigation with sterile saline is usually sufficient. Acetylcysteine and urokinase are the most commonly used mucolytic and thrombolytic agents, respectively. An *in vitro* study showed that urokinase decreased the viscosity of purulent material and increased drainage flow rates for all catheter sizes, suggesting that intracavitary urokinase may be useful if catheter drainage is inadequate [43]. Proteolytic enzymes (e.g., hyaluronidase) are potentially hazardous since their destructive effect on connective tissues of the abscess pseudocapsule may lead to the spreading of pus and toxic products [8].

Crude but effective debridement of large pieces of necrotic tissue and debris can be accomplished through a sheath using a Malecot catheter. Under fluoroscopic guidance and following contrast opacification of the cavity, the tip of the catheter is placed in the cavity and constant suction is applied to trap and retain fragments in the wings of the Malecot catheter. The catheter is then slowly removed through the sheath.

Recurrent or persistent collections

Recurrence or persistence of a collection suggests the presence of infection, neoplasm, or a communication (e.g., enteric, biliary, pancreatic, lymphatic, or urinary) [1,3,5,7–9,13,14]. During the course of percutaneous therapy, ongoing infection, reinfection of a fluid collection, or infection of an initially noninfected fluid collection may result in reaccumulation and recurrence. Maintenance of catheter patency, adherence to sterile technique during irrigation, and appropriate antibiotics should limit the occurrence of this complication.

Clues that a collection that has been drained is an undiagnosed neoplasm include nodularity within the cavity seen on imaging, failure of the cavity to diminish in size, hemorrhagic fluid output, persistent drainage, and recurrence. The interventional radiologist must determine that a cystic collection (e.g., pancreas) or a presumed enteric abscess are not cystic or necrotic neoplasms. If cancer is suspected, fluid is sent for cytologic analysis and biopsy of the wall of the abscess or collection is obtained. Biopsy alone does not rule out tumor; however, in a series of 16 patients who underwent PAD of *known* infected abdominal tumors, in no case ($n = 8$) did needle biopsy retrieve material positive for tumor; all eight cases showed only necrotic tissue [14].

Most commonly, a persistent or recurrent abscess or fluid collection is associated with a leak, communication, or fistula. Fistulous communications with abdominal abscesses are common, occurring in 44% of a series of 72 patients [12]. In another series of 38 infected pancreatic fluid collections, enteric fistulae were identified in 14 patients and pancreatic duct fistulae in nine patients [18]. Failure to recognize and/or adequately treat an abscess–fistula complex is a common cause of unsuccessful PAD.

A sudden increase in fluid drainage and/or change in fluid character should raise the suspicion of fistula or sometimes neoplasm [6,7,13]. Evaluation of fluid chemistries (e.g., bilirubin, amylase, urea, fat globules) and cytology might be of use. Immediate post-PAD sinography rarely demonstrates a communication [11–13,18]; however, this early step may help to determine optimal, dependent catheter position within a cavity. Some have speculated that the site of communication may be initially clogged with debris or obstructed by inflammation and edema, becoming detectable by retrograde contrast injection only after several days of drainage [11]. Most fistulae are demonstrated by delayed sinography several days to over 1 week post-PAD [11–13,18]. When a fistula is suspected and routine sinography is negative, some believe that the cavity and its recesses should be gently probed with a curved catheter and guidewire, combined with catheter injection of contrast material, to identify occult fistulae [12,13].

The diagnosis of *fistulous communication* following PAD is important for a number of reasons. First, it may suggest the underlying etiology of the abscess (e.g., enteric, biliary, pancreatic, lymphatic, or urinary communication). Second, the diagnosis of a fistula forewarns the radiologist and referring physician that drainage may be voluminous and protracted. Despite the presence of a fistula, eventual successful PAD usually can be expected [1,3,5,7–9,13,15,16,31,32]. Once a fistula is identified, the treatment course is prolonged and premature resignation to failure should be avoided. In one series, the mean duration of drainage was greater than 6 weeks, and up to 12 weeks if there was pancreatic involvement [13]. Communicating abscesses require greater attention to detail and closer patient monitoring to achieve cure [13]. Fistulous communications to the small bowel may require longer to drain than those to the colon, perhaps reflecting high- versus low-output status [3]. High-output fistulae are defined as having output greater than 200 ml in a 24-hour period and are easily recognized clinically. Low-output fistulae (< 200 ml/day) generally require sinography for identification [12]. Third, nasogastric suction to control secretions and hyperalimentation or distal enteral feeding have been advocated and may be indicated to allow fistula healing and closure [12]. In cases of biliary or urinary communication, biliary or urinary diversion with additional catheters may be necessary. Decreasing the volume of fistula drainage via antegrade drainage or diversion of secretions or fluid proximal to the fistula may be necessary for cure. For example, with enteric communication proximal or just distal to the ligament of Treitz, a nasojejunal tube or percutaneously, endoscopically, or surgically placed gastrojejunostomy/jejunostomy tube can control proximal intestinal contents to the communicating tract and achieve preferred enteral feeding distally. The potential for reflux into the tract should be assessed radiographically [13]. With distal small bowel and colonic perforations, hyperalimentation may be the only option. Finally, some believe that fistula detection requires repositioning the catheter tip adjacent to the fistula orifice and, optimally, the placement of an additional catheter through the fistulous tract to divert secretions; the PAD catheter tip is placed as close to the fistula orifice as possible, or cannulation of the fistulous tract achieved with an additional catheter to control and divert secretions [11,13]. A single catheter may be sufficient if the side holes are carefully positioned both to drain the abscess and suction the leak [11]. Overirrigation or -suction of the PAD catheter may maintain patency of a communicating tract and should be avoided.

Chronically diseased or inflamed bowel usually needs surgical resection for eventual cure [3,10,11,13,14] — presurgical PAD is almost always indicated and beneficial, however [10,13–15,17,18,31,32]. Essential modifications of simple PAD for effective treatment of a communicating abscess include a longer therapeutic trial, close attention to catheter drainage output, control of intestinal contents and peristalsis, ensuring that the patient receives nothing by mouth, nutritional supplementation, and monitoring of metabolic status [13].

Gastrostomy/gastroenterostomy

Introduction

Nutritional support is the most common indication for enteral feeding, usually because of esophageal disease. Neurologic deficits cause impaired swallowing, leading to aspiration risk. Abnormal peristalsis is associated with cerebrovascular accidents, anoxic brain injury, trauma, and neurosurgery. Severe aspiration of any etiology is an important indication for gastroenterostomy. Patients with primary, secondary, and recurrent head and neck neoplasms, and malignant esophageal obstruction may require nutritional support. Small bowel diseases like scleroderma, Crohn's disease, short-gut syndrome, and radiation enteritis may cause impaired intestinal absorption requiring nutritional support. Uncommonly, enteral nutritional support is used to manage anorexia nervosa, severe depression, and widespread metastatic disease.

Decompression of the stomach or small bowel is another indication for percutaneous gastrostomy/gastroenterostomy (PG/PGE). Patients with chronic small bowel obstruction from peritoneal carcinomatosis, usually of ovarian or gastric origin, may benefit from PG/PGE, obviating the discomfort and risk of long-term nasogastric tube placement and suction. Other uses for PG/PGE include retrograde stoma dilatation, simultaneous gastric suction and enteral feeding, and as a conduit for internal biliary drainage [44].

Gastrostomy and percutaneous gastrojejunostomy are well-established interventional radiologic procedures [44–50].

Contraindications

Contraindications include colonic or hepatic interposition and postoperative changes. PG/PGE is difficult or impossible after partial gastrectomy. However, almost all patients are amenable to PG when CT is utilized for guidance [51]. Coagulopathy is a relative contraindication and should be corrected prior to the procedure. Caution should be exercised in those patients with portal hypertension and gastric varices. The procedure may be performed successfully, even in the presence of marked ascites by utilizing the gastropexy technique after high-volume paracentesis. Additional relative contraindications include overlying paraphernalia on the abdomen, severe skin infection or burns, massive colonic dilatation (Ogilvie syndrome), large bowel obstruction, or flexion contracture whereby the patient's arm is the impediment.

Preprocedural technique

As with most interventional procedures, a variety of methods is workable for PG and PGE. The patient is given nothing by mouth 8–12 hours prior to the procedure with the exception of any orally administered drugs which may be taken with sips of water. A nasogastric tube is inserted and placed to low, continuous suction — the day before the procedure whenever possible — to aspirate gastric contents, to help minimize peritoneal spillage during the procedure, and to decrease gas in the small and large bowel [48,52]. The day before the procedure, the colon may be opacified by injecting a small amount of barium through the nasogastric tube before suction is applied or barium by mouth may be given. During the procedure, nasogastric tube position is important. Too distal positioning allows air to escape antegrade through the pylorus; too proximal and retrograde air leakage into the esophagus occurs [53,54]. Balloon occlusion of the gastro-esophageal junction or efferent loop in Billroth II surgery has been used to counter these problems [54]. To prevent explosive inflation, a pressure bulb may be utilized on the nasogastric tube instead of piped air [55]. The stomach should be well distended [46,53,56], especially if gastropexy is not planned. An air insufflation volume of 500 ml is advisable, and up to 1 l of air is optimal [53]. Although not essential, glucagon (1 mg) may be used prior to gastric insufflation to induce gastroparesis and decrease peristalsis [46,49,53,55].

If a nasogastric tube cannot be passed, an appropriate small catheter may be negotiated through the narrowed esophagus using conventional catheter and guidewire techniques (e.g., 5-F catheter with a 0.035 in Bentson wire) [52,57,58]. Effervescent granules may help to distend the stomach when a nasogastric tube cannot be positioned [46]. Under fluoroscopic or CT guidance, the stomach may be entered directly with a removable hub needle-set, through which air is instilled [59,60]. It is important to instill contrast medium through the needle prior to insufflation to prevent air embolism [51,53]. For esophageal obstruction, CT guidance may be used for PG alone, but PGE requires moving the patient to fluoroscopy [50,51,61]. Gastric insufflation with air is adequate in most cases, and balloon-assisted techniques for PG are not routinely necessary [54]. US may be used to puncture a fluid-filled (e.g., water) stomach or intragastric balloon. Thus, US guidance may be used for bedside placement of PG/PGE, although this is not commonly done.

Nontarget organ transgression

Catheter transgression of liver or colon should be avoided during PG/PGE. The colon can be identified with fluoroscopy with or without rectal contrast. C-arm fluoroscopy helps adequately to localize the colon and allows depth measurement [59]. Also, C-arm fluoroscopy allows identification of the anterior border of the inflated stomach lying close to the anterior abdominal wall, thus excluding interposition of the left lobe of the liver or transverse colon [58,61,62]. A cross-table lateral view of the stomach can also be obtained to evaluate bowel and liver interposition as well as distance from skin puncture site to the gastric wall.

US examination of the left upper quadrant shows the left lobe of the liver or a low-lying liver and allows depth measurement. In addition, US helps to avoid overlying vessels [53]. The superior epigastric artery lies at the junction of the medial two-thirds and lateral one-third of the rectus muscle. US is especially important if the patient has portal hypertension and upper abdominal varices. In patients with abdominal neoplasm, CT is valuable to avoid puncture through overlying or adjacent tumor [50].

If the colon is inadvertently punctured, a catheter colostomy should be performed as discussed under complications of PAD. If the liver is included in the gastrostomy tract, this is usually uneventful, particularly if only the periphery of the liver has been punctured. Transhepatic PAD is usually well tolerated.

Catheter insertion and catheter choice

Most PGs are performed with Seldinger technique [44]. The trocar method eliminates serial dilatation and has been advocated with the intragastric balloon support technique. Trocar technique is probably easier and safer if percutaneous gastropexy has been performed.

The incidence of hemorrhage may be kept to a minimum during PG by selecting a puncture site away from the curvatures of the stomach [47]. Initial puncture is made in an antegrade downhill fashion to facilitate duodenal cannulation [50]; however, needle entry should be as perpendicular to the stomach as possible (not tangential to the stomach) to avoid buckling out into the peritoneal cavity [46,62]. Unfavorable position and orientation of the transcutaneous tract may lead to difficult pyloric cannulation and even preclude jejunal intubation. Recoil of a successfully placed jejunal catheter back into the stomach may also occur [63].

Catheter and guidewire techniques

A stiff sheath or dilator, or a catheter over a metal cannula, aid in negotiating the pylorus. A rigid peelaway sheath helps to transmit axial forces more effectively to aid catheter movement, especially if jejunal cannulation is planned [57]. Placement of a cannula at the pylorus prevents buckling of the catheter in the stomach during advancement into the jejunum [61].

As discussed under complications of PAD, deep soft tissue dissection is important [59]. The entry needle and fascial dilators should be sharp, not blunt, to prevent the anterior stomach wall from backing away [53]. A rotatory movement of dilators during insertion prevents the gastric wall being pushed away from the dilator tip. A straight push of the dilator may displace the stomach back along the wire and result in loss of wire position [52,58]. This is less of a problem if gastropexy is performed. Resistance to puncture may be encountered due to firm fibrous tissue from prior upper abdominal surgery.

After each needle or catheter placement into the stomach, air is aspirated to confirm intraluminal position [51,64]. One may encounter resistance to passage through the stomach if a small-gauge needle (e.g., 22-gauge) is utilized [46]. Interestingly, it has been suggested that a rapidly performed procedure may decrease peritoneal irritation with consequent decreased likelihood of apposition of the stomach and anterior abdominal walls [46].

Many different types of catheters are used for PG and PGE [44,49,52,56,57,61]. Locking pigtail catheters are popular and large-bore Malecot catheters are also used. Hicks *et al.* [56] concluded that Foley catheters lead to more complications requiring surgery and more tube changes within 30 days of placement. Erosion of the gastric mucosa is a recognized complication of endoscopic gastrostomy, felt to be caused by the internal bumper-retaining device producing pressure necrosis [65,66]. A Foley balloon catheter may similarly cause pressure necrosis over time. For this reason, the loop of a Cope catheter or wings of a Malecot catheter should not be retracted tightly up against the gastric wall at the completion of the procedure. Likewise, extreme tension on T-fastener sutures is not indicated. Excessive traction on a gastrostomy tube may be related to gastric mucosal and/or skin erosion [66]. An increased wound infection rate has been noted with the use of endoscopically placed latex catheters [65].

Contrast examination through the tube is performed to confirm satisfactory catheter position. Catheter side holes should not be positioned within the percutaneous tract. Rotating a gastrostomy catheter after formation of the loop during fluoroscopic observation ensures that the catheter is intraluminal and not intraperitoneal or partially formed in the wall of the stomach [56].

Procedural technique modifications

Intragastric balloon support techniques have been advocated to reduce the compliance of the anterior gastric wall, which tends to retract from the puncturing needle, dilator, or advancing catheter [44,54,68]. The balloon-induced rigidity of the gastric wall facilitates trocar insertion, obviating the need for dilator and catheter exchanges. It is especially useful and usually reserved for special situations such as PG in patients with partial gastrectomy [54]. Intraenteral balloons have also been used for direct percutaneous jejunostomy [69]. Intragastric balloon techniques are not routinely used, however, because of the relative difficulty of fashioning and introducing the balloon [44]. Reported complications include premature balloon rupture and retrograde balloon migration into the fundus [59]. Migration can be corrected by further inflation in the body of the stomach.

The need for gastropexy is controversial and its routine use is a matter of preference. Many PGs are performed without gastropexy [44]. Several studies have shown that lack of anchoring and apposition of the serosa of the stomach to the parietal peritoneum are not related to intraperitoneal spillage [44,47−49]. The muscular coat of the stomach is self-sealing and probably allows for multiple punctures without leakage [48,56,58]. Ten to 12-F punctures through the stomach have closed without incident [44,58]. Gastropexy may produce its own complications such as tube angulation, gastric wall tension, and interference with peristalsis and emptying [52]. A possible shortcoming of gastropexy is that multiple needle punctures theoretically increase the risk of hemorrhage, but this is not borne out in multiple studies [55,64,70,71].

Proponents of gastropexy claim that lack of wall fixation increases the incidence of looping of catheters and guidewires within the peritoneum and loss of access [53,55,57,70], leakage of gastric contents [55,69,70], and delayed catheter dislodgment [55]. Loss of access without gastropexy can be prevented by adequate gastric insufflation and insertion of sufficient length of guidewire for adequate catheter support [52]. Although quite low with either technique, the reported minor and major complication rates are less in series of PG with gastropexy [55,64,71]. The tract is usually shorter following gastropexy and this may facilitate catheter manipulation and intubation of the duodenum [71]. Similarly, if access is lost, reentry of a shorter tract is usually less complicated.

Gastric versus jejunal placement of the catheter is also controversial. Small bowel position may be preferred for several reasons. Alimentation can be initiated sooner because the infusion site is far removed from the gastric puncture site so there is less risk of a gastric leak. There is an extra measure of anchoring safety with a more distally seated catheter [57,59]. Gastroenterostomy reduces the risk of aspiration and feedings can be performed during periods of ileus [58,59,67]. Little gastric reflux occurs when tube tip placement is distal to the ligament of Trietz; however, gastric reflux increases significantly if the catheter tip is at or proximal to the ligament of Trietz [72]. In patients with gastroparesis and a gastroenterostomy, enteral feedings may proceed with simultaneous low, intermittent wall suction through a gastrostomy port.

Complications during catheter management

When PG is performed with CT guidance, routine postprocedure scanning is not necessary. Usually, no postprocedure radiography is performed prior to feedings [64]. Follow-up plain radiographs may be useful to ascertain proper catheter position; a ruptured Foley balloon catheter has been identified [59].

The nasogastric tube may be removed immediately [55,64], or gastric suction can be maintained overnight through the nasogastric tube or the newly placed PG catheter [57,59,73]. The PG/PGE catheter is usually left to gravity overnight except for drugs which may be given through the tube [64]. Generally, feedings are delayed for 24 hours after the procedure. Prolonged ileus delayed tube feeding for 48 hours in only one out of 327 endoscopically placed gastrostomies [67]. A moderate rise in body temperature for 24–48 hours after the procedure is not uncommon [52].

There is a 98–100% success rate for PG with a low incidence of complications [44]. The overall procedure-related mortality involving 635 patients from four series, each with more than 100 patients, was 1% [44,52,56,64,74]. *Respiratory arrest* has been reported in a patient with emphysema felt to be related to gastric inflation causing restriction of diaphragmatic excursion [49], and in a sedated patient during difficult passage of a nasogastric tube [59]. *Retroperitoneal perforation*, at the duodenojejunal flexure [47] and involving the duodenum [57], has been reported without sequelae.

Peritonitis is an uncommon complication (1–2%) which usually results from leakage of gastric contents or from inadvertent infusion of enteral nutrients into the peritoneum [44,47,58,70,71]. This complication appears unrelated to the performance of gastropexy [52,56,64,74]. Intravenous antibiotics may be all that is necessary for treatment. Peritonitis requiring laparotomy is unusual (1%) [44]. Abdominal pain without evidence of infection or peritonitis occurred 3% of the time in the combined series noted above.

Hemorrhage requiring transfusion is uncommon (1%) and may be related to coagulopathy, vessel perforation, or gastritis [44]. Delayed bleeding raises the possibility of catheter erosion of an adjacent vessel or concomitant administration of an intravenous nonsteroidal antiinflammatory drug (e.g., Toradol), which may sometimes be given to relieve the pain of terminal cancer. Conservative measures including blood transfusion are usually adequate; surgical treatment is the exception [44,46,47]. Direct pressure, catheter/sheath/balloon tamponade of the tract, and/or angiography with embolization may also be useful. Pressure tamponade with a Foley balloon catheter within the stomach may be particularly helpful [47].

Infection

The use of prophylactic antibiotics is controversial with the PG method, however, their use is probably more important with the endoscopic method where the tube is passed through the contaminated oropharynx, into the stomach, and across the abdominal wound [50,64]. The endoscopic literature suggests that there is a decreased incidence of wound infection (e.g., necrotizing fasciitis) when a large gastrostomy incision is made [67,75]. The rationale, a surgical tenet, is that potentially contaminated fluid is less likely to accumulate under the skin if a generous incision is made.

Infection of the percutaneous tract is uncommon (1%) and is usually associated with peristomal leakage. Superficial pericatheter wound infection usually responds to local wound care (keeping the wound dry and application of an antiseptic) and sometimes antibiotics are used [44,47,49,57]. An iodophor ointment is preferred because fungal overgrowth is possible with antibiotic ointment alone. Leakage may be controlled with nasogastric or gastrostomy suction and/or replacement of the catheter with one of a size large enough to occlude the tract [76]. Skin irritation and chemical burns may occur due to leakage of gastric contents along the tube tract [59]. Placement of progressively larger tubes and ostomy appliances can be used to manage persistent leaks [52,77].

Necrotizing fasciitis has been described complicating endoscopic gastrostomies [75,78]. Fasciitis occurs typically 3–14 days postprocedure and radiographs are indicated to detect associated soft tissue gas [78]. Large incisions have been advocated to reduce the chances of this often fatal complication [67,75]. Subcutaneous air or intramural air are not normal findings postgastrostomy and should raise suspicion of mechanical problems with tube placement [73,76] if associated infection (e.g., fasciitis) has been ruled out. Treatment is by catheter repositioning and use of external fixation.

Postprocedure imaging

An understanding of normal postprocedural imaging findings should prevent inappropriate interventions [53,59,73]. Pneumoperitoneum detected by CT was found in more than 50% of a series of 18 post-PG patients [73]. The mean volume of intraperitoneal air was 40 ml. Benign and usually clinically inapparent abdominal wall (33%) and gastric wall (17%) hematomas were also described in this series. Pneumoperitoneum in association with subcutaneous emphysema has been described in a PG patient on a ventilator. Ventilator-induced gastric distension may have been contributory in this patient who died 48 hours after the procedure [46]. Pneumoperitoneum should only be of concern if associated with other symptoms or is increasing in volume [73]. *Subcutaneous air* is not normal and may alert one to a malpositioned catheter or necrotizing fasciitis. Finally, loculated or free *intraperitoneal fluid* are not normally seen post-PG and may suggest hemorrhage and/or abscess.

Catheter obstruction and dislodgment

A PG tube is susceptible to blockage and clogging [44,46,64] and it must be irrigated after each feeding [52]. A PG/PGE catheter usually remains patent for an average of 3−4 months with a range of 1−6 months. A catheter may kink or fracture requiring replacement [51,64]. If occluded, catheter exchange may be facilitated with various transcatheter and pericatheter manuevers as discussed above [40].

Catheter dislodgment is the most common potential complication of PG/PGE [44−47,52,58,59,64]. The PG tract is usually mature within 7 days [53,62] and external fixation is kept intact for at least 7−14 days in order to allow the PG tract to mature [76]. If catheter dislodgment does occur, the percutaneous tract is usually mature enough simply to withdraw the catheter and recannulate the tract [58,61]. Partial catheter dislodgment resulted in a case of subcutaneous emphysema associated with a cutaneous chemical burn from leakage of gastric acid [76]. Artificial ventilation may contribute to excessive movement between stomach and abdominal wall potentially resulting in dislodgment of a PG tube [58]. Catheter migration into the duodenum from peristaltic waves may also occur. Migration of a Foley catheter in this manner has caused duodenal obstruction [55,64]. Migration of self-retaining pigtail catheters also occurs [49] and may be corrected by simply withdrawing the catheter under fluoroscopic guidance. Occasionally, a patient may complain of vague abdominal pain which may be attributable to a migrated but nonobstructing PG catheter. The catheter may be marked or flagged with adhesive tape as an indicator of baseline position, thus allowing assessment of potential catheter migration.

Cholecystostomy

Introduction

Gall-bladder puncture and percutaneous cholecystostomy (PC) are commonly performed to diagnose and treat various gall bladder and bile duct disorders. Indications include diagnostic aspiration of bile, diagnostic transcholecystic cholangiography, drainage of acute calculous and acalculous cholecystitis, drainage of hydrops and empyema, drainage for obstructive jaundice or gall-bladder perforation, cholecystolithotomy, gall-bladder biopsy, gallstone dissolution, and gall-bladder ablation. The success rate of PC catheter placement for various indications in published series exceeds 95%, whether for elective or emergency indications; however, clinical benefit to the patient of establishing this access

to the gall bladder will vary, depending on the indication for PC [79−81]. In a series of 127 patients, diagnostic gall-bladder puncture or PC was successful in 125 patients, with a 98.4% success rate. Major and minor complication rates were 8.7% and 3.9%, respectively, with a 30-day mortality rate of 3.1% [82].

Contraindications

Relative contraindications to PC are an unsafe access route and uncorrectable coagulopathy. With coagulopathy, a prudent measure might be to insert the catheter transperitoneally rather than via the transhepatic approach; transhepatic puncture may not be preferred with a coagulopathy [82] (see below). The gall bladder must be distended to be a candidate for PC [83]. It is technically most difficult to insert a catheter into a small, scarred, shrunken, thick-walled, or contracted gall bladder [82,84]; PC and percutaneous cholecystolithotomy are relatively contraindicated in these situations [85,86].

Access route and technique

Initial needle puncture is usually made with realtime US guidance, followed by fluoroscopic monitoring of catheter insertion. CT may be a useful adjunct in the patient with a poorly distended gall bladder with a large stone burden, or a particularly thick-walled gall bladder in which US visualization is suboptimal and puncture may be difficult [79]. In most reported series, the transhepatic route is advocated [80,81, 83,87−89]. Usually, transhepatic access through the "bare area" of the gall bladder is chosen. The bare area is that portion of the gall bladder closely applied to the hepatic parenchyma. There is no peritoneal reflection involving this segment of the gall bladder, so the risk of bile leakage is minimized both at the time of initial puncture and after catheter removal. Percutaneous biliary drainage (PBD) has established the safety of the percutaneous transhepatic approach. The risk of major hemorrhage with transhepatic PC (and transhepatic PAD) is even less than with PBD since the liver periphery is traversed for PC (and PAD), and the larger vessels in the periportal region are avoided [88]. In a series of 100 patients undergoing CT of the abdomen, in only 17% of patients was there no interposition of colon or liver between the skin and the gall-bladder fundus, necessitating a transhepatic approach [88]. If large tracts (14−30-F) are used − often for cholecystolithotomy − a subhepatic, transperitoneal approach may be preferable [87]. The transperitoneal approach eliminates the hepatic trauma associated with the large sheaths often required for percutaneous gallstone removal. The transperitoneal approach may provide improved access for removing stones and cannulating the cystic duct because puncture is usually made along the long axis of the gall bladder. Invagination of the gall-bladder wall and loss of access are potential intraprocedural problems usually associated with the transperitoneal approach [79, 85,86]. When invagination of the gall-bladder wall is a problem, a second percutaneous transhepatic access has allowed successful tract dilatation, and retrievable T-fasteners which appose the gall-bladder wall to the peritoneum have been used as well [81,85]. Gall-bladder apposition to the abdominal wall is an option to prevent displacement or invagination of the gall-bladder wall after transperitoneal puncture and theoretically to avoid bile leakage [82,85]. Regardless of technique used, care should be taken not to puncture the back wall of the gall bladder, which could increase the risk of bile leakage.

Aspiration of bile confirms satisfactory position and a bile specimen is sent to the laboratory for Gram's stain and culture. The value of aspiration of gall-bladder bile to diagnose the presence of infection is limited; the diagnostic sensitivity of Gram stain or culture from percutaneous aspirates is less than 50% [90]. Sterile cultures of bile may not be helpful in excluding cholecystitis, especially in patients who have received broad-spectrum antibiotics, but abnormal Gram stain or positive cultures for enteric organisms suggest acute cholecystitis [91].

A catheter, usually 5–8-F, is delivered with either Seldinger or trocar techniques. Modified Seldinger technique (coaxial access set with a safety wire) is probably safer; some investigators have encountered difficulty with trocar insertion which may necessitate repeat punctures [89,91]. A theoretical advantage of the trocar puncture technique is the elimination of dilator exchanges during which bile may leak. The gall-bladder wall is quite resilient and a sharp entry device delivered with a quick thrust is necessary to penetrate the gall-bladder wall effectively [91]. Effective dilatation is achieved by performing adequate early dilatations and by introducing dilators with a smooth, rotary action [86]. Gillams *et al.* [86] found metal, telescopic dilators to be more effective than balloon dilatation during transperitoneal PC.

Additional tests may be performed, including cholecysto-cholangiography, gall-bladder biopsy, and manometry. Overdistension and manipulation of the gall bladder, biliary tree, or any initially decompressed, infected fluid collection is avoided for 24–48 hours to reduce the risk of *septicemia*. Additionally, during gall-bladder interventions, distension and manipulations are minimized to avert *vagal reactions* [92]. After initial PC, only small volume contrast injections should be made following removal of at least an equal amount of bile. All obtainable bile and contrast are aspirated from the gall bladder following needle puncture or catheter drainage.

Complications

Complications occur in 5–10% of patients [79,80,87]; primarily in patients with calculous or acalculous cholecystitis

[82]. A recent review of 231 emergent and elective cases of PC, reported in the English-language literature, yielded a complication rate of 7.8% [80]. Only one death directly attributable to PC has been reported; a result of a delay in recognition of catheter dislodgment in a moribund patient [79]. Complication rates of PC are remarkably low, given that the procedure usually is performed in patients who are poor operative risks. In comparative studies of surgical versus PC, potential selection bias would be expected to favor those patients considered healthy enough to tolerate surgery, yet mortality rates for emergency surgical cholecystostomy vary from 6 to 30% [79].

PC has the potential to cause general complications that might occur with any percutaneous procedure such as *hemorrhage*, infection of a noninfected system, inadvertent puncture of nontarget organs, and tube dislodgment (see below). Specific complications include *bile peritonitis, cholecystitis, hemobilia*, and *vagal effects* of bradycardia and hypotension. Bile peritonitis and vagal bradycardia with hypotension appear to have a proclivity to develop with PC, more than with other percutaneous procedures in the bile ducts [82].

Bile leakage is the most commonly reported complication of PC. A transhepatic puncture does not necessarily prevent bile leakage, although theoretically it protects against bile peritonitis [82]. Even a single needle puncture alone (transhepatic or peritoneal) may result in bile peritonitis [80,82]. Most cases of bile peritonitis have the common denominator of a hole in the gall bladder that was not being decompressed with a catheter [82]. A key to avoiding bile leak is adequate decompression of an obstructed biliary system. Because gall-bladder aspiration is nonspecific for the diagnosis of cholecystitis and needle puncture entails the risk of bile leak, a catheter should probably always be placed when performing gall-bladder interventions. Loss of access is a potential cause of bile leak; a safety wire should be used during PC catheter insertion [82,83]. A "protective" guidewire should be used with trocar punctures [30]. Because of the risk of bile peritonitis, retention devices on PC catheters are considered essential. Some early cases of catheter dislodgment were associated with the use of nonlocking catheters [82,93]. The catheter is also firmly attached to the patient's skin with a tape mesentery as previously described.

Any ongoing evidence of bile leakage from the gall bladder is treated with placement of additional catheter(s) and drainage to effect diversion and prevent further bile leakage [82,85,94]. However, many subhepatic bile collections can be managed with antibiotics alone [86]. Healing of the gall-bladder wall has occurred with catheter decompression and antibiotics alone, despite proved perforation and bile leakage [94].

Premature removal of a PC catheter may lead to leakage and bile peritonitis, even in a decompressed system. The catheter is left in place about 2–3 weeks, followed by cholecystocholangiography to ensure patency of the cystic and common bile ducts. Additionally or alternately, several days prior to anticipated removal, the PC tube may be clamped to effect a trial of internal drainage similar to the management of a surgical T-tube [89]. Tract maturation progresses slowly in the elderly, debilitated, and immunocompromised patients who come to PC; a tractogram should be performed on all patients during catheter removal to assess maturity of the tract and to exclude bile leakage [83,85,86]. A tractogram is performed by injecting contrast material through an end-hole dilator with a side adaptor over a thin guidewire; this allows simple catheter reinsertion if the tract is poorly formed. In one instance, however, bile peritonitis occurred where the tract was intact at radiography [85].

Vasovagal reactions such as bradycardia and hypotension occur infrequently but may be severe. Manipulation and/or distension of the gall bladder is usually the inciting event. Adverse vagal effects have been minimized by limiting manipulation of guidewires and catheters, removal of bile in small aliquots, and administration of atropine [92]. Cardiac, blood pressure, and oxygen saturation monitoring should be standard for all patients undergoing PC, along with ready availability of atropine, fluids, and resuscitative measures, should a reaction occur [82,86,92]. Preventive administration of atropine is controversial and generally has not been advocated, as myocardial work and oxygen consumption are increased which may be detrimental in high-risk elderly patients often referred for PC.

Percutaneous cholecystolithotomy

Percutaneous cholecystolithotomy can be used to remove any type, size, and number of stones — unlike other non-surgical alternates — in patients with both acute and chronic cholecystitis [85]. However, there are some disadvantages with percutaneous cholecystolithotomy. It is tedious and often requires several sessions for complete stone removal. Also, this gall-bladder preserving procedure entails the risk of *stone recurrence* and, rarely, *gall-bladder carcinoma* [85,95]. For these reasons, percutaneous cholecystolithotomy is usually restricted to those patients in whom the risk of surgery is substantial. It is controversial whether the post-cholecystolithotomy patient needs surveillance (usually with serial US) to detect the late complications of stone recurrence and carcinoma [85,95,96]. The incidence of carcinoma is very low and most patients with recurrent stones are asymptomatic [96]. In a study of gallstone recurrence after surgical cholecystostomy with either surgical or radiologic cholecystolithotomy, the stone detection rate was 27% (13 of 48 patients) by 4 years after stone removal. Seven (11%) of 61 patients complained of recurrent or residual biliary symptoms, but only three actually had recurrent calculi; one patient had an associated advanced gall-bladder carcinoma. The other nine patients with recurrent calculi were asymptomatic.

Other studies have shown gallstone recurrence rates of 50% or more and similar rates of recurrent biliary symptoms after cholecystolithotomy, ranging from 10 to 17%. Similarly, 30–50% of postcholecystectomy patients suffer "postcholecystectomy" symptoms. The study concludes that, despite the high frequency of stone recurrence, the low recurrence of symptoms after cholecystolithotomy appears to justify a conservative approach to the follow-up management of elderly patients, and that interval cholecystectomy need not be performed routinely [96].

In a later study, the same authors report five cases of gall-bladder carcinoma after cholecystolithotomy and assert that the question of interval cholecystectomy should be decided on an individual basis. The relative risks of development of gall-bladder carcinoma must be weighed against the potential complications of elective cholecystectomy for each patient [95]. Several studies have shown that the risk of development of gall-bladder carcinoma while harboring calculi for up to 20 years is less than 1%; there is a 1–2% prevalence of gall-bladder carcinoma in cholecystectomy patients. Most gall-bladder cancers occur in elderly women, and a high index of suspicion should be maintained. Imaging features that should preclude gall-bladder preserving therapies include porcelain gall bladder, gall bladder polyps that are 2 cm or greater in diameter, or focal gall-bladder wall thickening or irregularity. The feasibility and efficacy of total gall-bladder ablation is currently being investigated. Gall-bladder ablation offers a promising solution to gallstone recurrence and the development of gall-bladder carcinoma [82,89,95].

Gallstone dissolution

There are fewer indications for gallstone dissolution since the advent of laparoscopic cholecystectomy. Use of CT should be considered essential to characterize gallstone composition (cholesterol versus calcium or bilirubinate), and to avoid inappropriate catheterization and solvent infusion for non-cholesterol calculi [87]. Catheter material is important when the catheter is intended for contact dissolution of gallstones; some solvents can dissolve catheters [87]. Teflon, polyethylene, and polyurethane are resistant to methyl-tert-butyl ether (MTBE). Side-effects of MTBE include sedation, pain, duodenal ulceration, and renal failure. Complications can be minimized with techniques that keep MTBE in the gall bladder and prevent its escape into the duodenum; this is best achieved by using small volumes of MTBE or occluding the cystic duct [87].

Cecostomy

Introduction

Gross cecal distension may result from mechanical obstruction (e.g., carcinoma, volvulus, adhesions, fecal impaction), mesenteric ischemia, or, more commonly, from acute colonic pseudoobstruction (Ogilvie syndrome). The precise etiology of acute colonic pseudoobstruction is not known but afflicted patients often have severe medical illnesses that are postulated to be the inciting cause of the distension. The massive acute cecal dilatation (>10 cm diameter) that characterizes the syndrome can lead to ischemic injury and perforation of the cecum which are associated with a high mortality; over 50% [97,98]. The incidence of perforation in untreated acute colonic pseudoobstruction is not known, but is estimated to occur in up to 20% of cases [98–100]. The incidence of perforation has been shown to correlate with the duration of cecal distension and not necessarily with the diameter of the cecum [99]. The mean duration of cecal distension in most patients who perforate is greater than 6 days [99,100]. Conversely, chronic dilatation of the colon, as seen with constipation or colonic inertia, is rarely life threatening but may lead to acute symptoms [101].

The goal of therapy is to prevent bowel wall ischemia and perforation while the patient's associated medical problems are resolving. Mainstays of conservative therapy include cessation of oral intake, nasogastric tube suction, withdrawal of opiate and anticholinergic agents, rectal tube drainage, gentle enemas, and treatment of underlying sepsis and electrolyte abnormalities. Patients not responding to conservative management within 24–72 hours [98,99,101,102] are usually considered candidates for endoscopic, percutaneous, or (as a last resort) surgical decompression.

Decompression can be achieved by means of decompressive colonoscopy [97,98,101,102], decompressive colonoscopy with tube placement [98,101,102], percutaneous endoscopic cecostomy [103], percutaneous cecostomy (PCC) [104–108], fluoroscopically guided colonic tube placement [109], laparoscopic cecostomy [110], or surgical cecostomy [102]. Colonoscopic decompression is the most frequently used technique and has proved successful in approximately 85% of cases; however, there is a 20–40% chance or more of recurrence [97,98,102,110]. Concurrent endoscopic placement of a tube within the colon appears to decrease the recurrence rate but requires an endoscopist with considerable experience and may require additional fluoroscopy [98,102]. The colonoscopic method is not without risk; colonoscopy performed in this setting has a morbidity (3%) and mortality (1%) that is significantly higher than colonoscopy in patients without colonic pseudoobstruction (0.2 and 0.06%, respectively) [100]. Moreover, colonoscopy is not technically possible in some patients, usually due to fecal retention. Surgical cecostomy is fraught with higher morbidity and mortality [102].

When colonoscopic decompression is not available, not possible, or unsuccessful, PCC should be performed, obviating the high risk of laparotomy and general anesthesia in this very ill patient population [103,104]. PCC may be a curative alternate in cases of colonic pseudoobstruction or a tempor-izing or palliative measure in cases of mechanical obstruction [104–106].

Access route

Both transperitoneal and retroperitoneal routes have been used for PCC [104–108]. The retroperitoneal route has been described under CT guidance and has been advocated as possibly safer. The rationale is that potential spillage of fecal material would be contained in the retroperitoneum rather than contaminate the peritoneal cavity, resulting in peritonitis. Retroperitonitis is a possible result of spillage into the retroperitoneum, however, and most PCC cases have been performed via an anterior approach without reported peritonitis [104–106]. On anatomic and CT scan studies, the peritoneum bounded the cecum for at least 270° of circumference, precluding the theoretical advisability of retroperitoneal access [104]. In addition, the dilated cecum is often displaced anteromedially [99,105] and descends deeply into the right lower quadrant, and may be shielded by the iliac bone, preventing a posterior approach [104]. Moreover, in this debilitated patient population, often with multiple tubes and monitoring wires, it is easier to perform PCC on a supine patient under fluoroscopic guidance via an anterior approach. A posterior approach requires turning the patient on the side and using CT guidance [105].

Technique and catheter care

Both trocar and Seldinger techniques are feasible for PCC. Trocar technique via a single pass theoretically avoids any spillage of fecal material; this problem is felt more likely to occur during the dilator exchanges used with Seldinger technique [106]. Needle decompression is not advocated because of the risks of fecal spillage and of recurrent cecal distension [106]. Apposition of the cecum to the anterior abdominal wall using T-fasteners prior to catheter placement has been advocated [105]. This step is believed to decrease the chances of intraperitoneal fecal spillage during and after the procedure. Cecal fixation with T-fasteners allowed single-step Seldinger placement of large-bore catheters (24–30-F) [105]. For decompression of mechanical colonic obstruction, larger catheters may be preferred to facilitate irrigation and egress of colonic contents; obstruction of smaller catheters is more likely because of the viscosity of the fecal stream. For colonic pseudoobstruction, the goal of evacuation of gas has been accomplished successfully with 8–12-F catheters [104, 106].

Gas may audibly escape during colonic puncture and during wire and catheter insertion; fecal spillage does not necessarily occur [104]. PCC catheters equipped with a retention device are essential; Foley and Cope locking pigtail catheters have been used most frequently [104,106]. Balloon catheters may create a tight seal and prevent intraperitoneal fecal spillage. Excess tension on the catheter is avoided to prevent bowel wall necrosis. Aggressive pericatheter care is important to prevent wound infection. A generous skin incision might help reduce the chance of cellulitis or fasciitis by preventing accumulation of contaminated fluid under the skin. Intermittent irrigation of the catheter (e.g., 20 ml saline four times a day) will help prevent fecal occlusion of the catheter side holes [106]. In the largest reported series of PCC, catheters were removed uneventfully after 12–27 days [104]. If there is no distal colonic obstruction, the fistulous tract will heal spontaneously once the catheter is removed [106].

Complications

PCC has the potential to cause general complications that might occur with any percutaneous procedure such as hemorrhage, inadvertent puncture of nontarget organs, pericatheter infection, or tube dislodgment. Peritonitis is a specific complication which might be associated with PCC. However, there have been no major or minor complications of PCC reported. One patient had transient back leakage along a catheter that ceased when the Foley balloon catheter was retracted against the abdominal wall and taped more securely [104]. Another catheter inadvertently dislodged 11 days after insertion without consequence; colonic distension did not recur [106].

A 3-cm *vascular pseudotumor* was found at the site of prior surgical tube cecostomy in the only report of endoscopic findings after cecostomy [111]. Biopsy of the mass showed ulcerated, inflamed mucosa with granulation tissue compatible with ongoing healing. Attempted endoscopic snare removal of such a lesion might well be accompanied by increased risk of hemorrhage — our gastroenterology colleagues should be made aware of this potential finding.

References

1 vanSonnenberg E, D'Agostino HB, Casola G, Halasz NA, Sanchez RB, Goodacre BW. Percutaneous abscess drainage: current concepts. *Radiology* 1991;181:617–626.

2 Petit P, Bret PM, Lough JO, Reinhold C. Risks associated with intestinal perforation during experimental percutaneous drainage. *Invest Radiol* 1992;27:1012–1019.

3 Lambiase RE, Deyoe L, Cronan JJ, Dorfman GS. Percutaneous drainage of 335 consecutive abscesses: results of primary drainage with 1-year follow-up. *Radiology* 1992;184:167–179.

4 Hemming A, Davis NL, Robins E. Surgical versus percutaneous drainage of intraabdominal abscesses. *Am J Surg* 1991;161:593–595.

5 vanSonnenberg E, Mueller PR, Ferrucci JT. Percutaneous drainage of 250 abdominal abscesses and fluid collections. I. Results, failures, and complications. *Radiology* 1984;151:337–341.

6 Mueller PR, vanSonnenberg E, Ferrucci JT. Percutaneous drainage of 250 abdominal abscesses and fluid collections. II.

Current procedural concepts. *Radiology* 1984;151:343–347.

7 Lang EK, Springer RM, Glorioso LW, Cammarata CA. Abdominal abscess drainage under radiologic guidance: causes of failure. *Radiology* 1986;159:329–336.

8 van Waes PFGM, Feldberg MAM, Mali WPTM et al. Management of loculated abscesses that are difficult to drain: a new approach. *Radiology* 1983;147:57–63.

9 vanSonnenberg E, Ferrucci JT, Mueller PR, Wittenberg J, Simeone JF. Percutaneous drainage of abscesses and fluid collections: technique, results, and applications. *Radiology* 1982;142:1–10.

10 vanSonnenberg E, Wing VW, Casola G et al. Temporizing effect of percutaneous drainage of complicated abscesses in critically ill patients. *Am J Roentgenol* 1984;142:821–826.

11 Papanicolaou N, Mueller PR, Ferrucci JT et al. Abscess-fistula association: radiologic recognition and percutaneous management. *Am J Roentgenol* 1984;143:811–815.

12 Kerlan RK, Jeffrey RB, Pogany AC, Ring EJ. Abdominal abscess with low-output fistula: successful percutaneous drainage. *Radiology* 1985;155:73–75.

13 Lambiase RE, Cronan JJ, Dorfman GS, Paolella LP, Haas RA. Postoperative abscesses with enteric communication: percutaneous treatment. *Radiology* 1989;171:497–500.

14 Mueller PR, White EM, Glass-Royal M et al. Infected abdominal tumors: percutaneous catheter drainage. *Radiology* 1989;173:627–629.

15 vanSonnenberg E, Wittich GR, Casola G et al. Periappendiceal abscesses: percutaneous drainage. *Radiology* 1987;163:23–26.

16 Jaques P, Mauro M, Safrit H, Yankaskas B, Piggott B. CT features of intraabdominal abscesses: prediction of successful percutaneous drainage. *Am J Roentgenol* 1986;146:1041–1045.

17 vanSonnenberg E, Casola G, Varney RR, Wittich GR. Imaging and interventional radiology for pancreatitis and its complications. *Radiol Clin N Am* 1989;27(1):65–72.

18 Freeny PC, Lewis GP, Traverso LW, Ryan JA. Infected pancreatic fluid collections: percutaneous catheter drainage. *Radiology* 1988;167:435–441.

19 Hamper UM, Savader BL, Sheth S. Improved needle-tip visualization by color doppler sonography. *Am J Roentgenol* 1991;156:401–402.

20 Mueller PR, Ferrucci JT, Simeone JF et al. Lesser sac abscesses and fluid collections: drainage by transhepatic approach. *Radiology* 1985;155:615–618.

21 LeRoy AJ, Williams HJ, Bender CE, Segura JW, Patterson DE, Benson RC. Colon perforation following percutaneous nephrostomy and renal calculus removal. *Radiology* 1985;155:83–85.

22 vanSonnenberg E, D'Agostino HB, Casola G, Goodacre BW, Sanchez RB, Taylor B. US-guided transvaginal drainage of pelvic abscesses and fluid collections. *Radiology* 1991;181:53–56.

23 Sanchez RB, vanSonnenberg E, D'Agostino H, O'Laoide R, Oglevie S, Fundell L. Transvaginal drainage of pelvic fluid collections. *Semin Intervent Radiol* 1992;9(2):152–158.

24 Neff CC, Mueller PR, Ferrucci JT et al. Serious complications following transgression of the pleural space in drainage procedures. *Radiology* 1984;152:335–341.

25 Dawson SL, Neff CC, Mueller PR, Ferrucci JT. Fatal hemothorax after inadvertant transpleural biliary drainage. *Am J Roentgenol* 1983;141:33–34.

26 vanSonnenberg E, Wittenberg J, Ferrucci JT, Mueller PR, Simeone JF. Triangulation method for percutaneous needle guidance: the angled approach to upper abdominal masses. *Am*

J Roentgenol 1981;137:757−761.

27 Matalon TAS, Silver B. US guidance of interventional procedures. *Radiology* 1990;174:43−47.

28 vanSonnenberg E, Casola G, Maysey M. Simple apparatus to avoid inadvertent needle puncture. *Radiology* 1988;166:550.

29 Mueller PR, Silverman SG, Tung G *et al.* New universal precaution aspiration tray. *Radiology* 1989;173:278−279.

30 vanSonnenberg E, Polansky AD, Wittich GR, Cabrera OA. Guide wire protection for trocar puncture of fluid collections. *Am J Roentgenol* 1985;145:831−832.

31 Casola G, vanSonnenberg E, Neff CC, Saba RM, Withers C, Emarine CW. Abscesses in Crohn disease: percutaneous drainage. *Radiology* 1987;163:19−22.

32 Stabile BE, Puccio E, vanSonnenberg E, Neff CC. Preoperative percutaneous drainage of diverticular abscesses. *Am J Surg* 1990,159.99−105.

33 Quinn SF, Demlow TA. Large caliber (24−28-F) catheters for radiologically guided percutaneous procedures. *Radiology* 1993; 189:922−923.

34 vanSonnenberg E, Mueller PR, Ferrucci JT, Neff CC, Simeone JF, Wittenberg J. Sump catheter for percutaneous abscess and fluid drainage by trocar or seldinger technique. *Am J Roentgenol* 1982;139:613−614.

35 Eschelman DJ, Sullivan KL. Use of a Colapinto needle in US-guided transvaginal drainage of pelvic abscesses. *Radiology* 1993;186:893−894.

36 Dawson S, Papanicolaou N, Mueller PR, Ferrucci JT. Preserving access during percutaneous catheterization using a double-guide-wire technique. *Am J Roentgenol* 1983;141:407.

37 Jeffrey RB. A modified Cope introducer set for rapid insertion of a safety wire. *Am J Roentgenol* 1986;147:828−829.

38 D'Agostino HB, vanSonnenberg E, Sanchez RB, Goodacre BW, Casola G. Imaging of the percutaneous cholecystostomy tract: observations and utility. *Radiology* 1991;181:675−678.

39 Barth KH, Matsumoto AH. Patient care in interventional radiology: a perspective. *Radiology* 1991;178:11−17.

40 Lee AS, vanSonnenberg E, Wittich GR, Casola G. Exchange of occluded catheters with transcatheter and pericatheter maneuvers. *Radiology* 1987;163:273−274.

41 Vogelzang RL, Tobin RS, Burstein S, Anschuetz SL, Marzano M, Kozlowski JM. Transcatheter intracavitary fibrinolysis of infected extravascular hematomas. *Am J Roentgenol* 1987;148: 378−380.

42 Dawson SL, Mueller PR, Ferrucci JT. Mucomyst for abscesses: a clinical comment. *Radiology* 1984;151:342.

43 Park JK, Kraus FC, Haaga JR. Fluid flow during percutaneous drainage procedures: an *in vitro* study of the effects of fluid viscosity, catheter size, and adjunctive urokinase. *Am J Roentgenol* 1993;160:165−169.

44 Ho CS, Yeung EY. Percutaneous gastrostomy and transgastric jejunostomy. *Am J Roentgenol* 1992;158:251−257.

45 Ho CS. Percutaneous gastrostomy for jejunal feeding. *Radiology* 1983;149:595−596.

46 Wills JS, Oglesby JT. Percutaneous gastrostomy. *Radiology* 1983;149:449−453.

47 Ho CS, Yee ACN, McPherson R. Complications of surgical and percutaneous nonendoscopic gastrostomy: review of 233 patients. *Gastroenterology* 1988;95:1206−1210.

48 Wills JS, Oglesby JT. Percutaneous gastrostomy. *Radiology* 1988;167:41−43.

49 Deutsch LS, Kannegieter L, Vanson DT, Miller DP, Brandon JC. Simplified percutaneous gastrostomy. *Radiology* 1992;184:

181−183.

50 Foutch PG, vanSonnenberg E, Casola G, D'Agostino H. Nonsurgical gastrostomy: X-ray or endoscopy? (invited commentary). *Am J Gastroenterol* 1990;85:1560−1563.

51 Sanchez RB, vanSonnenberg E, D'Agostino HB, Goodacre BW, Moyers P, Casola G. CT guidance for percutaneous gastrostomy and gastroenterostomy. *Radiology* 1992;184:201−205.

52 O'Keeffe F, Carrasco CH, Charnsangavej C, Richli WR, Wallace S, Freedman RS. Percutaneous drainage and feeding gastrostomies in 100 patients. *Radiology* 1989;172:341−343.

53 vanSonnenberg E, Wittich GR, Brown LK *et al.* Percutaneous gastrostomy and gastroenterostomy: 1. Techniques derived from laboratory evaluation. *Am J Roentgenol* 1986;146:577−580.

54 Varney RA, vanSonnenberg E, Casola G, Sukthankar R. Balloon techniques for percutaneous gastrostomy in a patient with partial gastrectomy. *Radiology* 1988;167:69−70.

55 Brown AS, Mueller PR, Ferrucci JT. Controlled percutaneous gastrostomy: nylon t-fastener for fixation of the anterior gastric wall. *Radiology* 1986;158:543−545.

56 Hicks ME, Surratt RS, Picus D, Marx MV, Lang EV. Fluoroscopically guided percutaneous gastrostomy and gastroenterostomy: analysis of 158 consecutive cases. *Am J Roentgenol* 1990;154:725−728.

57 Alzate GD, Coons HG, Elliott J, Carey PH. Percutaneous gastrostomy for jejunal feeding: a new technique. *Am J Roentgenol* 1986;147:822−825.

58 Gray RR, St Louis EL, Grosman H. Percutaneous gastrostomy and gastrojejunostomy. *Br J Radiol* 1987;60:1067−1070.

59 vanSonnenberg E, Wittich GR, Cabrera OA *et al.* Percutaneous gastrostomy and gastroenterostomy: 2. Clinical experience. *Am J Roentgenol* 1986;146:581−586.

60 Tao HH, Gillies RR. Percutaneous feeding gastrostomy. *Am J Roentgenol* 1983;141:793−794.

61 Gray RR, St Louis EL, Grosman H. Modified catheter for percutaneous gastrojejunostomy. *Radiology* 1989;173:276−278.

62 Lindberg CG, Ivancev K, Kan Z, Lindberg R. Percutaneous gastrostomy: a clinical and experimental study. *Acta Radiol* 1991;32:302−304.

63 Lu DSK, Mueller PR, Lee MJ, Dawson SL, Hahn PF, Brountzos E. Gastrostomy conversion to transgastric jejunostomy: technical problems, causes of failure, and proposed solutions in 63 patients. *Radiology* 1993;187:679−683.

64 Saini S, Mueller PR, Gaa J *et al.* Percutaneous gastrostomy with gastropexy: experience in 125 patients. *Am J Roentgenol* 1990; 154:1003−1006.

65 Foutch PG, Woods CA, Talbert GA, Sanowski RA. A critical analysis of the Sacks−Vine gastrostomy tube: a review of 120 consecutive procedures. *Am J Gastroenterol* 1988;83:812−815.

66 Chung RS, Schertzer M. Pathogenesis of complications of percutaneous endoscopic gastrostomy: a lesson in surgical principles. *Am Surg* 1990;56:134−137.

67 Mamel JJ. Percutaneous endoscopic gastrostomy. *Am J Gastroenterol* 1989;84:703−710.

68 vanSonnenberg E, Cubberley DA, Brown LK, Wittich GR, Lyon JW, Stauffer AE. Percutaneous gastrostomy: use of intragastric balloon support. *Radiology* 1984;152:531−532.

69 Gray RR, Ho CS, Yee A, Montanera W, Jones DP. Direct percutaneous jejunostomy. *Am J Roentgenol* 1987;149:931−932.

70 Coleman CC, Coons HG, Cope C *et al.* Percutaneous enterostomy

with the Cope suture anchor. *Radiology* 1990;174:889−891.

71 Cope C. Suture anchor for visceral drainage. *Am J Roentgenol* 1986;146:160−161.

72 Gustke RF, Varma RR, Soergel KH. Gastric reflux during perfusion of the proximal small bowel. *Gastroenterology* 1970;59: 890−895.

73 Wojtowycz MM, Arata JA, Micklos TJ, Miller FJ. CT findings after uncomplicated percutaneous gastrostomy. *Am J Roentgenol* 1988;151:307−309.

74 Halkier BK, Ho CS, Yee ACN. Percutaneous feeding gastrostomy with the seldinger technique: review of 252 patients. *Radiology* 1989;171:359−362.

75 Greif JM, Ragland JJ, Ochsner MG, Riding R. Fatal necrotizing fasciitis complicating percutaneous endoscopic gastrostomy. *Gastrointest Endosc* 1986;32:292−294.

76 Wojtowycz MM, Arata JA. Subcutaneous emphysema after percutaneous gastrostomy. *Am J Roentgenol* 1988;151:311−312.

77 Lee MJ, Saini S, Brink JA, Morrison MC, Hahn PF, Mueller PR. Malignant small bowel obstruction and ascites: not a contraindication to percutaneous gastrostomy. *Clin Radiol* 1991;44: 332−334.

78 Cave DR, Robinson WR, Brotschi EA. Necrotizing fasciitis following percutaneous endoscopic gastrostomy. *Gastrointest Endosc* 1986;32:294−296.

79 Goodacre B, vanSonnenberg E, D'Agostino H, Sanchez R. Interventional radiology in gallstone disease. *Gastroenterol Clin N Am* 1991;20(1):209−227.

80 Teplick SK, Brandon JC, Wolferth CC, Amron G, Gambescia R, Zitomer N. Percutaneous interventional gallbladder procedures: personal experience and literature review. *Gastrointest Radiol* 1990;15:133−136.

81 Cope C. Percutaneous subhepatic cholecystostomy with removable anchor. *Am J Roentgenol* 1988;151:1129−1132.

82 vanSonnenberg E, D'Agostino HB, Goodacre BW, Sanchez RB, Casola G. Percutaneous gallbladder puncture and cholecystostomy: results, complications, and caveats for safety. *Radiology* 1992;183:167−170.

83 Lee MJ, Saini S, Brink JA *et al.* Treatment of critically ill patients with sepsis of unknown cause: value of percutaneous cholecystostomy. *Am J Roentgenol* 1991;156:1163−1166.

84 vanSonnenberg E, D'Agostino HB, Casola G, Varney RR, Taggart SC, May SR. The benefits of percutaneous cholecystostomy for decompression of selected cases of obstructive jaundice. *Radiology* 1990;176:15−18.

85 Picus D, Hicks ME, Darcy MD *et al.* Percutaneous cholecystolithotomy: analysis of results and complications in 58 consecutive patients. *Radiology* 1992;183:779−784.

86 Gillams A, Curtis SC, Donald J, Russell C, Lees W. Technical considerations in 113 percutaneous cholecystolithotomies. *Radiology* 1992;183:163−166.

87 vanSonnenberg E, D'Agostino HB, Casola G, Varney RR, Ainge GD. Interventional radiology in the gallbladder: diagnosis, drainage, dissolution, and management of stones. *Radiology* 1990;174:1−6.

88 Warren LP, Kadir S, Dunnick NR. Percutaneous cholecystostomy: anatomic considerations. *Radiology* 1988;168:615−616.

89 vanSonnenberg E, Wittich GR, Casola G *et al.* Diagnostic and therapeutic percutaneous gallbladder procedures. *Radiology* 1986;160:23−26.

90 McGahan JP, Lindfors KK. Acute cholecystitis: diagnostic accuracy of percutaneous aspiration of the gallbladder. *Radiology* 1988;167:669−671.

91 Lindemann SR, Tung G, Silverman SG, Mueller PR. Percutaneous cholecystostomy: a review. *Semin Intervent Radiol* 1988;5(3): 179−185.

92 vanSonnenberg E, Wing VW, Pollard JW, Casola G. Life-threatening vagal reactions associated with percutaneous cholecystostomy. *Radiology* 1984;151:377−380.

93 McGahan J. A new catheter design for percutaneous cholecystostomy. *Radiology* 1988;166:49−52.

94 vanSonnenberg E, D'Agostino HB, Casola G, Hoyt DB, Lurie A, Varney RR. Gallbladder perforation and bile leakage: percutaneous treatment. *Radiology* 1991;178:687−689.

95 So CB, Gibney RG, Scudamore CH. Carcinoma of the gallbladder: a risk associated with gallbladder-preserving treatments for cholelithiasis. *Radiology* 1990;174:127−130.

96 Gibney RG, Chow K, So CB, Rowley VA, Cooperberg PL, Burhenne HJ. Gallstone recurrence after cholecystolithotomy. *Am J Roentgenol* 1989;153:287−289.

97 Bode WE, Beart RW, Spencer RJ, Culp CE, Wolff BG, Taylor BM. Colonoscopic decompression for acute pseudoobstruction of the colon (Ogilvie's syndrome): report of 22 cases and review of the literature. *Am J Surg* 1984;147:243−245.

98 Harig JM, Fumo DE, Loo FD *et al.* Treatment of acute nontoxic megacolon during colonoscopy: tube placement versus simple decompression. *Gastrointest Endosc* 1988;34:23−27.

99 Johnson CD, Rice RP, Kelvin FM, Foster WL, Williford ME. The radiologic evaluation of gross cecal distension: emphasis on cecal ileus. *Am J Roentgenol* 1985;145:1211−1217.

100 Sloyer AF, Panella VS, Demas BE *et al.* Ogilvie's syndrome: successful management without colonoscopy. *Digest Dis Sci* 1988;33:1391−1396.

101 Strodel WE, Brothers T. Colonoscopic decompression of pseudoobstruction and volvulus. *Surg Clin N Am* 1989;69:1327−1335.

102 Vanek VW, Al-Salti M. Acute pseudoobstruction of the colon (Ogilvie's syndrome): an analysis of 400 cases. *Dis Colon Rectum* 1986;29:203−210.

103 Ponsky JL, Aszodi A, Perse D. Percutaneous endoscopic cecostomy: a new approach to nonobstructive colonic dilation. *Gastrointest Endosc* 1986;32:108−111.

104 vanSonnenberg E, Varney RR, Casola G *et al.* Percutaneous cecostomy for Ogilvie syndrome: laboratory observations and clinical experience. *Radiology* 1990;175:679−682.

105 Morrison MC, Lee MJ, Stafford SA, Saini S, Mueller PR. Percutaneous cecostomy: controlled transperitoneal approach. *Radiology* 1990;176:574−576.

106 Casola G, Withers C, vanSonnenberg E, Herba MJ, Saba RM, Brown RA. Percutaneous cecostomy for decompression of the massively distended cecum. *Radiology* 1986;158:793−794.

107 Crass JR, Simmons RL, Frick MP, Maile CW. Percutaneous decompression of the colon using CT guidance in Ogilvie syndrome. *Am J Roentgenol* 1985;144:475−476.

108 Haaga JR, Bick RJ, Zollinger RM. CT-guided percutaneous catheter cecostomy. *Gastrointest Radiol* 1987;12:166−168.

109 Bender GN, Do-Dai DD, Briggs LM. Colonic pseudo-obstruction: decompression with a tricomponent coaxial system under fluoroscopic guidance. *Radiology* 1993;188:395−398.

110 Duh QY, Way LW. Diagnostic laparoscopy and laparoscopic cecostomy for colonic pseudoobstruction. *Dis Colon Rectum* 1993;36:65−70.

111 Berg CL, Farraye FRA, Carr-Locke DL. Tube cecostomy as a cause of cecal pseudotumor. *Endoscopy* 1991;23:229−230.

112 vanSonnenberg E, D'Agostino HB, Sanchez RB, Casola G. Percutaneous abscess drainage: editorial comments. *Radiology*

1992;184:27−29.

113 D'Agostino HB, vanSonnenberg E, Sanchez RB, Goodacre BW, Casola G. A simple method to lock large mushroom-tip catheters. *Radiology* 1992;182:576−577.

114 vanSonnenberg E, Wittich GR, Schiffman HR *et al*. Percutaneous drainage access; a simplified coaxial technique. *Radiology* 1986;159:266−268.

115 Towbin RB, Ball WS, Bissett GS. Percutaneous gastrostomy and percutaneous gastrojejunostomy in children: antegrade approach. *Radiology* 1988;168:473−476.

116 Gray R, Rooney M, Grosman H. Use of t fasteners for primary jejunostomy. *Cardiovasc Intervent Radiol* 1990;13:93−94.

117 Cwikiel W. Percutaneous duodenostomy − alternative route for enteral nutrition. *Acta Radiol* 1991;32:153−154.

118 DiSario JA, Foutch PG, Sanowski. Poor results with percutaneous endoscopic jejunostomy. *Gastrointest Endosc* 1990;36: 257 260.

119 Wolfsen HC, Kozarek RA, Ball TJ, Patterson DJ, Botoman VA. Tube dysfunction following percutaneous endoscopic gastrostomy and jejunostomy. *Gastrointest Endosc* 1990;36:261− 263.

CHAPTER 31

Complications of gastrointestinal tract interventional endoscopy

Roger A. Frost

Introduction

Endoscopes, both rigid and flexible, have been available for examination of the gastrointestinal tract for several decades. However, the development of flexible, fiberoptic endoscopes in the 1960s heralded the endoscopy explosion of the 1970s and 1980s, fueled by the ability of the endoscopist to perform therapeutic as well as diagnostic procedures. Continuing improvements in instrument design, operative technique, and training have made modern endoscopy remarkably safe, considering the enormous numbers of procedures performed. However, endoscopy is invasive and necessary precautions must be taken to minimize risks.

The role of the radiologist

In the UK and Europe, some gastrointestinal radiologists perform endoscopy as an integral part of their radiologic practice. This is much less common in North America, but all radiologists have an important role in complementing endoscopy, both diagnostically and in the case of complications, in their prevention, diagnosis, and therapy. For example, anatomic abnormalities may be demonstrated by prior barium studies, thus preventing complications such as perforation of an unsuspected pharyngeal pouch. Complications of endoscopy can readily be diagnosed and investigated by radiologic means and interventional techniques have a role in treating them. This chapter will deal with general complications of

endoscopy, and then complications specific to diagnostic and therapeutic procedures including esophageal dilatation, sclerotherapy, endoscopic retrograde cholangiopancreatography (ERCP), and colonoscopy.

How safe is endoscopy today?

In assessing the relative safety of endoscopy, it must be remembered that many studies of endoscopic complications are up to 20 years old and have usually been retrospective and therefore prone to underreporting. Their results must be interpreted not only in the light of improvements in instruments and technique, but also of the increased length and complexity of procedures, now often performed on elderly and frail patients.

Early retrospective series of endoscopic complications reported mortality rates of between 1:5000 and 1:10 000 [1–4]. However, more recent studies indicate that the true incidence is higher. Benjamin et al. [5] found a mortality of 1:2600 in 26 008 upper and lower gastrointestinal endoscopies performed on 19 970 patients. A prospective study of endoscopy just carried out by members of the British Society of Gastroenterology [6], found seven deaths in 13 036 diagnostic upper gastrointestinal endoscopies, giving a mortality of 1:1862. Five deaths were cardiopulmonary, one was due to perforation, and one to hemorrhage. This confirms the earlier finding that 60% or more of endoscopy-related deaths have a cardiopulmonary cause [1,3,4].

General complications of endoscopy

Complications related to sedation

Complications related to anesthesia, analgesia, and sedation are fully described in Chapters 1 and 2. Intravenous sedation is used for many endoscopic procedures. The most commonly used drugs are diazepam and midazolam. Pethidine is often used in addition to a benzodiazepine for ERCP and colonoscopy. It must be remembered that all three drugs are respiratory depressants and oxygen desaturation can occur, particularly in the elderly and those with cardiopulmonary disease. The patient must be carefully observed by endoscopy assistants. Supplemental oxygen can effectively prevent hypoxia [7] and should be used routinely in patients at risk. I believe that all patients having endoscopy should be monitored by means of pulse oximetry. This is particularly important in a darkened room, such as during an ERCP. Use of pulse oximetry enables a drop in oxygen saturation of the blood to be detected long before it is clinically apparent. Specific antagonists, naloxone for pethidine and flumazenil for benzodiazepines, must be available at all times.

Cardiopulmonary complications

Electrocardiographic (EKG) changes, usually transient, occur in approximately 38% of patients undergoing upper gastrointestinal endoscopy [8,9], and include sinus tachycardia, atrial or ventricular premature contractions, and ST segment changes. Mathew *et al.* [9] showed much higher rates of EKG changes in patients with cardiac disease (55%), and chronic pulmonary disease (89%), than in normal patients (19%). Serious ventricular arrhythmias and cardiac arrest are less common. The 1974 American Society for Gastrointestinal Endoscopy (ASGE) survey reported eight cardiac arrests in 211410 procedures with a mortality of 50%. Six patients had a procedure-related myocardial infarction, with one death [10]. Hancy *et al.* [11] reported 12 cardiac arrests in 150000 endoscopies with nine deaths. However, in their recent prospective study of British endoscopists, Quine *et al.* [6] report five cardiopulmonary deaths in 13036 upper gastrointestinal endoscopies (0.04%).

Transient EKG changes also occur during colonoscopy [12]. Two early retrospective series reported one myocardial infarction each in 31512 and 20139 colonoscopies, respectively [10,13]. However, the true incidence is likely to be much higher. Macrae *et al.* [14] reported one death from myocardial infarction in 5000 colonoscopies. A large-scale prospective survey is required.

Several workers have shown that cardiac arrhythmias are more likely to occur at times of hypoxemia [8,9,15]. This emphasizes the importance of patient monitoring and confirms that the greatest care must be taken in endoscoping cyanosed patients with severe pulmonary disease [16]. It is my experience that these are the patients at greatest risk of cardiopulmonary complications. However, full resuscitation facilities should *always* be readily available when patients are undergoing endoscopy (see also p. 47).

Complications related to infection (see also Chapter 5)

Patient to patient transmission of infection

There have been several well-documented miniepidemics of infection by *Salmonella* spp. that have been traced back to transmission by endoscopes or ancillary equipment [17,18]. The infection has usually resulted in a mild illness, although a few patients have become seriously ill. Transmission of *Helicobacter pylori* has also been demonstrated [19]. This organism causes chronic gastritis and is important in the etiology and recurrence of peptic ulceration.

Two viruses have given rise to the most concern about possible transmission of infection by endoscopes, i.e., hepatitis B (HBV) and the human immunodeficiency virus (HIV). Despite the high parenteral infectivity of HBV, prospective longitudinal studies have failed to demonstrate its transmission by endoscopes subsequently found to have been used in an infected patient [20,21]. Indeed, there has only been one case in which endoscopic transmission of HBV has been convincingly demonstrated [22]. HIV is much less infective than HBV parenterally [23] and the risk of enteral infection is likely to be still lower. There has, as yet, been no report of endoscopic transmission of HIV.

Colonization by opportunistic organisms

Endoscopes, endoscopic washing machines, and ancillary equipment, such as water bottles, are all liable to become contaminated by opportunistic organisms including *Pseudomonas aeruginosa* and *Staphylococcus epidermidis* [24]. The patients who are most likely to develop complications after the use of contaminated equipment are those who are immunocompromised or those undergoing ERCP [25]. In the latter group, the infected material may be injected directly into the ductal systems. Moreover, duodenoscopes are more difficult to clean because of the presence of an elevating bridge channel. They are generally used less frequently than gastroscopes and colonoscopes so that there is more time for organisms to proliferate in the instrument channels during storage.

Cleaning and disinfection of endoscopes and ancillary equipment

In order to prevent patient to patient transmission of infection and patient infection by instrument contaminants, it is essential that all instruments and accessories are thoroughly cleaned, disinfected, and dried before lists, between patients, and after lists. Axon [25] has recently and comprehensively reviewed procedures for cleaning and disinfection. Equipment should be subject to regular microbiologic surveillance to audit the effectiveness of cleaning and disinfection procedures. Organisms multiply in damp, warm conditions. Therefore, in order to prevent multiplication, endoscope channels should be force air-dried for 10 minutes at the end of lists prior to storage in well-ventilated, dry cupboards [26]. This additional period of drying must, of course, take place after the standard process of cleaning and disinfection.

Bacteremia and endocarditis

It has been shown that bacteria can be cultured from the blood of a percentage of patients during and after endoscopy [27]. Timing and frequency of cultures has varied between studies, but the highest rates of bacteremia have been reported for esophageal dilatation and sclerotherapy of varices at 45% and 31%, respectively [27]. Gastroscopy, ERCP, and colonoscopy all have bacteremia rates of 4–6% (27,28]. Although these latter rates are probably an underestimate [29], the organisms are almost always quickly cleared from the blood with no clinical sequelae [27,28]. The incidence of endocarditis resulting from endoscopy-induced bacteremia is extremely low, with only five convincing cases in the literature [30]. There are incidentally no documented reports of endoscopy-related bacteremia leading to infection of prosthetic joints.

Antibiotic prophylaxis for endoscopic procedures has been much debated. The Working Party of the British Society for Antimicrobial Chemotherapy has recommended that, for gastrointestinal procedures, the risk of developing endocarditis is so small that antibiotics need only be given to patients with prosthetic cardiac valves [31]. This recommendation was made, not because there is evidence that prosthetic valves are more susceptible to infection than natural valves, but because prognosis in the case of an infected prosthetic valve is worse. For adult patients not allergic to penicillin and who have not had penicillin more than once in the previous month, the recommended regimen is amoxycillin 1 g together with gentamicin 120 mg given intravenously immediately before the procedure, followed by amoxycillin 500 mg orally at 6 hours. Other adults should receive teicoplanin 400 mg and gentamicin 120 mg intravenously immediately before the procedure.

Upper gastrointestinal endoscopy

The major complications of upper gastrointestinal endoscopy are aspiration, perforation, and hemorrhage.

Aspiration

Aspiration pneumonia has been reported in four large retrospective series in between 0.01 and 0.8%, with a median of 0.1% [1,2,11,32], and with a mortality of between 10 and 60%. Aspiration of gastric contents into the lungs may occur if the stomach is not completely empty. Endoscopy should always be carried out on fasting patients, but gastric outlet obstruction and upper gastrointestinal bleeding increase the risk of aspiration. Similarly, a patient with achalasia may have a good deal of fluid and solid residue in the dilated esophagus and thus be at risk of aspiration. Local anesthetic throat sprays and heavy sedation suppress the gag reflex and may increase the risk of aspiration, particularly in the elderly [32]. To prevent aspiration, a sucker must always be instantly available in case regurgitation occurs, and the endoscopy table or trolley must be able to be tilted head down. Aspiration may occur both during endoscopy and in the recovery period. Patients should be encouraged to cough when the procedure has finished and should be recovered in the left lateral or semiprone position.

Aspiration pneumonia is a potentially serious complication and if aspiration is suspected and confirmed by a chest X-ray, prompt treatment with broad-spectrum antibiotics is indicated, together with vigorous physiotherapy.

Esophageal perforation

Perforation can occur from the hypopharynx to the duodenum, but the majority of cases occur in the esophagus. Perforation of the esophagus is a potentially life-threatening condition. Although it can occur during diagnostic esophagoscopy, it is more common after dilatation, palliative intubation of malignant strictures, and sclerotherapy. The outcome of perforation is very much dependent on the delay between perforation and diagnosis, so that endoscopists and radiologists should be alert to its possibility.

The incidence of perforation of the esophagus during diagnostic fiberoptic endoscopy was reported in early series at 0.1%, 0.03%, and 0.018%, respectively [1,10,33]. A prospective study of endoscopies recently carried out by members of the British Society of Gastroenterology (BSG) [6], showed six perforations in 13 036 endoscopies (0.046%) with one death. Therapeutic endoscopy has a much higher incidence of perforation, reported at 0.9% for dilatation of esophageal strictures [33], between 2 and 5% for pneumodilatation of achalasia of the cardia [34], and from 7.9 to 11% for palliative intubation of malignant strictures [33,35]. In the recent multicenter study by the BSG [6] there were six perforations in 554 dilatations of benign strictures (1.1%) with three deaths, giving an overall mortality of 0.5%. Perforation was found in 14 of 220 dilatations for malignant strictures (6.4%), with five deaths (procedure related mortality 2.3%).

Perforation at diagnostic endoscopy usually occurs with difficult intubations, inexperienced endoscopists, and in elderly, frail patients with distorted anatomy [33,36]. Perforation is most common in the pharynx and upper esophagus, where predisposing factors include a pharyngeal pouch, cervical osteophytes, and benign strictures or cricopharyngeal hypertrophy [4,37]. The modern, narrow, forward-viewing gastroscope allows intubation under direct vision which should effectively prevent esophageal perforation during diagnostic endoscopy in experienced hands. The older, oblique-viewing instruments were widely regarded as more likely to cause perforation [38], but modern oblique viewers do not have a traumatic tip. Side-viewing instruments, no longer used for gastroscopy but used for ERCP, cannot be passed under direct vision. They have a smooth, atraumatic tip and perforation is very rare, but great care must be taken to avoid undue force as the instrument is passed.

Perforation of the middle and lower thirds of the esophagus is usually secondary to dilatation but has been described after biopsy [39] and in the presence of severe esophagitis or ulceration [4]. I do not dilate immediately after biopsy, and delay dilatation in the presence of severe esophagitis or peptic ulceration until healing is underway.

Diagnosis

Esophageal perforation [40] should always be suspected if a patient complains of neck or chest pain after endoscopy or dilatation. Cervical perforation may also lead to hoarseness and dysphonia. Subcutaneous emphysema may be apparent. Thoracic perforation causes chest pain which may be retrosternal, epigastric, or interscapular. Swallowing saliva may be painful.

After dilatation, or other therapeutic esophagoscopy, patients should be observed until pain-free and then given a few sips of cold water. If pain persists, or if swallowing causes pain (other than a sore throat), then investigation for possible perforation should be carried out immediately [41] (Figs 31.1 & 31.2). In cervical perforation, a lateral neck radiograph may show air as a prevertebral streak or as more marked surgical emphysema. The prevertebral soft tissue space may later become widened. For perforations below the cervical region, the chest radiograph must be carefully searched for signs of surgical emphysema in the neck and for pneumomediastinum and pneumoperitoneum [42,43]. Pneumothorax and pleural effusions only occur if there is a free pleural communication. If perforation is suspected and there is no plain-film evidence, then a low-osmolar water-soluble contrast swallow is performed, followed by a barium swallow if there is still no evidence of perforation [44,45]. The swallow will define the anatomic site and extent of perforation, demonstrating whether there is free communication with the pleural space.

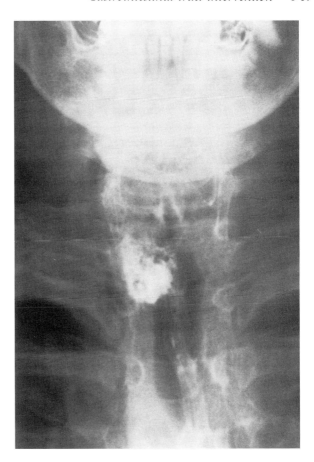

Fig. 31.1 Perforation of the cervical esophagus. A water-soluble contrast swallow 1 hour after esophageal dilatation shows a small perforation with a collection of contrast to the right of the esophagus. Note the streaks of surgical emphysema to the right of the spine.

Treatment

Endoscopic perforation of the esophagus is usually detected early [41]. For this reason, treatment can be instituted before significant contamination through the perforation occurs. Surgical treatment of all esophageal perforations has been advocated in the past, with an overall mortality of up to 30% [46]. However, conservative treatment has been shown to have a low mortality when careful patient selection is used and diagnosis takes place early [41,47]. Conservative treatment consists of: (i) keeping the patient strictly "nil by mouth" (spitting out all saliva if possible); (ii) administering broad-spectrum parenteral antibiotics; and (iii) intravenous hydration, together with parenteral nutrition. Some authors recommend continuous aspiration by nasoesophageal suction using a tube with multiple side holes placed across the level of the perforation [41].

Shaffer *et al.* [47] have refined the earlier criteria of Cameron *et al.* [48] for the selection of patients for conservative therapy. For thoracic perforation, they recommend

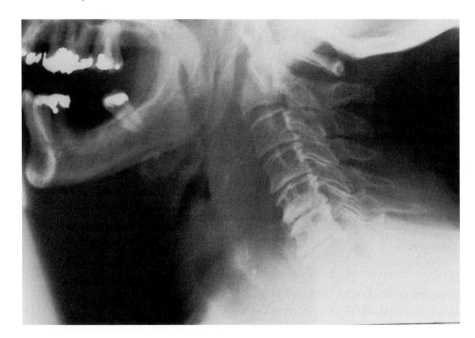

Fig. 31.2 Perforation of the cervical esophagus. Twenty-four hours after perforation, a lateral neck film shows widening of the prevertebral soft tissue space indicating a retropharyngeal collection.

conservative treatment if: (i) the patient is stable; (ii) perforation is diagnosed before major mediastinal contamination has occurred or after such a long delay that the patient has already demonstrated tolerance; and (iii) the disruption is demonstrated to be well contained within the mediastinum or a pleural loculus. Surgery remains the treatment of choice for unstable patients with sepsis, respiratory failure, or shock, for a large perforation with widespread contamination, for perforation of the intraabdominal esophagus, and for perforations with hydrothorax or pneumothorax.

In the case of cervical perforation, patients with a small perforation and little contamination may be managed conservatively. But, if there is a large tear with considerable contamination, then drainage via the neck, with or without repair, is advocated [49], in order to prevent retropharyngeal abscess formation which may extend to the mediastinum.

In patients who have had palliative intubation for an esophageal carcinoma, it is my practice to keep them nil by mouth until a water-soluble contrast swallow has been performed. If perforation is demonstrated, this is treated conservatively. It may be possible to adjust the position of the esophageal stent in such a way that the perforation is occluded [50], or it may be sealed by deploying a self-expanding, plastic-covered, metallic stent.

Hemorrhage

Bleeding is a rare complication of upper gastrointestinal endoscopy and usually settles spontaneously, or can be treated by endoscopic hemostasis. Its incidence is about 0.3% [10,39]. Bleeding occurs from biopsy of lesions in the stomach or duodenum, or from trauma to varices. Most endoscopists do not biopsy gastric or duodenal ulcers that have recently bled [4].

Miscellaneous complications

Transient, painful swelling of the parotid and of the submandibular glands has been reported after endoscopy [51–53]. The mechanism is unclear. Impaction of an endoscope is very rare and is usually caused by the instrument doubling back on itself in the esophagus or in a hiatus hernia [54,55]. The instrument can sometimes be disimpacted by gently advancing under fluoroscopic control, or it may be possible to grip the loop through the epigastrium, thus allowing the endoscope to be retracted straight [56]. If all else fails, laporotomy is required [55]. Incarcerated ventral hernia [57] and strangulated small intestinal obstruction [58] have both occurred as complications of endoscopy.

Percutaneous endoscopic gastrostomy (PEG)

PEG is a simple and safe means of establishing a feeding gastrostomy, which is now widely used. The technique is associated with a major complication rate of 3% and minor complication rate of 14% [59]. The major complications are intraperitoneal leak of gastric contents, gastrocolic fistula, infection around the stoma, pressure necrosis of the gastric wall by the retaining flange of the gastrostomy tube, and necrotizing fasciitis.

It is important to check the position of the retaining flange endoscopically at the end of the procedure. The flange should be pulled against the gastric wall to oppose the gastric serosa and peritoneum in order to prevent leakage, but there must not be sufficient traction to cause pressure necrosis [60]. The skin incision should be made slightly larger than the tube in order to prevent pressure ischemia of the skin and subsequent infection [61]. Although most authors recommend antibiotic prophylaxis with a broad-spectrum cephalosporin prior to PEG placement, trials have not clearly shown a benefit in reducing peristomal infection [62]. A purulent discharge commonly occurs around the tube. This does not indicate infection and should be treated with hydrogen peroxide and nonocclusive dressings.

Sclerotherapy

Endoscopic sclerotherapy of esophageal varices leads to a cumulative reported rate of complications of 20–40% [63–64], with a procedure-related mortality of 2%. There is no significant difference in complication rates between intravariceal and perivariceal injection. Ulceration is common, occurring in 31% [65] of patients and is so much a part of therapy that it cannot be considered a complication unless bleeding or perforation results, occurring in 9% and 2%, respectively [65]. Bronchopneumonia occurs in 6% [65]. Most procedure-related deaths are caused by perforation, aspiration, or bleeding.

Perforation may lead to pleural effusion, empyema, mediastinal collections, pericarditis, and even to cardiac tamponade [66,67]. A low-grade fever is common after sclerotherapy, but a mediastinal abscess must be considered if a spiking fever occurs. Perforation and tissue necrosis, usually due to deep injection of sclerosant, leads to abscess formation and periesophageal infection.

Intramural bleeding may occur leading to intramural hematoma. This can lead to the appearance of a mediastinal mass on the chest X-ray. A barium swallow will show a mural mass, which may be very extensive, deforming the esophagus and narrowing its lumen [68].

Stricturing of the esophagus occurs in up to 30% of cases after sclerotherapy [69], with a cumulative reported rate of 8% (65). The strictures are a result of cicatrization and fibrosis, which obliterates the varices. If dysphagia occurs, strictures may be dilated by means of bougies or balloons. The primary peristaltic wave in the distal esophagus may be impaired by sclerotherapy [70], but reflux is not increased [71]. Portal vein and mesenteric vein thrombosis have been reported [72,73].

ERCP

For the procedure of ERCP, a side-viewing duodenoscope is passed through the esophagus, stomach, and duodenum, to the papilla of Vater, where contrast is injected into the pancreatic and biliary systems. Therapeutic applications of ERCP include sphincterotomy and stone extraction, balloon dilatation, and stenting of biliary strictures.

ERCP is generally performed in the department of radiology. Although some radiologists perform ERCP, the procedures are usually undertaken by physicians or surgeons who are often regarded as unwelcome visitors to the department. The result is that all too often, screening for ERCP is left to the most junior radiologists or to inexperienced radiographers, resulting in the production of poor-quality films. Even if radiologists do not perform ERCP themselves, it is essential that gastrointestinal radiologists take an active interest in ERCP lists, thus ensuring high-quality films and interpretation. The presence of a skilled radiologist, or specialist radiographer, may prevent the occurrence of complications that can result from misinterpretation of the screening image by the endoscopist.

General complications are common to those of upper gastrointestinal endoscopy. However, the indications for ERCP and its therapeutic applications result in patients being examined with hepatic insufficiency, jaundice, and biliary sepsis. Hepatic insufficiency and jaundice increase the risk of sedation-related complications. Jaundiced patients, particularly in the presence of sepsis, often have an elevated urea and may readily develop renal failure. It is essential that they are not dehydrated prior to examination, so that intravenous fluid must be given to jaundiced patients being prepared for ERCP. The examination room is darkened for the procedure, so that careful patient monitoring, by means of pulse oximetry, is doubly important.

Contrast media

For many years, ERCP was exclusively performed using the then conventional, hyperosmolar, ionic contrast agents. More recently, nonionic, low-osmolar contrast agents have been increasingly used, the rationale being that the high osmolarity and ionic nature of the older agents is more likely to lead to pancreatic injury and pancreatitis.

Eight prospective, randomized studies have been performed to compare the quality of pancreatograms, and the incidence of hyperamylasemia and pancreatitis occurring with the use of ionic and nonionic contrast. Cunliffe *et al.* [74], Barkin *et al.* [75], and Banerjee *et al.* [76] all report a lower incidence of clinical pancreatitis in their nonionic, low-osmolar groups. Two studies [77,78] showed no difference in either pancreatitis or enzyme levels, while the remaining studies showed significantly higher pancreatic enzyme levels with ionic, high-osmolar agents. There was no difference in the quality of the pancreatogram between the ionic and nonionic groups.

Some authors have suggested that acinar filling may increase detection of small parenchymal lesions in the pancreas [79,80]. However, this technique has not gained popularity. Acinar filling increases the incidence of pancreatitis to about 26% for cases using ionic, hyperosmolar media compared to 6% using nonionic, low-osmolar media.

Although the numbers of patients in the above series are small, it now seems clear that the low-osmolarity agents are slightly safer for ERCP, although their considerably higher price has prevented many units from switching to them. Sherman and Lehman [81] recommend that the newer, more expensive agent should be reserved for high-risk patients with a history of post-ERCP pancreatitis or severe spontaneous pancreatitis. However, the cost of contrast is a very minor component of the overall cost of an ERCP service, and I believe that the advantages of the nonionic media considerably outweigh the extra cost. We use Omnipaque 240 (Nycomed (UK) Ltd, Birmingham) for all pancreatography and for cholangiography of nondilated bile ducts. If the bile ducts are dilated we switch to Omnipaque 140 to prevent the presence of small stones being obscured by dense contrast.

Allergy to contrast (see Chapter 13)

During ERCP, any contrast entering the bloodstream stems predominantly from the pancreas [82], via the pancreatic ductointerstitial venous pathway [83]. However, only small amounts of contrast agent are absorbed, with a very slow rise of concentration in the circulation. Probably for this reason, allergic reactions are rare. Moreira *et al.* [84] performed ERCP on 16 patients with a previous history of minor intravenous contrast reactions; no patient developed a subsequent reaction. Nevertheless, allergic reactions have occurred. One case of hypotensive shock has been reported [85], one grand mal seizure [81], and four cases of generalized rash [86,87]. Despite the very low risk of allergic reaction, it would seem prudent to use nonionic contrast for all patients with a history of reaction to intravenous contrast. If the previous reaction was severe, then extrapolating from the established protective value of pretreatment with steroids for intravenous contrast [88], two doses of methylprednisolone should be given 12 and 2 hours before the ERCP (see also p. 278).

Specific complications of ERCP

Pancreatitis and biliary sepsis are the main specific complications of diagnostic ERCP. Hemorrhage is the main complication of sphincterotomy, together with pancreatitis, biliary sepsis, and retroperitoneal perforation.

Diagnostic ERCP has an overall, generally retrospective, reported complication rate of 1–3%, with a mortality of 0.1–0.2% [89]. A British multicenter prospective study of 1928 patients undergoing ERCP showed a complication rate in 1980 of 2.4% with six deaths (0.3%) [90]. This same study found a complication rate of 10.8% in 855 patients undergoing endoscopic sphincterotomy with a mortality of 1% (Table 31.1).

Pancreatitis

Clinically significant pancreatitis occurs in 1–3% of patients undergoing ERCP and sphincterotomy [86,90–94]. Hyperamylasemia is practically universal after cannulation of the major duodenal papilla and pancreatography [95,96]. It can

Table 31.1 Prospective multicenter British study: complications of biliary sphincterotomy in 855 patients. (From Frost [90])

Complication	Patients	Surgery	Deaths
Hemorrhage	28 (3.3%)	9	3
Pancreatitis	26 (3%)	2	2
Cholangitis	19 (2.2%)	3	2
Perforation (retroperitoneal)	10	1	0
Impacted basket	4	4	0
Infected pseudocyst	1	0	1
Cardiopulmonary	3		1
Other	4		
Total	95 patients (11%)	19 (2%)	9 (1%)

occur following endoscopy without attempted cannulation [97] and some of the amylase may be salivary in origin [95]. Amylase should only be measured if a patient develops pain, suggestive of pancreatitis, that requires admission. It must be remembered that retroperitoneal perforation may cause pain very similar to that of pancreatitis and needs to be differentiated clinically from pancreatitis.

Etiology

The potential factors that may lead to pancreatitis are considered to be mechanical, hydrostatic, chemical, thermal, and microbiologic.

Clumsy cannulation technique, particularly pushing the cannula rather than gently lifting with the endoscope bridge, may traumatize the papilla and cause spasm and edema of the sphincters. Repeated attempts at cannulation may similarly lead to mechanical trauma and edema [98,99]. Fine-tipped catheters may cause submucosal injection of contrast, thus compromising drainage. Baskets and balloons, used to clear bile duct stones after sphincterotomy, may cause trauma to the pancreatic orifice. It has been observed that the incidence of hyperamylasemia and pancreatitis after ERCP is lower in patients who have a patent duct of Santorini draining via the minor duodenal papilla [100–101].

High volumes of contrast, high injection pressure, and repeated injections of contrast have all been implicated in causing pancreatitis. The repeated trauma of multiple attempts to cannulate the biliary tree is aggravated by multiple injections of contrast into the pancreatic duct [98]. Acinar filling occurs when the volume of contrast injected exceeds the capacity of the pancreatic duct (about 2 ml without spill). Rapid rate and high-pressure injection contributes to the development of acinar filling [102], which is associated with an increased incidence of pancreatitis [82,98,103]. Roszler and Campbell [104] showed a close correlation between acinar filling, subsequent opacification of the urinary tract, and the development of pancreatitis. It is thought that contrast is mainly absorbed from the pancreatic duct and that the appearance of a urogram suggests that sufficient volume and injection pressure of contrast has been used to cause acinar damage.

Pancreatic enzyme activation by pancreatography is a theoretical, but unproven, cause of pancreatitis due to auto-digestion. The chemical effects of contrast agents used for ERCP have already been discussed.

Thermal injury to the pancreatic duct may occur during sphincterotomy [105,106]. This occurs most profoundly if the sphincterotome lies in the pancreatic duct, rather than in the common bile duct, when a biliary sphincterotomy is performed (Fig. 31.3). It is essential to check the position of the sphincterotome in the common bile duct, by screening, before starting to cut. Excessive coagulation around the wire of the sphincterotome may lead to direct thermal damage to the pancreatic duct and to edema of the periductal tissues.

Microorganisms introduced into the pancreas from contaminated endoscopic equipment have, in rare cases, caused serious and sometimes fatal pancreatitis [107–109]. The

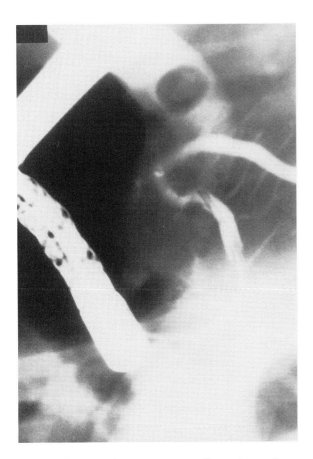

Fig. 31.3 Endoscopic sphincterotomy. A gallstone is seen in a dilated common bile duct. The sphincterotome lies in the pancreatic duct which is projected directly over the common bile duct, illustrating why it is essential to identify where the knife is before commencing a sphincterotomy.

organism that has been most often implicated is *Pseudomonas aeruginosa* due to its ability to colonize instruments [24,110]. The risk of complications of iatrogenic introduction of organisms is increased if there is obstruction of the duct system leading to stasis. *Staphylococcus epidermidis*, a skin or endoscope surface contaminant, has been isolated from blood cultures of patients after ERCP who have duct stasis [111]. Endoscopes must be scrupulously cleaned and disinfected before and between cases, and all ancillary equipment, including water bottles, biopsy valves, and catheters, must be thoroughly sterilized in order to minimize such complications [25].

Prevention

The risk of pancreatitis is lowered by careful technique and avoidance of the above risk factors. In particular, it is essential to ensure that all endoscopes and ancillary equipment are sterile. Overfilling of the pancreatic duct must be avoided by controlling the injection volume and injection pressure of contrast. This is best achieved by the endoscopist personally injecting by hand rather than by an assistant. I advocate the use of nonionic contrast media in preference to ionic. In the case of sphincterotomy, the use of cutting or a blend of cutting and coagulation diathermy current, together with careful selection of the length of wire in contact with the duct, prevents excessive heating and coagulation of tissue as the cut is made by short bursts of diathermy.

It is my practice to keep all patients on clear fluids for 6 hours after pancreatography. If significant trauma to the pancreatic orifice has occurred, due to repeated attempts at cannulation of the bile duct, intravenous fluids should be given overnight. Patients should not eat a large or fatty meal for 24 hours after ERCP.

Many pharmaceutical agents have been tried to prevent or to help resolve pancreatitis. However, clinical studies of antibiotics, glucagon, and aprotinin have failed to show significant benefit in preventing post-ERCP pancreatitis [81]. More recently, somatostatin has been shown to reduce the elevation of pancreatic enzymes, but not significantly to reduce the incidence of clinical pancreatitis [112].

Treatment

If pancreatic pain occurs in the first few hours after ERCP, the patient must be kept strictly nil by mouth and given intravenous fluids. Nasogastric suction is only necessary if nausea and vomiting are a problem. Pancreatitis will usually resolve over a few days (Fig. 31.4). After sphincterotomy, pancreatitis must be differentiated from retroperitoneal perforation. The latter may be diagnosed by the presence of retroperitoneal gas on the plain films or by retroperitoneal fluid or gas on ultrasound or computed tomography (CT) (Figs 31.5 & 31.6).

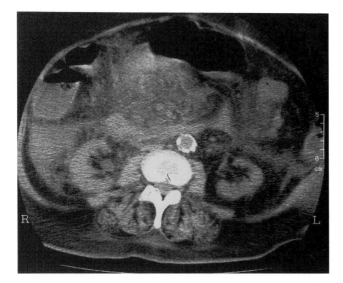

Fig. 31.4 Resolving post-ERCP pancreatitis. Computed tomography scan showing an extensive inflammatory mass. There is marked inflammatory change in the right pararenal and perirenal spaces.

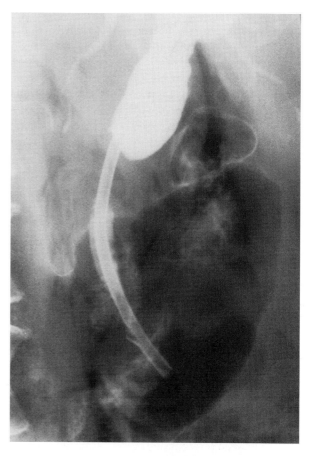

Fig. 31.6 Retroperitoneal perforation. The right kidney is again outlined by gas, but there are also curvilinear streaks of retroperitoneal gas projected over the pancreatic head. A sphincterotomy had been performed to facilitate stent placement.

Hemorrhage

Bleeding is the most frequent complication of endoscopic sphincterotomy, and the most common cause of death. Significant hemorrhage, requiring blood transfusion, occurs in 2.5–3.3%, with between 15 and 40% requiring laparotomy, and an overall mortality of around 10% [90,93,113, 114]. Bleeding usually occurs immediately, but may be delayed for a few hours. Secondary hemorrhage may rarely occur after a few days [115].

Brisk arterial hemorrhage only occurs with a large sphincterotomy as it is thought to stem from an aberrant branch of the retroduodenal artery. Large sphincterotomies are usually performed in an attempt to remove large stones. Profuse hemorrhage in early series required emergency surgery in 30% with a mortality of 50% [116]. The risk of bleeding is increased when an endoscopic sphincterotomy is enlarged [117], particularly at around 7 days when active granulation tissue has formed. The advent of effective mechanical lithotripters has now made very large sphincterotomies unnecessary [118]. In the rare case in which a stone cannot be

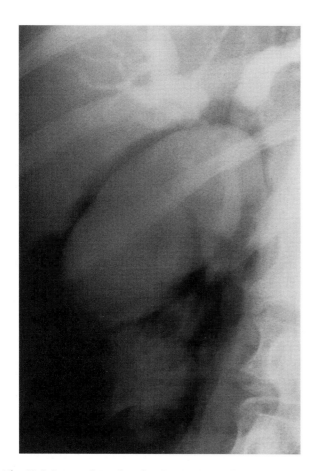

Fig. 31.5 Retroperitoneal perforation. A supine film shows gas in the perirenal space outlining the right kidney, following endoscopic sphincterotomy.

engaged in the lithotrite, it may be safer to place a biliary stent, without stone removal, rather than to enlarge an adequate sphincterotomy [119].

Bleeding more commonly takes place from small vessels in the edge of the sphincterotomy. The risk of bleeding is reduced by careful technique [94,120]. The incision should be made slowly with intermittent, blended diathermy current to ensure adequate, but not excessive, coagulation of the vessels in the edges of the cut. The wire of the sphincterotome should only be tightened a little and the power settings kept low in order to avoid a rapid "zipper" cut which is very likely to bleed. The patient's coagulation status must always be checked before sphincterotomy, and if deranged should be corrected with vitamin K if there is sufficient time or, if not, with fresh frozen plasma. There is an increased incidence of bleeding when tumors of the papilla of Vater are treated by means of sphincterotomy [114]. Complications, including hemorrhage, are no more common in patients with peripapillary duodenal diverticula, although the success rate of cannulation is reduced [121].

Treatment

Hemorrhage, other than brisk arterial bleeding, usually settles spontaneously and may be treated conservatively [90]. Balloon tamponade, using a dilatation balloon, can be effective with more profuse bleeding [122]. Injection of 1:10 000 adrenalin (epinephrine) into the edges of a bleeding sphincterotomy has been reported to stop hemorrhage [123], but is extremely difficult to perform if bleeding is profuse. If surgical treatment of bleeding becomes necessary, the edges of the sphincterotomy are oversewn with nonabsorbable sutures, even if bleeding has ceased when the duodenum is opened, and the sphincterotomy is converted into a formal sphincteroplasty. It may be necessary to consider ligation of the retroduodenal or gastroduodenal arteries [92,118].

Arteriography with selective cannulation and embolization has been reported to be effective [124]. However, the bleeding vessel is likely to be supplied by both sides of the pancreaticoduodenal arcade, so that this technique is only likely to prove effective if the vessel can be embolized very close to the site of bleeding.

Sepsis

Sepsis occurs after an ERCP, almost exclusively, if there is stasis within the biliary tree, the pancreatic duct, or within a pseudocyst in communication with the pancreatic duct [89]. Although iatrogenic introduction of microorganisms can occur (see Pancreatitis, p. 552), bacteria causing sepsis usually preexist within dilated, static ducts, particularly in the presence of stones. In the British multicenter study of sphincterotomy [90], cholangitis occurred in 2.2% with a mortality of 10%. The most important factor in the treatment and prevention of sepsis is the relief of obstruction and stasis. If obstruction is not relieved, or is only partially relieved, whether by endoscopic, percutaneous, or surgical drainage, then the incidence of sepsis will be very much higher [125,126].

Acute cholecystitis may occur after ERCP, usually if gallbladder stones are present, but is rare if prophylactic antibiotics are given [127]. However, the incidence increases to around 10% in patients who have cholangitis or in whom multiple procedures are required to clear the common bile duct of stones [128].

Early series reported a high mortality in those cases in which a pancreatic pseudocyst became infected after ERCP [86,129], which led to the general view that the presence of a pseudocyst was a contraindication to ERCP. However, it is now clear that pancreatography can be safely undertaken, provided that prophylactic antibiotics are given and that great care is taken to ensure that instruments and ancillary equipment are sterile. ERCP is a valuable predictor of the natural history of a pseudocyst in that it can establish whether or not a cyst connects with the duct system. Facilities should be available for surgical or percutaneous drainage of the pseudocyst within 24 hours, if required [89].

Prevention and treatment

As in all obstructed systems, injection of contrast into an obstructed, infected biliary tree, will increase pressure and lead to bacteremia. Every effort should be made to minimize the increase in pressure. If possible, bile should be aspirated from a dilated system before injecting contrast for cholangiography. Only enough contrast to establish the diagnosis should be injected, injecting with the catheter tip as close to the site of abnormality as possible. Great care should be taken not to distend the entire system with contrast.

By far the most important step in preventing and treating biliary sepsis is to provide good drainage as quickly as possible, preferably at the time of diagnostic ERCP, by means of sphincterotomy and stone extraction, placing a biliary stent, or insertion of a nasobiliary drain. If this is impossible, then the system should be drained percutaneously or surgically without delay. A sample of bile should always be taken for culture and sensitivity when an obstructed system is drained.

Prophylactic antibiotics are considered to be of value by most workers in reducing biliary and pancreatic sepsis [120,130,131]. The choice of antibiotic is important. Most broad-spectrum cephalosporins are poorly excreted into the bile. Excretion is further reduced in the presence of biliary obstruction [132]. However, the ureido penicillins — azlocillin, mezlocillin, and piperacillin — combine a very suitable broad-spectrum activity with high biliary excretion [133, 134]. I use piperacillin 2 g given parenterally 1 hour before the procedure for: all patients who have a gall bladder *in situ* containing stones; all patients with biliary obstruction; and all patients with common bile duct stones. The antibiotic is continued at 2 g three times daily for 24 hours in patients with gallstones, and for 48 hours in patients who have been stented for biliary obstruction. Patients with cholangitis may require 4 g three times daily. If bile culture shows an organism resistant to piperacillin, it will usually be sensitive to ciprofloxacin.

Retroperitoneal perforation

A long sphincterotomy, a short intramural segment of the distal common bile duct, and incisions outside the range of 11−1 o'clock, may lead to perforation and leakage of gas, duodenal fluids, and contrast into the retroperitoneum. This complication occurs in about 1% of sphincterotomies [90,94]. The reported mortality ranges from 0 [90 135] to 35% [116]. The risk of perforation in increased in patients with undilated ducts and papillary stenosis [136]. If perforation occurs, patients usually develop pain, tenderness, and fever, but may remain asymptomatic [135]. Perforation can usually be recognized at the time of the ERCP by the presence of gas or contrast in the retroperitoneum on a supine film [135]. CT or ultrasound scan may also demonstrate gas and fluid in the retroperitoneum, differentiating the complication from pancreatitis [137]. Surgical emphysema and even pneumothorax may occur.

Treatment

If the perforation is small and recognized early, then conservative management is usually successful [90,135,137]. Adequate biliary drainage will normally have been ensured by sphincterotomy, but if stones remain in the duct then it may be prudent to place a nasobiliary tube or a stent. The patient is kept nil by mouth, nasogastric suction is instituted, and intravenous fluids and antibiotics given. The progress of retroperitoneal collections can be monitored by CT or ultrasound and may require percutaneous drainage. Larger perforations may require surgical drainage, particularly if stones remain in the common bile duct which would be difficult to remove endoscopically. In addition to drainage of the retroperitoneum, the common bile duct is explored, stones removed and the duct closed over a T-tube.

Basket impaction

All early series of sphincterotomy reported cases of stones caught in baskets that could not be pulled through the sphincterotomy or released from the basket. This complication can generally be avoided by checking the size of a sphincterotomy by means of an occlusion balloon prior to using a basket to extract stones. However, with the advent of mechanical lithotripters, impaction need no longer be a problem. When impaction occurs, the basket is cut outside the biopsy valve and the endoscope is removed over the wire. The plastic sheath of the basket is replaced by a flexible, spiral, metal rod. Traction is applied to the wire, thus breaking the stone or the basket. There are reports of impacted stones in baskets being broken up by extracorporeal shock wave lithotripsy [138].

Long-term complications of endoscopic sphincterotomy

Patients have now been followed up for more than 10 years after sphincterotomy [114,139]. Hawes *et al.* [139] reviewed 148 postcholocystectomy patients, who underwent successful endoscopic sphincterotomy and duct clearance, over a period of 6−11 years. Fifteen patients (13%) had further biliary problems, including new stones and cholangitis. Five patients developed stenosis of the sphincterotomy. Three failed to respond to conservative and endoscopic treatment.

Miscellaneous complications

Guidewires and catheters may occasionally perforate biliary strictures or the ductal systems themselves. However, such perforation is hardly ever associated with significant sequelae [135,140]. Gallstones larger than about 24 mm in diameter may lead to gallstone obstruction (ileus) after sphincterotomy [141]. One 29-mm stone, after causing gallstone obstruction, fistulated from the bowel, leading to necrotizing fasciitis [142]. Traumatic rupture of the gastroepiploic artery, leading to hemoperitoneum, has been reported during an ERCP with sphincterotomy and stone removal [143].

Endoscopic biliary stent placement

The procedure of placement of a biliary stent, by means of ERCP, in the palliation of malignant obstructive jaundice, has a complication rate of 10%, with a procedure related mortality of 4%, and a 30-day mortality of 7% [144]. This compares favorably with palliative bypass surgery, particularly in elderly, frail patients. The complications of stenting are those of general endoscopy and ERCP, together with those of sphincterotomy if this is required for stent placement.

The main specific complication is blockage of the lumen of the stent by a sludge derived from protein, bilirubin, food particles, and bacteria [145]. Early signs of stent blockage include itching, darkening of the urine, right hypochondrial pain, and pyrexia. Rigors and cholangitis can rapidly follow [89]. At the first indication of blockage, the stent must be extracted as soon as possible and replaced with a new stent. A sample of bile should be obtained for culture and a broad-spectrum antibiotic given.

Colonoscopy

The colonoscope has become a very powerful diagnostic and therapeutic tool in the large bowel, allowing the detection and treatment of polypoid tumors and angiodysplasia. Colonoscopy is more difficult to perform than upper gastrointestinal endoscopy and can be uncomfortable for the patient. However, its ability to diagnose and treat small lesions, particularly those that are flat and cannot be reliably shown by barium enema, gives colonoscopy a strong and ever-growing place, with great potential for the detection and treatment of adenomas, so preventing the development of carcinoma.

Diagnostic colonoscopy

There are two major complications of diagnostic colonoscopy, perforation, and bleeding, with incidences from the literature of 0.17% and 0.03%, respectively [146].

Perforation

Perforation [147–150] can occur due to: (i) direct penetration or stretching trauma by the instrument tip or shaft; (ii) penetration by ancillary instruments such as biopsy forceps; or (iii) by pneumatic pressure. Perforation by pneumatic pressure is less common than by mechanical trauma and is due either to overdistension of the whole colon by insufflated gas, or overdistension of a closed segment. Impaction of the instrument tip in a diverticulum may either cause perforation directly or by pressure of insufflated gas [151]. The serosa is damaged more easily than the mucosa by overdistension or stretching. Serosal tears without mucosal injury can be regarded as incomplete perforations. They are thought to occur more commonly than is suspected and usually heal spontaneously [152,153].

The rectosigmoid junction and sigmoid colon are the most common sites of perforation [147,148], probably because they are the most difficult sites to intubate, particularly in the presence of diverticular disease or after pelvic surgery which leads to fixation of loops in the pelvis. However, the cecum is the segment of the colon most susceptible to pneumatic injury [154]. The incidence of perforation is increased by the presence of colonic strictures and colitis [147,149]. The risk of perforation is also increased by heavy sedation and general anesthesia [155].

Intraperitoneal perforation usually leads to immediate pain, abdominal distension, and gradual onset of peritonism, although silent perforation does occur [156], particularly in elderly patients. Free intraperitoneal air will be seen on the abdominal film. Acute tension pneumoperitoneum has been described, leading to elevation of both diaphragms and respiratory distress [157], which was rapidly relieved by placement of a percutaneous catheter.

Retroperitoneal perforation [39,148] is considerably less common than intraperitoneal and usually occurs from the rectum or posterior wall of the descending colon. It may not become apparent for hours or days after the procedure [146]. Due to the division of the retroperitoneum into compartments by fascial planes, the pattern of gas on abdominal films and CT will depend on the site of perforation. A rectal perforation allows gas to pass into the posterior pararenal space, with possible extension into the scrotum, mediastinum, and abdominal wall, while a sigmoid perforation allows gas to pass into the anterior pararenal space [148,158]. Subcutaneous emphysema may be palpable and patients may develop pneumothorax, pneumomediastinum, and pneumopericardium [159,160].

Immediate surgery is indicated for a frank, clinically apparent perforation [146]. Local debridement, primary closure of the perforation, and drainage of the peritoneal cavity or retroperitoneum are performed. If surgery is delayed, or there is gross contamination, then a colostomy may be required. Associated diverticulitis, carcinoma, or colitis will require resection. If the patient is asymptomatic, or has a small perforation with minimal pneumoperitoneum, or only a little retroperitoneal emphysema, treatment can be conservative [161], consisting of nil by mouth, intravenous fluids, and parenteral antibiotics.

Hemorrhage

Bleeding due to diagnostic colonoscopy is rare and usually stops spontaneously. It may occur from a biopsy site or due to avulsion of a polyp by biopsy forceps. Bleeding may occur without biopsy [162].

Miscellaneous complications

Bleeding may occur outside the colonic lumen and results from tearing of the mesentery or colonic ligaments by pushing, pulling, or twisting forces [146]. There are reports of hematoma of the sigmoid mesocolon [148], laceration of the mesentery [13], ruptured spleen [161], laceration of the liver and spleen [163], and even avulsion of the spleen [148].

There have been 12 reports of splenic injury secondary to colonoscopy [164,165]. Most patients experience left upper quadrant pain with referral to the left shoulder within a few hours, but the diagnosis is sometimes delayed. Splenic hematoma, capsular tear, and rupture must be considered in the differential diagnosis of left-sided abdominal pain after colonoscopy and may be readily investigated by ultrasound or CT.

Pneumatic perforation of the ileum has been described [166]. Colonoscopy may rarely cause dissection of gas into the wall of the bowel and thus to *Pneumatosis coli* [167]. Volvulus of the cecum with gangrene [168] and volvulus of the sigmoid [13] have occurred. Colonoscopy can be hazardous in patients with acute colitis. The risk of perforation has been discussed, but toxic megacolon may also complicate colonoscopy [150], as may the appearance of portal vein gas [169]. A colonoscope may become impacted in a hernia [170], or the procedure may cause a hernia to become incarcerated [171]. These latter complications can be avoided if the presence of a hernia is regarded as a contraindication to colonoscopy, or if reduction of the hernia is maintained during the procedure by external pressure.

Therapeutic colonoscopy

The main complications of colonoscopic polypectomy are hemorrhage, perforation, and the postpolypectomy coagulation syndrome.

Hemorrhage has a reported incidence of about 1.4% with a mortality of 0.03% [146], although this incidence is very much dependent on the experience of the endoscopist and will be higher in the learning phase [155]. Primary hemorrhage usually occurs immediately but secondary hemorrhage may be delayed for days or even 1–2 weeks [162]. Bleeding occurs at the time of polypectomy if the vessels in the stalk are not fully coagulated before the polyp separates. If bleeding occurs, the pedicle should be snared just tightly enough to stop bleeding. Pressure is maintained for several minutes to allow coagulation to occur. It is preferable to avoid diathermy as this makes it difficult to remove the snare without producing further bleeding [172]. Other hemostatic maneuvers, such as injection of 1 : 10 000 epinephrine into the bleeding site, use of the heater probe, and selective mesenteric artery cannulation with infusion of vasopressin have all been used, but bleeding will often settle spontaneously [30,146]. Surgery is only rarely required [155,162]. Delayed hemorrhage can be effectively treated by repeat colonoscopy and endoscopic hemostatic therapy [173].

Perforation during therapeutic procedures is more than twice as common than at diagnostic colonoscopy, with an incidence of about 0.44% [146]. It usually occurs due to mechanical damage from the snare or accidental entrapment of bowel wall within the snare [146]. Alternately, excessive coagulation of the bowel wall may lead to perforation which can be delayed [174]. Frank perforation will require surgery, the management being essentially the same as that for perforation occurring at diagnostic colonoscopy.

Postpolypectomy coagulation syndrome [175] occurs as a result of transmural thermal injury to the colon without perforation. The patient suffers abdominal pain, pyrexia, and localized peritonitis. There is no plain-film evidence of perforation and recovery takes place with conservative treatment, again including nil by mouth, intravenous fluids, and parenteral antibiotics.

Miscellaneous complications

A 10% solution of mannitol is a very effective bowel preparation for colonoscopy. However, it can lead to production of hydrogen in the colon with the risk of explosion during the use of diathermy [176]. An intussuscepted appendix may mimic a polyp. Endoscopic "polypectomy" of the appendix may lead to perforation and peritonitis [177]. Accidental removal of the stoma of a ureterosigmoidostomy has also been reported [178], leading to renal sepsis and nephrectomy.

References

1 Schiller KFR, Cotton PB, Salmon PR. The hazards of digestive fibre-endoscopy: a survey of British experience. *Gut* 1972;13: 1027.

2 Colin-Jones DG, Cockel R, Schiller KFR. Current endoscopic practice in the United Kingdom. *Clin Gastroenterol* 1978;7: 775–786.

3 Silvis SE, Nebel O, Rogers G, Sugawa C, Mandelstam P. Endoscopic complications. Results of the 1974 American Society for Gastrointestinal Endoscopy Survey. *J Am Med Assoc* 1976;235: 928–930.

4 Katon RM. Complications of upper gastrointestinal endoscopy in the gastrointestinal bleeder. *Digest Dis Sci* 1981;26:47S–54S.

5 Benjamin S, Kruss DM, Fleischer DE. Cardiopulmonary complications are not increased during therapeutic EGD and colonoscopy. *Gastrointest Endosc* 1990;36:186A.

6 Quine MA, Bell GD, McCloy RF, Charlton JE, Devlin HB, Hopkins A. Prospective audit of upper gastrointestinal endoscopy in two regions of England: safety, staffing, and sedation methods. *Gut* 1995;36:462–467.

7 Griffin SM, Chung SCS, Leung JWC, Li AKC. Effect of intranasal oxygen on hypoxia and tachycardia during endoscopic cholangiopancreatography. *Br Med J* 1990;300:83–84.

8 Levy N, Abinader E. Continuous electrocardiographic monitoring with Holter electrocardiocorder throughout all stages of gastroscopy. *Am J Digest Dis* 1977;22:1091–1096.

9 Mathew PK, Ona FV, Damevski K, Wallace WA. Arrythmias during upper gastrointestinal endoscopy. *Angiology* 1979;30: 834–840.

10 Mandelstam P, Sugawa C, Silvis SE, Nebel OT, Rogers BH. Complications associated with esophagogastroduodenoscopy and with esophageal dilation. An analysis of the 1974 ASGE Survey. *Gastrointest Endosc* 1976;23:16–19.

11 Hancy A, Condat M, Cougard A *et al.* Les accidents de la fibroscopie oeso-gastro-duodenuale. Enquete nationale portant sur 150 000 fibroscopies oeso-gastro-duodenales. *Ann Gastroenterol Hepatol* 1977;13:101–110.

12 Vawter M, Ruiz R, Alaama A, Aronow WS, Dagradi AE. Electrocardiographic monitoring during colonoscopy. *Am J Gastroenterol* 1975;63:155–157.

13 Smith LE. Fiberoptic colonoscopy: complications of colonoscopy and polypectomy. *Dis Colon Rectum* 1976;19:407–412.

14 Macrae FA, Tan KG, Williams CB. Towards safer colonoscopy: a report on the complications of 5000 diagnostic or therapeutic colonoscopies. *Gut* 1983;24:376–383.

15 Lieberman DA, Wuerker CK, Katon RM. Cardiopulmonary risk of esophagogastroduodenoscopy: Role of endoscope diameter

and systemic sedation. *Gastroenterology* 1985;88:468−472.

16 Rostykus PS, McDonald GB, Albert RK. Upper intestinal endoscopy induces hypoxaemia in patients with obstructive pulmonary disease. *Gastroenterology* 1980;78:488−491.

17 O'Connor HJ, Axon ATR. Gastrointestinal endoscopy: infection and disinfection. *Gut* 1983;24:1067−1077.

18 Dwyer DM, Klein G, Istre GR, Robinson MG, Neumann DA, McCoy GA. *Salmonella* newport infections transmitted by fiberoptic colonoscopy. *Gastrointest Endosc* 1987;33:84−87.

19 Langenberg W, Rauws EA, Oudbier JH, Tytgat GNJ. Patient-to-patient transmission of *Campylobacter pylori* infection by fiberoptic gastroduoendoscopy and biopsy. *J Inf Dis* 1990;161: 507−511.

20 Villa E, Pasquinelli C, Rigo G *et al.* Gastrointestinal endoscopy and HBV infection: no evidence for a causal relationship. A prospective controlled study. *Gastrointest Endosc* 1984;30: 15−17.

21 Kok ASF, Lai CL, Hui WM *et al.* Absence of transmission of hepatitis B by fibreoptic upper gastrointestinal endoscopy. *J Gastroenterol Hepatol* 1987;2:175−180.

22 Birnie GG, Quigley EM, Clements GB, Follett EAC, Watkinson G. Endoscopic transmission of hepatitis B virus. *Gut* 1983;24: 171−174.

23 McEvoy M, Porter K, Mortimer P, Simmons N, Shanson D. Prospective study of clinical, laboratory and ancillary staff with accidental exposures to blood or body fluids from patients infected with HIV. *Br Med J* 1987;294:1595−1597.

24 Noy MF, Harrison L, Holmes GK, Cockel R. The significance of bacterial contamination of fibreoptic endoscopes. *J Hosp Infect* 1980;1:53−61.

25 Axon ATR. Disinfection of endoscopic equipment. *Baillieres Clin Gastroenterol* 1991;5:61−77.

26 Alfa MJ, Sitter DL. In-hospital evaluation of contamination of duoendoscopes: a quantitative assessment of the effect of drying. *J Hosp Infect* 1991;19:89−98.

27 Botoman VA, Surawicz CM. Bacteremia with gastrointestinal endoscopic procedures. *Gastrointest Endosc* 1986;32:342−346.

28 Shorvon PJ, Eykyn SJ, Cotton PB. Gastrointestinal instrumentation, bacteraemia and endocarditis. *Gut* 1983;24:1078−1093.

29 Pelican G, Hentges D, Butt J, Haag T, Rolfe R, Hutcheson D. Bacteremia during colonoscopy. *Gastrointest Endosc* 1977;23: 33−35.

30 Taylor MB. Complications of upper endoscopy and colonoscopy. In: Taylor MB, ed. *Gastrointestinal Emergencies.* Baltimore: Williams & Wilkins, 1992;551−561.

31 Report of a Working Party of the British Society for Antimicrobial Chemotherapy. The antibiotic prophylaxis of infective endocarditis. *Lancet* 1990;335:88−89. (Updated in *Lancet* 1992; 339:1292−1293.)

32 Gilbert DA, Silverstein FE, Tedesco FJ and 277 members of the American Society for Gastrointestinal Endoscopy. National ASGE survey on upper gastrointestinal bleeding: complications of endoscopy. *Digest Dis Sci* 1981;26:55S−59S.

33 Dawson J, Cockel R. Oesophageal perforation at fibreoptic gastroscopy. *Br Med J* 1981;283−583.

34 Vantrappen G, Hellemans J. Treatment of achalasia and related motor disorders. *Gastroenterology* 1980;79:144−154.

35 Ogilvie AL, Dronfield MW, Ferguson R, Atkinson M. Palliative intubation of eosophagogastric neoplasms at fibreoptic endoscopy. *Gut* 1982;23:1060−1067.

36 Wesdorp ICE, Bartelsman JFW, den Hartog Jager FCA, Huibregtse K, Tytgat GN. Results of conservative treatment of

benign oesophageal strictures: a follow-up study in 100 patients. *Gastroenterology* 1982;82:487−493.

37 Wright RA. Upper-esophageal perforation with a flexible endoscope secondary to cervical oestophytes. *Digest Dis Sci* 1980;25: 66−68.

38 Starlinger M, Dinstl K, Schlessel R. Perforation of the oesophagus with an oblique-viewing endoscope in a patient with caustic stenosis. *Endoscopy* 1978;10:209−210.

39 Shahmir M, Schuman BM. Complications of fiberoptic endoscopy. *Gastrointest Endosc* 1980;26:86−91.

40 Ajalat GM, Mulder DG. Esophageal perforations. The need for an individualized approach. *Arch Surg* 1984;119:1318−1320.

41 Wesdorp ICE, Bartelsman JFW, Huibregtse K, den Hartog Jager FCA, Tytgat GN. Treatment of instrumental oesophagal perforation. *Gut* 1984;25:398−404.

42 Parkin GJ. The radiology of perforated oesophagus. *Clin Radiol* 1973;24:324−332.

43 DeMeester TR. Perforation of the esophagus. *Ann Thorac Surg* 1986;42:231−232.

44 Dodds WJ, Stewart ET, Vlymen WJ. Appropriate contrast media for evaluation of esophageal disruption. *Radiology* 1982;144: 439−441.

45 Foley MJ, Ghahremani GG, Rogers LF. Reappraisal of contrast media used to detect upper gastrointestinal perforations: comparison of ionic water-soluble media with barium sulfate. *Radiology* 1982;144:231−237.

46 Bergdahl L, Henze A. The treatment of oesophageal perforations. *Scand J Thorac Cardiovasc Surg* 1978;12:137−141.

47 Shaffer HA, Valenzuela G, Mittal RK. Esophageal perforation. A reassessment of the criteria for choosing medical or surgical therapy. *Arch Int Med* 1992;152:757−761.

48 Cameron JL, Kieffer RF, Hendrix TR, Mehigan DG, Baker RR. Selective nonoperative management of contained intrathoracic esophageal disruptions. *Ann Thorac Surg* 1979;27:404−408.

49 Prinsley PR, Murrant NJ. Cervical esophageal perforation caused by diagnostic flexible esophagoscopy. *J Otolaryngol* 1989;18: 314−316.

50 Fulton RL, Garrison RN, Polk HC. The nonoperative approach to esophageal perforation due to Celestin tube placement. *Arch Surg* 1979;114:90−91.

51 Shields HM, Soloway RD, Long WB, Weiss JB. Bilateral recurrent parotid swelling after endoscopy. *Gastroenterology* 1977; 73:164−165.

52 Gardon MJ. Transient submandibular swelling following esophagoduodenoscopy. *Am J Digest Dis* 1976;21:507−508.

53 Nijhawan S, Rai RR. Parotid swelling after upper gastrointestinal endoscopy. *Gastrointest Endosc* 1992;38:94.

54 Braucher RE, Kirschner JB. Case-report: impacted fibrescope. *Gastrointest Endosc* 1965;12:20.

55 Barrett B. New instruments, new horizons, new hazards. The impaction injury. *Gastrointest Endosc* 1970;16:142.

56 Gronlund B, Svendsen LB. Management of endoscopic impaction using "the gastric grip." *Endoscopy* 1993;25:375−376.

57 Patel NM, Marks LM. Incarcerated ventral hernia — a complication after oesophagogastroduodenoscopy. *J Clin Gastroenterol* 1982;4:257−258.

58 Pollard EJ, Roberts RK, Nye JA. Strangulated small intestinal obstruction following upper gastrointestinal panendoscopy. *Gastrointest Endosc* 1977;23:166−167.

59 Foutch PG, Haynes WC, Bellapravalu S, Sanowski RA. Percutaneous endoscopic gastrostomy (PEG). A new procedure comes of age. *J Clin Gastroenterol* 1986;8:10−15.

60 Chung RS, Schertzer M. Pathogenesis of complications of percutaneous endoscopic gastrostomy. A lesson in surgical principles. *Am Surg* 1990;56:134−137.

61 Steffes C, Weaver DW, Bouwman DL. Percutaneous endoscopic gastrostomy. New technique − old complications. *Am Surg* 1989;55:273−277.

62 Kozarek RA, Ball TJ, Patterson DT. Prophylactic antibiotics in percutaneous endoscopic gastrostomy (PEG): need or nuisance? *Gastrointest Endosc* 1986;32:147−148.

63 Schuman BM, Beckman JW, Tedesco FJ, Griffin JW, Assad RT. Complications of endoscopic injection sclerotherapy: a review. *Am J Gastroenterol* 1987;82:823−830.

64 Kahn D, Jones B, Bornman PC, Terblanche J. Incidence and management of complications after injection sclerotherapy: a ten year prospective evaluation. *Surgery* 1989;105:160−165.

65 Sauerbruch T, Fischer G, Ansari H. Variceal injection sclerotherapy. *Baillieres Clin Gastroenterol* 1991;5:131−153.

66 Saks BJ, Kilby AE, Dietrich PA, Coffin LH, Krawitt EL. Pleural and mediastinal changes following endoscopic injection sclerotherapy of esophageal varices. *Radiology* 1983;149:639−642.

67 Tabibian N, Schwartz JT, Smith JL, Graham DY. Cardiac tamponade as a result of endoscopic sclerotherapy: report of a case. *Surgery* 1987;102:546−547.

68 Jones DB, Frost RA, Goodacre RL. Intramural hematoma of the esophagus − a complication of endoscopic injection sclerotherapy. *Gastrointest Endosc* 1986;32:239−240.

69 Haynes WC, Sanowski RA, Foutch PG, Belapravalu S. Esophageal strictures following endoscopic variceal sclerotherapy: clinical course and response to dilatation therapy. *Gastrointest Endosc* 1986;32:202−205.

70 Reilly JJ, Schade R, Van Thiel DS. Esophageal function after injection sclerotherapy: pathogenesis of esophageal stricture. *Am J Surg* 1984;147:85−88.

71 Sauerbruch T, Wirsching R, Holl J, Grobl J, Weinzierl M. Effects of repeated injection sclerotherapy on acid gastro-oesophageal reflux. *Gastrointest Endosc* 1986;32:81−83.

72 Hunter GC, Steinkirchner T, Burbige EJ, Guernsey JM, Putnam CW. Venous complications of sclerotherapy for esophageal varices. *Am J Surg* 1988;156:497−501.

73 Goldberg H, Fabry TL. Mesenteric thrombosis following sclerotherapy during vasopression infusion: mechanism and therapeutic implications. *J Clin Gastroenterol* 1989;11:56−57.

74 Cunliffe WJ, Cobden I, Lavelle MI, Lendrum R, Tait NP, Venables CW. A randomised, prospective study comparing two contrast media in ERCP. *Endoscopy* 1987;19:201−202.

75 Barkin JS, Casal GL, Reiner DK, Goldberg RI, Phillips RS, Kaplan S. A comparative study of contrast agents for endoscopic retrograde pancreatography. *Am J Gastoenterol* 1991;86:1437−1441.

76 Banerjee AK, Grainger SL, Thompson RPH. Trial of low versus high osmolar contrast media in endoscopic retrograde cholangiopancreatography. *Br J Clin Pract* 1990;44:445−447.

77 Hannigan BF, Keeling PWN, Slavin B, Thompson RPH. Hyperamylasemia after ERCP with ionic and non-ionic contrast media. *Gastrointest Endosc* 1985;31:109−110.

78 Hamilton I, Lintott DJ, Rothwell J, Axon ATR. Metrizamide as contrast medium in endoscopic retrograde cholangiopancreatography. *Clin Radiol* 1982;33:293−295.

79 Lavelle MI, Tait NP, Walsh T, Anderson D, Record CO. Demonstration of pancreatic parenchyma by digital subtraction techniques during endoscopic retrograde cholangiopancreatography. *Clin Radiol* 1985;36:405−407.

80 Twomey B, Wilkins RA, Levi AJ. Pancreatic parenchymography using metrizamide. *Gut* 1982;23:462A.

81 Sherman S Lehman GA. ERCP − and endoscopic sphincterotomy − induced pancreatitis. *Pancreas* 1991;6:350−367.

82 Sable RA, Rosenthal WS, Siegel J, Ho R, Jankowski RH. Absorption of contrast medium during ERCP. *Digest Dis Sci* 1983;28:801−806.

83 Waldron RL, Luse SA, Wollowick HE, Seaman WB. Demonstration of a retrograde pancreatic pathway: correlation of roentgenographic and electron microscopic studies. *Am J Roentgenol* 1971;111:695−699.

84 Moreira VF, Merono E, Larraona JL *et al.* ERCP and allergic reactions to iodised contrast media. *Gastrointest Endosc* 1985;31:293.

85 Gmelin E, Kramann R, Weiss H-D. Kontrastmittelzwischenfall bei einer endoscopischen retrograden Cholangiopankreatographie. *Munch Med Wschr* 1977;119−1439.

86 Bilbao MK, Dotter CT, Lee TG, Katon RM. Complications of endoscopic retrograde cholangiopancreatography (ERCP). A study of 10 000 cases. *Gastroenterology* 1976;70:314−320.

87 Lorenz R. Allergic reaction to contrast medium after endoscopic retrograde pancreatography. *Endoscopy* 1990;22:196.

88 Lasser EC, Berry CC, Talner LB *et al.* Pretreatment with corticosteroids to alleviate reactions to intravenous contrast material. *New Engl J Med* 1987;317:845−849.

89 Cotton PB. Complications of ERCP and its therapeutic applications. In: Taylor MB, ed. *Gastrointestinal Emergencies.* Baltimore: Williams & Wilkins, 1992:562−567.

90 Frost RA. Prospective multicentre study of British Sphincterotomy: initial results and complications. *Gut* 1984;25:A549.

91 Cotton PB, Frost RA, Shorvon PJ. Computer analysis of a decade of ERP. *Gut* 1982;23:A432.

92 Leese T, Neoptolemos JP, Carr-Locke DL. Successes, failures, early complications and their management following endoscopic sphincterotomy: results in 394 consecutive patients from a single centre. *Br J Surg* 1985;72:215−219.

93 Vaira D, d'Anna L, Ainley C *et al.* Endoscopic sphincterotomy in 1000 consecutive patients. *Lancet* 1989;ii:431−434.

94 Geenen JE, Vennes JA, Silvis SE. Resume of a seminar on endoscopic retrograde sphincterotomy (ERS). *Gastrointest Endosc* 1981;27:31−38.

95 Skude G, Wehlin L, Maruyama T, Ariyama J. Hyperamylasaemia after duodenoscopy and retrograde cholangiopancreatography. *Gut* 1976;17:127−132.

96 Weaver DW, Sugawa C, Bouwman DL, Altshuler J. Isoamylase analysis in patients undergoing ERCP. *Gastrointest Endosc* 1983;29:175A.

97 Lifton L, Brooks C, Rosson R, Scheig R. The effect of UGI endoscopy on serum amylase. *Gastroenterology* 1975;68:936A.

98 Hamilton I, Lintott DJ, Rothwell J, Axon ATR. Acute pancreatitis following endoscopic retrograde cholangiopancreatography. *Clin Radiol* 1983;34:543−546.

99 Podolsky I, Haber CB, Kortan P, Gray R. Risk factors for pancreatitis following ERCP: a prospective study. *Am J Gastroenterol* 1987;82:972A.

100 Mairose UB, Wurbs D, Classen M. Santorini's duct − an insignificant variant from normal or an important overflow valve? *Endoscopy* 1978;10:24−29.

101 Arakawa S, Ueno F, Iwamura K. Evaluation of the role of Santorini's duct by digital subtraction endoscopic retrograde pancreatography. *Am J Gastroenterol* 1988;83:1072A.

102 Kivisaari L. Contrast absorption and pancreatic inflammation

following experimental ERCP. *Invest Radiol* 1979;14:493−497.

103 LaFerla G, Gordon S, Archibald M, Murray WR. Hyperamylasaemia and acute pancreatitis following endoscopic retrograde cholangiopancreatography. *Pancreas* 1986;1:160−163.

104 Roszler MH, Campbell WL. Post-ERCP pancreatitis: association with urographic visualization during ERCP. *Radiology* 1985; 157:595−598.

105 Sivak MV. Endoscopic management of bile duct stones. *Am J Surg* 1989;158:228−240.

106 Classen M. Endoscopic papillotomy. In: Sivak M, ed. *Gastroenterologic Endoscopy*. Philadelphia: WB Saunders, 1987;631−651.

107 Doherty DE, Falko JM, Lefkovitz N, Rogers J, Fromkes J. *Pseudomonas aeruginosa* sepsis following retrograde cholangiopancreatography (ERCP). *Digest Dis Sci* 1982;27:169−170.

108 Classen DC, Jacobson JA, Burke JP, Jacobson JT, Evans RS. Serious *Pseudomonas* infections associated with endoscopic retrograde cholangiopancreatography. *Am J Med* 1988;84: 590−596.

109 Godiwala T, Andry M, Agrawal N, Ertan A. Consecutive *Serratia marcescens* infections following endoscopic retrograde cholangiopancreatography. *Gastrointest Endosc* 1988;34:345−347.

110 Axon ATR, Phillips I, Cotton PB, Avery SA. Disinfection of gastrointestinal fibre endoscopes. *Lancet* 1974;i:656−658.

111 Dutta SK, Cox M, Williams RB, Eisenstat TE, Standiford HC. Prospective evaluation of the risk of bacteremia and the role of antibiotics in ERCP. *J Clin Gastroenterol* 1983;5:325−329.

112 Bordas JM, Toledo V, Mondelo F, Rodes J. Prevention of pancreatic reactions by bolus somatostatin administration in patients undergoing endoscopic retrograde cholangiopancreatography and endoscopic sphincterotomy. *Horm Res* 1988;29: 106−108.

113 Ostroff JW, Shapiro HA. Complications of endoscopic sphincterotomy. In: Jacobson I, ed. *ERCP: Diagnostic and Therapeutic Applications*. New York: Elsevier, 1989;61−73.

114 Seifert E. Long term follow up after endoscopic sphincterotomy (EST). *Endoscopy* 1988;20:232−235.

115 Finnie IA, Tobin MV, Morris AI, Gilmore IT. Late bleeding after endoscopic sphincterotomy for bile duct calculi. *Br Med J* 1991; 302:1114.

116 Safrany L. Endoscopic treatment of biliary tract diseases. An international study. *Lancet* 1978;ii:983−985.

117 Goodall RJR. Bleeding after endoscopic sphincterotomy. *Ann Roy Coll Surg Engl* 1985;67:87−88.

118 Siegel JH, Ben-Zvi JS, Pullano WE. Mechanical lithotripsy of common bile duct stones. *Gastrointest Endosc* 1990;36:351−356.

119 Cairns SR, Dias L, Cotton PB, Salmon PR, Russell RCG. Additional endoscopic procedures instead of urgent surgery for retained common bile duct stones. *Gut* 1989;30:535−540.

120 Safrany L, Cotton PB. Endoscopic management of choledocholithiasis. *Surg Clin N Am* 1982;6:825−836.

121 Vaira D, Dowsett JF, Hatfield ARW *et al*. Is duodenal diverticulum a risk factor for sphincterotomy? *Gut* 1989;30:939−942.

122 Staritz M, Ewe K, Goerg K, Meyer zum Buschenfelde KH. Endoscopic balloon tamponade for conservative management of severe hemorrhage following endoscopic sphincterotomy. *Z Gastroenterol* 1984;22:644−646.

123 Griim H, Soehendra N. Unterspiritzung Behandlung der Papillotomieblutung. *Deutsch Med Wochenschr* 1983;108:1512−1514.

124 Saeed M, Kadir S, Kaufman SL, Murray RR, Milligan F, Cotton PB. Bleeding following endoscopic sphincterotomy: angiographic management by transcatheter embolisation. *Gastrointest*

Endosc 1989;35:300−303.

125 Vennes JA, Jacobson JR, Silvis SE. Endoscopic cholangiography for biliary system diagnosis. *Ann Int Med* 1974;80:61−64.

126 Deviere J, Motte S, Dumonceau JM, Serruys E, Thys JP, Cremer M. Septicemia after endoscopic retrograde cholangiopancreatography. *Endoscopy* 1990;22:72−75.

127 Escourrou J, Cordova JA, Lazorthes F, Frexinos J, Ribet A. Early and late complications after endoscopic sphincterotomy for biliary lithiasis with and without the gall bladder "*in situ*." *Gut* 1984;25:598−602.

128 Davidson BR, Neoptolemos JP, Carr-Locke DL. Endoscopic sphincterotomy for common bile duct calculi in patients with gall bladder *in situ* considered unfit for surgery. *Gut* 1988;29: 114−120.

129 James EC, Collin DB. Sepsis complications in endoscopic retrograde cholangiopancreatography. *Am Surg* 1976;42:229−232.

130 Ferguson D, Sivak MV. Indication, contraindication and complications in ERCP. In: Sivak MV, ed. *Gastroenterologic Endoscopy*. Philadelphia: WB Saunders, 1987;581.

131 Cotton PB. Critical appraisal of therapeutic endoscopy in biliary tract diseases. *Ann Rev Med* 1990;41:211−222.

132 Leung JWC, Chan RCY, Cheung SW, Sung JY, Chung SCS, French GL. The effect of obstruction on the biliary excretion of cefoperazone and ceftazidime. *J Antimicrob Chemother* 1990;25: 399−406.

133 Eliopoulos GM, Moellering RC. Azlocillin, mezlocillin and piperacillin: new broad-spectrum penicillins. *Ann Int Med* 1982;97:755−760.

134 Brogard JM, Kopferschmitt J, Arnaud JP, Dorner M, La Villaureix J. Biliary elimination of mezlocillin: an experimental and clinical study. *Antimicrob Agents Chemother* 1980;18:69−76.

135 Martin DF, Tweedle DEF. Retroperitoneal perforation during ERCP and endoscopic sphincterotomy: causes, clinical features and management. *Endoscopy* 1990;22:174−175.

136 Sherman S, Ruffolo TA, Hawes RH, Lehman GA. Complications of endoscopic sphincterotomy. A prospective series with emphasis on the increased risk associated with sphincter of Oddi dysfunction and nondilated bile ducts. *Gastroenterology* 1991;101:1068−1075.

137 Byrne P, Leung JWC, Cotton PB. Retroperitoneal perforation during duodenoscopic sphincterotomy. *Radiology* 1984;150: 383−384.

138 Merrett M, Desmond P. Removal of impacted endoscopic basket and stone from the common bile duct by extracorporeal shock waves. *Endoscopy* 1990;22:92.

139 Hawes RH, Cotton PB, Vallon AG. Follow-up 6 to 11 years after duodenoscopic sphincterotomy for stones in patient with prior cholecystectomy. *Gastroenterology* 1990;98:1008−1012.

140 Jayaprakash B, Wright R. Common bile duct perforation − an unusual complication of ERCP. *Gastrointest Endosc* 1986;32: 246−247.

141 Halter F, Bangerter U, Gigon JP, Pusterla C. Gallstone ileus after endoscopic sphincterotomy. *Endoscopy* 1981;13:88−89.

142 Welch NT, Ellis DJ, Bradby GVH. Necrotizing fasciitis − a complication of "successful" endoscopic sphincterotomy. *Gastrointest Endosc* 1990;36:425−426.

143 Risher WH, Smith JW. Intraperitoneal haemorrhage from injury to the gastroepiploic artery: a complication of endoscopic retrograde sphincterotomy. *Gastrointest Endosc* 1990;36: 426−427.

144 Hatfield ARW. Palliation of malignant obstructive jaundice − surgery or stent? *Gut* 1990;31:1339−1340.

145 Groen AK, Out T, Huibregtse R, Delzenne B, Hoek FJ, Tytgat GNJ. Characterisation of the content of occluded biliary endoprostheses. *Endoscopy* 1987;19:57−59.

146 Habr-Gama A, Waye JD. Complications and hazards of gastrointestinal endoscopy. *World J Surg* 1989;13:193−201.

147 Schwesinger WH, Levine BA, Ramos R. Complications in colonoscopy. *Surg Gynecol Obstet* 1979;148:270−281.

148 Meyers MA, Ghahremani GG. Complications of fiberoptic endoscopy. II. Colonoscopy. *Radiology* 1975;115:301−307.

149 Rankin GB. Indications, contraindications and complications of colonoscopy. In: Sivak M, ed. *Gastroenterologic Endoscopy*. Philadelphia: WB Saunders, 1987;868−880.

150 Ghazi A, Grossman M. Complications of colonoscopy and polypectomy. *Surg Clin N Am* 1982;62:889−896.

151 Brayko CM, Kozarek RA, Sanowski RA, Howells T. Diverticular rupture during colonoscopy. Fact or fancy? *Digest Dis Sci* 1984; 29:427−431.

152 Livstone EM, Kerstein MD. Serosal tears following colonoscopy. *Arch Surg* 1976;111:88.

153 Kozarek RA, Earnest DL, Silverstein ME, Smith RG. Air-pressure-induced colon injury during diagnostic colonoscopy. *Gastroenterology* 1980;78:7−14.

154 Reeve T, Kukora JS. Pneumatic perforation of the colon during colonoscopy: is the hypermobile right colon a risk factor. *Dis Colon Rectum* 1984;27:751−753.

155 Fruhmorgen P, Demling L. Complications of diagnostic and therapeutic colonoscopy in the Federal Republic of Germany. Results of an inquiry. *Endoscopy* 1979;11:146−150.

156 Ecker MD, Goldstein M, Hoexter B, Hyman RA, Naidich JB, Stein HL. Benign pneumoperitoneum after fiberoptic colonoscopy. A prospective study of 100 patients. *Gastroenterology* 1977;73:226−230.

157 Barnett T, McGeehin W, Chen C, Brennan EJ. Acute tension pneumoperitoneum following colonoscopy. *Gastrointest Endosc* 1992;38:99−100.

158 Meyers MA. Radiological features of the spread and localisation of extraperitoneal gas and their relationship to its source. An anatomical approach. *Radiology* 1974;111:17−26.

159 Schmidt G, Borsch G, Wegener M. Subcutaneous emphysema and pneumothorax complicating diagnostic colonoscopy. *Dis Colon Rectum* 1986;29:136−138.

160 Bakker J, van Kersen F, Bellaar Spruyt JB. Pneumopericardium and pneumomediastinum after polypectomy. *Endoscopy* 1991; 23:46−47.

161 Smith LE, Nivatvongs S. Complications in colonoscopy. *Dis Colon Rectum* 1975;18:214−220.

162 Rogers BHG, Silvis SE, Nebel OT, Sugawa C, Mandelstam P. Complications of flexible fiberoptic colonoscopy and polypectomy. An analysis of the 1974 ASGE survey. *Gastrointest Endosc* 1975;22:73−77.

163 Ellis WR, Harrison JM, Williams RS. Rupture of spleen at colonoscopy. *Br Med J* 1979;1:307−308.

164 Ong E, Bohmler U, Wurbs D. Splenic injury as a complication of endoscopy: two case reports and a literature review. *Endoscopy* 1991;23:302−304.

165 Rockey DC, Weber JR, Wright TL, Wall SD. Splenic injury following colonoscopy. *Gastrointest Endosc* 1990;36:306−309.

166 Razzak IA, Millan J, Schuster MM. Pneumatic ileal perforation: an unusual complication of colonoscopy. *Gastroenterology* 1976; 70:268−271.

167 Wertkin MG, Wetchler BB, Waye JD, Brown LK. *Pneumatosis coli* associated with sigmoid volvulus and colonoscopy. *Am J Gastroenterol* 1976;65:209−214.

168 Anderson JR, Spence RAJ, Wilson BG, Hanna WA. Gangrenous caecal volvulus after colonoscopy. *Br Med J* 1983;286; 439−440.

169 Haber I. Hepatic portal vein gas following colonoscopy in ulcerative colitis: report of a case. *Acta Gastroenterol Belg* 1983; 46:14−17.

170 Koltun WA, Coller JA. Incarceration of colonoscope in an inguinal hernia. "Pulley" technique of removal. *Dis Colon Rectum* 1991;34:191−193.

171 Rees BI, Williams LA. Incarceration of hernia after colonoscopy. *Lancet* 1977;i:371.

172 Hunt RH. Towards safer colonoscopy. *Gut* 1983;24:371−375.

173 Rex DK, Lewis BS, Waye JD. Colonoscopy and endoscopic therapy for delayed post-polypectomy hemorrhage. *Gastrointest Endosc* 1992;38:127−129.

174 DeGerome JH. Late perforation following colonoscopic polypectomy. *Gastrointest Endosc* 1977;24:44.

175 Waye JD. The postpolypectomy coagulation syndrome. *Gastrointest Endosc* 1981;27:184.

176 Bigard MA, Gaucher P, Lassalle C. Fatal colonic explosion during colonoscopic polypectomy. *Gastroenterology* 1979;77: 1307−1310.

177 Falzio RA, Wickremesinghe PC, Arsura EL, Rando J. Endoscopic removal of an intussuscepted appendix mimicking a polyp — an endoscopic hazard. *Am J Gastroenterol* 1982;77:556−558.

178 Williams CB, Gillespie PE. Accidental removal of ureteral stoma at colonoscopy. *Gastrointest Endosc* 1979;25:109−110.

CHAPTER 32

Complications of urinary tract diagnostic procedures

Mohamed Amin, Marilyn A. Roubidoux, Richard H. Cohan and N. Reed Dunnick

Introduction

Diagnostic uroradiology includes procedures that image the adrenal glands, the urinary tract, and the male and female genital systems. Interventional techniques and magnetic resonance imaging are considered in other areas. Tests included here are those involving intravenous contrast material, such as excretory urography, cystography, or contrast-enhanced computed tomography (CT), and those in whom the contrast material is introduced in a retrograde fashion such as retrograde pyelography, retrograde urethrography, or cystourethrography.

The most common complications are those related to injection of intravascular contrast media for urography. However, other complications may arise as a result of needle or catheter manipulation during the performance of any of these other procedures.

Intravascular contrast studies (see also Chapter 13)

Adverse contrast reactions

Types of reactions

Adverse contrast reactions may be classified as idiosyncratic or nonidiosyncratic. *Idiosyncratic* reactions produce signs and symptoms that mimic true anaphylaxis and are independent of dose [1]. Since anticontrast media immunoglobulin E (IgE) antibodies have been isolated from only a small number of reacting patients, these reactions are considered to be anaphylactoid or "allergic-like" rather than truly anaphylactic. While their etiology remains unknown, possible mechanisms include activation of the complement and/or contact systems. Manifestations of idiosyncratic reactions include hives, itching, facial and laryngeal edema, bronchospasm, and even respiratory or circulatory collapse.

Nonidiosyncratic reactions are thought to result from direct chemotoxic or hyperosmolar effects of contrast material. They produce pathophysiologic abnormalities and are usually dose related. Symptoms include nausea, vomiting, cardiac arrhythmias, renal failure, pulmonary edema, and cardiovascular collapse.

Incidence

The incidence of adverse contrast reactions reported varies with the criteria for determining a reaction, the risk factors of the patient population, and the diligence with which they are sought. Furthermore, the type of contrast media (CM) used has a significant influence on whether or not the patient will experience an adverse reaction.

Mild, moderate, and severe reactions of both idiosyncratic and nonidiosyncratic types occur less frequently with low-osmolar contrast media (LOCM) than high-osmolar contrast media (HOCM) [2–5]. Palmer [2] in a series of 109 546 patients, Wolf et al. [3] in a series of over 6000 patients, and Katayama et al. [4] in a series of 337 647 patients reported the incidence of all adverse reactions to HOCM as 3.8%, 4.17%, and 12.66%, respectively. The rate of reactions to nonionic LOCM was only 1.2% [2], 0.69% [3], and 3.13% [4] in these three studies.

Katayama et al. [4] reported severe adverse reactions in 0.22% of patients injected with ionic media, but in only 0.04% of patients receiving nonionic media. Very severe reactions (requiring hospitalization) decreased from 0.04

(HOCM) to 0.004% (nonionic LOCM) in the same study (Table 32.1).

Although a patient may die from an adverse reaction to either HOCM or LOCM [6], it is rare. In the study by Katayama *et al.* [4], only one patient receiving HOCM and one patient receiving nonionic LOCM died, but there was no definite relationship of the death to the contrast injection. These data indicate that HOCM and LOCM are both very safe agents.

Risk groups

Patients who have had prior reactions to iodinated CM are at increased risk for another reaction. Repeat reactions to HOCM occur in 16–44% of patients [4,7], while repeat reactions to nonionic LOCM occur in only 4.1–11.24% of patients [4]. History of allergy to drugs, food, or other substances, and asthma are other risk factors for adverse reactions. Katayama *et al.* [4] noted reactions in 23.35% of patients with allergies who received HOCM, but in only 6.85% of patients with allergies who received nonionic LOCM. In patients with asthma, adverse reactions occurred in 19.68% of patients receiving HOCM, but only 7.75% of patients receiving LOCM.

Delayed reactions

Most adverse reactions to iodinated CM occur within 1 hour of injection [8]. Recently, a number of articles assessing delayed reactions (occurring more than 1 hour, but within 24 hours after contrast injection) have appeared. In one study, an incidence of up to 30% for delayed reactions was observed [9].

Reported manifestations of delayed reactions include erythematous rashes, fever, chills, flu-like symptoms, joint pain, pruritis, loss of appetite, headache, abdominal pain, constipation, diarrhea, fatigue, depression, and taste disturbance [9–11]. The incidence of delayed reactions does not appear to be reduced markedly by using LOCM.

Contrast nephropathy

Contrast-induced renal failure is usually defined as an increase in serum creatinine of 1 mg/dl or more [12] and/or of 25–50% of the baseline creatinine level after intravascular contrast administration [13,14]. The reported incidence of acute renal failure after the use of intravascular CM varies widely from as low as 0% to as high as 12% [15,16].

The rise in serum creatinine is usually seen within 1–2 days after contrast injection, peaks in approximately 4–7 days, and returns to normal by 10–14 days [17,18]. Oliguria (urine volume of <400 ml/day) is less frequently observed than nonoliguric renal failure [18]. Essentially all patients with contrast nephropathy will have persistent nephrograms on plain radiographs or CT (Fig. 32.1). Recently, Love *et al.* [19] found that measurements of the attenuation of a persistent nephrogram on CT may be used to predict the likelihood of a patient developing clinically significant contrast nephropathy. Cortical attenuation under 110 Hounsfied units (HU) on scans obtained 24 hours after contrast injection identified a group of patients with subclinical renal impairment who did not develop serum creatinine elevations. Cortical attenuation over 140 HU was always associated with an eventual rise in the serum creatinine level [19].

Mechanism of contrast nephropathy

No mechanism of contrast-induced renal failure has been completely accepted [20]. One favored possibility, however, involves a combination of preexisting hemodynamic alterations and of CM toxicity.

Table 32.1 Comparison of the prevalence of severe reactions and relative risk with parenteral uses of HOCM and LOCM

Reference	Cases with ionic contrast media		Cases with nonionic contrast media		Relative risk ionic/nonionic
	Total number	Number with ADRs	Total number	Number with ARDs	
Katayama *et al.* [4]					
Total number of ADRs	169 284	21 428 (12.66%)	168 363	5276 (3.13%)	4.10
Severe	169 284	367 (0.22%)	168 363	70 (0.04%)	5.50
Very severe	169 284	63 (0.04%)	168 363	6 (0.004%)	10.00
Palmer [2]					
Total number	79 278	2982 (3.8%)	30 168	351 (1.2%)	3.20
Low risk	77 910	2841 (3.6%)	15 088	161 (1.1%)	3.20
High risk	1368	141 (10.3%)	15 080	190 (1.3%)	7.90
Wolf *et al.* [3]	6006	24 (0.4%)	7170	0 (0.0%)	—

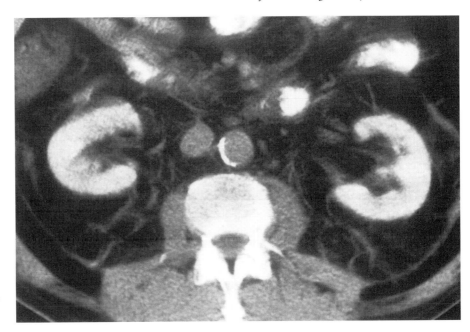

Fig. 32.1 Contrast-induced renal failure. This unenhanced CT scan demonstrates a persistently dense renal cortex from contrast injected more than 24 hours earlier. Note absence of contrast in the collecting system.

Risk groups for contrast nephropathy

Patients with preexisting renal insufficiency and diabetes mellitus (DM) (particularly when insulin dependent), have been consistently identified as being at increased risk of developing contrast nephropathy, especially when these two etiologies are combined [14,21,22]. Other potential risk factors for contrast-induced renal failure include concomitant administration of other nephrotoxic drugs (such as aminoglycoside antibiotics and nonsteroidal antiinflammatory agents), American Heart Association class IV congestive heart failure, and hyperuricemia.

It is believed that the greater the volume of CM injected, the more likely a patient will develop contrast nephropathy [23]. In the past, patients with multiple myeloma have been considered to be at increased risk for developing contrast-induced renal failure. This issue has recently been reexamined [24]. It is now felt that contrast-induced renal failure in myeloma is not seen with greatly increased frequency, although when it occurs it may be associated with significant morbidity [24–26].

Some factors such as dehydration, hypertension, proteinuria, peripheral vascular diseases, and age over 65 years are believed not to predispose patients to contrast nephropathy unless other risks are present.

The role of LOCM in patients with contrast nephropathy

While older studies failed to show any difference between HOCM and LOCM with respect to their likelihood of inducing contrast-induced renal failure [21,27,28], more recent series have suggested that LOCM is indeed safer [29–31]. In light of the current reports, use of LOCM, at least in those patients at risk for developing contrast-induced renal failure, is probably indicated.

It is also prudent to minimize the dose of contrast material administered to high-risk patients [32], although the safest alternative remains avoiding intravascular CM injection entirely by performing alternate studies such as ultrasound and/or retrograde pyelography.

Premedication for prevention of idiosyncratic reactions

Oral administration of corticosteroids, H_1 and H_2 antihistamines, and ephedrine have all been used as premedication for patients at high risk for an idiosyncratic contrast reaction. In the only controlled, prospective, and randomized study to date, Lasser *et al.* [33] found that a 2 day, two-dose pretreatment regimen using methylprednisolone (32 mg orally) 12 and 2 hours before CM administration had a significant beneficial effect on patients undergoing examinations using HOCM. The incidence of all reactions was reduced from 9.4% in patients receiving just a single dose of steroids 2 hours before CM injection or one (9.9%) or two doses (9.0%) of placebo, to 6.4% when two doses of steroids were administered.

Greenberger *et al.* [34] showed that ephedrine further decreases recurrent contrast reaction rates in high-risk patients treated with steroids and H_1 antihistamines (from 9 to 3.1%). Ephedrine sulfate is administered as a single 25 mg oral dose 1 hour prior to the procedure (Table 32.2). It is not an innocuous drug, however, and must be used with caution in patients with heart disease, hypertension, or hyperthyroidism.

Table 32.2 Effect of various pretreatment regimens on the prevalence of anaphylactoid reactions in patients with previous reaction to intravascular CM

Pretreatment drug	Regimen	Number of procedures	Number of reactions	Reference
Prednisone	50 mg p.o./6 h for three doses beginning 18 hours before injection	86	4 (4.7%)	Zweiman *et al.* [35]
Prednisone	50 mg p.o./6 h for three doses beginning 13 hours before injection			
Diphenhydramine	50 mg p.o. or i.m. 1 hour before injection	415	45 (9.2%)	Greenberger *et al.* [34]
Prednisone	Same as above			
Diphenhydramine	Same as above			
Ephedrine	25 mg p.o. 1 hour before injection	180	9 (5.0%)	Greenberger *et al.* [34]
Prednisone	Same as above			
Diphenhydramine	Same as above			
Ephedrine	Same as above			
Cimetidine	300 mg p.o. 1 hour before injection	100	14 (14.0%)	Greenberger *et al.* [34]
Methylprednisolone (32 mg p.o.)	Two doses 12 and 2 hours before injection. One dose 2 hours before injection	1759	166 (9.4%)	Lasser *et al.* [33]
Prednisolone	Same as above			
Diphenhydramine	Same as above			
Ephedrine plus LOCM	Same as above	200	1 (0.5%)	Greenberger and Patterson [38]

i.m., intramuscular; p.o., oral administration.

The role of any pretreatment regimen has been less clear since LOCMs have become widely used. For example, Wolf *et al.* [37] found that steroid premedication and use of HOCM was not as effective (severe reaction rate = 0.25%) as was use of nonionic media alone (severe reaction rate = 0.01%) in high-risk patients. Furthermore, corticosteroids are not without side-effects in some patients. They should be used with caution in patients with a history of active tuberculosis, DM, or peptic ulcer disease.

Perhaps the safest alternate in most patients is to provide high-risk patients with both steroid pretreatment and non-ionic CM. Zweiman *et al.* [35] demonstrated a reduction of the incidence of repeat reactions to LOCM in 141 pretreated high-risk patients. Prophylaxis was performed with prednisone 50 mg, 13, 7, and 1 hour before, and diphenhydramine 1 hour before CM infusion. Ephedrine, 25 mg (1 hour before CM infusion) was also added in 41 cases. Only one urticarial reaction occurred (in a patient who had not received ephedrine). Total incidence of repeated reactions was 0.5%, compared with a reaction rate of 9.1% with the same pretreatment regimen in 800 intravascular procedures in previous reactors who received HOCM [36].

At the present time, we recommend that LOCM should be used for urography in patients who have had previous idiosyncratic contrast reactions of any type, or who have a history of significant allergies or asthma. Corticosteroid prophylaxis should be added in patients whose previous reactions included a respiratory component or in patients who have severe asthma.

Selective use of nonionic CM

The higher costs of LOCM are due to a variety of factors and is the most critical factor retarding the universal use of LOCM. Guidelines and rationale for use of LOCM have been suggested by various specialty societies. In 1990, the American College of Radiology's Committee on Drugs and Contrast Media [38] suggested that LOCM should be used in the following situations.

1 Patients with a history of previous adverse reactions to contrast material (with the exception of a sensation of heat, flushing, or a single episode of nausea or vomiting).
2 Patients with a history of asthma or allergy.
3 Patients with known cardiac dysfunction, including recent or potentially imminent cardiac decompensation, severe arrhythmias, unstable angina pectoris, recent myocardial infarction, and pulmonary hypertension.
4 Patients with generalized severe debilitation.

5 Any other circumstances where, after due consideration, the radiologist believes there is a specific indication for the use of LOCM (with examples including patients with sickle cell disease, pheochromocytoma, multiple myeloma, DM, increased risk for aspiration, much anxiety about the contrast procedure, patients with whom communication cannot be established in order to determine the presence or absence of risk factors, patients who request or demand the use of LOCM, patients who are to receive high doses of CM [39].

The Society of Cardiovascular and Interventional Radiology (SCVIR) also has proposed guidelines for selective use of LOCM [40]; some absolute indications are included here.
1 Patients who have had prior reactions and strong allergic diathesis or asthma.
2 Hemodynamic instability or limited cardiac reserve (patients with tight aortic stenosis, severe cardiomyopathy, or severe three-vessel or left main stem coronary artery disease or who are hemodynamically unstable).
3 Inability to tolerate a marked osmotic load (patients with oliguric or anuric renal failure, markedly dehydrated patients).
4 Patients with marked anxiety, risk.

The SCVIR has also suggested that some conditions should be considered as only relative indications for the use of LOCM such as age over 65–70 years, patients with multiple myeloma, polycythemia vera, or renal failure.

Treatment of CM reactions

The vast majority of reactions occur within 20 minutes of receiving CM. Therefore, any physician who is responsible for injection of contrast agents (ionic or nonionic) should be able to identify and respond to any reaction that may occur.

When a patient has a reaction, the patient's vital signs, including blood pressure, pulse, and respirations, should be immediately assessed. Tachycardia (pulse >100 bpm) and hypotension (systolic pressure <80 mmHg) usually indicate an anaphylactoid or cardiogenic reaction. Bradycardia (pulse <60 bpm) and hypotension are manifestations of vasovagal reactions, although this may also be seen in patients on β-adrenergic blockers who are having an anaphylactoid reaction [41,42]. The various types of reactions and suggested treatment (with normal adult dosages) are summarized in the discussion here and in Table 32.3.

Table 32.3 Acute reactions to CM: primary treatment outline

Reaction	Manifestation	Degree	Primary treatment	Adult dose/route
Vasomotor effect	Warmth		Reassurance	
	Nausea/vomiting	Mild	Reassurance	
		Severe	Patient position, prochlorperazine	5–10 mg i.m., i.v.
Anaphylactoid	Cutaneous urticaria "hives"	Scattered	Supportive/observation	
		Protracted	Diphenhydramine	25–50 mg i.v., i.m.
		Severe	Cimetidine	300 mg (diluted 10 ml) i.v. (slowly)
			Ranitidine	50 mg (diluted to 20 ml) i.v. (slowly)
	Bronchospastic "prolonged expiration," "wheezing"	Mild–moderate	Subcutaneous, epinephrine 1:1000	0.1–0.3 mg (0.1–0.3 ml) s.c.
		Severe	Intravenous, epinephrine 1:10 000	0.1 mg (1 ml) i.v.
		Isolated/protracted	Inhaled β-adrenergics, albuterol metaproterenol, terbutaline	Two deep inhalations/metered dose inhaler
	Isolated hypotension "Normal sinus rhythm/ tachycardia"		Intravenous fluid (normal saline or Ringer's solution)	1–2 l i.v. (rapid)
Vasovagal	Hypotension and bradycardia		Intravenous fluid (normal saline or Ringer's solution) plus atropine	1–2 l i.v. (rapid) 0.6–1 mg i.v. (push)
Systemic	Seizures	Mild +/− vasovagal Continuous/ repeated	Same as hypotension plus patient protection, diazepam	5–10 mg i.v.

i.m., intramuscular; i.v., intravenous; s.c., subcutaneous.

Nausea and vomiting

Nausea and/or vomiting are frequently encountered after ionic CM is injected for urography. If a patient's nausea or vomiting is determined to be mild and self-limiting, he or she should be reassured that a serious reaction is not occurring. If these symptoms are severe and persistent, and there are no other manifestations, an antinausea drug may be administered (prochlorperazine, 5−10 mg intramuscularly) [43]. It is important to support the patient in a sitting or lateral recumbent position to avoid aspiration of vomitus. If the patient loses consciousness, one should clear the airway by turning the patient's head to one side and promptly using suction.

Anaphylactoid reactions

An anaphylactoid reaction often involves multiple organ systems including the skin, cardiovascular, and respiratory systems, but it may be limited to one. Specific manifestations include laryngeal edema, bronchospasm alone or with asthma, and hypotension. Even apparently mild anaphylactoid reactions should be closely monitored, as they may progress and even become life threatening.

Urticaria

Scattered "hives" (blotchy reddening of the skin with itching) require close observation. For many patients, urticaria is the only manifestation of allergy, and may be so slight as not to need treatment. However, it may be the forerunner of a more serious reaction. If pruritis is severe and troublesome to the patient, H_1 antihistamines, such as diphenhydramine (25−50 mg orally) are often effective [44,45].

Prominent urticaria or diffuse cutaneous reactions occurring independently of generalized systemic or anaphylactoid reactions often respond to a combination of H_1 and H_2 antihistamines such as diphenhydramine and cimetidine (300 mg intravenously, diluted in 5% dextrose, slowly), or ranitidine (50 mg intravenously, diluted slowly) [45].

Bronchospasm

Bronchospasm presents a shortness of breath or difficulty breathing. Prolonged *expiration*, wheezing, and musical rales are typical auscultatory findings and help to distinguish bronchospasm from the (predominantly *inspiratory*) stridor of laryngeal edema. As a reaction to CM, it begins early and abruptly. It is most common in patients with a history of asthma.

A patent airway must be maintained. Oxygen is administered by nasal prongs or mask at a rate of 2−3 l/min. Inhalation of β-agonist inhalers (metaproterenol, terbutaline, or albuterol) is often effective in reversing mild to moderate isolated bronchospasm [45,46].

Epinephrine should be used if response to inhalers is inadequate or if initial bronchospastic reaction is severe or rapidly worsening. Epinephrine has both α- and β-agonist effects. α-Agonist actions produce vasoconstriction, primarily increasing blood pressure by reversing peripheral vasodilatation [41]. Angioedema and urticaria may also be decreased. The β-agonist effects of epinephrine are most desirable because they reverse bronchoconstriction and also have positive inotropic and chronotropic function [47]. Patients with asthma who take β-agonists may show a refractory response at the β-receptor site, and this can encourage the utilization of an epinephrine dose to the point that they may experience hypertensive crises, resulting in stroke or myocardial ischemia [48]. Patients on β-blockers may have only an α-adrenergic response to epinephrine, also greatly increasing the likelihood of a hypertensive reaction or cardiac damage [48]. In this circumstance, isoproterenol, a β-agonist, may be considered [48]. Hypertensive crises can occasionally also be seen in patients who are not receiving β-blockers.

Epinephrine can be given subcutaneously in a dosage of 0.1−0.2 ml of 1:1000 concentration. Subcutaneous dosages can be repeated every 5−15 minutes up to three times, if needed [49]. For the most severe or rapidly accelerating reactions, epinephrine should be given intravenously, but at lower doses. Intravenous epinephrine can be administered at a rate of 10 μg/min (0.1 ml/min of 1:10 000 dilution). Antihistamines can be added if the response to epinephrine is not complete and can be administered every 6 hours for 1−2 days to prevent symptoms from recurring [49]. Aminophylline can also be used for treatment of bronchospasm not relieved by epinephrine [50]. The suggested dose is 250 mg in 10 ml of 5% dextrose as a loading dose. Aminophylline is administered slowly to minimize the severity of any hypotensive effects. Subsequently, it is infused at a rate of 0.4−1.0 mg/h.

Facial and/or laryngeal edema

Laryngeal edema may be manifested by predominantly *inspiratory* stridor, a sensation of swelling or tightness in the throat, difficulty in swallowing and speaking, croupy cough (persistent, relatively nonproductive), or edema of the throat and/or face. Laryngeal edema may be so marked as to seriously impair breathing.

Oxygen (by nasal prongs or mask at 2−3 l/min) and intravenous fluid (normal saline or Ringers lactate) should be given immediately. If laryngeal edema is becoming severe, prompt intubation should be considered, as this procedure becomes increasingly difficult. If rapid intubation is not possible, transcrycothyroid puncture or tracheostomy may be required.

Epinephrine is the drug of choice for treatment of airway edema [48]. Subcutaneous administration can be used in all but the most severe reaction. If epinephrine is not therapeutic, H_1 and H_2 antihistamines can also be administered [50,51].

Corticosteroids

Corticosteroids do not have an immediate effect on CM reactions; however, they may confer some delayed protection, especially when severe reactions extend over hours rather than minutes [44]. Steroids may also prevent recurrence of symptoms once the acute episode has been successfully treated. Steroids are administered slowly in large dosages. For example, 500 mg hydrocortisone can be given over several minutes, or 2000 mg over 30 minutes. Steroids can be continued for 1–2 days [44].

Isolated hypotension

The treatment regimen of patients with hypotension, but without bradycardia, bronchospasm, or airway edema, consists of rapid administration of isotonic fluid (0.9% saline, or Ringers lactate). Vasopressors should be used when patients do not respond to initial infusion of fluid. In such cases 2–5 µg/kg per min of intravenous dopamine is often helpful [45,51]. Epinephrine and antihistamines are not recommended as they may produce unwanted side-effects.

Vasovagal reactions

Identification of vasovagal reaction by the combination of sinus bradycardia (pulse <60 bpm) and hypotension (systolic pressure <80 mmHg) is essential because treatment is specific. Syncope rarely occurs as the patient is recumbent, but light headedness, visual difficulties, and weakness may occur in response to the insertion of the needle or fear of the procedure. Vasovagal attack induces arterial and venous dilatation. Because of peripheral pooling, cardiac output falls and hypotension ensues.

Patients often respond to leg elevation, placement of the patient in the Trendelenburg position, and rapid infusion of isotonic fluid. Atropine (0.6–1.0 mg intravenously) is often effective when fluid alone is not. The initial dose can be repeated every 3–5 minutes to a maximum of 3.0 mg [41,42]. Patients with coronary artery disease should be monitored closely because positive chronotropic effects of atropine may induce angina or even myocardial infarction.

Seizures

Seizures may be the end result of a severe hypotensive episode or a vagal reaction, or they may be chemotoxic. A seizing patient should be protected from self-inflicted injury. If seizure activity is continuous or repeated, 5–10 mg diazepam intravenously is often therapeutic [51].

Exacerbation of cardiac disease

Exacerbation of heart disease (acute myocardial infarction or ischemia and/or congestive heart failure) must be appropriately recognized and not misdiagnosed as an anaphylactoid reaction, because the drugs used to treat the latter can seriously stress the heart and can cause significant morbidity. Cardiac disease should be considered in any patient who complains of chest pain or tightness or shortness of breath, especially if there is a history of angina [52].

Extravasation injuries

The contrast material used for excretory urography is intended for intravenous use. In some instances, intravenous access may be difficult and/or the patient may be uncooperative. This can result in at least a partially extravascular injection. Most often, volumes of extravasated CM are small (<5 ml) (Fig. 32.2), and the minor amount of local soft tissue swelling, erythema, and/or pain that may result resolves without any morbidity to the patient. Larger amounts of extravasation may occur when a power injector is used for dynamic CT examinations (Fig. 32.3). The incidence of extravasations during excretory urography has not been estimated. It is known, however, that accidental extravasations can be encountered in as many as 22% of adults receiving intravenous fluids of all kinds [53].

Rarely, significant complications may result from extravascular injections of contrast agents. These include skin and subcutaneous tissue ulceration and necrosis, as well as damage to adjacent blood vessels, nerves, and tendons. Deformities can be permanent and disfiguring and multiple reparative operations may be required, including surgical debridements and skin grafting [54]. While adverse reactions can rarely result from extravasations of as little as 10 ml of 60% by weight CM [55], it is generally believed that the larger the volume injected, the more likely the local tissues will be seriously damaged. For this reason, intravenous sites should be closely monitored (i.e., not obscured by tape or bandages) when contrast material is being injected for urography. Injections should be terminated immediately if they produce any local swelling or pain.

Incidence of serious injuries caused by extravasation of CM

It is difficult to determine the incidence of significant extravasation injuries. They are certainly infrequent. Skin necrosis has been observed in 0.4–0.5% of patients undergoing

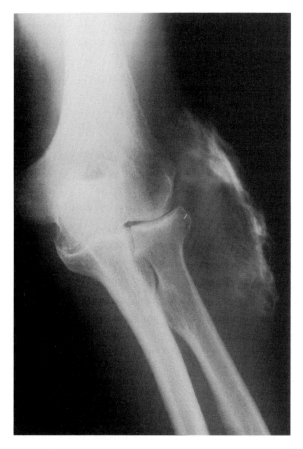

Fig. 32.2 Contrast extravasation. A small amount of contrast material is seen in the soft tissues after an antecubital fossa injection for an excretory urogram.

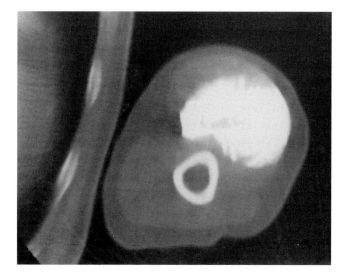

Fig. 32.3 Contrast extravasation. A large amount of contrast within the soft tissues of the arm is the result of contrast injected by a mechanical pump injector during a dynamic CT examination.

venography with 60% by weight contrast material [56,57]. Presumably, necrosis would be encountered in considerably fewer patients having excretory urograms, since venous access is usually less of a problem in these patients, and tourniquets are always released prior to injection.

Mechanism

The mechanism of injury from CM extravasation is not known with certainty; however, it is suspected that hyperosmolality is primarily responsible [1,58,59]. In addition, simple mechanical compression, direct cytotoxicity, and possibly even viscosity may have a role [1].

Risk factors

Certain patients have been identified as being at increased risk for extravasations and, therefore, extravasation injuries. These patients should be injected with extreme caution. This includes:

1 patients at the extremes of age or who are unconscious, as these individuals are less likely to complain about injection site pain [54];

2 patients who have had prior radiation therapy to an injection site;

3 patients with abnormalities of circulation (either venous or arterial insufficiency) such as patients with atherosclerosis, peripheral vascular complications of DM, connective tissue diseases (such as Raynaud phenomenon), and central or peripheral venous thrombosis are all at increased risk [54].

A few clinical situations are more likely to result in extravascular accumulations of contrast material. The first involves the use of indwelling intravenous lines. The catheter tip may be dislodged in the course of a patient being transferred to the radiology department [60]. While backflow of blood should be demonstrated through tubing connected to an intravenous site prior to contrast material injection, its presence does not guarantee adequate position of the intravenous line [61].

Second, multiple attempts to establish intravenous access through the same vein can also be a problem in some instances. Contrast material that is properly instilled through a distal vein may leak out through a defect that has just been created more centrally. It is therefore preferable to proceed centrally or to a site that has different venous drainage when initial punctures that traverse one or both walls of a vein are not usable.

Third, injections into the dorsum of the hand, foot, or ankle are more likely to result in local damage when extravasations occur because of the smaller amount of subcutaneous tissue and the close proximity of many important tendons, blood vessels, and nerves in these patients [54]. For this reason, the antecubital fossae or forearms should be checked first when searching for a suitable location for venipuncture.

Lastly, it has been noted that extravasations are more likely to result after injections through metal needles (such as butterflies) than plastic cannulae [61]. Although this may in part reflect an intrinsic technical advantage of the latter over the former, it is also possible that metal needles are more likely to be used in patients whose intravenous access sites are more tenuous (i.e., smaller veins). Nevertheless, we recommend using plastic cannulae whenever practical.

Treatment

Although a wide variety of regimens have been investigated, no nonsurgical treatment has been accepted as being effective in mitigating the severity of damage produced by extravascular CM. Animal studies assessing the potential role of immediate topical cooling [62,63] and local injections of hyaluronidase (an enzyme that breaks down the connective tissue mucopolysaccharide hyaluronic acid) [62,64] have had conflicting results. Topical heat [62] and local installation of corticosteroids [63,65] or propranolol [65] have not been of any benefit in these cases, although these agents may be beneficial when other substances (such as chemotherapeutic agents) are extravasated [66,67]. Two studies have found that local dilution with saline [63,65] or sterile water [65] modestly but significantly reduces the severity and/or frequency of skin necrosis produced by extravasation of CM in rats. A third however, concluded injection of both of these agents was ineffective [64]. Even if local dilution is helpful in humans, the volumes used in animal studies are so large (up to 50% of the volume of extravasated CM), that such treatment may often not be practical. For example, a radiologist might be reluctant to inject a 50-ml contrast extravasation site with an additional 25 ml of saline.

While topical application of dimethylsulfoxide (which may function as a free-radical scavenger) has been observed to lessen injuries resulting from extravascular injections of chemotherapeutic agents [68,69], this agent has not been assessed in animals or patients with CM extravasations.

Surgical decompression has been recommended [60] and is effective for CM extravasation in excess of 20 ml. We do not advocate such aggressive therapy at least for smaller volume extravasations, since many extravasations resolve without any problem. Such a treatment policy may result in many patients having an unnecessary invasive procedure.

At the present time, we believe that an acute extravasation injury can be treated initially with ice packs* (to reduce swelling) and elevation. Heat can be employed later for pain (if needed). Local injections are not indicated. Close observation until all local signs and symptoms resolve is imperative, so that the patient can be promptly referred to a plastic surgeon if this becomes necessary. If an outpatient is involved, the referring physician should be notified. The

patient should be contacted at the least on the following day by telephone. This is important, since there is a tendency (at least initially) to underestimate the severity of an extravasation injury. Both laboratory [64] and clinical [54] studies have shown that the extent of damage may not become apparent for 48–72 hours.

Prevention

Since treatment remains controversial and, except for surgery, may be ineffective, the best way to limit the severity of an extravasation injury is to prevent it from occurring in the first place. High-risk patients should be injected with extra care. High-risk situations should be avoided whenever possible.

It has recently been shown [58,59] that LOCM is better tolerated than conventional ionic CM when extravasated in animals. Anecdotally, extravascular nonionic CM is felt to be extremely safe in humans as well. All of four intermediate or large volume (20–150 ml) extravasations during dynamic CT reported by Cohan *et al.* [70] resolved uneventfully. Twenty-eight extravasations of nonionic media observed by Sistrom *et al.* [71] during dynamic CT did not produce any lasting damage to the skin or subcutaneous tissues, and seven of these involved volumes of 50 ml or more. To date, there have only been two reports of injuries produced by extravasated nonionic CM. One involved skin ulceration developing after extravasation of 150 ml from an upper extremity injection site [72]. This extravasation occurred while an automatic blood-pressure cuff (on the same arm, more cephalically) was inflated. In the second instance, a compartment syndrome resulted from injection of over 100 ml of a nonionic agent into a patient's forearm [73]. Despite these two recent problems, we believe that use of LOCM (especially nonionic) should be strongly considered in patients in whom an extravasation is more likely to occur or when an extravasation injury is more likely to be severe.

Extravascular contrast studies

Like the excretory urogram, retrograde pyelography, retrograde urethrography, and cystourethrography also require contrast material. However, CM is not given intravenously, but is instead injected directly into the ureter, urethra, or bladder. Since some CM may be absorbed through the urothelium, or from the adjacent tissues in the case of extravasation, idiosyncratic reactions may occur. However, the incidence of adverse reactions is much lower than with intravenous contrast injections, occurring in only 0.26% of cases [74]. In addition to adverse contrast reactions, several other types of complications occur.

---

* Care should be exercised to avoid "cold burns."

Retrograde pyelography

Extracollecting system injections: perforations

The complications of retrograde pyelography include local contrast extravasations, ureteral perforation, systemic contrast material reactions, and, rarely, renal failure.

Extravasation may occur as a result of either mechanical injury from the catheter or backflow. Extravasation from catheter injury to the bladder, ureters, or renal pelvis is uncommon. Catheter-induced ureteral injury occurs most often at the ureterovesical junction where the ureter is cannulated during cystoscopy (Fig. 32.4). Less commonly the ureteropelvic junction may be injured during catheter manipulation necessitated by angulation of the ureter at this location.

Ureteral perforation is reported in only 0.16% of cases [75], and can be divided into two types. One is a perforation of the wall, resulting in complete tear. The second, more common type, is a splitting of the wall, resulting in a subintimal tear. Both types are more common in diseased ureters, particularly in the ureter above an obstructing stone or stricture.

In most patients, injuries seal without further extravasation or therapy. Sequelae resulting from perforations are more likely when the injured ureter becomes superinfected. While many infected periureteral fluid collections become walled-off and can be treated with percutaneous drainage, occasional perforations do not seal and require surgical drainage. Rarely, overwhelming sepsis and death may result [75].

Extracollecting system injections: backflow

Extravasation from back pressure is common. Pyelosinus extravasation or backflow is the most common, resulting from mucosal tears at the fornix of the calyx (Fig. 32.5). CM tracks through the renal sinus into the perirenal space adjacent to the renal pelvis, or into the pararenal space along the ureter [76]. Rupture at the caliceal fornix may also result in contrast entering a renal vein (pyelovenous backflow) or lymphatic (pyelolymphatic backflow). This contrast is quickly carried away by the vein and more slowly by the lymph vessel, and the fornix heals spontaneously (Fig. 32.5). Intrarenal backflow allows contrast to enter the collecting ducts (of Bellini) and interstitium (pyelotubular backflow). A contrast "stain" is seen within the kidney and is slowly resorbed (Fig. 32.6). Occasionally, this may extend into the subcapsular space.

The etiology for all types of backflow is increased pressure

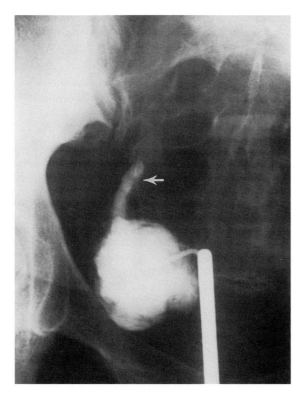

Fig. 32.4 Contrast extravasation during retrograde pyelography. The distal ureter was perforated during attempted cannulation for a retrograde pyelogram. A small amount of contrast can also be seen in the distal right ureter (arrow).

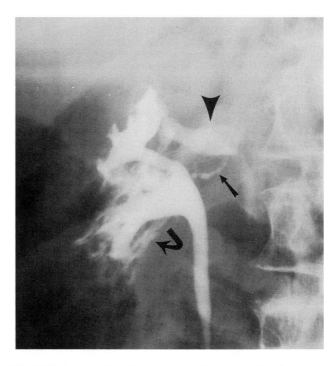

Fig. 32.5 Extravasation during retrograde pyelography. Forniceal rupture has resulted in pyelosinus (curved arrow), pyelovenous (arrowhead), and pyelolymphatic (straight arrow) extravasation.

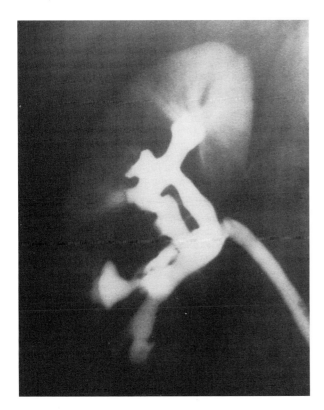

Fig. 32.6 Extravasation during retrograde pyelography. Contrast has entered the collecting ducts (pyelotubular backflow) and is creating an intrarenal contrast "stain."

in the renal pelvis. This may occur during pressure injection of contrast during retrograde pyelography or during intravenous urography from a distal obstructing stone or stricture, especially when higher doses of contrast are administered [77–79]. Backflow serves as a protective mechanism for the release of abnormally high pressure in the renal pelvis. When pressure equalizes, the site of leak is tamponaded and the extravasation ceases.

The typical outcome of backflow is resorption and resolution without further complication. However, intrarenal backflow may provide an access route for bacteria into the renal parenchyma, resulting in pyelonephritis. Infection from pyelosinus backflow is rare but perinephric abscess has been reported. Pyelosinus backflow may also result in a urinoma if persistent obstruction is present. Using small, nonocclusive catheters for retrograde pyelography may decrease the likelihood of backflow and its complications.

Systemic contrast reactions

Life-threatening and fatal systemic reactions to CM injected during retrograde pyelography have been reported [80]. The mechanism is absorption of contrast material either directly from the bladder or after extravasation. Although contrast reactions from retrograde pyelography are rare, an allergic

history to assess the risk of contrast allergy should be elicited from the patient before beginning the procedure.

Renal failure

The rarest complication of retrograde pyelography is renal failure. This may occur from catheter trauma to ureters, resulting in ureteral edema and obstruction [80]. Acute tubular necrosis has also been reported, and is postulated to be from backflow [81].

Retrograde urethrography

Potential complications from retrograde urethrography include extravasation, reflux, systemic contrast reactions, trauma from catheterization, and neurologic complications.

Extravasation

Extravasation of contrast material may occur into the penis, bladder, or vagina. Penile extravasation occurs into the soft tissues of either of the corpora cavernosa, the corpus spongiosum, or into the penile vein. The most common setting is a urethral stricture with prior urethral instrumentation. A preexisting iatrogenic injury with downstream obstruction to the flow of contrast material from the stricture causes urethral extravasation [82]. Urethral mucosal inflammation is another risk factor for extravasation [83]. In most patients, the extravasated contrast material is resorbed and subsequent complications from penile extravasation are very rare [82].

Cystography and cystourethrography

Extravasation

Extravasation from the bladder most commonly occurs as an intramural perforation of the wall by the catheter, or less commonly by complete perforation of the bladder [84]. Extravasation may also occur if the bladder is overfilled with CM and ruptures. This is more common when hand injections of contrast are performed than when the bladder is filled by gravity [84,85].

Reflux

A second complication of cystourethrography is reflux, which may occur into the ureters or into the male ejaculatory system via the ejaculatory ducts [82,84]. Ureteral reflux is common and may result in pyelosinus or intrarenal backflow. If the urine is infected, pyelonephritis and sepsis may occur. Therefore, cystourethrography is contraindicated when urinary tract infection is present. Death due to sepsis has been reported in patients with reflux and hydronephrosis.

Reflux may also cause severe pain [84]. Reflux may be prevented by tilting the table into a semiupright position during the procedure. Extravasation into the vagina often occurs during voiding, but generally results in no further complications. The vagina may also be inadvertently catheterized and filled with contrast material, which in turn may lead to dispersal of vaginal flora into the uterus and peritoneum [84].

Reflux of contrast into the ejaculatory ducts, seminal vesicles, and vasa deferentia occurs more commonly in patients who have had transurethral prostatectomy. Epididimitis may result from this reflux but is very uncommon, occurring in only 0.1% of patients [82].

Systemic contrast reactions

As with retrograde pyelography, risk for contrast reactions should be assessed in all patients [74,82,86]. The etiologies are the extravasation mechanisms previously described for direct absorption of contrast from the bladder [87,88]. Absorption from the bladder is more likely when concentrated CM is used. This may also induce localized inflammation. Also, administration of CM under pressure, large volumes of CM which creates greater distension, and retention of contrast for longer than 15 minutes are more likely to result in CM being absorbed [74].

Trauma from bladder catheterization

Catheterization may cause new or recurrent infections, and mechanical trauma from the catheter may cause mucosal erosions in the bladder or urethra and resultant hematuria [85]. Severe edema may occur in the urethra or bladder and cause bladder obstruction [85,86]. Another traumatic catheter complication is tearing of the mucosa at the meatus or fossa navicularis, resulting from excess dilatation of the catheter balloon.

Autonomic dysreflexia

A neurologic complication of retrograde urethrography may occur in spinal cord injury patients who have lesions above T5. Autonomic dysreflexia, manifest by hypertension, sweating, and bradycardia occurs when the bladder is filled and the neck is opened. This complication may be prevented by administration of α-adrenergic antagonists prior to cystography or urethrography [89].

References

1 Cohan RH, Dunnick NR. Intravascular contrast media: adverse reactions. *Am J Roentgenol* 1987;149:665–670.
2 Palmer FG. The RACR survey of intravenous contrast media reactions: final report. *Australas Radiol* 1988;32:426–428.
3 Wolf GL, Arenson RL, Cross AP. A prospective trial of ionic vs nonionic contrast agents in routine clinical practice: comparison of adverse effects. *Am J Roentgenol* 1989;152:930–944.
4 Katayama H, Yamaguchi K, Kozuka T *et al.* Adverse reaction to ionic and nonionic contrast media. Report from the Japanese Committee on the Safety of Contrast Media. *Radiology* 1990; 175:621–628.
5 Caro JJ, Trindade E, McGregor M. The risk of death and of severe nonfatal reactions with high- vs low-osmolarity contrast media: a meta-analysis. *Am J Roentgenol* 1991;156:825–832.
6 Curry NS, Schabel SI, Reiheld CT *et al.* Fatal reaction to intravenous nonionic contrast material. *Radiology* 1991;178:361–362.
7 Shehadi WH. Adverse reaction to intravascularly administered contrast media. *Am J Roentgenol* 1975;119:832–840.
8 Netzel MC. Anaphylaxis: clinical presentations, immunological mechanisms, and treatment. *J Emerg Med* 1986;4:227–236.
9 Panto PN, Davis P. Delayed reaction to urographic contrast media. *Br J Radiol* 1986;59:41–44.
10 Higashi TS, Takizawa K, Nagashima J *et al.* Prospective two-phase study of delayed symptoms after intravenous injection of low-osmolality contrast media. *Invest Radiol* 1991;26:S37–S39.
11 Choyke PL, Miller DL, Lotze MT *et al.* Delayed reactions to contrast media after interleukin-2 immunotherapy. *Radiology* 1992;183:111–114.
12 Talierico CP, Vliestra RE, Fisher LD, Burnett JC. Risk for renal dysfunction with cardiac angiography. *Ann Int Med* 1986;104: 501–504.
13 Parfrey PS, Griffiths SM, Barrett BJ *et al.* Contrast material-induced renal failure in patients with diabetes mellitus, renal insufficiency, or both. *New Engl J Med* 1989;320:143–149.
14 Lautin EM, Freeman NJ, Schoenfeld AH *et al.* Radiocontrast-associated renal dysfunction: incidence and risk factors. *Am J Roentgenol* 1991;157:49–58.
15 Cochran ST, Wong WS, Roe DJ. Predicting angiography-induced acute renal function impairment: clinical risk model. *Am J Roentgenol* 1983;141:1027–1033.
16 Harris KG, Smith TP, Cragg AH, Lemke JH. Nephrotoxicity from contrast material in renal insufficiency: ionic versus nonionic agents. *Radiology* 1991;179:849–852.
17 Porter GA. Experimental contrast-associated nephropathy and its clinical implications. *Am J Cardiol* 1990;66:18F–22F.
18 Teruel JL, Marcen R, Onaindia JM, Serrano A, Quereda C, Ortuno J. Renal functional impairment caused by intravenous urography: a prospective study. *Arch Int Med* 1981;141:1271–1274.
19 Love L, Lind JA, Olson MC. Persistent CT nephrogram: significance in the diagnosis of contrast nephropathy. *Radiology* 1989; 172:125–129.
20 Bettmann MA. The evaluation of contrast-related renal failure. *Am J Roentgenol* 1991;157:66–68.
21 Schwab SJ, Hlatky MA, Pieper KS *et al.* Contrast nephropathy: a randomized controlled trial of a nonionic and an ionic radiographic contrast agent. *New Engl J Med* 1989;320:149–153.
22 Porter GA. Contrast-associated nephropathy. *Am J Cardiol* 1989; 64:22E–26E.
23 Mansake C, Sprafka J, Stony J, Wang Y. Contrast nephropathy in azotemic patients undergoing coronary angiography. *Am J Med* 1990;89:615–619.
24 McCarthy CS, Becker JA. Multiple myeloma and contrast media. *Radiology* 1992;183:519–521.
25 Baez-Diaz L, Martinez-Maldolando M. Paraproteinemic disorders. In: Massry SG, Glassock RJ, eds. *Textbook of Nephrology,*

2nd edn. Vol. 1. Baltimore: Williams & Wilkins, 1989:738–745.

26 DeFronzo RA, Humphrey RL, Wright JR, Cooke CR. Acute renal failure in multiple myeloma. *Medicine* 1975;54:209–223.

27 Kinnison ML, Powe NR, Steinberg EP. Results of radiologic controlled trials of low vs high osmolality contrast media. *Radiology* 1989;170:381–386.

28 Moore RD, Steinberg EP, Powe NR *et al.* Nephrotoxicity of high-osmolality contrast media: randomized clinical trial. *Radiology* 1992;182:649–655.

29 Lautin EM, Freeman NJ, Schoenfeld AH *et al.* Radiocontrast associated renal dysfunction: a comparison of lower-osmolality and conventional high-osmolality contrast media. *Am J Roentgenol* 1991;157:59–65.

30 Harris KG, Smith TP, Cragg AH *et al.* Nephrotoxicity from contrast material in renal insufficiency: ionic versus nonionic agents. *Radiology* 1991;179:849–852.

31 Katholi RF, Taylor GJ, Wood WT *et al.* Nephrotoxicity of nonionic low-osmolality versus high-osmolality contrast media: a prospective double-blind randomized comparison in human beings. *Radiology* 1993;186:183–187.

32 Mudge GH. Nephrotoxicity radiocontrast drugs. *Kidney Int* 1980;18:540–552.

33 Lasser EC, Berry CC, Talner LB *et al.* Pretreatment with corticosteroids to alleviate reactions to intravenous contrast material. *New Engl J Med* 1987;317:845–849.

34 Greenberger PA, Patterson R, Radin RC. Two pretreatment regimens for high-risk patients receiving radiographic contrast media. *J Allergy Clin Immunol* 1984;74:540–543.

35 Zweiman B, Mishkin MM, Hildreth EA. An approach to the performance of contrast studies in contrast material-reactive persons. *Ann Int Med* 1975;83:159–163.

36 Greenberger PA, Patterson R. The prevention of immediate generalized reactions to radiocontrast media in high-risk patients. *J Allergy Clin Immunol* 1991;87:867–872.

37 Wolf GL, Mishkin MM, Roux SG *et al.* Comparison of the rates of adverse drug reactions: ionic contrast agents, ionic agents combined with steroids, and nonionic agents. *Invest Radiol* 1991:26:404–410.

38 American College of Radiology, Committee on Drugs and Contrast Media, Commission on Education. In: Bettman MA, Bueguer RE, Gelfaud DW *et al.*, eds. *Manual on Iodinated Contrast Media.* Boston, VA: American College of Radiology, 1991:28–29.

39 McClennan BL. Ionic versus nonionic contrast media: safety, tolerance, and rationale for use. *Urol Radiol* 1989;11:200–202.

40 Bettmann MA. Guidelines for use of low-osmolality contrast agents. *Radiology* 1989;172:901–903.

41 Montgomery WH, Donegan J, Mcintyre KM (Chairperson). Standards and guidelines for cardiopulmonary resuscitation (CPR) and emergency cardiac care (ECC). Part III. *J Am Med Assoc* 1986;225:2936–2942.

42 Bagenstose AH, Tennenbaum JI. Anaphylaxis: a medical emergency. *Compr Ther* 1980;6(4):6–10.

43 Bush WH. Treatment of systemic reactions to contrast media. *Urology* 1990;33:145–150.

44 Cohan RH, Dunnick NR, Bashore TM. Treatment of reactions to radiographic contrast media. *Am J Roentgenol* 1988;151:263–270.

45 Bush WH, Swanson DP. Acute reaction to intravascular contrast media: types, risk factors, recognition, and specific treatment. *Am J Roentgenol* 1991;157:1153–1161.

46 Lehr D, Guideri G. More on combined beta-agonist and methyl-

47 Barach EM, Nowak RM, Lee TG *et al.* Epinephrine for treatment of anaphylactic shock. *J Am Med Assoc* 1984;215(16):2118–2122.

48 Katzberg RW. *The Contrast Media Manual*, 1st edn. Baltimore: Williams & Wilkins, 1992.

49 Mayumi H, Kimura S, Asano M *et al.* Intravenous cimitidine as an effective treatment for systemic anaphylaxis and acute allergic skin reactions. *Ann Allergy* 1987;58:447–450.

50 Netzel MC. Anaphylaxis: clinical presentation, immunologic mechanisms, and treatment. *J Emerg Med* 1986;4:227–236.

51 Bielory L, Kaliner MA. Anaphylactoid reactions to radiocontrast materials. *Int Anesthesiol Clin* 1985;23(3):97–118.

52 Borish L, Matloff SM, Findley SR. Radiographic contrast media induced noncardiogenic pulmonary edema: case report and review of literature. *J Allergy Clin Immunol* 1984;74:104–107.

53 Burd DAR, Santis G, Milward TM. Severe extravasation injury: an avoidable iatrogenic disaster. *Br Med J* 1985;290:1579–1580.

54 Upton J, Mulliken JB, Murray JE. Major intravenous extravasation during peripheral phlebography. *Am J Surg* 1979;137:497–506.

55 Ayre-Smith G. Tissue necrosis following extravasation of contrast media. *J Can Assoc Radiol* 1982;33:104.

56 Lea Thomas J. Gangrene following peripheral phlebography of the legs. *Br J Radiol* 1970;43:528–530.

57 Berge T, Bergqvist D, Efsing HO, Hallbook T. Local complications of ascending phlebography. *Clin Radiol* 1978;29:691–696.

58 Cohan RH, Leder RA, Bolick D *et al.* Extravascular extravasation of radiographic contrast media. Effects of conventional and low-osmolar agents in the rat thigh. *Invest Radiol* 1990;25:504–510.

59 Kim SH, Park JH, Kim YI, Kim CW, Han MC. Experimental tissue damage after subcutaneous injection of water soluble contrast media. *Invest Radiol* 1990;25:678–685.

60 Loth TS, Jones DEC. Extravasations of radiographic contrast material in the upper extremity. *J Hand Surg* 1988;13:395–398.

61 Gothlin J. The comparative frequency of extravasal injection at phlegraphy with steel and plastic cannula. *Clin Radiol* 1972;23:183–184.

62 Elam EA, Dorr RT, Lagel KE, Pond GD. Cutaneous ulceration due to contrast extravasation: experimental assessment of injury and potential antidotes. *Invest Radiol* 1991;26:13–16.

63 Park KS, Kim SH, Park JH, Han MC, Kim DY, Kim SJ. Methods for mitigating soft-tissue injury after subcutaneous injection of water soluble contrast media. *Invest Radiol* 1993;28:332–334.

64 McCallister WH, Palmer K. The histologic effects of four commonly used media for excretory urography and an attempt to modify the responses. *Radiology* 1971;99:511–516.

65 Cohan RH, Leder RA, Hertzberg AJ, Hedlund LW, Beam CA, Dunnick NR. *Treatment of Injuries Induced by Extravasation of Radiologic Contrast Media.* Presentation at the Association of University Radiologists 38th Annual Meeting. Minneapolis MN, April, 1990.

66 Bellone JD. Treatment of vincristine extravasation. *J Am Med Assoc* 1981;245:343.

67 Dorr AT, Alberts DS. Modulation of experimental doxorubicin skin toxicity by beta-adrenergic compounds. *Cancer Res* 1981;41:2428–2432.

68 Oliver IN. The optimal management of cytotoxic-drug extravasation: solving the burning question. *Med J Aust* 1988;149:405.

69 Lawrence JH, Walsh D, Zapotowski KA, Denham A, Goodnight

SH, Gandara DR. Topical dimethylsulfoxide may present tissue damage from anthracycline extravasation. *Cancer Chemother Pharmacol* 1989;23:316−318.

70 Cohan RH, Dunnick NR, Leder RA, Baker ME. Extravasation of nonionic radiologic contrast media: efficiency of conservative treatment. *Radiology* 1990;174:65−67.

71 Sistrom CL, Gay SB, Peffley L. Extravasation of Iopamidol and Iohexol during contrast-enhanced CT: report of 28 cases. *Radiology* 1991;180:707−710.

72 Pond GD, Dorr RT, McAleese KA. Skin ulceration from extravasation of low-osmolality contrast medium: a complication of automation. *Am J Roentgenol* 1992;158:915−916.

73 Memolo M, Dyer R, Zagoria RJ. Extravasation injury with nonionic contrast material. *Am J Roentgenol* 1993;160:203.

74 Weese DL, Greenberg HM, Zimmerman PE. Contrast media reactions during voiding cystourethrography or retrograde pyelography. *Urology* 1993;41(1):81−83.

75 Goldstein AG, Conger KB. Perforation of the ureter during retrograde pyelography. *J Urol* 1965;94:288−290.

76 Dunnick NR, McCallum RW, Sandler CM. *A Textbook of Uroradiology*. Baltimore: Williams & Wilkins, 1991.

77 Gold IW, Sternbach GL. Spontaneous urinary extravasation during intravenous pyelography. *Ann Emerg Med* 1982;11:485−486.

78 Bernardino ME, McClennan BL. High dose urography: incidence and relationship to spontaneous peripelvic extravasation. *Am J Roentgenol* 1976;127:373−376.

79 Baker JS, Carlin MR, Hammerman H. Pyelosinus extravasation in the acute renal colic patient. *Ann Emerg Med* 1981;10:437−440.

80 Imray TJ, Lieberman RP. Retrograde pyelography. In: Pollack HM, ed. *Clinical Urography: An Atlas and Textbook of Urological Imaging*. Philadelphia, PA: WB Saunders Co, 1990:244−255.

81 Whalley DW, Ibels LS, Eckstein RP, Alexander JH, Smith RD. Acute tubular necrosis complicating bilateral retrograde pyelography. *Aust N Z J Med* 1987;17(5):536−538.

82 McCallum RW, Colapinto V. *Urological Radiology of the Adult Male Lower Urinary Tract: Anatomy, Physiology, Pathology and Sequelae Diagnosis and Management*. Springfield, IL: Charles C Thomas Publisher, 1976.

83 Gupta SK, Kaur B, Shulka RC. Urethro-venous intravasation during retrograde urethrography (report of 5 cases). *J Postgrad Med* 1991;37(2):102−104.

84 McAlister WH, Cacciarelli A, Shackelford GD. Complications associated with cystography in children. *Radiology* 1974;111:167−172.

85 Hertz M. Cystourethrography. In: Pollack HM, ed. *Clinical Urography: An Atlas and Textbook of Urological Imaging*. Philadelphia, PA: WB Saunders Co, 1990:256−295.

86 McClennan BL, Becker JA, Robinson T. Venous extravasation at retrograde urethrography: precautions. *J Urol* 1971;106:412.

87 Castellino RA, Marshall WH Jr. The urinary mucosal barrier in retrograde pyelography: experimental findings and clinical implications. *Radiology* 1970;95:403−409.

88 Bettenay F, de Campo J. Allergic reaction following micturating cystourethrography. *Urol Radiol* 1989;11:167−168.

89 Friedland GW, Perkash J. Neuromuscular dysfunction of the bladder and urethra. *Semin Roentgenol* 1983;18:255−266.

Complications of interventional uroradiology

Michael J. Kellett

Cyst puncture

Diagnostic aspiration of suspected cysts is only required when the diagnosis is in doubt. This may be in an obese patient where ultrasound (US) may be equivocal, and a simple diagnostic aspiration under local anesthesia will give a rapid and accurate diagnosis avoiding a more costly computed tomography (CT) scan. Alternately, the CT scan may be equivocal if there has been a recent bleed into the cyst or if the wall of the cyst is slightly irregular or thickened.

Cyst aspiration is usually performed with direct US guidance under local anesthesia. For a diagnostic tap a fine 22-gage needle is adequate as the aim is not to aspirate the cyst "dry", merely to confirm clear straw-colored fluid and send a sample for cytologic screening. Occasionally, large cysts may be symptomatic, in which case a Seldinger technique is used to insert a multiple side-hole catheter for complete aspiration. The complications of this procedure are similar, but less common, to those of a needle nephrostomy.

Ablation of cyst

Instillation of irritant substances such as tetracycline or Myodil in an attempt to close off a cyst is very rarely indicated, as cyst recurrence is still likely in over 50% of cases. Alcohol has been used with greater success, but as

with embolization it does carry the danger of any liquid embolizing agent in that it may intravasate and reach other parts of the kidney or other organs. Care must be taken to inject contrast first to ensure that the cyst is not communicating with the collecting system or the vascular tree before instilling a small quantity of alcohol. After 1–2 minutes the alcohol should be reaspirated.

Antegrade pyelography

The most rapid and accurate method to demonstrate the presence and site of an obstruction is by antegrade pyelography. This is usually combined with a percutaneous nephrostomy if obstruction is present. If there is good renal function, intravenous contrast may be given first in order to use fluoroscopic guidance for the antegrade puncture. Problems can be encountered if there is poor visualization of the pelvicaliceal system. A suitable dose of intravenous contrast (up to 2 ml/kg body weight of a 300–350 mgI/ml contrast medium) should be given. If there is diminished renal function the puncture is performed under US guidance. In general, the complications of renal puncture for any purpose are the same and these will be covered under Percutaneous needle nephrostomy.

Antegrade pressure-flow studies (Whitaker test)

When an obstruction is suspected but diuretic intravenous urography or diuretic isotopic scans have been equivocal, the kidney may be tested by a pressure-flow study. This involves inserting two needles or a double-lumen pigtail catheter into the pervicaliceal system. The kidney can then be perfused at a known flow rate with dilute contrast medium, while the intrarenal pressure is simultaneously recorded from the second needle or down the second lumen of the catheter. Clearly, if there is obstruction and the contrast flow is continued without care the high intrarenal pressure that may result would give *intravasation*. If there is any infection present this may give rise to *bacteremia* or possibly *septicemia*. The complications of the test are otherwise very low, similar care being required as is taken for a needle nephrostomy.

Percutaneous needle nephrostomy

Patient positioning

The prone oblique position is the most comfortable for the patient and gives the radiologist the best access. The arm on the side to be punctured should be lifted up on to the pillow, thus increasing the gap between the ribcage and the iliac crest. A pad placed under the flank will prevent a very mobile kidney from rotating anteriorly in the prone position. This will later facilitate the manipulation of a guidewire from a posterior calix into the renal pelvis and possibly down the ureter. The contralateral arm should be resting by the side of the patient to prevent shoulder strain. The head is turned to the side to be punctured to avoid neck strain. A pillow under the ankles gives a comfortable position to the patient's feet. All these points will reduce patient movement during the renal puncture, facilitating the nephrostomy placement, and avoiding many of the complications caused by loss of the track.

Anesthesia and sedation

Simple local anesthesia (1–2% lignocaine) is sufficient for most needle nephrostomies. Up to 20 ml of 1% lignocaine can be given for the average 70-kg patient, concentrating the anesthesia in the skin and around the capsule of the kidney. It is often impossible to anesthetize the calix and patients do feel pain when the fornix to a calix is distorted by a needle tip or guidewire. This should be anticipated by the operator and simple forewarning to the patient (e.g., "you may feel some pressure in the kidney now...") will usually encourage an anxious patient. Indeed, a quiet running commentary during the procedure results in a cooperative patient and the dividends are far greater than with a sedated but restless patient or heavy sedation with its added risks.

When bilateral nephrostomies are being inserted, or in the very anxious patient or child, sedation pre- or peroperative may be helpful. An intravenous cannula should be inserted into the back of the hand which is on the pillow. A small dose of sedative (e.g., 2 mg of midazolam in an adult, diluted with saline, and given slowly will usually have adequate calming effects on the patient and give good postoperative amnesia, but not heavy sedation with the consequent risk of respiratory depression. Sedation during radiologic procedures is fully covered in Chapters 1 and 2. Anesthetists are justifiably anxious that the radiologist is following the dental surgeon and becoming an operator anesthetist [1]. It is dangerous to sedate patients heavily and then proceed to operate in a radiology department without full patient monitoring equipment, including a pulse oximeter and an assistant monitoring the patient. Close consultation with the anesthetic department is advised. At the very least, a nurse trained in anesthesia should be present when intravenous sedation is used.

Needles

Many nephrostomy needles have a beveled cutting edge which can cut blood vessel walls. Diamond tipped and conical-ended needles are probably less traumatic, pushing the vessels to one side (Fig. 33.1). To allow a guidewire to be

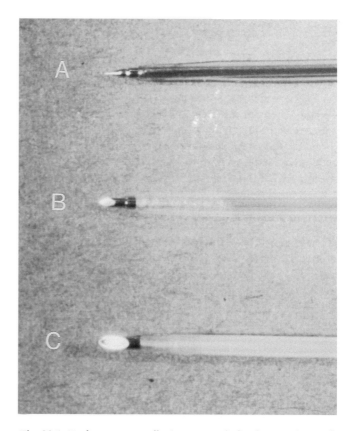

Fig. 33.1 Nephrostomy needle tips: (A) conical stylet; (B) diamond point; and (C) beveled cutting needle. All have flexible Teflon sheaths.

inserted, the needles have either a rigid cannula or a soft sheath. A cannula may cause trauma to the parenchyma during respiratory movements of the kidney: this, however, is minimal. More important, a rigid sheath is more easily displaced from a calix. A flexible sheath is less likely to "cheese-wire" the parenchyma and less likely to be displaced from the collecting system during respiratory movement of the kidney.

Hemorrhage

Bleeding is the most common complication of any renal puncture and in a mild form is unavoidable. A clotting screen should be performed before needle nephrostomy, to ensure that no coagulation defect is present [2]. However, occasionally with an emergency nephrostomy it is more important to relieve the obstruction than to worry about the remote chance of a bleeding disorder. To avoid bleeding from a major vessel, the site of renal puncture is more important than the type of needle used. A central puncture towards the renal pelvis, and therefore near the hilum of the kidney, is obviously more likely to damage a large hilar vessel than a needle approaching the lateral border of the lower pole. A calix should be pierced, thus crossing the least depth of parenchyma and tracking parallel to the interlobular vessels. Such "peripheral" punctures cause the least trauma [3]. A "central" puncture between calices is more likely to hit interlobular vessels and cause hemorrhage (Fig. 33.2). If a large vessel is punctured, the needle should be withdrawn and angled more toward the periphery of the calix or possibly a different calix. The anterior calices tend to be more lateral on fluoroscopy and the posterior calices, which should be the target as they will result in a correct peripheral puncture, are situated more medially.

It should be remembered that after a few unsuccessful passes, there may be hematuria. When aspirating to confirm that the needle is in the collecting system, hematuria can be confused with venous blood. If in doubt, gentle probing with a "J"-guidewire may confirm a good puncture, the wire passing freely into the renal pelvis under fluoroscopy. A little dilute contrast could be injected to confirm a correct puncture, but if in the renal sinus, the resultant contrast "smudge" may cause imaging problems for subsequent punctures.

When advancing Teflon fascial dilators or a small pigtail nephrostomy over the guidewire, a little venous ooze is to be expected to start with. The catheter itself will tamponade such bleeding from the track. Decompression of a tense hydronephrosis will result in bleeding from capillaries in the urothelium, similar to that seen when decompressing an obstructed bladder by catheterization. Hematuria for between 6 and 24 hours is to be expected following the insertion of a needle nephrostomy into a hydronephrosis. Serious hemorrhage requiring transfusion or prolonged hospitalization occurs in less than 5% of cases [4]. In comparison, up to 25% of patients require transfusion after surgical nephros-

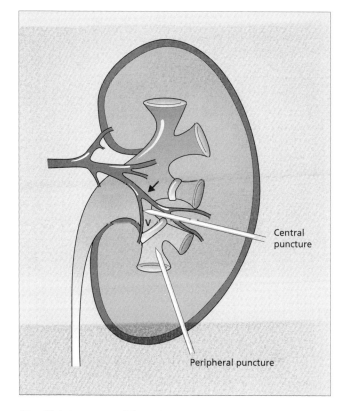

Fig. 33.2 Punctures of the collecting system. A peripheral puncture is less traumatic as it enters the papilla. A central puncture may pierce the complex veins around the caliceal necks (V) or interlobular arteries (arrow).

tomy [5]. Renal hemorrhage following the placement of a percutaneous needle nephrostomy, is now managed by selective percutaneous arterial embolization with extremely good results and low morbidity [6].

Damage to other organs

Fluoroscopic or US-guided punctures performed with forethought of the anatomy, should avoid damage to organs adjacent to the kidney. However, occasionally the kidney is difficult to image. A poorly functioning kidney may not excrete intravenous contrast sufficiently to visualize it at fluoroscopy, or US may be difficult in very obese patients. If the system has not been entered after three passes with the nephrostomy needle, a second puncture with a fine 21-gage Chiba needle to locate and opacify the collecting system may be used. Such fine needles cause negligible trauma to the kidney or adjacent organs.

Very oblique lateral approaches with a nephrostomy needle should be avoided as the colon, liver, or spleen may be pierced *en route* to the kidney [7]. In particular, lateral punctures in women may pass through the colon [8]. The lack of retroperitoneal fat compared to subcutaneous fat in women allows the descending colon to drop into the pararenal gutter (Fig. 33.3a). In men, on the other hand, there is

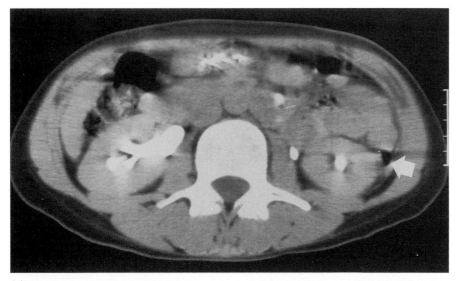

(a)

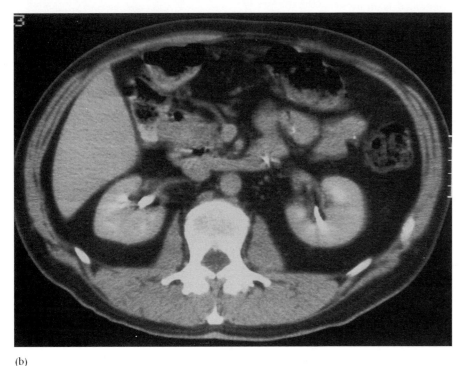

(b)

Fig. 33.3 (a) Female descending colon (arrow) lying close to left kidney — little retroperitoneal fat interposed. (b) Compare male abundant retroperitoneal fat displacing descending colon anterior to lateral border of left kidney.

a high ratio of retroperitoneal fat to subcutaneous fat and the descending colon is often displaced out of the left pararenal gutter (Fig. 33.3b).

If a transcolonic puncture is only appreciated after the nephrostomy has been inserted, conservative management is recommended allowing the track to heal around the catheter [9]. A second nephrostomy can be inserted and the first catheter removed later, after allowing 5–10 days for the track to heal. The catheter should first be withdrawn to lie within the lumen of the bowel, thus draining the bowel for a few days before being fully withdrawn. Such conservative

staged removal allows time for the track to heal which may prevent spillage of bowel contents and allow the small perforation to close, avoiding an open operation (S. Petterrson, personal communication).

A nephrostomy needle advanced too far may puncture the small bowel or gall bladder. If a gall-bladder puncture is made, a catheter must be inserted as a drain. This should then be left in the gall bladder for 7–10 days to allow the track to heal before being withdrawn, thus avoiding bile leakage and biliary peritonitis.

Intercostal punctures

A supra twelfth rib puncture should, if possible, be avoided because of the danger of catching pleura and causing a pneumothorax [10]. If the kidney is too high and an intercostal route is unavoidable, a puncture can safely be made over the tip of the twelfth rib [11]. The parietal pleural reflection usually leaves the twelfth rib two-thirds of the way along its length to ride up to the eleventh rib. Thus, there is a safe triangle of access over the tip of the twelfth rib (Fig. 33.4).

Such high punctures are usually only necessary for access to an upper calix for percutaneous nephrolithotomy. A simple drainage nephrostomy through a lower calix can nearly always be performed angling up underneath the twelfth rib. Punctures very close to the ribs should be avoided because intercostal vessels and nerves may be damaged. A nephrostomy can cause severe pain if it is irritating an intercostal nerve.

Guidewires

A floppy J-guidewire introduced into a lower calix will slide into the renal pelvis causing the least trauma. A straight guidewire might snare the urothelium or, if the puncture was initially too deep and there is a small track through the anterior wall of the calix, a straight guidewire may enter the parenchyma through this track.

Once a guidewire is coiled in the renal pelvis, the track needs some dilatation before introducing a pigtail nephrostomy. One of the most common causes of a failed needle nephrostomy is losing the track because of a kinked guidewire. When advancing Teflon fascial dilators over a floppy wire, it is very easy to angle the dilator slightly which will tug on the guidewire. To persist in advancing the dilator will either kink the guidewire or twist the wire out of the collecting system. Controlling the guidewire with one hand, while gently advancing the dilator will prevent this happen-

ing, because a warning tug will be felt if the track is being angled at all [12]. Heavy duty guidewires or stiff Amplatz wires may be helpful if the track is being dilated for endoscopy, but they are rarely necessary for a simple nephrostomy.

Insertion of nephrostomy

The track needs to be dilated up to, or slightly larger than the size of the nephrostomy, particularly when there is scar tissue, otherwise the softer nephrostomy catheter will kink as it is being advanced. The coil of the pigtail should be seated in the pelvis or upper calix. If it is passed down the ureter, the coil may open and the tip may traumatize or even perforate the ureter [10]. Adequate fixation of the catheter to the skin is essential to prevent it subsequently being pulled out by a restless patient. It is safer to use two skin sutures with multiple slip knots wrapped firmly around the catheter. Adhesive disks are generally less secure. Dressings should be applied to prevent the nephrostomy from kinking at the skin or at the catheter hub. Coiling the nephrostomy underneath an adhesive dressing prevents an accidental tug pulling on the skin sutures. A loose rubber connector to the drainage bag is also safer than a tight luer lock, so that any accidental tug results in a disconnected bag rather than a displaced nephrostomy.

Pyonephrosis and septicemia

An important indication for an emergency needle nephrostomy is the presence or suspicion of a pyonephrosis. When pus is encountered it is very important that the pressure in the collecting system should not be raised by injection of large volumes of contrast medium. Injecting contrast medium before aspirating the pus will increase intrarenal pressure and cause intrarenal reflux of infected urine. This may lead to a Gram-negative septicemia, the very complication of a pyonephrosis that one is trying to avoid by performing a nephrostomy. For this reason, a single-puncture technique is preferable using US guidance. A double puncture, injecting contrast through a Chiba needle first, may cause intravasation of infected urine before the nephrostomy needle can decompress the system. Dilatation of the track to insert a large catheter may also cause septicemia. Such large nephrostomies are not necessary even with thick pus in the urine. Gentle intermittent irrigation with saline can help to clear catheters when pus is very thick [4]. Once the pressure in a system has been relieved, a diuresis will occur diluting and thinning the pus and washing it out even through small holes in a 7-F catheter. If a pyonephrosis is suspected, a broad-spectrum antibiotic, such as gentamicin, should be given before the procedure. Approximately 2% of patients with pyonephrosis will have septicemia as a result of a needle nephrostomy [4]. A diagnostic nephrostogram to show the site and possible nature fo an obstruction should

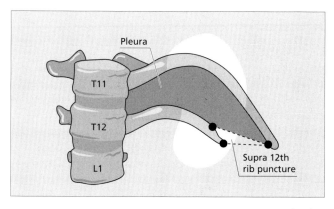

Fig. 33.4 Pleura leaves the twelfth rib early, allowing triangle of access to the kidney over the tip of the twelfth rib (●).

be postponed for several days. Stables *et al.* [4], in reviewing 1207 patients who had had needle nephrostomies, reported two deaths (0.2%). In comparison, open renal surgical mortality rates range from 1 to 6% [13].

Long-term nephrostomies

The length of time a single nephrostomy can be left without blocking is very variable. Some become encrusted within 1 week, while others may last several months. Silastic catheters are less irritant than polyethylene or polyurethane catheters. They are also less likely to kink. Sutures or other surface anchors are not practicable for securing long-term nephrostomies. A self-retaining loop mechanism, as in the Cope catheter, is preferable to prevent displacement of the nephrostomy. A fine thread passing down the catheter once pulled maintains a fixed loop to the pigtail within the pelvis of the kidney. An attempt to remove these catheters, without releasing the cord closing the loop, can severely traumatize the kidney.

The mechanism of the catheter should be explained to patients in case they are admitted to another hospital unfamiliar with such nephrostomies. Replacing kinked or blocked catheters may be difficult if a guidewire cannot be advanced through the lumen of a nephrostomy. The track may well be mature enough for gentle probing with a guidewire or soft catheter once the nephrostomy has been withdrawn. If the track is mature, a small soft Foley catheter may be passed into the kidney as a nephrostomy. If this is used, a further side hole should be cut proximal to the balloon so that the calix through which the catheter passes can drain, and is not obstructed by the inflated balloon. An alternate method of exchanging a blocked nephrostomy is to insert a Teflon sheath over the catheter into the renal pelvis and, after withdrawing the old nephrostomy, insert a fresh catheter through the sheath [14].

Percutaneous nephrolithotomy (PCNL)

Anesthesia

PCNL is usually performed as a one-stage procedure under general anesthesia. Because the patient will be lying prone, controlled ventilation via an endotracheal tube is preferred. The patient's shoulders, elbows, and knees must be adequately padded to prevent pressure effects from the hard X-ray table. When draping the patient, adequate drainage bags to catch the irrigant used for the endoscopy are required to prevent irrigant fluid (saline) from seeping into the mechanisms of the table, causing rust and electric hazards.

The initial procedure of puncturing the collecting system carries the same complications as already described for a simple needle nephrostomy.

Retrograde ureteric catheter

Prior to renal puncture for PCNL, a retrograde catheter is usually passed up the ureter at cystoscopy. The tip of this should be seated at the pelviureteric junction to allow distension and opacification of the system for percutaneous puncture. At the same time, it will prevent large fragments of stone passing down the ureter at endoscopy. Regular blind-ending retrograde catheters can traumatize a tortuous ureter. The least traumatic method of inserting a retrograde is to first pass a straight guidewire. Extremely tortuous ureters can be negotiated with Bentson or Terumo wires. The cystoscope can then be used and a straight 5-F or 7-F catheter fed over the wire. The bladder should be drained by a parallel Foley catheter, as large quantities of irrigant saline may pass down the ureter during a prolonged endoscopic nephrolithopaxy.

Track dilatation

The use of serial fascial dilators exchanged over a guidewire is probably the most common method of dilating a track. Because of the danger of kinking the guidewire, a Lundequist wire with a stiff shaft and floppy tip is recommended. However, care must be taken not to advance this guidewire with the dilators, or the stiff portion will perforate the renal pelvis. An Amplatz extra-stiff wire has a longer more gradual junction between the stiff and floppy wire and is thus safer. Scar tissue needs to be cut first with a scalpel blade, and care should be taken not to damage intercostal vessels or nerves. Extravasation of urine occurs when dilators are exchanged (Fig. 33.5). When dilating a track into a hydronephrosis, aspirating urine first will prevent a large leak of urine which could displace the kidney anteriorly. Aspiration via the retrograde catheter can also help. Each time a dilator is exchanged, there is bleeding into the track, and blood clots collect in the pelvicaliceal system making the subsequent endoscopy difficult. For this reason, metal telescopic dilators, which continually tamponade the track, were developed.

Metal dilators

Metal telescopic dilators designed by Alken fit together like a car aerial, each dilator fitting snugly over the previous one (Fig. 33.6). A shoulder at the tail end of each dilator prevents it advancing further than the previous one, thus limiting the depth. If one dilator is inadvertently missed out and a step is jumped, the larger dilator will not be arrested and could be advanced right through the kidney like a cork bore, causing a severe perforation. Therefore, care must be taken when assembling and using these rigid metal dilators.

It is generally safer to limit the dilatation just to the calix and not attempt to dilate through the caliceal neck into the renal pelvis. This may well split the caliceal neck and cause

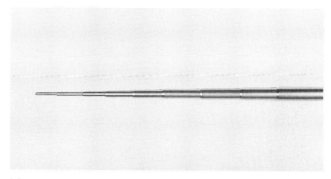

(a)

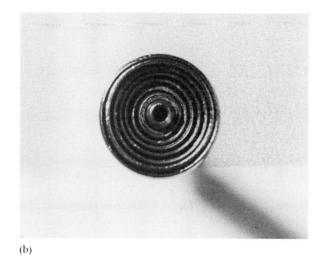

(b)

Fig. 33.6 (a) Metallic aerial dilators snugly fitting over each other. (b) End-on view when fully assembled.

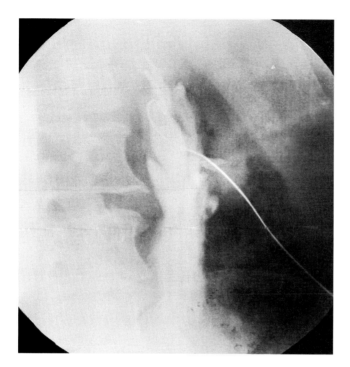

Fig. 33.5 Leakage of contrast and urine from the track during exchange of dilators. Guidewire enters via lower calix to coil in pelvis.

venous bleeding from the veins around the calix. It is better to be slightly short with the dilatation: if the endoscopist cannot quite negotiate a way through into the collecting system, a tapered Teflon dilator the same size as the Amplatz can be used to dilate and advance the Amplatz sheath through the last few millimeters of parenchyma into the calix. The usual difficulty is when a staghorn calculus completely fills the calix being punctured. Any dilator passed over a guidewire between the stone and the urothelium will split the caliceal neck. Provided the endoscopist has a view adequate to reach the tip of the stone with the US or electrohydraulic lithotripter probe, they can create their own space in which to work.

Balloon dilatation

The use of purpose-built balloon catheters is probably the least traumatic method of dilating a track [15], but it does take time and they are expensive. The complication of bursting a balloon is not serious, merely a nuisance. A fixed dilatation of a balloon has been described, requiring needle decompression to remove the catheter [16].

Once a track has been dilated, an Amplatz Teflon sheath is introduced to protect the track through which intrarenal manipulations can be performed.

Endoscopic complications

Rigid nephroscopes combine optimal optics with the best operating instruments, but being rigid they can traumatize the kidney.

Hemorrhage

Tears in the parenchyma can occur if a rigid scope is not handled with care. Toothed alligator forceps can snare the urothelium and cause bleeding. Serious venous or arterial bleeding is rare with a simple nephrolithotomy [17], and is usually due to disintegrating larger stones either with US probes or, more often, electrohydraulic probes. If a stone suddenly moves during disintegration, the probe may slip against the pelvis and damage a vessel just under the urothelium (Fig. 33.7).

Bleeding requiring transfusion following percutaneous renal manipulation is rare, with most reports quoting an incidence of about 3%; about 0.5% of patients may require balloon tamponade of the track or arterial embolization [18]. In a series of the first 500 PCNLs at the Institute of Urology,

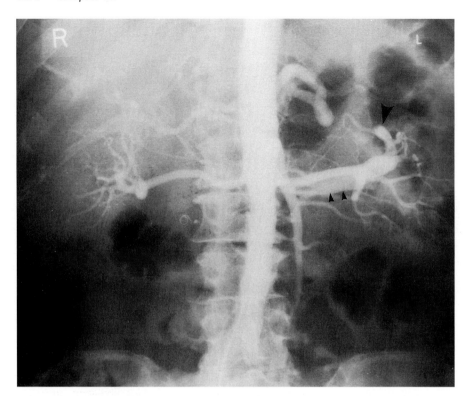

Fig. 33.7 Arteriovenous fistula caused by electrohydraulic probe slipping off staghorn calculus. Renal vein, small arrows.

London, the incidence of bleeding requiring embolization was similar (0.6%), but 6% required transfusion (mean 2.6 U) [19]. However, most of these were in patients with large staghorn calculi, 50% of whom were transfused, whereas transfusion was very rare in patients with small calculi. Bleeding does not appear to be related to the size of the track, which should encourage radiologists dilating tracks. Bleeding is related to the size of the stone treated and thus to methods of stone disintegration. Since having a lithotripter at the Institute of Urology, PCNL has been reserved for complicated large calculi; in the last 1000 cases we have again had an incidence of bleeding requiring embolization of approximately 0.5%.

Extravasation

Any tear in the pelvicaliceal system will result in some extravasation of the irrigant fluid. It is important, therefore, that normal saline is used as the endoscopic irrigant. Water or glycine can cause fluid intoxication because they are absorbed from the retroperitoneum [20].

As mentioned previously, a supra twelfth rib puncture should be kept lateral to avoid the pleura. If a stone is inadvertently pushed out of the collecting system or lost in the track, further endoscopy may retrieve it, but this may also cause further trauma. Calculi left outside the kidney do not appear to cause any serious problems [21,22].

Pleural complications

If an intercostal puncture is performed to reach an upper caliceal calculus, the pleura may be entered and either a minor pleural reaction seen or, following endoscopy, there could be a massive collection of irrigant fluid and air within the thoracic cavity [23].

If the pleural space has been entered, the nephrostomy should be left in to allow a sealed track to form from the calix to the skin [11]. Removing all catheters at the end of PCNL has the theoretical rationale that, provided the kidney is draining freely down the ureter, the parenchymal hole will close and there will not be a fistula to the pleura. However, although this has worked in the majority of our intercostal approaches, we have had one severe pleural empyema from a urinary fistula (Fig. 33.8), and now advocate a more conservative approach with a nephrostomy tamponading and forming a track to the skin. Only when there is no demonstrable leak into the pleural cavity at nephrostogram should the catheter be removed.

Infection

The most serious complication that must be guarded against is infection. A mid-stream specimen of urine must be taken before any manipulation, and any infection found must be treated with the appropriate antibiotic. If an obstruction is present with a pyonephrosis, then a simple nephrostomy should be carried out first, and intrarenal manipulations delayed until the urine is sterile.

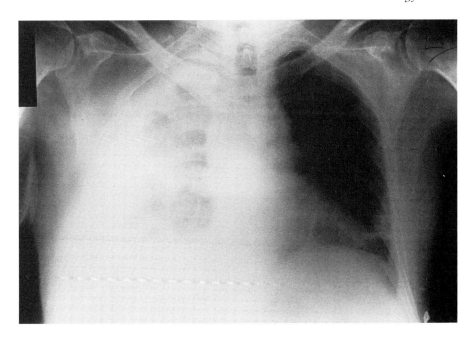

Fig. 33.8 Gross urine collection in the thorax following an upper pole puncture between the eleventh and tenth rib to gain access for PCNL.

Prophylactic antibiotics (see also Chapter 5)

Most surgical procedures in the sterile urinary tract do not require prophylactic antibiotics. However, stones containing bacteria may be disintegrated during PCNL, releasing bacteria into the urine and potentially, therefore into the blood-stream; prophylactic antibiotics should therefore be used routinely. In a series of the first 1000 patients at the Institute of Urology, 10 patients (1%) had serious infections despite prophylactic gentamicin (80–120 mg) given intravenously at the time of PCNL [24].

Bacteremia is unavoidable, but the time of endoscopy should be limited. If a large struvite stone is being disintegrated and infection is clearly present, the endoscopy should be limited to 1 hour. With hard cystine stones, which are not as likely to be infected, endoscopy may be continued for up to 1.5 hours.

Gram-negative septicemia

The classic signs of bradycardia, fever and shivering, nausea, confusion, and hyperventilation, are only present in about two-thirds of patients with Gram-negative septicemia. Old or debilitated patients with septicemia may only exhibit hypothermia, and because of the lack of clear clinical signs mortality may be as high as 83% [25]. Therefore, early treatment of septicemia is vital, with good results to be expected in the initial hyperdynamic phase. If early signs are missed, the subsequent phase is that of hypotension and shock.

Immediately septicemia is suspected, cardiac output and central venous pressure should be monitored, together with arterial blood pressure and urine output. Treatment with

intravenous antibiotics should be commenced. As urinary tract infection can be due to a wide range of organisms, appropriate antibiotics should be used, e.g., gentamicin 80–120 mg intravenously and a cephalosporin. Subsequent doses must be regulated depending upon the renal function. Once culture and sensitivity results have been obtained, treatment can be modified accordingly. Aggressive intravenous fluid replacement should be given initially, this being modified by the central venous pressure monitoring.

Post-PCNL nephrostomy

After an uneventful PCNL it is not always necessary to insert a nephrostomy. At the Institute of Urology a nephrostomy is placed if:
1 there has been perforation of the renal pelvis;
2 there is bleeding requiring tamponade;
3 there is edema at pelviureteric junction or other cause for poor ureteric drainage;
4 there are any retained fragments.

The removal of the nephrostomy is usually dependent upon a normal postoperative nephrostogram at 1–3 days. A modification of a Whitaker pressure-flow study can be performed to ensure free flow into the bladder [26], or one can merely clamp the nephrostomy and judge by the patient's symptoms before removing the nephrostomy.

Treatment of ureteric stones

The use of baskets introduced via a nephrostomy track into the ureter for the removal of small calculi under X-ray control is widely practised [18]; in expert hands the results are excellent. However, the urothelium may be snared by the baskets and a perforation created. More seriously, the ureter may be torn or avulsed by excessive tugging with a basket. When the ureteric stone has only been in the ureter for 1–2 weeks, it can usually be flushed back to the kidney using a retrograde catheter and saline. The stone can then be removed by PCNL under the same anesthesia, or a JJ-stent can be inserted to prevent the stone reentering the ureter and extracorporeal shock wave lithotripsy (ESWL) performed on the calculus. Alternately, fluoroscopically guided ESWL can be used to treat the ureteric stone *in situ*.

The problem stones are those found in the ureter with severe surrounding bullous edema. They may not disintegrate with ESWL if not surrounded by urine in a dilated ureter, and the edema may prevent retrograde flushing of the stone back to the kidney. Retrograde ureteroscopy is indicated here with disintegration of the stone either with laser [27] or with small electrohydraulic probes. The latter can cause severe ureteric trauma with perforation [28]. A safety guidewire should be manipulated past the stone first, either by the ureteroscopy or, if a needle nephrostomy has already been performed to relieve obstruction, the guidewire can be gently manipulated past the ureteric stone by the antegrade route using local anesthetic before the ureteroscopy.

Occasionally, stones jammed high in the ureter require an antegrade ureteroscopic approach. A high upper caliceal puncture can allow the endoscopist to use a rigid ureteroscope but care must be taken not to involve the pleura, as has already been stressed. Small flexible ureteroscopes can overcome this problem using laser to disintegrate the ureteric stone.

Following all these maneuvers, ureteric edema and possibly perforation may well be present: a ureteric stent should therefore be inserted at the end of each procedure.

The main complications of ureteroscopy are perforation, urine leakage, or edematous stricture. If the endoscopist has not anticipated these and failed to insert a JJ-stent, the radiologist may be left with the job of diverting the urine and stenting the ureter (Fig. 33.9) (see below).

ESWL

Small renal calculi lying within a normally draining pelvi-caliceal system are eminently suitable for fragmentation by ESWL [29]. There are virtually no complications with these small calculi.

Calculi over 2 cm in diameter will almost certainly give rise to an obstructing steinstrasse after ESWL (Fig. 33.10); retrograde JJ-stents should therefore be inserted in the ureter prior to lithotripsy to avoid the dangers of obstruction and septicemia [30]. Once the stone has been adequately fragmented, which may take several ESWL sessions, and provided the bulk of fragments have passed alongside the stent, the latter is removed. This can be done with sedation and local anesthesia, particularly if using flexible cystoscopes.

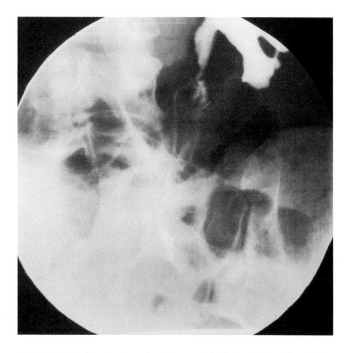

Fig. 33.9 Nephrostogram showing partial obstruction and ureteric leak following ureteroscopic lithotripsy. A stent inserted percutaneously for 2 weeks allowed it to heal.

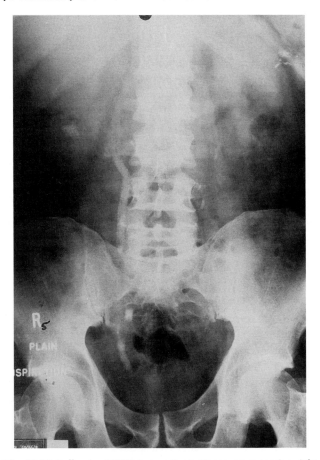

Fig. 33.10 Following ESWL to two 3-cm stones, an extensive right steinstrasse is obstructing the right kidney.

For partial or complete staghorn calculi, ESWL alone has been attempted — so-called monotherapy. However, the number of sessions required and the high incidence of obstruction, even with JJ-stents *in situ*, have led to most centers adopting a debulking PCNL first, leaving ESWL for the small caliceal fragments that cannot be reached with the one session of PCNL. ESWL has been researched and tested perhaps more than any other new treatment modality and the complications are well documented [31,32].

With the basic approach laid out above, complications should be avoidable. The acute problems are subcapsular hematoma or, very rarely, rupture of the kidney. This may be due to using too long a session with a poorly focused shock wave. Bacterial release at lithotripsy is to be expected; adequate antibiotic cover should always be given. Obstruction by an infected steinstrasse must always be kept in mind with prophylactic ureteric stenting for any stone larger than 2 cm.

Late effects are still being checked. In particular, hypertension probably secondary to subcapsular hemorrhage and increased capsular pressure have been implicated, but the incidence appears to be no greater than in the general population and, in particular, no greater than following open surgery for renal calculi.

By combining ESWL, PCNL, and ureteroscopy, over 98% of urinary tract calculi can be treated without open surgery. With careful consideration of the position and size of the calculi, and the anatomy and drainage of the pelvicaliceal system, the appropriate treatment can be selected with an overall complication rate that is extremely low [32,33].

Ureteric stent insertion

Ureteric stents may be inserted via a retrograde or antegrade route. When the patient is having cystoscopy anyway, the retrograde route is attempted first under the same general anesthesia. If a needle nephrostomy is indicated, then the anterior route may be used with local anesthesia only. It can be difficult to maneuver a JJ-stent around the bend of the pelviureteric junction, but tortuous ureters are more easily negotiated from above than below. The use of a stiffer wire can ease the tight bend at the pelviureteric junction, but such wires may be traumatic unless care is taken. Salazar *et al.* [34] have described a JJ-stent perforating a renal pelvis, but this must be quite rare. A fistula between the ureter and the iliac artery following stricture dilatation and stent insertion has also been described [35].

The main complication of percutaneous insertion of JJ-stents is incorrect positioning. If the distal end is short of the ureteric orifice it will not function as a ureteric drain. If too long a stent is used, the distal end coiled against the trigone can give severe irritation (Fig. 33.11). It is often difficult to see the position of the pusher catheter tip and for this reason the JJ-stent may be advanced too far. If the proximal end of the stent is not advanced sufficiently, there is the possibility

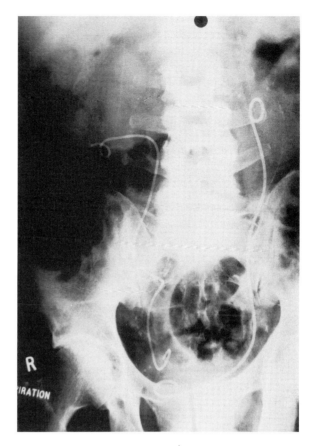

Fig. 33.11 Left JJ-stent too long, with the lower end irritating the trigone. Right stent also too long and the proximal end is in renal parenchyma.

of a retrograde leak through the parenchyma, giving rise to a perirenal collection.

Dilatation of ureteric strictures

Benign ureteric strictures may be dilated with graduated Teflon dilators (van Andel William Cook Ltd) or with purpose-built balloon catheters. Rupture or perforation of the ureter often occurs and is unavoidable. It may be more serious in transplant patients on immunosuppression, with strictures at the ureteric anastomosis to the bladder; careful follow-up with US is recommended here, with appropriate antibiotic cover during and after the procedure.

A false passage may be created by the guidewire attempting to pass a ureteric stricture. A careful ureterogram with dilute contrast to define the anatomy and direction of the ureteric stricture should first be performed, so that an appropriate catheter (straight-tapered 5-F van Andel or cobra catheter) can be chosen. A floppy Bentson wire or a straight or bent Terumo wire should then be used; these wires give the best chance of passing a tortuous stricture without ureteric trauma. If a stricture cannot be passed, or if a perforation is made, it is worth leaving a nephrostomy draining for 1 week, repeating the procedure after the ureter has healed and perhaps some of the edema at the stricture site has subsided. It may well prove feasible to cross the stricture at this second attempt.

Rendezvous procedures

Complete strictures of the ureter can be approached by combined antegrade (radiologic) and retrograde (uretero-scopic) manipulations. A nephrostomy is first performed and a catheter and guidewire passed down to the blocked ureter. The patient is then turned onto the supine position for ureteroscopy. The proximal limit of the stricture is distended with dilute contrast and methylene blue via the nephrostomy. A guidewire is then inserted to probe the ureter from above. The endoscopist may then see some blue dye and the movement of the guidewire and, using the ureteroscope and a guidewire, can probe his/her way through. The upper guidewire is then grasped by the ureteroscope, or the radio-logist manipulates the guidewire down the ureter into the bladder. This is then grasped via a cystoscope so that a wire passes through from the nephrostomy track to the urethra. This gives stability for stricture dilatation and the insertion of a JJ-stent.

Perforation of the ureter is part of the procedure and adequate antibiotic cover is needed. A nephrostomy is required for a few days, until the ureteric leak has healed, in order to divert urine away from this area.

Pyelolysis

Obstruction of the pelviureteric junction may now be treated by balloon dilatation percutaneously or by using a retrograde balloon catheter. An antegrade cut in the pelviureteric junc-tion can be performed over a bridging guidewire using a urethrotome and a tapered JJ-stent (pyelolysis or endo-pyelotomy) [36]. A retrograde ureteroscopic method has been used to cut the pelviureteric junction with diathermy [37]. More recently, a Holmium laser has been used to cut the pelviureteric junction from above and via a ureteroscope. All these methods that involve cutting may damage vessels. The incision should be made posteriolaterally on the side of the pelviureteric junction towards the kidney, avoiding any aberrant vessels found anteriorly in 25–30% of patients.

If a patient has already had an open pyeloplasty the vessels may have been transposed, and this should be checked by CT before attempting pyelolysis (Fig. 33.12).

Thus, apart from vessel damage the procedure has a very low morbidity compared with open pyeloplasty. The results are now more encouraging also: some reports showing 90% success rates at long-term follow-up.

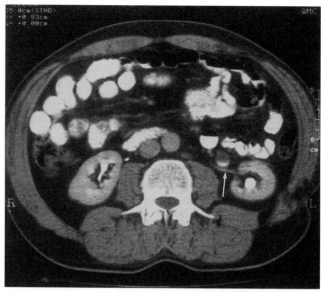

(a)

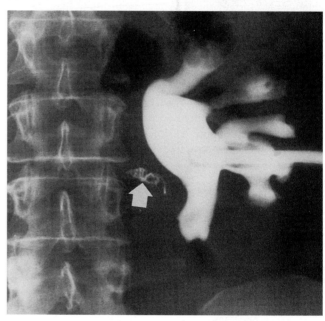

(b)

Fig. 33.12 (a) CT scan showing lower polar vessel crossing behind the pelviureteric junction after previous pyeloplasty with replacement of vessel. A pyelolysis here resulted in lower polar vessel bleed — treated by embolization. (b) Coils used to embolize lower polar vessel (arrow). Nephrostomy track *in situ* later had balloon dilatation of pelviureteric junction.

Percutaneous treatment of upper tract urothelial tumors

Low-grade transitional cell carcinoma (TCC) of the upper urinary tract can be treated in exactly the same way as it is in the bladder, i.e., by local resection. Using a percutaneous

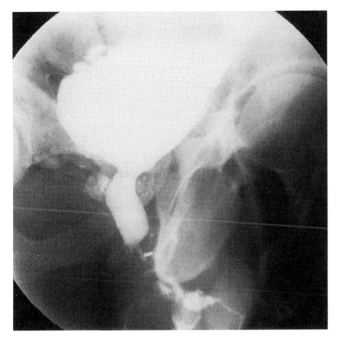

(a)

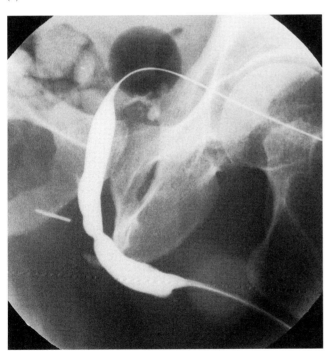

(b)

Fig. 33.13 (a) Long irregular stricture of the bulbar urethra.
(b) Dilatation by balloon via suprapubic catheter, but complicated
by septicemia.

track, the tumor of the pelvicaliceal system can be resected,
and the track "sterilized" afterwards by inserting an iridium
wire down the nephrostomy [38]. Perforation of the renal
pelvis may be a complication, and healing may be delayed if

the irradiation is given to the track. "Tumor seeding" has not
been encountered in series where low-grade tumors have
been resected and when the track has been irradiated, but it
has been described without track irradiation (D.R. Webb,
personal communication).

The complications of track dilatation and endoscopy are,
otherwise, exactly the same as for PCNL.

Interventional procedures in the lower urinary tract

Dilatation of urethral strictures

Occasionally, the endoscopist will insert metallic stents after
dilating or incising a urethral stricture. These strictures
harbor infection and it is imperative to cover the dilatation
with adequate antibiotics. Difficult strictures can be negotiated by the radiologist using guidewire techniques and the
stricture may then be dilated. Again, it is stressed that
antibiotic cover is required (Fig. 33.13).

References

1 Casey WF. *Anaesthetic Aspects (Abstract). Anaesthesia for Growth
Points in Surgery.* Paper presented at Symposium Faculty of
Anaesthetists, London, November, 1985.
2 Wickham JEA, Miller RA (eds). *Percutaneous Renal Surgery.*
London: Churchill Livingstone, 1983:138.
3 Webb DR, Fitzpatrick JM. Percutaneous nephrolithotripsy: a
functional and morphological study. *Urology* 1985;134:587−591.
4 Stables DP, Ginsberg NJ, Johnson ML. Percutaneous nephrostomy: a series and review of the literature. *Am J Roentgenol*
1978;130:75−82.
5 Gunter R, Alken P. Percutaneous nephropyelostomy and
endourological manipulations. In: Baert AL, Duijsen E, Fuchs
WA, Heuck FHW, eds. *Frontiers in European Radiology*, Vol. I.
Heidelberg: Springer-Verlag, 1982:33−35.
6 Peene P, Wilms G, Baert AL. Embolisation of iatrogenic renal
hemorrhage following percutaneous nephrostomy. *Urol Radiol*
1990;12:84−87.
7 Barbaric ZL. Percutaneous nephrostomy for urinary tract
obstruction. *Am J Roentgenol* 1984;143:773−776.
8 Hadar H, Gadoth N. Positional relations of the colon and kidney
determined by peri-renal fat. *Am J Roentgenol* 1984;143.
803−809.
9 Fernstrom I. Complications of percutaneous nephrostomy. *Br J
Urol* 1983;23(Suppl.):11−13.
10 Saxton HM. Percutaneous nephrostomy technique. *Urol Radiol*
1981;2:131−139.
11 Narasimham DL, Jacobsson B, Vijayan P, Bhuyan BC, Nyman U,
Holmquist B. Percutaneous nephrolithotomy through an intercostal approach. *Acta Radiol* 1991;32:162−165.
12 Kellett MJ. Percutaneous access to the kidney: radiology and
ultrasound. In: Wickham JEA, Miller RA, eds. *Percutaneous
Renal Surgery.* London: Churchill Livingstone, 1983:17−31.
13 Gonzales-Serva L, Weinnerth JL, Glenn JF. Minimal mortality of
renal surgery. *Urology* 1977;9:253−255.
14 Baron RL, McClennan BL. Replacing the occluded percutaneous

nephrostomy catheter. *Radiology* 1981;141:824.

15 Clayman RV, Castaneda-Zuniga WR, Hunter DW *et al.* Rapid balloon dilatation of the nephrostomy track for nephrostolithotomy. *Radiology* 1983;147:884–885.

16 Gray RR, St Louis EL, Jewett MAS. Aneurysm of the dilation balloon catheter: an unusual complication of percutaneous nephrolithotomy. *Urol Radiol* 1989;11:165–166.

17 Marberger M, Stackl W, Hruby W. Percutaneous litholopaxy of renal calculi with ultrasound. *Eur Urol* 1982;8:236–237.

18 Pollack HM, Banner MP. Percutaneous extraction of renal and ureteral calculi, technical considerations. *Am J Roentgenol* 1984; 143:778–784.

19 Payne SR, Ford TF, Wickham JEA. Endoscopic management of upper urinary tract stones. *Br J Surg* 1985;72:822–824.

20 Schultz PE, Hanno PM, Wein AJ *et al.* Percutaneous ultrasonic lithotripsy: choice of irrigant. *J Urol* 1983;130:858–860.

21 Verstandig AG, Banner MP, Van Arsdalen KN, Pollack HM. Upper urinary tract calculi. Upper urinary tract calculi: extrusion into perinephric and periureteric tissues during percutaneous management. *Radiology* 1986;158:215–218.

22 Moretti KL, Miller RA, Kellett MJ, Wickham JEA. Extrusion of calculi from the upper urinary tract into perinephric and periureteric tissues during endourologic stone surgery. *Urology* 1991;38(5):447–449.

23 Young AT, Hunter DW, Castaneda-Zuniga WR *et al.* Percutaneous extraction of urinary calculi: use of the intercostal approach. *Radiology* 1985;154:633–638.

24 Jones DJ, Russell GL, Kellett MJ, Whitfield HN, Wickham JEA. The changing practice of percutaneous stone surgery: review of 1000 cases 1981–1988. *Br J Urol* 1990;66:1–5.

25 Kreber BF, Craven DE, McCabe WR. Gram negative bacteriuria. Re-evaluation of clinical features and treatment in 612 patients. *Am J Med* 1980;68:344.

26 Özgök IY, Erduran R, Sağlam R, Dayanç M. Intrarenal pressure following pyeloplasty or percutaneous surgery. *Br J Urol* 1991;

23:251–252.

27 Watson GF. Laser fragmentation of urinary calculi. In: Smith JA, Stein BS, Benson RC, eds. *Lasers in Urological Surgery.* Chicago: Year Book Medical Publishers, Inc., 1985;120–137.

28 Raney AM. Electrohydraulic ureterolithotripsy. *Urology* 1978; 12:284.

29 Fuchs G, Miller K, Bub P, Eisenberger F. *Extra-corporeal Shockwave Lithotripsy: Clinical Experience and Results (Abstract).* Second World Congress on Percutaneous Renal Surgery, University of Mainz, Mainz, 1984:53.

30 Silber N, Kremer I, Gaton DD, Servadio C. Severe sepsis following extracorporeal shock wave lithotripsy. *J Urol* 1991;145:1045–1046.

31 Evan AP, Willis LR, Conners B, Reed G, McAteer JA, Lingeman JE. Shock wave lithotripsy-induced renal injury. *Am J Kidney Dis* 1991;XVII(No. 4):445–450.

32 Chandhoke PS, Albala DM, Clayman RV. Long term comparison of renal function in patients with solitary kidneys and/or moderate renal insufficiency undergoing extracorporeal shock wave lithotripsy or percutaneous nephrolithotomy. *J Urol* 1992;147: 1226–1230.

33 Krysiewicz S. Complications of renal extracorporeal shock wave lithotripsy reviewed. *Urol Radiol* 1992;13:139–145.

34 Salazar JE, Johnson JB, Scott RL. Perforation of renal pelvis by internal ureteral stents. *Am J Roentgenol* 1984;143:816–818.

35 Adams PS Jr. Iliac artery – ureteral fistula developing after dilatation and stent placement. *Radiology* 1984;153:647–648.

36 Ramsay JWA, Miller RA, Kellett MJ, Blackford HN, Wickham JEA, Whitfield HN. Percutaneous pyelolysis; indications, complications and results. *Br J Urol* 1984;56:586–588.

37 Meretyk I, Meretyk S, Clayman RV. Endopyelotomy – comparison of ureteroscopic, retrograde and antegrade percutaneous techniques. *J Urol* 1992;148(3):775–782.

38 Nurse DE, Woodhouse CR, Kellett MJ. Percutaneous removal of upper tract tumours. *World J Urol* 1989;7:131–134.

Complications of gynecologic diagnostic and interventional procedures

Amy S. Thurmond

Introduction

Obstetric and gynecologic radiology consists of the diagnostic techniques and interventional procedures used for conditions that occur in women and, generally, not in men. Complications of mammography and complications in pregnant women are dealt with elsewhere in this book. I will limit my discussion to pelvic inflammatory disease, female infertility, and neoplasms of the female reproductive organs which may require a multimodality approach for diagnosis and treatment. For most conditions plain films, fluoroscopy, ultrasound, computed tomography (CT), and magnetic resonance imaging (MRI) will have the same side-effects and complications as generally described. Hysterosalpingography (HSG), Fallopian tube catheterization, and vaginal ultrasound, however, are unique techniques for examining women and I will describe the current known complications of these modalities in detail.

HSG

Technique

The patient is examined usually without cardiac monitoring or anesthesia. She is placed in the dorsal lithotomy position, and a vaginal speculum is used to expose the cervix. The cervix is swabbed with an antiseptic, and a cervical cup, a cervical acorn with tenaculum, or an intrauterine balloon is placed [1]. The speculum can then be removed. Using fluoroscopic guidance, room-temperature contrast medium is instilled until the uterus and Fallopian tubes are filled.

When the anatomy has been documented, the device can be removed and the patient allowed to leave the department.

Minor complications (Table 34.1)

Pain

There is usually some pain associated with HSG, and the severity varies widely. The discomfort is similar to menstrual cramps and is presumably due to distension of the cervical canal and/or uterine cavity by the HSG device or the contrast medium. There is some evidence to suggest that when the Fallopian tubes are patent, discomfort may also be caused by peritoneal irritation from the contrast medium. Sinografin (diatrizoate methylglucamine and iodipamide methylglucamine, Squibb) may cause more discomfort than other water-based media [2] and oil may cause less discomfort than water-based media [3], otherwise there does not seem to be a significant difference in contrast media including the low-osmolar nonionic contrast agents. Rapid, skillful, and gentle completion of the examination are probably the best way of preventing unnecessary discomfort. The pain associated with HSG usually subsides within about 10 minutes of concluding the procedure and does not require treatment.

Bleeding

There is usually very mild vaginal bleeding for about 24 hours after completion of HSG. Bleeding that is heavier than a menstrual period is unusual and may indicate underlying pathology which requires treatment such as endometrial

591

Table 34.1 Common or severe complications of HSG

Complications	Incidence	Prevention
Minor		
Pain	Varies widely	Reassuring and competent demeanor
		Skilled technique:
		topical anesthetic when using tenaculum
		slow inflation when using balloon
		slow application of vacuum when using cervical cup
		slow injection of contrast media
Intravasation	Up to 7%	Careful fluoroscopic monitoring
Severe bleeding	Very low	
Contrast reaction	Very low	(Be prepared to treat)
Vasovagal reaction	1–2%	(Be prepared to treat)
Radiation of early pregnancy	Very low	Perform examination in follicular phase
		Question all patients about recent menstrual flow
		Request pregnancy test in patients with absent or irregular cycles
Ovarian radiation exposure > 1 mGy	Very low	Judicious use of fluoroscopy and films
Major		
Pelvic infection	1–2%	Doxycycline prophylaxis for high-risk patients

polyp or submucosal leiomyoma. If a tenaculum was used, then heavy bleeding may indicate a cervical laceration which needs cauterization.

Intravasation

Intravasation into the myometrial veins and subsequently into pelvic veins and lymphatics occurs in up to 7% of patients having HSG [4] (Fig. 34.1). This complication is usually related to underlying pathology, such as a submucosal leiomyoma or blocked Fallopian tubes combined with vigorous pressure of injection. Intravasation can, however, occur with normal anatomy. Venous intravasation of water-soluble contrast media has not been associated with adverse effects; however, the potential for an idiosyncratic reaction from the contrast medium exists. Intravasation of oil contrast media, however, results in oil emboli and can be associated with shortness of breath, dizziness, coma, and even death [5]. Adverse effects of intravasation can be prevented by ceasing injection as soon as early intravasation is recognized. Myometrial intravasation of contrast agent usually does not require treatment; however, massive intravasation of oil contrast medium may require supportive therapy for the organs affected.

Contrast reaction

Contrast reactions following HSG are either extremely rare or underreported. In addition to a reaction at the time of the

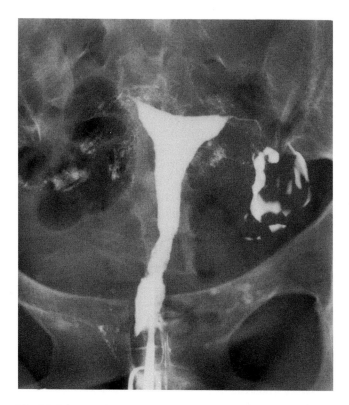

Fig. 34.1 HSG performed with oil contrast media shows a patent left tube, obstruction of the right tube 5 mm from the uterine cavity, and intravasation of oil into the uterine muscle and into right-sided pelvic veins.

examination, which could occur from venous intravasation as described above, there is the possibility of a delayed reaction as a result of resorption of the contrast medium from the peritoneal surfaces into the venous system [6]. As with other procedures that use iodinated contrast medium, it is imperative that the benefits of the procedure outweigh the risks in each individual. Treatment of contrast reaction is described in detail elsewhere in this book (see p. 281).

Vasovagal syncope

This complication is familiar to most radiologists, however it deserves mention here because it does seem to occur anecdotally more often in young healthy women, particularly with cervical manipulation. The etiology and mechanism of vasovagal syncope are poorly understood. It appears to be caused by a parasympathetic response that results in decreased blood pressure followed by inappropriate cardiac slowing which lowers the blood pressure even further [7]. The incidence is not known, although vasovagal symptoms probably occur in 1–2% of patients undergoing HSG. It almost always occurs at the conclusion of the procedure, and is heralded by the patient yawning, appearing pale, and complaining of "not feeling very good." Patients should be watched closely for about 10 minutes after HSG, and if these warnings signs occur, the patient should be placed in the Trendelenburg position. The vasovagal symptoms are usually self-limited; however, if the patient loses consciousness while supine one may give 0.6 mg atropine by intravenous push.

Irradiation of early pregnancy

Inadvertent irradiation of an early pregnancy can occur, particularly if implantation bleeding is mistaken for a normal menstrual period. The incidence of this complication is probably underreported but still very low. Based on the small number of cases that have been reported, there is nothing to suggest that performance of HSG during early pregnancy causes spontaneous abortion or fetal malformation [8]. In one case, it was thought that HSG caused displacement of an early intrauterine pregnancy into the Fallopian tube [8]. Performance of HSG in patients who are pregnant is prevented by allowing patients to schedule the procedure only in the follicular phase of their cycle, i.e., about 10 days after they have started bleeding. Patients should also be questioned about their last period. If the period was late and/or light, then the HSG should be postponed until after the next period or until after a serum pregnancy test has been obtained.

Ovarian radiation exposure

The radiation dose to the ovaries during HSG is approximately 1 mGy, which is well-below accepted limits [9].

Major complication

Pelvic infection

Pelvic infection following HSG can be very severe and refractory to antibiotic therapy, sometimes necessitating hysterectomy and, in the days before antibiotics, even resulted in death. The incidence of pelvic infection in a population not taking prophylactic antibiotics is about 1–2% [10]. Infections occur in patients with abnormal tubes, particularly tubes that are dilated but still patent (Fig. 34.2). Presumably these tubes harbor indolent infection which is then forced into the peritoneal cavity by the HSG procedure. Many gynecologists have their patients take prophylactic antibiotics, particularly if there is a history of pelvic inflammatory disease. If the patient is not already taking antibiotics prescribed by her gynecologist, and the examination reveals she has abnormal tubes, she should be given doxycycline 200 mg by mouth while in the department, as well as a prescription for 100 mg by mouth, twice daily for 5 days. There is nothing to suggest that women who have normal appearing tubes need prophylactic antibiotics [10]. All patients should be warned of the symptoms of pelvic infection.

Fallopian tube catheterization

Technique

Fallopian tube catheterization is usually performed with fluoroscopic guidance for the purpose of relieving proximal tubal obstruction. It is an interventional extension of HSG and, therefore, complications of HSG are also potential complications of Fallopian tube catheterization (Table 34.2). The discussion below is limited to those complications that are in addition to those of HSG or which may be more severe because of the interventional techniques. Fallopian tube catheterization can also be performed with ultrasound guidance, which avoids the problems of radiation and iodinated contrast media. At this point, however, the applications of this method are limited because of the poor definition of tubal anatomy [11].

Fallopian tube catheterization may take as long as 30–45 minutes, therefore intravenous sedation may be used but is not necessary. The patients receive 5 days of doxycycline 100 mg orally, twice daily, which ideally is started 2 days before the procedure. Fallopian tube catheterization is performed after a conventional HSG [12] (Fig. 34.3). Using fluoroscopic guidance a catheter is advanced into the tubal ostium. I use a J-guidewire to get around the bend at the fundus, followed by a straight wire for wedging the catheter in the tubal ostium. Once this larger catheter is wedged in the ostium, smaller catheters and wires can be advanced into the Fallopian tube [13]. When the procedure is completed and anatomy has been documented, catheters and HSG

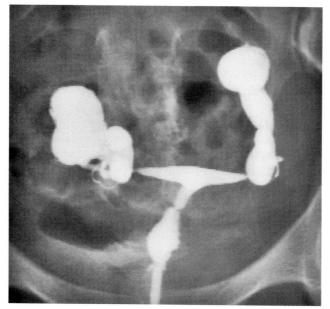

(a)

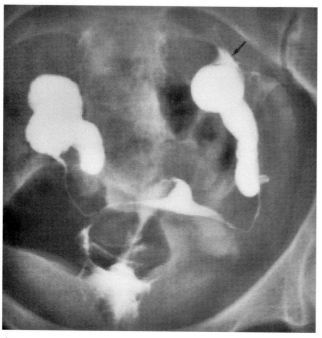

(b)

Fig. 34.2 HSG in a patient with patent but dilated tubes. She should receive doxycycline at the time of the examination and continue with a 5-day course. (a) Both tubes are dilated in the ampullary portions, without definite spill of contrast medium into the peritoneal cavity. (b) After removing the HSG and rolling the patient, a small amount of spill into the peritoneal cavity is visualized (arrow), indicative of a pinpoint opening.

device are removed and the patient is discharged from the department.

Minor complications

Pain, bleeding, vasovagal syncope, intravasation

All of these complications are more frequent and more severe than with HSG because of the manipulation of the guidewires and catheter in the uterus. Pain, bleeding, and vasovagal symptoms occur with pushing the guidewire or catheter against or into the uterine fundus. Intravasation occurs if instead of wedging the catheter into the tubal ostium one "misses" and wedges it into the myometrium. The tubal ostium has a characteristic location and offers less resistance to advancement of the straight wire than does the myometrium, and one soon learns to recognize the difference.

Tubal perforation

Tubal perforation occurs in about 3% of tubes. This complication may be related to technique, i.e., using too stiff a guidewire or catheter in an angulated or tortuous Fallopian tube (Fig. 34.4). Perforation can also be related to the underlying tubal pathology. Perforation occurs more often in patients with salpingitis isthmica nodosa and is presumably due to the guidewire exiting through one of the isthmic diverticulae (Fig. 34.5). In these patients, it is better to use a soft flexible guidewire and to probe the tube carefully. The other tubal condition that may result in perforation is occlusion due to dense fibrosis, which often occurs at the site of a previous tubal anastomosis (see Fig. 34.3). The guidewire will take the path of least resistance, which in these cases is the tubal wall.

Bleeding may occur when there is tubal perforation, since branches of the uterine and ovarian artery course along the Fallopian tube in the mesosalpinx (Fig. 34.6). If perforation is recognized when the hole is small then any bleeding will be self-limited. If perforation occurs during blind catheterization or ultrasound-guided catheterization, however, it would not be recognized and potentially significant trauma and bleeding could occur.

Ovarian radiation exposure

The average radiation dose during fluoroscopically guided Fallopian tube catheterization is less than 10 mGy, which is in the same range as a barium enema or excretory urogram [15].

Table 34.2 Common or severe complications of fluoroscopic Fallopian tube catheterization

Complications	Incidence	Prevention
Minor		
Pain	Varies widely	Avoid pushing on uterine fundus with catheters
		Intravenous pain drugs for lengthy procedures
Intravasation	Low	Careful fluoroscopic monitoring
		Avoid impaling uterine wall with catheter
Severe bleeding	Very low	Avoid pushing on uterine fundus with catheters
Vasovagal reaction	Low	Avoid pushing on uterine fundus with catheters
Tubal perforation	3%	Use softer, tapered catheters and guidewires for tortuous tubes, isthmic obstructions
Ovarian radiation exposure > 10 mGy	Low	Judicious use of fluoroscopy and films
Major		
Pelvic infection	Very low	Give prophylactic doxycycline antibiotic
Tubal pregnancy	Depends on tubal status	Advise patients of warning signs

Major complication

Tubal pregnancy

This is a late complication that ironically results from a successful procedure. If one opens a diseased Fallopian tube which may have disturbed motility from peritubal adhesions or intrinsic disease, this exposes the patient to the risk of tubal pregnancy (see Fig. 34.5). If the patient has no evidence of tubal abnormalities once the tube is opened, then the risk of tubal pregnancy is very small [12]. If, however, there is known or suspected peritubal or distal tubal disease, the chance that a pregnancy is in the tube and not in the uterus is probably 10–20%. This is a life-threatening condition which thankfully now, because of improvements in the assays for the β-subunit of human chorionic gonadotropin and improvements in ultrasound, can be detected as early as 5 weeks from the last menstrual period. If it is detected early, the patient may be a candidate for local or systemic methotrexate therapy or laparoscopic linear salpingotomy with salvage of the tube. If the tubal pregnancy is not detected until later, the tube may rupture and have to be removed.

Vaginal ultrasound diagnosis

Technique

The vaginal probe is usually placed in the vaginal fornix and, because it is closer to the uterus and ovaries, it gives a higher resolution image of these structures. Ultrasound gel is placed on the end of the probe, the probe is covered with a condom, and lubricating jelly is put on the end outside of the condom to allow easier insertion. The probe can be inserted by the patient or by the examiner.

Minor complication (Table 34.3)

Misconduct charges

Because of the nature of the examination, a physician or technologist who performs a vaginal ultrasound examination on a patient without a chaperone in the room, exposes him- or herself to accusations of molestation. This is obviously more of a risk for males, however I am aware of five instances where a patient has accused her examiner of molestation, and one of the accused was a female gynecology resident (R. Sanders, personal communication).

Major complications (Table 34.4)

Pregnant women with vaginal bleeding or ruptured membranes

Vaginal ultrasound can be helpful in determining the cause of vaginal bleeding during pregnancy, particularly if the internal os of the cervix is not visible by transabdominal or transperineal ultrasound because of fetal position or maternal obesity. The rules that apply to manual pelvic examination under these circumstances also apply to vaginal ultrasound examination. The probe should be inserted carefully and vigorous contact of the probe with the cervix should be avoided, particularly if there is a placenta previa.

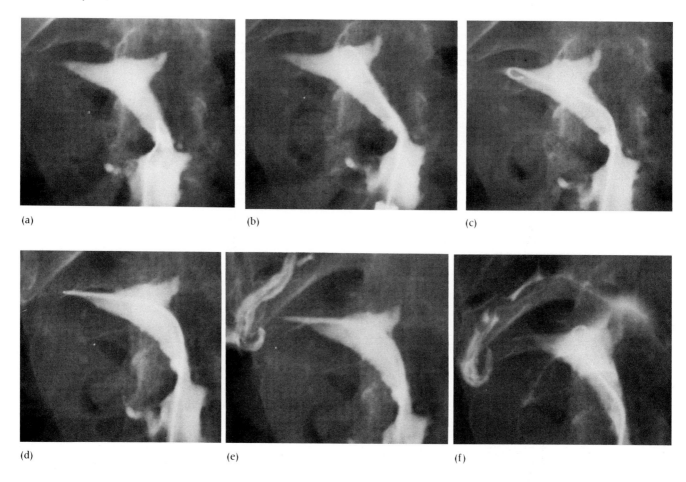

(a)   (b)   (c)

(d)   (e)   (f)

Fig. 34.3 Successful bilateral Fallopian tube recanalization, complicated by contained and free perforation on the left side, in a patient with previous ligation-reversal tubal anastomoses. The patient conceived 2 months after this procedure and delivered a healthy infant. (a) Following initial HSG, the J-guidewire is advanced through the cervical canal. (b) Using the 5.5-F catheter, the J-guide is directed to the uterine cornu. Looping of the guidewire in the uterus (as shown here), or pushing or stretching of the uterus should be avoided since this causes pain, bleeding, and sometimes vasovagal syncope. (c) Satisfactory placement of the J-guide and 5.5-F catheter in the right uterine cornu. (d) A straight guide is used to wedge the catheter into the tubal ostium. (e) Direct injection reveals a patent tube that is short, consistent with the prior ligation-reversal surgery. (f) The catheter is pulled back, the J-guide reinserted, and the catheter directed to the opposite side, again trying to avoid stretching the uterus.

Table 34.3 Common or severe complications of vaginal ultrasound diagnosis

Complications	Incidence	Prevention
Minor		
Misconduct charges	Low	Chaperone in examining room
Major		
Complications in pregnant women	Low	Avoid cervical contact if there is bleeding Avoid examination if membranes could be ruptured
Rupture of adnexal structures	Low	Careful examination
Transmission of disease	Unknown	Follow manufacturers' instructions for sterilizing probe
Misdiagnosis	Potentially high	Consider all possibilities Discuss the findings with the referring physician

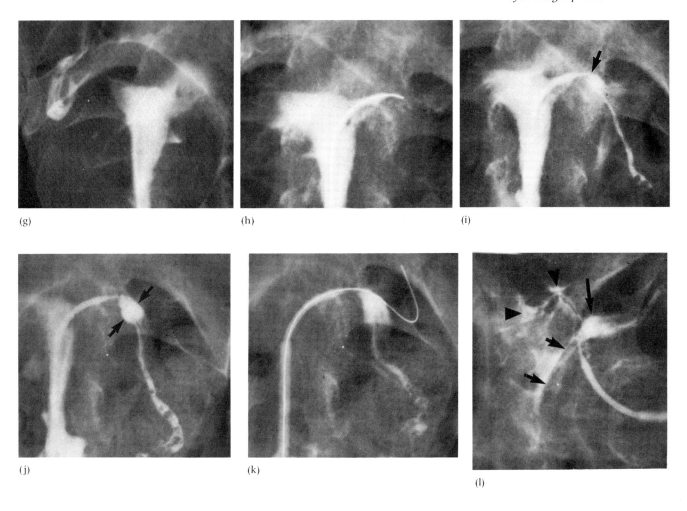

(g)　　　　　　(h)　　　　　　(i)

(j)　　　　　　(k)

(l)

Fig. 34.3 *Continued.* (g) Careful manipulation of the catheter and guidewire avoids unnecessary pushing on the uterine fundus. (h) Direct injection via the 5.5-F catheter did not open the tube, therefore a smaller guidewire and 3-F catheter are used to probe the obstruction in the left tube. (i) Direct injection through the 3-F catheter (tip indicated by arrow) reveals a contained tubal perforation, as well as some filling of the left Fallopian tube beyond the perforation. (j) Continued injection enlarges the perforation cavity (arrows), and shows the tube is patent. (k) In an attempt to dilate the tube further, the small guidewire was reinserted, but instead of following the course of the Fallopian tube it exited the antimesenteric border of the Fallopian tube. (l) Injection reveals contrast media free in the peritoneal cavity (arrowheads). Both the free perforation and the contained perforation (long arrow) occurred at the serosal margin of the uterus (short arrows), probably at the surgical anastomosis.

Table 34.4 Common or severe complications of vaginal ultrasound-guided procedures

Complications	Incidence	Prevention
Minor		
Pain	High	Adequate analgesia
Bleeding	Very low	
Pelvic infection	Very low	Prophylactic antibiotics
Spread of tumor	Very low	Careful technique
Major		
Misdiagnosis	Potentially high	Consider all possibilities
		Discuss the findings with the referring physician
Untreated disease	Around 20%	Long-term patient follow-up
		Adequate communication with the referring physician

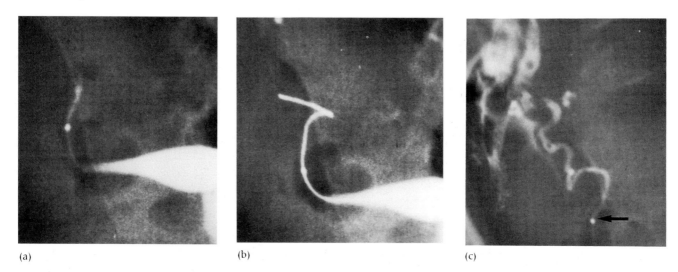

(a)   (b)   (c)

Fig. 34.4 A soft, tapered catheter and guidewire are used in the isthmic portion of a tube. (a) Injection via a 3-F catheter (tip indicated by radioopaque bead), reveals obstruction about 2 cm from the uterine cavity. (b) The guidewire is carefully advanced beyond the obstruction and reveals that the tube is tortuous. (c) Direct injection confirms successful recanalization (tip of catheter indicated by arrow) with free spill evident.

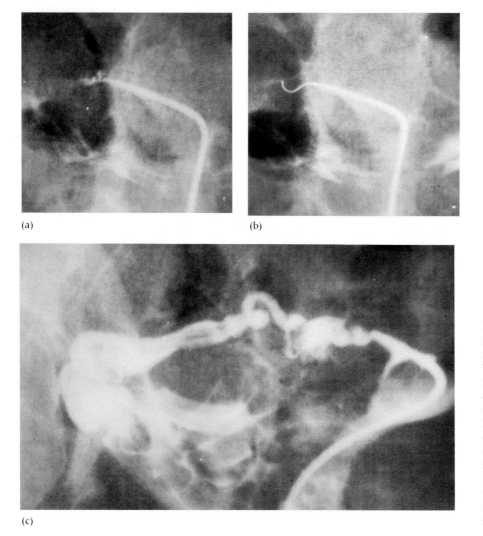

(a)   (b)

(c)

Fig. 34.5 Successful catheterization in a patient with bilateral salpingitis isthmica nodosa (SIN) and 3 years of infertility. The patient conceived 1 month after the procedure; however, the pregnancy was a right tubal pregnancy, treated medically with systemic methotrexate. Recanalization of an abnormal tube exposes the patient to the risk of an ectopic pregnancy. (a) Right ostial selective salpingogram reveals SIN. (b) The guidewire is carefully advanced through the area of diverticulae and nodules. (c) Ostial selective salpingogram reveals a patent right tube.

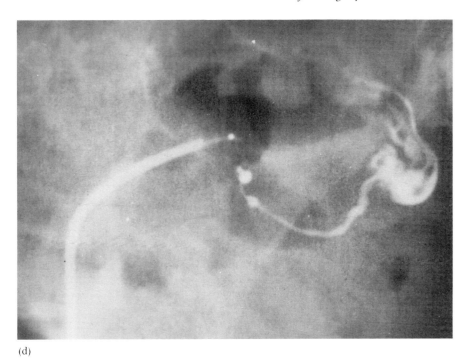

(d)

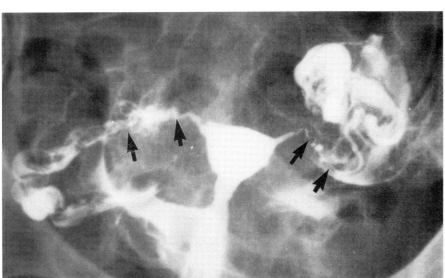

Fig. 34.5 *Continued.* (d) Successful recanalization on the left side also reveals SIN. (e) HSG at the conclusion of the procedure shows bilateral SIN (arrows) with patent tubes.

(e)

If there is a chance that the amniotic membrane is ruptured, then vaginal ultrasound should be avoided.

Rupture of adnexal structures

As with physical examination, it is possible to rupture a tense ovarian cyst with the vaginal probe (R. Sanders, personal communication), or rupture an ectopic pregnancy (M. Novy, personal communication).

Transmission of disease

Condoms are used to cover the probe to avoid contamination. Occasionally, however, the condoms may break or slip off the probe. It is important to sterilize the probe between patients according to the manufacturer's instructions to avoid transmitting herpes, condylomata, or other vaginally transmitted infections.

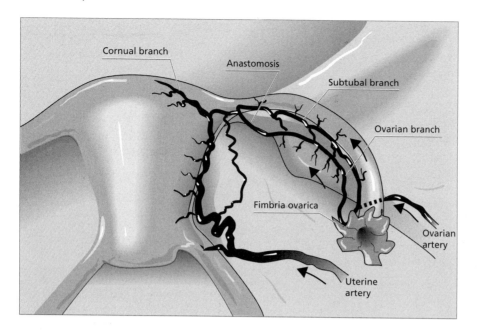

Fig. 34.6 Diagram of the blood supply to the Fallopian tube, which shows that the vessels are small branches from the uterine and ovarian arteries. (From Hunt [14].)

Misdiagnosis

A wide variety of pelvic conditions may unfortunately look similar by imaging studies. The most difficult category of pelvic pathology are those conditions that are manifest as a complex mass by transvaginal ultrasound, i.e., the mass has cystic and solid components. This category includes hemorrhagic ovarian cysts, cystadenoma, cystadenocarcinoma, teratoma, tuboovarian abscess, endometrioma, ectopic pregnancy, and bowel (Figs 34.7–34.10). Each of these lesions requires different management, therefore discussion with the referring physician is mandatory so that the differential diagnosis can be narrowed and appropriate follow-up planned [16].

Vaginal ultrasound-guided procedures

Technique

Masses or fluid collections in the pelvis are usually deep and may be surrounded by bowel. For this reason, interventional techniques in the past usually utilized CT guidance and a transabdominal or transgluteal route. Vaginal ultrasound has emerged as a better technique for guiding most procedures in the pelvis, since it gives a detailed view of the

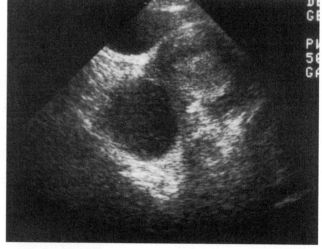

(a)

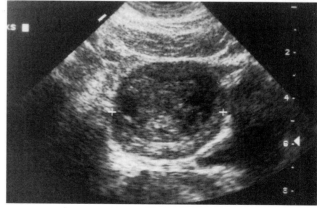

(b)

Fig. 34.7 Persistent, complex right adnexal mass which on exploratory laparotomy was a stool within a normal low-lying cecum. (a) Cross-sectional view through the uterus and right adnexa using transabdominal ultrasound. (b) Right adnexal mass using transvaginal ultrasound.

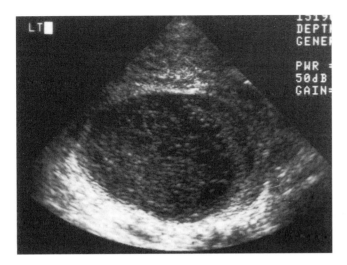

Fig. 34.8 Transvaginal ultrasound view of a complex left adnexal mass which was a hemorrhagic corpus luteum.

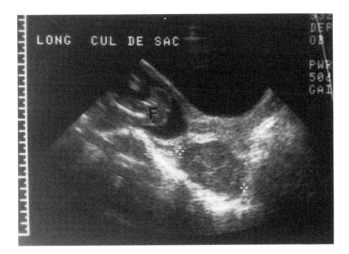

Fig. 34.9 Sagittal view using transabdominal ultrasound of a complex mass (cursors) in the cul-de-sac of a pregnant woman. This was a malignant ovarian dysgerminoma. F, fetus.

female pelvic organs, allows realtime visualization, provides a more direct route to most lesions through the vaginal fornix, and is less costly. Some of the procedures that can be performed using this technique include transvaginal intra-tubal methotrexate treatment for ectopic pregnancy [17], percutaneous drainage of tuboovarian abscesses and other fluid collections [18,19], and percutaneous biopsy of pelvic masses [16,20].

Minor complications

Pain

The tissue of the vaginal fornix can be difficult to penetrate and attempts to place a large needle or catheter through it

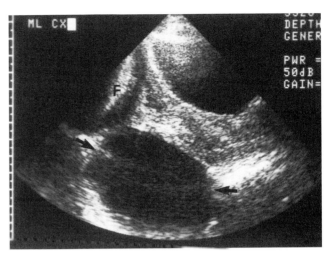

Fig. 34.10 Sagittal view using transabdominal ultrasound of a complex mass (arrows) in the cul-de-sac of a pregnant woman. This was fecal material in the rectum. F, fetus.

can be painful (Fig. 34.11). Intravenous sedation may help, but occasionally a lengthy or difficult procedure cannot be performed because of patient discomfort [19].

Bleeding

Vessels from the broad ligament are located just deep to the vagina (see Fig. 34.6), however, no increased risk from bleeding due to the vaginal route has been reported.

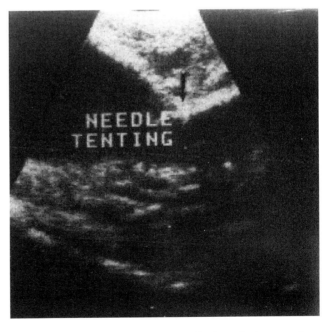

Fig. 34.11 Attempts to introduce a needle through the vaginal fornix may be quite painful and result in "tenting" of this tough tissue. (From Bret *et al.* [20].)

Pelvic infection

The vagina normally harbors a mixed flora of microorganisms that potentially could be introduced into the peritoneal cavity. Transient bacteremia has been described [18]; however, no major septic complications have been reported following percutaneous procedures using the vaginal route. Copious swabbing of the vagina with a suitable antiseptic such as povidone — iodine, and avoidance of contamination with the external genitalia presumably minimize this risk.

Peritoneal spread of tumor

Benign and ovarian epithelial tumors spread via the peritoneal route. Benign mucinous tumors may rupture and cause pseudomyxoma peritonei, while malignant tumors metastasize via peritoneal implants. There have been scattered reports of these complications occurring at the time of laparoscopy or laparotomy, and there is a fear that this might occur more frequently with percutaneous drainage or biopsy. So far, this is an unsubstantiated fear and there is probably minimal if any risk of disseminating disease via careful drainage or biopsy of an ovarian epithelial tumor [16,20].

Major complications

Misdiagnosis

As described above, a wide variety of pelvic conditions may look quite similar by imaging studies. If one is asked to treat a lesion such as a tuboovarian abscess or ectopic pregnancy, one should be sure that the laboratory tests, clinical course, and ultrasound findings are consistent with that disease process. Any discrepancies should be discussed with the patient's gynecologist and the risks of misdiagnosis determined. If there is any chance that the lesion might be bowel, then a CT scan is helpful. If one is asked to biopsy a possible ovarian neoplasm, careful consideration must be given to all the diagnostic possibilities, and the risks of misdiagnosis and sampling error must be discussed. Many mucinous ovarian tumors contain only focal areas of high-grade neoplasia amid otherwise benign tissue [16].

Untreated disease

Eighty-six per cent of patients who received interventional radiology treatment for tuboovarian abscess [18], and 70% of patients who received interventional radiology treatment for tubal pregnancies [17,21] had a long-term response. The majority of the remainder required surgery after the interventional treatment failed. One of the patients treated for tubal pregnancy ruptured her tube 41 days after treatment [17], therefore, these patients need to be counseled and followed closely for complications related to untreated disease.

References

1 Winfield AC, Wentz AC. *Diagnostic Imaging in Infertility* Baltimore: Williams and Wilkins, 1992:13—38.

2 Winfield AC, Henderson-Slayden R, Wentz AC, Harding DR. Hysterosalpingography: comparison of Conray 60 and Sinografin. *Am J Roentgenol* 1982;138:559—560.

3 Lindequist S, Justesen P, Larsen C, Rasfussen F. Diagnostic quality and complications of hysterosalpingography: oil- versus water-soluble contrast media — a randomized prospective study. *Radiology* 1991;179:69—74.

4 Nunley WC, Bateman BG, Kitchen JD, Pope TL. Intravasation during hysterosalpingography using oil-based media — a second look. *Obstet Gynecol* 1987;70:309—312.

5 Uzi D, Oelsner G, Gruberg L, Ezra D, Menczer J. Cerebral embolization and coma after hysterosalpingography with oil-soluble contrast medium. *Fertil Steril* 1990;53:939—940.

6 Schuitemaker NWE, Helmerhorst FM, Tjon A, Tham RTO, vanSaase JLC. Late anaphylactic shock after hysterosalpingography. *Fertil Steril* 1990;54:535—536.

7 vanLieshout JJ, Wieling W, Karemaker JM, Eckberg DL. The vasovagal response. *Clin Sci* 1991;81:575—586.

8 Justesen P, Rasmussen F, Anderson PE. Inadvertently performed hysterosalpingography during early pregnancy. *Acta Radiol Diagn* 1986;27:711—713.

9 vanderWeiden RMF, vanZijl J. Radiation exposure of the ovaries during hysterosalpingography. Is radionuclide hysterosalpingography justified? *Br J Obstet Gynecol* 1989;96:471—472.

10 Pittaway DE, Winfield AC, Maxson W, Daniell J, Herbert C, Wentz AC. Prevention of acute pelvic inflammatory disease after hysterosalpingography: efficacy of doxycycline prophylaxis. *Am J Obstet Gynecol* 1983;147:623—626.

11 Thurmond AS, Patton PE, Hector DM, Jones MK. US-guided fallopian tube catheterization. *Radiology* 1991;180:571—572.

12 Thurmond AS, Rosch J. Nonsurgical fallopian tube recanalization for treatment of infertility. *Radiology* 1990;174:371—374.

13 Thurmond AS, Rosch J. Fallopian tubes: improved technique for catheterization. *Radiology* 1990;174:572—573.

14 Hunt RB. *Atlas of Female Infertility Surgery*. St Louis: Mosby Year Book, 1992:390.

15 Hedgpeth PL, Thurmond AS, Fry R, Schmidgall JR, Rosch J. Radiographic fallopian tube recanalization: absorbed ovarian radiation dose. *Radiology* 1991;180:121—122.

16 Cohen DJ, Kucera PR. Percutaneous biopsy of pelvic masses. *Semin Intervent Radiol* 1992;9:138—151.

17 Tulandi T, Atri M, Bret P, Falcone T, Khalife S. Transvaginal intratubal methotrexate treatment for ectopic pregnancy. *Fertil Steril* 1992;58:98—100.

18 Casola G, vanSonnenberg E, D'Agostino HB, Harker CP, Varney RR, Smith D. Percutaneous drainage of tubo-ovarian abscesses. *Radiology* 1992;182:399—402.

19 vanSonnenberg E, D'Agostino HB, Casola G, Goodacre BW, Sanchez RB, Taylor B. US-guided transvaginal drainage of pelvic abscesses and fluid collections. *Radiology* 1991;181:53—56.

20 Bret PM, Guibaud L, Atri M, Gillett P, Seymour RJ, Senterman MK. Transvaginal US-guided aspiration of ovarian cysts and solid pelvic masses. *Radiology* 1992;185:377—380.

21 Risquez F, Forman R, Maleika F *et al*. Transvaginal cannulation of the fallopian tube for the management of ectopic pregnancy: prospective multicenter study. *Fertil Steril* 1992;58:1131—1135.

Complications of interventional procedures in the breast

Elsie Levin and Norman Sadowsky

Introduction

The role of the radiologist in breast imaging is changing from passive film reader to someone who is actively involved in management decisions, including the appropriate use of interventional techniques. As more women participate in mammographic screening, the detection of both benign and malignant disease has increased. The psychologic and economic costs of surgical biopsies should not be underestimated, and can account for 50% of the total costs of screening programs. Periodic mammographic follow-up for probably benign lesions has been established as a safe and reasonable alternate to surgical biopsy [1–4]. If the lesion cannot be confidently categorized as probably benign, or if patient anxiety level is high, cytologic or histologic diagnosis can be obtained either through fine needle aspiration (FNA) or core biopsy. Cyst aspiration and galactography are interventional techniques that are also employed to aid in the diagnosis of breast diseases. Wire localization is used for preoperative localization of nonpalpable breast lesions. No life-threatening complications have been reported with any of the interventional procedures involving the breast. These procedures have gained acceptance by both patients and physicians because of their diagnostic value and low rate of complications. Despite their low morbidity, the use of these procedures should never be a substitute for a thorough mammographic and ultrasonographic evaluation.

Galactography

Introduction

Galactography or ductography is a contrast examination of the lactiferous duct system which is performed after a significant nipple discharge has been identified. In general, significant discharge is usually unilateral, from one duct orifice, and most often is spontaneous, although an elicited discharge (by the patient, physician, or during compression for mammography) can be significant if it satisfies other criteria. Nipple discharge should be tested for occult blood; a reading beyond trace positive is significant. The color and consistency of the discharge is important; serus, serosanguinous, bloody (red, brown, black), and clear watery discharge should be investigated further. Bilateral milky discharge is usually physiologic or related to drugs. Thick green, yellow, or brown discharge is usually associated with duct ectasia, is frequently nonspontaneous and often occurs from multiple ducts.

After it is determined that a significant discharge is present, a galactogram is often performed to identify the cause of the discharge, and the location of the lesion. Prior to a galactogram, high-quality preliminary mammograms are obtained in the craniocaudal and mediolateral projections. The procedure is usually performed with the patient in an oblique supine position, but some prefer to have the patient seated. Meticulous cleansing of the nipple and areola with Betadine and alcohol as well as aseptic technique should be observed to prevent infection. A 30-gauge blunt tip galactography cannula (similar to a sialogram cannula, but with a 90° bend, Ranfac, Avon, MA) is connected to a 1-ml tuberculin syringe. Some radiologists use the 30-gauge blunt tip sialography needle. A coaxial technique using a guidewire and either a 22- or 24-gauge Abbocath catheter has also been described [5]. It is important to fill the system completely to eliminate air bubbles which can appear as filling defects on galactograms and simulate pathology. If there is a strong allergic history, nonionic contrast can be employed. The duct openings are not readily visible but use of a florescent lamp with a magnifying lens will facilitate the examination. Following cleansing of the nipple, a tiny drop of discharge is produced to identify the duct orifice. The nipple is gently probed until the cannula engages the duct orifice. Contrast material (usually <0.5 ml) is slowly injected until either the patient experiences fullness, pain, or burning, or there is reflux of contrast. We prefer to withdraw the cannula and apply steristrips to prevent leakage of contrast while others advocate taping the cannula in place. Mammograms are then obtained in the craniocaudal and mediolateral projections followed by spot craniocaudal and 90° compression manification views once the location of the duct system has been identified.

Galactography is a safe, well-tolerated procedure with few complications. It is contraindicated, however, in patients with acute mastitis or breast abscess, since it may worsen the inflammatory process [6–10]. Rare complications from galactography are duct perforation, mastitis, or infection, but their exact incidence is not well documented [5–10]. No significant contrast reactions have been reported with the use of water-soluble contrast agents [9,10], but the theoretical possibility exists. In three cases, we have recorded a mild erythematous skin eruption over the anterior chest beginning 2–3 days after the examination. This may be a delayed sensitivity reaction which resolved with antihistamine treatment.

Duct perforation

Perforation of the duct is reported to be the most serious complication of galactography, but the exact incidence is not widely known. In our experience of over 1000 galactograms, it probably occurs in less than 2%. Perforation of the duct leads to extravasation of contrast material which may be painful, but in many cases it is asymptomatic and recognized only mammographically. Care should be taken not to overdistend the duct, and the injection should be stopped at the first complaint of burning or fullness. No long-term complications have been reported, and the galactogram can be successfully performed after allowing time for the contrast to be absorbed, or at a later date.

Mastitis/infection

Mastitis or infection can occur following a galactogram if careful aseptic technique is not used. Like duct perforation, this complication is uncommon. In over 1000 galactograms, we have had two cases of mastitis, one case occurred 2 days after the procedure. Occasionally, cannulation of the duct may be difficult and one should discontinue further attempts before traumatizing the nipple which could lead to potential infection.

Conclusion

If significant pathology is demonstrated on a galactogram, presurgical localization galactography can be performed either with a 1:3 mixture of contrast and methylene blue or insertion of a length of prolene suture material. If the lesion is peripheral in location, the preoperative galactogram can be supplemented with a wire localization. These preoperative localization procedures allow for a more conservative surgical excision while ensuring complete removal of the lesion and affected duct. In one study, six of 30 lesions (20%) shown by galactography were not seen on histopathologic examination, but in these women preoperative localization procedures were not performed [11].

Currently, galactography is the only diagnostic study available for evaluation of nipple discharge. Despite the fact that it is an extremely low-risk procedure that is well tolerated by patients, it has not gained widespread acceptance by physicians [8,10,12]. Some surgeons advocate excision of the major subareolar ducts in postmenopausal women or solitary duct excision in premenopausal women without preoperative diagnostic imaging [9,12]. This will treat the symptom of nipple discharge in most cases but does not ensure that the lesion causing the discharge has been excised. Excision of the major subareolar ducts can also cause significant breast deformity. Surgery can be avoided altogether if the galactogram shows terminal duct cysts or duct ectasia [9]. As more physicians are educated regarding the clinical utility of galactography, we hope that its use will increase.

Cyst aspiration/pneumocystography

Introduction

Breast cysts occur commonly in perimenopausal women and can be seen in postmenopausal women on hormone replacement therapy or other drugs. If strict criteria are applied, ultrasound is extremely accurate in the diagnosis of breast cysts.

Indications for cyst aspiration include: (i) atypical cysts on ultrasound (irregular or thickened margins, internal echoes, or lack of posterior acoustic enhancement); (ii) symptomatic relief of pain or anxiety; or (iii) to clarify mammographic findings [13,14]. Ultrasound guidance is useful when a palpable mass that is suspected to be a cyst does not yield fluid when aspiration is performed using clinical guidance, or to avoid complications (e.g., lesions near the chest wall or in patients with implants) [13].

Pneumocystography can be performed following cyst aspiration for evaluation of mural abnormalities, definitive correlation of a mammographic abnormality, or as a marker for subsequent localization or aspiration [8,13,14]. Some studies advocate pneumocystography as a method to prevent cyst recurrence by inducing sclerosis of the cyst wall, although its mechanism as well as its effectiveness remains unclear [8,14–16]. In our experience, completely aspirating a cyst is even more effective in preventing recurrence, but this is unproven.

Cyst aspiration can be performed using clinical guidance for palpable masses, although we prefer ultrasound guidance to ensure complete aspiration. For nonpalpable lesions, the choice of image guidance (mammographic/stereotaxic or ultrasound) depends on the location of the lesion, availability of equipment, and preference of the radiologist. Ultrasound guidance is well tolerated by patients since they are supine, the breast is not compressed, and the procedure is fast due to the realtime capability of ultrasound. Regardless of the guidance method chosen, the technique is similar and involves cleansing of the skin, local anesthesia at the discretion of the patient and radiologist, and advancement of a 22-gauge needle into the cyst. Occasionally, the cyst fluid is very thick and requires an 18-gauge needle and/or irrigation to aspirate the cyst. If a diagnostic pneumocystogram is to be performed, the needle is left in the cyst and the fluid is replaced with approximately two-thirds of the volume of fluid removed [8,16]. Following injection of air, craniocaudal and mediolateral mammograms are obtained.

Cyst aspiration is a frequently performed procedure for both diagnostic and therapeutic reasons. Many patients present to our breast center specifically for this procedure. Although there are potential complications from cyst aspiration and pneumocystography, it is a well-tolerated procedure. Complications are listed in Table 35.1, but as with galactography, their exact incidence is not well documented in the radiologic literature. The complication rate is probably similar to the rate for FNA, although it may actually be lower since it usually involves only a single puncture.

Table 35.1 Complications from cyst aspiration/ pneumocystography

Vasovagal reactions
Bleeding
Infection
Localized pain
Pneumothorax

Vasovagal reactions

Vasovagal reactions are possible, particularly when aspiration is performed using mammographic guidance with the fenestrated compression plate, since the patient is sitting upright. These reactions should be less frequent when the patient is placed in the prone position on a stereotactic table, or supine when ultrasound guidance is used. Vasovagal reactions are usually minor and rarely require therapy. Patients should never be left unattended during any interventional procedure.

Bleeding

Interstitial hemorrhage may occur, but significant hematoma formation is uncommon and responds well to compression and ice packs.

Infection

This complication is possible as with any procedure that involves a skin puncture. Using aseptic technique, with proper skin cleansing it is rare. We have had one infection in thousands of cyst aspirations.

Localized pain

Pain is one of the common indications for cyst aspiration and this procedure usually provides symptomatic relief. Rarely, pain can occur following cyst aspiration. It usually responds well to ice packs and nonaspirin-containing analgesics.

Pneumothorax

Pneumothorax is a potential complication, which can be avoided when image guidance is used and the needle approach is parallel to the chest wall.

Conclusion

Cyst aspiration is performed commonly for both diagnostic and therapeutic purposes. Pneumocystography for diagnostic purposes is less commonly employed since the advent of high-resolution ultrasound equipment but may be employed for therapeutic purposes as some feel it may reduce the risk of cyst recurrence. Complications related to these procedures are infrequent and rarely of clinical significance.

FNA

Introduction

FNA cytology has been applied for the diagnosis of palpable breast lesions for many years with variable results. Grant *et al.* [17] reviewed 15 separate studies involving 10 197 patients and found the sensitivity ranged between 53 and 99% with an average of 87.5% and the specificity ranged between 99 and 100% with an overall acurracy between 85 and 99% (average 95.7%). The rates of unsatisfactory specimens were reported to be between 0 and 47% [17]. FNA cytology of breast lesions was advocated by Swedish researchers in the 1970s and has been used extensively in Europe. The relative lack of expertise in breast cytology in the USA is one of the reasons cited for its lower use.

FNA cytology is now used for the diagnosis of nonpalpable breast lesions. This can reduce the number of surgical biopsies for benign disease which is a major cost of screening. If a diagnosis of cancer is made by FNA, the patient can be counseled appropriately and have a one-stage surgical procedure. The advantages of FNA include that it can be performed quickly and is well tolerated by patients with few complications. The disadvantages of FNA include the need for an expert cytopathologist, the risk of insufficient specimens, the inability to distinguish between *in situ* and invasive disease, and the inability to obtain a specific benign diagnosis consistently.

Nonpalpable breast lesions can be sampled using FNA cytology with mammographic guidance with a fenestrated coordinate grid compression paddle, stereotactic guidance (prone table or add-on device), or with ultrasound guidance. The technique has been well described [8,14,18,19]. FNA is a safe procedure as shown by the low complication rates listed in Table 35.2.

Vasovagal reactions

In a prospective study performed by Helvie *et al.* [20], the most common complication was vasovagal reactions, which occurred in 7% of patients ranging from mild lightheadedness to syncope. It is interesting to note that the use of local anesthesia did not affect the frequency of reactions and many radiologists do not routinely administer local anes-

thesia prior to performing FNA. Of the four patients who experienced syncope, two fainted while the breast was compressed prior to needle insertion, one fainted after the first pass, and one fainted at the completion of the procedure [20]. It is clear that there are contributing factors other than pain that can lead to a vasovagal reaction, including anxiety which may be the most significant. One would expect a lower rate when the FNA is performed with the patient supine with ultrasound guidance or when the patient is prone on a stereotactic table.

The patient should never be left unattended. Both the radiologist and technologist must be aware of the potential for vasovagal reactions and be prepared to treat these reactions.

Bleeding

Although bleeding is a potential complication, it is rarely clinically significant. Occasionally, we have performed FNA in patients on anticoagulant therapy without sequelae. As reported by Fajardo *et al.* [8], there was evidence of minor local hematoma formation in 35% of patients at surgical biopsy immediately following FNA, but it did not interfere with pathologic evaluation or receptor analysis, and no serious bleeding complications have occurred in over 250 biopsies. If bleeding occurs during FNA, it is readily treated by applying direct compression and ice packs. We have had only one patient who bled enough to cause us to terminate the procedure; bleeding started as the local anesthesia was injected using a 25-gauge needle. The patient was a heavy aspirin user.

Other

Although post-FNA infection is a theoretical complication, there have been no reported cases. One pneumothorax was reported following FNA performed with clinical guidance out of a total of 285 patients [22]. Pneumothorax is unlikely when imaging guidance is used since the mammographic approach is parallel to the chest wall, and with ultrasound guidance the needle tip is continuously monitored.

Conclusion

Although FNA is clearly a safe procedure, one must consider the issues of insufficient specimens, sensitivity, and specificity before incorporating this procedure in one's own practice. The rates of insufficient specimens vary from 7 to 54% with mammographic guidance [21,23−25]; 0−27% with stereotactic guidance [25−32]; and 3−20.8% with ultrasound guidance [32−34]. Evaluation of sensitivity and specificity is difficult as some authors exclude their insufficient specimens while others treat them as negative. In his review, Fornage [19] found: "claimed values for specificity of 91%, 95%, 94%, 97% and 94% drop after correction to 80%, 74%,

Table 35.2 FNA complications

Technique/reference	Vasovagal reactions	Bleeding
Mammographic guidance		
Helvie *et al.* [20]	7/107	0
Hann *et al.* [21]	2/101	Not reported
Stereotactic guidance		
Helvie *et al.* [20]	4/45	0
Ultrasound guidance		
Helvie *et al.* [20]	1/15	1/15 (no Rx required)

78%, 76% and 75%, respectively and the overall accuracy drops from 92% to 83%." Sensitivity values range from a low of 68% to a high of 97% [22–34].

A false-negative cytology report can lead to a delay in diagnosis unless the cytology results are carefully correlated with the mammographic/ultrasonographic findings. The patient should be rebiopsied (repeat FNA, core biopsy, or surgical excision) if the specimen is inadequate or benign when the imaging findings are suspicious.

In order to establish a successful program of FNA cytology of the breast, a team approach is required [35]. A compulsive mammographer, experienced cytopathologist, and supportive breast surgeon must work together to achieve satisfactory results.

FNA biopsy, when used appropriately, can contribute to the cost-effective management of nonpalpable breast lesions by identifying benign lesions that do not require excisional biopsy. If a suspicious lesion is confirmed to be malignant, the patient can have a single surgical procedure [36,37].

As wisely stated by Kopans [38]:

> before any physician embarks on a triage program involving fine-needle aspiration that might result in delayed diagnosis of breast cancer, the practitioner should be certain that the necessary skills are mastered and that the techniques have been demonstrated in the setting to be used. It would be prudent to perform at least 100 fine-needle aspiration studies … and to compare their results with those of an open biopsy in the same patients in order to establish the predictive values for the particular practice setting.

Core biopsy

Introduction

Since the introduction of large-core needle biopsy of the breast in 1990 by Parker *et al.* [39], its technique has been refined and its use has expanded [19,39,40]. Subsequently, ultrasound guidance was described and in many centers it is the preferred guidance method [14,41].

The appropriate role of core biopsy in the evaluation and management of nonpalpable breast lesions has been the subject of great debate [42–49]. Large-core needle biopsy is not a substitute for meticulous mammographic and ultrasonographic evaluation. The "probably benign" lesion can be followed safely [1–4], but if the patient is unavailable for close follow-up, or is anxious, core biopsy is a valid alternate. If a malignant lesion is suspected, core biopsy can establish the diagnosis and the patient can have a single surgical procedure.

The advantages of core biopsy over FNA are related to the fact that tissue is obtained for histologic evaluation, eliminating the need for expert cytopathology. Core biopsy has a lower insufficiency rate and can distinguish between *in situ* and invasive carcinoma, although microinvasion within an area of ductal carcinoma *in situ* (DCIS) can be missed due to sampling error. Core biopsy takes longer than FNA and the larger gauge needle is thought to be associated with a higher complication rate. As the number of core specimens obtained increases, the risk of histologic evidence of hemorrhage increases, although clinically significant hemorrhage is unusual. The most common complications associated with core biopsy are listed in Table 35.3, and rare complications are listed in Table 35.4.

Table 35.3 Core biopsy complications

Guidance method	Bleeding	Infection	Vasovagal	Reference
Upright/prone stereo	Minor oozing	3/103*	2/30 upright	Parker *et al.* [39]
Prone stereo	Minor oozing	0	0	Parker *et al.* [40]
Prone stereo	1/100†	0	0	Elvecrog *et al.* [50]
Upright stereo	Minor oozing	0	4/254‡	Caines *et al.* [51]
Prone stereo	—	1/160§		Gisvold *et al.* [52]
Prone stereo	5/450¶			Jackman *et al.* [53]
Prone stereo	8% histologically**	0		Liberman *et al.* [54]
Prone stereo/ultrasound	3/3765††	3/3765‡‡		Parker *et al.* [55]

* Three cases of cellulitis reported, but unclear whether related to core biopsy, wire localization, or surgical biopsy.
† One hematoma which precluded open biopsy.
‡ The four vasovagal reactions occurred in the first 125 patients.
§ One case of a serious systemic infection (?from core or surgical biopsy).
¶ Three cases of arterial bleeding which occurred during procedure, which subsequently was completed successfully; two patients had delayed gross bleeding 6–12 hours after biopsy which was controlled with manual pressure.
** Although 8% of patients showed histologic evidence of bleeding, there were no clinically significant hematomas.
†† Required surgical drainage.
‡‡ Required drainage/antibiotics, or both.

Table 35.4 Rare complications of core biopsy

Complication	Reference
Malignant seeding of the needle track	Harter *et al.* [56]
Milk fistula	Shackmuth *et al.* [57]

In the largest series of core biopsies involving a consortium of 20 institutions, the data from 6152 lesions were gathered [55]. Follow-up was available for 3765 cases and clinically significant complications (requiring additional surgical or medical intervention) occurred in only six patients (0.2%).

Bleeding

Histologic evidence of hemorrhage was evident in core biopsy specimens [54] and in surgical specimens obtained immediately following core biopsy [50,52], but clinically significant hematomas are rare. Some radiologists have noted there is less bleeding when the patient is in the supine position for ultrasound-guided core biopsy than in the prone position for stereotactic guidance, most likely due to the venous engorgement of the breast in the dependent position.

Infection

Using aseptic technique, infection is an uncommon complication following core biopsy. In four of the reported infections [39,52], the patient also underwent wire localization followed by surgical biopsy, and the source of infection was unclear.

Vasovagal reactions

Vasovagal reactions have not been reported with core biopsies performed with the patient in the supine position for ultrasound-guided core biopsy, or with the dedicated prone stereotactic table. With the add-on stereotactic unit, the patient is seated and a few vasovagal reactions have been reported [39,51]. As with any interventional breast procedure, the patient should not be left unattended.

Malignant seeding of the needle track

As the needle gage used for breast core biopsy increased from 18- to 14-gauge, the concern about malignant seeding was raised. There has been a single case report documenting seeding of the needle track following a 14-gauge core biopsy of a mucinous carcinoma [56]. In patients undergoing mastectomy, tumor seeding of the needle track is not insignificant. Seeding of the needle track is a theoretical concern in patients choosing conservative surgery followed by radiation therapy. It has not been proven to be clinically significant, although a longer follow-up will be needed to see if there is an increase in local recurrence rates [56].

Milk fistula

A single report of a milk fistula following core biopsy was reported in 1993 [57]. A milk fistula is a track that develops between a lactiferous duct and the skin overlying the biopsy site, and is a known complication of surgical intervention in a lactating female. In the case reported, four cores were performed using a 14-gauge needle when the patient was 8 weeks postpartum since a previous FNA was equivocal. The patient was successfully treated by weaning her child over a 2-week period. If it is necessary to perform a core biopsy in a lactating female, the patient should be informed of the potential risk of milk fistula. Smaller gauge needles and fewer passes may reduce the risk of this complication.

Conclusion

Large-core needle biopsy has been shown to be a safe, cost-effective alternate to surgical biopsy. An additional advantage of core biopsy over surgery is that there is no permanent scarring or deformity of the breast which could interfere with subsequent mammographic evaluation [58]. The same principles apply to core biopsy as with FNA, including a team approach and careful mammographic/pathologic correlation.

Needle localization

Introduction

Nonpalpable breast lesions that require excision must be accurately localized to facilitate surgical removal. The techniques available for preoperative localization have been described and include needle/hook wire systems and localizing dyes [14,59–62]. Which system is employed should be chosen in consultation with the surgeon. Most radiologists employ a fenestrated paddle for mammographic guidance. With this method, the needle remains parallel to the chest wall and eliminates the risk of pneumothorax, which is a concern with the freehand technique when the approach is perpendicular to the chest wall. Mammographic guidance has been shown to be extremely accurate and, in a series of 100 consecutive needle-directed biopsies, the wire was placed within 2 mm of the lesion in 96 cases [63]. The realtime capability of ultrasound also allows for even more accurate needle placement, and has other advantages over mammographic placement.

The risks associated with localization procedures are listed in Table 35.5 and relate to the needle. Rare complications listed in Table 35.6 are secondary to the wires employed.

Needle-related complications

Vasovagal reactions

See previous discussion in Cyst aspiration/pneumocystography and FNA sections, pp. 604, 605.

Table 35.5 Needle localization complications

Vasovagal	Bleeding	Pain	Reference
2/60*	NR	NR	Urrutia *et al.* [60]
15/203	2/203	2/103	Helvie *et al.* [20]

* One patient had a similar episode after a standard mammogram 1-week earlier and one patient (diabetic on oral agents) was found to be hypoglycemic during the vasovagal reaction.
NR, not reported.

Table 35.6 Rare complications of wire localization

Complication	Reference
Transgression of localizing wire into the pleural cavity	Bristol and Jones [64]
Migration of breast biopsy localization wire	Davis *et al.* [65], Owen and Kumar [66]
Spontaneous fracture of the wire tip	O'Doherty [67]
Transection of the localization hook wire	Homer [68]
Fragmentation of a braided hook wire	D'Orsi *et al.* [69]

Bleeding

See previous discussion in Cyst aspiration/pneumocystography and FNA sections, pp. 604, 605.

Pain

Significant pain is uncommon with needle localization procedures. The use of local anesthesia is variable among radiologists. In the series reported by Helvie *et al.* [20], the two patients who experienced "an unusual amount of pain" had been given local anesthesia. One study addressed this question and found that the group of patients who received local anesthesia actually had a significantly higher pain score, although overall it was not judged to be a particularly painful procedure [70].

Wire-related complications

One case was reported of a localizing wire passing into the pleural space without causing a pneumothorax [64]. The Frank needle was placed using a free-hand technique with 5 cm left protruding from the skin. Prior to confirming the position with mammography, the patient complained of chest pain after sitting up.

Four cases of wire migration have been reported where the wire retracted into the breast, followed by migration [65, 66]. In one case using the Frank needle, the wire migrated into the supraclavicular fossa with the wire tip terminating in the posterior muscles of the neck. Three cases of retraction and migration occurred in a series of 158 patients [66]. The wires were found in the subcutaneous tissues of the left flank and gluteal region, the infraclavicular fossa, and in the soft tissues of the left axilla. This complication can be avoided if a sufficient length of wire protrudes from the skin and is properly secured.

A single case of spontaneous fracture of a localizing wire has been reported, presumably due to a defective wire [67].

In a series of 100 breast localizations, three intraoperative transections of the localizing wire occurred [68]. The wire may be difficult to palpate during surgery, but use of a stiffening cannula protects the wire and renders it palpable.

Fragmentation of a braided hook wire with deposition of fine metallic fragments was identified on a postbiopsy follow-up mammogram [69].

Conclusion

Needle localization of nonpalpable breast lesions is a safe procedure with few complications. Accurate placement is imperative so that the surgeon can successfully excise the lesion and establish the dianosis. If the lesion is benign, a minimal volume of tissue can be removed, which reduces the risk of cosmetic deformity.

Summary

Needle-guided procedures of the breast including galactography, cyst aspiration, FNA, core biopsy, and wire localization are low-risk procedures with few complications. Vasovagal reactions, one of the most common complications, are not always related to the needle itself, and the anxiety produced when any woman is faced with the possible diagnosis of breast cancer may be relevant. Bleeding occurs infrequently and responds well to local pressure and ice packs. Infection can be avoided when proper aseptic technique is employed. As stated previously, needle biopsies (FNA or core) should not be a substitute for a complete mammographic/ultrasonographic evaluation, but when used appropriately can reduce the cost of screening. The role of the radiologist in breast imaging is in a state of evolution. The radiologist is now becoming an integral member of the breast care team.

References

1 Brenner RJ, Sickles EA. Acceptability of periodic follow-up as an alternative to biopsy for mammographically detected lesions as probably benign. *Radiology* 1989;171:645–646.
2 Helvie MA, Pennes DR, Rebner M, Adler DD. Mammographic follow-up of low suspicion lesions: compliance rates and diagnostic yield. *Radiology* 1991;178:155–158.
3 Sickles EA. Periodic follow-up of probably benign mammographic lesions: results in 3184 cases. *Radiology* 1991;179:463–468.

4　Varas X, Leborgne F, Leborgne JH. Nonpalpable probably benign lesions: role of follow-up mammography. *Radiology* 1992;184: 409–414.

5　Berna JD, Guirao J, Garcia V. A coaxial technique for performing galactography. *Am J Roentgenol* 1989;153:273–274.

6　Threatt B. Ductography. In: Bassett LW, Gold RH, eds. *Breast Cancer Detection: Mammography and Other Methods in Breast Imaging*, 2nd edn. Orlando, FL: Grune & Stratton, 1987:119–129.

7　Tabar L, Dean PB, Pentek Z. Galactography: the diagnostic procedure of choice for nipple discharge. *Radiology* 1983;149: 31–38.

8　Fajardo LL, Jackson VP, Hunter TB. Interventional procedures in diseases of the breast: needle biopsy, pneumocystography, and galactography. *Am J Roentgenol* 1992;158:1231–1238.

9　Cardenosa G, Doudna C, Eklund GW. Ductography of the breast: technique and findings. *Am J Roentgenol* 1994;162:1081–1087.

10　Jones MK. Galactography: procedure of choice for evaluation of nipple discharge. *Semin Intervent Radiol* 1992;9:112–119.

11　Baker KS, Davey DD, Stelling CB. Ductal abnormalities detected with galactography: frequency of adequate excisional biopsy. *Am J Roentgenol* 1994;162:821–824.

12　Woods ER, Helvie MA, Ikeda DM, Mandell SH, Chapel KL, Adler DD. Solitary breast papilloma: comparison of mammographic, galactographic and pathologic findings. *Am J Roentgenol* 1992; 159:487–491.

13　Mendelson EB. Breast sonography. In: Rumack CM, Wilson SR, Charboneau JW, eds. *Diagnostic Ultrasound*. St Louis: Mosby-Year Book Inc., 1991:541–563.

14　Fornage BD, Coan JD, David CL. Ultrasound-guided needle biopsy of the breast and other interventional procedures. *Radiol Clin North Am* 1992;30:167–185.

15　Tabar L, Pentek Z, Dean PB. The diagnostic and therapeutic value of breast cyst puncture and pneumocystography. *Radiology* 1981;141:659–663.

16　Ikeda DM, Helvie MA, Adler DD, Schwindt LA, Chang AE, Rebner M. The role of fine-needle aspiration and pneumo-cystography in the treatment of impalpable breast cysts. *Am J Roentgenol* 1992;158:1239–1241.

17　Grant CS, Goellner JR, Welch JS, Martin JK. Fine-needle aspir-ation of the breast. *Mayo Clin Proc* 1986;61:377–381.

18　Jackson VP. The status of mammographically guided fine needle aspiration biopsy of nonpalpable breast lesions. *Radiol Clin North Am* 1992;30:155–166.

19　Fornage BD. Percutaneous biopsies of the breast: state of the art. *Cardiovasc Intervent Radiol* 1991;14:29–39.

20　Helvie MA, Ikeda DM, Adler DD. Localization and needle aspir-ation of breast lesions: complications in 370 cases. *Am J Roentgenol* 1991;157:711–714.

21　Hann L, Ducatman BS, Wang HH, Fein V, McIntire JM. Non-palpable breast lesions: evaluation by means of fine needle aspiration cytology. *Radiology* 1989;171:373–376.

22　Goodson WH III, Mailman R, Miller TR. Three year follow-up of benign fine needle aspiration biopsies of the breast. *Am J Surg* 1987;154:58–61.

23　Helvie MA, Baker DE, Adler DD, Andersson I, Naylor B, Buck-walter KA. Radiographically guided fine-needle aspiration of nonpalpable breast lesions. *Radiology* 1990;174:657–661.

24　Teixidor HS, Wojtasek DA, Reiches EM, Santos-Buch CA, Mitnick CR. Fine-needle aspiration of breast biopsy specimens: correlation of histologic and cytologic findings. *Radiology* 1992;184:55–58.

25　Evans WP, Case SH. Needle localization and fine-needle aspiration biopsy of nonpalpable breast lesions with use of standard and stereotactic equipment. *Radiology* 1989;173:53–56.

26　Lofgren M, Andersson I, Lindholm K. Stereotactic fine-needle aspiration for cytologic diagnosis of nonpalpable breast lesions. *Am J Roentgenol* 1990;154:1191–1195.

27　Azavedo E, Svane G, Auer G. Stereotactic fine-needle biopsy in 2594 mammographically detected non-palpable lesions. *Lancet* 1989;1:1033–1036.

28　Ciatto S, Rosselli DelTurco M, Bravetti P. Nonpalpable breast lesions: stereotactic fine-needle aspiration cytology. *Radiology* 1989;173:57–59.

29　Fajardo LL, Davis JR, Wiens JL, Trego DC. Mammography-guided stereotactic fine needle aspiration cytology of nonpalpable breast lesions: prospective comparison with surgical biopsy results. *Am J Roentgenol* 1990;155:977–981.

30　Dowlatshahi K, Gent HJ, Schmidt R, Jokich PM, Bibbo M, Sprenger E. Nonpalpable breast tumors: diagnosis with stereo-taxic localization and fine needle aspiration. *Radiology* 1989;170: 427–433.

31　Mitnick JS, Vazquez MF, Roses DF, Harris MN, Gianutsos R, Waisman J. Stereotaxic localization for fine-needle aspiration breast biopsy. *Arch Surg* 1991;126:1137–1140.

32　Ciatto S, Catarzi S, Morrone D, Rosselli DelTurco M. Fine-needle aspiration cytology of nonpalpable breast lesions: US versus stereotaxic guidance. *Radiology* 1993;188:195–198.

33　Fornage BD, Faroux MJ, Simatos A. Breast masses: US-guided fine-needle aspiration biopsy. *Radiology* 1987;162:409–414.

34　Gordon PB, Goldenberg SL, Chan NHL. Solid breast lesions: diagnosis with US-guided fine-needle aspiration biopsy. *Radiology* 1993;189:573–580.

35　Jackson VP, Bassett LW. Stereotactic fine-needle aspiration biopsy for nonpalpable breast lesions. *Am J Roentgenol* 1990;154: 1196–1197.

36　Dowlatshahi K, Yaremko ML, Kluskens LF, Jokcih PM. Non-palpable breast lesions: findings of stereotaxic needle-core biopsy and fine-needle aspiration cytology. *Radiology* 1991;181:745–750.

37　Franquet T, Cozcolluella R, DeMiguel C. Stereotaxic fine-needle aspiration of low suspicion, nonpalpable breast nodules: valid alternative to follow-up mammography. *Radiology* 1992;183: 635–637.

38　Kopans DB. Fine needle aspiration of clinically occult breast lesions. *Radiology* 1989;170:313–314.

39　Parker SH, Lovin JD, Jobé WE *et al.* Stereotactic breast biopsy with a biopsy gun. *Radiology* 1990;176:741–747.

40　Parker SH, Lovin JD, Jobe WE, Burke BJ, Hopper KD, Yakes WF. Nonpalpable breast lesions: stereotactic automated large-core biopsies. *Radiology* 1991;180:403–407.

41　Parker SH, Jobe WE, Dennis MA *et al.* US-guided automated large core breast biopsy. *Radiology* 1993;187:507–516.

42　Meyer JE. Value of large-core biopsy of occult breast lesions. *Am J Roentgenol* 1992;158:991–992.

43　Burbank F, Belville J. Core breast biopsy, research, and what not to do. *Radiology* 1992;185:639–644.

44　Sickles EA, Parker SH. Appropriate role of core breast biopsy in the management of probably benign lesions. *Radiology* 1993; 188:315.

45　Logan-Young WW, Janus JA, Destounis SV, Hoffman NY. Appro-priate role of core breast biopsy in the management of probably benign lesions. *Radiology* 1994;190:313–314.

46　Kopans DB. Caution on core. *Radiology* 1994;193:325–328.

47　Parker SH, Burbank F, Jackman RJ. Response to "caution on core." *Radiology* 1994;193:326–327.

48 Sullivan DC. Needle core biopsy of mammographic lesions. *Am J Roentgenol* 1994;162:601–608.

49 Lindfors KK, Rosenquist CJ. Needle core biopsy guided with mammography: a study of cost-effectiveness. *Radiology* 1994; 190:217–222.

50 Elvecrog EL, Lechner MC, Nelson MT. Nonpalpable breast lesions: correlation of stereotaxic large-core needle biopsy and surgical biopsy results. *Radiology* 1993;188:453–455.

51 Caines JS, McPhee MD, Konok GP, Wright BA. Stereotaxic needle core biopsy of breast lesions using a regular mammographic table with an adaptable stereotaxic device. *Am J Roentgenol* 1994;163:317–321.

52 Gisvold JJ, Goellner JR, Grant CS *et al.* Breast biopsy: a comparative study of stereotaxically guided core and excisional techniques. *Am J Roentgenol* 1994;162:815–820.

53 Jackman RJ, Nowels KW, Shepard MJ, Finkelstein SI, Marzoni FA. Stereotaxic large-core needle biopsy of 450 nonpalpable breast lesions with surgical correlation in lesions with cancer or atypical hyperplasia. *Radiology* 1994;193:91–95.

54 Liberman L, Dershaw DD, Rosen PP, Abramson AF, Deutch BM, Hann L. Stereotaxic 14-gage breast biopsy: how many core biopsy specimens are needed. *Radiology* 1994;192:793–795.

55 Parker SH, Burbank F, Jackman RT *et al.* Percutaneous large-core breast biopsy: a multi-institutional study. *Radiology* 1994; 193:359–364.

56 Harter LP, Curtis JS, Ponto G, Craig PH. Malignant seeding of the needle track during stereotaxic core needle breast biopsy. *Radiology* 1992;185:713–714.

57 Shackmuth EM, Harlow CL, Norton LW. Milk fistula: a complication after core breast biopsy. *Am J Roentgenol* 1993;161:961–962.

58 Kaye MD, Vicinanza-Adami CA, Sullivan MC. Mammographic findings after stereotactic biopsy of the breast performed with large-core needles. *Radiology* 1994;192:149–151.

59 Gisvold JJ, Martin JK. Prebiopsy localization of nonpalpable breast lesions. *Am J Roentgenol* 1984;143:477–481.

60 Urrutia EJ, Hawkins MC, Steinbach BG *et al.* Retractable-barb needle for breast lesion localization: use in 60 cases. *Radiology* 1988;169:845–847.

61 Kopans DB, Swann CA. Preoperative imaging-guided needle placement and localization of clinically occult breast lesions. *Am J Roentgenol* 1989;152:1–9.

62 Homer MJ, Smith TJ, Safaii H. Prebiopsy needle localization. *Radiol Clin North Am* 1992;30:139–153.

63 Gallagher WJ, Cardenosa G, Rubens JR, McCarthy KA, Kopans DB. Minimal-volume excision of nonpalpable breast lesions. *Am J Roentgenol* 1989;153:957–961.

64 Bristol JB, Jones PA. Transgression of localizing wire into the pleural cavity prior to mammography. *Br J Radiol* 1981;54:139–140.

65 Davis PS, Wechsler RJ, Feig S, March D. Migration of breast biopsy localization wire. *Am J Roentgenol* 1988;150:787–788.

66 Owen AWMC, Kumar EN. Migration of localizing wires used in guided biopsy of the breast. *Clin Radiol* 1991;43:251.

67 O'Doherty AJ. Spontaneous fracture of the wire tip during breast localization. *Br J Radiol* 1991;64:1154–1156.

68 Homer MJ. Transection of the localization hooked wire during breast biopsy. *Am J Roentgenol* 1993;141:929–930.

69 D'Orsi CJ, Swanson RS, Moss LJ, Reale FR, Wetheimer MD. A complication involving a braided hook-wire localization device. *Radiology* 1993;187:580–581.

70 Reynolds HE, Jackson VP, Musick BS. Preoperative needle localization in the breast: utility of local anesthesia. *Radiology* 1993; 187:503–505.

Orthopedic complications

Iain W. McCall

Musculoskeletal imaging involves the use of all imaging modalities including plain radiographs, computed tomography (CT), technetium-99m methylene diphosphonate (MDP) scanning, ultrasound, and magnetic resonance imaging (MRI). Intravenous contrast enhancement of CT and MRI may be undertaken, but the complications that result are similar to their use in all other systems. Invasive diagnostic techniques in musculoskeletal disorders are limited and mainly involve the examination of the internal structure of the joints and the intervertebral disks using contrast injections. Percutaneous bone biopsy and intradiskal therapy are, however, also undertaken by radiologists. Complications are unusual but must be recognized so that they are limited in frequency and are treated adequately if they occur.

Arthrography

Newberg *et al.* [1] conducted a survey of 57 radiologists experienced in arthrography who had performed more than 126 000 arthrographic procedures. There were no deaths, three cases of infection, and 61 cases of urticaria. Other acute reactions, all of which were extremely rare, included hypotensive seizures, air embolism, and laryngeal edema.

Infection

Infection caused by the needle puncture of a joint may rarely occur. This is usually avoided by careful skin preparation and by the use of disposable prepack sterilized needles. In a series of 25 000 knee arthrograms, only one case of septic arthritis was reported [2]. Symptoms of pain and swelling

developed 48 hours following the arthrogram in this case, and the diagnosis was confirmed by aspiration and culture of *Staphylococcus aureus*. Some swelling and discomfort may follow a double-contrast knee arthrogram for 2 or 3 days due to the slow absorption of the air and sometimes the presence of a mild synovitis. These changes should not be misdiagnosed as infection but careful assessment is required before excluding infection. The continued presence of fluid in the joint can be demonstrated by CT, and aspiration should be performed if infection is considered. The fluid should be submitted to microscopy and culture. Treatment with antibiotics, as soon as the diagnosis of a septic arthritis is made, should avoid residual damage to the joint.

An arthrogram should not be performed on a normal joint if the needle is required to traverse infected tissue before it enters the joint. There are no contraindications to aspiration of an infected joint and arthrography following aspiration is not known to cause any further complication.

Synovial irritation

Rarely, a sterile effusion may occur following the investigation. There will be persistent pain and some stiffness of the joint may be present, due to distension of the joint capsule. The effusion has a rapid onset, which assists in differentiation from a septic arthritis. The joint should be aspirated, and microscopy with culture of the fluid will confirm its aseptic nature. This acute local irritative synovitis has been reported with both water-soluble contrast agents and air alone.

Histologic abnormalities in the synovial membrane are encountered following the injection of most agents in experimental situations. These show mild focal proliferation of surface synovial cells and stromal mononuclear cells, eosinophilia, and dilatation with congestion of vascular channels [3]. The low-grade synovial inflammatory process may also be accompanied by eosinophilia in the synovial fluid [4]. Air may produce less patient discomfort than carbon dioxide [5,6]; this may be related to a reduced decrease in pH of joint fluid [7].

Allergic reactions

Allergic reactions during arthrograms are also rare. This is in the form of urticaria occurring usually within 20 minutes of the injection of contrast medium. A history of a previous severe allergic reaction to contrast agents may be relevant, but sensitivities to other substances have no known association with contrast reaction in arthrography. The incidence of allergic reactions using nonionic contrast agents is not known (see also Chapter 13, pp. 280, 285).

Syncope

Syncope following needle placement in a joint, or during injection of contrast or air, may occur; it is more common in teenagers or athletic males. The patient is usually horizontal during arthrography and elevation of the feet with manipulation of the calves is usually sufficient to restore consciousness.

Air embolism

The potential danger of inducing air embolus exists when a double-contrast technique is employed in a knee with acute hemarthrosis but only when gas is injected directly under pressure. If this should occur, the patient should be placed in the left lateral, head-down position.

Persistence of gas within the joint some 3–4 days following the arthrogram often occurs, and high-altitude flying is not recommended for this period following the injection. Accidental extravasation of air or contrast degrades the images but has not other consequence.

Diskography

Spinal diskography involves the injection of contrast into the nucleus pulposus of intervertebral disks. It is most commonly undertaken in the lower lumbar spine and is less often performed in the midcervical region. Thoracic and upper lumbar disks are rarely investigated. The examination is indicated for the evaluation of diskogenic pain and is usually undertaken prior to surgical intervention.

Complications are primarily due to either misplacement of the needle or to the introduction of infection. Allergies to contrast agents may very rarely occur as contrast may occasionally enter the venous system through a defect in the end plate, which enables a direct link with the vertebral venous system.

Misplacement of the needle

In the cervical spine the needle approach to the disk is lateral to the midline at approximately 45°. The needle passes between the common and internal carotid arteries laterally, and the pharynx or esophagus medially. The needle is inserted just medial to the sternomastoid muscle. Inadequate lateral displacement of the carotid artery may lead to direct puncture. The needle used is only 21-gage and damage to the artery is unlikely. This complication is avoided by digital pressure down to the vertebra, which pushes the carotid laterally.

A puncture site that is too medial, or incorrect needle angulation, may result in puncture through the pharynx or esophagus. There are no direct sequelae but an increased risk of infection may result.

Neural structures should not be at risk in the cervical spine, although overzealous insertion of the needle can result in its passage through the disk and into the spinal cord. Careful monitoring with lateral screening during needle insertion is essential to avoid such a complication, and the hand should brace the hub of the needle during injection to avoid accidental advance of the needle.

In the thoracic spine, the needle passes between the vertebral posterior elements and the pleura. Penetration of the pleura may occur and pneumothorax may result. Needle insertion, that is too lateral, or misangulation of the needle, may result in this complication. Careful biplane fluoroscopy during needle placement should avoid this complication. Needle placement under CT control may also avoid this complication but the process of needle placement may be more laborious and the radiation dose higher with this method.

In the thoracic and lumbar spine, striking the ventral ramus is a potential hazard but is avoided by careful technique. Patients must be conscious during the investigation and contact of the needle with the ventral ramus will be heralded by severe, sharp lancinating pain in the distribution of the nerve, which indicates that the needle should be withdrawn and redirected. If the approach to the lumbar spine is too lateral, greater than 60°, or one hand's breadth lateral to the midline at the point of insertion, penetration of the peritoneum and bowel lateral to the paraspinal muscles may result. Puncture of lateral lumbar veins may occur but no sequelae have been reported as hemorrhage is rapidly arrested by local tissue pressure.

Needle placement that is too vertical may transgress the dural sac. No specific sequelae are related and transdural midline needle insertion into the disk is an accepted technique, although its use has diminished in favor of the

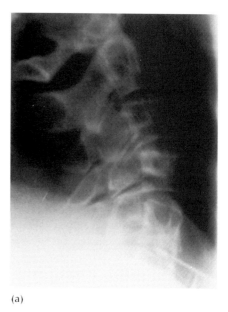

(a)

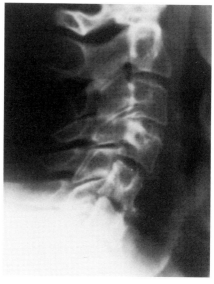

(b)

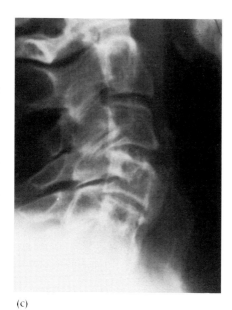

(c)

Fig. 36.1 (a) Cervical diskography. The contrast injection into the C5–6 disk space is demonstrated. (b) Widening of the prevertebral soft tissue and irregularity of the end plate, with some sclerosis of the vertebral body, indicating an active infection. (c) Bony fusion of the vertebral bodies has occurred with ossification extending upwards anteriorly to the level above.

posterolateral approach. Contrast agents should only be injected when the needle tip lies in the center of the nucleus pulposus in both AP and lateral planes. Nonionic contrast media should be used, as inadvertent intrathecal leak or injection of ionic agents at diskography have resulted in myoclonic spasms [8], and inadvertent ionic contrast injected into the dural sac at myelography has resulted in ascending tonic-clonic seizure syndrome and death in some cases [9].

Contraindications

Diskography is contraindicated in the presence of significant neurologic deficit. In the cervical and thoracic spine, any clinical evidence of cord compression or significant nerve root compression is an absolute contraindication. This may be due to osteophyte narrowing of the canal or the presence of a large disk herniation. In the lumbar spine, diskography should be avoided if there is likelihood of a large disk prolapse being present, since this could result in a complete spinal block and a cauda equina lesion following intranuclear contrast injection. MRI examination prior to diskography will avoid such a complication.

Infection

The main complication is postdiskography infection and disk infection. This complication was initially considered to be rare [10,11] and was attributed to a chemical or aseptic reaction [12]. More recent assessment has suggested that this complication may be more common, and in one series an incidence of 2.7% has been reported for the lumbar spine [13]. However, most large series report an incidence of between 0.1 and 0.7% of patients investigated [13,14].

In the cervical spine, the incidence was again initially considered rare [11,15]. However, a recent series has indicated an incidence of 1.38% [14]. An incidence of 7% has been reported but this would seem to be much higher than other investigators [16].

The cardinal clinical feature is a marked increase or sustained acute pain at the site of the diskographic investigation. Intense muscle spasm may occur. In the cervical region, *retropharyngeal abscess* may also occur with difficulty in swallowing. The erythrocyte sedimentation rate or C reactive protein will be consistently raised. In plain radiographs the onset of bone changes is delayed but prevertebral soft tissue widening in the cervical region may be demonstrated. In the cervical, thoracic, and lumbar spine, erosion of the end plate will occur after 3 weeks and disk space narrowing follows. Fusion is a common end point in the cervical spine (Fig. 36.1).

Technetium-99m MDP scanning may provide an earlier diagnosis of infection, with increased activity being seen at around 18 days [14]. Spinal infection may be diagnosed at an earlier stage by MRI, with a decreased signal in disk and adjacent end plate on T1 and an increase in signal of the end plate on T2 (Fig. 36.2). Experimental studies suggest that these changes are present before technetium studies become positive [17]. Guyer *et al.* [14], however, did not find a consistently positive finding in the early stages of infection, with negative appearances in one case at 48 days; this was positive on a follow-up scan 6-months later.

Disk changes may result from an inoculation of relatively small numbers of bacteria, and a positive culture from the disk after 6 weeks is rare [13]. Because of its isolation from

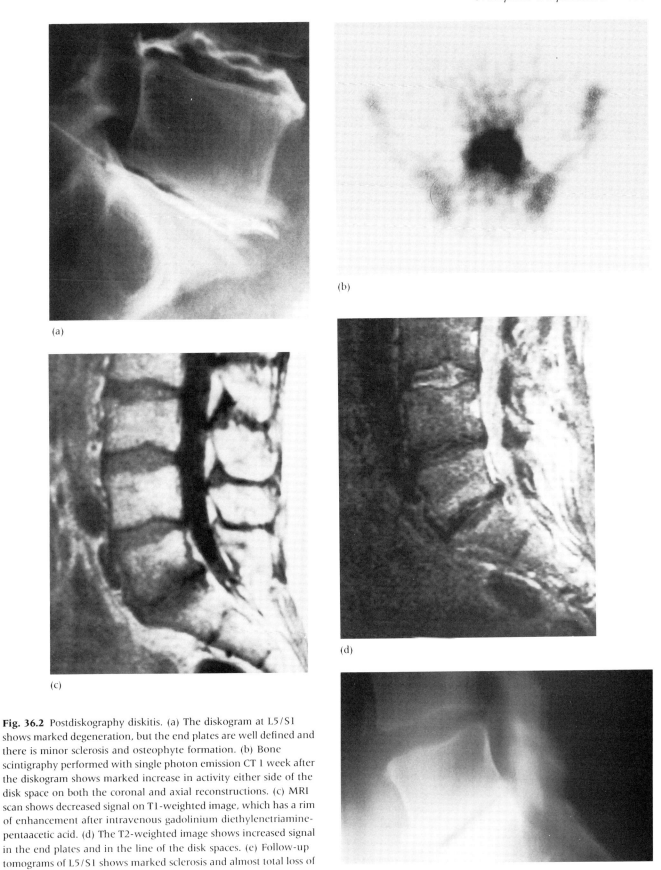

Fig. 36.2 Postdiskography diskitis. (a) The diskogram at L5/S1 shows marked degeneration, but the end plates are well defined and there is minor sclerosis and osteophyte formation. (b) Bone scintigraphy performed with single photon emission CT 1 week after the diskogram shows marked increase in activity either side of the disk space on both the coronal and axial reconstructions. (c) MRI scan shows decreased signal on T1-weighted image, which has a rim of enhancement after intravenous gadolinium diethylenetriamine-pentaacetic acid. (d) The T2-weighted image shows increased signal in the end plates and in the line of the disk spaces. (e) Follow-up tomograms of L5/S1 shows marked sclerosis and almost total loss of disk space 1-year later.

vascular tissue, the normal nucleus pulposus may be considered an ideal culture medium but once the end plate is breached the bacteria are rapidly removed by the body defences [18]. When culture is positive the organisms are usually *S. aureus, S. epidermis* or *Escherichia coli,* suggesting inoculation with surface or bowel organisms.

Neurologic sequelae have not been reported in the lumbar spine, but *epidural abscess* may occur in the cervical spine and three cases of *quadriplegia* have been reported, due to cord damage from epidural or subdural abscess [16,19,20].

Careful assessment is necessary of patients in whom significant pain persists following diskography. Antibiotics are unlikely to affect the outcome in the lumbar spine, and the absence of a positive culture in most cases makes it difficult to choose an appropriate antibiotic. In the cervical spine, early antibiotic therapy is indicated, although culture may be difficult and a MRI scan should be undertaken to exclude an epidural abscess.

Infection may be avoided by careful examination technique. Careful skin cleansing and a full aseptic technique, with the operator fully gowned and protection of radiographic equipment, are indicated. The use of single 18-gauge needles has been shown to be related to the highest reported incidence of infection [13]. A two-needle technique is therefore recommended, with a 21-gauge outer needle inserted into the annulus followed by the passage of a 26-gauge needle into the disk. The operator should avoid touching the needle tip and a separate needle should be used for each disk level. The angle of the needle should be carefully assessed to avoid passage through pharynx or peritoneum.

Prophylactic antibiotics have been suggested to decrease the risk of infection. Evidence suggests that intravenous broad-spectrum cephalosporins immediately prior to the diskogram, or the injection of these antibiotics into the nucleus at the time of the contrast injection may provide increased security [21]. The intradiskal levels of antibiotic rapidly decrease after the intravenous injection and are of little value at 60 minutes.

Percutaneous vertebral biopsy

The percutaneous approach to obtain a sample of tissue for histologic and bacteriologic study prior to therapy, is both easy and safe and avoids the morbidity associated with open surgery. The success rate for histologic diagnosis approaches 90% [22], but positive cultures are less commonly obtained, particularly in cases of tuberculosis.

Complications may be caused by misplacement of the biopsy needle or directly from the biopsy site. Accurate localization can be achieved either by screening, which usually requires a biplane screening system, or by guidance of the needle using CT. The former is perfectly satisfactory for some spinal and most appendicular lesions, but if the lesion is small or the anatomy is complex, such as the pelvis

or posterior arch of the spine. CT is the system of choice.

Pneumothorax may result from biopsy of the thoracic spine if passage of the biopsy needle is too laterally placed. A chest X-ray should always be undertaken following a thoracic vertebral biopsy *Nerve root damage* may occur during vertebral body biopsy and, again, this is more likely to occur in the thoracic spine, where the approach to the vertebra is restricted by the transverse processes and the articular processes of the ribs. In the lumbar spine, biopsy of the vertebral end plate may require close approximation to the lumbar nerve roots.

In the thoracic spine, angulation of the biopsy needle should be carefully assessed to avoid cord damage. In the cervical spine, *cord damage* may occur if undue pressure is applied anteriorly to the vertebral body. In the appendicular skeleton, nerve trunks and main vessels must be avoided and the normal anatomic line of these structures should be considered before the needle approach is decided.

The main complication from bone biopsy is *hemorrhage.* This is usually transient and stops spontaneously, although it may result in hematoma formation (Fig. 36.3). Although very vascular lesions may be regarded as relative contraindications to needle biopsy, in practice, the relatively narrow needle track preserves the supporting tissue, thus limiting local hemorrhage [22]. Overall, the incidence of complications is low at 0.2% [23].

Chemonucleolysis

Although the level of complications arising from chemonucleolysis is very low, consideration must be given to it during the treatment of disk herniation by chymopapain injection. There have been two substantial reviews of the complication rate in the USA and in Europe, involving over 60 000 patients in whom the injections have been performed by doctors from a number of specialties including orthopedic, neurosurgery, radiology, rheumatology, and other medical teams [24,25].

Allergic reactions

The majority of allergic reactions are mild with a rash being the most common, while facial edema and a drop in blood pressure of less than 20 mmHg may also occur. The overall incidence in Europe was 1.75% [25]. *Severe anaphylaxis* predominantly involved a profound drop in blood pressure, whereas respiratory manifestation ranging from bronchospasm to pulmonary edema were less common. The incidence of anaphylaxis in the USA was 0.67% and was more frequent in women than men, whereas in Europe 0.14% of patients had anaphylactic shock and all were treated satisfactorily without sequelae [25].

Sensitivity to chymopapain is thought to be mediated through chymopapain specific serum immunoglobulin E

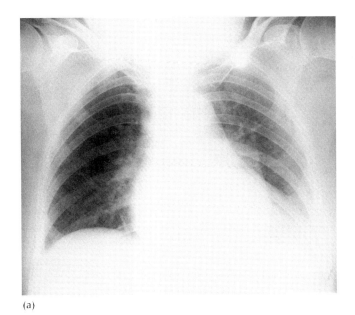

(a)

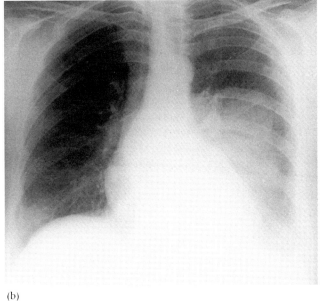

(b)

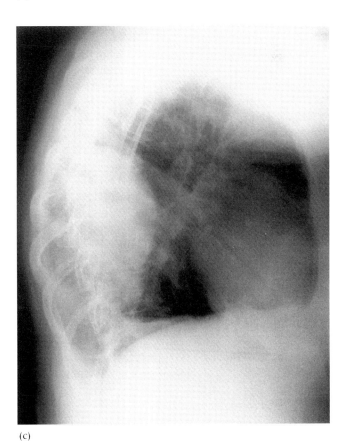

(c)

Fig. 36.3 (a) Chest X-ray shows a moderate paravertebral shadow on both sides of the spine. (b, c) Following the biopsy, there was a rapid and dramatic increase in size of the paravertebral shadow, consistent with a paravertebral hematoma.

(IgE). This has been the base of preinjection testing by measuring the IgE level. Skin testing has also been advocated for preinjection testing with a successful reduction in reactions being reported [26]. Pretreatment with H_1 and H_2-histamine blocking agents, corticosteroids, or both has frequently been used to reduce the potential severity of anaphylactic reaction, although Bouillet [25] found no difference in the incidence of anaphylaxis between the group who used premedication and those who did not.

The anaphylactic reaction usually occurs within minutes of the chymopapain injection and rarely develops beyond 30 minutes from the time of the injection.

Disk infection

Diskitis following chymopapain injection may cause severe backache and spasm for a few days to many weeks following the injection. Cultures may not always be positive and a presumptive diagnosis may be required in some cases. An elevated sedimentation rate may be a valuable clue as this only rises a few millimeters after a normal chemonucleolysis.

The incidence varies between 0.1 and 0.25% and may require antibiotics for treatment. It should not be difficult to differentiate infection from the normal postinjection backache, which may be intense in the first day following the injection, but settles with rest and antiinflammatory drugs.

Neurologic complications

Review of the reported neurologic complications following chymopapain injection suggests that a number of reported events may be coincidental. Three cases of cerebral hemorrhage were due to preexisting aneurysm or vascular malformation. Others, however, were clearly related to needle-puncture techniques. It is known that injection of chymopapain into the epidural space is innocuous [27], but *intrathecal injection* is toxic producing immediate *capillary bleeding*, with resultant *increased intracranial pressure* [28]. Compromise of the dural sac may occur if the needle technique is inadequate: some of the patients who subsequently became paraplegic had multiple needle approaches or had transdural injections. The latter are absolutely contraindicated, either prior to or for the purposes of chemonucleolysis. *Paraplegia* has, however, been reported 2−3 weeks following the injection in two cases in the series by Agre *et al.* [24] and one by Bouillet [25], and this would seem to be due to transverse myelitis.

Cauda equina syndrome occurred in three out of 10 000 patients in the European series [25]. This was due primarily to extruded disk fragments following the injection and was manifest by substantial aggravation of symptoms a few hours after the injection. Immediate surgical intervention resulted in a reversal of symptoms, although in two cases this was achieved by conservative therapy. One case developed due to diffusion of chymopapain and contrast media into the intradural space following a posterior transdural approach.

General complications

Despite the relatively short period of hospitalization following chemonucleolysis, 0.12% of patients developed *deep vein thrombosis* or had mild *pulmonary emboli* [25]. *Paralytic ileus* has also been reported to occur [25].

The overall severe complication rate for chemonucleolysis is low at 0.44%, in the series by Bouillet [25]. Careful techniques avoiding the dura and maintaining a high standard of asepsis will reduce this to a very low level. Local anesthetic injected around the disk after the injection of chymopapain into the disk, has been reported to improve the postinjection back pain and spasm.

Automated percutaneous diskectomy

This procedure involves the placement of a suction and cutting device into the nucleus pulposus to remove part of the nuclear material in a protruded or herniated intervertebral disk. The procedure would seem to have a high margin of safety, but *nerve root injury*, *diskitis* and *vessel injury* are known possible complications. The performance of the procedure under local anesthesia allows the patient to respond to an inadvertent trocar penetration of the nerve root.

Retroperitoneal bleeding resulting in enlargement of the psoas muscle and associated muscle pain and spasm may result from damage to veins in the posterolateral portion of the spine directly adjacent to the entry site of the percutaneous probe into the annulus fibrosis. Bleeding may occur until a tamponade effect develops, and careful observation must be undertaken for 1−2 days in such circumstances [29]. Blankstein *et al.* [30] have reported a case of *staphylococcal diskitis* and osteomyelitis following percutaneous diskectomy, but the risk of infection is low.

Finally, posterior bowel may overlap the desired needle tract in up to 3% of the population, and careful assessment of the preoperative procedure, CT, or MRI axial scans, should be made to check the location of the abdominal contents.

Conclusion

The advent of MRI scanning has significantly reduced the requirement for invasive procedures in orthopedic radiology. It can, however, be seen from the literature that the complication rate in orthopedic radiology is low provided particular attention is taken to the aseptic procedures during the investigation.

References

1 Newberg AH, Muhu CS, Robbins AH. Complications of arthrography. *Radiology* 1985;155:605.
2 Frieberger RH, Kaye JJ. *Introducing Arthrography PZ in Arthrography*. New York: Appleton-Century Crofts, 1979.
3 Pastershank SP, Resnick D, Niwayama G, Danzigi L, Haghighi P. The effect of water soluble contrast media on the synovial membrane. *Radiology* 1982;143:331.
4 Hasselbacher P, Schumacher HR. Synovial fluid eosinophilia following arthrography. *J Rheumatol* 1978;5:173.
5 Goldberg RP, Hall FM, Wyshak G. Pain in knee arthrography. Comparison of air vs CO_2 and respiration vs no respiration. *Am J Roentgenol* 1981;136:377.
6 Mink JH, Dickerson R. Air or CO_2 for knee arthrography. *Am J*

Roentgenol 1980;134:991.

7 Goldberg RP, Hall FM. Pain and PH. *Am J Roentgenol* 1980;135:875.

8 Wollin DG, Lamon MD, Cawley AJ, Wortzman G. The neurotoxic effect of water soluble contrast media in the spinal canal, with emphasis on appropriate management. *J Can Assoc Radiol* 1967;19:296–303.

9 Bohn HP, Reich L, Suljaga-Petchel K. Inadvertent intrathecal use of ionic contrast media for myelography. *Am J Neuroradiol* 1992;13:1515–1519.

10 Collis JS, Gardiner WJ. Lumbar discography. An analysis of one thousand cases. *J Neurosurg* 1962;19:452–461.

11 Simmons EH, Segil CM. An evaluation of discography and the localisation of symptomatic levels in discogenic disease of the spine. *Clin Orthopaed* 1975;108:57–68.

12 Brodsky AE, Binder WF. Lumbar discography. Its value in diagnosis and treatment of lumbar disc lesions. *Spine* 1979;4:110–120.

13 Fraser RD, Osti OL, Vernon Roberts B. Discitis after discography. *J Bone Joint Surg* 1987;69B:26–35.

14 Guyer RD, Collier R, Stilh NJ *et al.* Discitis after discography. *Spine* 1988;13:1352–1354.

15 Cloward RB. Cervical discography technique, indications and use in diagnosis of rupture of cervical discs. *Am J Roentgenol* 1958;79:563–574.

16 Connor PM, Darden BV. Cervical discography complication and clinical efficacy. *Spine* 1993;18:2035–2038.

17 Szypryt EP, Hardy JG, Hinton CE, Worthington BS, Mulholland RC. A comparison between magnetic resonance imaging and scintigraphic bone imaging in the diagnosis of disc space infection in an animal model. *Spine* 1988;13:1042–1048.

18 Fraser RD. Chymopapain for the treatment of intervertebral disc herniation. A preliminary report of a double blind trial. *Spine* 1982;7:608–612.

19 Lowrie SP, Ferguson GG. Spinal subdural empyema complicating cervical discography. *Spine* 1989;14:1415–1417.

20 Eismont FJ, Bohlmann HH, Prasanna L *et al.* Pyogenic and fungal vertebral osteomyelitis with paralysis. *J Bone Joint Surg* 1983;65A:19–29.

21 Fraser RD, Osti OL, Vernon Roberts B. Iatrogenic discitis. The role of intravenous antibiotics in prevention and treatment. An experimental study. *Spine* 1989;14:1025–1031.

22 Stoker DJ, Kissin CM. Percutaneous vertebral biopsy. A review of 135 cases. *Clin Radiol* 1985;36:569–577.

23 Moore TM, Meyers MH, Patzakis MJ, Terry R, Harvey JP. Closed biopsy of musculoskeletal lesions. *J Bone Joint Surg* 1979;61A:375–379.

24 Agre K, Wilson RR, Brim M, McDermott DJ. Chymodiactin post marketing surveillance, demographic and adverse experience data in 29 075 patients. *Spine* 1984;9:479–485.

25 Bouillet R. Treatment of sciatica. A comparative survey of complications of surgical treatment and nucleolysis with chymopapain. *Clin Orthopaed Related Res* 1990;251:144–152.

26 McCulloch JA. Skin testing for Chymopapain sensitivity. *Acta Orthop Belg* 1987;53:221–224.

27 Ford LT. Experimental study of chymopapain in cats. *Clin Orthopaed Related Res* 1969;67:68.

28 Garvin PJ, Jennings RB, Smith L, Gesler RM. Chymopapain: a pharmacologic and toxicologic evaluation of experimental animals. *Clin Orthopaed Related Res* 1965;42:204–223.

29 Gill K. Retroperitoneal bleeding after automated percutaneous discectomy. *Spine* 1990;15:1376–1377.

30 Blankstein A, Rubinstein E, Ezra E, Lokier F, Caspi I, Horoszowski H. Disc space infection and vertebral osteomyelitis as a complication of percutaneous lateral discectomy. *Clin Orthopaed Related Res* 1987;225:234–237.

CHAPTER 37

Complications in pediatric radiology

Anne E. Boothroyd and Helen Carty

General considerations

One of the pleasures of practising pediatric radiology is that radiologically induced complications are fewer than in adult practice, and most that do occur are minor and require no specific treatment. However, this presumes that meticulous attention is paid to the detail of a procedure both from the radiologic and radiographic viewpoint, and to the nursing care of the child. This is particularly important in neonates. There are numerous iatrogenic complications described in the radiologic literature related to modern therapeutic techniques associated with intensive care — prolonged intravenous feeding — but, these are outside the scope of this chapter, which will be confined to those complications induced in the radiology department.

Over the past 5–10 years there have been major changes in the workload of pediatric radiology departments which have paralleled changes in adult departments. These changes comprise an increase in the number of noninvasive diagnostic investigations and in interventional techniques. Thus, complications due to intravenous urography and myelography have decreased with the increased use of renal ultrasound and magnetic resonance imaging (MRI), and new complications are reported with the increasing use of interventional and therapeutic procedures in children. However, the general principles described in the previous edition of this book still apply and are important to reduce the risks of radiologic complications.

Temperature

Heat loss is particularly a problem in neonates and young infants. It is important to maintain the body temperature by keeping the infant well wrapped or in an incubator prior to the procedure and by warming all contrast media and cleansing fluids before use.

Pediatric environment

In addition to being warm, the environment should be "child friendly" and safe. Ideally, more time should be allocated to a pediatric examination to allow a clear explanation of the procedure and time for the child to settle, reducing the risks of complications in a struggling, uncooperative child.

Fluid volumes

Careful attention should also be paid to the volumes of fluid injected, particularly during the flushing of arterial or venous catheters. The blood volume of a baby is 80 ml/kg. For the same reason, the volume of aspirated blood in sampling procedures should also be carefully monitored.

Resuscitation

Medical preparation of the sick infant or child is important in reducing complications. Therefore, even in "urgent" procedures such as intussusception reduction, it is important to make sure that body temperature, dehydration, and biochemical derangement have been corrected. These are the responsibility of the referring medical staff, but the radiologist should have sufficient familiarity with these problems to insist that he or she is delivered a child to investigate in the best condition possible. Adequate analgesia reduces the need for general anesthesia in many invasive procedures.

Sedation

The increasing use of imaging techniques such as computed tomography (CT), MRI, and radionuclide scintigraphy, all of which require stillness during imaging, has led to an increase in the use of sedation. It is important for the radiologist to satisfy him- or herself that the child is fit for sedation. Sedation regimens must be agreed with pediatric and anesthetic staff of the hospital and there must be agreed protocols for monitoring and resuscitation. In general, single drugs are preferable to "cocktails" as it is easier to identify appropriate antagonists in case of difficulty. Analgesia will be needed in addition to sedation for invasive procedures done under local anesthesia. With all sedation regimens, care must be taken to avoid respiratory depression. Sedated children must recover in safe circumstances, such as on a day ward, and be medically checked prior to discharge.

An increasing number of invasive procedures are being carried out on outpatients and with appropriate selection this can be done safely. Many parents are anxious to avoid hospitalization of their children and are capable of managing minor problems (see also p. 7).

Radiation

There is increasing concern about the potential long-term effects of irradiation in childhood. The concerns include the possibility of cancer induction and potential genetic effects. The overriding principle of ALARP — as low as reasonably possible — applies in all pediatric examinations. Techniques to reduce the dose include the use of fast film/screen combinations, e.g., two-speed systems, the use of carbon fiber or its equivalent for tables and cassettes, removal of the grid during screening [1], and the use of 100-mm camera film instead of conventional film. Computed radiography is playing an increasing role in dose reduction, especially where it replaces a system using slow film/screen combinations, such as 400 speed systems. The radiologist must satisfy him- or herself about the choice of the appropriate procedure to investigate the child's problem and choose the one with minimum dose, bearing in mind available facilities. CT represents a major source of radiation, accounting for only 2% of radiology examinations but 20% of the radiation dose [2]. Low-dose techniques and careful consideration of slice widths and intervals are important in reducing exposure.

Patient dose monitoring should be part of the quality assurance programs in radiology departments [3].

Medical and drug-related complications

The imaging features of drug-related and intensive-care-related complications are frequently described in the radiological literature, but are not strictly radiologic complications and will not be described in this chapter [4].

Contrast media (see also Chapter 13)

The complications of iodinated contrast agents are similar in pediatric to adult practice. These include: (i) minor reactions such as arm pain, sneezing, and coughing; (ii) intermediate reactions such as hypotension, bronchospasm, and abdominal pain; and (iii) severe fatal reactions, including cardiac arrest, laryngeal edema, and anuria [5].

The advent of newer nonionic contrast agents has reduced the cellular effects and the increase in intravascular volume associated with conventional agents [6]. Ideally, nonionic contrast agents should be exclusively used in children, even though the incidence of acute reactions of all degrees of severity is lower in children than in adults. The low-osmolar media are more comfortable for the child and do not cause pain if extravasated. More importantly, they do not cause hemodynamic disturbance as they are low osmolar. Fluid overload may still occur with excess volume of contrast. For most procedures, a dose of 2 ml/kg is appropriate (this dosage is safe) but more may be needed in cardiac catheterization.

Deterioration of renal function is well recognized following high-dose urography with ionic contrast, but rare with low-osmolar media [7]. Children who are dehydrated, diabetic, or with a preexisting renal disorder are most at risk of this complication. Urography or angiography should be avoided until biochemical stability is optimum.

Aqueous Dionosil has been widely used for bronchography. However, bilateral bronchograms, general anesthesia, and "alveolarization" of the contrast media should be avoided. Death following the use of heated Dionosil has been reported due to the "alveolarization" associated with a lowered viscosity [8]. Selective bronchography with small quantities of nonionic contrast is safe, but the examination should be carried out by skilled personnel.

With the development of MRI, gadolinium diethylenetriaminepentaaceticacid (DTPA) has been increasingly used in children and has proved extremely helpful in characterizing tumors and other lesions. The absence of enhancement is also helpful in excluding tumor recurrence. There were no adverse reactions in a prospective study of 65 consecutive children for cranial MRI in whom 50% were under 10 years and 15% under 2 years [9].

Adverse reactions associated with the administration of

radioisotopes are extremely rare, but care must be taken to inject methyliodobetaguanidine (MIBG) slowly as it may precipitate a hypertensive crisis.

The hazards of barium and other contrast media in the gastrointestinal tract are discussed in the next section.

Gastrointestinal tract

The choice of contrast media to evaluate the gastrointestinal tract lies between three major groups: barium, Gastrografin (meglumine diatrizoate 66% w/v, sodium diatrizoate 10% w/v), and the low-osmolality water-soluble agents. Barium sulfate suspension is the most frequently used of these and since it is insoluble in water and almost totally inert it has little physiologic effect on the gastrointestinal tract [10]. In addition, it is cheap and provides excellent contrast. The major disadvantages relate to extravasation from bowel into the peritoneum, retroperitoneum, and mediastinum, where it may occasionally result in the formation of granulomas and fibrosis. Clinical experience, however, indicates that the reported complications of barium extravasation are not experienced in practice and the reports exaggerate the hazards [11, 12]. Barium may inspissate within the bowel to form a barolith and cause partial or complete obstruction. Children particularly at risk include those with cystic fibrosis, defunctioned segments of bowel, blind loops, and ileus [13]. Barium should be avoided in these children and water-soluble contrast should be used if possible. There are infrequent reports of allergic reactions to barium but these are thought to be due to the additives rather than the barium itself [14].

Small amounts of aspirated barium are nontoxic and may be cleared by coughing or physiotherapy. In the deaths that have been reported, it is felt that the volume of material aspirated was more important than its nature [10].

Since the advent of low-osmolality contrast agents, the use of Gastrografin has been virtually restricted to neonates with suspected meconium ileus, where it is used therapeutically because of its hypertonicity which draws fluid into the bowel and causes disimpaction of the sticky meconium. It has also been used orally in older children with meconium ileus equivalent. Due to the marked fluid shift that may occur, it is imperative that the infant or child is well hydrated with an intravenous line *in situ* before commencing the study. Older children, taking Gastrografin for meconium ileus equivalent, should be advised to increase oral fluids [15]. They do not need intravenous rehydration. The fluid shift dilutes the contrast agent with consequent poor visualization of the bowel, rendering it less suitable than nonionic contrast media for most other purposes. Severe toxic effects on bowel mucosa may result from prolonged contact with undiluted Gastrografin [16].

Low-osmolality contrast agents provide excellent bowel opacification without the disadvantages of barium and Gastrografin. They are rapidly absorbed from the peritoneum if extravasated from the bowel [17]. Because of their low osmolality there is no fluid shift and better bowel opacification compared with Gastrografin. Good delayed images may be obtained. They do not damage bowel mucosa [18] and are much less irritating to the lining than other agents [19]. They are the contrast media of first choice in examining the sick neonate. One relative disadvantage is cost, but the volumes used are small. The indications for their use include suspected esophageal or bowel perforation, aspiration, and most neonatal gastrointestinal examinations.

The side-effects of anticholinergic and hypotonic agents [20] are rarely encountered in pediatric practice as they are rarely used to reduce intestinal peristalsis.

In addition to selecting an appropriate contrast agent, it is important to perform all gastrointestinal studies carefully with fluoroscopic control. If there is a risk of aspiration, e.g., pharyngeal incoordination, fistula, or cleft palate, then the study should be commenced with small volumes of contrast and suction should be immediately available. Contrast studies are contraindicated in the initial assessment of tracheo-esophageal fistula where the upper pouch may be delineated by a plain film with an opaque tube.

All requests for a contrast enema should be vetted by a radiologist to prevent inappropriate preparation. The risk of water intoxication in children with Hirschsprung's disease has been documented [21], but since the diagnosis is now usually made in the neonatal period it is rarely a problem.

The risks of inspissation of barium in partial colonic obstruction are probably quite small, although studies of defunctioned bowel or the distal bowel in patients with imperforate anus should be done with water-soluble contrast media to avoid the formation of barium concretions in the distal bowel [22] or bladder in the presence of a rectovesical fistula.

Tube complications

The enema tip may injure the rectal wall, causing superficial abrasions or deep lacerations with dissection of barium beneath the mucosa, submucosa, or perianal skin [23]. The use of a balloon catheter may cause overdistension and subsequent bowel rupture. For this reason, balloon catheters are not recommended routinely in infants and children, but may sometimes be needed for intussusception reduction when failure to retain contrast prevents the desired therapeutic effect of the enema.

Premature neonates are particularly at risk of complications from catheter misplacement. One report describes the development of gastric pneumatosis secondary to an intramural feeding catheter [24]. Further reports have documented perforation at other sites, including the lamina cribrosa, with the tip of the nasogastric tube in a cerebral hemisphere [25].

The balloon tip of a gastrostomy tube may occasionally migrate distally and has resulted in cases of pancreatitis, bowel obstruction, and intussusception [26]. It is important to check catheters for an abnormal course or associated collection on the plain film and, if misplacement is suspected, to instil a small amount of nonionic contrast to confirm the position of the catheter tip (Fig. 37.1).

Intussusception

Hydrostatic reduction of an intussusception is a well-described alternative to surgical reduction. An absolute contra-indication to the technique is evidence of perforation, and a relative contraindication is a shocked child with circulatory shutdown. Following resuscitation and rehydration, the child should be reviewed to see whether nonoperative reduction is possible. Radiologic signs such as the "dissection sign" have not been found to be good prognostic indicators [27]. Ultrasound is extremely helpful in making the diagnosis of intussusception prior to reduction and to detect free intra-peritoneal fluid, of which moderate to large quantities generally indicate peritonitis. More recently, the use of color Doppler has been described to assess the viability of the bowel in children presenting late with an intussusception [28], but this is not widely accepted at the time of writing. In addition to careful selection of children for enema reduction, technique is also important. Good analgesia prior to the procedure increases the ease of reduction, while gentle and slow filling of the colon provides better retention of barium with sustained pressure, than attempts at rectal occlusion. A balance has to be struck between achieving successful re-duction and causing perforation because of too high a pressure in the colon. Traditionally, it has been taught that occlusion of the rectum by balloon catheters, and raising the barium reservoir more than 1 m above tabletop height, are unsafe procedures and increase the risk of perforation (Fig. 37.2). While great care must be exercised during hydrostatic or gas reduction, it is increasingly accepted that rectal occlusion by balloon, handholding of the buttocks, and higher reduction pressures may be used safely and will achieve an increased nonsurgical reduction rate.

A comparison between the hydrostatic pressures and flow rates achieved by hydrostatic versus pneumatic intus-susception reduction showed that experienced pediatric radiologists significantly underestimated the height at which contrast should be placed. This may account for the apparent improvement in intussusception reduction rates with pneumatic reduction [29].

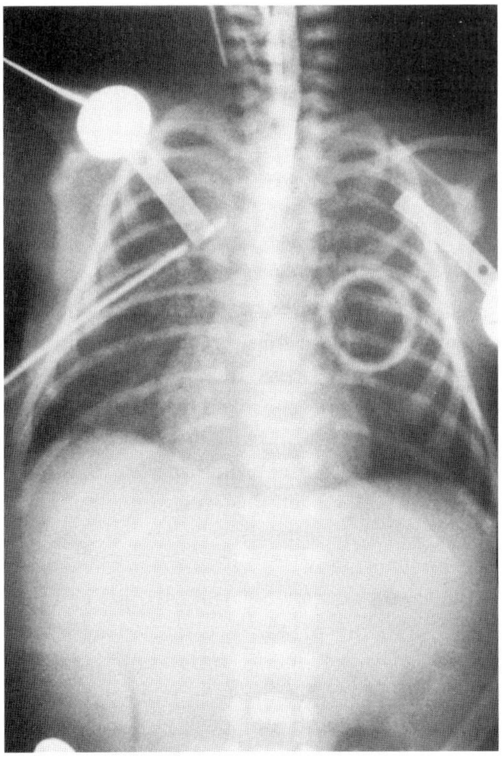

Fig. 37.1 Perforation of esophagus by a nasogastric tube.

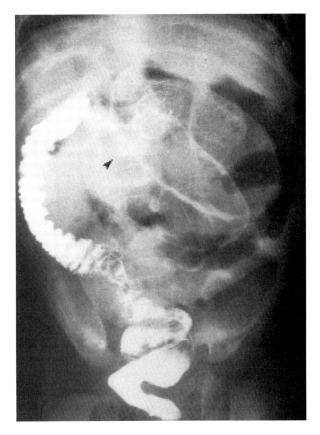

Fig. 37.2 Perforation of the bowel occurred during attempted reduction of an intussusception (prone film).

There is an increasing use of pneumatic reduction of intussusception using oxygen or air and a greater success rate with fewer complications has been claimed [30, 31], but in unselected groups of patients in skilled hands the success rate of barium and gas reduction is about equal. The debate is not yet resolved and both reduction techniques are still acceptable [32, 33]. These authors describe oxygen flow rates of 2 l/min and a maximum pressure of 80 mmHg, but pressures of up to 120 mmHg are used in practice. Should perforation occur, the tension pneumoperitoneum should be relieved by peritoneal puncture with an 18-gauge needle placed midway between the xiphisternum and the umbilicus [34]. This must always be available before starting the procedure. Perforation rates are higher with air reduction than barium reduction.

Catheter removal of esophageal foreign bodies

The use of a balloon catheter under fluoroscopic guidance to remove esophageal foreign bodies is a generally accepted technique. Perforation of the esophagus due to overinflation of the balloon and laceration during manipulation of a sharp foreign body are recognized complications. Aspiration into the larynx and impaction in the nasopharynx have also been described. These latter hazards can be avoided by introducing the catheter through the mouth and by withdrawing the foreign body with the patient in the prone oblique position. Some authors [35] attempt catheter extraction only for smooth, rounded foreign objects in patients with no previous esophageal disease or surgery. They also consider the presence of the foreign body for more than 7–10 days to be a relative contraindication to removal, and mediastinal widening to be an absolute contraindication. Magnetic catheters have been used to remove ferromagnetic foreign bodies from the stomach. Complications are the same as for esophageal foreign bodies.

Balloon dilatation of esophageal strictures

Balloon dilatation is increasingly used in pediatric practice and has been found to be both effective and safe in the treatment of stenoses caused by postoperative stricture, restrictive Nissen fundoplication, and esophagitis [36]. Balloon dilatation is thought to be safer than traditional bouginage since only radially directed forces are used without additional longitudinal and shearing forces. It is also a safe procedure for the treatment of strictures occurring following esophageal replacement [37]. There is a small risk of perforation which may be reduced by not stretching the esophagus to more than twice its resting diameter and by discontinuing dilatation if blood densely coats the balloon [38].

Genitourinary tract

Cystography

Micturating cystourethrography is a widely performed and generally safe examination in children [39]. Careful technique is required to minimize trauma of an unpleasant examination. Catheterization should be carried out aseptically using the smallest diameter straight catheter — pediatric nasogastric feeding tubes, 5–8-F gauge are ideal. Catheterization is performed in the X-ray department immediately prior to the procedure to allow the use of simple catheters and to minimize the time the catheter remains in the bladder. Adequate lubricating jelly should be used to minimize urethral trauma and no force should be used to pass the catheter for fear of urethral trauma or creation of a false passage. The catheter position should be checked before filling, using fluoroscopy, and care should be taken to prevent overdistension of the bladder.

Complications

Infection is the major potential hazard causing fever sepsis, renal scarring, and occasionally death. Glynn and Gordon [40] reported a 6% incidence of postprocedural infections which they defined as a new infection or an exacerbation of an existing one. For this reason, cystourethrography should be avoided in the presence of infected urine. Many children are taking prophylactic antibiotics at the time of the study and this is usually adequate to prevent infection. If reflux is detected in a child not already on antibiotics, these should be prescribed. Routine antibiotic cover is not required in non-refluxing children.

Local damage to the urethra or bladder during catheterization may result in dysuria, hematuria, or urinary retention. Advice to parents following the procedure to minimize these complications includes increased oral fluids and putting the child into a bath if dysuria or retention occur. Occasionally, inadvertent catheterization of a dilated ureteric orifice may occur with associated ureteral trauma. Reflux of contrast into the vagina occurs frequently in girls. This is normal and not a complication. Very rarely, contrast refluxes from the vagina into the uterus and peritoneal cavity, providing a means of peritoneal contamination, and is more likely in children with adrenogenital syndrome and ambiguous genitalia [41].

Contrast may be absorbed from the bladder and can cause the same allergic reactions as intravenous contrast media. In addition, all contrast agents can elicit an inflammatory response in the bladder, particularly at high concentrations: transient vesicoureteric reflux following cystography is probably a contrast-related complication in some cases [42]. These contrast-related complications do not occur with isotope cystography.

Interventional techniques

Renal biopsy, percutaneous nephrostomy, and Whitaker tests are now part of established investigation of the pediatric urinary tract. Complications occur infrequently and are similar to those encountered in adult practice [43]. The use of ultrasound guidance allows accurate placement of needles and catheters in the smaller pediatric organs and the smallest size of needle or catheter should be used, commensurate with obtaining adequate biopsy samples.

Neuroradiology

The complications of neuroradiology procedures have been markedly reduced by the increasing use of CT and MRI, and the use of nonionic low-osmolar contrast in myelography. Pneumoencephalography has become an investigation of the past, and the numbers of cerebral angiograms and myelograms have been markedly reduced.

Myelography is still indicated when there is limited access to MRI or when a severe scoliosis or the presence of rods and metal hooks renders MRI and CT technically difficult due to metal artifacts. Transient side-effects include headache, nausea, and low-grade fever, which are thought to be due to the lumbar puncture. More severe reactions, including persistent nausea, and severe leg and back pain are thought to be due to neurotoxicity since they are associated with larger amounts of contrast and high extension in the spinal canal [44]. However, the overall incidence of complications in myelography is low [45].

Cerebral angiography is still a relatively common procedure in children and is performed for the diagnosis of aneurysms, arteriovenous malformations, or prior to interventional procedures. The most serious complication is ischemic brain damage which may be due to embolization, arterial spasm, or mechanical occlusion. All cerebral complications of angiography are more common in children with reduced cerebral blood flow and, thus, hypotension, dehydration, and anemia should be corrected prior to the procedure. Good technique may also reduce the risk of complications, including the use of small, soft catheters, never advancing the catheter against resistance, and a careful flush technique [46].

Angiography

Most angiograms are now performed by a percutaneous transfemoral technique, even in neonates. Many of the complications of angiography such as hematoma at the puncture site and dissection, perforation, or thrombosis of a vessel are common to both children and adults (Fig. 37.3). Spasm is more common in children, partly due to the relatively large catheter size as compared with the arterial diameter. Other factors including age, a high hematocrit,

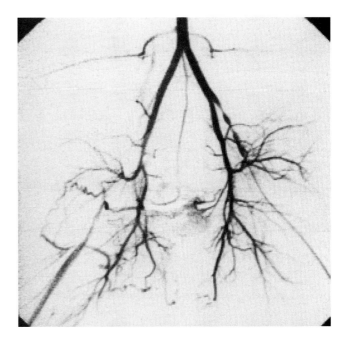

Fig. 37.3 Femoral artery occlusion following previous angiography.

and prolonged catheterization time are also implicated [47]. Systemic heparinization (100 U/kg) is indicated in prolonged procedures and children with a high hematocrit to reduce thrombotic complications. The smallest gauge catheter suitable for the procedure should be used. Thin-walled catheters that can tolerate high flow rates are ideal. Careful technique is particularly important in angiographic and interventional procedures, which should only be done in children by those skilled in pediatric examinations. Simple measures such as increased obliquity of the vessel puncture will increase the likelihood of the guidewire advancing entirely within the lumen of very small caliber vessels and reduces the risk of dissection.

Aortic thrombosis is a particular risk associated with umbilical artery catheterization in neonates. Despite recanalization of the thrombus, renovascular hypertension and leg-growth discrepancy may occur [48]. Other complications include renal and gastrointestinal infarction from intimal aortic tears or thrombotic emboli.

A review of 33 children with suspected iatrogenic arterial injuries, revealed that nonoperative treatment comprising Doppler assessment and systemic heparinization produced better results than thrombectomy [49].

Many procedures have now been extended from adult to pediatric practice such as splenoportography in children with portal hypertension. A significant reduction in the traditional complications has been attained by embolization of the needle track [50].

Cardiac catheterization

In addition to the complications associated with angiography, cardiac catheterization is more likely to result in excessive contrast use and blood loss. Contrast-medium overdosage may cause seizures, cerebral edema, acute renal shutdown, and progressive deterioration in a patient whose cardiac function is already impaired [51]. Larger contrast volumes are required than in other areas of the body because of the high flow rates, and the volumes of test injections are often forgotten. Similarly, a surprisingly large volume of blood may be lost if frequent samples are taken for blood-gas analysis. A careful record of the volumes of contrast and flushing solution used, and volumes of blood samples taken is mandatory.

Particular complications of cardiac catheterization include death, arrhythmias, cardiac perforation, and myocardial "staining" due to intramyocardial contrast injection (Fig. 37.4). Uncorrected acidosis and the morbidity of the cardiac lesion undoubtedly contribute to the deaths. Cardiac perforation and myocardial staining may be minimized by the use of soft, side-hole only catheters and by ensuring that the catheter tip is free prior to pressure injection.

An increasing number of cardiac catheterizations are now being performed to carry out therapeutic techniques. Balloon dilatation, embolization, and the insertion of occlusion devices account for most of the interventional work. Larger catheters and sheaths are usually required, and the procedure times are increased when compared with diagnostic studies. A study of 417 such interventions found that serious arrhythmias and complications of vascular access are more frequent in infants younger than 6 months and that pulmonary artery rupture is a life-threatening risk in dilatation of peripheral pulmonary stenosis [52]. They also emphasize that only a small number of thoroughly trained cardiologists or radiologists should perform these procedures.

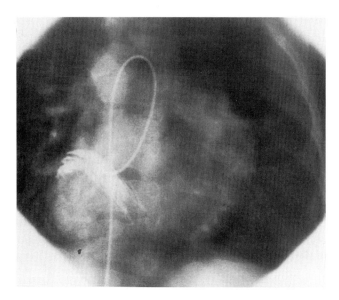

Fig. 37.4 Myocardial staining due to catheter tip abutting the ventricular wall.

Interventional procedures

Interventional procedures are now common in pediatric practice. The diagnostic accuracy and therapeutic efficiency of guided biopsy aspiration and drainage techniques in children, mirror the results in adults [53, 54]. The main differences are the need to modify equipment so that the smallest needles and catheters are used and the increased use of sedation or general anesthesia [55]. In addition, there are usually less routine interventional procedures and more complex, "one-off" procedures such as the percutaneous transhepatic dilatation of a membranous obstruction in Budd–Chiari syndrome [56].

Careful discussion with the parents is essential to explain the relative benefits and risks of the procedure. This should be recorded in the case sheet. The radiologist should personally check the preprocedure investigations such as a clotting screen, and that informed consent has been obtained.

The complications of interventional procedures that are specific to pediatrics will be discussed below.

Congenital heart disease

Cardiac and femoral arterial complications following diagnostic catheter procedures, particularly in infants weighing less than 15 kg, have been well documented [57]. To avoid these complications, techniques such as systemic heparinization, smaller catheters, and venous cannulation have been developed. However, the incidence of femoral arterial complications has again risen with the use of transfemoral balloon catheter techniques for treating systemic cardiovascular obstructive lesions. The complications include arterial disruption and thrombosis. The incidence of these complications may be reduced by the use of smaller low-profile catheters introduced through a femoral artery sheath, and possibly using a bifemoral technique with the catheters rather than a single large catheter [58].

Another interventional technique used in children with congenital heart disease is the embolization of systemic to pulmonary collateral vessels. These vessels develop in children with right ventricular outflow or pulmonary artery obstruction and may result in heart failure and pulmonary hemorrhage. Embolization of the collateral vessels is now used to reduce the time of operation and minimize the risks of bypass. The procedure may be prolonged and the general risks of angiography apply. However, pulmonary infarction may also occur in segments of the lung that do not have a dual arterial supply [59.]

Vascular malformations

Congenital lesions such as hemangiomas and venous malformations may require intervention. The development of a new sclerosing agent (Ethibloc), which is an alcoholic solution of a corn protein, has allowed direct percutaneous sclerotherapy of soft tissue venous malformations [60]. This has produced a technically good result in most cases and may facilitate future surgery. There is a marked inflammatory reaction in all cases, with swelling of the lesion, pain, and mild fever, which usually resolves within 48 hours. When the lesion is close to an airway, facilities for intensive care and ventilation must be available before embarking on the procedure. No major complications have been recorded. This technique has major advantages over the use of absolute alcohol which may cause neuropathy and tissue devitalization and requires extremely careful superselective use [61].

Routine resection of hemangiomas is not advocated since most involute spontaneously with a good cosmetic result. However, occasionally a hemangioma may result in deformity of adjacent structures, or the large physical size restricts activity or blocks an orifice. In such cases, superselective embolization may be employed with or without other techniques such as laser ablation [62]. As with adults, careful patient selection is important. The complications of migrating coils, thrombosis of adjacent vessels, necrosis, and gangrene may all occur but are similar to those in adult practice.

Varicocele

Percutaneous sclerotherapy of idiopathic varicoceles is indicated in patients with testicular discomfort and/or abnormal seminal analysis. Following demonstration of testicular vein insufficiency by reflux of contrast medium, sclerotherapy is performed. A small percentage suffer acute swelling and pain in the scrotal sac and groin but this usually resolves within days [63].

Intracavitary sclerotherapy

Percutaneous aspiration of cysts and subsequent instillation of a sclerosing agent such as tetracycline has proved effective for lesions such as lymphangiomata and simple renal cysts [64, 65].

References

1 Drury P, Robinson A. Fluoroscopy without the grid: a method of reducing the radiation dose. *Br J Radiol* 1980;53:93–99.

2 National Radiological Protection Board. *Protection of the Patient in Computed Tomography*, Vol. 3 (4), Documents of the NRPB 1992.

3 National Radiological Protection Board. *National Protocol for Patient Dose Measurements in Diagnostic Radiology*. Documents of the NRPB, 1992.

4 Kassner EG. Drug related complications in infants and children: imaging features. *Am J Roentgenol*. 1991;157:1039–1049.

5 Kassner EG. *Iatrogenic Disorders of the Fetus, Infant and Child*. Berlin Springer-Verlag, 1985:3.

6 Wood BP, Smith WL. Pulmonary edema in infants following injection of contrast media for urography. *Radiology* 1981;139: 377–379.

7 Older RA, Korobkin M, Cleeve DM, Schaaf R, Thompson W. Contrast induced acute renal failure: Persistent nephrogram as clue to early detection. *Am J Roentgenol* 1980;134:339–342.

8 McAlister WH. Death associated with bronchography. *Pediat Radiol* 1989;19:458–460.

9 Elster AD, Reiser GD. Gd-DTPA-enhanced cranial MR imaging in children: initial clinical experience and recommendations for its use. *Am J Roentgenol* 1989;153:1265–1268.

10 Gelfand DW. Complications of gastrointestinal radiologic procedures. Complications of routine fluoroscopic studies. *Gastrointest Radiol* 1980;5:293–315.

11 Cohen MD. Choosing contrast media for the evaluation of the gastrointestinal tract of neonates and infants. *Radiology* 1987; 162:447–456.

12 Eklof O, Hald J, Thomasson B. Barium peritonitis. Experience of five pediatric cases. *Pediat Radiol* 1983;13:5–9.

13 Ratcliffe JF. The use of low osmolality water soluble (LOWS) contrast media in the pediatric gastro-intestinal tract: a report of 115 examinations. *Pediat Radiol* 1986;16:47–52.

14 McAvoy M, Young JWR, Keramati B. Hypersensitivity reaction to barium suspension. (Letter to editor). *Am J Roentgenol* 1985; 144:1316.

15 O'Halloran SM, Gilbert K, McKendrick OM, Carty HML, Heaf DP. Gastrografin in acute meconium ileus equivalent. *Arch Dis Child* 1986;61:1128–1130.

16 Gallitano AL, Kondi ES, Phillips E, Ferris E. Near fatal hemorrhage following Gastrografin studies. *Radiology* 1976;118:35–36.

17 Cohen MD, Weber TR, Grosfield JL. Bowel perforation in the newborn: diagnosis with metrizamide. *Radiology* 1984;150: 65–69.

18 Schwartzentruber D, Billmire DF, Cohen M, Block T, Gunter M, Grosfield JL. Use of Ioxhexol in the radiographic diagnosis of ischaemic bowel. *J Pediat Surg* 1986;21:525–529.

19 Ginai AZ, ten Kate FJW, ten Berg RGM, Hoornstra K. Experimental evaluation of various available contrast agents for use in the upper gastrointestinal tract in case of suspected leakage: effect on lungs. *Br J Radiol* 1984;57:895–901.

20 Kassner EG. *Iatrogenic Disorders of the Fetus, Infant and Child*. Berlin: Springer-Verlag, 1985:13.

21 Steinback HL, Rosenberg RH, Grossman M, Nelson TL. The potential hazard of enemas in patients with Hirschsprung's disease. *Radiology* 1955;64:45–50.

22 Kassner EG. *Iatrogenic Disorders of the Fetus, Infant and Child*. Berlin: Springer-Verlag, 1985:12.

23 Kassner EG. *Iatrogenic Disorders of the Fetus, Infant and Child*. Berlin: Springer-Verlag, 1985:17.

24 Mandell GA, Finkelstein M. Gastric pneumatosis secondary to an intramural feeding catheter. *Pediat Radiol* 1988;18:418–420.

25 van den Anker JN, Quak JME, Robben SGF, Meradji M. Iatrogenic perforation of the lamina cribrosa by a nasogastric tube in an infant. *Pediat Radiol* 1992;22:545–546.

26 Panicek DM, Ewing DK, Gottlieb RH, Chew FS. Gastrostomy tube pancreatitis. *Pediat Radiol* 1988;18:416–417.

27 Barr LY, Stansberry SD, Swischuk LE. Significance of age, duration, obstruction and the dissection sign in intussusception. *Pediat Radiol* 1990;20:454–456.

28 Lam AH, Firman K. Value of sonography including color Doppler in the diagnosis and management of long standing intussusception. *Pediat Radiol* 1992;22:112–114.

29 Sargent MA, Wilson BP. Are hydrostatic and pneumatic methods

of intussusception reduction comparable? *Pediat Radiol* 1991; 21(5):346−349.

30 Phelan E, de Campo JF, Malecky G. Comparison of oxygen and barium reduction of ileocolic intussusception. *Am J Roentgenol* 1988;150:1349−1352.

31 Stein M, Alton DJ, Daneman A. Pneumatic reduction of intussusception: 5 year experience. *Radiology* 1992;183:681−685.

32 Katz ME, Kolm P. Intussusception reduction 1991: an international survey of pediatric radiologists. *Pediat Radiol* 1992;22: 318−322.

33 Markowitz RI, Meyer JS. Pneumatic versus hydrostatic reduction of intussusception. *Radiology* 1992;183:623−624.

34 Zhang J, Wang Y, Wei L. Rectal inflation reduction of intussusception in infants. *J Pediat Surg* 1986;21:30−32.

35 Kassner EG. *Iatrogenic Disorders of the Fetus, Infant and Child.* Berlin: Springer-Verlag, 1985:23.

36 Sato Y, Frey EE, Smith WL, Pringle KC, Soper RT, Franken EA. Balloon dilatation of esophageal stenosis in children. *Am J Roentgenol* 1988;150:639−642.

37 Tam PKH, Sprigg A, Cudmore RE, Cook RCM, Carty H. Endoscopy-guided balloon dilatation of esophageal strictures and anastomotic strictures after esophageal replacement in children. *J Pediat Surg* 1991;26(9):1101−1103.

38 Hoffer FA, Winter HS, Fellows KE. The treatment of postoperative and peptic esophageal strictures after esophageal atresia repair. *Pediat Radiol* 1987;17:454−458.

39 McAlister WH, Cacciarelli A, Shackleford GD. Complications associated with cystography in children. *Radiology* 1974;111: 167−172.

40 Glynn B, Gordon IR. The risk of infection of the urinary tract as a result of micturating cystourethrography in children. *Ann Radiol* 1970;13:283−287.

41 Bolich PR, Babbitt DP. Reflux into vagina, uterus and fallopian tubes and peritoneal cavity during voiding cystourethrography: case report. *Pediat Radiol* 1975;3:242−243.

42 Kassner EG. *Iatrogenic Disorders of the Fetus, Infant and Child.* Berlin: Springer-Verlag, 1985:7.

43 Pfister RC, Newhouse JH, Yader IV *et al.* Complications of pediatric percutaneous renal procedures: incidence and observations. *Urol Clin N Am* 1983;10:563−567.

44 Petersson H, Fitz CR, Harwood-Nash DCF, Armstrong E, Chuang SH. Adverse reactions to myelography with metrizamide in infants, children and adolescents. *Acta Radiol* 1982;23:323−329.

45 Dube LJ, Blair IG, Geoffroy G. Paediatric myelography with Iohexol. *Pediat Radiol* 1992;22:290−292.

46 Kassner EG. *Iatrogenic Disorders of the Fetus, Infant and Child.* Berlin: Springer-Verlag, 1985:72.

47 Mortensson W, Hallbrook T, Lundstrom NR. Percutaneous catheterisation of the femoral vessels in children. Thrombotic occlusion of the catheterised artery: frequency and causes. *Pediat Radiol* 1975;4:1−9.

48 Seibert JJ, Northington FJ, Miers JF, Taylor BJ. Aortic thrombosis after umbilical artery catheterisation in neonates. *Am J Roentgenol* 1991;156:567−569.

49 Klein MD, Coran AG, Whitehouse WM, Stanley JC, Wesley JR, Lebowitz EC. Management of iatrogenic arterial injuries in infants and children. *J Pediat Surg* 1982;17:933−939.

50 Brazzini A, Hunter DW, Darcy MD *et al.* Safe splenoportography. *Radiology* 1987;162:607−609.

51 Lalli AF. Contrast media reactions: data analysis and hypothesis. *Radiology* 1980;134:1−12.

52 Fellows KE, Radtke W, Keane JF, Lock JE. Acute complications of catheter therapy for congenital heart disease. *Am J Cardiol* 1987;60:679−683.

53 vanSonnenberg E, Wittich GR, Edwards DK *et al.* Percutaneous diagnostic and therapeutic interventional radiologic procedures in children. Experience in 100 patients. *Radiology* 1987;162: 601−605.

54 Baran GW, Haaga JR, Shurin SB, Alfidi RJ. CT guided percutaneous biopsies in pediatric patients. *Pediat Radiol* 1984;14: 161−164.

55 Hansen ME, Kadir S. Elective and emergency embolotherapy in children and adolescents. *Radiology* 1990;30:331−336.

56 Lois JF, Hartzman S, McGlade CT *et al.* Budd−Chiari syndrome: Treatment with percutaneous trans-hepatic recanalisation and dilatation. *Radiology* 1989;170:791−793.

57 Hurnitz RA, Franken EA, Girod DA, Smith DA, Smith WL. Angiographic determination of arterial patency after percutaneous catheterisation in infants and small children. *Circulation* 1977;56:102−105.

58 Burrows PE, Benson LN, Williams WG, *et al.* Ileofemoral arterial complications of balloon angioplasty for systemic obstructions in infants and children. *Circulation* 1990;82:1697−1704.

59 Lois JF, Gomes AS, Smith DC, Laks H. Systemic to pulmonary collateral vessels and shunts: treatment with embolisation. *Radiology* 1988;169:671−676.

60 Dubois JM, Sebag GH, De Prost Y, Teillac D, Chretien B, Brunelle FO. Soft-tissue venous malformations in children: percutaneous sclerotherapy with Ethibloc. *Radiology* 1991;180:195−198.

61 Yakes WF, Luethke JM, Parker SH. *et al.* Ethanol embolization of vascular malformations. *Radiographics* 1990;10:787−796.

62 Apfelberg DB, Lane B, Marx MP. Combined (team) approach to haemangioma management: arteriography with superselective embolization plus YAG laser/sapphire-tip resection. *Plastic Reconstr Surg* 1991;8:71−82.

63 Sigmund G, Bahren W, Gall H, Lenz M, Thon W. Idiopathic varicocoeles: feasibility of percutaneous sclerotherapy. *Radiology* 1987;164:161−168.

64 Edmonds CJ, Tellez M. Treatment of thyroid cysts by aspiration and injection of a sclerosant. *Br Med J* 1987;275:529.

65 Reiner I, Donnell S, Carty HML, Rickwood AMK. Percutaneous sclerotherapy for simple renal cysts in children. *Br J Radiol* 1992;65:281−282.

Part 5
Risk Identification
and Management

Malpractice, risk management, and quality improvement in radiology

James B. Spies

Few subjects have caused more concern among physicians, patients, regulatory and payer groups than the related subjects of medical malpractice and the quality of health care. From the first malpractice "crisis" of the mid-1970s, there has been growing demand for quality care; demand fueled by highly publicized individual examples of flagrant malpractice or Medicare fraud. These isolated incidents have received such publicity that they have helped to undermine the public's confidence in the medical treatment they receive. The public has become concerned that physicians care more about money than about their patient's well-being.

At the same time, researchers and academic medical centers have promoted new research findings and new services to the lay media. The public has been barraged with news of "new breakthroughs" and "dramatic advances" in health care, and this has led to the mistaken belief that current medical practice is near perfect. Coincidently, because of its increasing complexity, medical practice has become more specialized. Patients may see two or three physicians before they are diagnosed or treated. This shuffling between specialists has frustrated patients, who seek simple answers to complex complaints. They look for a single doctor who they can trust to solve their problems. By allowing increasingly fragmented care, physicians have allowed their relationships with patients to suffer. There are fewer stable physician–patient relationships than in the past and, therefore, a diminution in the trust patients place in the physicians that they see.

All these factors have resulted in more technically advanced but less personal medical care. Patients have less trust in physicians and may question their motivations. With high expectations but little trust, patients may readily believe that a poor outcome or a complication represents malpractice rather than the uncertainty inherent in medicine. With no personal relationship to fall back on, patients often simply do not believe the explanations that their doctors give them.

It is in this uneasy atmosphere that we address the related problems of medical malpractice, risk management, and quality improvement in health care. In the first portion of this chapter, the current state of malpractice is reviewed, including the underlying causes of claims, the incidence of negligence in medicine, and the range of claims in diagnostic radiology. In the second section, the principles of risk management are discussed, with emphasis on the areas of specific concern to radiologists. In the final section, the broader issues of how health care quality may be improved will be discussed and the current mandated quality improvement programs will be reviewed. We will conclude with a discussion of more recent initiatives in continuing quality improvement, practice parameters, and malpractice reform.

Medical malpractice

Physicians are being accused of substandard or negligent care with growing frequency, and claims are becoming more detailed, more sophisticated, and more frustrating. From the perspective of the physician, the most terrifying, depressing, and outraging experience in medicine is the receipt of an attorney's letter notifying them of a claim against them. Usually, there is no warning and the patient and the event may not be recalled. Most commonly, there has been no malpractice [1]. But, the feelings of uncertainty, fear, guilt (for acts unknown), and hurt are very real. Medical malpractice litigation may be considered an honorable pursuit for attorneys, a just redress for grievances or injuries by patients, an expense to be managed by health administrators and insurance carriers, but for physicians it is a terrible blow to self-esteem, professional standing, and confidence. Despite the fact that the majority of claims do not result in settlement or adverse jury verdict [2], when a malpractice claim appears, agonizing uncertainty is the immediate reaction; a reaction that lasts for weeks or months until the allegations and substance of the claim are known. Then follows the slow, costly, and time-consuming process of discovery, depositions, and eventual trial. While the majority of claims do not reach trial, every claim has that potential, and also the potential for the damaging of reputation, self-confidence, and relationships with patients. For most physicians, the costs of malpractice insurance and claims are not the primary motivation for avoiding suits. It is the pain and uncertainty of the legal process.

The current status of malpractice claims

According to the American Medical Association (AMA), in 1990 the average annual rate for malpractice claims for all physicians was 7.7 claims per 100 physicians, essentially unchanged from the previous year [3]. This has decreased since 1985, when there were 8.9 claims per 100 physicians. However, the premiums for malpractice insurance have continued to climb at an average annual rate of 12.1% since 1982, reflecting the increasing size of awards and the cost of the litigation process. The average liability premium for all physicians in 1990 was $14 500. Approximately 39% of all physicians have had at least one malpractice claim against them during their careers, with the career experience of certain specialties somewhat higher (obstetrician–gynecologists 57%, surgeons 52%).

There are other costs of the current malpractice system. In a study using data from 1984, the direct and indirect costs of professional liability and defensive medicine were estimated. Using two different methods of calculation, it was determined that 15% of physician's services could be attributed to professional liability [4]. More significantly, 60% of the increase in cost of physician services each year were due to professional liability. In addition, this study does not calculate the cost of hospitalization, diagnostic testing, and other nonphysician services that are ordered for defensive medicine reasons. The direct costs of malpractice in the USA are $7 billion/year, with the bulk of this amount spent on administrative costs, not on compensating patients [5]. The cost of defensive medicine is at least another $15 billion/year: not only is this system of compensation expensive, but it is also slow. From the time of the alleged negligence to compensation is an average of 6 years.

Negligence in medical practice

Until recently, there was very little data on the incidence of adverse events in medical practice and the portion of those events that were due to negligence care. The Harvard Medical Practice Study was undertaken, in cooperation with the state of New York, to provide current and reliable estimates of the incidence of adverse events and negligence in practice in a large sampling of hospitalizations [1]. The project included the review of 30 121 randomly selected records from 51 acute care hospitals. Adverse events, defined as injuries caused by medical management, were detected in 3.7% of hospitalizations. Of these, 27.6% were judged to be due to negligence. Of all the adverse events, 2.6% resulted in permanently disabling injuries and 13.6% led to death. The incidence of adverse events was higher in older patients. There was variation in the number of adverse events among different specialties, with surgery being the highest. However, the percentage of events caused by negligence was not significantly different between the specialties. This reflects the higher risk of complications associated with procedure-oriented specialties, most of which are *not* due to negligence. The single most common adverse event was a drug complication (19%), followed by wound infections and technical complications [6]. The most common site of occurrence for an adverse event was the operating room, but these were less likely due to negligence than those associated with non-surgical events (17% versus 37%). The most common site for *negligent* events was the emergency room. The proportion of adverse events due to negligence was highest for errors in diagnosis (diagnostic mishaps) at 75%, errors of omission (noninvasive therapeutic mishaps) at 77%, and events occurring in the emergency room at 70%. In this sample, severe adverse events were more likely to be due to negligence. In discussing the results, the authors noted that although standards of practice may not be clearly defined, perfection can never be the standard. Many adverse events are unavoidable and there must always be acceptance of some error.

Using the same database, Localio *et al.* [7] studied the actual incidence of malpractice in the same population. Among the 31 675 charts reviewed, 1133 adverse events were identified, with 280 of these judged to be due to negligence. The authors then used malpractice claims data to determine the number of malpractice claims among the same group of 31 675 hospitalizations. There had been 51 claims filed. Of the negligent events, only eight had malpractice claims filed. It was estimated that the statewide ratio of adverse events to malpractice claims was 7.6:1, indicating that the great majority of negligent acts do not result in suits. Conversely, 43 of the malpractice claims were in cases in which negligence was *not* identified, indicating that in only 15% of malpractice claims was negligence identified. The authors conclude that malpractice infrequently compensates patients injured by negligence and rarely identifies or holds responsible providers of substandard care, i.e., only in a small minority of malpractice claims has negligence actually occurred.

Legal definition of malpractice

Medical malpractice cases are generally tried under the law of negligence. There are four elements that must be proven under the tort of negligence.

1 A duty to the patient must be established. This is met when a physician agrees to render services to a patient. In the case of a radiologist, this occurs when he or she agrees to provide radiologic services to the patient.

2 A breach of the standard of care must occur.

3 There must be significant injury to the patient.

4 The breach of care must be the proximate cause of the injury [8].

In the past, the standard of care was defined as the local standard, i.e., the care that a physician or reasonable skill would provide under similar circumstances in the same locality. This was defined by the testimony of local expert witnesses. The local standard arose when there were significant differences in the availability of medical technology and opportunities for continuing education in various regions. More recently, as more uniform care and educational opportunities have become available, the courts have moved toward using a national standard of care [9]. Defining the standard of care still requires the use of expert witnesses, but now allows the use of experts from other regions. Unfortunately, this has led to the development of a cottage industry of "expert" witnesses, often individuals with inferior ability. According to Gagliardi [9], a pool of physicians who allow themselves to be manipulated, have made themselves available to plaintiff's attorneys. A particularly ominous development has been the role of the academic expert witness, who bears the imprimatur of a university medical center and whose testimony, as a result, carries considerable weight with juries. There has been a recent call for the development of guidelines by academic chairmen to govern the actions of faculty, in order to reduce abuses [9]. This sentiment has been echoed by Berlin in reporting the circumstances of a radiologic "miss" [10]. In depositions, two of the plaintiff's expert witnesses made remarks that clearly were inflammatory and exaggerated the nature of the error ("an orthopedic student could have seen the abnormality," "I saw the lesion cold, immediately, and without a history"). These types of remarks are unnecessary and fail to take account of the ease of diagnosis in retrospect as compared to the difficulty prospectively. It would seem that the facts could speak for themselves without gratuitous embellishment.

While the four elements of negligence appear to demand substantive grounds for bringing a claim, the reality is different. As noted, the large majority of malpractice claims are for events where there is no negligence [7]. Furthermore, claims are often made when there is no injury or minimal injury. Thus, defense in malpractice often becomes a pragmatic decision of cost of complete and active defense versus cost of settlement. Given the inevitability of claims, attention to risk management becomes the primary means of both avoiding claims and of successfully defending them once they occur.

Malpractice in radiology

The first suit for damages in diagnostic radiology most likely occurred in 1896, within a year of the time that Conrad Roentgen discovered X-rays. A patient sued two physicians for burns that occurred during an exposure for a diagnostic roentgenogram of his ankle. The exposure caused erythema, ulceration, and pain of such severity that amputation was eventually required [11]. Most claims for damages in the early years of diagnostic radiology were for burns that resulted from diagnostic studies. The early problems with excessive radiation exposure claims have been solved in the modern era [12].

In 1990, the annual professional liability claims rate in radiology was 8.7 claims per 100 physicians, having declined from 12.8 in 1985 [3]. The career claims rate is 39.4% of radiologists. Berlin [13] reviewed the radiology related claims from 1980 to 1986 in Cook County, Illinois. They accounted for 12% of all medical malpractice suits. In decreasing order, the most common claims were for missed radiologic diagnosis, complications from procedures, failure to order diagnostic tests (mostly nonradiologists), and miscellaneous injuries (slip and fall) in radiology departments. In this group of claims, the most common missed diagnosis was fracture, but missed malignancy was the next most common and appeared to be increasing. The author noted the difficulty in reducing missed diagnoses, as many studies had shown miss rates in approximately 30% of abnormal radiographs. The most common complications occurred in angiographic procedures, followed by myelograms. Failure properly to communicate radiographic reports was also noted in 10 cases.

Spring and Tennenhouse [14] reviewed lawsuits in California, using data from lawsuit verdicts between 1971 and 1985. The authors estimated that one in every 50 000 examinations resulted in a lawsuit. Of the 144 cases reviewed, 66 were for failure to diagnose, most commonly missed fractures and neoplasms of the chest. There were also six cases of missed or incorrectly identified surgical sponges, which resulted in settlements or verdicts for the plaintiff in five. Forty-five suits were for complications with 22 angiography cases and 11 for myelography. Most of the procedure-related suits included allegations of lack of informed consent. The average award in those verdicts against radiologists was $125 000, but approximately three-quarters of the verdicts favored the radiologist.

A review of settled claims in the military medical system had similar findings to those above [15]. Missed diagnoses were again the most common cause, although malignancy was the most frequently missed abnormality. This result may be skewed because this data was from the military medical system. Active duty military members are not allowed to sue the government, and therefore the majority of the suits are filed by military retirees who are older. Complications were the second most common cause for claim with 14% of cases, the majority due to angiographic procedures. In the miscellaneous category, failure to inform a referring physician in a timely manner was the cause of action in 9% of cases. Sixty-three per cent of claims resulted in compensation, with the median payment $57 000. In a follow-up report on the same patient population, missed malignancies of the lung and colon were again the most frequent causes for malpractice claim [16]. It was noted that there had been an increase in the rate of claims and an increase in the percentage of cases in which radiologists were named.

A review of the database of the Physician's Insurance Association of America (PIAA) reveals that, with few exceptions, the overall pattern of claims had not changed in 1992 [17]. These again showed that missed diagnosis on plain radiographs was the most common source for alleged error leading to suit. The major recent change has been the growth of suits involving mammography, which has become the second most common source for litigation and the most costly in terms of awards.

In reviewing any set of data on claims, it should be remembered that fewer than 1% of allegations reach trial and that radiologists win eight out of 10 court cases [2]. However, it seems likely that when obvious negligence has occurred a settlement will be reached prior to trial. Thus, the percentage of claims that result in no payment to plaintiffs is likely to be lower.

Lest we think that only radiologists in the USA face the risk of litigation, medical malpractice is an issue in other countries, including those with nationalized health systems. The causes for claims are similar to those experienced in the USA [18,19] (see Chapter 40).

Risk management

There has been a tremendous effort made in the last 15 years to understand the causes for medical malpractice claims. The field of medical risk management has developed as a response to the cost of malpractice claims, and may be defined as the process of developing systems, procedures, and practice patterns that minimize the risks of errors that commonly form the basis of suits. As has been outlined in the sections above, the types of claims that occur in radiology relate primarily to errors in diagnosis, procedural complications, faulty communications, and poor documentation. In this section, the primary strategies for avoiding malpractice claims in radiology will be reviewed.

The AMA has developed materials to assist physicians in improving patient relations, practice management, communication, and documentation of patient care [20]. Many of these lessons apply to radiologic practice. It is important to be courteous in patient contacts, and listen to the patient's concerns and questions. A few minutes of conversation can put the patient at ease and may be the source of valuable history that may help in interpreting the radiologic study. For the physician, it is an opportunity to show the patient the care and interest that is taken in their diagnosis. There are few opportunities to meet with patients in general diagnostic radiologic practice and those contacts that do occur should be positive. It is also important that technologists and other ancillary personnel are encouraged to be friendly, polite, and helpful to patients. They should assist those that need assistance to and from dressing areas. They should be alert for hazards that might result in patient injury. The members of the radiology department should work together to provide an efficient, pleasant, and safe environment for patients to visit.

There are general rules that should be applied each time a radiographic study is performed and interpreted [2,13]. First, do not attempt to perform or interpret studies without adequate knowledge or training. Seek the assistance of other radiologists in areas of uncertainty, and have a sufficient number of references available to allow consultation in difficult or unfamiliar studies. Spend enough time with each study to be sure that a careful interpretation is possible. Do not try to interpret any study, no matter how simple, without careful review. Use hot lights and other aids liberally. Try to maintain a quiet comfortable reading area that will minimize distractions. Use old films and reports as tools to improve the accuracy of your reading. Old reports are very helpful in trying to address questions raised in earlier interpretations and to assist you in avoiding interpretative errors. Obviously, prior films are essential in evaluating most radiologic studies and failure to use comparisons is a primary cause of both undercalling and overcalling abnormalities. Review other types of radiologic examinations that have been performed to "put it all together" for a final diagnosis. The differential diagnosis for most findings can be limited to just a few possibilities when an examination is correlated with previous studies. Be sure to have quality films; if a study is of poor quality, find out why and decide whether a repeat will result in improved diagnostic efficacy. If a study is of limited quality because of factors beyond your control, such as patient size or inability to cooperate sufficiently, state the limitations in the report and what possible errors could occur as a result of the limitations. Most of these recommendations seem self-evident and universally practiced. It is surprising how frequently these suggestions are not followed, however and how often this results in diagnostic errors [21].

By using common sense and following the above rules, the number of suits you are subjected to will be reduced and those that do occur will be in the best position to be defended. In the following sections, specific areas of concern in radiology will be reviewed in detail. They should be viewed within the framework of these rules, which should be the basis of all risk management programs.

Communication in radiology

Communication is fundamental to everything that a radiologist does. Our utility to physicians and to patients is predicated on our ability accurately to communicate the findings of our studies in a timely manner. As mentioned previously, a significant number of malpractice claims allege a failure of communication [15]. The American College of Radiology (ACR) has sought to address this problem with a standard for communication [22]. Kline and Kline [23] have reviewed this standard and the legal implications of failure to communicate. The ACR standard is becoming recognized as the national standard. Case law has held that written communication alone is not adequate in certain circumstances. The degree of urgency of the finding and its seriousness should dictate the level of communication that is undertaken. The ACR has stated four principles of direct communication (verbal communication) of radiologic findings.

1 The radiologist should coordinate his or her efforts with referring physicians in order best to serve the patient's well-being. That may require direct communication of unusual, unexpected, or urgent findings to the referring physician in advance of the formal written report.

2 In these circumstances, the radiologist or his or her representative should attempt to communicate directly with the referring physician, or his or her representative; the timeliness of direct communication should be based upon the immediacy of the situation.

3 Documentation of actual or attempted direct communication is appropriate.

4 Any discrepancy between an emergency or preliminary report and the final written report should be promptly reconciled by direct communication. The direct communication should be documented in the written report.

The radiologist has a duty to communicate to the referring physician, but not to the patient. However, in an emergency and when the physician cannot be contacted, the radiologist may inform the patient. The ACR standard appears to answer most of the questions raised in case law. There have been exceptions: in one case, a radiologist called the emergency room and gave a verbal report to a nurse and not to the physician himself. In a suit related to the case, this level of communication was considered insufficient. However, this type of exception is unusual and by using the ACR communication standard, which is clear, simple, and attainable, radiologists can both ensure adequate communication and avoid the large majority of litigation related to inadequate communication.

In a related issue, the lack of adequate history is a common source of misinterpretation of radiologic studies [21]. Hall [24] has advocated documentation of this fact with the inclusion of a statement that no clinical history was given. While this is likely to be perceived as a confrontation with referring physicians, it should also prompt better compliance and it provides a defensive medicolegal posture. Another means of improving compliance for clinical history would be a monitoring program with reporting of the results to referring physicians and hospital staff. This type of monitoring program will be discussed in greater depth in the section on quality improvement (p. 641).

Finally, it is important to review the essentials of the radiographic report itself. Again, the ACR standard provides a useful guide [22]. The report should include the patient's name and another identifier, the name of the referring physician, the name of the examination, and the dates of the examination and transcription, and the time of the examination for intensive care unit — coronary care unit (ICU — CCU) patients. The body of the report should include a description of the procedures performed and any contrast media, drugs, catheters, and devices. The body should include a concise description of the findings, and any limitations of the examination. The body of the report should also answer any specific clinical questions that are raised in the history. Comparison studies should be noted and the conclusions based on the comparison should be included. Each report should have a conclusion or impression, unless the body of the report is brief and no changes have occurred. A precise diagnosis should be given when possible and a differential diagnosis should be included, when appropriate. The report should also recommend follow-up and additional radiologic studies, when appropriate. The written report remains the primary medical record that will be used in the management of the patient's care and also will be the center of any litigation that is brought against you for failure to diagnose or failure to communicate. Given its importance in patient care and in risk management, great care should be exercised in ensuring that it reflects your opinion and your recommendations accurately.

Informed consent

Proper informed consent is essential to risk management efforts in procedural specialties. Most malpractice claims related to procedural complications also include allegations of lack of informed consent. Since complications will always be a possible outcome from medical procedures, one of the primary means to avoid losing verdicts in malpractice is adequate informed consent. The other means of reducing malpractice claims, by reducing the incidence of complications, represents a goal of quality improvement programs which will be discussed later in this chapter.

Detailed reviews of the legal principles of informed consent have been published [25,26]. Reuter [26] provides a particularly comprehensive overview for radiologists. The following represents a summary of informed consent based primarily on Reuter's work and the original article is recommended for those interested in further detail.

Modern informed consent rests on legal principles first set out by Judge Cardozo when he wrote that: "every human being of adult years and sound mind has a right to determine what shall be done with his own body" [25]. Until the 1950s, lack of consent was tried under a claim of *battery*, or unwanted touching. Beginning in the 1950s, states began to consider these claims, negligence regarding *disclosure* and battery is generally not used in these circumstances any longer. Originally, the standard used to judge the adequacy of the informed consent was the "community of physician peers" or the "reasonable physician" standard. This was defined as the information a reasonable physician would give a patient in similar circumstances. This standard requires expert witnesses to establish the standard for any particular case. Because of this requirement, beginning in the 1970s, some states began to adopt the "reasonable man" standard, i.e., what a reasonable person would want to know prior to consenting to a procedure. This standard has the practical effect of eliminating the need for expert testimony to determine the adequacy of consent. The other effect of the "reasonable man" standard is that the range of information given to the patient is probably greater than required by the "reasonable physician" standard. The required elements of informed consent discussed below assume the "reasonable man" standard. The majority of states adhere to either the "reasonable physician" or the "reasonable man" standards. There are states that use other standards or where the standards are unclear, and the reader should discuss local requirements with hospital attorneys or malpractice carrier risk managers.

Informed consent using the "reasonable man" standard, represents a process rather than a signature on a form or a patient agreeing to a procedure. It includes a discussion in which the procedure is explained, including its purpose, risks, and complications. It should also include a discussion of the alternate procedures, their risks, and the risk of doing nothing at all. The patient's questions should be answered. All this information allows the patient to decide whether to undergo the procedure, i.e., to give informed consent. In addition to a signature on a consent form, the consent should be documented with a note in the medical record that details the elements of the discussion with the patient (and his or her family, if present), and should include the specific complications that were mentioned.

A negligence suit claiming lack of informed consent must have the following four elements.

1 The physician must have a duty to the patient to obtain informed consent, which is the case when he or she is performing a procedure that has significant risks.

2 There needs to be a breach of that duty; having provided inadequate information for the patient to make an informed decision.

3 An injury is required, which can range from pain to severe injury to death.

4 There must be a causal relationship between the breach of duty and the injury, meaning that if the patient had known of the potential risks they would not have consented to the procedure.

To summarize, the plaintiff must be injured in a procedure, must show that the information they were given was inadequate, and that if they had known the risks they would have rejected the procedure and therefore would not have sustained the injury. It has been suggested that each consent should include mention of the possibility of death, paralysis, or organ damage [2]. This is viewed as an ironclad consent, because consent for the procedure with these potential risks precludes any claim of inadequate information. The assumption is that any patient who agrees to a procedure with these severe risks cannot make a claim that they would have refused it when a less severe complication occurs. This approach seems an extreme length to go to, particularly when one thinks of mentioning these terrible outcomes when obtaining consent in all radiologic procedures. When trying to decide which potential complications should be mentioned, a rule of thumb is to mention the potential severe complications and the common complications. This follows the legal concept of informing the patient of the material risks. The formula for material risks might be stated as the product of serious risks and their incidence, with the emphasis on serious. If death or paralysis are unusual but potential risks they should be mentioned. However, only common minor complications need be discussed and those that are rare need not necessarily be mentioned. To provide informed consent, the patient should understand the *range* of potential complications that might occur.

There are several basic concepts that relate to consent. We have already discussed informed consent. Another is simple consent, which is when a patient simply agrees to a procedure. This type of consent may be expressed or implied. Most of diagnostic radiology uses implied consent; the patient's agreement is implied by the fact that he or she climbs on the table and allows the radiograph to be done. Implied consent is also used when an emergency occurs and the patient is not able to give consent. In this circumstance, if a reasonable person in similar circumstances would have given consent, consent is implied.

There are potential problems associated with consents. The first is when there is withdrawn consent. This is when a patient asks for the procedure to stop after initially giving consent. The physician should stop and discuss it with the patient. If the patient cannot be convinced to reconsent, the procedure should be stopped. Failure to do so can result in a claim of civil battery. The second is exceeded consent, when more is done than the patient consents for. A common setting is when only an angiogram is consented to and a lesion is found that can be treated with angioplasty. The consent would be exceeded if the procedure is done. If the patient is not heavily sedated and is alert enough, the appropriate consent can be obtained with the patient on the table. This should be appropriately documented and witnessed. Otherwise, the procedure should be delayed until another day. A third potential problem is the curbstone consult. If the operating physician calls in an associate to assist during a procedure, the patient must give consent for the second physician's participation. This can be handled in one of two ways. The initial consent can include the operating physician's associates which would satisfy the doctrine of consent. The other way is for the second physician to introduce him- or herself to the patient and ask permission to participate in the procedure, and to document the patient's assent in the chart. Without consent obtained by one of these two means, the second physician may be subject to a claim of civil battery.

There are circumstances when informed consent is not necessary. If a patient states that they do not want to know the risks of the procedure, they do have to be informed. However, this should be documented in the medical record. Another exception to the need for informed consent is therapeutic privilege, which is when the physician believes that information regarding the risks of the procedure would harm the patient, and therefore is withheld. It should be obvious that this is a rare occurrence and could be difficult to defend in court.

The operating physician or their designate should obtain consent. The referring physician should not. The operating physician is in the best position to discuss all the potential problems associated with the procedure. For radiologists, this may be the only time to establish rapport with the patient, which allows the basis for forming a patient–physician relationship. With the exception of consent for intravenous contrast injections which will be discussed in the next section, the radiologist should obtain consent from the patient. The radiologist will be held responsible for the adequacy of the information that is given by his or her designate, and therefore can best guarantee the result by doing it themselves.

When the patient is not competent to give consent for elective procedures, consent should be obtained as follows: if the patient has a court-appointed guardian or conservator, consent may be obtained from that individual. If there is no legal representative, most states recognize the use of substituted consent by the spouse or nearest relative. If there are no relatives, the local court may be petitioned. This may be done with the assistance of the hospital attorney. These rules only apply in elective procedures; emergencies do not require this process to be followed, although discussion with the family or spouse is still advised, if possible. For children, the parents may give consent. In the absence of parents, adult siblings or relatives may give consent. If the minor is emancipated, they may give consent for themselves.

The requirements for the consent form itself will vary, depending on the jurisdiction. The local requirements should be reviewed with the hospital or malpractice carrier risk managers. In general, blanket consent forms agreeing to all procedures are poor protection, and should be avoided. If using a detailed form, there should be inclusion of some key points:

1 that the patient has read and understands the information provided;
2 that the patient has had the opportunity to ask any questions of the physician about information that is not understood;
3 it should state that the patient gives consent to the operating physician's associates to participate in the procedure.

Contrast material

Bettman *et al.* [27] reviewed all malpractice claims for an 11-year period at the Harvard Medical Group. There were 100 radiology claims, only 10 of which were related to radiographic contrast material. Only four resulted in financial settlement. Anaphylaxis was not a cause of any claim; rather local infiltration and nonfatal injuries were the issues. All these claims were for the period before the availability of low-osmolality agents. Key factors in the successful defense of these cases included adequate informed consent, adequate screening of patients for prior reactions, treatment efforts performed, documentation, communication with the patient, and adequate follow-up. The authors concluded that suits involving contrast material that lead to settlement or trial are rare.

Despite the rarity of claims related to contrast material, one of the central debates in radiology policy in recent years has been the appropriate use of the new low-osmolality contrast agents [28]. It is generally agreed that the use of these agents results in fewer minor reactions than more traditional high-osmolality agents, but there is controversy regarding more serious reactions. While it appears that there are fewer serious reactions with the new agents, these reactions are also very rare for high-osmolality agents [29]. The difficulty in the development of policy using these agents has been the cost of the newer agents, which ranges from 10 to 20 times as much as high-osmolality agents [30]. The ACR has issued guidelines on the use of these agents, suggesting their use in high-risk patients only [31]. This provides a framework for the decisions required in daily practice.

The legal implications of decisions in the use of the contrast agents remain unresolved [28]. There has been concern in the radiology community that any reaction that may occur when using high-osmolality agents may become the basis for malpractice claims. While there are not yet any precedents for this concern, this fear has been fostered by the marketing campaigns by some of the suppliers of the low-osmolality agents. The primary defense against suits in the use of contrast agents is the use of informed consent. The legal basis of informed consent is detailed in the previous section. With regard to informed consent in the use of contrast agents, a suggested form has been published, and the means of using it in a busy practice have been detailed [32]. Because of the large number of patients that will receive intravenous contrast each day in a radiology department, this is one circumstance where consent may be obtained by the technologist. The consent form should include a discussion of the risks of intravenous contrast, those patients who might be at high risk for reactions, and the alternate use of more expensive, low-osmolality agents in these cases. The radiologist should be available to answer any questions the patient may have. Reuter [26] recommends inclusion of a statement that the patient has read and understood the information that has been presented and that they have had the opportunity to have their questions answered.

The use of consent forms for contrast has been growing in practice in the USA in the past 12 years, from 34% in 1984 to approximately 70% today [33,34]. This trend appears to be in response to the current controversy concerning the different classes of contrast agents, as well as a part of general risk management efforts.

The other major emphasis in reducing risks in the use of contrast is ensuring that the contrast reactions that do occur are appropriately treated. This includes the regular review of proper treatment of reactions with physicians and technologists. Maintenance of certification in basic life support for personnel in this area is very helpful. Physicians who regularly administer intravenous contrast or who perform invasive procedures should strongly consider being trained and certified in advanced cardiac life support. Drugs and equipment needed for resuscitation should be regularly checked and replaced or repaired as required. Personnel should be trained to operate the emergency equipment, including defibrillators, cardiac monitors, oxygen equipment, and intravenous supplies. These efforts are essential to quality patient care and also are fundamental for risk management efforts.

Mammography

The detection and treatment of breast cancer is becoming a leading cause of malpractice claims [35]. Certainly for radiologists, mammography has recently emerged as a common and costly source of malpractice settlements and verdicts [17]. Radiologists were named in 40 of 273 cases reported by the PIAA [35]. Thirty-five per cent of claimants had a negative mammogram report, and this was the second most common cause for delay in diagnosis. Physician to physician communication was also a contributing cause for delay in diagnosis. The mammogram was misread in only 8.9% of cases. Other less common issues included poor-quality mammograms and failure to react to a mammogram reading. In this study, the claims against radiologists resulted in settlements or awards totaling $8.1 million. The average patient age of plaintiffs was 44 years, with 69% of claims below the age of 50 years. This study points out the difficulties in diagnosing breast cancer in younger patients. Certainly, this study also highlights the misunderstanding of many referring physicians regarding a negative mammogram report.

In reviewing the medicolegal aspects of screening mammography, the extent of the radiologist's duty is clear [36]. The radiologist has a duty to perform a proper mammogram and to provide a reasonable interpretation. Inadequate mammograms will subject a radiologist to liability, and the mammographic films will be accepted as evidence. In addition, the radiologist must apply diligent and reasonable standards in the evaluation of a mammographic lesion. The report should reflect the abnormalities discovered and the appropriate additional studies required. A diagnosis is not required for an indeterminant lesion detected on a screening study. However, the need for follow-up views must be communicated to the referring physician. Theoretically, only a reasonable evaluation of any abnormality is required by law. Unfortunately, when a screening process is done annually and the screening eventually detects a cancer, immediate attention is directed to the preceding studies. Expert witnesses for plaintiffs have the benefit of retrospective evaluation not available to the radiologist at the time of the original examination.

The duty of the radiologist is different for screening and diagnostic studies, and for self-referred patients [37]. Screening mammography is designed to identify the small segment of patients with mammographic abnormalities from those with normal studies. The duty then is appropriately to inform the referring physician of the results of the study, including the need for further views. Diagnostic mammograms, i.e., those obtained to evaluate a clinically palpable lesion or an abnormality previously seen on a screening study, require a reasonable effort using appropriate views, technology, and interpretation to evaluate the abnormality. The report should be more definitive and come to conclusion about the mammographic characteristics of the abnormality. Self-referred patients present another level of duty. In addition to informing the patient of the results of the study, the radiologist probably has a duty to perform a breast examination or to ensure that one is performed. In addition, the radiologist must refer the patient to a surgeon when the evaluation concludes that surgical consultation is needed. Documentation and record-keeping in this circumstance is essential.

There are other problems with communication that can arise. Robertson and Kopans [38] reviewed the responses to mammographic reports that included recommendations for further views or biopsy made to referring physicians. They found that no action had been taken within 2.5 months by 63% of patients, which had been reduced to 6% by 4.5 months. However, the compliance level achieved required a concerted effort at recalling referring physicians during that period. Failure to receive the report or the report sent to the wrong address were significant reasons for the delays.

Brenner [37] notes one further potential problem in mammography, that of informal consultations on films obtained at another facility. These informal consultations open the radiologist to liability from that interpretation. Verbal communication can be misinterpreted, misrecorded in the medical record, or misrepresented to the patient. The only potential for defense in this circumstance is to record the consultation either formally with a radiographic report or informally in a log.

Potchen *et al.* [8] recommend several concrete steps that can be taken. The mammography department should obtain certification by the ACR. This certification, or its equivalent, is clearly becoming the national standard and has been included in legislation regarding reimbursement at both the federal and state level. While it has yet to occur, it may be that lack of certification will be represented as a breech of the standard of care. Certainly, certification can be a positive defense of film quality. The department should also develop practices that ensure the proper performance of the equipment and the technologists, and a standard set of recommendations to be used in the conclusion of the reports. These may be based on the standard reporting language that is being developed by the ACR. This helps to reduce ambiguity and misunderstanding of the report and the recommendations. It is also suggested that surgical consultation, rather than biopsy, be the recommendation when biopsy may be required. This allows the surgeon latitude for decisions other than biopsy, due to unusual clinical circumstances not known to the radiologist. Any recommendation for surgical consultation should be made both verbally and in writing. The verbal communication should be documented in the written report. It is important to develop a reliable means for communicating reports to physicians, including requests for further views, etc. Potchen *et al.* [8] also advise the addition of a standard disclaimer in each report. This should include that a normal mammogram does not exclude cancer in the presence of a palpable mass. Also, it can be added that the sensitivity of mammography is reduced in the presence of dense breasts.

Routine use of practice audits are recommended to determine the relative sensitivity and specificity of the program, and methods to perform such an audit have been published [8,39−42]. Potchen *et al.* [8] give guidelines of the results for such audits. They suggest one in every six to eight biopsies should be positive for malignancy, i.e., 13−17 cancers per 100 recommended biopsies. The number of negative biopsies continues to be controversial. A report of a large series of biopsies revealed a subset of lesions that are almost certainly benign. The authors indicate that obtaining a second opinion to screen out these lesions would reduce the number of unnecessary biopsies and suggest that they may be followed at 6-month intervals with only a 1% chance of malignancy

[43]. In response, Darios [44] states the worry of many radiologists: in a year where 100 second opinions are given, one cancer will be missed and may represent the basis of a suit. Unfortunately, many patients are not comfortable waiting with a 1% chance of malignancy and often want a biopsy regardless of what the overall health policy implications are.

Practice audits may represent a primary defense in the event of litigation [36]. As any case could result in a suit, particularly when repetitive screening studies are obtained over time, having data to support the quality of the program overall may be the only means of convincing the jury that negligence has not occurred.

Finally, there is evidence that continuing medical education has a positive impact on the results of screening mammography [45]. Even the most experienced mammographers can benefit from regular refresher courses.

Ultrasound

The greatest potential for litigation in ultrasound is in obstetric and gynecologic studies. While all ultrasound examinations are subject to the potential of missed diagnosis, the failure to diagnose ectopic pregnancy and fetal abnormalities can result in devastating injuries and, as a result, large malpractice awards.

Ectopic pregnancies do result in claims, although more commonly against nonradiologists. The radiologist can help improve the care of patients with this diagnosis by including a statement that ectopic pregnancies are often not visualized, and that the primary goal of ultrasound is to exclude an intrauterine pregnancy [46]. A woman of the appropriate menstrual age with a positive pregnancy test with no intrauterine pregnancy by ultrasound must be considered as having an ectopic pregnancy. The early diagnosis of intrauterine pregnancy has been aided by the recent introduction of transvaginal ultrasonography.

The realm of obstetric sonography is more complicated from a medicolegal point of view [47]. Suits in obstetric ultrasound often involve one of three legal concepts, *wrongful pregnancy*, *wrongful birth*, and *wrongful life*. *Wrongful pregnancy* represents the failure to prevent a pregnancy that results in the birth of a normal child. This would be the case when there was an unsuccessful sterilization procedure or abortion. In ultrasonography, failure to diagnose a pregnancy or twin pregnancy may result in a liability claim, if the couple could prove that they would have terminated the pregnancy. In this type of case, awards are usually limited to the cost of pregnancy and childbirth costs. *Wrongful birth* represents the failure to diagnose a fetal defect and the baby is born defective. Ultrasonographers are vulnerable to these types of claims when performing fetal surveys. These can be costly settlements, including pregnancy costs, extraordinary medical expenses, and occasionally, child rearing. *Wrongful life* is the final concept, and is similar to wrongful birth in that the child is defective. However, the suit is brought by the child. This type of suit is an ethical, legal, and moral morass. It requires the judgment of which is better; an impaired life or no life at all. Wrongful life and wrongful birth suits may be filed by the family and the child simultaneously.

Another legal principle applicable in ultrasound is that of the technologist as the agent of the radiologist. In medicine, a technologist under the supervision of a physician is considered his or her agent, and the physician may be held liable for the actions and errors made by the technologist. In ultrasound, this is particularly pertinent. Since the images obtained are very operator dependent, relying on the technologist alone for the examination, without scanning the patient themself, opens a great risk for the radiologist.

The primary risk management strategies in ultrasound are those that also lead to quality care. These are best stated in reviews by Macones *et al.* [47] and Leopold [48]. Both authors recommend the adherence to the ultrasound standards published by the ACR. These detail the elements of the fetal survey, studies of the abdomen, scrotum, female pelvis, and others.

The radiologist is responsible for the quality and thoroughness of the examination. After reviewing preliminary images obtained by the technologist, the radiologist should rescan the patient to be certain of the major findings and to be sure no significant findings have been missed. If a significant fetal abnormality is detected in an obstetric study, it may be prudent to obtain a second opinion or a repeat examination before action is undertaken based on the study [47]. Adequate images should be obtained to document any abnormalities.

Missed fractures

In many studies, missed fractures are the most common cause of claims and even in the PIAA data, missed fractures represent four of the 10 most common claims [13,14,17]. The most common fractures missed are cervical fractures, carpal navicular fractures, and hip and pelvis fractures. These diagnoses are also a problem for emergency room physicians, and missed fractures on radiographs remain a primary focus of risk management efforts in both radiology and emergency departments [49,50]. The key to reducing the risk of error in the emergency department is a positive relationship between the emergency room (ER) staff and the radiology department. Both groups have a contribution to make. The emergency physician should provide adequate clinical information, perform the initial interpretation, and when necessary ask for repeat films to ensure good quality films. Radiologists should provide timely review of emergency films, and communicate discordant interpretations directly to the ER. If the radiologist is the first physician to interpret the study, it is their responsibility directly to communicate those results that will have an immediate impact on the patient's well-being.

Missed malignancies

Along with breast malignancy, colon and lung malignancies are the most frequently missed cancers that result in litigation. The colon cancer study of 151 closed malpractice claims revealed that misinterpretation of barium enema examination was the cause of delayed diagnosis in 18% of cases [51]. Radiologists were the fourth most commonly named specialty and suffered the third highest indemnity payments. A recent PIAA study of lung cancer offered a bleaker picture, with radiologists the most commonly sued physicians in relation to lung cancer [52]. In this group of claims, prior films were suggestive of lung cancer in 70% of cases, emphasizing the need for careful review of the films in relation to old films. However, it is clear that small peripheral lung lesions are frequently missed on initial evaluation. In a screening study of high-risk patients, chest radiographs were obtained at 4-month intervals [53]. Films were interpreted by two experienced readers aware that this was a high-risk population. Even under these circumstances, 90% of small peripheral cancers that developed were missed initially and when discovered were visible on prior radiographs.

Others have commented that radiographic "misses" are common and discuss some of the factors that lead to error [13,54]. In addition to the obvious causes of poor viewing areas, noise, and distractions, a lesion must have sufficient conspicuity, or sufficient contrast related to the surrounding structures, to be detectable. Despite what logic would say, it is unclear that double reading would be effective or practical in reducing errors. Experience may also have no bearing on error rate, and the length of time spent in interpreting a radiograph may also not significantly reduce misses [13]. It appears that while vigilance should be maintained to reduce errors in interpretation, errors in diagnosis or misdiagnosis will remain a continuing problem in radiology.

Interventional radiology

Often thought of as the greatest source of radiology malpractice claims, interventional procedures constitute only a minority of suits. The relatively risky nature of these procedures would seem to leave great room for claims. It may be that the informed consent process succeeds in detailing the risks sufficiently to avert many claims. There may also be the general realization among patients and their attorneys that a complication does not usually result from negligence.

Twenty to thirty per cent of radiology claims are for procedural complications [13,14]. The majority are for angiographic complications, particularly cerebral angiograms [13,14,17]. These suits are the fourth most expensive among radiology claims. The next most common invasive procedures resulting in claims are myelography and venography. Most claims for negligence in radiologic procedures are also accompanied by claims of lack of informed consent.

Many of the best risk management strategies for interventional radiology are the same that have been recommended for all medical practitioners [20]. It is important to develop a relationship with patients, beginning with the initial history and physical examination. Patients referred to an interventional radiologist expect the same evaluation that any specialist would provide. They expect the physician to take a history of the clinical problem, to perform a problem oriented examination, and to discuss the diagnosis and recommended diagnostic or therapeutic procedures. The patient has this expectation, whether the radiologist realizes it or not. Therefore, the traditional radiologist's role as a consultant to physicians with minimal patient contact must be changed to meet the patient's expectations. The interventional radiologist is becoming a clinical subspecialist, not an expert in handling all the medical problems of their patients, but willing to assume responsibility in certain aspects of patient care [55]. The interventional specialist should be an activist in evaluating patients, rather than a passive recipient of requests for radiologic studies. The radiologist will be held accountable for the procedures performed, and the decision to perform a study should be based on his or her evaluation of the patient. This evaluation will confirm or refute the basis of the request and is a key step in assuring the patient of the active interest the radiologist has in their well-being. For example, requests are regularly received for peripheral arteriography to evaluate leg pain unrelated to vascular disease. It is the radiologist's responsibility to ensure that there is adequate documentation of the indications prior to proceeding.

From the discussion on informed consent that preceded this section, it is clear that this represents a primary risk management focus. Procedures in medicine will always be associated with complications: it is therefore important that patients have a complete understanding of the risks, potential benefits, and alternates. Very few patients refuse procedures after informed consent, and in the event of a complication it may be the only defense that is available. It is particularly important that the informed consent be adequately documented in the medical record, with a written note detailing the essentials of the discussion, including the specific risks mentioned.

There are other areas in clinical care that are important in interventional radiology. Regularly "rounding" on hospitalized patients that have had interventional procedures can significantly reduce the number of problems associated with drainage catheters. While only one visit to some patients after a diagnostic procedure may be needed, regular visits to those patients with drainage catheters or who have had other interventions are important in avoiding complications. In one study, 59 catheter-related problems were detected in 268 patient visits [56]. The authors conclude that rounding resulted in preventing significant complications related to tube drainage.

In addition to inpatient care, postdischarge care may be needed. The interventionalist can help avoid many problems by providing information on tube care at home, arranging visiting nurses, or predischarge instruction by ancillary personnel. The radiologist should also help coordinate follow-up care and tube checks for patients. This can be facilitated by regularly communicating with primary care physicians who will be following the patient. The radiologist should develop means of informing other physicians involved in care via letter or by sending copies of radiographic reports. Finally, it is prudent to provide patients with the emergency number for nights and weekends, or to arrange for an answering service. All these measures will enhance the access to care for patients and improve communication among the health care providers involved in the case.

Receipt of a malpractice claim

If you receive a notification of a malpractice claim, it is important to follow these guidelines to avoid prejudicing the outcome of the case [2].

1 Contact your malpractice carrier immediately.

2 Do not contact the plaintiff or the plaintiff's attorney yourself. All communication with the plaintiff should be through your attorney. It is important to remember that the case is no longer a medical issue, it is a legal issue. Right or wrong, the case will be decided by the legal system and its rules apply.

3 Do not destroy or alter films or medical records. Ensure that all records related to the claim are held in a secure place.

4 Do not discuss the case with anyone other than your attorney or your spouse. Any other conversations about this claim are not privileged and can be used against you at trial. Any questions related to the case and its conduct should be directed to your attorney.

The shock of receiving a notification of a malpractice claim is often followed by an intense desire to know the reasons for the claim. This is particularly true for radiologists who may not recall the case and may be completely in the dark. It is your attorney who will investigate and will make the details available to you. Do not try to bypass the process by contacting the plaintiff or the patient yourself. Do not try to propose a settlement with anyone other than through your attorney. Such a settlement proposal, although possibly motivated by the best of intentions, may be portrayed as efforts to sweep the issue under the rug by the plaintiff in court. Unfortunately, the legal process is slow, agonizing, expensive, and inefficient, but must be allowed to run its course within the rules of the system.

Methods for health care quality improvement (QI)

Malpractice litigation

Medical malpractice litigation and the threat of litigation is often cited as a means of ensuring health care quality.

Malpractice attorneys claim that physicians are unable or unwilling to "weed out" bad practitioners. They portray themselves as the means of enforcing the standard of care.

A review of the facts would indicate otherwise. As mentioned earlier, the Harvard Medical Practice study found two striking facts [7]. Of the 280 adverse events deemed due to negligence, only eight resulted in suits for a weighted rate of 1.53%. The investigators estimated that there is a ratio of 7.6 negligent events for each malpractice claim in New York, leading them to conclude that medical malpractice litigation infrequently compensates patients injured by medical negligence and rarely identifies and holds providers accountable for substandard care. What is not emphasized in the study is that in the Harvard Medical Practice study group, they identified 51 malpractice claims of which only eight were in cases where negligence had occurred. This suggests that only 15% of malpractice claims are filed in cases where negligence has occurred, and the overwhelming number are in instances when there has been no negligence. Therefore, the claim that malpractice is only directed towards physicians practicing substandard care appears to be legal hyperbole. Most malpractice claims are directed toward physicians who have not deviated from the standard of care.

Even the use of malpractice claims data as a tool to direct QI has little validity. Kravitz *et al.* [57] used reviewed cases or those in which negligence was admitted to try to determine root causes for medical negligence. They found that cognitive errors were the most common among all specialties. They found only 15% of cases were for failure to order tests, which the authors conclude indicates that tests ordered for defensive medicine purposes may not be justified. Unfortunately, the authors studied a system in which defensive medicine is already deeply entrenched, so it is not surprising that there are few claims for failure to order tests. In a related study [58], the use of malpractice data only slightly aids in identifying physicians prone to malpractice, and they were unable to identify characteristics of physicians that might make them subject to suits. The conclusion is that the use of malpractice claims data to identify substandard care has no basis, because prior malpractice settlements are generally not an indicator of future behaviors. Considering that the data source used by these authors is malpractice cases in which negligence *had* occurred and that the majority of malpractice claims occur in cases where no negligence has taken place, the notion that malpractice serves any role in enforcing the standard of care or identifying "bad doctors" is completely discredited.

Nonetheless, Congress has created the National Practitioner Data Bank as part of the Health Care Quality Improvement Act (HCQA) of 1986. Prompted by some well-publicized suits filed by physicians who had had their privileges revoked or limited by hospital peer review groups, the HCQA provided protection for all involved in legitimate peer review activities. Because of the protection for hospital staffs that the bill provided, organized medicine supported the bill. The "trade-off" was the development of the National Practitioner Data Bank. The databank was intended to prevent "bad doctors" from moving from hospital to hospital or from state to state. It requires the reporting of all adverse actions taken against individual physicians, dentists, and other health care providers who are licensed and otherwise authorized to provide health care services by hospitals, state medical boards, and professional medical societies. In addition, all payments by malpractice carriers for settlements or judgments against individual physicians or dentists must also be reported [59]. The legislation also required all hospitals to query the databank when considering applications for privileges by health care providers, and every 2 years for its entire staff. Only hospitals, professional medical societies, state medical boards, and other health care organizations with formally constituted peer review processes are allowed access to the database records. Physicians and other providers are allowed access to their own files only. Plaintiffs and their legal counsel are not allowed access to the data.

There was initially great concern about the security of the data and the AMA sought to run the databank. This was denied and a contract was let to Unisys Corporation in Camarillo, California. In the first year of operation, 85% of the data entered was for malpractice payments, with the rest for adverse actions by state medical boards and hospitals. There has also been concern that the requirement for *all* malpractice payments to be reported will significantly impede the claims resolution process and that a floor should be placed at $30 000 or $50 000 to allow the settlement of nuisance claims without requiring a databank record. Congress directed the Public Health Service (PHS) to study this issue and also to recommend whether open malpractice claims should be reported to the databank. Recently, the Office of the Inspector General of the Department of Health and Human Services (DHHS) has recommended that there no change in the current regulations, i.e., that no floor level should be placed on the malpractice reporting and open claims should not be reported [60]. The PHS has not issued a final decision on this issue as of this date.

The practitioner databank was intended to identify "bad doctors", but at the conclusion of its first year it is unclear who it has identified [59]. It was created at a time when it was assumed that the number of malpractice claims payments would correlate with a physician's skill or lack of it. As the earlier discussion has pointed out, malpractice data is a poor predictor of incompetence and the majority of malpractice claims occur in cases where there is no negligence. With the databank now in place, the physician unfortunate enough to be sued when no negligence has occurred faces a difficult choice. Settling such a claim for a small amount carries with it a record that will be carried with him or her for life; on the other hand, not settling requires considerable expense and time, and may not result in vindication.

QI programs

Before health care quality can be improved, the term quality must be defined. In his review of QI in radiology, Cascade [61] describes the definition of quality used by the Joint Commission on the Accreditation of Health Organizations (JCAHO). Quality is defined in terms of outcome, i.e., the degree to which patient care increases the probability of desired patient outcomes and reduces the possibility of undesired outcomes. Simply stated, the care that patients receive should result in improvement in their condition and not worsening in that condition.

How can health care be improved? This problem is the subject of volumes, and clear answers are not yet available. There are a wide variety of proposed solutions, ranging from individual physician initiative to central planning by government agencies. The JCAHO has mandated development of a QI program by each health care organization, programs that will be reviewed during periodic accreditation. They have outlined the elements required for QI programs in their Agenda for Change [62]. These must meet several requirements for monitoring and evaluation activities, including that they be planned, systematic, and comprehensive. They should be based on indicators and criteria that are agreed on by the staff of the department, and accomplished by routine collection and periodic evaluation of data, and result in appropriate actions to resolve identified problems. These efforts must be continuous and integrated with those of the rest of the facility.

These somewhat daunting requirements have been distilled to 10 essential steps in monitoring and evaluation. These are as follows.

1 Assign responsibility for the department's monitoring and evaluation efforts.

2 Delineate the scope of care or service that the department provides.

3 Having reviewed the range of the department's activities, identify the important aspects of its services, i.e., those aspects that should be monitored.

4 Identify indicators of quality and appropriateness for the identified important aspects of care. Indicators are measures of quality, i.e., specific measures that are objective, quantifiable, and statistically reliable. So, if safety is the important aspect of care that is to be monitored, complication rates are the indicators. These are quantifiable and objective.

5 Establish the criteria that will be used to evaluate the indicators. The criteria are thresholds, i.e., levels that if exceeded will trigger a review to determine the cause of the problem.

6 Collect and organize the data. The sources can be procedure logs, pathology reports, incident reports, etc.

7 If a threshold is exceeded, evaluate care to determine the cause of the problem.

8 Take actions to solve identified problems, which includes who or what is expected to change, what action will be taken, and how the change will be achieved.

9 Assess the actions and document improvement, by continuing to monitor and reevaluate the care.

10 Communicate the relevant information to the organizationwide quality assurance program.

With this framework each department can develop their program using the same format, but targeted to the specific needs and concerns of that department. The problems monitored might include missed diagnoses, inadequate clinical history on requests, lost X-ray reports, complications, etc. QI is a means of solving problems, an organized approach to detect deficiencies and address them. It has the means of improving the department's systems and policies to provide safer, more efficient service. Rather than viewing QI programs as an imposed bureaucratic burden (which they are), they can be viewed as a positive tool truly to change and improve the care we provide.

Several radiology organizations have developed model QI programs that can be used by practicing radiologists to meet JCAHO requirements. In 1990, the ACR published a model QI program that encompasses all the areas of the department, including the technical areas of the department [63]. The Society of Cardiovascular and Interventional Radiology (SCVIR) has published a detailed program for vascular and interventional procedures and provides a specific example applied to the 10 steps of the Agenda of Change [64]. It has been suggested that these programs have the potential to provide information for a national database of procedure success rates and complications by integration into registries [65].

There are also concrete examples of missed cases that can be used to improve the quality of care a department provides [21,66]. A problem case conference can become a major portion of a department's quality program. A recent review of such a program discovered several causes for error, including failure to consult old films or reports, incomplete history, failure to search for abnormalities after the first is found, and lack of knowledge [21]. It also noted that errors in communication are common. The parallel between the errors brought to light by these types of conferences and the causes for malpractice claims are striking. By bringing an openminded and candid attitude to self-evaluation, the goals of improved patient care and effective risk management are furthered. As one author notes, a recognized mistake is the best teacher [66].

There are problems with QI programs as currently mandated. In order to meet JCAHO requirements, they require extensive documentation for the reviewers to audit during a site visit. As a result, they generate disproportionate paperwork for the information gained and for the improvements made. It is not even known if such programs really affect care at all. By their very nature, they concentrate on identifying outlyers, the events that exceed the thresholds. While these should, in theory, identify problem areas, they may in fact only identify sporadic events. For example, in the model program for interventional radiology that the SCVIR has developed, angioplasty is one of the procedures that is monitored. One of the complication thresholds is distal embolization causing tissue damage in less than 0.5% of cases. This number was derived using a consensus process, after reviewing reported complication rates from the literature. While this may be a valid threshold to choose, distal embolization is a very rare event and its use in a typical community hospital practice points up an immediate problem. If that practice performs 100 angioplasties/year, the semi-annual QI report will show this threshold exceeded with the occurrence of a single event, i.e., one case in 50 or 2%. If the same complication occurs in a practice performing 500 angioplasties per year, then the threshold is not exceeded (one in 250 or 0.4%). It is obvious that the problem is magnified when fewer procedures are done, and if the same threshold is applied to an individual in such a practice the margin that the threshold is exceeded is even greater. If the physician continues to monitor him- or herself, using the same nominator of one complication, and an increasing denominator of 20 or 30 or 40 cases that are accumulated over time, it may take 1−2 years or longer for that rate to return below the threshold. Distal embolization during an angioplasty can be due to negligence or incompetence, but also is a sporadic complication that all angiographers will experience. What value then is it to identify a single event, when we do not have the ability to distinguish negligence or incompetence from a sporadic event? While recurrence of the same complication over and over clearly points to a serious problem, the individual event is much more common and more difficult to evaluate. It also focuses a spotlight on a single practitioner, and gives that practitioner an incentive to be less than candid in discussing the case or similar cases in the future. This type of system tends to reward those who hide complications and penalizes those who are honest in their reporting. The SCVIR has attempted to address this problem in more recent documents by grouping all the complications experienced by a single physician, and using a threshold of 5% [67]. While this type of QI program is mandated by the JCAHO, and this is the reason the SCVIR and the ACR have developed models for use by their members, the primary utility of the programs may be satisfying the needs of a regulatory body and not improving the quality of care. Certainly, when adhered to and actively participated in by the department, such a program can identify the outliers; those procedures or practitioners that have problems. But, it concentrates on the exception and does nothing to improve the average care that is given to patients. The goal of QI should be to improve the overall level of care, and current monitoring and evaluation programs fail to examine the root causes of problems that are inherent in the system and fail to develop the means to solve them.

Continuing QI (CQI)

In recent years, health policy researchers have discovered considerable variation in practice patterns, utilization of resources, and outcome of treatments for the same illnesses [68]. The results of these studies have generated considerable interest to reduce the variation in practice and, as a result, to improve care and reduce utilization of resources. Among proposed systems are computerized diagnostic systems and automated patient records that will decrease the incidence of errors. There is considerable interest in the development of practice algorithms by medical specialty societies and regulatory agencies. Practice algorithms are designed to assist in patient care decisions by formulating a common pattern of evaluation and management of specific clinical problems.

In an effort to address the limitations of the current QI programs, health planners have begun to explore the application of industrial CQI methods to health care [68]. In medicine, these methods are called total quality management or, perhaps more commonly, CQI. These programs rely on statistical measurement of variation in systems, with variations often meaning substandard or poor-quality work. Multidisciplinary teams try to determine the root causes of the variations and propose solutions to them. The solutions are then evaluated by continued analysis, thus the continuous efforts at improvement. There are several basic precepts of this type of program [69]. The first is that individuals are generally not the cause of problems or errors in a system, but that the system itself is the problem. A second is that the patient is treated as a customer for the purposes of determining needs. The needs of the patient, those things that will provide customer satisfaction, are the focus of the program. This is achieved by evaluating a system using a nonblaming, open evaluation by a team with representatives from all levels of the departments involved. By identifying the most likely causes of error in a system, the team can perform a statistical analysis of the system to determine the true causes. By then directing efforts to the most common causes of error, the system can be improved. These general concepts form the basis of a virtual revolution in QI in industrial and manufacturing processes. These concepts have long been championed by Deming, Juran, and others. In particular, the efforts of Deming have been the major cause of the wide acceptance and application of these policies in Japanese industry and have been a primary reason for their economic success in the past 30 years. These methods have also been applied in this country by Ford, Motorola, and other major corporations with substantial increases in quality.

CQI is now being embraced throughout the health care system in this country, particularly by hospitals, health maintenance organizations, and others. The National Demonstration Project for Quality Improvement served as a pilot program to test the methods in the health setting [69]. This project was a great success, resulting in improvement in service and efficiency. There are also examples of successful application of these techniques in radiology departments [70,71].

However, the majority of CQI programs in medicine to date have been used to improve administrative systems, such as admissions, records, and ancillary services. There are few examples of the use of these principles in the physician's care of patients. It is unclear how these methods·will be applied to decisions in patient care, but most likely it will be through use of practice guidelines. Variation from established guidelines will form the basis of evaluation for care in individual hospitals. This plan has been outlined recently in the Health Care Quality Improvement Initiative by the Health Care Financing Administration (HCFA) [72]. This initiative uses the CQI model as a foundation of a system to improve the average quality of care provided for Medicare patients. The emphasis of the proposed program is on evaluating the patterns of care in each hospital and comparing its care and outcomes with the national average and a benchmark standard (defined as the care and outcomes of the best 10% of institutions). This information will be shared with the hospital and its medical staff by the local peer review organization (PRO). The areas that require improvement will be addressed by the medical staff itself, which will try to identify the root causes of the problems and attempt solutions. The emphasis will be on the institution and not on the individual practitioner's occasional error. While this approach has potential for engaging physicians actively in the process (a necessary element for the success of the program), it has been met with some skepticism [73]. The obstacles to be overcome include repairing the strained relationship between physicians and HCFA, which has suffered from the recent enactment of the relative value scale reimbursement changes. More important, such a plan would require cooperation between local PROs and physicians, which would entail a complete reversal of the current adversarial relationship. In addition, the proposed system will use very complex and as yet unproven databases, including the Patient Care Algorithm System (PCAS) and Uniform Clinical Data Set (UCDS). Implementation will require introducing the entire health care system to these new and unfamiliar concepts. However, the goal of trying to improve the system and not singling out or punishing individual practitioners is likely to have greater support from doctors and is therefore more likely to succeed.

It is clear that the demands of patients and Congress for measurable systems to improve the quality of care will continue and are unavoidable. The tool of CQI will play a prominent part in the process and offers incentives to physicians actively to participate and lead in the changes that are certain to come. At the same time, the efforts to improve average care given to patients may result in real improvement in the system.

Practice parameters

Another major effort to improve the quality of health care has been the development of the practice parameters, a generic term the AMA has used to describe practice guidelines, standards, algorithms, and other authoritative statements on patient care. The practice parameters movement has been developed by medical societies over the last decade in response to both internal and external pressures for guidelines to help standardize practice and to define the minimum standards of care. For physicians, practice parameters have the potential to guide practice decisions and to distill the conflicting data in the literature into a usable document that represents the consensus of the specialty. These can be of great assistance to physicians in dealing with the tremendous growth of medical knowledge and technology. In addition, they provide a defense against claims of inappropriate care by PROs, and insurance carriers, as well as a theoretical defense against claims of malpractice. For patients, health care analysts, and legislators, the development of practice guidelines is a concrete message that medical societies are taking positive steps to improve care. They are an effective response to the rising demands for documentation of the quality of care.

Whether practice standards may be effective in decreasing the number and costs of malpractice claims is not known [5]. There are several prerequisites in order for practice parameters to be effective in reducing malpractice costs: (i) guidelines must be available for conditions or problems that frequently lead to negligence claims; (ii) they must be widely accepted by the medical profession; (iii) they must be fully integrated into practice; and (iv) they must be straightforward and readily interpretable in a litigation setting. Practice parameters are a long way from meeting all these requirements, but their development and acceptance does represent a major shift in medical culture. The hope that practice parameters will result in dramatic malpractice savings is overly optimistic, but they may result in raising the overall level of care and thus result in fewer adverse events and thus fewer claims.

The use of practice standards by plaintiff's attorneys as evidence of a breach of standard care is a fear often expressed by physicians, but it appears that practice parameters will not be allowed as *prima facie* evidence of breach of care. However, there are examples where these have been used by plaintiffs to build a case against physicians. A review of the potential use of practice parameters in medical litigation by the AMA legal counsel reveals that their application faces several problems [74]. There is no agreed process for the development or format of these statements. The vocabulary used to describe them is not even standardized. The diversity of the practice of medicine also presents a challenge to their applicability because there are so many variables in patient care that guidelines are by necessity general. In addition, there are varying purposes and goals for practice parameters.

Some are designed as patient care standards to improve the level of care, while others are utilization standards or appropriateness criteria to try to decrease the number of unnecessary procedures. In order significantly to decrease the cost and frequency of malpractice claims, a standard must be easily applicable and universally applied. A good example is the anesthesiology standard on patient monitoring, which has resulted in reduced malpractice premiums. This standard is simple, easy to interpret, and prescriptive. The standard was initially developed by the Harvard Anesthesia Department after review of malpractice claims data. The standard applies to almost all patients undergoing general anesthesia. Because it is so straightforward, it has been universally accepted. It does not address the more complex issues of which anesthetic to use or how to handle emergencies. The AMA counsel concludes that there are drawbacks to the use of standards as evidence of the standard of care because there may be disagreements among specialties regarding appropriate care [74], but believes that testing of practice parameters should be done by HCFA or the federal PROs.

There are experiments that are underway in the use of practice guidelines as a shield against malpractice claims. The best known is the Maine Demonstration Project, which involves four subspecialties: anesthesiology, emergency medicine, radiology, and obstetrics and gynecology [74–76]. The project will allow the use of specific practice guidelines as a positive defense to allow some suits to be dismissed before reaching court. In this project, the standards cannot be used by plaintiffs. As a result, this project has been opposed by the trial lawyers and may be challenged constitutionally.

Among radiology organizations, the ACR, the SCVIR, and others have been active in the development of standards. Early standards of these organizations were training standards, detailing the requirements for obtaining hospital privileges for certain procedures. The SCVIR has also been active in encouraging the development of a multispecialty statement on training for angioplasty by the American Heart Association. The more recent statements of radiology organizations have been performance standards for procedures, appropriateness criteria, and patient care standards. These documents are all intended to improve quality of diagnosis and treatment. As with other medical organizations, organized radiology has addressed the major areas of practice and written documents that guide decisions or performance in daily practice. Because they represent the consensus of practicing radiologists, they are widely accepted. Despite initial reluctance, practicing radiologists are now enthusiastic about guidelines to aid them in practice. It truly represents a "cultural" change.

The federal government has also entered the standards development field. Congress created the Agency for Health Policy and Research (AHCPR), with the charge to develop means to improved the quality of health care. They have commissioned several practice studies, and have now de-

veloped their first practice algorithms. The first, on urinary stress incontinence, has been formulated in the form of an annotated algorithm, with references to the appropriate support from the literature [77]. It is designed to maintain clinical flexibility, but also allow its use as a tool to monitor quality and appropriateness of care. Such practice algorithms do represent "cookbook medicine", in that they are prescriptive. However, following them may represent a defense against malpractice litigation. In the near future, the AHCPR will begin to address areas of medicine that will generate considerable controversy, such as coronary artery disease, and the algorithms that are developed may result in significant changes in practice patterns.

Conclusions and future directions

The past decade has witnessed a tremendous growth in malpractice claims, defensive medicine, disillusionment among physicians, and clamor for reform of health care delivery. The Congress, and through them the public, have demanded an accounting in health care and creation of a means of measuring the quality of care. These demands came, and regulation was imposed, before there were even definitions of quality care. No system or discipline existed to measure quality or outcomes. There were cries for proof of the efficacy of our care based on outcomes research before methods to perform such research were available.

In the past few years there has been considerable progress in the efforts to improve care, primarily by the development of practice standards, and these will become more sophisticated and thorough. As they are developed, they will be used by HCFA and others to monitor care and to attempt to improve the process of care. The practice of medicine will become more systematized and regulated. The trade-off *may* be that we will be subject to less malpractice litigation and with it, the need for defensive medicine and the fear of litigation will decrease in daily practice.

Unfortunately, the regulation of medical practice and the imposition of algorithms are not linked to malpractice reform. This is subject to the vagaries of the political process. Malpractice reform has become a part of the debate on the reform of both the health care and civil justice systems [78]. As of this writing, there are over 14 major medical liability reform proposals that have been introduced in Congress. Most do not address the central issue of reducing malpractice claims, but rather are intended to limit the awards that may be obtained [79]. For example, the one proposal would place a $250 000 limit on noneconomic damages, bar duplicate or collateral source payments, eliminate lump sum payments of malpractice awards, implement procedures to enhance the quality of care, and promote alternate dispute resolution. Whether this type of reform occurs remains to be seen. There are even more sweeping plans proposed by health policy makers, including no-fault insurance for compensation for all iatrogenic injuries [80]. A feasibility study found that the cost of such a system would be about the same as the current system, and would compensate many more patients who have suffered injury.

The scrutiny that physicians will undergo in practice in the years ahead will continue to grow. There will be significant changes in the way we practice and the way we monitor our care. It is only with the active involvement of physicians and their specialty societies that they will be able to shape the process to reflect the state of the art in medical care and thus assure that patients do have the best outcome.

References

1 Brennan T, Leape L, Laird N *et al*. Incidence of adverse events and negligence in hospitalized patients: results of the Harvard Medical Practice Study I. *New Engl J Med* 1991;324;370−376.

2 Brice J. Simple tactics to minimize exposure to malpractice. *Diagn Imag* 1992;March:43−46.

3 Gonzalez M. Medical professional liability claims and premiums, 1985−1990. In: *American Medical Association Center for Health Policy Research*. Chicago: AMA, 1992.

4 Reynolds R, Rizzo J, Gonzalez M. The cost of medical professional liability. *J Am Med Assoc* 1987;257:2776−2781.

5 Garnick D, Hendricks A, Brennan T. Can practice guidelines reduce the number and costs of malpractice claims? *J Am Med Assoc* 1991;266:2856−2860.

6 Leape L, Brennan T, Laird N *et al*. The nature of adverse events in hospitalized patients: results of the Harvard Medical Practice Study II. *New Engl J Med* 1991;324:377−384.

7 Localio A, Lawthers A, Brennan T *et al*. Relation between malpractice claims and adverse events due to negligence; results of the Harvard Medical Practice Study III. *New Engl J Med* 1991;325:245−251.

8 Potchen E, Bisese M, Sierra A, Potchen J. Mammography and malpractice. *Am J Roentgenol* 1991;156:475−480.

9 Gagliardi R. The academic medical expert witness: a new confrontation between town and gown. *Invest Radiol* 1988;23:636−638.

10 Berlin L. Is a radiologic "miss" malpractice? An ominous example. *Am J Roentgenol* 1983;140:1031−1034.

11 Halperin E. X-rays at the bar. *Invest Radiol* 1988;23:639−646.

12 Ross W. Medicolegal aspects of medical radiation exposure. *Br J Radiol* 1990;63:313−314.

13 Berlin L. Malpractice and radiologists, update 1986: and 11.5 year perspective. *Am J Roentgenol* 1986;147:1291−1298.

14 Spring D, Tennenhouse D. Radiology malpractice lawsuits: California jury verdicts. *Radiology* 1986;159:811−814.

15 Hamer M, Morlock F, Foley H, Ros P. Medical malpractice in diagnostic radiology: claims, compensation, and patient injury. *Radiology* 1987;164:263−266.

16 Dahlen R, Foley H. Medical malpractice claims in diagnostic radiology: update. *Radiology* 1989;170:277.

17 PIAA. PIAA database of malpractice claims. Unpublished data.

18 Craig J. The Knox Lecture: radiology and the law. *Clin Radiol* 1989;40:343−346.

19 Morrish H, Messenger O. Medicolegal encounters in Canadian radiology. *J Can Assoc Radiol* 1990;41:259−263.

20 AMA. Risk management principles and commentaries for the medical office. In: *Medical Liability Project*. Chicago: American Medical Association, 1990.

21 Renfrew D, Franken E, Berbaum K, Weigelt F, Abu-Yousef M. Error in radiology: classification and lessons in 182 cases presented at a problem case conference. *Radiology* 1992;183:145−150

22 ACR. ACR standard for communication − diagnostic radiology. Unpublished data.

23 Kline T, Kline T. Radiologists, communication, and resolution 5: a medicolegal issue. *Radiology* 1992;184:131−134.

24 Hall F. Clinical history, radiographic reporting, and defensive radiologic practice. *Radiology* 1989;170:575−576.

25 Mazur D. What should patients be told prior to a medical procedure? Ethical and legal perspectives on medical informed consent. *Am J Med* 1986;81:1051−1054.

26 Reuter S. An overview of informed consent for radiologists *Am J Roentgenol* 1987;148:219−227.

27 Bettman M, Holzer J, Trombly S. Risk management issues related to the use of contrast agents. *Radiology* 1990;175:629−631.

28 Jacobson P, Rosenquist J. The introduction of low-osmolar contrast agents in radiology: medical, economic, legal and public policy issues. *J Am Med Assoc* 1988;260:1586−1592.

29 Katayama H, Yamaguchi K, Kozuka T, Takashima T, Seez P, Matsuura K. Adverse reactions to inonic and nonionic contrast media: a report from the Japanese committee on the safety of contrast media. *Radiology* 1990;175:621−628.

30 Powe N. Low- versus high-osmolality contrast media for intravenous use: a health care luxury or necessity. *Radiology* 1992;183:21−22.

31 ACR. Current criteria for the use of water soluble contrast agents for intravenous injections. In: American College of Radiology, 1990.

32 Bush W. Informed consent for contrast media. *Am J Roentgenol* 1989;152:867−869.

33 Spring D, Akin J, Margulis A. Informed consent for intravenous contrast-enhanced radiology: a national survey of practice and opinion. *Radiology* 1984;152:609−613.

34 Lambe H, Hopper K, Matthews Y. Use of informed consent for ionic and nonionic contrast media. *Radiology* 1992;184:145−148.

35 PIAA. Breast cancer study. In: 1990.

36 Brenner R. Medicolegal aspects of screening mammography. *Am J Roentgenol* 1989;153:53−56.

37 Brenner R. Medicolegal aspects of breast imaging: variable standards of care relating to different types of practice. *Am J Roentgenol* 1991;156:719−723.

38 Robertson C, Kopans D. Communication problems after mammographic screening. *Radiology* 1989;172:443−444.

39 Sickles E. Quality assurance: how to audit your own mammography practice. *Radiol Clin N Am* 1992;30:265−275.

40 Sickles E, Ominsky S, Sollitto R, Galvin H, Monticciolo D. Medical audit of a rapid-throughput mammography screening practice: methodology and results of 27 114 examinations. *Radiology* 1990;175:323−327.

41 Spring D, Kimbrell-Wilmot K. Evaluating the success of mammography at the local level: how to conduct an audit of your practice. *Radiol Clin N Am* 1987;25:983−992.

42 Moseson D. Audit of mammography in a community setting. *Am J Surg* 1992;163:544−546.

43 Meyer J, Eberlein T, Stomper P, Sonnenfeld M. Biopsy of occult breast lesion: analysis of 1261 abnormalities. *J Am Med Assoc* 1990;263:2341−2343.

44 Darios R. Biopsy of occult breast lesions and professional liability. *J Am Med Assoc* 1990;264:1948.

45 Linver M, Paster S, Rosenburg R, Key C, Stidley C. Improvement

in mammography interpretation skills in a community radiology practice after dedicated teaching course: 2-year medical audit of 38 633. *Radiology* 1992;184:39−43.

46 James A, Fleischer A, Sacks G, Greeson T. Ectopic pregnancy: a malpractice paradigm. *Radiology* 1986;160:411−413.

47 Macones A, Lev-Toaff A, Macones G, Jaffe J, Williams V. Legal aspects of obstetric sonography. *Am J Roentgenol* 1989;153: 1251−1254.

48 Leopold G. Responsibilities associated with obstetric sonography. *Am J Roentgenol* 1989;153:1255−1257.

49 George J, Espinosa J, Quattrone M. Legal issues in emergency radiology: practical strategies to reduce risk. *Emerg Med Clin of N Am* 1992;10:179−203.

50 Stone P, Hilton C. Medicolegal aspects of emergency department radiology. *Radiol Clin N Am* 1992;30:495−501.

51 PIAA. Colon cancer study. Unpublished data.

52 PIAA. Lung cancer study. Unpublished data.

53 Muhm J, Miller W, Fontana R, Sanderson D, Uhlenhopp M. Lung cancer detected during a screening program using four-month chest radiographs. *Radiology* 1983;148:609−615.

54 Potchen E, Bisesi M. When is it malpractice to miss lung cancer on chest radiographs? *Radiology* 1990;175:29−32.

55 Picus D. Angiography in the 1990's: diagnosis and therapy. *Radiology* 1990;175:33.

56 Goldberg M, Mueller P, Saini S *et al.* Importance of daily rounds by the radiologist after interventional procedures of the abdomen and chest. *Radiology* 1991;180:767−770.

57 Kravitz R, Rolph J, McGuigan K. Malpractice claims data as a quality improvement tool. 1. Epidemiology of error in four specialties. *J Am Med Assoc* 1991;266:2087−2092.

58 Rolph J, Kravitz R, McGuigan K. Malpractice claims data as a quality improvement tool. 2. Is targeting effective? *J Am Med Assoc* 1991;266:2093−2097.

59 Mullan F, Politzer R, Lewis C, Bastacky S, Rodak J, Harmon R. The national practitioner data bank: report from the first year. *J Am Med Assoc* 1992;268:73−79.

60 OIG. National Practitioner Data Bank: malpractice reporting requirements. Department of Health and Human Services, 1992.

61 Cascade P. Quality improvement in diagnostic radiology. *Am J Roentgenol* 1990;154:1117−1120.

62 JCAHO. Monitoring and evaluation of the quality and appropriateness of care: a hospital example. Joint Commission on the Accreditation of Health Organizations. *Quality Rev Bull* 1986; 326−330.

63 ACR. Quality improvement manual, a model program for radiology. American College of Radiology, 1990.

64 SCVIR. Guidelines for establishing a quality assurance program in vascular and interventional radiology. Society of Cardiovascular and Interventional Radiology, 1989.

65 Cascade P, Kastan D. Monitoring and evaluating the quality and appropriateness of angiographic/interventional radiologic procedures. *Radiology* 1990;174:926−928.

66 Wheeler P. Risk prevention, quality assurance, and the missed diagnosis conference. *Radiology* 1982;145:227−228.

67 SCVIR. Standard of practice for diagnostic angiography. *J Vasc Intervent Radiol* 1993;4:385−395.

68 Laffel G, Berwick D. Quality in health care. *J Am Med Assoc* 1992;268:407−409.

69 Berwick D, Godfrey A, Roessner J. *Curing Health Care, New Strategies for Quality Improvement*, 1st edn. San Francisco: Jossey-Boss, 1991:281.

70 Chopra PS, Kandarpa K, Aliabadi P. Improving the patient evaluation process in a cardiovascular and interventional radiology department. *Qual Manag Hlth Care* 1992;1:21−28.

71 ACR. X-ray processing time cut 81 percent. *Am Coll Radiol* 1992:18.

72 Jencks S, Wilensky G. The health care quality improvement initiative: a new approach to quality assurance in medicare. *J Am Med Assoc* 1992;268:900−904.

73 Nash D. Is the quality cart before the horse? *J Am Med Assoc* 1992;268:917−918.

74 Hirshfield E. Should practice parameters be the standard of care in malpractice litigation. *J Am Med Assoc* 1991;266:2886−2891.

75 Dakins D. Practice standards offer defense against lawsuits. *Diagn Imag* 1992:25−26.

76 ACR. Maine begins five-year medical guidelines experiment. *Am Coll Radiol Bull* 1992:8−9.

77 Hadorn D, McCormick K, Diokno A. An annotated algorithm approach to clinical guideline development. *J Am Med Assoc* 1992;267:3311−3314.

78 Gerson S. *Malpractice Reform*. Washington, DC: Society of Cardiovascular and Interventional Radiology, 1992.

79 Harr D. Federal interest in malpractice tort reform intensifies. *Radiol Today* 1992:16.

80 Johnson W, Brennan T, Newhouse J *et al.* The economic consequences of medical injuries: implications for a no-fault insurance plan. *J Am Med Assoc* 1992;267:2487−2492.

Informed consent and liability: controversies for the 1990s

Yuri R. Parisky and Catherine Dring*

Although informed consent is not a new doctrine, it has recently gained new relevance due to the expanding right of patient autonomy. Informed consent, or lack of it, is becoming a critical element in today's medical malpractice crisis. Patients frequently bring malpractice suits in situations where they claim they were not involved in the decision-making process; hence, as a result, their expectations were not tempered to medical realities.

The legal doctrines underlying informed consent coupled with the mechanics of cost containment will be examined in light of a perplexing yet practical problem radiologists face daily. The development and introduction of low-osmolar contrast media (LOCM) used in contrast studies has presented significant medical and legal problems, in addition to potential conflict between health care reimbursement, patient autonomy, and sound medical practice.

Informed consent

Individuality and autonomy have long been important values in American society and law. As John Stuart Mill stated: "Over himself, over his own body and mind, the individual is sovereign" [1]. Using history as a guide, it appears that the more intense and personal the consequences of a choice, and the less direct or significant the impact that choice has on others, the more compelling the individual's claim to autonomy becomes. If one applies these criteria to patient

decision making, it would seem that there is a strong case for respecting patient autonomy in decisions about health and body. The informed consent doctrine requires the physician to discuss and explain to patients the significance of their ailments, the nature of the proposed treatment or operation, the probability of success, alternate methods of treatment, and the foreseeable risks [2]. Lack of informed consent can lead to a cause of action for either battery or negligence.

The legal requirement of informed consent has become a point of conflict between the medical and legal professions. At work are conflicting goals: paternalistic views of social and medical policies versus respect for the individual's autonomy. Some physicians view informed consent as a restrictive requirement that infringes on their professional judgment as to what is best for the patient. Lawyers and legal theorists, however, are more concerned with the individual right of self-determination. Although judges and legal scholars have long asserted the importance of patient autonomy in medical decision making, patient autonomy by itself has yet to be recognized as a legally protected interest.

Physician paternalism is encouraged by the very fact that health care choices carry great significance and tend to be complicated. The doctrine of informed consent is both a product of, and the basis for the physician–patient relationship. Their communications to each other establish the relationship, but once established, heightened degrees of expectations on the patient's part have dictated the need for

---

* A study of the issues presented in this paper was undertaken by Ms Catherine Dring during her senior year of Law School at USC 1990–1991. Ms Dring passed her bar in 1991 and is in private practice in San Diego.

a more sophisticated level of communication. Advancing medical technology has greatly expanded the options available to the patient. With this, the law should protect the patients' growing autonomy to make choices concerning their bodily integrity.

History of informed consent

The doctrine of informed consent originated under a theory of battery, the cause of action for the unconsented touching of one's person. Physicians were held liable for the unconsented touching of a patient's body under this theory. One of the earliest cases applying this doctrine was *Mohr* v. *Williams* [3], an action involving lack of consent for an operation. In this case, plaintiff consulted the defendant physician concerning difficulties with her hearing, and subsequently consented to an operation on her right ear. While the patient was under anesthesia, the physician found the left ear to be in worse condition, and chose to perform the unconsented surgery on the left ear. The plaintiff brought a suit claiming that the unconsented operation on her left ear seriously impaired her sense of hearing, was wrongful, and unlawful.

The Minnesota Supreme Court held that even though the operation was skillfully performed, the plaintiff did not consent and, therefore, the surgery was unlawful and wrongful, constituting an assault and battery. The court in *Mohr* v. *Williams* went on to state the proposition that the patient, the final arbiter, is the one who decides whether he/she will take his/her chances with the operation, or take chances without it. However, the court noted that while there is no rule or principle of law that extends to a physician-free license respecting operations, the physician must be given reasonable latitude. The court expressed reluctance to lay down any law that would unreasonably interfere with the exercise of a physician's discretion, or would prevent them from taking measures as judgment dictated in a case of emergency.

After *Mohr* v. *Williams*, any procedure performed on a patient without his/her consent constituted an action for battery. Since battery is a cause of action whose aim is to deter antisocial conduct, many courts were reluctant to hold physicians liable under this theory. This prompted most jurisdictions to limit this action to the relatively unusual situation where a medical procedure is carried out without any type of consent, rather than where the consent has merely been insufficiently informed. "We agree with the majority trend. The battery theory should be reserved for those circumstances when a doctor performs an operation to which the patient has not consented" [4]. The modern allegation of battery now typically arises only where consent to a particular procedure is given, and a different or additional procedure is carried out. Although infrequently used today to bring informed consent-claims, the theory of battery was critical in the move to protect patient autonomy in medical decision making.

Modern doctrine

Today, most litigation claims involving informed consent occur over the physicians' nondisclosure, or incomplete disclosure of information regarding patient care. The majority are brought as elements of general medical negligence claims. Informed consent has become a subcategory of the medical malpractice doctrine. The standard negligence analysis protects the patient's interest in physical well-being. The doctrine of informed consent injects into the established framework of negligence a concern with patient choice that would otherwise be absent. The courts recognize that actionable physical injury may occur through failure to disclose information that would have resulted in nonconsent to treatment. Unfortunately, the concern for patient autonomy does not give rise to a fully protected legal interest, because informed consent is strongly tied to the dominant interest in physical well-being. This most likely reflects society's tendency to assume that reasonable people choose as their physicians tell them to. Therefore, the importance of separately protecting patient autonomy has been greatly diminished.

The trend towards analyzing lack of informed consent under a negligence theory began with the case of *Natanson* v. *Kiline* [5]. Plaintiff brought this cause of action after suffering side-effects from radiation therapy, alleging that the physician had failed to disclose the risk of injury she subsequently suffered. The plaintiff was able to show from evidence presented that had she been properly informed of the treatment's inherent risks, she would not have consented. The Kansas Supreme Court began its analysis by stating that the sufficiency of the physician's disclosure is to be determined by the standards of the profession. If the physician fails to perform up to the professional standard of adequate disclosure of risk, he or she is liable for medical malpractice. Under this rule, the plaintiff has the burden to prove deviation from this standard by expert medical testimony. The professional standard established in *Natanson* v. *Kiline* is now adopted by a majority of jurisdictions, and is referred to as the *reasonable physician standard*.

The jurisdictions that follow the reasonable physician standard require the physician to disclose to his or her patients those risks and alternatives that a reasonable physician would disclose under the same or similar circumstances. The plaintiff will not recover unless the omission forsakes a practice prevalent in the profession. The plaintiff must present expert medical testimony to show that the professional standard of disclosure for the eventuated risk was violated, and that had the risk been disclosed, consent to the proposed therapy would not have been forthcoming.

The growing minority trend, as manifest in California, is to adopt the patient oriented approach, also known as the *reasonable patient standard*. This standard is based on what a reasonable patient would want to know, rather than what the average competent doctor would disclose. As opposed to the reasonable physician jurisdictions, plaintiffs in reasonable patient jurisdictions are given a significant procedural advantage because they no longer require expert testimony by physicians in the area. The reasonable person standard gained prominence with the decision of *Canterbury* v. *Spence* [6]. In this case, the plaintiff consented to a back operation without being informed of a 1% possibility of paralysis. When the paralysis resulted, plaintiff brought suit against the surgeon and hospital, which included a claim for lack of adequate disclosure. The court in *Canterbury* v. *Spence* emphasized the accepted principle that due care demands the physician to warn the patient of any risks to their well-being that the proposed treatment may involve. The court then rejected the reasonable physician standard, and held that a patient's cause of action for lack of informed consent is not dependent upon the existence and nonperformance of a relevant professional tradition.

The court in *Canterbury* v. *Spence* went on to state that since the patient's right of self-decision shapes the boundaries of the duty to disclose, that right can be effectively exercised only if the patient possesses enough information to make an intelligent choice. The court determined that a particular risk must be divulged if it is material to the patient's decision. Therefore, all risks potentially affecting the decision must be unmasked. A particular risk is material when a reasonable person, in what the physician knows or should know to be the patient's position, would be likely to attach significance to the risk or cluster of risks in deciding whether or not to forego the proposed therapy. These risks include the inherent and potential hazards of the proposed treatment, the alternates to that treatment, and the consequences of nontreatment.

The court in *Canterbury* v. *Spence* refused to accept the notion that a physician's obligation to disclose is either created or limited by medical practice. Respect for the patient's autonomy, in regard to choosing a particular therapy, demands a standard set by law for physicians, rather than one which physicians may or may not impose upon themselves. Any definition of scope solely in terms of a professional standard, is at odds with the patient's own predilection to decide on a projected therapy.

The *reasonable patient jurisdictions* divide into two camps: (i) those that judge materiality and consent by an *objective* standard; and (ii) those that judge materiality and consent *subjectively*. The latter jurisdictions imply that the physician should be able to read the patient's mind in order to determine what this patient believes is material to an informed decision. For this reason, the objective standard is the majority rule in reasonable patient jurisdictions. However, this majority rule is not as beneficial to a patient's autonomy, especially if the patient has views substantially different from the reasonable person.

Advocates of autonomy argue that the correct standard for disclosure in informed consent cases is what a reasonable patient would want to know, rather than what the average competent physician would actually disclose [7]. Their argument is that a reasonable patient standard should always be used because it gives substance to the idea of self-determination, yet it does not impose as tremendous a burden on the physician as a subjective standard would. When physicians evaluate the adequacy of disclosure, they naturally respond with reluctance to disclose risks and share decision making. Physician training reinforces the duty to take active responsibility, and stresses first and foremost the concern with outcomes. Therefore, professional expertise is not the appropriate determinant of how much disclosure is desirable or adequate for purposes of patient choice. The reasonable patient standard may also help to eliminate any alleged conspiracy of silence that exists throughout the medical community, since no expert testimony is needed to establish what a reasonable physician would have disclosed.

Causation

To bring a successful informed consent case, the plaintiff must show that had the contested disclosure been made, a reasonable person would not have consented to the proposed treatment. This objective standard prevents plaintiffs from presenting self-serving testimony, which is often biased by hindsight. There must be a causal relationship between the physician's failure adequately to divulge, and the damage to the patient. A causal connection is found to exist when disclosure of the significant risks incidental to the treatment would have resulted in a decision against it. The plaintiff obviously has no complaint if he or she would have submitted to the therapy, not withstanding awareness that the materialized risk was one of its perils.

Proponents of this objective standard argue that it is necessary because the answer to the hypothetical question: "Viewed from the point at which he or she had to decide, would the patient have decided differently had he/she known something he/she did not know?" represents little more than a guess, tinged by hindsight and personal bias. The *Canterbury* v. *Spence* court framed this objective standard in terms of what a prudent person in the plaintiff's position would have decided if suitably informed of all perils bearing significance. Such a standard eases the fact-finding process, and better assures the truth as its product. Although the plaintiff's testimony is still relevant to the issue of cause, it does not dominate the findings.

Critics of the objective standard testify that it invites juries and physicians to make the too easy and superficial assumption that reasonable people do what their competent physicians tell them to do. Choices made by reasonable others should not substitute as appropriate screening criteria, where the value at stake is personal autonomy. Instead, a narrow factual cause issue should be proposed: "Has the patient's right to choose been encroached upon as a result of a doctor's failure to disclose?" [7]. Some standard of materiality is needed. However, the question would then become whether it should be determined objectively or subjectively. The solution to this is precarious, due to the problems of uncertainty, prediction, and credibility faced in determining what the patient would have done if given a more informed choice.

Defenses to the informed consent doctrine

Three exceptions exist to the doctrine of informed consent: *emergency*, *waiver*, and *therapeutic privilege*. These exceptions recognize society's interest in promoting health, protecting others, and protecting the individual. An emergency is presumed in circumstances where immediate action is required and consent is implied. This occurs when the individual is incapable of giving and/or receiving information, and time is critical.

Patients may waive their right to informed consent. Patients may be so apprehensive of what they might hear, that they would prefer the doctor to make the decision for them. To waive the right of informed consent, the patient must be aware that the right exists. Patients need to be aware of the doctor's duty to disclose, their own right to make a decision, by either consenting to or refusing the treatment, and the doctor's inability to do anything without this consent.

A physician may also withhold information, if in his or her opinion it would be harmful to the patient. This is known as the therapeutic privilege. When risk disclosure poses such a threat of detriment to the patient as to become unfeasible or contraindicated from a medical point of view, the physician has no duty to disclose. The patient may become so ill or emotionally distraught on disclosure as to foreclose a rational decision, or complicate or hinder the treatment, or perhaps even pose psychological damage to the patient. "The critical inquiry is whether the physician responded to a sound medical judgment that communication of the risk information would present a threat to the patient's well-being" [8]. The standard for this exception is determined by what the competent and responsible physician would have done in similar circumstances.

Courts do not apply the therapeutic privilege too liberally. Physicians should not be able to invoke the therapeutic privilege simply because they believe the patient will refuse the treatment. Physicians that rely on the therapeutic privi-

lege should advise the patient's spouse or close family members of the proposed treatment.

Informed consent today

Informed consent remains a controversial and often poorly understood topic among physicians. However, in reality the doctrine rarely provides the sole cause of action for a prevailing plaintiff. The claim is usually coupled with a cause of action in negligent malpractice. Yet, the importance of the doctrine should encourage increased interpersonal relationships between the physician and patient. The litigation potential alone should encourage all physicians to secure some form of informed consent from their patients themselves. At least 26 states have adopted some type of informed consent statute. Twelve follow a professional standard, six a lay standard, and eight are silent on the standard of disclosure.

Many physicians do not obtain an informed consent from their patients. Physicians' arguments against obtaining informed consent break down into several categories:
1 physicians argue that patients want their doctors to decide for them;
2 patients would not understand or might misuse the information;
3 such information would emotionally harm the patient and lead to refusals;
4 the informed consent procedure itself is too burdensome [9].
Their main complaint is that it takes too much time, and it is not cost effective adequately to inform patients. This resistance to obtaining informed consent undermines the doctrine. Courts have strongly stated that competent adults have the right to decide what is medically done to their bodies. While legally valid informed consent dialog may be time consuming, medical care providers and patients will both benefit from its observance.

Informed consent in California

The dispositive case for California's treatment of informed consent is *Cobbs* v. *Grant* [10]. This case examined the physician's scope of duty to disclose information regarding proposed medical procedures. The plaintiff went to the hospital, seeking treatment for a duodenal ulcer. Although the physician/defendant explained the nature of the operation to the plaintiff, he did not disclose the inherent risks of the surgery. After he was released from the hospital, the plaintiff began to experience severe pain, and was later readmitted. The plaintiff subsequently underwent three additional operations, his spleen was removed, and he developed another ulcer. The resultant injuries the plaintiff suffered were all inherent risks of the original operation. The California Supreme Court held that as

[A]n integral part of the physician's overall obligation to the patient there is a duty of reasonable disclosure of the available choices with respect to proposed therapy and of the dangers inherently and potentially involved in each [10].

The court in *Cobbs* v. *Grant* identified certain characteristics of the physician–patient relationship that necessitate a fully informed consent.

1 Patients are generally persons unlearned in the medical sciences and therefore, except in rare cases, courts may safely assume the knowledge of the patient and the physician are not in parity.

2 A person of adult years and in sound mind has the right, in the exercise of control over his or her own body, to determine whether or not to submit to lawful medical treatment.

3 The patient's consent to treatment, to be effective, must be an informed consent.

4 The patient, being unlearned in medical sciences, has an abject dependence upon and trust in his or her physician for the information upon which he/she relies during the decisional process, thus raising an obligation in the physician that transcends arms-length transactions.

The court concluded that from these ingredients emerged the necessary and resultant requirement that the physician divulge to his or her patient all information relevant to a meaningful decision-making process. Therefore, the duty reasonably to disclose the available choices with respect to a proposed therapy, and of the dangers inherently and potentially involved in each, is an integral part of the physician's overall obligation to the patient.

The court in *Cobbs* v. *Grant* went on to address the issue of what standard to apply when determining the reasonableness of disclosure. While noting that the majority's rule professional standard was too broad, the court adopted the standard announced in *Canterbury* v. *Spence*. The court reasoned that allowing unlimited discretion to the physician is irreconcilable with the basic right of the patient to make the ultimate informed decision regarding the course of treatment to which they knowledgably consent to be subjected. The court clarified their holding, stating that the patient's interest in information does not extend to a mini course in medical science, and the physician has no duty to discuss the relatively minor risks inherent in common procedures. "The scope of the physician's communications to the patient, then, must be measured by the patient's need, and that need is whatever information is material to the decision" [10].

The court in *Cobbs* v. *Grant* applied the objective test of what a prudent person in the patient's position would have decided if adequately informed of all significant perils. On the issue of causality, they found this standard would better serve justice by not placing the physician in jeopardy of the patient's bitterness and disillusionment. The court concluded

their analysis by setting out the defenses available to a physician who fails to make the disclosure required by law: patient waiver, emergency situations, therapeutic privilege, and no need to disclose if the procedure is simple and the danger remote, and commonly appreciated to be remote.

The California Supreme Court has extended informed consent to diagnostic tests, giving rise to the "informed refusal" doctrine. This doctrine was first enunciated in *Truman* v. *Thomas* [11], a medical malpractice action brought for the wrongful death of decedent (patient). The pertinent issue before the court, was whether the failure to inform the patient of the material risks of refusing a recommended pap smear may have breached the physician's duty of due care to his or her patient, who subsequently died from cancer of the cervix. During the 6-year period that the defendant physician saw the decedent, he recommended a pap smear to her several times, which she refused, stating she could not afford the cost. The defendant testified that he did not specifically inform his patient of the risk involved for failure to undergo a pap smear.

The court in *Truman* v. *Thomas* reaffirmed their holding in *Cobbs* v. *Grant*, defining materiality as any information that the physician knows or should know would be regarded as significant by a reasonable person in the patient's position, when deciding to accept or reject the recommended medical procedure. The court extended their rule in *Cobbs* v. *Grant*, that states that a patient must be apprised not only of the risks inherent in the procedure, but also the risks of a decision not to undergo the treatment, to apply whether the procedure involves treatment or a diagnostic test. Under *Cobbs* v. *Grant*, it appears that if a patient indicates that he or she is going to decline a risk-free test or treatment, the physician has the additional duty of advising the patient of all material risks of which a reasonable person would want to be informed of before deciding not to undergo the treatment or test. If the recommended test or treatment is itself risky, then the physician should always explain the potential consequences of declining to follow the recommended course of action.

The defendant physician in *Truman* v. *Thomas*, argued that the rules laid down in *Cobbs* v. *Grant* did not apply to him because the duty to disclose applies only where the patient consents to the recommended procedure. This rationale would require patients who reject their physician's advice, to shoulder the burden of inquiring as to the possible consequences of their decision. The majority found this argument inconsistent with *Cobbs* v. *Grant*, which held that the duty to disclose is to be imposed so that patients might meaningfully exercise their right to make decisions about their own bodies. "The importance of this right should not be diminished by the manner in which it is exercised. Furthermore, the need for disclosure is not lessened because patients reject a recommended procedure" [11]. To hold otherwise would imply that patients who reject their physician's advice have the burden of inquiry as to the potential consequences of their decisions.

The dissent in *Truman* v. *Thomas* argued that the majority's holding will impose upon physician's the intolerable burden of having to inform healthy patients about existing diagnostic tests. They found this burden undesirable because physicians will have to spend the greater part of their day not examining or treating patients, but explaining to them all information relevant to the purposes of diagnostic examinations and tests. "In short, today's ruling mandates doctors to provide each such patient with a summary course covering most of his or her medical education" [11]. The dissent hypothesized that by requiring physicians to spend a large portion of their time teaching medical science, the cost of medical diagnosis would greatly increase, and would ultimately be borne by an unwanting public.

> Persons desiring treatment for specific complaints will be deterred from seeking advice once they realize they will be charged not only for treatment, but also for lengthy lectures on the merits of their examination [11].

The dissent further criticized the majority's ruling, finding nothing in *Cobbs* v. *Grant* that warranted the imposition of such an onerous duty. The dissent interprets Cobbs as expressly rejecting any such duty, because the decision circumscribed the duty of the physician, holding that a: "mini-course in medical science is not required," and that:

> there is no physician's duty to discuss the relatively minor risks inherent in common procedures, when it is common knowledge that such risks inherent in the procedure are of very low incidence [12].

The dissent went on to comment that the holding in *Cobbs* v. *Grant* is not useful to the majority, because the duty of disclosure in that case was imposed to assure that consent to the intrusion would be effective. The dissent concluded that this new duty to explain, imposed by the majority as a matter of law, creates an undue burden on both the physician and society, and should be rejected.

> The great educational program the majority embarked upon, even if justifiable, is a question of public policy for the Legislature to determine whether the cost warrants the burden, and whether the duty to educate rests with doctors, schools, or health departments [13].

Physicians practicing in California must be made aware that they practice in a full disclosure or reasonable patient jurisdiction. Subsequent courts have followed *Truman* v. *Thomas*, and now, as a matter of law, physicians have a duty to disclose to their patients all material information that will enable them to make an informed decision regarding the acceptance or refusal of a recommended procedure or diagnostic test [14]. Physicians should also keep in mind that California maintains the traditional three exceptions to the informed consent doctrine (i.e., emergency, waiver and therapeutic privilege).

Iodinated contrast media
(see also Chapter 13)

A study in 1988 [15] on the frequency and severity of malpractice claims reported that informed consent was a major factor in the increased number of malpractice claims that led to the malpractice crisis of the 1970s. Radiologists have numerous brief patient encounters each day; therefore, it is essential that they comply with the informed consent doctrine for the jurisdiction in which they practice. The diagnostic radiologist is routinely faced with the issue of informed consent, due to the performance of angiography and interventional procedures which warrant the obtaining of informed consent. One of the most controversial topics in radiology today involves the use of informed consent prior to the intravascular administration of radiopaque iodinated contrast media.

Each year in the USA alone, approximately 10 million radiographic procedures are performed that require an intravascular injection of contrast media. Until recently, all contrast injections were made with iodinated high-osmolality contrast media (HOCM). Iodinated contrast media have been utilized by radiologists for intravascular injections over 60 years. The evolution and acceptance of these agents was predicated on the continued introduction of newer and better tolerated iodinated high-osmolality contrast agents. These iodinated compounds are of great diagnostic value. However, the incidence of minor, severe, and fatal reactions following injection cannot be ignored [15]. The first LOCM was developed in Europe in the late 1960s. Following clinical trials in the USA, three LOCM were approved by the Food and Drug Administration in 1986. LOCM were touted as safer alternates to HOCM, with fewer side-effects and potentially fewer fatal reactions. Numerous studies in the USA and Europe have demonstrated essentially equal efficacy of HOCM and LOCM for producing diagnostic contrast examinations, with LOCM demonstrating reduction of both minor and major adverse reactions when compared to HOCM. Reactions are classified as mild, moderate, or severe. Mild reactions, such as heat sensation and nausea, usually do not require treatment; moderate reactions require some sort of treatment and pharmaceutical intervention; and severe reactions, such as cardiovascular collapse, cardiopulmonary arrest, or severe respiratory arrest require intensive treatment and may result in fatality. Numerous studies indicate that LOCM cause fewer nonsevere reactions than HOCM [16]. Patients who receive LOCM have been shown to experience decreased heat sensation, fewer episodes of nausea and vomiting, and less anxiety than those receiving HOCM. However, most patients in the studies experienced some form of discomfort regardless of the media used. The studies also indicate a lower incidence of severe reactions in those patients injected with LOCM as compared to those patients injected with HOCM. The incidence of severe reactions ranged from 0 to

0.26% in patients who received LOCM, compared to 0.06–1.73% in patients who received HOCM [16].

Studies have also shown that the incidence of death associated with the administration of HOCM averages approximately one in every 40 000 patients [17]. A difference of opinion remains as to what is the incidence of death after injection of LOCM. One study indicates that the death rate is probably closer to one in 300 000 [18]. However, many authors feel that the death rate data for LOCM compared to HOCM is insufficient to make conclusions about whether the use of LOCM leads to a reduction in fatal reactions. A statistically large data pool is needed to quantify differences in death rates. The marked decrease in severe reactions while using LOCM theoretically should lead to fewer LOCM-related fatalities. This is the conumdrum radiologists should keep in mind.

Radiologists seem to agree, were it not for the 10–15-fold greater cost of LOCM compared to HOCM, all intravascular contrast examinations would be performed with LOCM. Based on sales of contrast agents in 1988, it was estimated that LOCM were used in 15–20% of all intravascular contrast injections [17]. Usage today exceeds 60%, with a number of medical facilities converting to 100% LOCM usage for intravascular contrast administrations (personal communication).

Because of the high cost of LOCM, compromises between health cost containment forces and sound medical usage doctrine have been urged. Identification of high-risk patients who may benefit from the selective administration of LOCM has been central to numerous comparative contrast studies. Confusing this attempt at compromise between fiscal and medical policies was the discovery of a paradox; high-risk patients receiving LOCM were less likely to suffer adverse reactions than low-risk patients receiving HOCM [19]. Current guidelines of The Committee on Drugs and Contrast Media of the Commission on Education of the American College of Radiology advise the use of LOCM under the following circumstances [20]:

1 patients with a history of a previous adverse reaction to contrast material, with the exception of a sensation of heat, flushing, or a single episode of nausea or vomiting;
2 patients with a history of asthma or allergy;
3 patients with known cardiac dysfunction, including recent or potentially imminent cardiac decompensation and pulmonary hypertension;
4 patients with generalized severe debilitation;
5 any other circumstances where, after due consideration, the radiologist believes there is a specific indication for the use of LOCM.

Some radiologists recommend the use of LOCM for all patients undergoing contrast studies. Some studies have suggested that a patient previously considered to be at high risk for a severe contrast reaction, was less at risk for a severe adverse reaction if given LOCM, than a low-risk individual given HOCM [21]. One study concluded that a high-risk patient is anybody who receives HOCM [19].

The doctrine of informed consent raises two issues concerning the use of contrast media. First, must the radiologist inform his or her patients of the risk for severe and fatal reactions? Second, should the radiologist inform his or her patients of the existence of LOCM, a safer, yet more expensive alternate?

Informed consent for all contrast-media injections

Until recently, the issue of informed consent central to a malpractice case most often arose in vascular or interventional procedures that were complicated by adverse or unexpected results. Successful malpractice actions centered on lack of sufficient informed consent related to the administration of contrast media were few and far between. The rarity of successful lawsuits, coupled with the volume of radiologic examinations requiring the administration of contrast media and the radiologist's time required to obtain the informed consent, has resulted in significant divisiveness among practicing radiologists about the importance of obtaining informed consent from patients before administering intravenous contrast material. Some radiologists feel that by informing their patients of the risks involved they will cause anxiety, and this will affect the success of the procedure. Studies suggest otherwise. One study surveyed 902 patients to learn their opinions about the use of written informed consent for intravenous contrast-enhanced procedures [22]. The results indicated that only 23% of the patients reported feeling more anxious about the procedure following a risk disclosure that included a description of moderate reaction symptoms and the slight possibility of death. Ninety per cent of the patients indicated a preference for having information about the risks, while an overwhelming majority of the patients (98–99%) who were informed of the risks and the benefits elected to receive the contrast-material injection.

A key issue is, to what degree should the patient be informed about the dangers inherent in contrast agents? An obvious problem is whether the patient needs to be informed of the approximately one in 40 000 to one in 300 000 risk of death associated with intravenous injection of the various types of contrast media. There also exists the one in 10 000–20 000 risk of a major nonfatal cardiopulmonary or renal reaction. The answer to this question depends on whether the radiologist practices in a "reasonable physician" or a "reasonable patient" jurisdiction. While these risks appear remote, the decision whether they are "material risks" which mandate informed consent, is determined state by state.

In a *reasonable physician jurisdiction*, the radiologist needs to inform the patient of the risks and complications that reasonable physicians under similar circumstances in a similar locality would elucidate. This issue was raised in *Hook* v.

Rothstein [23]. In this case, an action was brought for the wrongful death of a patient, allegedly caused by the radiologist's failure to inform the patient of the potential fatal risks involved in an intravenous pyelogram (IVP). The court of appeals affirmed the lower court's judgment in favor of the radiologist, holding that the radiologist's duty to disclose material risks is governed by those communications a reasonable radiologist would have made under the same or similar circumstances.

In *Hook* v. *Rothstein*, the patient was advised to undergo an IVP. Although the patient suffered from many allergies, he did not inform the radiologist when asked if he suffered any (patients with a history of either asthma or allergies have a greater risk of reaction to contrast media). The radiologist testified that he did not inform the patient about the approximate one in 40 000 possibility of suffering a fatal reaction, because he was convinced that the patient's apprehension would play a significant role in causing a contrast reaction. Shortly after the injection, the patient suffered a severe reaction and died.

The court in *Hook* v. *Rothstein* began its analysis by noting that under the doctrine of informed consent, the physician has a duty to disclose: (i) the diagnosis; (ii) the general nature of the contemplated procedure; (iii) the material risks involved in the procedure; (iv) the probability of success; (v) the prognosis if the procedure is not carried out; and (vi) the existence of any alternates to the procedure [23]. The court emphasized what they viewed as the weakness of the reasonable patient standard: the notion that the decision to disclose is a nonmedical one, and can be appraised by the jury without the aid of, or in opposition to, expert medical testimony. The court decided that the scope of the radiologist's duty to disclose risks is measured by those communications a reasonable radiologist would have disclosed under the same or similar circumstances. The plaintiff has the burden to establish the standard of care by expert testimony.

If most radiologists believe it is not in the patient's best interest to be made aware of the possibility of an adverse reaction to contrast media, the *reasonable physician standard* will not require physicians to inform their patients of these risks. The requirements of disclosure could be quite different in a *reasonable patient jurisdiction*, because a reasonable person could well want to know about a one in 40 000 chance of death. They would even more likely want to be informed of the one in 10 000 chance of a severe nonfatal reaction. A jury would determine whether a reasonable person would want these risks disclosed. However, in *Smith* v. *Shannon* [23], the court held that every minute risk does not need to be disclosed, because the informed consent doctrine does not place upon the physician a duty to elucidate upon all of the possible risks.

Smith v. *Shannon* involved a medical malpractice action where the plaintiff claimed negligent treatment and failure to obtain informed consent. Prior to an IVP examination, the defendant physician informed the plaintiff that she might become nauseous, flushed, or unconscious. However, the radiologist did not inform her of the 10 other risks listed in a widely used physician drug reference (*The Physician's Desk Reference*). The Washington Supreme Court allowed the jury's verdict, which found that lack of disclosure of these risks was not material under the reasonable patient standard.

HOCM versus LOCM: should the patient be informed?

The issue of informed consent has become an even more important consideration for radiologists with the introduction of LOCM. While it is generally agreed that LOCM lessen the frequency and severity of reactions, many radiologists do not feel that there is a need for routine use in all patients. This is solely because of greater cost compared to HOCM. Two schools of thought for the use of LOCM have emerged: one advocates universal usage of LOCM, thereby decreasing the risk of adverse reactions in all patients; the other advocates the use of LOCM for patients who are identified as high risk for having an adverse reaction to contrast media. The latter standard begs the following question: "If an alternate is limited to high-risk patients, can a physician be held liable for failure to inform a low-risk patient of the alternate?"

All states require that the physician obtains the patient's simple consent before proceeding with a procedure or treatment. In jurisdictions that use the *reasonable physician* approach, the radiologist should inquire as to whether his or her colleagues are informing their patients about the risks and complications of intravenous contrast injections, and if they are, what complications or alternates are being disclosed. If most radiologists are not informing their low-risk patients about LOCM, there should be no liability for failure to do so. However, the court could decide that the risk of suffering an adverse reaction is so great, that the radiology profession as a whole is behaving unreasonably for failing to advise patients about LOCM.

When LOCM is used on a selective basis in *reasonable patient* jurisdictions for high-risk patients only, low-risk patients who are to receive HOCM should, in our opinion, be informed that an alternate contrast agent is available. In California, the courts have made it clear that alternates must be disclosed [24]. Based on such direction from the court, radiologists may be obligated to inform the patient about the availability of LOCM, and how, at a greater expense, the already small risk of an adverse reaction may be further reduced by use of LOCM. A reasonable patient would likely want to know relative-risk information, i.e., information on how much potentially lower their risk of having a major or minor adverse reaction to the contrast media would be.

Studies indicate that very few patients refuse the contrast

injection altogether or request LOCM when they are designated low risk, after being fully informed of the relative-risk information [25]. In a survey of 500 patients who received intravenous contrast, fewer than 1% of the patients refused the examination, and less than 1% of the low-risk patients requested LOCM after reviewing a detailed consent form. The consent form contained the following information:

1 the minor and major adverse effects that could occur;
2 the fact that some patients are at higher risk for contrast reactions;
3 that LOCM can lower this risk;
4 that LOCM is used for high-risk patients;
5 why routine HOCM use is recommended for low-risk patients;
6 that LOCM is more expensive and that the patient's insurance may not cover LOCM use.

So far, the courts that have considered whether alternates need be disclosed have not addressed the issue when procedures are limited by cost or customary practice. Some commentators argue that alternates that are prohibitively expensive or restricted to certain high-risk categories should not be a part of informed consent [15]. Their argument is based on the premise that although the patient must be informed of all anticipated material risks and other reasonably available therapeutic alternates, it is doubtful that every potential alternate, regardless of its proven safety, effectiveness, or cost, should be noted in obtaining informed consent. This assumption is based on the premise that patients will have no incentive to reject LOCM as an alternate. They argue that such a result would stretch the concept of informed consent well beyond that which is necessary for a patient to evaluate the range of medical practice decisions and maintain self-determination.

It is doubtful that every potential alternative, regardless of its proven safety, effectiveness or cost, should be evaluated by the patient. Otherwise, the patient's right to be informed compromises the medical profession's responsibility for medical practice decisions and resource allocating, and is a severe limitation on cost containment. Some commentators feel that the legal system should not act as a barrier to a strategy that limits LOCM to high-risk patients. "The ability to define and limit what is acceptable medical innovation rests first, as it should, with the medical profession itself" [26]. To us this reasoning appears contrary to the foundation of the informed consent doctrine in a reasonable patient jurisdiction.

Cost containment

The problem of social justice and access to health care is essentially moral and political. There are those who feel that professional medical and legal expertise cannot, and should not provide society with answers about how scarce resources should be distributed, any more than it should provide answers about individual utilization regarding medical choice [7]. For decades, medicine has been dominated by a "spare-no-expense" philosophy that fostered an ethic of providing all the care that was of any conceivable benefit regardless of the cost [27]. However, this situation is now changing rapidly. The progress achieved during the past 30 years in improving the quality and availability of medical care has been accompanied by a drastic increase in the overall cost of health care delivery. Today, the public's attention is focused on cost containment. Before the 1980s, quality and access to medical care were the chief concerns of USA health care law. Recently, another concern has emerged as the primary focus of health care policy: controlling the exorbitant and escalating costs of providing access to high-quality health care. The rising costs in health care have threatened the viability of both public and private health care programs, prompting vigorous efforts by government, health insurers, and corporations to contain their expenditures. As a result, the financial structure of health care delivery is being overhauled with such changes as prospective payment plans, managed care plans, and subtle restriction of access to costly medical intervention by medical review and utilization programs.

In 1965, Americans spent $41.9 billion on health care. By 1985, this amount had risen more than 10-fold to $425 billion, and by 1990 almost 15-fold to $600 billion. Six per cent of the country's gross national product was devoted to health care in 1965. Today, the figure is over 11% [28]. The governmental component of health care expenditures has increased even more dramatically. In 1965, the federal government spent $5.5 billion on health care. In 1985, the amount was over $124 billion. Over 10% of the federal budget is devoted to health care. Federal Medicare payments today account for 40% of all hospital revenues [28].

The explosion in health care expenditures can be attributed to increases in physicians' fees, high profit overhead of private insurance companies, the expansion of expensive medical technology, the corporatization of health care, and the overconsumption of health care by patients [29]. Economists argue that conventional health insurance systems intrinsically encourage the overutilization of health care. Patients are not sensitized to costs because they bear little of the increased costs associated with high consumption of health care. As expensive technologies emerge, virtually unlimited third-party reimbursement encourages physicians to provide their patients with all services that promise potential benefit. Conventional third-party retrospective payment plans encourage the waste of health care resources by allowing physicians to practice "defensive medicine", the ordering of necessary and unnecessary diagnostic treatments as potential protection from malpractice claims in a litigious society. How many diagnostic procedures of questionable merit would not be performed if insurance companies refused to reimburse for them?

For the first time, hospitals, physicians, and other health

care providers are being pressured to do less for patients, to perform more procedures on an outpatient basis, and to discharge hospitalized patients earlier. A variety of cost-containment programs have emerged on the scene as potential policies for deterring the continued escalation of health care costs. Congress responded to the problem of rising costs by implementing a new system of prospective payment in 1983. Reimbursement for treating a Medicare patient is no longer retrospectively based on the hospital's actual costs and the physician's reasonable charges. Under this prospective payment system (PPS), hospital reimbursement for patient care is calculated prospectively by formula [28].

The reimbursement formula used by Medicare is determined by the hospital's case mix, as defined by the federally mandated Diagnosis-Related Group (DRG). Each Medicare patient admitted into a facility is assigned a DRG and the hospital's reimbursement is determined by this classification, regardless of the patient's actual length of stay or resource consumption. The reimbursement paid to the provider bears no relationship to the costs actually incurred, but directly corresponds to the patient's particular diagnosis and illness. If the patient ultimately consumes more resources than the amount reimbursed under the assigned DRG, the hospital must absorb the additional cost. On the other hand, if the patient requires less treatment than the DRG allots, the facility keeps the profit. The permissible pocketing by the provider of any reimbursement payment that exceeds its cost of care is a greatly needed incentive for the provider to implement cost-containment policies. To survive financially, hospitals and physicians must operate within the bands of prospective reimbursement levels: real costs must not exceed the current DRG reimbursement rates overall. The PPS has proven effective in reducing the amount of hospital services consumed by Medicare patients [29]. More drastic, wider changes, focussing on stricter, population-based capitation, are currently occurring.

The legal implications of cost containment

The new systems of reimbursement may significantly alter the physician's financial incentives regarding the provision of health care. Under the traditional fee-for-service reimbursement system, the more services the physician performed, the more he or she would be paid. Under Medicare's PPS, where the reimbursement rate is predetermined, the physician's allegiance to the patient's best medical interest is no longer undivided. Today, physicians are often forced to make cost/benefit trade-offs in many patient treatment decisions. The important issue now is the possibility of patient injury because of inadequate health care due to cost containment.

Medical malpractice actions have grown tremendously in recent years, both in number and in expense. One reason why physician liability for malpractice has burgeoned is that the standard of care in malpractice cases has grown more exacting. This higher standard can be attributed to several factors. Among these factors are physicians' training and professional outlook, advances in medical technology, incentives created by third-party payments, and the public's high expectation of medical success and cure with an exaggerated perception of the nature of medical care. The added perception is that medical malpractice actions are a recourse for the medical consumer who's expectations were not met. As the medical profession's technologic capability increases, the legal standard of care becomes more stringent. An egalitarian ethic regarding access to health services influences standards of care, which require hospitals and physicians to adhere to a unitary standard, regardless of the patient's financial position. Juries may take a dim view of a physician's and/or a hospital's decision to forego available means of care because of financial constraints.

Pressure to conform to the existing standard of care, induced by the fear of being sued and found liable, may have led some physicians to practice defensive medicine in order to guard against liability. The American Medical Association estimates that the annual cost of defensive medicine has grown to roughly $15 billion [30]. The ceiling placed by Medicare on patient care reimbursement will force hospitals to bear overutilization costs, and may discourage the practice of defensive medicine. Cost-cutting measures are sure to bring about tension between the hospital and the physician, as health care providers attempt to bring their aggregate costs within prospective rate setting guidelines, while maintaining professional standards of care in individual cases.

The elimination of unnecessary services poses no ethical dilemma. However, reducing services of marginal benefit, potential or real may threaten the quality of care and the patient's best interests. The quality of patient care will largely be determined by the professional standard of care applicable under the physician's duty to treat. Any compromise of the quality of care in a given situation will have to be resolved within the corresponding standard of care applicable to that situation. The question remains: "How should health care's economic revolution affect the legal standard of care that physicians owe to their patients?" The four elements the patient—plaintiff must prove against the physician—defendant in malpractice litigation are:

1 the physician owed a duty to the patient to ensure that his or her medical care measured up to certain standards of quality;
2 the physician's care violated this standard;
3 the patient suffered an injury;
4 the breach of duty caused the injury.

Do cost constraints provide sufficient grounds for exonerating physicians of their responsibilities to meet the standard of care? What about physicians in inner city public hospitals who may be so economically strapped that they are compelled to use costly interventions more sparingly than their better-funded colleagues in private hospitals?

Medical malpractice law is designed to achieve quality assurance and victim compensation. Cost-containment policies have an impact on the standard of care as physicians and hospitals seek to implement cost-saving policies such as early discharge of patients, and restrictions on costly diagnostic tests and treatment. The physician who, by keeping within the hospital's guidelines, declines to order certain costly tests or treatments that are routinely ordered by other physicians, runs a calculated risk that a harmed patient will successfully recover damages in a malpractice suit. Unless the physician can show that a respectable minority of practitioners practice similar rationing of health care resources under similar circumstances, a decision to ration may expose the practitioner to the risk of malpractice liability [31].

Some commentators hypothesize that the pressures of cost containment will cause medical care standards to shift downward, reflecting a diminished intensity of resource use. The tort system, viewed as a mirror of this standard of practice, will simply reflect this downward shift [32]. If this is the case, the physician may be at no more risk for liability after cost-containment policies, such as PPS, are implemented, than he or she was before. However, this transition period worries many physicians and commentators since the risk of liability may be temporarily increased until equilibrium is achieved. It is equally likely that new standards will not emerge, because these standards would have to replace or undo the large body of medical law that embraces such medicolegal issues as misdiagnosis, failure to diagnose, informed consent, and patient abandonment. This would require a change in the professional norms upon which these standards rest and it is highly unlikely that the medical profession will subscribe to norms that might threaten patient care or endanger the deeper sense of medical professionalism [33].

E. Haavi Morreim [34], a leading commentator on the legal and ethical impact of health care cost containment, has proposed the use of cost constraints as a malpractice defense. She suggests that the legal concept of "rebuttable presumption" be used to reconceive the traditional requirement of a uniform standard of care. She bases her arguments on the premise that so long as society refuses to provide fully adequate resources for the health care of the poor, yet demands that adequate care be rendered, physicians as primary medical decision makers stand to be held personally liable for a problem not of their own making.

Morreim points out the inadequacy of traditional medical malpractice law. She first examines the locality rule, which holds that it is unfair to apply the same standards of care to physicians who practice in rural areas, and have limited access to the opportunities for learning that are available to professionals in larger cities. Today, the locality rule has been for the most part abandoned, since standardized education and board certification have largely eliminated the regional differences of competence within various medical specialties. However, when there exists a difference in physical facilities, services, and resources, physicians are not held to a nationwide standard of care.

This bifurcated locality rule does not address the issue of cost constraints. Where the indigent patient is denied desirable diagnostic procedures or treatments on the grounds of cost, the locality rule would have to cover both the unavailability of resources and the conscious decision to refrain from using available resources. Morreim argues that the locality rule was never intended to stretch this far. Contrary to Morreim's argument, application of the locality rule to today's health care crisis would be consistent to the way it was applied historically. The locality rule was based upon the realistic appraisal of limits under which physicians practice, and the ways in which these limits constrain the care.

The second legal concept Morreim discusses concerns physician standard of care. This standard is usually specified by the prevailing custom of practice. She proposes the idea that since physicians set their own standards, they can collectively trim them. It is not clear how a reduction in the standard of care could be initiated. The courts will accept new standards only if they serve patient welfare at least as well as prevailing practices. Physicians who dare to compromise the quality of care in the name of cost, do so at their peril, because the law currently does not accept a direct economic justification for substandard care. Besides, the plaintiff will surely be able to find expert testimony of what a reasonable physician would have done.

Morreim concluded that existing legal concepts are not adequate to resolve the conflict brought on by cost-cutting measures; therefore, she proposed that the uniform legal standard of care should give way to a rebuttable presumption. Current case law stipulates that physicians give all patients the same basic standard of care, regardless of their financial resources. Morreim suggests that the law offer economically pressed physicians some opportunity to rebut this presumption, by demonstrating the particular nature and severity of their financial constraints. Physicians would be able to eliminate useless and highly marginal interventions in order to extend limited resources as far as possible. The physician would be required under this rebuttable presumption standard to justify the general allocation policies that guided his or her decision, and the appropriateness of applying those principles to this patient. The ruling concept in describing the physician's burden of rebuttal would be reasonableness, the central value in tort law.

Morreim's rebuttable presumption doctrine can be criticized on several grounds. First, it allows the issue of cost constraint to be an element of the primary standard of care.

When this cost issue is raised, there is a shift of inquiry from the prevailing custom, to a direct assessment of the net social welfare of performing a particular test or procedure. This approach is at odds with the current state of the law, which maintains that anyone who undertakes to provide health care assumes the absolute duty to provide adequate health care [35].

When Morreim assessed the current state of medical malpractice law, she assumed that it was incapable, within its present framework, of responding to changed social circumstances. On the contrary, since the law mimics the medical profession, as the health care sector is forced to take costs seriously, the law will reflect this concern. Physicians as a group are better qualified than judges or juries to address technical and scientific questions of medical appropriateness. Certain forces will constrain the health care sector from departing too far from what is medically best for the patient. These include:

1 professional ethics;
2 professional prestige;
3 competition for patients [27].

While Morreim feels that the current state of medical malpractice law will not accept a diminution of care in response to financial constraints, there are others who feel that existing law is perfectly capable of incorporating cost-sensitive medical decisions within its existing doctrinal framework. They argue that significant savings are possible without departure from existing practice patterns [27]. The existing standards are broad enough; all that is needed is a relative shift toward the more conservative end. The primary mechanism for incorporating cost constraints into the malpractice standard would be to redefine the concept of fault [36]. Cost-cutting behavior that was previously considered "negligent" might now be deemed socially desirable. Studies that establish the legitimacy of certain efforts to cut costs might be admitted as evidence of due care. This change would place the burden of cost-associated quality reduction on patients who might have won malpractice awards if not for the new cost-responsive standard of care.

Modifying the standard of care might intensify social inequities because the individuals most affected by modification would be the poor or the elderly. This goes against the basic premise that a single malpractice standard should govern the care of the rich and poor, the old and the young alike. If injuries would otherwise be compensatable under medical malpractice law, victims of medical mishaps should not, and probably will not, be denied compensation on the ground that their injuries resulted from cost-cutting measures, no matter how reasonable.

Current case law

A recent and much discussed case, *Wickline* v. *State of California* [37], portrayed the difficult circumstances phys-

icians must now face as they try to reconcile the conflict between adequate care and cost containment. This case represents the first attempt to tie a health care payor into the medical malpractice causation chain. In this case, a patient brought action against Medi-Cal, California's medical assistance program, following the amputation of her leg as a result of an alleged premature hospital discharge. The trial court entered judgment on jury verdict in favor of the patient, and the State appealed. The Court of Appeal reversed the judgment.

Plaintiff—patient was admitted to the hospital for problems associated with her back and legs. A specialist determined that her condition was so far advanced that it was necessary to bypass a part of an artery, using a synthetic graft. Since plaintiff was eligible for medical benefits under Medi-Cal, her physicians requested and received authorization for the surgical procedure, with 10 days of hospitalization. On the day before she was to be released from the hospital following the successful operation, her physician concluded that it was medically necessary for the plaintiff to remain in the hospital for an additional 8 days. To secure an extension of hospital stay under Medi-Cal, the hospital had to complete and file a request form stating the reasons for the extension. The patient's diagnosis, significant medical history, clinical status, and treatment plan were then evaluated by a Medi-Cal representative. The Medi-Cal Consultant, a board certified general surgeon, rejected the physician's request for an 8-day hospital extension and, instead, authorized an additional 4 days. After this extension, plaintiff was discharged against her stated wishes. She returned to the hospital 9 days later, and subsequently had her leg amputated. It was her treating physician's opinion that had she remained in the hospital for the 8 additional days requested she would not have suffered the loss of her leg.

The plaintiff claimed that the State of California, as third-party payor, was legally responsible for her harm, because its cost-containment program was applied in such a manner that it affected the implementation of the treating physician's medical wishes. The principal issue before the court was: "Who is to bear the responsibility for allowing the patient to be discharged from the hospital, her physicians or the health care payor?" At the outset the court pointed out that stakes are much higher when a prospective cost-containment review process is utilized. An erroneous decision in the prospective review process may result in the withholding of necessary care which may lead to a patient's permanent disability or death [37].

The court in *Wickline* v. *State of California*, stated that third-party payers of health care services can be held legally responsible when medically inappropriate decisions result from defects in the implementation of cost-containment mechanisms. The court applied Title 22 of the California Administrative Code, Section 51110, which provides in part that the determination of need for acute care should be made in accordance with the usual standards of medical practice in the community. The expert testimony presented by both sides agreed that the physician's decision to discharge plaintiff met the standard of care applicable at the time. The Medi-Cal Consultant's decision, regarding the request to extend the patient's hospitalization, was in accord with the existing statutory law. Since Medi-Cal was not a party to the medical decision, it cannot be held liable for the harm resulting if such a decision was negligently made [37].

The court in *Wickline* v. *State of California*, stated in dicta:
[T]he physician who complies without protest with the limitations imposed by a third-party payer, when his medical judgment dictates otherwise, cannot avoid his ultimate responsibility for his patient's care. He cannot point to the health care payor as the liability scapegoat when the consequences of his own determinative medical decisions go sour [37].

The court emphasized that while cost consciousness has become a prominent feature of the health care system, it is essential that cost-limitation programs not be permitted to corrupt medical judgment. The court concluded, in this instance, that medical judgment was not corrupted [37].

According to the dicta stated in *Wickline* v. *State of California*, the pressures and constraints of a prospective evaluation of medical care costs will not be taken into account when the court assesses physician liability. The treating physician retains ultimate responsibility for the care of the patient. Jurors will tend to be unsympathetic towards physicians who have discharged a patient prematurely, or who have mismanaged a patient due to a concern for keeping costs down. The practice of medicine will be seen as subordinate to profit maximization. After *Wickline* v. *State of California*, physicians must carefully examine the terms and conditions of the agreements which they enter into with health insurers. Regardless of the conduct of the hospital policy makers or insurers, the physician's actions will be independently scrutinized to determine whether he or she did anything to jeopardize the quality of the patient's care. Physicians who permit an erosion of the quality of health care do so at their own peril. Physicians should be advocates for their patients through all levels of utilization review.

After *Wickline* v. *State of California*, the question remained as to what impact this decision would have on private insurers and the utilization review personnel who carry out similar cost containment procedures. *Wilson* v. *Blue Cross of Southern California* [38], provides a tentative answer to this question. In this case survivors of patient–decedent brought suit against the physicians, hospital, insurer, and the utilization review organization to recover damages for the patient who committed suicide after being involuntarily discharged due to discontinuation of insurance benefits. The lower court granted summary judgment for the defendants, and an appeal followed. The facts indicated that decedent was admitted to a hospital in Los Angeles, suffering from major depression, drug dependency, and anorexia. His treating physician determined that he needed 3–4 weeks of inpatient hospital care. At the recommendation of an independent utilization review organization, defendant Blue Cross refused to pay for the decedent to continue his hospital stay. Because the decedent could not afford to pay for additional care he was discharged. He committed suicide 20-days later.

At trial, the hospital, insurer, and utilization review organization prevailed on summary judgment motions, arguing that *Wickline* v. *State of California* stated a general rule that cost-containment procedures support important policy goals. The court of appeal held that the trial court incorrectly granted the summary judgment motions, because a triable issue existed as to whether the conduct of the decedent's insurance company and related entities was a substantial factor in causing the decedent's death. The key legal issue before the court was whether *Wickline* v. *State of California* extends beyond the context of Medi-Cal patients, to an insured under an insurance policy issued in the private sector. The court began its analysis by analyzing the holding in *Wickline* v. *State of California*. The court pointed out the three key legal components of *Wickline* v. *State of California*:
1 as a matter of law, the discharge decision in *Wickline* v. *State of California* met the standard of care for physicians;
2 the funding process was not pursuant to a contract, but to statutes and provisions of codes;
3 the cost-limitation program was not found to have corrupted medical judgment.

The utilization review organization relied on language in *Wickline* v. *State of California*, which stated that the exclusive responsibility for a discharge decision rests with the physician, even though an insurance company refuses to pay benefits. The court in *Wilson* v. *Blue Cross* disagreed, declaring that: "This broadly stated language was unnecessary to the decision and in all contexts does not correctly state the law relative to causation issues in a tort case" [38]. The holding relied on by defendants was dicta. Also, the evidence in *Wickline* v. *State of California* showed that the denial of benefits was consistent with the standard of care at the time, and was different from the present lawsuit. The court in *Wilson* v. *Blue Cross*, held that in this instance, there was substantial evidence that the decision not to approve further hospitalization was a substantial factor in the decedent's demise.

Since *Wilson* v. *Blue Cross* reversed a summary motion, its holding is limited. It is a triable issue of fact whether a private insurer breached its insurance contract by conducting utilization review. If an insured can prove he or she was injured as a result of a premature discharge or restrictive treatment, an issue of fact arises as to whether cost containment was conducted carefully and skillfully. It is also important to note that the court in *Wilson* v. *Blue Cross* held the language concerning physician liability in *Wickline* v. *State of California* to be dicta. The *Wilson* v. *Blue Cross* court failed to note the objectives and importance of cost containment in the private sector. The extension of a corporate negligence theory to private insurers would likely have a cooling effect on needed private cost-containment efforts.

The impact of cost containment on informed consent

The decision to contain medical costs raises difficult legal and ethical issues concerning informed consent. The physician's new incentive to limit medical resource consumption may tempt him or her to not inform patients about possible tests or procedures. The physician may determine that the cost of a procedure outweighs the potential benefits to the patient. However, consumers should participate in the implementation of cost-control measures as part of informed consent. When fully informed, patients may decline many types of recommended procedures or drugs, feeling that they are unnecessary or undesirable based on cost. Full patient autonomy might never be achieved if the physician alone is allowed to determine whether a procedure is too costly for any given patient.

Physicians who simply say nothing about potential treatments could find themself liable for failure to disclose information. The issue becomes: "Should the law protecting patient choice under informed consent theory change to accommodate the new cost-cutting incentives placed on physicians and hospitals?" Prospective reimbursement should increase, not decrease the physician's disclosure duties. When the decision to perform or omit treatment is based primarily on cost considerations rather than medical judgment, who is in a better position than the patient to make the final choice? The patient, not the physician, should decide what he or she can afford. Respect for personal autonomy requires physicians to disclose potentially beneficial treatments or procedures regardless of their cost. Let the patient decide whether the cost outweighs the benefit.

The fundamental values that underlie informed consent, patient self-determination and well-being, dictate that patients should have access to information they need to help them understand their condition, and to appreciate the medical options available. There is no reason to suggest that cost-containment policies that affect these medical options should not be an essential part of this information. The courts have recognized that nonmedical factors that are important to the patient's decision whether to undergo treatment exist. In *Truman* v. *Thomas* [11], the doctor failed to inform his patient of the medical cost or potential benefit of undergoing a pap smear test. Had the patient been made aware of the risks involved in foregoing such a test, she may have decided differently. These difficult personal financial choices must be made by the patient, on the basis of fully disclosed costs and benefits.

Any consideration of the content of the information to be disclosed, and a decision by the physician to adhere to an institution's cost-containment guidelines, must focus on the nature of the physician's duty to the patient [33]. In a *reasonable patient* jurisdiction, which focuses solely on the information a reasonable patient would want to know in order to make a decision, it is likely that patients would want to know about every alternate course of treatment, regardless of the cost-containment program established by the hospital. A failure on the part of the physician and hospital to disclose these alternates, could expose them to potential liability. Therefore, it would seem prudent for the physician under these circumstances carefully to explain to the patient the full ramifications of the hospital's guidelines, and to what extent available alternatives exist. In a reasonable physician jurisdiction, where the physician has to disclose information that a reasonable medical professional would deem to be material to the patient's decision, it is unlikely that cost-containment policies would influence the scope of the physician's duty to disclose.

Some commentators argue that the informed consent doctrine will exert powerful pressure on providers of health care to furnish patients with nonwasteful technology [39]. When cost information is furnished to patients as part of the informed consent process the patients must also be informed of the extent of their financial obligations, if any, for the available alternates. Burden should be placed on the provider to identify and disclose to the patient the conflicts cost constraints have created. This would give those patients who could afford it the option of paying for the technology themselves, and would facilitate patient challenges to prospective denials of treatment or reimbursement by third-party payers.

Cost constraints and contrast media

The introduction of LOCM is an issue ripe for cost-containment debate. The only major criticism of LOCM is cost. Contributing to the cost are the fees that must be paid to European pharmaceutical companies holding patents on LOCM, and the complexity of the process required for synthesis and purification [21]. Since they are expensive to produce, it is unlikely that their price will decrease drastically, even after USA companies are able to develop their own. Cost-conscious analysts paint a gloomy picture of the soaring costs a hospital might incur in just 1 year of exclusive LOCM use. Because LOCM is 10−20 times more expensive than HOCM, this problem is critical to radiologists and hospitals as reimbursement shrinks nationwide. LOCM raise a number of medical, economic, legal, and public policy questions relating to cost and benefit. One central issue is whether LOCM should be limited to identified high-risk patients, or adopted in all contrast injections. There is general agreement that, were it not for the huge cost increment of LOCM, all intravascular injections would be performed with LOCM.

The aggregate costs for complete LOCM conversion are considerable.

If LOCM were used for all contrast studies in the USA, the annual additional cost would be almost $1 billion [15]. If one performs a cost per saved life analysis, assuming a decrease in fatal reactions from one in 30 000 studies using HOCM, to one in 250 000 using LOCM, 293 fatal reactions would be prevented, and the cost per death averted would be $3.4 million. With a mean patient age of 46 years, and a life expectancy of 32 years, the cost per year of life saved would be $106 000. This cost per year of life saved is considerably higher than that of most screening or treatment programs in the USA, including hypertension ($30 000), hemodialysis for end-stage renal disease ($32 000), and coronary artery bypass grafting ($10 000). A similar cost−benefit analysis was done using LOCM exclusively on high-risk patients (15−20% of patients having contrast injections will fall in this category). The cost per year life saved for this group amounts to $31 250 [15]. The cost effectiveness of LOCM for this group is more reasonable.

This cost-effectiveness analysis suggests that LOCM should be limited in use to high-risk patients. Many medical commentators agree with this line of thinking. However, studies suggest that high-risk patients who receive LOCM are actually in a safer position than low-risk patients receiving HOCM [19,21]. A hospital's true cost for switching to exclusive use of LOCM is not just equal to the amount spent for the contrast agent. The marginal cost is the amount paid for LOCM, minus the cost that would have been incurred to treat side-effects had HOCM been used, minus whatever reimbursement is received for the additional cost of the agent. The cost of treating adverse reactions to contrast media should not be overlooked. When LOCM are used, the incidence of adverse reactions decreases, therefore, the cost incurred in treating these reactions will also decrease.

Some commentators feel that the exclusive use of LOCM will become a legal necessity. They argue that "cost considerations" will not hold up in court as a defense for using HOCM [21]. It would be hard to defend the case where a serious reaction occurred following the injection of HOCM, because of a $100−200 difference in cost. Whether a physician will be held liable for not using the safer LOCM depends on the standard dictated by the field of radiology. The radiologist who does not use LOCM for procedures on high-risk patients, could be held liable for medical negligence as this practice deviates from the standard of care. The problem is whether radiologists should use LOCM for their patients who are at low risk for suffering an adverse reaction. This issue is likely to be determined by the existing standard in the radiology community. Since the medical profession essentially sets its own standard of care, the customary and usual medical practice, it is important for radiologists to know what this standard is, and not just what their hospital allows.

If LOCM are limited in availability to high-risk patients, a low-risk patient may bring suit against the radiologist after suffering an adverse reaction, arguing that the radiologist was negligent in not using LOCM. The court will have to determine whether this usage falls within the customary bounds of practice. The patient may argue that the established custom falls below standards of negligence. The court will then have to determine whether the alternate standard of using LOCM for all injections is likely to provide additional protection to a degree justifying the costs. Even though low-risk patients would derive some additional benefit, this additional protection may not justify the costs. The courts must look at the aggregate costs, and not just the cost of a single episode. Applying the rationale of *Wickline* v. *State of California* [38], as long as cost containment does not corrupt medical judgment, limiting LOCM to high-risk patients is an appropriate balancing of cost limitations and medical judgment. It must be kept in mind that, after more than a decade of use in the USA, a claim based on such an argument has still not been put forward.

The standard of care could change as reimbursement levels change. If third-party payers are willing to reimburse for LOCM, radiologists will be more likely to use it exclusively. Would radiologists then appear guilty of practicing defensive medicine? They will use LOCM for low-risk patients to protect themselves from possible lawsuits, even though a cost−benefit analysis renders this use an unduly expensive expenditure. Radiologists may order the use of LOCM only for their low-risk patients who can either afford it, or for those patients whose insurers will reimburse for its use. This discriminating practice will deny other low-risk patients potential benefit.

Currently, most third-party payers cover LOCM use for certain indications. Reimbursement varies based on conditions set by individual insurance carriers. For instance, reimbursement by Medicare for LOCM depends on where the procedure takes place. Since Medicare reimbursement for hospital inpatients is based on DRGs, no distinction is made between the use of LOCM or HOCM in a given radiologic procedure. It is left to the hospital to set guidelines for its use. Payments to a hospital will not increase because it routinely uses LOCM for all procedures; however, frequent use of LOCM overall will be taken into account in recalibrating the DRGs. Blue Cross/Blue Shield plans reimburse the cost of LOCM for patients in certain risk factor categories. Kaiser health plans in Southern California after switching to 100% usage of LOCM, have changed to a policy of limited use in certain indications. In the current cost-containment environment, most insurers will probably follow the trend of Blue Cross/Blue Shield and require evidence of indication for LOCM use.

Informed consent

The threat of malpractice looms over the radiologist each time he or she must decide whether to use LOCM or HOCM for his or her patients. Should the radiologist inform the patient who is to receive HOCM of the costly alternative of LOCM, even though its use may not be reimbursable and the medical profession wishes to limit its use because of resource constraints? Since the frequency and severity of adverse reactions to HOCM are not always predictable, it is important for the radiologist to provide patients with the appropriate information so that they can make informed decisions regarding their health care. Some commentators feel that in view of current cost constraints, it is inappropriate to use informed consent to expand the range of medical practice beyond customary practice. "Alternatives that are prohibitively expensive or restricted to certain high risk categories should not be a part of informed consent" [15]. The choice becomes that of autonomy in medical decision making versus controlling escalating medical costs. So far, the courts have not answered this particular question in regard to contrast agents.

In jurisdictions using a reasonable patient standard, low-risk patients need to be informed that an alternate contrast agent exists, if LOCM is used on a selective basis only. Case law supports this proposition. One could hypothesize that informing these patients about LOCM is tantamount to giving it to them, especially if they are cost insensitive due to third-party reimbursement. However, several studies actually contradict this belief. A study was conducted at Johns Hopkins to determine the patient's willingness to pay to receive LOCM instead of HOCM. They found that the majority of patients studied were unwilling to pay the minimum extra per procedure price of LOCM ($50), in return for a reduced risk of minor side-effects, such as pain, nausea, hives, and flushing. However, patients were willing to pay the increased cost of LOCM in order to reduce major side-effects, such as severe allergic reactions and death [40].

Conclusion

Informed consent and cost-containment strategies pose difficult problems for the radiologist in regard to choosing whether to administer HOCM or LOCM. The use of LOCM for designated high-risk patients is strongly recommended by professional standards. If more and more radiologists and hospitals switch over to usage of LOCM for all patients, the standard of care will change. Radiologists may be held negligent for administering HOCM. This will lead to increasing expenditures for the hospital, especially if the use of LOCM goes unreimbursed. More studies should be done to determine the efficacy of administering LOCM for all patients.

Informed consent should be obtained from all patients before they undergo a procedure involving contrast media.

The content depends on the jurisdiction. If LOCM is to be used on a selective basis, radiologists are advised to inform low-risk patients of its availability, and to explain to them why they are being given HOCM instead. This will go a long way in protecting the radiologist from liability.

References

1　Mill J. *On Liberty* 6. (1873).
2　Burwell. Informed consent. *Med Trial Tech* Q 439. (1989).
3　95 Minn. 261, 104 NW 12 (1905).
4　*Cobbs* v. *Grant*, 8 Cal.3d 229, 240, 104 Cal. Rptr. 505, 512 1972.
5　186 Kan. 393, 350 P.2d 1093 (1960).
6　464 F.2d 772 (D.C. Cir.), cert. denied, 409 U.S. 1064 (1972).
7　Shultz. From: Informed consent to patient choice: a new protected interest. 95 *Yale Law J* 219 (1985).
8　Burwell. *Med Trial Tech.* Q 442.
9　Seidelson. Medical malpractice actions based on lack of informed consent in "full-disclosure" jurisdictions: the enigmatic affirmative defense. 29 DUQ. *Law Review* 1990;39.
10　8 Cal.3d 229, 104 Calif. Rptr. 505, 502 P.2d 1 (1972).
11　27 Cal.3d 285, 165 Calif. Rptr. 308, 611 P.2d 902 (1980).
12　8 Cal.3d 229, 244 (1972).
13　27 Cal.3d 285, 165 (1980).
14　*Moore* v. *Preventive Medicine Medical Group*, Inc., 178 Cal. App.3d 728, 223 Calif. Rptr. 859 1986.
15　Jacobson & Rosenquist, The introduction of low-osmolar contrast agents in radiology. *J Am Med Assoc* 1988;260:1586.
16　Environ Corp., *Perspectives on Adverse Reaction Rates Associated with the Use of High Osmolar Ionic and Low Osmolar Nonionic Contrast Media*, vol. 1. May 23, 1990.
17　McClennan. Low osmolality contrast media: a practical approach *Diagn Imag* 1987;9:16–18.
18　Katayama H, Yamaguchi K, Kozuka T, Takashima T, Seez P, Matsuura K. Adverse reactions to ionic and nonionic contrast media. *Radiology* 1990;175:621–628.
19　Palmer F. The RACR survey of intravenous contrast media reactions: final report. *Aust Radiol* 1988;32:426–428.
20　*Report from the Committee on Drugs and Contrast Media of the Commission on Education of the American College of Radiology.* (1990).
21　Zelch. Can we afford not to use nonionic contrast media? *Diagn Imag* 1989;April:67–73.
22　Reuter. An overview of informed consent for radiologists *Am J Roentgenol* 1987;148:219–227.
23　316 S.E.2.d 690 (S.C. 1984).
24　100 WASH.2d 26, 666 p2.D 351 (1983).
25　Bush W. Informed consent for contrast media *Am J Roentgenol* 1989;152:867–869.
26　Jacobson. The availability of low osmolar contrast media: analysis of an emerging technology. *Diagn Imag* (Suppl.) December 1987.
27　Hall. The malpractice standard under health care cost containment. *L Med Health Care* 1989;17:347.
28　Gregory. Hard choices: patient autonomy in an era of health care cost containment. *Jurimetrics J* 1990;30:483.
29　O'Neal. Safe harbor for health care cost containment. *Stan L Rev* 1991;43:399.
30　Note. Rethinking medical malpractice law in light of medical cost-cutting. *98 Harvard Law Rev* 1985;1004:1012.

31 Schuck. Malpractice liability and the rationing of care. *Texas L Rev* 1981;59:1421.

32 Furrow. Medical malpractice and cost containment: tightening the screws. *36 Case West Res Law Rev* 1986;985:1009.

33 Marsh.

34 Morreim. *Cost Constraints as a Malpractice Defense*. 18 Hastings Center Report 5 (1988).

35 Boyd. Cost containment and the physician's fiduciary duty to the patient. *39 DePaul L Rev* 1989;131:152.

36 Note.

37 192 Cal.App.3d 1630, 239 Cal.Rptr. 810 (1986). The California Court of Appeal filed published opinion, 183 Cal.Ap.3d 1175, 228 Cal.Rptr. 661 (1986). The California Supreme Court granted review, 231 Cal. Rptr. 560, and subsequently dismissed, remanded, and ordered published 192 Cal.App.3d 1630, a republication of 183 Cal.App.3d 1175.

38 222 Cal. App.3d 660, 271 Cal. Rptr. 876 (1990).

39 Mehlman. Health care cost containment and medical technology: a critique of waste theory. *36 Case W Res Law Rev* 1986;778:857.

40 Joint Commission on Accreditation of Hospitals: The 1990s: the critical decade for medical technology. *QRB* 1990;16:218−222.

CHAPTER 40

Medicolegal problems in the UK involving diagnostic radiology

J. Oscar M.C. Craig

The present situation

A Department of Health Circular HC(89)34 [1] effective from January 1, 1990, introduced new arrangements for dealing with medical negligence claims. With these arrangements, the responsibility for handling and funding existing and new claims, arising from the act or omission of medical and dental staff in the course of their National Health Service employment, passed from the medical defence organizations (The Medical Protection Society, Medical Defence Union, and the Medical and Dental Defence Union of Scotland) to the health authorities. It is no longer a contractual requirement for hospital doctors working for health authorities to belong to one of the medical defence organizations. This does not apply to those working in general practice or those engaged in private practice. A letter was issued by the National Health Service Management Executive [2] which was dated February 11, 1991, and stated that the responsibility to pay the costs and awards in medical negligence cases has moved to the providers of health care, i.e., directly managed units and hospital trusts. These changes have had a profound effect on many aspects of medical litigation. As the responsibility for dealing with National Health Service cases shifted from a few central bodies down to many local hospital units, the statistics regarding litigation, compiled and held by the medical defence organizations, ceased to be complete.

The incidence of litigation has been increasing at a steady rate in the UK since 1947. In that year the Medical Defence Union reported 49 cases (involving all specialties). Anxiety was expressed when in 1957 the number of cases alleging medical negligence involving the Medical Defence Union

had risen to 92. By 1983, the Medical Protection Society considered 3100 cases relating to standards of care. This had risen to 4200 in 1987. There can be no doubt that there is an upward trend in claims for medical negligence. It was pointed out in a report by the National Association for Hospital Authorities and Trusts (NAHAT) [3] in February, 1992, that the cost of negligence claims to the medical defence organizations in 1987 was £40 million, but that the cost to the health authorities in 1990–1991 was £53 million.

A graph produced by D. Murray of the Medical Protection Society some years ago, showed that the average cost of settlement of medical negligence claims had risen over 400% from 1976 to 1985. The source of the information was from the Medical Protection Society actuarial reports. We can conclude that the number of cases concerning medical negligence is still increasing and the costs are still rising. The question must be asked, as to what effect this trend will have on the delivery of health care, on the attitudes and reactions of individual doctors, on recruitment into medicine, and especially recruitment into specific specialties.

In the report of the working party of the NAHAT [3], concern was expressed by members that the new arrangements for dealing with medical negligence claims at a unit or trust level will result in an increase in prices for services, and this will certainly adversely affect facilities and the provision of health care for patients. The report points out that the health service providers, both directly managed units and hospital trusts, are not permitted to insure for clinical negligence. Increase in litigation is one of the factors responsible for a growing disillusionment among young doctors. Doctors find themselves liable to multiple jeopardy. A single doctor may find him- or herself answerable for one particular mistake to:

1 the coroner;
2 a hospital enquiry;
3 a Health Service Commissioner;
4 General Medical Council;
5 employment law officers;
6 criminal court.

There has been a falling off in recruitment into medical schools as reported by deans. There has also been a falling off in graduates entering obstetrics and gynecology (President, Royal College of Obstetricians and Gynaecologists, UK, personal communication). At the same time, there has been an increase in the practice of defensive medicine. This is reflected by an increase in the incidence of Cesarean sections and by an increase in laboratory and radiologic investigations.

Medical negligence in Europe

The late Dr Ivor Quest of the Medical Protection Society presented the European malpractice scene at a conference held in July 1990 at St Bartholomew's Hospital, London. This was reported in a document *Standards of Excellence 1992* [4]. Dr Quest contrasted the means for patients to complain regarding medical negligence in the UK with that in Continental Europe. Whereas there are many routes in the UK, such as directly to hospital management, to Health Service Commissioners, to Family Practitioner Committees, and assisted by such bodies as the Citizens' Advice Bureau and the legal aid system, there were fewer such systems elsewhere in Europe. Dr Quest pointed out that there were social and cultural differences between the UK and other European Community countries. Holland and Belgium offered injured citizens higher social insurance benefits than the UK did and had many fewer negligence claims. The Latin nations also had fewer claims than the Anglo–Saxon nations. In Western Germany as the standard of living rose, so did the claims for medical negligence. Since the 1970s demands for claims in excess of DM 100 000 have increased 10-fold.

In Spain from 1975–1984, only 43 cases had been heard by the Spanish Supreme Court. Analysis since 1984 showed a fourfold increase in claims for medical negligence. A questionnaire sent by Dr Quest to eight European countries (Spain, Denmark, Greece, Norway, Italy, West Germany, Hungary, and East Germany prior to union) asked if negligence claims were increasing and the answer was yes for each country. In Continental Europe all malpractice cover is controlled by the insurance industry and there are no medically controlled bodies concerned in litigation that would equate with the medical defense organizations that exist in the UK.

Factors influencing claims

There are a number of reasons for the increase in medical negligence claims.

1 There is more public awareness of medical matters by means of the press and media, and patients have greater expectations from the medical profession. If these expectations are not fulfilled, patients and their relatives feel that negligence must be the cause.
2 Patients cannot distinguish between the genuine complications of a procedure and those that result from negligence.
3 Today, there is a greater willingness to challenge authority in all its forms, and in cases of possible negligence, the doctor's authority.
4 There is easier access to litigation than previously, e.g., Citizens' Advice Bureau, Family Practitioners' Committees, Community Health Councils, legal aid schemes.
5 Awards in personal injury cases have been escalating.

Definition of medical negligence

We should understand what we mean by medical negligence and there are many definitions. My favorite understanding comes from Chief Justice Tindal [5] who, over 100 years ago, in the case of *Lanphier* v. *Phipos*, imposed a legal duty to exercise skill and care. In his judgment of the case he said:

> Every person who enters into a learned profession undertakes to bring to the exercise of it a reasonable degree of care and skill. He does not undertake, if he is an attorney, that at all events you will gain your case, nor does a surgeon undertake that he will perform a cure, nor does he undertake to use the highest degree of skill. There may be persons who have higher education and greater advantages than he has, but he undertakes to bring a fair, reasonable and competent degree of skill.

This means that in the UK, at the present time, a doctor is liable only if he or she fails to exercise that standard of skill and care that would be expected of a normal prudent doctor of similar status and experience. That which might be considered negligent for a senior surgeon, might not be so in a house surgeon. In diagnostic radiology, the interpretation of a radiograph by a radiologist that might be considered negligent, might not be considered negligent if so interpreted by a casualty officer. Today, to bring a successful claim of medical negligence against a health authority or a named medical defendant, involves the law of tort and there is a necessity to establish a breach of a duty of care. The following are necessary under this law of tort.

1 There must be a duty of care owed to the patient by the named defendants.
2 The standard of care appropriate to that duty must not have been achieved and as a result the duty breached, either by action or inaction, advice given, or failure to advise.
3 Such a breach must be shown to have caused the injury

and therefore the resulting loss complained about by the patient.

4 Any loss sustained as a result of the injury and complained about by the patient, must be of a kind that the court recognizes and for which they allow compensation.

Many of the disagreements and much of the controversy in medicolegal cases relates to the third of these criteria, i.e., causation.

The most common specialties to be involved in medical litigation in the UK are obstetrics and gynaecology, followed by general surgery, orthopedics, and accident and emergency medicine. This league table was calculated from the number of claims handled by the Medical Protection Society between 1983 and 1986. It is interesting to compare this with the incidence of litigation in the US, where in obstetrics and gynaecology 26.6% of specialists were sued annually; second in line was surgery including orthopedics, where 16.5% were sued annually; and third was radiology, where 12.9% were sued annually. These figures relate to 1985 and all showed a dramatic increase since 1981 when the figures were 7.1, 4.1, and 2.4%, respectively. At the time of writing, clinical radiology does not appear high in the specialties involved in litigation in the UK. It seems possible that this may change, especially as radiologists are now so heavily involved in high-risk interventional procedures.

The radiologic case mix in litigation

A personal analysis of 360 cases where radiologic errors were central to the claim for negligence, amounted to 9% of all the cases heard in the cases committee of the Medical Protection Society between 1985 and 1988. Although there was an error related to film interpretation, these did not all involve radiologists. (Also, only a relatively small number of cases reach the cases committee; more minor problems are dealt with directly by the secretariat.) Of these 360 cases, 78% were related to trauma. The most commonly missed fractures were neck of femur, cervical spine, and scaphoid and the most commonly missed dislocations were the posterior dislocation of the shoulder, dislocations of the metatarsus, and the carpus. The most serious and the most expensive claims were missed spinal fractures, and in this series there were eight patients with spinal injuries, three of whom became paraplegic. Among the strong lessons to be learned is that whoever examines the cervical spine radiographs, must do so carefully and must ensure that all seven cervical vertebrae are seen clearly, especially the C7/D1 level where traumatic lesions are common. Scaphoid fractures still pose a problem, even though it is still taught clearly that if a scaphoid fracture is suspected, then the patient should be treated as having a scaphoid fracture, and reradiographed in 10–14-days time. It is important to ask for scaphoid views and not a wrist radiograph. If there is serious anxiety about a fracture which cannot be seen on a radiograph, then an isotope bone scan can be helpful.

It is especially important that an injury involving glass is radiographed. Missed glass foreign bodies are common and glass is radiopaque. Injuries to the eye that could be due to foreign bodies also deserve radiograph. Fractures involving the orbit or elsewhere in the skull are difficult to detect and junior doctors should be ready to seek further advice.

Of the 278 cases of trauma in this series, there was no radiologic report in 32%. The interpretation of these radiographs was performed by accident and emergency staff, most often junior doctors who had received no radiologic training. The reasons for the absence of a radiologic report are many, but most of them are related to the lack of radiologic staff and the alarming increase in radiologic workload. A paper by Vincent *et al.* [6] dealt with the ability of junior doctors in accident and emergency departments to detect radiographic abnormalities. Each assessment by a senior house officer was compared with the subsequent diagnosis of a radiologist of senior registrar or consultant status. For abnormalities with clinically significant consequences, the error rate was 39% for the accident and emergency doctors. No improvement was found in the performance of the senior house officers over the 6-months tenure of the post. The paper concludes that it is unrealistic to expect accident and emergency senior house officers to acquire the complex skill of image interpretation simply through experience over that time. Radiologists, despite an increasing workload, should give special priority to the reporting of accident and emergency radiographs if the incidence of litigation in trauma is to decrease. It would certainly be helpful if formal training and guidance could be given to accident and emergency doctors, but this, too, would add an additional burden to departments of clinical radiology.

In the Medical Protection Society series, 22% of the medical negligence cases involving radiology were non-traumatic in origin. These cases included the following.

1 *Contrast reactions* — two arrests, two deaths, several minor reactions, and one extravasation.

2 *Barium examinations* — there were five falls from the X-ray table. There were a number of barium extravasations during barium enema examinations (four cases over the previous 6 years).

3 *Myelography* — these included fits, missed tumors, and negligent injections. Since 1988, there have been many claims referring to Myodil. These claim the development of arachnoiditis, secondary to the use of Myodil and its incomplete removal after the procedure.

4 *Computed tomography* (CT) complaints referred to missed diagnoses.

5 *Ultrasound* errors included missed ectopic pregnancy, missed spina bifida, and there was one death from hemorrhage following biopsy under ultrasound control.

6 *Angiography* — in this group there was a failed angioplasty, an intimal tear, a hemorrhage, a postarteriography embolus, and one case of injection of surgical spirit in error.

New regulations have been produced concerning exposing

patients to ionizing radiation [7], which will be discussed later in this chapter. Efforts to reduce the number of ill-advised requests for radiographic examinations are being made, but in this series of 360 cases, the absence of radiography was central to the litigation in 32% of cases. This failure to radiograph included injuries with glass, intra-ocular foreign bodies, retained swabs and drains, fractures, and one case of failure to radiograph for a slipped femoral epiphysis.

Duty to provide a service

The duty to provide a radiologic service rests with the hospital authorities, be they health authorities, directly managed units, or hospital trusts. This duty is delegated to the radiologist in charge of the department. Most departments are directed by a consultant radiologist but he or she in turn delegates responsibilities to others, e.g., business manager, superintendent radiographer. There is a medicolegal responsibility resting with each, concerning their duties and their delegation. Providing a service involves the taking and reporting of radiographs and the clinical and physical directing of these examinations; in many places it also involves providing a radiologic interventional service. There is a responsibility in many departments related to ultrasound, isotope imaging, CT, and magnetic resonance imaging. There is a responsibility to see that the equipment is safe and adequate for its required use for patients.

If a radiologist considers that the apparatus is inadequate for the task required, it is his or her duty to report this to the health authorities. In certain circumstances, it may be justifiable for the radiologist to refuse to perform a particular procedure if he or she considers the equipment inadequate. Health and Safety Regulations must be observed within the department, especially concerning ionizing radiation. All personnel in the department should have read and noted the Code of Practice [8].

The duty to provide a service includes the duty to provide an opinion on the radiographic examinations. When this duty cannot be met satisfactorily, the employing authorities should be notified.

Standing orders

The consultant in charge of a radiologic department is responsible for the standing orders relating to the efficient and safe running of the department. These standing orders should include the protocols to be followed in radiographic examinations, i.e., the particular views to be taken in each examination carried out by a radiographer. This protocol can be drawn up following discussions between radiologic and radiographic staff. Standing orders are necessary to deal with emergency procedures, be they a cardiac arrest or a departmental fire. Instructions regarding the aftercare of patients following complicated radiologic procedures should be clearly understood by radiologic, radiographic, and departmental nursing staff. The aftercare of a patient is invariably a shared responsibility with the referring doctor and this should be agreed beforehand and known to all medical and nursing staff both in the department and on the wards.

Myodil litigation

Since 1988, a large number of claims appeared referring to the alleged development of arachnoiditis following the use of Myodil for myelography and its incomplete removal after the procedure. In the USA, large volumes of Myodil, even up to 100 ml, were used, but in the UK it was customary only to inject 6 ml. The size of the litigation problem and its potential for anxiety to the profession was sufficient for the Royal College of Radiologists and the British Society of Neuroradiologists to issue a joint statement in 1991 [9] concerning the use of Myodil. This statement addressed the following questions.

1 Was the use of any contrast medium for myelography justified?

2 Was the use of Myodil justified in the light of other contrast media available?

3 Should Myodil have been aspirated after the examination had been completed?

4 What was the relevance of informed consent in the Myodil era?

The conclusions were the following.

1 We consider that where clinical features of possible spinal pathology indicated the need for a definitive diagnosis and precise localization of a lesion, radiculography or myelography was essential.

2 We consider it correct that in 1944–1972 Myodil was the contrast medium of choice for radiculography and full myelography.

3 During the Conray/Dimer-X era, the use of Myodil was still acceptable for radiculography and it remained the medium of choice for run-up myelography.

4 Following the introduction of Metrizamide, despite its advantages, a decision had to be made balancing the quality of the images against the potential severity of immediate complications. It became widely accepted as a contrast medium for myelography in the early 1980s.

5 Despite the recommendations in the data sheet that Myodil should be removed after examination, unless it was required for a further study, it was common practice in the UK not to aspirate the relatively small volumes used here. This practice is supported by work which showed that aspiration failed to prevent the development of arachnoiditis, and we consider nonaspiration of the contrast medium to have been an acceptable practice.

6 Current practice regarding "informed consent" did not apply in the Myodil era and, in any case, there are reports indicating that the rate of symptomatic post-Myodil arachnoiditis was not greater than 1%.

The joint publication included 33 literature references to support the stated opinions.

Ionizing radiation regulations (protection of persons undergoing medical examination or treatment, POPUMET) (see also Chapter 7)

These regulations (POPUMET) [7] refer to "clinically directing" and "physically directing". Clinically directing is the clinical responsibility for the decision to effect the medical exposure. The medical exposure is the exposure of a person to ionizing radiation for diagnostic or therapeutic purposes. Physically directing is the act of effecting the exposure. In most cases, the radiologist is clinically directing and the radiographer is physically directing. However, during fluoroscopic examinations the radiologist may be both clinically and physically directing; a surgeon in theater using fluoroscopy can be doing either or both. The regulations require that those persons clinically directing medical exposures should have received "adequate training". This requires instruction in the "core of knowledge" regarding competence in radiation protection. It is also a requirement that the smallest possible irradiation dose should be used to obtain a satisfactory medical result. These regulations are not related to the request for a radiologic examination, but to the clinical decision to effect that examination. Thus, with regard to clinically directing, the responsibility usually falls on the radiologist who must make the decision whether or not the examination is justified and whether or not the correct examination has been requested. Radiographic examinations performed by the radiographers when the radiologist is not present are physically directed by the radiographer but are still clinically directed by the radiologist, e.g., a chest radiograph. This clinical direction is made possible through the standing orders of the department. It is the responsibility of the person clinically directing an examination to ensure that the requirements of the ionizing radiation regulations are satisfied. Failure to do so can lead to criminal prosecution by the Inspectorate of the Secretary of State under the Health and Safety Regulations.

Medicolegal aspects of delegation

Delegation is a necessity in the management of a department of radiology and in the training of medical and nonmedical personnel, and this is recognized by the General Medical Council (Fitness to Practice Document [10]). There are serious medicolegal consequences accompanying the delegation of tasks and the Royal College of Radiologists is issuing guidelines [11] to point out these aspects of delegation that need to be understood clearly and observed fully. However good the guidelines, any case that leads to the courts will be decided on its own individual circumstances.

To delegate is to entrust or empower a colleague to perform a particular task. A radiologist may delegate a task to: (i) a junior doctor, e.g., a radiologist in training; (ii) to a nonradiologic medical colleague; or (iii) to a nonmedical colleague.

It is essential for the delegator to know that the task delegated is within the training and the competence of the delegatee. If so, then this is a "proper delegation". If not, then it is an "improper delegation". It is incumbent on the delegatee to state if he or she thinks that the task delegated is outside his or her competence.

If a proper delegation has been made and a mishap occurs, it is likely, depending on the individual circumstances, that the responsibility will lie with the delegatee. If an improper delegation is made and a mishap occurs, it is likely, again depending on the varying circumstances, that the responsibility will lie with the delegator, who may be liable for medical negligence. In a personal communication with R. Palmer of the Medical Protection Society, he said that, were a death to occur following an improper delegation, the delegator might be liable to a charge of manslaughter. R. Palmer also said he would not wish to alarm the profession, but there had been an increasing number of manslaughter charges brought against medical practitioners, where even one decade ago no such criminal prosecution would have been considered. Practitioners should be aware of their potential liability.

The delegator must be aware of the ease or the difficulty of a case he or she delegates and must be aware of the need for supervision or the need to be contactable. A task may be delegated to a nonradiologically trained medical colleague, e.g., the interpretation of a radiograph. This is common and most often the radiologist knows that it is within the competence of the colleague, e.g., an orthopedic film interpreted by an orthopedic surgeon. This occurs when unreported films leave the department for chest clinics, intensive care units, fracture clinics, and the like. There are medicolegal consequences when this happens, falling on both the radiologist and those that interpret the radiograph. The latter is responsible for any mishap that flows from the interpretation.

Increasingly, tasks are delegated to nonmedical colleagues, e.g., radiographic and nursing staff. Here also, the delegator must be satisfied that the task delegated is within the training and competence of the delegatee. The General Medical Council recognizes the need to delegate tasks to paramedical colleagues, but a medical opinion cannot be given by a nonmedical practitioner, and it is considered serious professional misconduct, by the General Medical Council, to delegate a task requiring the skill and knowledge of a medical practitioner to persons not medically qualified.

Ultrasound

Ultrasound examinations may be performed by radiologists, obstetricians, radiographers, nurses, midwives, and physicists. Doppler examinations are often performed by surgeons or cardiologists. Delegation is an important aspect of every ultrasound department, and it is essential to see that each delegation is a proper one in legal terms. The issue that would most likely be addressed if a legal case did arise would be the training and the experience of the ultrasonographer and whether or not the conduct of the procedure was accepted practice.

The radiologist has responsibilities when he or she is in charge of an ultrasound service to the patient, but often also to provide the appropriate instruction and supervision of radiographers and other paramedical staff. Appropriate delegation must be observed and the protocol for delegated examinations must be understood clearly. The radiologist may find it necessary to issue a report on an examination performed to his or her satisfaction by a radiographer or another paramedical colleague. In these cases, it is necessary to include on the report the name and the status of the ultrasonographer.

Radiographers and other paramedical colleagues may make observations on an ultrasound examination conducted by them, and it is necessary in these cases that the name and status of the ultrasonographer appears on the report.

The consultant in charge of the department bears the final clinical responsibility to the patient.

Requests for unreported films

A document on this issue was published in 1992 by the Royal College of Radiologists [12]. The aim in every department of radiology should be that unreported films never leave that department, but the manpower shortage and the increasing workload make this goal difficult to achieve. The patient's interests are paramount, and the release of films without reports may be necessary at times to fulfil this obligation.

It is necessary to distinguish between films that leave the department without a report but for which there is an established mechanism for their return, and those that leave with the knowledge that a report will never be produced. The report issued by the Royal College of Radiologists advises that when issuing films without reports, the following conditions should be met.

1 There should be an overriding patient need.

2 If on a non-*ad hoc* basis, there should be a formal agreement with the consultant radiologist in charge of the department, and there should be a clear understanding by the radiologist and the referring clinician of the medicolegal consequences of this action.

3 The employing authorities should be aware of the agreement.

4 The radiologist will usually be responsible for clinically directing the examination.

5 If the nonradiologist interprets the radiograph, he or she takes on the medicolegal responsibilities that accompany that interpretation.

6 There should be an agreement to document the interpretation on the patient's notes.

The department should always know to whom a film has been sent. There should be an agreement that films are returned to the department for reporting.

Low-osmolar intravascular contrast agents (see also Chapter 13)

There is concern among radiologists regarding the continuing use of conventional high-osmolar contrast agents and the need to use low-osmolar contrast agents.

R. Grainger drafted guidelines [13] for the selective use of low-osmolar contrast in 1984, but it was considered necessary to review the problem and further guidelines were issued by the Royal College of Radiologists with help and advice from Grainger and Dawson [14]. These guidelines stated that the ultimate objective was to replace conventional high-osmolar media by low-osmolar media as soon as the necessary finance is available. Until this is possible, guidelines are necessary. The main recommendations are the following.

1 Nonionic agents should be used intravascularly in all patients thought to be at higher risk of an anaphylactoid reaction, e.g., previous reactors, asthmatics, atopic patients, and those allergic to other drugs or agents.

2 Nonionic agents should be used generally in all procedures anticipated to be high-dose procedures. This would include patients unable to tolerate a high osmotic load.

3 Infants and babies should be given nonionic media.

4 Ioxaglate may be used to best advantage in arteriography. Low-osmolar media, either ionic or nonionic, should be used in all arteriography expected to be painful.

5 Nonionic media should be used if there is difficulty in monitoring the patient or when machinery makes vomiting a particular hazard, e.g., CT scanning.

6 Patients with known hemodynamic instability or limited cardiac reserve, merit the use of low-osmolar contrast.

7 Although there is no convincing evidence that elderly patients are at significant risk, many authorities argue that the use of less stressful low-osmolar contrast is advisable.

8 Either type of low-osmolar contrast should be used in sickle cell disease or trait. Ideally, this should be diluted 1:2 to render them isosmolar to plasma.

9 In angioplasty low-osmolar agents should be used.

10 An argument has been made that in patients with pre-existing renal impairment, the most inert agent should be used, i.e., nonionic in the smallest possible dose.

If a legal case were to occur concerning the use of contrast medium and its type, to have followed these guidelines would be a reasonable defense.

Informed consent

Lack of informed consent for a procedure is a recurring medicolegal problem. Scarman [15] said in a lecture delivered to a forum on medical communication in 1985, that medical paternalism was no longer acceptable in English law, and that the sovereignty of the patient had been reinstated. He also said that information of risk that the doctor judges to be significant must be given to the patient. This appears to leave room for the doctor to use his or her clinical judgment as to the risks he or she details to the patient. Unfortunately, many arguments in court occur between expert witnesses as to whether this or that complication should be considered significant. It has often been said that a figure above 1% is significant, but some would argue that the serious nature of a possible complication may make it prudent to discuss it with the patient, even though the incidence may be less than 1%.

Problems arise in radiology regarding what procedures require written informed consent. The decision is affected by logistics as well as by common sense. All doctors should be guided by the premise that good communication and good relationships with the patient take precedence even over a signed document. It is not advised that all examinations require written consent, e.g., excretion urography, barium examinations, and the like. It is advised, however, that each patient is consulted sufficiently to understand exactly what any procedure entails, why it is being done, what it is hoped to learn from it, and what alternate choices there may be. The radiologist must be ready and willing to answer any questions that the patient thinks significant.

Vascular and interventional procedures do require written consent following a meaningful discussion with the patient. It is also prudent to enter into the patient's notes an account of what was said, which the radiologist should date and sign. It is a great help if a witness to this discussion is present, e.g., a junior colleague, radiographer, or nurse. It is recommended that the radiologist performing the procedure should obtain the consent personally. There are times when this must be delegated, but this must be a "proper delegation". It is unwise for any person to obtain consent on behalf of the radiologist, if that person, be they consultant surgeon or house surgeon, is unfamiliar with the procedure, its performance, and its complications. Some patients do not wish to know about the complications of a procedure or alternate procedures. When this is the case, it is more important than ever that a record of this fact is kept in the patient's notes.

Consent must be obtained at a reasonable time prior to the procedure, so that the patient can be given sufficient time to arrive at a considered opinion. It must certainly not be obtained when the patient is in the department just prior to the procedure, or when the patient has had premedication.

These recommendations are not overzealous in the present climate of litigation. The increasing involvement of radiologists in complex procedures, makes it necessary for them to give informed consent detailed consideration.

The radiologist is responsible for any complications that arise as the result of a procedure that he or she performs. So, the duty of care continues when the patient leaves the department or returns to the wards. This aftercare is usually shared with clinical colleagues, but this should be clearly understood and standing orders should include these arrangements and must be available for all medical and nursing staff.

Guidelines

The number of radiologic investigations has increased enormously over the past few decades. It has been stated, in a publication by the National Radiological Protection Board and the Royal College of Radiologists in 1990 [16], that 20% of radiologic examinations had no clinical justification. The Royal College of Radiologists issued guidelines in 1989 and 1993 [17], detailing the clinical indications and the appropriate radiologic examination in the 12 most commonly requested examinations, which constituted 95% of radiologic examinations in National Health Service hospitals. These were guidelines which could be modified to accommodate local circumstances. However, they should be followed as closely as possible by all doctors. All radiologic examinations should be based on sound clinical justification and it is not acceptable to irradiate a patient without this clinical justification. To follow the guidelines would be a reasonable defense in a court of law.

It is distressing that medical litigation is today a fact of medical life. However, to practise defensive medicine is not necessarily the same as to practise good medicine.

The greatest antagonists to medical litigation are good communication with the patient, establishing a good doctor–patient relationship, and basing all of one's decisions on that which is in the patient's best interests.

References

1 *Department of Health Circular HC(89)34*. London: HMSO, 1989.
2 *National Health Service Management Executive EL(91)*. London: HMSO, 1991.
3 NAHAT. *Just Finance in Medical Negligence Cases*. National Association for Hospital Authorities and Trusts, 1992.
4 *Standards of Excellence*. Summary of first conference at St. Bartholomew's Hospital 1990 on European Standards, 1992.
5 Tindal 1838. *Lanphier* v. *Phipos C & P 475*.
6 Vincent CF, Driscoll PA, Audley RJ *et al*. Accuracy of detection of radiographic abnormalities by junior doctors. *Arch Emerg Med* 1988;5:101–109.
7 Protection of Persons Undergoing Medical Examination or Treatment (POPUMET). London: HMSO, 1988:EC(88)29.
8 NRPB. *Guidance Notes for the Protection of Persons Against Ionizing Radiation Arising from Medical and Dental Use*. National Radiological Protection Board, 1988.

9 Royal College of Radiologists. *Statement on Myodil*. December, 1991.

10 GMC. *Professional Conduct and Discipline: Fitness to Practice*. London: General Medical Council, 1985.

11 RCR. *Medico-Legal Aspects of Delegation*. London: Royal College of Radiologists, 1993.

12 RCR. *Requests for Unreported Films*. London: Royal College of Radiologists, FCR/4/, 1992.

13 Grainger RG. The clinical and financial implications of low osmolar media. *Clin Radiol* 1984;35:251−252.

14 Grainger RG, Dawson P. Low osmolar contrast media: an appraisal. Editorial. *Clin Radiol* 1990;42:1−5.

15 Scarman (Lord). Consent, communication and responsibility. *J Roy Soc Med* 1986;79:697−700.

16 Report by National Radiological Protection Board and Royal College of Radiologists. *Patient Dose Reduction in Diagnostic Radiology*, Vol. 1, 3. 1990.

17 RCR. *Making the Best Use of a Department of Radiology. Guidelines for Doctors*. London: Royal College of Radiologists, 1989, 1990, 1991, 1993.

Legal considerations and quality assurance in the USA

A. Everette James, Jr

The interrelationships of law and medicine

This chapter will attempt to provide an environmental context for the reader. From many points of reference or inquiry, medicine and law may seem to be in conflict. However, their ultimate goals are often quite similar.

Medicine grew from man's instinct to assist and heal fellow human beings, while the law was designed to provide persons living in a social circumstance with a structured methodology to protect, preserve, and maintain their rights. These two professions seem to have origins in laudable instincts and are, thus, praiseworthy in concept. They have in common certain traits by which each could be judged as concerned, dedicated, and highly skilled. The complexity of present society tends to stress the differences between law and medicine. These may appear unduly important even though the differences may be small compared with the similarities in the two professions.

In considering the inherent characteristics of medicine and law, the fact is that the approaches and techniques of achieving their purposes are fundamentally different. Medicine emphasizes the use of a body of data such as the content of a radiographic image to determine the proper course of action. The aim is to render the data absolute. Additionally, the practice of medicine occurs in an environment designed to promote collaboration and good will among one's colleagues. Group activities and attitudes work to incur favor among one's peers and are stated and tacit goals throughout the training, experience, and the conduct of a physician's medical career. The discipline of radiology is a consultative specialty where this collegiality is greatly emphasized.

The legal profession promotes utilization of a body of rules, facts, and opinions as guidelines for professional conduct, which is often adversarial in nature. Attorneys are trained to use the data they acquire to establish the validity of a particular line of reasoning. Their responsibility includes dealing with data similar to that utilized by their colleagues, but to employ it in certain ways that are intended to lead to different conclusions. This process often occurs in a public forum — the courtroom.

Attorneys are also taught to emphasize the validity of the available data to the benefit of their clients. By this fundamental difference in process, attorneys will place little emphasis upon cooperation and collaboration with their adversarial colleague in any particular and specific litigation procedure.

"Truth" is the decision of the trier of fact and not an immutable conclusion arrived at by the inherent sanctity of fact. Both law and medicine have a purpose and investment in public welfare. While this might provide a natural common ground, the differences in attitudes and approach by each profession may be manifest by a lack of understanding and acceptance of each for the activities of the other. Medicine and law promote well-being. However, the legal profession is oriented to the well-being of society, while medicine is primarily directed to the well-being of the individual. The law is process directed, whereas medicine is effort directed.

The fundamental principle of medical practice is the relationship of trust between physician and patient. In legal terms, the patient is the jury, while the physician is the initiator of thought and provider of evidence. Medicine tends to approach patients and their ailments as a scientific endeavor, but with human compassion. The law focuses upon the complaint or defense of the client as a fundamental truth and accepts an adversarial relationship as part of the process.

The relevance of law in the practice of radiology would have been problematic to both professions only a few decades ago. However, such considerations now assume an ever-increasing role which may be traced to several developments, which will be discussed. As a paradigm, we will examine the involvement of antitrust law in medicine and devote considerable discussion to this endeavor. Historically, antitrust and medicine have less than two decades of interactivity. Until the USA Supreme Court's decision and opinion by Chief Justice Burger in the case of *Goldfarb* v. *the Virginia State Bar* in 1974 [1], it was generally accepted that the "learned professions" of law and medicine were exempt from antitrust considerations. The courts held that there was no intention in the initiation and application of antitrust policy to provide such an exemption. In addition, antitrust laws had been felt to apply only to interstate commerce. The delivery of health care, if to be considered a business at all, was characterized as an intrastate business only. Subsequent rulings by federal agencies and the courts that quickly followed showed that this position was no longer to be accepted.

In the landmark case of *Hospital Building Company* v. *Trustees of Rex Hospital*, it was found that if in the conduct of a health care facility's normal activity there exists a potential for use of goods, services, or assistance rendered to persons or firms that reside outside of a state, then interstate commerce is involved. The complexity of radiology obviously makes the practice of this discipline an interstate endeavor. The Federal Trade Commission (FTC) took the position that the delivery of health care is a major USA industry, and one and a half decades ago the FTC launched a major investigation of the degree of competition within the medical industry. Radiology has not been exempt; antitrust scrutiny of radiologic practices has been intense, because of the nature of the conduct of practice, the value of the technology involved, and the contractual arrangements.

Antitrust legislation is sometimes difficult to apply to the health care industry for several fundamental reasons. These will be considered in detail in the discussion of exclusive contracts and "turf". A general consideration of antitrust law usually begins with the Sherman Act of 1890, which has two important sections. Section One of this legislation proscribes contracts, combinations, or conspiracies which restrain trade. The mandate for Section One is broad and at times difficult to define accurately.

Section Two of the Sherman Act is more circumscribed and forbids all activities that could lead to monopolization. Both sections have profound implications for our specialty. The latter components of antitrust legislation such as the Clayton Act of 1914 forbade certain tie-in arrangements and exclusive dealing group policies, whereas the Robinson–Patman Act proscribes predatory pricing and price discrimination. As the economics of medicine become more important in health policy, these will acquire greater significance. The Federal Trade Commission Act, passed subsequent to the Sherman legislation, forbids unfair methods of competition. This latter mandate has often been interpreted by the FTC, and sometimes by the courts, to include anything prohibited by either the Sherman or Clayton Acts. The FTC has expanded even further their mandate to forbid whatever is deemed contrary to the public's best interest.

Self-determination as a public policy has received great recent interest. The posture that licensing, certification, and the granting of professional privileges are sacrosanct and that internal activities of professional groups are exempt from outside influence or control are also no longer appropriate in today's social climate [2–5]. As noted, trends in American society appear to be oriented to the promotion of the rights and privileges of the individual with emphasis upon self-determination, relating principally to body and person. Accepting the premise that adequate health care is a public right implies that the public should also have a significant role in ensuring the availability of medical care and in determining what compensation levels are to be considered reasonable.

Recent activities of federal agencies suggest that they are orienting their activities to operate under this concept [6]. Diagnosis-related groups (DRGs) and relative value scales (RVS) are just such examples. Many observers of health policies argue that a change in philosophy and public attitudes has occurred; from health needs being provided for the public good, to a public right of adequate health care, to the concept that health care is a limited and very expensive resource that must be controlled for public protection.

The issue of quality

Universal agreement exists that good-quality health care is desirable. Who determines what high-quality health care represents and who is to decide how this is to be administered constitute controversial issues for present policy makers. Physicians no longer make these judgments alone; in fact, they may not have a major role in this endeavor in the future.

The issue of quality control is a concept appreciated at many different levels, especially in radiology. It may, however, be interpreted in different terms by those who have or believe they have the responsibility to make such determinations. Organized professional groups often evaluate high-quality care in terms of sophistication of technology, accuracy of diagnosis, specificity of treatment, and percentage of cures. Administrators of medical institutions tend to emphasize such parameters as length of hospital stay, cost effectiveness of radiologic equipment usage, documentation of health care delivered and the results achieved, efficiency of department or staff function, and adequacy of maintenance of archives such as X-ray reports.

Health planners consider quality in general performance terms, such as ratios of physicians to patients, number of inpatient versus outpatient visits, availability of services to various population groups, and other criteria which they consider to be even more objective. Any quality assurance program will apply different judgmental criteria and will have different goals, depending upon which group initiates or judges the performance of the program.

Radiologists often object to their performance being judged in quantifiable terms, such as the timeliness of X-ray reports, without due regard to their value or accuracy. The character of medical practice and the determination of quality have historically been the province of physicians. Administrative personnel in health care systems and those responsible for medical policy were either entirely physicians or groups with significant physician representation.

Physicians traditionally have had the responsibility of determining the prerequisite intelligence and experience necessary for entry into medical schools. It is mainly physicians who have formulated entrance criteria and were largely responsible for the conduct of the entry process at every level. The body of knowledge felt necessary to assure that the student acquires an adequate database for practice has been almost entirely determined by physicians. Our discipline has set standards for their practice and the requirements to be met before one can be a candidate for board examination.

The clinical experience obtained in an internship and radiology residency attempts to ensure that the facts required are made applicable in the practice of the discipline and provide experiences to assure competence on the part of the trainee. The radiology training programs, therefore, are periodically evaluated to determine the adequate availability of resources and personnel. However, specialty competency is not judged by a simple evaluation of the training environment and experience. Rather, availability of resources and personnel and suitable exposure to them are prerequisites for a trainee being permitted to "stand" for the radiology certifying specialty board examination. In many of our newer subspecialties, the appropriate resources are an evolving determination. Thus, no legal standard exists.

The public as consumer is usually not represented during specialty board examinations, nor are the physicians from other disciplines, previously unsuccessful candidates of that specialty examination, or representatives from government agencies or regulatory groups. Given this circumstance, the fundamental issues of certification by licensure and specialty board examination rest on the consideration of what is to be achieved by such accrediting procedures and the problem of appropriate administration of these activities to reach determined goals [7]. At issue are the judgmental quality of the examination versus representation from all interested groups in the accrediting process. In subspecialty discussions, professionals generally maintain that only they have prerequisite training, experience, and knowledge properly to define quality in reference to their own specialty and discipline. Thus, if only they have the appropriate qualifications, then it is proper that they establish the certifying requirements as well as the process by which the evaluation and examination are administered.

One recognizes that this entire methodology eliminates candidates at every level in the qualifying process, from undergraduate college or university to medical school admission and completion, through internship and residency experience (including fellowship), and ultimately through the final steps of board examination and state licensure [8]. Most physicians believe that these methods have historically served the public well, but firm data are often lacking.

Stringent requirements exclude a great number of individuals desiring entry into the marketplace in all medical disciplines, especially in certain subdisciplines of radiology. The imposed entry requirements may not have such exclusion as their goal (either implicit or explicit) but do, indeed, work to ensure that only a select number of candidates will be successful in their attempts to become qualified to practice a particular medical discipline. Combining the limitation of available providers with a relatively high cost of the service and high compensation for this selected group of physicians (medical practitioners), has caused concerns at many levels about the structure and intent of the certification and licensure system [9]. A number of years ago, to ensure that specialty board examinations are administered fairly and in such a manner as to protect the public, the FTC subpoenaed the records of several of these bodies including radiology [4].

Specialty groups maintain that the circumstances created by this form of licensure and certification constitute the most reasonable method to guarantee that quality medical care will be delivered to the public, even though the system may be selective and costly. By preventing uncontrolled entry into the marketplace of specialty practitioners, the public is to be protected from incompetent physicians who might engage, through ignorance or intent, in substandard practices detrimental to the general public welfare. Although such "safeguards" may tend to increase the cost of medical care, the proponents of the specialty certifying system believe that the expenditure is justified and proper. This is especially true if the alternative is truly substandard medical care [10–12]. The additional cost to the individual patient at present is proposed to be offset by the financial implications of poor health care delivery to a substantial segment of the population. Certainly, radiology will be among those specialties challenged first; it is expensive and often poorly understood by the public.

Many patient-advocate groups claim that these entry restrictions work effectively to exclude minority groups and the financially disadvantaged. Specialty board examinations are regarded by these groups as an extension of the medieval "guild system", denying entry of a large number of individuals into a particular skill, profession, or discipline, in order to maintain the limited availability of expensive compensation structures.

Lack of disclosure regarding details of the examination process, exclusion of the public as consumers from the licensing bodies, and lack of public review of certifying criteria are regarded by many groups as evidence that the intent is not that of public protection. This appears to be a predictable legal challenge for interventive radiology in the future. Can radiologists determine what the training should be and who should be trained to provide "radiologic" services? These answers may require mutual agreement between many groups in the future.

Determining the characteristics of a suitable individual for training and methodology of the process is a difficult problem, especially in a field where the procedures and technology are changing so rapidly. Many would concede that the consumer must have a role in this undertaking, but would reason that most appropriately this should be in the "front end of the system". Thus, policies that set forth requirements for entry into our complex training programs should be established by joint decisions of the providers and consumers. The length of training and the methods involved would, under this logic, require this same cooperative mode.

Should content of the examination for certification following radiologic training have consumer input for assurance of protection of the public interests? Whether or not it is appropriate to have public representation of all interested parties at the time of the examination process remains problematic. Accountability of the professional specialty group may be effected by some observation of consumer representatives. Active participation by the consumer representative has the potential risk of disruption of the certification process and compromise of the stated intent. As long as the public representation in the standards, requirements, and the planning is assured, with consumer accountability by the certifying body as well, many believe that public welfare will be protected.

The cost of a finite service or product must be controlled in relation to the resources available for delivery of health care. Consumer representation is perceived as vitally important in this regard [13]. Third-party compensation plans have been a major determinant in decreasing accountability and engendering appropriate professional response. Displacement of the cost, charge, and even of service rendered from the compensation level has led to such an indirect audit trail that identification of areas of abuse and misuse has been difficult. This is one of the major goals of health care reform.

The relation of the costs of medical care with licensure and certification is not direct, and the inference that such an association exists may not be tenable. Identification of the actual causes of expenditures will allow focus upon other mechanisms in the total system. For these reasons, we have had the Tax Equity Financing Responsibility Act, the initiation of DRGs and the RVS in the past, and health care reform on our future policy agenda. Physicians are being asked to provide an environment wherein documented claims

accruing to public good by maintenance of high standards and strict requirements can be more readily perceived. "Outcomes research" is part of this process. Such an approach is a more rational concept for public protection than regulation, in response to the "guild theory" interpretation with its attendant abuses.

Many believe that capital expenditures for medical instrumentation are a major factor in the rapid escalation of health care costs. Certainly, the equipment employed for radiology is expensive. Some type of regulation of expenditures for and distribution of certain medical services is believed to be necessary to control costs [14].

Federal legislation enacted to attempt to control health care costs has in the past mandated state government to require certificates of need (CON) for utilization of expensive new medical technology in hospitals. It was believed that this control legislation would ensure that patient requirements would then greatly influence the purchase and distribution of costly instrumentation [15]. If appropriate criteria to determine the correct distribution of expensive medical technology could be established, it was felt that the public interest could be protected.

The free enterprise system historically has not offered sufficiently effective safeguards, given the public's appetite for expensive new procedures and the technology to perform them. With the enactment of certain regulations, useful criteria for approval of the CON can be developed and economic guidelines for individual hospitals enacted. Although these policies would sometimes create quasimonopolies and restraint of trade circumstances for certain hospitals in specific locations, pragmatically it has been perceived that the general proposed benefits would outweigh the potential undesired local effects.

The concept that regulation should govern the supply of institutional health services is based upon several assumptions. If supply is controlled, private enterprise will be forced to ration services, and the resulting demand for these rationed services will more closely approximate actual clinical need. The health care industry, if unregulated, will soon acquire excess capacity because it does not function competitively in the traditional sense [16,17]. An informed choice by the consumer (patient) may be precluded by the uncertainties of and the technical complexity attendant to both diagnosis and treatment. Usually, the physician, rather than the patient, makes the determinant choice. In radiology, the patient may not even be fully aware that a choice has been made.

One should examine whether CON considerations achieved the intended outcome. In small, isolated communities, a single provider can dominate the supply curve. The dominant provider can then promote the initiation of new technology with little constraint from considerations of previous levels of demand. If an institutional provider is satisfied with the market share it is granted, the provider may use the CON to regulate its competition. If entry barriers are established by

CON regulations, this may create a circumstance where the self-interest of the provider, as opposed to the consumer, is protected. CON appeared to have achieved some accommodation with X-ray computed tomography (CT) scanners, but the advent of magnetic resonance imaging (MRI) technology again made CON important.

Regulation and competition have been viewed as mutually exclusive. Although certain effects of this health care regulation are well recognized, methodologies for structuring regulation to achieve coordination of objectives are not generally accepted or understood. In the health care industry, analysis of the effects of regulation is often undertaken only after implementation. For example, one should examine the combined effects of changing criteria for hospital practice privileges and the interrelationship with CON regulation and implementation for the equipment to perform the interventive procedures. This is merely an initiating point for the changes invoked by DRGs, RVS, analysis of diagnostic imaging centers, and financial negotiations of health maintenance organizations (HMSOs), preferred provider organizations (PPOs), etc.

The granting of hospital and practice privileges to physicians has traditionally been a simple process undertaken without emphasis of the liability implications. Recently, hospital trustees and governing bodies have had reason to investigate the issue of "due process". The ultimate responsibility for decisions related to the access to a particular hospital must be considered. Litigation has been instituted by unsuccessful applicants; the courts no longer accord the decision maker great latitude in setting criteria for admission to the staff of hospitals.

If the methodology employed is either faulty by design or the agreed-upon mechanisms were not being respected, a challenge to denial of privileges might be sustained. With present extension of liability under the expansion of agency logic to be discussed, boards of trust and hospital administrations have become much more aware of the liability implications arising from the granting of physician hospital privileges.

In considering the combined effects of these initiatives, the interrelationships achieve great importance. With the quasimonopoly effect created by the application of CON legislation, associated with the constraint of free entry due to changes in granting hospital privileges, the effect upon radiologic practice is significant [18]. CON effects upon instrument location can result in limited distribution of a particular costly and sophisticated technology such as X-ray CT, a positron emission tomography (PET) device, single photon emission CT (SPECT), MRI, or an angiographic suite [19]. Patients, in order to have diagnostic studies and therapy utilizing many of these instruments, will often be admitted to the hospital requiring hospital admission privileges for their physicians.

The traditional posture of granting of hospital privileges has been a relaxed one, with only general attention given to due process. There was little inquiry regarding the procedures and process, criteria, and effects of the decisions, and a rather accepting posture by the professionals requesting hospital privileges for themselves. As long as the criteria appeared even potentially reasonable, the courts have given wide latitude to the decision makers. Activities relating to the discharge of this responsibility were generously interpreted to represent "due process". The denial of hospital privileges was usually accepted by unsuccessful physicians. Today, they may no longer be as reluctant to use the legal process to seek redress.

The technologic opportunities offered by the department of radiology of a particular hospital are a significant factor in the type and character of patient care possible in that institution [20]. Exclusion from a specific hospital in the past might have denied use of certain technologies to both physicians and their patients, but these were of lesser importance, or viewed as such by both the provider and consumer. This is not the prevailing attitude today. The reasons for this change in consumer expectations and attitudes are numerous. Adequate medical care in the USA is viewed by the public and their policy-making representatives as a right that must be ensured, monitored, and protected [19]. Methods to ensure this right to quality health care are therefore justified as regulation of a necessary resource.

Improved therapeutic capabilities by radiology have changed the character of our practice. The general trends of specialization and subspecialization have been associated with heightened expectation of patients. Medical practice in the USA has become increasingly dependent upon sophisticated and costly technology. Issues of "turf" can be expected both from without and within medicine in general, the radiological specialty, and from the public at large. These issues will be considered in further detail.

As more definitive radiologic techniques have evolved, the desire by both the provider of health care and consumer of services to be able to utilize these developments has increased commensurately. When the denial of hospital privileges effectively precludes access to the desired service, patients and physicians are aware of the implications. They have become increasingly aggressive in seeking legal means to overcome this perceived constraint.

A more substantive role of physicians and hospital privileges review processes has offered protection of the providers [21–23]. Is this process sufficiently immune from provider manipulation that the distribution of services and technology is in concert with patient needs? Should methods be developed for granting limited hospital privileges for the expressed purpose of gaining access to a specific resource such as an interventive study? Guidelines for limited liability would, of necessity, have to be established if we have limited hospital privileges. Technologic and biomedical instrumentation trends in USA medicine, regulation of this technology, and more rigorous and difficult requirements for hospital staff privileges could have a combined effect that is both unintended and unexpected.

Society must question whether or not regulation assures a more appropriate distribution of services at less total cost [24]. Determinations must be made as to whether consumer desires are reflected by limited access justified by resource limitation. Stiffened requirements for hospital privileges can certainly be viewed as a method to promote professional quality assurance. Certain specific issues will be considered in greater detail.

Agency relationships

The basis of the legal system in the USA is that of traditional English common law, which represents the alternate to codification of legal decisions as exist in many other nations. The former structure, while somewhat unpredictable, allows modification and, ideally, appropriate interpretation to meet changing circumstances, and permits adaptation to social progress and contemporary societal concerns. Case-made law theoretically provides an imperfect but flexible system in which temporary inequities and departures from fairness can be addressed [5]. Of particular importance to radiology are relationships that relate not only to nonprofessional employees but to our trainees at all levels.

In any radiology department, there are complex relationships that represent the manner of modern health care delivery [25,26]. Diagnostic as well as therapeutic radiology are particularly appropriate disciplines to consider because the interdependence of employees and physicians is as fundamental as any in the health care system [27]. Most of these relationships can be characterized in the nature of agency arrangements.

What is an agency? An agency relationship exists when an individual or group of individuals performs a service for the benefit of another — the principal. In radiology, there are both expressed and implied agency relationships. Expressed relationships may be memorialized in departments by a document such as a contract. Implied relationships may exist when a circumstance is created in which a third party would logically assume that the agent is acting on behalf of and for the benefit of the principal. The mere appearance of an agency relationship may well create one in the legal sense. This occurs daily in angiography and other subspecialties such as interventional radiology.

Compensation is not necessary for an agency relationship to be formed, but some identifiable benefit to both parties is. For the principal, this may be as ill-defined as increased efficiency and capability. For the agent, it may be as seemingly unrelated a benefit as educational opportunities, added prestige from a clinical appointment to the institution, or one as fundamental as maintenance of employment. The fact that financial reward is not part of an agreement does not mean that an agency relationship does not exist.

Agency relationships may be so complex in radiology departments that subagencies can be formed even without the knowledge of the principal. Both agency and subagency relationships are characteristic of diagnostic and therapeutic radiology and are very common in the newer subspecialty of interventive angiography. What may be unusual, even unique in the entire health care field, are the medical responsibilities accorded the technologic staff in certain subspecialties of radiology. Almost nowhere else in medicine is the technical (nondoctorate of medicine) employee delegated the decisional latitude given the angiographic technologist in the usual practice of performing these studies. Many functions and activities, if they occurred in other disciplines, would be outside the usual scope of nonphysician employment and might well be considered, in themselves, "the practice of medicine".

In common law, each case is decided upon its own merits with legal precedent offering weight to the testimony and line of reasoning given. The principal is liable for the actions of the agent as long as these activities are a natural and logic consequence of the "scope of employment". Documents such as descriptions of scope of employment in a contract, notwithstanding actions, provide evidence of intent both in the limits of performance and liability. New procedures in the radiological sciences or medical imaging discipline are almost always characterized as a corporate effort with an inherent agency bias. Analysis of agency responsibility often involved determination of "scope of employment".

Scope of employment may be modified greatly by those activities assumed by the agents and permitted by the principals. If, in the conduct of the delivery of a particular radiologic service, agents assume expanded responsibilities that are allowed by the principal, those activities will then legally fall within the scope of employment. For example, if a technologist or junior resident is allowed routinely to provide the major effort for a particular interventive study, the principal staff radiologist becomes liable for those injuries in which proximate cause in relation to that examination by the resident can be established. This responsibility may well occur even if the principal was physically absent at the time of the study, the acquired images were not recorded for subsequent review, or, if obtained, were not even analyzed by the principal [28,29]. Nonpermanent recording during angiography, depending upon the image on the cathode-ray tube monitor, or observing at fluoroscopy obviously provides significant problems with establishment of responsibility in agency relationships in the documented absence of the principal.

According to "captain of the ship" logic, the principal is responsible for the actions of the agent — not only those under his or her control, but also those that he or she should have controlled. Vicarious or extended liability is a concept that the courts have expanded greatly in recent years for medical circumstances. Medical delivery is regarded as a complex effort in which many persons may interact with patients.

One must understand that it is difficult for lay persons to identify clearly the roles and responsibilities of the individual participants of a medical team, especially in radiology departments where all levels of expertise exist. Extension of the vicarious liability concept has been a response to this lack of clearly defined roles of each member. When a diagnostic imaging study is performed, the patient may have personal contact with only the technologist; therefore, the staff radiologist, resident, or fellow's role may not be apparent to or understood by the patient. Given this circumstance, there is a tendency to accord extended liability to the principal for the actions of the agent. The ultimate responsibility rests with the principal — the radiologist in charge of the activity in question.

Agency relationships between technologists and physicians depend to some extent upon the customs of practice in a particular locality. As part of the technologists' oath in the USA, they agree not to render interpretations regarding studies generated by themselves or others. In the UK, certain technologists may render opinions regarding the findings on diagnostic studies and may issue official reports without designating whether they are qualified physicians. Liability for harm due to negligence in performing or interpreting the study belongs to the physician.

In all localities in the USA, agency law is interpreted similarly by the courts, but differences in practice customs can change significantly who is accorded the final responsibility. By independently engaging in the "practice of medicine", someone who does not have a medical degree no longer acts as the agent for the principal. There appears to be no legal impediment in certain locales to having a nonradiologist purchase instrumentation, perform the imaging studies, and ultimately render interpretations. The financial guidelines and constraints of reimbursement may, indeed, preclude this as a practical possibility. Rendering interpretations by technologists in the USA would be restricted by certification agreement but not entirely prevented by law. Licensure requirements in certain states may well preclude the operation of the equipment by nonmedical groups. CON legislation and ruling of antitrust in the USA have controlled to some degree the numbers and distribution of expensive and sophisticated instrumentation [14]. These barriers, in addition to restriction of hospital privileges, have limited both acquisition of, use of, and access to certain medical devices [17].

Agency relationships in the USA for purchase of costly instrumentation have been established through venture capital arrangements, partnerships (both limited and general), and specifically constituted corporations. The liability of each group in this agency relationship may be determined largely by the language and specifications of the agreement document. Obviously, recent decisions by the Inspector General's office and certain "health reforms" may render this all moot.

Exclusive contracts have created problems of access and also distribution, and may dramatically alter the possibilities of establishing agency relationships [30]. If a particular radiology group has an exclusive contract to perform studies in a particular hospital or group of medical institutions, radiologists can perform studies at that location only if they are employed by the group. Additionally, radiologists can interpret and charge for studies if they are members of the practice group. To provide interventive services, specialized contracts have been employed. This provides a circumstance in which issues of "turf" become quite important and subcontracts may necessarily have certain cardiac, vascular, or therapeutic procedures rendered by anyone except, e.g., the radiologic partnership group that holds the imaging contract for that hospital.

Agency relationships and training requirements may be in conflict. If certain studies such as cardiac angiography, coronary dilatations, and vascular stents are performed by other disciplines, a subagency may have to be created for residents in radiology to receive the proper training experience. With displacement of certain technology by imaging centers, the radiology department, if excluded, may need to form an agency relationship by contract on behalf of their trainees.

Often, agency relationships are affected and even determined by compensation schemes. In certain locales, reimbursement for self-referral is less than that paid for comparable procedures rendered under a consultant (independent contractor) relationship. A consultant acts as an independent contractor and exposes the referring physician to less malpractice exposure than in cases of self-referral [31].

In the USA, the health care system has moved from the concept of a retrospective reimbursement system to a prospective one. This policy decision will alter practice patterns fundamentally in ways that have legal implications for agency relationships. Alternates of studies and procedures likely will favor those characterized as "safe, simple, and inexpensive" [32]. Emphasis will be placed upon procedures with minimal physician involvement and, if possible, will be performed by nonphysician agents to make them more financially rewarding. For example, physicians may be replaced by an agent in time-consuming diagnostic studies such as pulsed Doppler realtime study of the carotid circulation [33]. Agency relationships may well achieve increasing importance in this circumstance of substitution of nonprofessional for professional personnel [25].

As angiographers expand their activities in the area of "interventive medicine", their malpractice exposure will increase. Intrauterine treatment using ultrasound for hydrocephalus, cardiac abnormalities, and urinary obstruction have been described in the literature [34]. Therapeutic angiographic procedures have placed radiologists at much greater legal risk just by the nature of the studies themselves. It may become exceedingly difficult to determine legally when the radiologist is acting as a consultant (independent contractor) or as an agent of the surgeon. When summoned by the surgeon to perform interventive studies, is the technologist the agent of the surgeon, the radiologists, or both? There are no precedent decisions in this regard to date. These procedures are being performed more frequently, and litigation should be expected. We must provide our trainees with some experience in interventive procedures, recognizing that our legal exposure will be much greater than with more traditional training circumstances. Where standard of practice analysis is obviated by experimental procedures, the legal implications are particularly important.

Untoward events during angiographic procedures can result from a variety of etiologies. Technologists may act outside their scope of employment, trainees and staff radiologists may not perform to the level of standard care, or the equipment may fail. If a patient is injured due to equipment failure, is the manufacturer liable, the radiologist as ensurer of a good result, or is the principal on whose behalf the agent performed the study at legal risk? In the USA, courts have ruled that the instrument manufacturer is the most responsible party to ensure the appropriate performance of the machine itself and is, therefore, liable for harm to patients for faulty design or fabrication [35]. Since many departments performing interventive procedures use prototype equipment, instruments loaned by manufacturers for "clinical testing", and other complex arrangements, these determinations are quite problematic.

If the technology is applied inappropriately, the radiologist will be found liable for any injury in which proximate cause can be established. In this circumstance, radiologists are not agents of the manufacturer. Whether the instrumentation is on loan or has been purchased by the radiology department does not substantially change the facts. However, new guidewires, stents, balloons, and pharmacologic agents carry an enhanced risk.

Many areas of the law of agency in medical imaging are founded on common law theory. Circumstances in one locale may result in the existence of precedent cases prior to their litigation in another. These precedent decisions may serve as instructive in anticipating legal ramifications to continuing developments in therapeutic radiology. Agency law is particularly appropriate to consider as interventive radiology continues to increase in complexity and sophistication, necessitating a team approach. The previous lack of invasiveness has made medical imaging traditionally immune from concerted legal inquiry. Interventive radiology will predictably extend the questions of agency relationships.

In many radiology departments composed of staff members with specialty and subspecialty interests, trainees at varied levels of expertise, and research associates, "standard of care" and "scope of employment" will be difficult to determine. The graduated responsibilities of trainees will make it quite difficult to determine whether any particular behavior is appropriate. For example, the question of supervision during any particular invasive procedure may be the determinant factor in assessing liability. It appears prudent for the angiographer to consider that the final responsibility will rest with the principal in any interventive radiology procedure.

Antitrust and turf

As noted, the general area of antitrust and exclusive contracts has become an increasingly important one for the discipline of radiology and radiologic sciences, especially in the new and dramatic subspecialties. Intrusion of regulation into the health care industry has been a phenomenon of the 1980s and appears to be a trend that will continue through the 1990s and beyond. Our discipline has experienced the application of antitrust regulation in resource allocation and distribution, determination of exclusivity and market capture of delivery contracts, and the fairness of compensation schemes. Through the analysis of certain landmark cases involving the application of antitrust principles to health care situations, we can enhance our understanding of the implications of these decisions [30,36,37] and possibly anticipate their future effects [14,38,39].

Among the more fundamental issues in a service, hospital-based specialty such as medical imaging is the determination of the scope and limits of this service as established by an exclusive contractual arrangement. The colloquial expression for this arrangement is couched in terms of "turf". The case of *White* v. *Rockingham Radiologists, Ltd.* [40] is an important one in which the issues of concern are quite well articulated, the legal analysis is sufficiently broad to reveal potential future applications for other areas such as interventional radiology, and the explanation of the decision process significant enough to make this a landmark case.

In *White* v. *Rockingham Radiologists, Ltd.*, the plaintiff neurologist sued both the hospital, a shared service organization, and the radiology group because the hospital mandated that the radiologists render all interpretations of the X-ray CT head scans. According to the plaintiff, this exclusive arrangement resulted in a variety of legal issues including conspiracy in restraint of trade, a group boycott, tying arrangement, monopolization, attempted monopolization, and conspiracy to monopolize. The district court granted the defendant's motions for summary judgment on all claims and the Fourth Circuit affirmed this decision. The court held that there existed no conspiracy or group boycott, because the evidence showed that the decision concerning who would render official interpretations was made unilaterally by the hospital governing body. The radiologists did no more than to lobby the board, and the shared service organization played no role in the decision process at all.

The plaintiff also claimed that the hospital tied the sale

of medical and surgical services to CT scanning services. However, the hospital neither owned the scanner (which was owned by the shared service organization), nor forced all its patients to purchase the particular service, a CT scan. The court rejected the tying arrangement allegations that the hospital tied the sale of CT scans to its patients' purchasing CT scan interpretations from only the radiologists. The court emphasized that the seller of the tying product (the CT scans) was not a competitor in the market for the tied product (interpretations) because it had no economic interest in the sale of those interpretations. The radiologists paid no part of their fees for their interpretations to the hospital, which has been viewed in other instances as a "kickback". The professional and technical charges were separate and distinct in the arrangement between the hospital and the radiology group.

The court affirmed dismissal of the plaintiff's claim that the hospital had monopolized the market for hospital services because the hospital was neither a provider nor consumer of those particular services. The court also dismissed the claim that the hospital monopolized the market for the CT scan interpretations because the hospital was not a competitor in that market. Moreover, there was found to be no "willful acquisition" of monopoly power because the hospital placed at the court's disposal valid business and efficiency reasons for the decision about who should interpret the diagnostic scans.

Testimony emphasizing the advantage of allocative efficiency and improved quality assurance control is standard and traditional in defense of exclusive contracts. From the trial testimony it became apparent that the radiologists lacked monopoly power in the market for CT interpretations because, according to the terms of their contract, the hospital — showing due cause and process — could replace them as official interpreters whenever they wished [41].

White v. *Rockingham Radiologists, Ltd.*, is an instructive and important case for radiology as it embodies many elements of an exclusive medical contract dispute analysis as well as the evolving issue of turf conflicts for elements of health care service delivery. Radiology and radiologic science departments must continually compete to maintain the institutional approval to provide the clinical service in nuclear cardiology, obstetric ultrasound, cardiac angiography, pulsed Doppler realtime carotid sonography, X-ray CT, MRI, as well as interventive radiology.

As the delivery of health care becomes increasingly competitive, as the effects of physician oversupply or conversely maldistribution become more important, and cost considerations resulting in reduction of technology as well as distribution control initiatives, more effective designation of providers by contract will assume an ever-increasing importance. This is not simply an economic issue but has implications for specialty and subspecialty relationships, control of patient care, the standing of various disciplines within the institutional hierarchy, and even for prestige

and media attention. All of these issues are important for radiology.

The legal issues in *White* v. *Rockingham Radiologists, Ltd.*, are more complicated than those in several often cited precedent cases such as *Harron* v. *United Hospital Center, Inc.*, [9], but these merit analysis. The contractual arrangement of the radiology group with the hospital in *White* v. *Rockingham Radiologists, Ltd.*, was more complex, and the plaintiff neurology group was seeking to provide only a specialized part of a particular service (X-ray CT interpretations of studies involving the central nervous system). As interventive radiology grows in size and complexity, specialization will occur to a much greater extent than at present.

In the antitrust analysis of any exclusive contract case a pivotal element is in defining the relevant market and to determine whether it is geographic or product related. The standards and techniques for market definition in health care cases are now being equated to those involving other industries. The results are specific to health care, of course, because market definition depends on the facts of the industry at issue. This will be quite problematic in a changing field such as radiology. Market definition remains significant in health industry cases because of certain characteristics of the endeavor. This is because of the prominence of third-party payers and economic regulation, which deprive health care markets of many nonshare factors that temper the interpretation of market shares [42–44]. Determination of the market for a new radiologic procedure will be difficult and subject to modification over time.

A review of antitrust principles may place *White* v. *Rockingham Radiologists, Ltd.*, in perspective for our discipline. The central concern embodied in antitrust laws is the fear of exercise or abuse of market power (i.e., power to control price or exclude competitors). In principle, market power may be exercised by a single dominant contracting group or by a group of firms acting collectively. In either case, market definition is described as central to the assessment of market power. In assessing single-firm exercise or acquisition of market power, market definition is characterized as "an analytical construct enabling one to compensate the inability to measure market power directly" [45].

> Market definition becomes crucial only when there are no other discoverable facts establishing the existence and degree of market power more directly and with accuracy. One would never need to define the market if they could accurately establish the firm's demand and cost curves — the quantities that could be sold at various prices, and the costs of producing those quantities. That information would directly establish both the presence of market power and the magnitude of potential monopoly profits. The firm's demand curve would reflect the availability of any substitutes, without further need for identifying them or their closeness [46].

One can easily recognize the problem in *White* v. *Rockingham*

Radiologists, Ltd. Market definition is an aid for determining whether power exists. A characteristic of relevant terms of product and geographic market is the relationship such that if prices were appreciably raised or volume appreciably curtailed for the product within a given area, while demand remained constant, supply from other sources could not be expected to enter quickly enough or in sufficient amounts to restore the former price or volume. A "relevant market" consists of all services rendered that directly affect the pricing decisions of the defendant. It is the narrowest market that is wide enough so that products from adjacent areas or from other producers in the same area cannot compete on substantial parity with those included in the market. Something as specialized as medical imaging can effectively exclude and capture all of the market. As the present administration and health policy groups attempt to assess the economic factors in the cost of health care, these issues may become paramount.

Because of the difficulties in measuring market power directly, an indirect measurement process has evolved. This is to define the relevant market, and subsequently infer power within the market through the use of proxies such as market shares and other factors. Economists have recently developed techniques that show progress toward enabling direct econometric estimation of market power, but substantial application in court decisions will be necessary before the techniques can be widely employed to our discipline. In general, markets are defined in medical antitrust cases when the circumstances of market power are at issue and cannot be established by presumption.

Markets must be defined in cases brought under most monopoly-related theories under Section Two of the Sherman Antitrust Act [47]. When actual or attempted monopolization has been alleged, a relevant market must be defined. In *Walker Process Equipment, Inc.* v. *Food Machinery & Chemical Corp.* [48], the Supreme Court noted that:

> to establish monopolization or attempt to monopolize a part of trade or commerce under § 2 of the Sherman Act, it is necessary to appraise the exclusionary power in terms of the relevant market for the product involved. Without a definition of that market one is not able to measure (the defendant's) ability to lessen or destroy competition.

When combination or conspiracy to monopolize has been alleged, definition of a relevant market may not be necessary. Most authorities support the proposition that a plaintiff is not required to establish a relevant market in such circumstances "because proof of the agreement to commit an illegal act and proof of an overt act establishes the violation". This exception did not appear to be applicable in *White* v. *Rockingham Radiologists, Ltd.*

Markets must be defined in restraint of trade cases brought under Section One of the Sherman Antitrust Act [47]. This is very important when market power is at issue and cannot be presumed as a matter of law or on the basis of an in-depth analysis. Determining whether such a presumption applies and how it is to be structured, however, is often a crucial issue in Section One cases.

Under traditional doctrine, restraints of trade have been categorized into two alternate methods of analysis: (i) the per se rule; or (ii) the Brandeis "rule of reason". Whether market definition was necessary in a particular case has turned on the categorization of a particular restraint. In the per se cases are agreements whose nature and necessary effect are so plainly anticompetitive that no elaborate study of the industry is needed to establish their illegality — they are "illegal per se". These violations are proscribed in the language of the Sherman Antitrust Act [47].

In the non-per se category are agreements whose competitive effect can only be evaluated by analyzing the facts peculiar to the business, the history of the restraint, and the reasons why it was imposed [49]. Most radiology cases fall under this analysis [50]. Under the per se rule, the "market impact" of a practice has historically been presumed, thus obviating the need for market definition. Under the non-per se rule of reason, the market impact of a practice has historically been determined by its effect in a relevant market.

In recent years, the dichotomy between the per se rule and the rule of reason has become less defined, and alternate modes of analysis have shifted from two distinct categories towards a spectrum.

> While the "reasonableness" of a particular alleged restraint often depends on the market power of the parties involved, because a judgment about market power is the means by which the effects of the conduct on the market place can be assessed, market power is only one test of "reasonableness." And where the anticompetitive effects of conduct can be ascertained through means short of extensive market analysis, and where no countervailing competitive virtues are evident, a lengthy analysis of market power is not necessary [51].

For example, with new techniques such as certain procedures in the subspecialties of radiology, an extensive analysis would seldom be necessary.

Basic Section One, Sherman Antitrust Act analysis determines whether an agreement between competitors unreasonably restrains trade. The Act provides "that every contract, combination or conspiracy in restraint of trade or commerce among the several States, or with foreign nations ... is illegal" [47]. This section of the Sherman Antitrust Act includes two preliminary requirements: (i) at least two firms or economic units must be involved; and (ii) there must be some form of agreement or collaboration between the two or more parties such as an exclusive contract to perform the interventive procedures and to be compensated for this service.

Market definition to prove the existence of market capture becomes necessary only if these threshold requirements are satisfied. Depending upon the type of agreement and its anticompetitive effects, the court will either commence a "rule of reason" analysis [52], or will declare the agreement per se illegal.

Market definition is generally unnecessary in discrimination cases brought under the Robinson–Patman Act [53]. Although competitive injury must be proven under the principal statutory provision, courts typically assess competitive injury with little regard to market power or market effect. Instead, courts commonly look to the nature and degree of harm suffered by the injured party. In *White* v. *Rockingham Radiologists, Ltd.* [40], the neurologists failed to convince the trier of the fact that their claimed potential injury was real.

The relevant market normally must be identified along two dimensions: (i) the trade in products or services affected (the relevant product market); and (ii) the geographic areas within which such trade may be affected (the relevant geographic market) [54]. Because most radiologic procedures have possible substitutes, one cannot give "that infinite range" to the definition of the alternates. In considering what is the relevant market for determining the control of price and competition, no more definite rule can be declared than that commodities reasonably interchangeable by consumers for the same purpose make up this "part of the trade or commerce", monopolization of which may be illegal [55]. Medical procedures leading to images could well be considered in this manner.

When the market is viewed from the production rather than the consumption standpoint, the degree to which substitution can be made in production is measured by crosselasticity of supply. The ability to substitute in production refers to the capacity of firms in a given line of commerce to turn their productive facilities towards the production of commodities in another line because of similarities in technology between them. Where the degree of substitutability in production is high, such as CT or MRI of the abdomen, crosselasticities of supply will also be high, and again the two commodities in question should be treated as part of the same market. In medicine, cross-substitution is often impossible. However, would studies such as X-ray CT, MRI, or PET be considered equivalent in all circumstances?

In some instances, courts have found a narrow relevant market — a "submarket" — within a larger market. In a broad market such as medical imaging, well-defined submarkets such as interventive procedures may exist which, in themselves, may constitute product markets for antitrust purposes. The boundaries of such a submarket may be determined by examining such practical indicia as industry or public recognition of the submarket as a separate economic entity, the product's peculiar characteristics and uses, unique production facilities, unique customers, distinct prices, sensitivity to price changes, and specialized vendors. These characteristics may very well apply to the newer areas of radiology.

The USA Department of Justice Merger Guidelines and Vertical Restraints Guidelines define a market as a group of products and associated geographic area in which the exercise of market power would be feasible. Formally, a market was defined as a product or group of products and a geographic area in which the product is sold. According to this definition, a hypothetical, profit-maximizing firm such as a group of interventive radiologists not strictly subject to price regulation, was the only present and future seller of those products in that patient area. This firm could impose a "small but significant and nontransitory" increase in charges above the prevailing ones for similar but not identical services or likely future levels [56,57].

Obviously, marketplace analysis and determination in a complex field such as radiology and radiologic sciences is exceedingly difficult. The trier of fact often will be perplexed by the implications of the technology at issue. While X-ray CT has been clinically available in the USA since 1973, its relative efficacy to alternate procedures such as radionuclide brain scans, digital angiography, or MRI is an evolving determination which will be crucial to accurate assessment of the product marketplace. Some of the newer subspecialties of radiology have even fewer standards, credentials, and practice precedents to judge the value or to determine appropriate compensation for these procedures.

In *White* v. *Rockingham Radiologists, Ltd.* [40], the neurologists accused the radiologist and the hospital of conspiring to effect a group boycott. Although the radiologists may well have influenced the decision of the hospital board by their lobbying effort, no conspiracy was found because the neurology group was given an equal opportunity to lobby the hospital (and on advice of counsel declined), and the hospital board reached their decision about the radiology group without the presence of a representative of that legal entity.

Tying arrangements in antitrust suits are often alleged when it appears that choice or selection of one product is tantamount to selecting a second and different product. Such a circumstance is felt *de facto* to preclude choice or potential rejection by the consumer (patient) of the tied product. Clearly, violation of antitrust is possible if both products are controlled by the same person, group, or entity accused. In the *White* v. *Rockingham Radiologists, Ltd.* analysis, the court deemed that the tying product was the CT scan and that the tied product was the interpretation. In so doing, the seller of the tying product became the shared service organization that owned the CT instrumentation, and the control of the tied product rested in the radiology group. Given this arrangement, the claim of conspiracy to monopolize, naming the hospital and the radiology group, would be inherently flawed. The arrangement of ownership of the CT scanner and the clear separation of technical and professional charges have removed the hospital from a great deal of the usual microeconomic analysis regarding monopolization and market capture. In instances where a comingling of the technical and professional charges exists, or having the professional charges included as an institutional contribution or return for privileges, the hospital's exposure to culpability relating to these claims would be substantially increased. Therefore, the contract to perform radiologic procedures should be based upon training, experience, and merit, and never upon some primarily financial impetus.

Exclusive contracts for radiologic services must be finite. The importance of termination clauses in exclusive contracts depends upon the language of the justification, the length of the documented contract, and the options and alternates of service available to all appropriate parties. In *White* v. *Rockingham Radiologists, Ltd.* the court was convinced that the hospital could actually void the exclusive services contract and dismiss with proper cause the radiology group. According the contracting institution a defined ability and stated methodology to replace their privileges and services with another group can often afford the contracting radiologists a measure of protection from challenges of active monopolization or conspiracy to monopolize. *White* v. *Rockingham Radiologists, Ltd.* is an instructive case in that regard, and essentially demonstrates that if a contracting radiology group does not display standard of care in providing their services then their contract can be terminated.

White v. *Rockingham Radiologists, Ltd.* is an important precedent case to the discipline of radiology as well as to all of medicine from several viewpoints. This case is fundamentally instructive regarding the elements of marketplace determination in the health care area. Also, *White* v. *Rockingham Radiologists, Ltd.* demonstrates the legal implications resulting from an issue of medical "turf." It provides insight into the various arrangements of instrumentation ownership such as angiography suites, compensation for professional services as in specialized procedures, technical charges, and elements of legal concern in the language, duration, and implications of exclusive contracts.

One can view *White* v. *Rockingham Radiologists, Ltd.* as one of what promises to be a series of future legal challenges to the delivery of radiologic services, especially those that are technique oriented and have a high degree of specificity such as interventive procedures. Only by improving our understanding of these precedent decisions can we hope to respond in a sufficiently appropriate manner so that the delivery of diagnostic services will remain intact and our role in health care will be delivered in the most expert and efficient manner. To segment the various elements of an interventive service does not appear to be in the patient's best interests which, in the end, should be our paramount concern.

The most pervasive challenge of medicine in the remainder of this century and the decades to follow will be decreasing health care costs. The impact upon the overall economy is believed to be exceedingly important. There is increasing awareness that decisions must be made that will limit availability of certain services, and those involving large unit cost

such as medical imaging technology will attract intense scrutiny and analysis. Quality may well be judged mainly in terms of efficiency and effectiveness. These are social issues of unprecedented magnitude. Radiologists will need to understand the issue in a societal context. "Legal" concerns will assume a more ethical characterization. While these challenges are truly monumental, the discipline has a historic tradition of appropriate responses. Hopefully, this communication will provide a framework to achieve a useful understanding.

Acknowledgments

The author is grateful for the advice, ideas, and support of colleagues such as Sy Perry, Clark Havighurst, Terry Calvani, Jeff Miles, Joe Sims, Phil Posner, Bill Blumenthal, Toby Singer, Jim Blumstein, Elizabeth Gee, Paul Gephart, and Tom Greeson.

References

1 *Goldfarb* v. *Virginia State Bar*, 497 F.2d 1, 421 U.S., 773, 787. 1974.
2 Shryock R. *Medical Licensing in America*. Baltimore: Johns Hopkins Press, 1967.
3 Gelhorn W. The abuse of occupational licensing. *Univ Chicago Law Rev* 1976;44:6.
4 *FTC* v. *American College of Radiology*, CCH Trade Case 21, 236. 1977.
5 James AE Jr. Medical imaging technology in a societal context. *Am J Roentgenol* 1985;144:1109−1116.
6 Posner R. *Antitrust Law: an Economic Perspective*. Chicago: University of Chicago Press, 1976.
7 Roemer M, Shain M. *Hospital Utilization Under AHA*. Chicago, 1959.
8 *Datillo* v. *Tucson General Hospital, Inc.*, 533 P.2d 700, Ariz. 1975.
9 *Harron* v. *United Hospital Center, Inc.*, 522 F.2d 1133, 424 U.S. 916. 1975.
10 *Bank Building and Equipment Corporation of America* v. *National Council of Architectural Registration Board*, CCH Trade Case 60108, Calc.D. 1975.
11 *Report on Health Manpower*. Washington, DC: Department of Health, Education and Welfare, 1977.
12 Calvani T, James AE. Antitrust law and the practice of medicine. *J Leg Med (Chicago)* 1980;1:147−172.
13 Gibson RM, Fisher CR. National health expenditures. *Soc Secur Bull* 1977;41:7.
14 James AE Jr, Sloan FA, Blumstein JF *et al*. Certificate-of-need in an antitrust context. *J Health Polit Policy Law* 1983;8:314−319.
15 Havighurst C. Health care cost-containment regulation: prospects and an alternative. *Am J Law Med* 1977;3:309.
16 James AE Jr. Certain legal aspects of medical imaging. In: Margulis AR, Gooding CA, eds. *Diagnostic Radiology*. San Francisco: University of California, 1985:309−315.
17 James AE Jr, Winfield AC, Rollo FD *et al*. An analysis of the combined effects of certificate of need legislation (CON) and changes in the granting of hospital privileges. *Radiology* 1982; 145:299−331.
18 Greenberg W. *Competition in the Health Care Sector: Past, Present, and Future*. FTC Conference Proceedings, Washington, 1978.

19 Calvani T, James AE. Antitrust and medicine. In: James AE, ed. *Legal Medicine*. Baltimore: Urban and Schwarzenberg, 1980: 149–173.

20 Coulam C, Erickson J, Rollo FD, James AE. *The Physical Basis of Medical Imaging*. New York: Appleton-Century-Crofts, 1981.

21 *Parker* v. *Brown*, 417, U.S. 350–351.

22 *Eastern Railroad Presidents Conference* v. *Noerr Freight Inc.*, 365 U.S. 127. 1961.

23 *United Mine Workers* v. *Pennington*, 381 U.S. 657. 1965.

24 Blumstein J. Redefining government's role in health care. Is a dose of competition what the doctor should order? *Vanderbilt Law Rev* May 1981.

25 James AE Jr, Sherrard TJ. The law of agency as applied to radiology. *Radiology* 1978;128:257–260.

26 James AE Jr, Bundy AL, Fleischer AC *et al*. Legal aspects of diagnostic sonography. *Semin Ultrasound CT MR* 1985;6:207–216.

27 James AE Jr, Fleischer AC, Thieme G, Bundy AL, Sanders RC, Johnson B, Boehm FH. Diagnostic ultrasonography: certain legal considerations. *J Ultrasound Med* 1985;4:427–431.

28 James AE Jr, Hall DJ, Johnson BA. Some applications of the law of evidence to the specialty of radiology. *Radiology* 1977;124: 845–848.

29 James AE Jr, Waddill WB III, Feazell GL *et al*. The new medical imaging technologies as evidence. *J Contemp Law* 1984;11:105–130.

30 James AE Jr, Sloan FA, Hamilton RJ *et al*. Antitrust aspects of exclusive contracts in medical imaging. *Radiology* 1985;156: 237–241.

31 James AE Jr, Sherrard TJ. Agency. In: James AE Jr, ed. *Legal Medicine with Special Reference to Diagnostic Imaging*. Baltimore: Urban and Schwarzenberg, 1980:135–146.

32 James AE Jr, Sloan FA, Carroll FE *et al*. Hospital cost regulation: some cumulative effects from certificate of need and diagnostic related groups. *Noninvas Med Imag* 1984;1:259–263.

33 James AE Jr (ed.). *Medical/Legal Issues for Radiologists*. Chicago: Precept Press, 1987.

34 James AE Jr, Thieme GA, Price RR. Ultrasound instrumentation and its practical applications. In: Sanders RC, James AE Jr, eds. *The Principles and Practice of Ultrasonography in Obstetrics and Gynecology*. Norwalk, CT: Appleton-Century-Crofts, 1985.

35 *Dubin* v. *Michael Reese Hospital*, 83 Ill 2nd 277. 1980.

36 James AE Jr, Pendergrass HP, Robinson R, Hamilton RJ, Rollo FD, Hollowell E. Exclusive physician contracts in hospitals: precedent cases for radiologic practice. *Admin Radiol* May 1987; 6(5):28–31.

37 James AE Jr, Price RR, Sloan F, Zaner R, Chapman J. Certain social considerations in abandoning high technology medical imaging. *Health Matrix* 1987;5:31–34.

38 James AE Jr, Chapman J, Carroll F *et al*. Ethical choices in high technology medicine: Current dilemmas in diagnostic imaging. *Health Care Instr* 1986;1(5):158–167.

39 James AE Jr, Curran WJ, Pendergrass HP, Chapman JE. Academic radiology, turf conflict and antitrust laws. *Invest Radiol* 1990;25:200–202.

40 *White* v. *Rockingham Radiologists, Ltd.*, 820 F.2d 98. 4th Cir., 1987.

41 *Collins* v. *Associated Pathologists, Ltd.*, 1987–1 Trade Cas. (CCH) ¶67, 603, C.D. Ill. 1987.

42 James AE. *Medical Administration*. WH Green, 1994.

43 Alpert G, McCarthy TR. Beyond Goldfarb: applying traditional antitrust analysis to changing health markets. *Antitrust Bull* 1984;29:165.

44 Proger. *Relevant Market*, 55 Antitrust L.J. 613. 1986.

45 Baker, Blumenthal. *The 1982 Guidelines and Preexisting Law*, 71 Calif. L. Rev. 311, 323. 1983.

46 Areeda P, Turner D. *Antitrust Law* ¶507, at 330–31. 1978.

47 Sherman Antitrust Act, 15 U.S.C. § 2. 1982.

48 *Walker Process Equipment, Inc.* v. *Food Machinery & Chemical Corp.*, 382 U.S. 172. 1965.

49 *National Society of Professional Engineers* v. *United States*, 435 U.S. 679. 1978.

50 *Arizona* v. *Maricopa County Medical Society*, 457 U.S. 332, 343. 1982.

51 *National Collegiate Athletic Association* v. *Board of Regents of the University of Oklahoma*, 468 U.S. 85. 1984.

52 *National Society of Professional Engineers* v. *U.S.* 1978.

53 Robinson–Patman Act, 15 U.S.C. §§ 13–13b, 21a. 1982.

54 ABA Antitrust Section, Monograph No. 12. *Horizontal Mergers: Law and Policy*. 1986:68–69.

55 *United States* v. *E.I. du Pont de Nemours & Co. (Cellophane)*, 351 U.S. 377. 1956.

56 Antitrust Div., U.S. Department of Justice, Merger Guidelines § 2, 49 Fed. Reg. 26 823, 26 827. June 19, 1984.

57 Antitrust Div., U.S. Department of Justice, Vertical Restraints Guidelines § 6.1, 50 Fed. Reg. 6263, 6272. February 14, 1985.

CHAPTER 42

General considerations

Satish C. Muluk and John A. Kaufman

Many potential complications can be identified and prevented before a procedure begins. The preprocedural evaluation of the patient is as important as the technical ability to perform the procedure. In this chapter we describe a general approach to this aspect of diagnostic and interventional radiology. The actual process may vary according to physician preferences and institutional needs. Specific recommendations regarding management of patients with such issues as contrast allergies, renal failure, and pregnancy can be found in appropriate chapters.

Patient assessment should always begin with a history and physical examination that is pertinent to the anticipated procedure. Specific systems will be individually discussed below, but a few general comments are in order. Completion of a preprocedural worksheet for each patient may be useful in order to ensure consistent, thorough evaluations (Fig. 42.1). Except in emergency situations, a proper environment, free of distractions and haste, should be selected for obtaining the history and physical examination. An interpreter may be necessary to overcome a language barrier. The patient should be questioned carefully regarding prior complications with similar past procedures. Identification and documentation of allergies is crucial.

The physical examination should include assessment of vital signs, examination of the skin for easy bruising, as well as a routine examination of the heart and lungs. Special attention should be directed to evaluation of pulses, skin integrity over anticipated sites of percutaneous access, and the ability of the patient to assume procedure-specific positions.

For elective major cases, current laboratory data should be available. This typically consists of a hematocrit, platelet count, prothrombin time (PT), partial thromboplastin time (PTT), creatinine, and in patients over 35 years or those undergoing cardiac or pulmonary angiography, an electrocardiogram (EKG).

Risk and benefit assessment

A clear understanding of the natural history and stage of each patient's disorder, the planned procedure, and alternate therapies is the foundation upon which the assessment of risks and benefits is based. Consultation with the referring physician is essential to ensure that the expected goals of the procedure are appropriate and realistic. It is in this context that the potential benefits should be weighed against the procedure-specific risks. Disregard for clinical issues may result in a narrow, technical perspective, and performance of inappropriate procedures.

Patient preparation

Informed consent requires that the above risk/benefit considerations be clearly conveyed to the patient. A frank explanation of the procedure and the expected postprocedure course is essential, as is an open discussion of the major potential complications. Discussion of special preparatory measures, such as insertion of urinary or nasogastric catheters, should not be overlooked. Written, accurate descriptive materials are useful when explaining the procedure and for the patient's later reference. Many patients benefit from the preprocedural administration of anxiolytics (e.g., 5–10 mg of diazepam given orally the night before and/or the morning of the procedure). Upon the patient's arrival in the radiology department, members of the interventional team should introduce themselves. Every attempt should be made to keep the patient informed and reassured while awaiting the procedure.

Name:	Inpatient ☐	Emergency ☐	Patient stamp here
Hosp›:	Outpatient ☐	Day ☐	
DOB:_____ M ☐ F ☐	Scheduled ☐	Night ☐	
Ref MD:	Add-on ☐	Weekend ☐	
Service:			
Pt location:	Procedure requested:		

Clinical history:

Prior studies:

Allergy   No ☐   Yes ☐   Unknown☐
Describe:

Cr:_____   BUN:_____   PT:_____   PTT:_____
HCT:_____   PLT:_____   Other:_____

Meds: Heparin☐   Warfarin ☐   Insulin ☐
Others (list):

Premeds:

Pulse examination

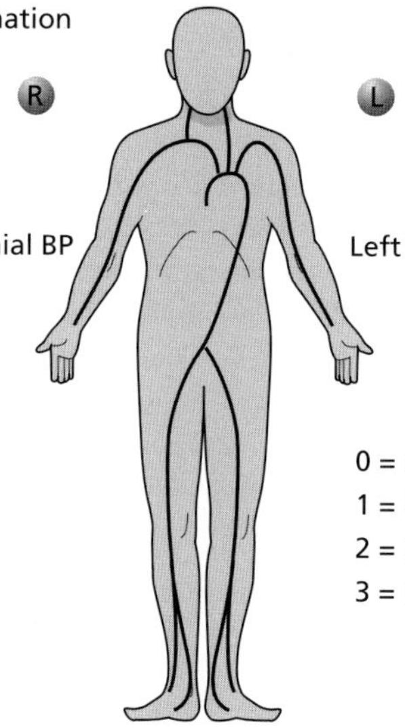

Ⓡ   Ⓛ

Right brachial BP   Left brachial BP

0 = Absent
1 = Diminished
2 = Normal
3 = Increased

Non-invasive studies: No ☐ Yes ☐ Results:_____

Prior vascular surgery: No ☐ Yes ☐ Type:_____

Prior contrast: No ☐   Yes ☐   Unknown☐
                HOCA ☐   LOCA ☐   Unknown☐

Reaction: No ☐   Yes ☐
Type and RX:_____

Peripheral vascular disease: No ☐   Yes ☐
Claudication: R ☐   L ☐   Rest pain ☐
        Tissue loss ☐   Known AAA☐
Renal failure: No ☐   Yes ☐   Dialysis ☐

Coronary artery disease: No ☐   Yes ☐
MI ☐   When:_____   CABG ☐   When:_____
Angina ☐   How often_____   x's per_____
CHF ☐   HPTN ☐   LBBB ☐

CVA/TIA: No ☐ Yes ☐ Most recent_____
Neurosurgery: No ☐ Yes ☐   When:_____
Able to give consent?:   No ☐ Yes ☐

Diabetes: No ☐ Yes ☐
Smoker: No ☐ Yes ☐ Quit☐ COPD ☐ Asthma ☐
Hx PE: No ☐ Yes ☐   Hx DVT: No ☐ Yes ☐
Malig: No ☐ Yes ☐ Primary:_____   Mets ☐

Fig. 42.1 Sample pre-procedural worksheet.

Specific systems

Volume and electrolyte status

It is important to achieve a euvolemic state prior to many diagnostic and interventional procedures. For example, hypovolemia may be an important contributor to contrast-induced renal failure. Conversely, volume overload can lead to intolerance of the supine position or even to overt pulmonary edema. Careful evaluation of fluid status is important in patients with a history of cardiac or renal insufficiency, and in those with a history of uncompensated losses (e.g., severe diarrhea, vomiting, or hemorrhage). Volume status is best assessed by: (i) checking the patient's vital signs (especially looking for tachycardia and hypotension as indicators of hypovolemia); (ii) observing the urine output, since oliguria is generally a sensitive indicator of hypovolemia; and (iii) examining the patient for distended neck veins, peripheral edema, pulmonary rales, and an S3 gallop (all indicators of volume excess). Once volume excess or deficit has been diagnosed, correction with diuresis or intravenous infusion is generally straightforward. The physician should keep in mind that most patients cease oral intake around the time of invasive procedures. Therefore, maintenance intravenous infusion is often indicated. Significant electrolyte disturbances, most commonly hyper- or hypokalemia, should be corrected if possible prior to major interventional procedures.

Prevention of infection

Prophylactic antibiotics are not indicated for the majority of radiologic interventions. Exceptions include biliary tract manipulations, embolizations, transrectal biopsies, Fallopian tube interventions, and implantation of venous access devices. Appropriate chapters should be consulted for recommended regimens. When hair removal is necessary, it is best done in the radiology department immediately prior to the procedure.

Cardiac

Although many studies have shown the feasibility and importance of cardiac risk stratification before surgical procedures, such extensive evaluation is not necessary prior to most radiologic procedures. However, a cardiac history should be routinely obtained, and patients should be examined to evaluate for congestive heart failure or arrhythmias. An EKG should be obtained in patients over the age of 35 years, in cases of suspected active myocardial ischemia, and prior to pulmonary angiography. Specific cardiac conditions that require corrective therapy prior to a procedure are unstable angina, congestive heart failure, and uncontrolled arrhythmias.

The great majority of oral cardiac drugs can simply be continued around the time of the procedure. Although an empty stomach at the time of the procedure is desirable, there is little risk in allowing patients to continue their drugs with a small sip of water. It is especially important that cardiac drugs, digoxin, and β-blockers not be interrupted around the time of the procedure. In the unusual event that oral administration of drugs must be stopped, many of the critical drugs can be converted to a parenteral or transcutaneous form.

Respiratory

The majority of radiologic procedures do not adversely affect respiratory reserve. However, the effects of the intravenous sedatives and analgesics required for many procedures must be kept in mind. Patients who may tolerate sedation poorly should be identified during the preprocedure evaluation. A history of chronic lung disease, severe asthma, or smoking may be indicators of compromised pulmonary function. Examination may reveal evidence of chronic lung disease, such as clubbing of the digits or increased anteroposterior chest size. In selected cases, further assessment of respiratory status includes review of the chest X-ray, pulmonary function tests, or consultation with an anesthesiologist. Because sedation and other factors can alter an individual's ability to protect him- or herself from aspiration, patients should have either clear liquids, or nothing by mouth (NPO), starting on the night before a major interventional procedure. Patients who are made NPO should receive intravenous hydration; important oral drugs can be continued with a sip of water.

Renal

Radiologic procedures that involve administration of iodinated contrast should not be performed without prior assessment of renal function. In most instances, a recent serum creatinine (within 4 weeks) is sufficient. If the patient has had a recent iodinated contrast load, or exposure to nephrotoxic drugs, the creatinine should be rechecked. Insertion of a urinary catheter should be considered in patients with marginal renal function to permit accurate monitoring of urinary output. Measures for prevention of contrast-induced acute renal failure are discussed in Chapter 13, p. 257.

Coagulopathies

Patients should routinely be questioned about prior problems with abnormal bleeding (after, e.g., dental extractions or minor trauma). Examination may reveal easy bruising or unusual hematomas. Although routine laboratory tests of coagulation in young, healthy patients may be unnecessary, most centers obtain a platelet count, PT, and PTT prior to invasive procedures. Abnormalities suspected based on the above evaluation require further evaluation, often with the help of hematologist.

Special note should be made of patients on heparin or warfarin. The half-life of heparin is approximately 1–2 hours, so that procedures can be safely performed 4 hours after stopping heparin administration, without any need to recheck the PTT. Most angiographic procedures performed from a femoral approach can be begun shortly after stopping heparin, as the procedures usually last long enough to permit return of normal coagulation. Axillary and translumbar punctures should not commence until abnormal coagulation parameters are corrected. A useful measure of the degree of heparinization is the activated clotting time (ACT), which can be measured quickly in the radiology suite with inexpensive, but specialized equipment. When rapid correction of an abnormal PTT is required, slow administration of intravenous protamine sulfate in appropriate doses should be considered.

In contrast to heparin, warfarin must generally be stopped 3–4 days prior to an invasive procedure. In such cases, most invasive procedures can be safely performed when the PT is less than 2–3 seconds over control. Two units of fresh frozen plasma should be available if the procedure is initiated while the PT is still prolonged. In some cases, such as patients with mechanical heart valves, a period of loss of anticoagulation may be unacceptable. These patients should be admitted and placed on intravenous heparin as the effect of the warfarin diminishes. Heparin can be resumed at a suitable time after the procedure, and continued as warfarin is resumed, until the PT is once again in a therapeutic range. This method minimizes the time that the patient is not anticoagulated.

No special measures are required in the patient who is on aspirin or nonsteroidal agents, despite the known antiplatelet activity of these drugs. However, nonsteroidal agents may increase the risk of contrast nephropathy.

Endocrine

Special measures are indicated in diabetic patients who are taking either oral hypoglycemic agents or insulin, when the procedure causes a significant period of cessation of oral intake. The long half-life of many oral hypoglycemic agents requires that a continuous glucose infusion be maintained, even if the patients are not given the oral hypoglycemic on the day of the procedure. Insulin-dependent patients can be suitably managed by halving their morning insulin dose on the day of the procedure, with administration of continuous glucose infusion. For adults, a 5% glucose solution given at 80–100 ml/h is adequate. Intermittent fingerstick checking of glucose levels is indicated in some cases.

Patients who may have suppression of the pituitary–adrenal axis (most commonly related to the exogenous administration of glucocorticoid agents) should receive periprocedure steroid coverage (e.g., intravenous hydrocortisone 100 mg every 8 hours around the time of the procedure).

Conclusion

The preprocedural evaluation of the patient is an integral part of the procedure itself. The majority of radiologic procedures are performed as referrals from nonradiologists. These physicians may be unfamiliar with the technical aspects of the procedure which they have ordered. The preprocedural evaluation allows the radiologist to introduce him- or herself to the patient, review the history and physical examination, explain the procedure, assess the appropriateness of the request, and obtain consent. This encounter also provides an opportunity to identify patients at increased risk of complications. Although the anticipation of a complication will not necessarily prevent it from occurring, the severity may be diminished. A thoughtful, careful evaluation of the patient should be the first step in any procedure.

Index